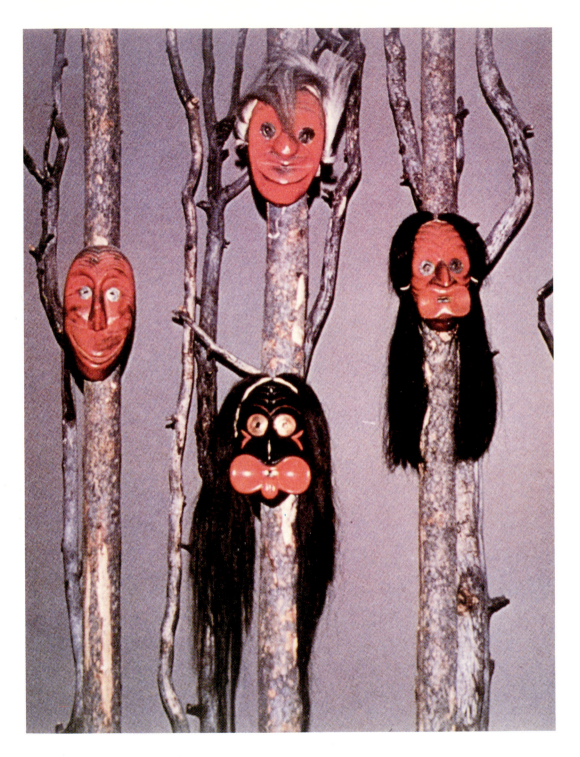

Masks worn by members of the Iroquois False Face Society to visit sick friends. Masks represent cheerful spirits invoked to aid the patient's recovery. Contemporary pain management includes similar behavioral modification techniques to control the patient's pain. (Courtesy of the Denver Art Museum.)

PRACTICAL MANAGEMENT OF PAIN

PRACTICAL MANAGEMENT
OF PAIN

With Special Emphasis on Physiology of Pain Syndromes and Techniques
of Pain Management

P. PRITHVI RAJ, M.D., F.A.C.A., F.F.A.R.C.S. (Engl.)

Director, Pain Control Center
Professor of Anesthesiology
University of Cincinnati College of Medicine
Cincinnati, Ohio

YEAR BOOK MEDICAL PUBLISHERS, INC.
Chicago • London

1 2 3 4 5 6 7 8 9 CK 8 9 8 8 8 7 8 6

Library of Congress Cataloging-in-Publication Data
Main entry under title:

Practical management of pain.

    Includes bibliographies and index.
    1. Pain—Treatment.   2. Intractable pain—Treatment.
3. Analgesia.   4. Pain, Postoperative—Treatment.
I. Raj, P. Prithvi. [DNLM: 1. Pain—therapy.
WL 704 P895]
RB127.P73 1986   616′.0472   85-26634
ISBN 0-8151-7013-0

Sponsoring Editors: Daniel J. Doody, Susan M. Harter, David K. Marshall
Manager, Copyediting Services: Frances M. Perveiler
Production Project Manager: Max Perez
Proofroom Supervisor: Shirley E. Taylor

To my wife, Susan, and my children, Mark, Maya, and Sarah

Contributors

STEPHEN E. ABRAM, M.D.
Professor and Vice Chairman
Department of Anesthesiology
The Medical College of Wisconsin
Milwaukee, Wisconsin
(Chapters 16A, 16B, 16C, 16D, 25C, 34F)

PATRICIA ARNOLD, B.S.Ed.
Associate Editor
Current Reviews Publications
Miami, Florida
(Chapter 22)

MICHAEL BEHBEHANI, Ph.D.
Associate Professor of Physiology and
    Biophysics
University of Cincinnati College of
    Medicine
Cincinnati, Ohio
(Chapter 11)

RICHARD G. BLACK, M.D.
Associate Professor of Anesthesia and
    Critical Care Medicine
Assistant Professor of Neurological
    Surgery
The Johns Hopkins University
Baltimore, Maryland
(Chapter 13)

MARK BROWN, M.D.
Staff Anesthesiologist
Mount Sinai Medical Center of Greater
    Miami
Miami Beach, Florida
(Chapter 22)

ELIZABETH BULLITT, M.D.
Assistant Professor of Neurosurgery
Department of Surgery
Division of Neurosurgery
University of North Carolina–Chapel Hill
Chapel Hill, North Carolina
(Chapters 7, 39A, 39C)

SANJAY DATTA, M.D., F.F.A.R.C.S.
    (ENGL.)
Associate Professor
Harvard Medical School
Senior Staff Anesthesiologist
Associate Director of Obstetric
    Anesthesia
Brigham and Women's Hospital
Boston, Massachusetts
(Chapter 18)

DONALD D. DENSON, Ph.D.
Associate Professor of Anesthesia
University of Cincinnati College of
    Medicine
Associate Professor of Pharmacology
University of Cincinnati College of
    Pharmacology
Cincinnati, Ohio
(Chapters 27, 28, 29, 30, 32, 36)

RUDOLPH H. DE JONG, M.D.
Deputy Commander, Chemical Institute
U.S. Army Medical Institute of Chemical
    Defense
Aberdeen Proving Ground, Maryland
Formerly Professor of Anesthesiology,
    and Senior Consultant, Pain Clinic
University of Cincinnati College of
    Medicine
Cincinnati, Ohio
(Chapter 31)

VICKIE M. FAIRCHILD, B.S., L.P.T.
Supervisor, Physical Therapy
Pain Control Center
University of Cincinnati Medical Center
Cincinnati, Ohio
(Chapters 5, 47)

THERESA FERRER-BRECHNER, M.D.
Professor, Department of Anesthesiology
Director, Pain Management Center
University of California Center for Health
    Sciences
Los Angeles, California
(Chapter 20A)

vi

ALLAN H. FRIEDMAN, M.D.
Assistant Professor
Duke University Medical Center
Chief, Division of Neurosurgery
Veterans Administration Hospital
Durham, North Carolina
(Chapter 39A, 39C)

CRAIG T. HARTRICK, M.D.
Assistant Director, Pain Control Center
Providence Hospital
Southfield, Michigan
(Chapter 19)

CHRISTINE HOVANITZ, Ph.D.
Assistant Professor of Psychology
Department of Psychology
University of Cincinnati
Cincinnati, Ohio
(Chapter 46)

JENNIFER HOWELL TROTT, R.N.
Coordinator, Pain Control Center
University of Cincinnati
Ambulatory Administrative Nurse
Nursing and Anesthesia
University Hospital
Cincinnati, Ohio
(Chapter 4)

KATHY S. JOHNSON, R.N.
Clinical Nurse
University Hospital
Cincinnati, Ohio
(Chapters 34A, 42, Appendix II)

MATT J. LIKAVEC, M.D.
Assistant Professor
Case Western Reserve University
Attending Physician
Division of Neurosurgery
Cleveland Metropolitan General
  Hospital
Cleveland, Ohio
(Chapters 16A, 16E, 16F, 23A)

LAURENCE E. MATHER, Ph.D.,
  F.F.A.R.A.C.S.
Reader in Anaesthesia and Intensive
  Care
Flinders University of South Australia
Clinical Associate
Flinders Medical Centre
Adelaide, South Australia
(Chapters 27, 28, 29, 38)

GLORIA E. MAYNE, M.D.
Attending Physician
Department of Anesthesiology
Associate, The Pain Center
Mount Sinai Medical Center
Miami Beach, Florida
(Chapters 3, 22)

JOHN S. MCDONALD, D.D.S., M.S.
Assistant Professor, Otolaryngology and
  Maxillofacial Surgery, Anesthesia,
  Pediatrics, and Surgery
University of Cincinnati College of
  Medicine
Cincinnati, Ohio
(Chapters 23B, 23D, 23E, 23F, 23G, 37)

WILLIAM MEISSNER, B.S., R.Ph.
Pharmacy Department
University Hospital
Cincinnati, Ohio
(Appendix I)

GERALD MORIARTY, M.D.
Assistant Professor of Neurology
University of Cincinnati College of
  Medicine
Cincinnati, Ohio
(Chapter 7)

FRANK MOYA, M.D.
Clinical Professor
Department of Anesthesiology
University of Miami School of Medicine
Chairman, Department of
  Anesthesiology
Director, The Pain Center
Mount Sinai Medical Center
Miami Beach, Florida
(Chapters 3, 22)

TERENCE M. MURPHY, M.B., Ch.B.,
  F.F.A.R.C.S.
Professor, Department of Anesthesiology
University of Washington School of
  Medicine
Seattle, Washington
(Chapters 34C, 34D)

J. STEPHEN NAULTY, M.D.
Assistant Professor of Anaesthesia
Harvard Medical School
Director, Clinical Obstetric Anesthesia
  Research
Brigham and Women's Hospital
Boston, Massachusetts
(Chapter 18)

HANS NOLTE, PROF., DR. MED.,
   M.D., D.A.
Professor of Anesthesiology
Department of Anesthesiology
Klinikum Minden
Federal Republic of Germany
(Chapter 34F)

GERARD W. OSTHEIMER, M.D.
Associate Professor in Anaesthesia
Harvard Medical School
Director of Obstetric Anesthesia
Brigham and Women's Hospital
Boston, Massachusetts
(Chapter 18)

THOMAS E. OXMAN, M.D.
Assistant Professor of Psychiatry
Community and Family Medicine
Dartmouth Medical School
Associate Director of Psychiatric
   Consultation—Liaison Service
Mary Hitchcock Memorial Hospital
Hanover, New Hampshire
(Chapters 14, 15E, 30, 44)

ROBERT E. PAWLICKI, Ph.D.
Professor of Psychology
Department of Anesthesiology
University of Cincinnati College of
   Medicine
Cincinnati, Ohio
(Chapters 45, 46, Appendices IIB and
   IV)

JAMES C. PHERO, D.M.D.
Assistant Professor of Surgery
Associate Professor of Clinical
   Anesthesia
Department of Anesthesia
University of Cincinnati Medical Center
Assistant Director, Pain Control Center
University Hospital
Cincinnati, Ohio
(Chapters 23B, 23D, 23E, 23F, 23G, 37)

CHARLES E. PITHER, M.B.B.S.,
   F.F.A.R.C.S.
Senior Registrar
St. Thomas' Hospital
London, England
(Chapter 19)

P. PRITHVI RAJ, M.B.B.S., F.A.C.A.,
   F.F.A.R.C.S. (ENGL.)
Director, Pain Control Center
Professor of Anesthesiology
University of Cincinnati College of
   Medicine
Cincinnati, Ohio
(Chapters 1, 2, 6, 8, 9, 10, 12, 15B, 15D,
   16B, 25A, 25B, 32, 33, 34A, 34B, 34D,
   35, 36, 38, 40, 41, 43, Appendices II
   and IV)

SOMAYAJI RAMAMURTHY, M.D.
Professor of Anesthesiology and
   Physical Medicine and Rehabilitation
University of Texas Health Science
   Center at San Antonio
Chief, Pain Management Clinic
Medical Center Hospital
Audie Murphy VA Hospital
San Antonio, Texas
(Chapters 15D, 24, 26A, 26B)

GARY S. ROBINS, D.M.D.
Adjunct Assistant Professor of Pharmacy
University of Cincinnati College of
   Pharmacy
Assistant Clinical Professor of Oral
   Surgery
University Hospital
Cincinnati, Ohio
(Chapters 23B, 23D, 23E, 23F, 23G)

RICHARD M. ROSENBLATT, M.D.
Clinical Faculty
UCLA
Staff Physician
Cedars-Sinai Medical Center
Beverly Hills, California
(Chapters 20B, 21)

LYNNE M. SALERNO, B.S., L.P.T.
Administrator and Director of Satellite
   Office for Rehabilitative Health
   Services
Anchorage, Alaska
(Chapters 5, 47)

LALIGAM N. SEKHAR, M.D.
Assistant Professor of Neurological
   Surgery
University of Pittsburgh
Attending Neurosurgeon
Presbyterian-University Hospital
Pittsburgh, Pennsylvania
(Chapters 15A, 39B)

SARJIT SINGH, M.D.
Assistant Professor of Clinical Neurology
Presbyterian-University Hospital
University of Pittsburgh School of
  Medicine
Pittsburgh, Pennsylvania
Chief-of-Staff
St. John Hospital
Steubenville, Ohio
(Chapter 15A)

MICHAEL STANTON-HICKS, M.B.B.S.,
  M.D., F.F.A.R.C.S.
Professor and Acting Chairman
University of Colorado Health Sciences
  Center
Chief of Anesthesiology
University of Colorado Hospital
Denver, Colorado
(Chapters 17, 34D, 34E, 34F)

JOHN STEINER, M.D.
Associate Clinical Professor of
  Neurology
University of Cincinnati College of
  Medicine
Cincinnati, Ohio
(Chapter 23C)

P. SEBASTIAN THOMAS, M.D.
Assistant Professor
State University of New York
Director, Pain Treatment Center
Upstate Medical Center
Syracuse, New York
(Chapter 15C)

STACY L. WEDDING, B.S., L.P.T.
Field Service Instructor
Department of Orthopedics
University of Cincinnati Medical Center
Formerly Physical Therapy Supervisor
University of Cincinnati Hospital
Cincinnati, Ohio
(Chapters 5, 47)

ELLIOTT WEINBERG, B.S., L.P.T.
Instructor in Clinical Physical Therapy
Director, Department of Physical
  Therapy
University of Cincinnati Medical Center
Cincinnati, Ohio
(Chapters 5, 47)

WILLIAM C. WESTER, II, Ed.D.
Clinical Professor
Wright State University
School of Professional Psychology
Cincinnati, Ohio
(Chapter 45)

HOWARD L. ZAUDER, M.D., Ph.D.
Professor of Anesthesiology and
  Pharmacology
Interim Vice President and Dean for
  Clinical Affairs
State University of New York—Upstate
  Medical Center
Attending Anesthesiologist
State University Hospital
Syracuse, New York
(Chapter 15C)

Foreword

Much has been written about pain and its teleological purpose in limiting injury as well as its supposed benefits for strengthening moral fiber, but to the sufferer it is an unmitigated evil. To the physician, pain is a redoubtable enemy that wreaks physical and mental havoc in his patients by destroying sleep, impairing function, and sometimes producing secondary deterioration in tissues through an overactive sympathetic nervous system. Mental changes of despondency, depression, and occasionally suicidal depression, march in the footsteps of unrelenting and unrelieved pain.

Historically, pain relief has always been one of the highest aims of the medical profession, but one of the most elusive, and current interest in hypnosis and behavior modification hark back to a time when there was little else to offer. Practical control of pain, as we understand it today, only began with the advent of general anesthesia a century ago. Since then, enormous advances have been made at accelerating pace and in many disciplines.

This book brings together the practical wisdom of 45 experts working in the field of pain management, all with a solid foundation in the basic principles underlying individual areas of their clinical expertise. The editor, Dr. P. Prithvi Raj, has devoted his professional life to the control of pain, and like all true professionals, he and his collaborators have the courage to face the shortcomings of their chosen art, and to admit limitations where they exist. And so, this work has a refreshing frankness that is not afraid to say: "We think we know and can do so much, but beyond that point we cannot go with assurance." This is what our patients want to hear from us, as a sign that they are not the victims of quackery, and it is what we as physicians need to know so that we can deserve that trust that has always been so essential to the healing art. The end result of this book is what was planned: a practical, no-nonsense guide to pain management.

PHILIP BROMAGE, M.B.B.S., F.F.A.R.C.S.
PROFESSOR AND CHAIRMAN
DEPARTMENT OF ANESTHESIA
UNIVERSITY OF COLORADO HEALTH SCIENCES
  CENTER
DENVER, COLORADO

Preface

Even though numerous books have been published in the past on the subject of pain, they have either covered specific regions or have been compilations of successful symposia or international conferences. This book attempts to cover practical aspects of pain management currently in use in pain clinics across the United States. In general, the authors were chosen for their specialized and active interests in treating pain. Their experience is fully recognized by my request that they write on all aspects of pain that interest them. Their contributions are appropriately placed in relevant sections to maintain the format and minimize duplication.

The purpose of *Practical Management of Pain* is to present in one volume the current practice of pain management. It is directed toward the practitioner-in-training who is specializing in the subspeciality of pain. The book is also of interest to the practicing physician who wishes to embark on managing pain patients but has had little experience treating pain patients.

In this book the *practical* management of pain is emphasized. Recent advances and significant basic researches are mentioned only for thoroughness. The chapters are grouped into six parts, each illustrating a specific aspect of pain management. For example, Part I deals with organization of pain clinics and role of personnel, while Part VI deals with the details of techniques of pain management. Black-and-white and color illustrations have been used to enhance the impact of the text. The Appendix, which includes a directory of pain clinics, inventory of equipment, and information on educational material in pain management, may be useful to the reader.

I hope that physicians-in-training will find this book informative. I further hope that their enthusiasm and interest will remain high after their training. We look forward to the coming generation of trained physicians who will treat and manage the pains of the future. They will have the opportunity to discover new horizons in dealing with *pain*, the oldest affliction of mankind.

P. PRITHVI RAJ, M.B.B.S., F.F.A.R.C.S. (ENGL.)

Acknowledgment

A work of the size of *Practical Management of Pain* is never accomplished without hard work and dedication of many people. I have been fortunate to get the dedicated support of my family to complete this book. My wife Susan took on the onerous task of coordinating various aspects of the book. This book would have been impossible to complete without her help.

I would like to thank the Department of Anesthesia of the University of Cincinnati for its unqualified support of this project. The innumerable hours spent by the secretarial staff in researching, word processing, and preparing illustrations were never questioned.

It would be impossible to complete a task such as this without some people making major contributions. Marilyn Schwier's word processing and editing have been an important contribution to this book. I sincerely thank her for her tireless work, especially in the evenings and on weekends. Mary Ann Cost made similar contributions at a lesser scale. During the last 2 years, my secretary, Mary Therese Dixon, has kept the work flowing from me to the contributors, to the publishers, to the coordinator, and to the word processor. She has done this without complaint. I am grateful to her. Some of the illustrations in this book are drawn by my good friend, Tom Sims. For these brilliant illustrations, I am indebted to him. I also acknowledge the efforts of Kelly Hsu in editing the chapter on acupuncture.

Many authors and publishers gave permission for their work to be quoted or reproduced in this book. Due acknowledgment is given to them here and in the respective chapters. At the outset, my interest in pain was aroused by the brilliant teachings of John Bonica. It is no wonder that during the writing of this book I have called on many of his works, especially from his classic book, *The Management of Pain*. I have used excerpts from his book in the chapters on history and pharmacology of neurolytic agents. I am grateful to him. From the book, *Chronic Low Back Pain*, edited by Stanton-Hicks and Boas and published by Raven Press, excerpts and illustrations have been used from chapters on epidemiology, assessment and management planning, the radiologic evaluation of back pain, and epidural steroid therapy. I am grateful to authors G. G. Steinberg, J. McLennan, David J. Berg, H. Carron, and T. Toomey for the use of their material from that book. From the textbook, *Medical Physiology*, by Guyton and published by W. B. Saunders Co., excerpts and illustrations have been used in Part II. The chapter on neurological examination uses material published in *Clinical Neurology*, Vol. I, Chapter I, by Russell and DeJong, edited by A. B. Baker, L. H. Baker and published by Harper & Row in 1983. The writings of Travell and her new book, *Myofascial Pain and Dysfunction, The Trigger Point Manual*, published by Williams & Wilkins in 1983, have been a source of excerpts and illustrations for chapters of musculoskeletal pain and trigger point injections. Excerpts are used in the chapter on neurolytic agents from an excellent review on phenol by K. Wood, published in the journal *Pain*, Vol. 5, 1978. In the chapter on chemonucleolysis, excerpts and illustrations were used from the book *Intradiscal Therapy Chymopapain or Collagenase*, by Mark D. Brown and published by Year Book Medical Publishers. In the chapter on management of pain due to peripheral nerve problems, Dr. Aage Moller performed all the intraoperative neurophysiological studies, without which sophisticated nerve surgery is impossible. Mary Ann Polakovic prepared the manuscript. The illustrations were made by William R. Filer. The technique of D. Coombes has been excerpted from his published work and described in the chapter on spinal narcotics. I am grateful to all of them for allowing me to borrow their work.

The text was originally planned after extensive discussion between me and Daniel J. Doody, then Medical Editor at Year Book Medical Publishers. However, the table of contents has changed somewhat since then and Daniel J. Doody has progressed in his career. Susan Harter and David K. Marshall became constant sources of help to get this book published. I am grateful to all of them in keeping the faith in all of us.

Acknowledgments would not be complete without thanking all the contributors who worked very hard to conform to the objective of the book. They sacrificed individuality and accepted breaking of their contributions to maintain the format of the book. Some of them were asked to rewrite. They did this without any complaints. I am grateful to all of them.

P. Prithvi Raj, M.B.B.S., F.F.A.R.C.S. (Engl.)

Contents

PLATE 1

Thermograms (Chapter 15)

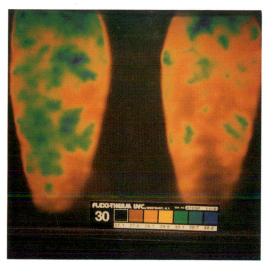

Fig 15C–1.—Thermogram obtained prior to epidural steroid block showing decrease in temperature in the right posterior thigh.

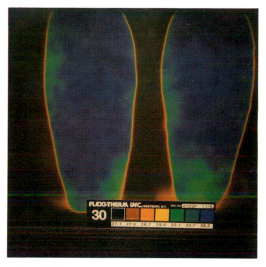

Fig 15C–2.—Thermogram obtained after epidural block showing increase in temperature in both legs, indicating effectiveness of sympathetic block.

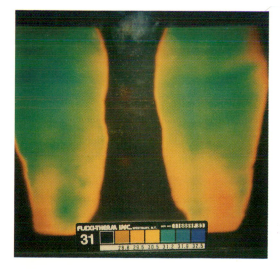

Fig 15C–3.—Thermogram obtained 2 weeks after epidural steroid blocks. Temperature distribution pattern indicates the efficacy of epidural steroid injections.

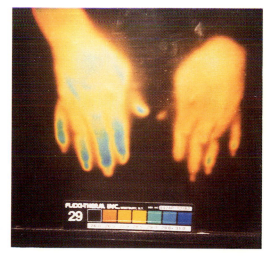

Fig 15C–4.—Case 1. Thermogram of left hand, dorsal view, shows uniform decrease in temperature.

PLATE 2

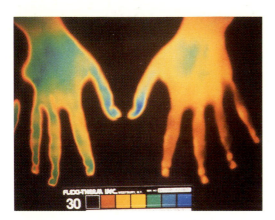

Fig 15C–5.—Case 1. Thermogram of left hand, dorsal view, shows decrease in temperature compared to right hand.

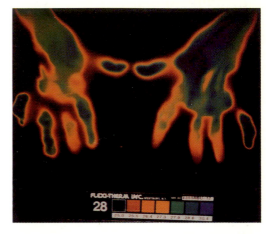

Fig 15C–6.—Case 2. Patient had rheumatoid vasculitis with ischemic ulcers on the tips of the index, middle, and ring fingers of the left hand.

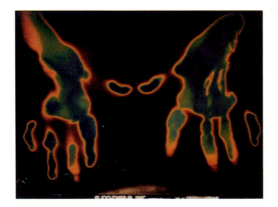

Fig 15C–7.—Case 2. Note increased temperature elevation in the affected extremity after the initial stellate ganglion block.

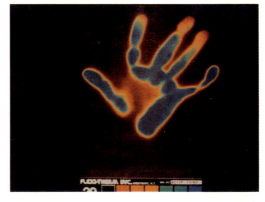

Fig 15C–8.—Case 2. Thermograms of the same hand after a series of sympathetic blocks. Patient was discharged home with intact fingers.

PLATE 3

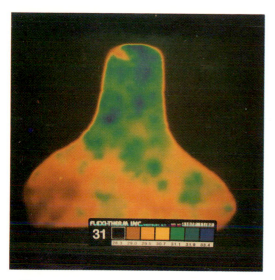

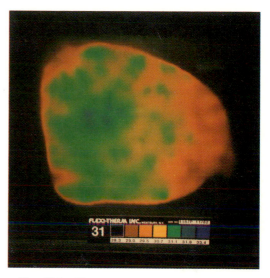

Fig 15C–9.—Case 3. Thermogram shows trigger points in the left scapular and paravertebral regions. Thermographically, trigger points often appear as hot areas, occasionally as cold areas.

Fig 15C–10.—Case 3. Trigger points appear as well-circumscribed hot areas in the right scapular region.

Herpes Zoster (Chapter 22)

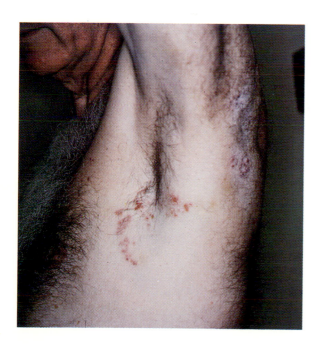

Fig 22–3.—A 55-year-old man complained of shooting pain and itching in the axilla for 3 days. This was followed by appearance of skin lesions in the axilla, confirming the diagnosis of acute herpes zoster.

PLATE 4

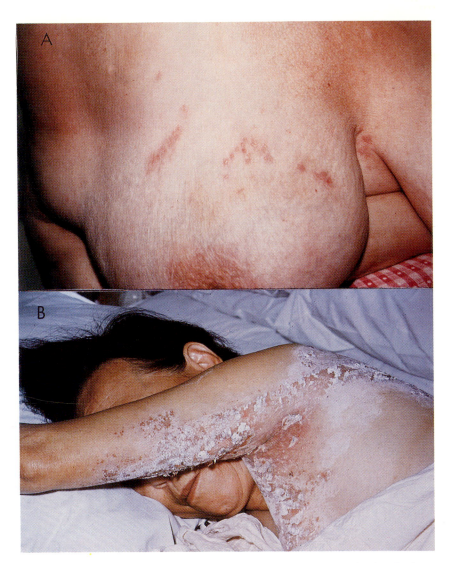

Fig 22—4.—A, a 60-year-old woman had radicular pain for 2 days, followed by local redness, swelling, and red papules due to acute herpes zoster. **B,** 3-week-old acute herpes zoster in the crusting stage.

PLATE 5

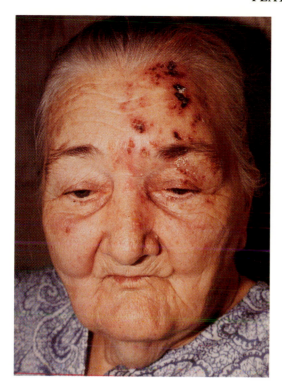

Fig 22–5.—Acute herpes zoster of 1 week's duration affecting the left ophthalmic division of the trigeminal nerve.

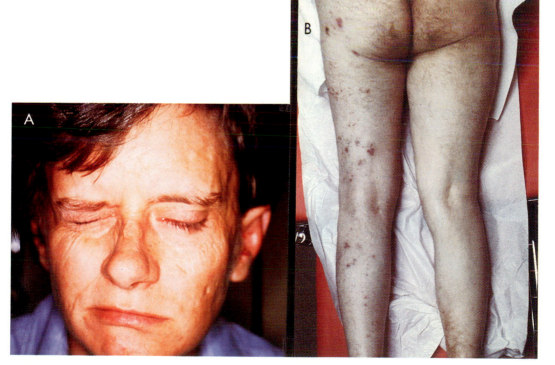

Fig 22–6.—A, acute geniculate neuralgia (Ramsay Hunt syndrome) in a 50-year-old woman. Note the redness of the left external ear, the vesicular lesion, and the left facial palsy. **B,** acute herpes zoster affecting the ᴸ4ᴸ5 dermatome in the lower extremity.

PLATE 6

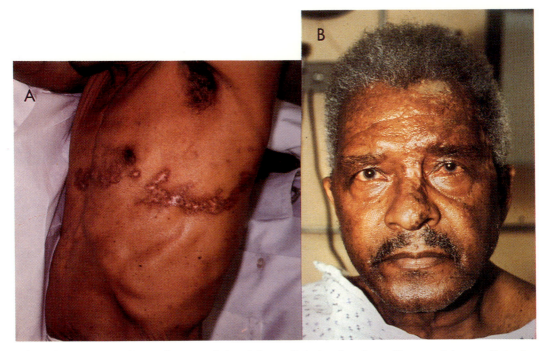

Fig 22–7.—A, postherpetic neuralgia of 6 months' duration in a 49-year-old man. Note the healed vesicular scabs with skin discoloration in the radicular fashion affecting the intercostal nerve. **B,** postherpetic neuralgia in the right ophthalmic division of the trigeminal nerve. Note the redness of the left eye. The patient had burning pain in the eyeball with crawling feelings in the forehead.

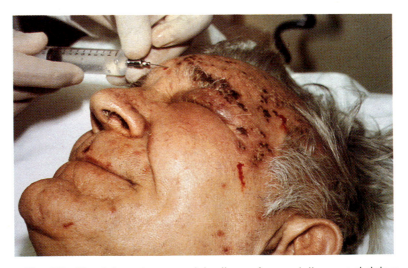

Fig 22–11.—Intracutaneous injection of a solution containing 0–25% bupivacaine and dexamethasone for the treatment of acute herpes zoster of the ophthalmic division of the trigeminal nerve.

PLATE 7

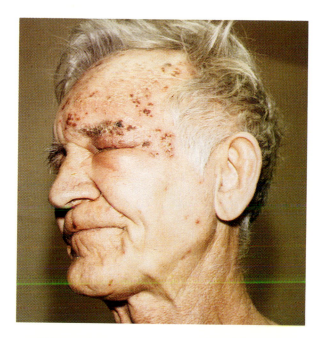

Fig 22—12.—Four days after intra-cutaneous injection, vesicular lesions dry and disappear.

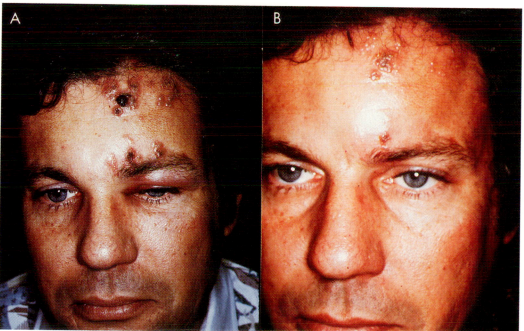

Fig 22—13.—**A,** acute herpes zoster of the left eye and forehead prior to treatment with intralesional injection and left stellate ganglion block. **B,** appearance 3 days after left stellate ganglion block. Note the clearing of the eye and the lesions of the forehead.

PLATE 8

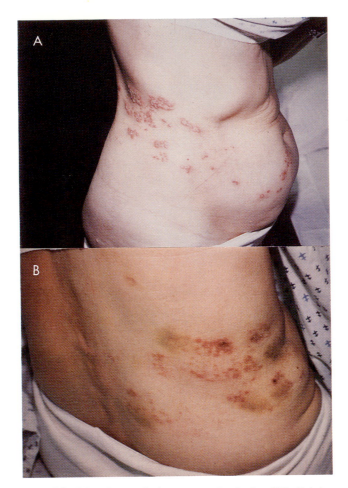

Fig 22–14.—A, acute herpes zoster in the T10–11 inter-costal distribution prior to the intracutaneous injection of a steroid–local anesthetic mixture. **B,** note healing of the vesicular lesions 3 days after the intracutaneous injection. Subcutaneous bruising is frequently seen for a few days after the injection.

PLATE 9

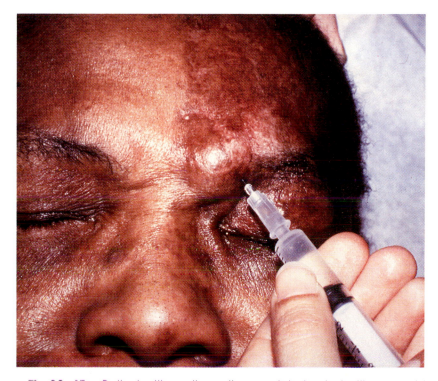

Fig 22–15.—Patient with postherpetic neuralgia treated with supraorbital nerve block.

PLATE 10

Pain of Neurogenic Origin (Chapter 25A)

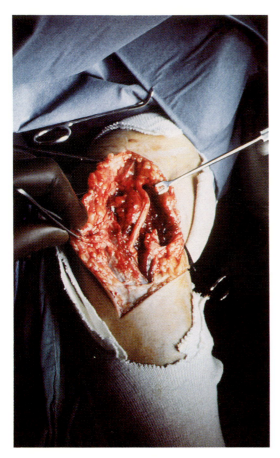

Fig 25A–9.—Even following ulnar nerve transposition for ulnar neuralgia, there was entrapment of the nerve in the muscle which required reexploration as shown here.

Pain of Sympathetic Origin (Chapter 25C)

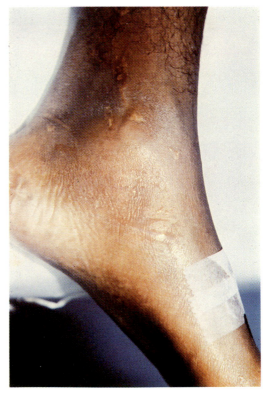

Fig 25C–6.—A young patient with trauma to the ankle followed by multiple surgical procedures in the region developed severe reflex sympathetic dystrophy. Note hyperhidrosis in the area.

PLATE 11

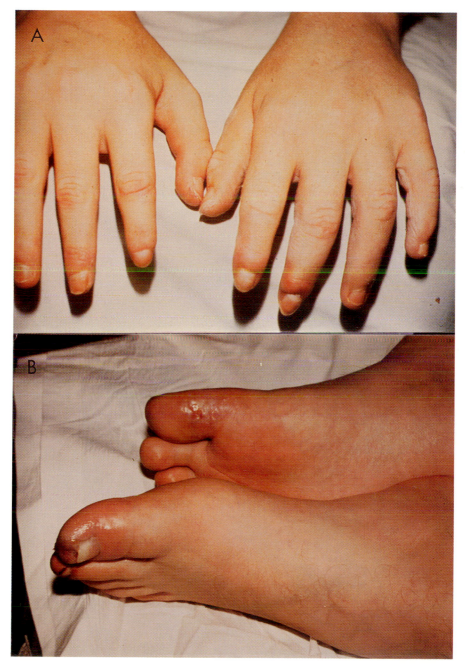

Fig 25C—8.—Raynaud's disease in an 18-year-old boy. The disease first manifested in the hands with pain, synostosis, and ulceration. Treatment with stellate ganglion blocks brought relief. Later, ulceration and pain appeared in both great toes; treatment was with sympathetic blocks and hyperbaric oxygen.

PLATE 12

Neurolytic Agents (Chapter 32)

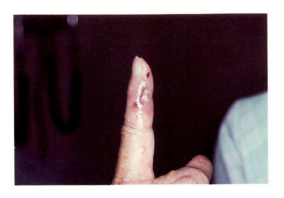

Fig 32–4.—Patient had severe pain in the index finger following development of a neuroma after surgery on the fingers. Ulceration of the skin developed 10 days after 6% phenol was injected into the digital nerve. With conservative management the ulcer healed in 2 weeks.

Sympathetic Block (Chapter 34F)

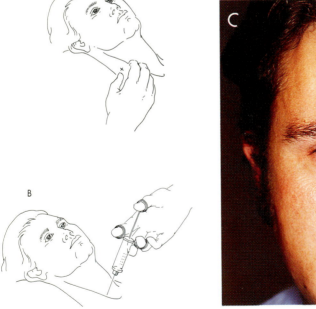

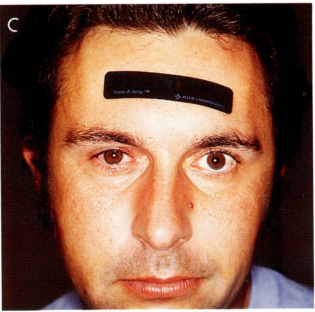

Fig 34F–3.—Stellate ganglion block. **A,** position of the fingers between the trachea and the carotid sheath at level of the sixth and seventh transverse processes prior to needle insertion. **B,** correct position of syringe and needle. **C,** appearance of patient with Horner's syndrome after right stellate ganglion block. Note the conjunctivitis and meiosis with slight ptosis in the right eye.

PLATE 13

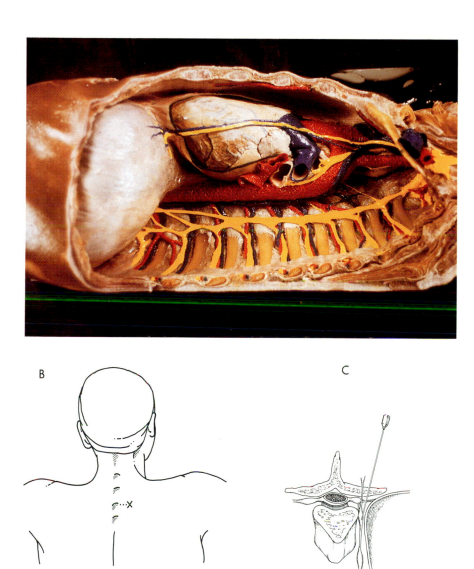

Fig 34F–4.—A, anatomy of thoracic sympathetic chain. The sympathetic chain lies at the junction of anterior and middle thirds of the lateral aspect of the vertebral body. (Courtesy of U. Pai, M.D., Department of Anatomy, University of Manipal, India.) **B,** position of the patient on the x-ray table showing point of needle at insertion. **C,** position of needle at the sympathetic chain.

PLATE 14

Neurological Procedure for Cancer Pain (Chapter 39C)

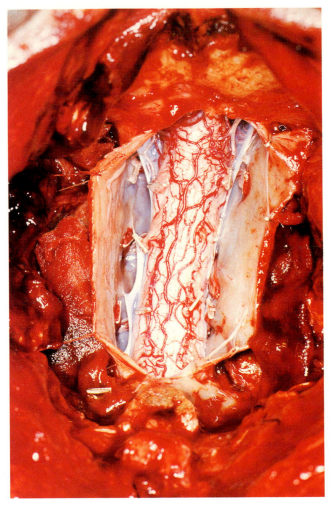

Fig 39C–1.—Open surgical dorsal rhizotomy at levels C2–5 following laminectomy. Note the section of dorsal nerve roots intradurally.

PLATE 15

TENS (Chapter 42)

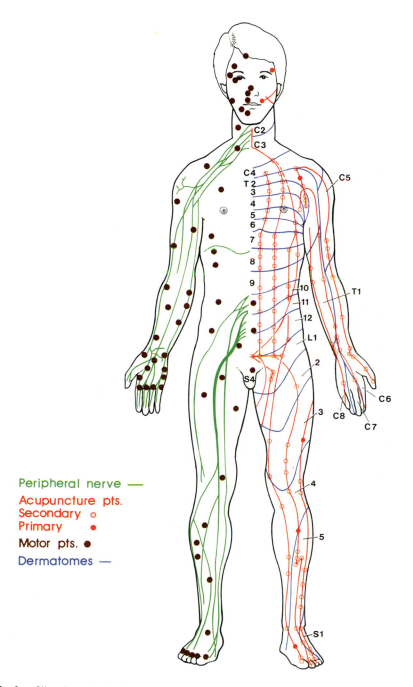

C2
C3
C4
T2
3
4
5
6
7
8
9
C5
T1
10
11
12
L1
2
3
4
5
S4
S1
C6
C8
C7

Peripheral nerve —
Acupuncture pts.
Secondary o
Primary •
Motor pts. •
Dermatomes —

Fig 42—4.—Sites for electrode placement *(front)*. These sites may be based on dermatomes, major peripheral nerves, acupuncture points, or motor points. *(Continued)*.

PLATE 16

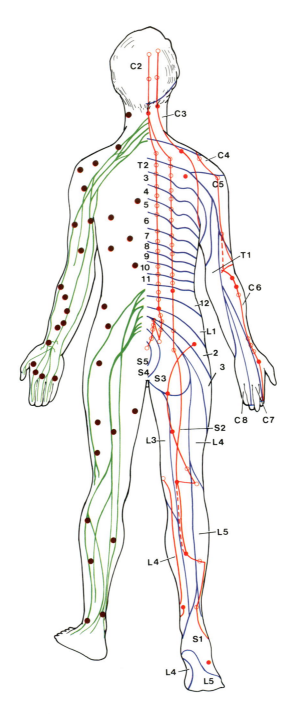

Fig 42–4 (cont.).—Sites for electrode placement *(back)*. These sites may be based on dermatomes, major peripheral nerves, acupuncture points, or motor points.

PART I

General Considerations

1 / History of Pain Management

P. PRITHVI RAJ, M.D.

MAN HAS BEEN AFFLICTED with pain since his beginning. In the records of every civilization one finds testimonials to the omnipresence of pain. On Babylonian clay tablets, in Egyptian papyri, in Persian leathern documents, in inscriptions from Mycenae, on parchment rolls from Troy, and all down through the ages, in every civilization, in every culture, are found prayers, exorcisms, and incantations that bear testimony to the dominance of pain (Figs 1–1 and 1–2). The unearthing of prehistoric human skeletons has added millions of years to man's recorded history, including the history of pain, for many of these bones bear signs of painful diseases.

It is therefore natural that since its beginning mankind should have engaged its energies to appease such an evil force, and as long as pain has existed there have been efforts to find means of controlling it. Its management has always taxed the diagnostic acumen and therapeutic skill of physicians.

Early indications of man's continuous struggle to alleviate pain are found in myths and oral histories, which describe man groping in the darkness of superstition and religious mysticism. Later, as knowledge increased, medicine was based more or less on reason, but almost all attempts to ease pain were futile and the desired end was attained only to a limited degree.

EARLY PAIN MANAGEMENT

Perhaps the earliest attempts at managing pain included physical therapeutic methods. Ancient man sensed relief from pain when the injured part was rubbed or exposed to the cold water of streams or lakes, the heat of the sun, and later that of fires.[1] Pressure was also used to benumb the part and thus lessen the pain, and probably in time primitive man learned that pressure over certain regions, such as the nerves and arteries, had a more pronounced effect, though he did not know why.[2] Psychotherapy in the form of autosuggestion was also employed by our aboriginal forefathers, who considered pain an evil spirit and made many efforts to appease or frighten away these pain demons with rings worn in the ear and nose, talismans, amulets, tiger claws, and similar charms. In addition, the skin was tattooed with exorcist signs to keep these evil spirits outside the body. Above all, conjurations, spells, and words of might were used by the injured man, enabling him to put the pain demons to flight.

When a primitive man could not relieve his own suffering, he called on the head of the family who, according to anthropologists, in prehistoric times was the woman—the Great Mother—who acted as priestess and sorcerer in one, perhaps because the maternal instinct made her better qualified than anyone else to protect the life she had given (Fig 1–3). Even in the subsequent patriarchal state, women remained preeminent as healers. Gradually, however, their duties of banishing pain were taken over by the medicine man, conjurer, or shaman of the tribe, who, having no maternal instinct and having the same shape as all other men of the village, had to rely on the art of conjuring. It was therefore necessary for him to change his shape by dressing as an antidemon and make his house a special ''medicine hut'' where he muttered incantations and fought and wrestled with the invisible pain demons.

Change in the Meaning of Pain

Gradually man's idea of the cause of pain underwent a change; what had been interpreted as the sport of evil spirits was then seen as punishment

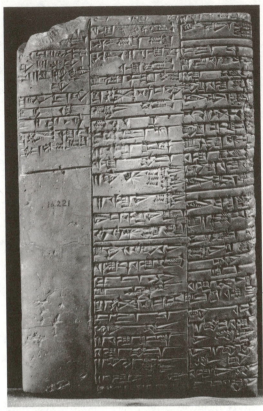

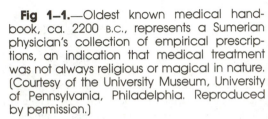

Fig 1–1.—Oldest known medical handbook, ca. 2200 B.C., represents a Sumerian physician's collection of empirical prescriptions, an indication that medical treatment was not always religious or magical in nature. (Courtesy of the University Museum, University of Pennsylvania, Philadelphia. Reproduced by permission.)

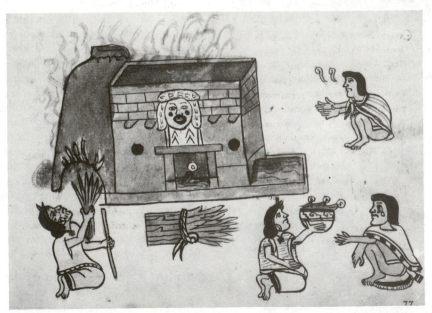

Fig 1–2.—Aztec temascal, or steam bath, was headquarters for massage specialists, who treated rheumatism, paralysis, and neuralgia. (Courtesy of the Biblioteca Nazionale Centrale, Florence. Reproduced by permission.)

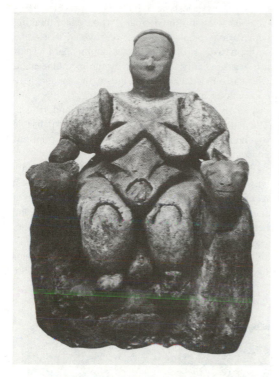

Fig 1–3.—Seated female figure, ca. 6500–5700 B.C., found in excavations of Catal Huyuk in Central Turkey, thought to be a fertility goddess shown giving birth, one of the earliest representations of delivery in this position. (Courtesy of the Archaeological Museum of Ankara, Ankara, Turkey. Reproduced by permission.)

inflicted by an offended deity. The methods of alleviating pain changed likewise, and the medicine man was replaced by the priest, servant of the gods (Fig 1–4). Along with the natural remedies, the priest relied on prayers usually made at the shrines of the deities, whether these shrines were the ziggurats of the Babylonians and Assyrians, the pyramids of the Pharaohs, the pillared temples of the Greeks, or the teocallis of the Aztecs. In holy ecstasy, the priests besought the deity to enlighten them as to the offense for which the sufferer had been smitten with a painful illness, using charms and sacrifices to propitiate the immortals. When the sacrifices had been duly made, the gods might be ready to listen to the supplications of the priests and perhaps to grant relief. Classical medicine was based on such belief, and even Hippocrates believed that *divinum est opus sedare dolorum* ("divine is the work to subdue pain").

Influence of Christianity

With the birth of Christianity, there developed a new concept of relief of pain based on divine healing through the laying on of hands and through prayer. One of the tasks of the Son of God and His

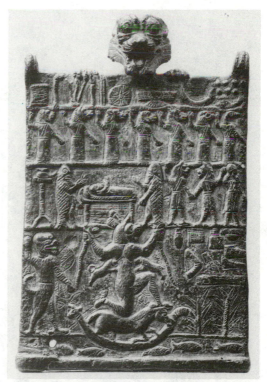

Fig 1–4.—Assyrian bronze amulet showing details of exorcism. The sick person is in the center, the priests are in the guise of fish, symbolizing Ea, the god of water, and the female demon Labartu is shown about to depart on a boat, possibly to flee the exorcism. (Courtesy of the Louvre, Paris. Reproduced by permission.)

disciples was to heal the sick and banish pain and suffering. Consequently the church of the Early and Middle Ages laid great stress on, and devoted much attention to, the alleviation of pain by its clergy by means of prayer (Fig 1–5). Faith in prayer could turn every action into a remedy, and its efficacy in relieving pain through psychotherapeutic effects has always been appreciated by physicians.

Use of Herbs and Medicines

In addition to prayer, priests employed natural remedies consisting mostly of herbs. The origin of the medicinal use of herbs is lost in the obscurities of antiquity. In the Rig-Veda of the ancient Hindus it is written, "such herbs come to us from the most ancient times, three eras before the gods were born" (Fig 1–6). It is most probable that before they were employed by priests as adjuvants to prayers, herbs were used by primitive man, who, experimenting with various plants as foods, discovered that some of them were efficacious in assuaging pain. Their use was gradually taken over by the medicine man, who surrounded his knowledge of the mystic herb concoctions handed down to him by sorcerers and magicians with mystery, incantations, and rituals. The latter were and continued to be indispensable psychotherapeutic adjuvants to the prescriptions concocted by the early physicians.

The use of analgesic drugs derived from plant life was prominent in all ancient cultures. The earliest records relate legends of pain relieving effects of such plants as the poppy, mandragora, hemp, and henbane.[1] Aesculapius, the Greek god of medicine, was said to have used a potion made from herbs called nepenthe to produce relief of pain. Perhaps the first written records on the use of analgesia are

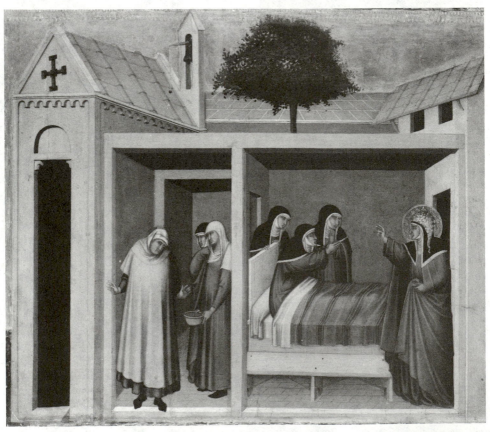

Fig 1–5.—Detail from a predella (ca. 1316?) by Pietro Lorenzetti, in which St. Humilitas miraculously heals a nun as the doctor leaves, feeling he has done everything he can for the patient. (Courtesy of the Gemäldegalerie, Staatliche Museen Preussischer Kulturbesitz, West Berlin. Reproduced by permission.)

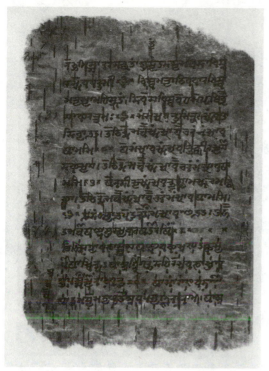

Fig 1–6.—Manuscript page from Atharva-Veda, the earliest Indian text to give much medical information. It was one of several vedas (meaning "knowledge") of Aryan invaders, on which Ayurvedic or traditional Indian medical practice was based, along with later commentaries by Charaka, Sushrata, and Vagbhata. (Courtesy of Universitätsbibliothek, Tübingen, West Germany. Reproduced by permission.)

those contained in an ancient Babylonian clay tablet from Nippur, which dates back to 2250 B.C.[3] One of these describes the remedy for the pain of dental caries by means of a cement consisting of henbane seeds mixed with gum mastic which was applied to the cavity in the tooth. The Ebers Papyrus, written about 1550 B.C., includes an early Egyptian pharmacopoeia which contains many prescriptions on the use of opium, one of which was a remedy of divine origin prescribed by Isis for Ra's headaches.[4] Surgical methods, such as trephining the skull for headaches, and physical procedures, such as exercise, massage, and the application of heat or cold, were also used by the ancient Assyrians, Babylonians, and particularly the Egyptians (Fig 1–7).[5]

The first authentic reference to the use of opium for pain relief is found in the writings of Theophrastus, who lived in the 3d century B.C.[3] The works of such famous physicians as Hippocrates, Dioscorides, Pliny, Pien Ch'iao, and Hua T'o contain many references on the use of drugs for the relief of pain.

Among the earlier references to the use of pain-relieving drugs is found in a passage of Homer's *Odyssey:* Ulysses and his comrades are treated by Helen of Troy, daughter of Zeus, who "cast into the wine whereof they drank a drug to lull pain and anger and bring forgetfulness to every sorrow."[6]

Celsus, in his *De Medicine,* written during the first century A.D., makes early reference to analgesic pills. At about the same time lived Dioscorides, a Greek army surgeon in the services of Nero, Pliny the Elder, and Scribonius Largus, all of whom wrote extensively on the preparation and use of mandragora, opium, henbane, hemp, and other drugs for the relief of pain. Largus and Dioscorides also advocated electrotherapy, in the form of shocks from torpedo fish, for neuralgia and headache,[5] and probably also practiced surgical methods for the relief of pain. A century later Galen spoke enthusiastically of the analgesic effects of opium and mandragora. He also recommended the use of electrotherapy and other physical methods,[5] and no doubt performed operations for the relief of pain (Fig 1–8).

INFLUENCE OF THE DARK AGES

As the ignorance and superstition of the Dark Ages settled over Europe, many of the methods that had been employed for the relief of pain were forgotten. During this period, the center of medicine shifted to Arabia, where Avicenna, "the Prince of Physicians," became the dominant figure. Avicenna was particularly interested in pain and the means for relieving it. In his *Canon of Medicine,* in which he codified all available medical knowledge, he described 15 types of pain and suggested such methods for its relief as exercise, heat, and massage, in addition to the use of opium and other natural drugs. This became the authoritative medical textbook of Europe for six centuries.

Paracelsus (1490–1540), who did much to overthrow the dominance which Galen had exercised over European medicine, advocated the use of various methods of analgesia, including natural drugs and such physical therapeutic methods as electrotherapy, massage, and exercise.[5] During the latter part of the Middle Ages, somniferant sponge, a sea sponge saturated with a concoction of the juices

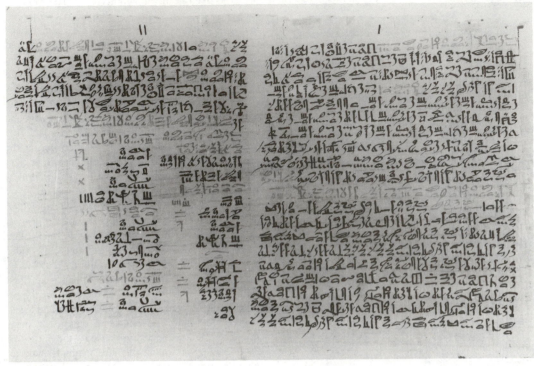

Fig 1–7.—Section of medical papyrus (ca. 1550 B.C.), one of seven extant, discovered by Georg Ebers at Thebes in 1872. The papyrus contains recipes, treatments, and magical and religious incantations. (Courtesy of Universitätsbibliothek der Karl-Marx Universität, Leipzig. Reproduced by permission.)

of opium, hyoscine, mandragora, and other plants, became quite popular in Europe. This method, which was probably based on the ancient custom of inhaling fumes produced by burning hemp, practiced by the Scythians, Egyptians, and Arabians, was employed to afford relief of pain by inducing sleep.[8]

THE RENAISSANCE

The hundreds of years of the Middle Ages contributed little to man's knowledge of alleviating pain. The Renaissance fostered a scientific spirit that enabled remarkable advancements to be made in other sciences, particulary in chemistry and physics, but there were few developments in medicine. Thus, at the end of the 18th century, one finds that opium, henbane, mandragora, and a few other natural drugs were still used much as the Egyptians, Chinese, Greeks, and Romans had used them two thousand years earlier.

CONTEMPORARY ERA

The contemporary era in pain management began in 1772 with Joseph Priestley's discovery of nitrous oxide[9] and the subsequent observation by Sir Humphrey Davy of the analgesic properties of this gas.[10] This was followed by scientific investigations on animals of the anesthetic properties of nitrous oxide and ether by Faraday[11] and Hickman,[9] and subsequent sporadic use of these agents in man by Stockman,[12] Clarke,[9] Colton,[13] Jackson,[9] Long,[9] and Wells,[9] who either did not realize the importance of their observations at the time they were made or did not publish them. This period culiminated in the first public demonstration of surgical anesthesia at the Massachusetts General Hospital on Oct. 16, 1846, by William T. G. Morton. Figure 1–9 is a wood engraving, made in 1858, showing a young woman with a chloroform inhaler attached to her face.

Soon after Davy observed the analgesic effect of nitrous oxide, another important event took place in

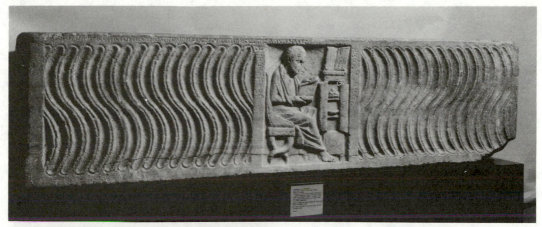

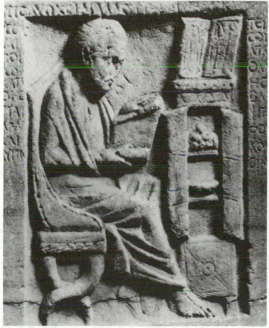

Fig 1–8.—A, Greco-Roman bas-relief of the first century A.D. showing **(B)** a physician at his desk and a case of surgical instruments on top of the cabinet. (Courtesy of the Metropolitan Museum of Art, New York. Gift of Earnest and Beata Brummer, 1948, in memory of Joseph Brummer (48.76.1). Reproduced by permission.)

man's fight to conquer pain when Frederick Sertuner,[14] an apothecary's assistant, isolated the active constituents of opium. Following isolation and preliminary testing on animals and on himself and friends, Sertuner in 1806 published his first paper, "Principium Somniferum." This important discovery was ignored, however, until 1817, when Sertuner published his second paper, in which he renamed the new active alkaloid of opium, morphine, after Morpheus, the Greek god of dreams. This ushered in a most prolific scientific period characterized by the extraction and purification of many important alkaloids employed not only for analgesia, but also for other therapeutic purposes.

Development of Anesthesia

At the time that inhalation analgesia and anesthesia was being introduced into surgical practice, another new method was being initiated by Lafargue of France (1836), Taylor and Washington of the United States (1839), Rynd of Ireland (1844), and Wood of Scotland (1843–1853),[9] all of whom began to practice hypodermic injection of a medication by various techniques. The introduction of the metallic hollow needle by Rynd[15] in 1843 and the syringe by Wood[16] in 1853 (and by Pravaz of France in the same year[17]) advanced this method, to provide analgesia for neuralgia and other types of intractable

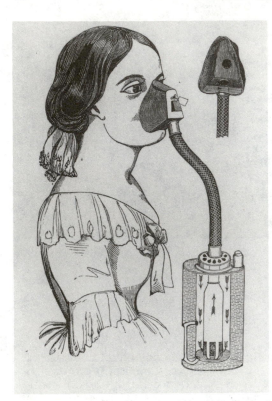

Fig 1–9.—Chloroform inhaler, as illustrated in *On Chloroform and Other Anaesthetics* (1858) by John Snow, who was influential in making anesthesiology a specialty of medicine. (Courtesy of the National Library of Medicine, Bethesda, Md. Reproduced by permission.)

pain. Spessa of Italy in 1871 advocated the injection of morphine into fistulous tracts prior to surgical excision.[18] The isolation of cocaine by Gaedeke in 1855 and the subsequent demonstration of its anesthetic properties by Bennet in 1873 and Anrep in 1878 were important, though ignored, milestones in the conquest of pain, which preceded Karl Koller's historical 1884 report on the efficacy of cocaine as a local anesthetic.[19] Though Fauvel, Saglia, and others had already learned the use of cocoa leaves and their extracts in the treatment of painful disorders of the larynx and pharynx,[20] it was Koller's work that was responsible for the development and use of cocaine as a local anesthetic.

Development of Surgical Techniques for Pain Relief

The 19th century was to produce still another great advance in the conquest of pain: surgical

methods for its eradication. Although surgery for pain was practiced in ancient times and sporadically during the Middle Ages (Fig 1–10), it did not come into its own until the advent of the Listerian era. As soon as it became possible to operate without the fear of infection, a number of surgeons throughout the world began to attack pain by a new method—the permanent interruption of its afferent pathways. Among those who pioneered surgery for pain were Horsley of England, who originated the operation for trigeminal neuralgia. The Americans Abbe, the originator of posterior rhizotomy, and Spiller and Frazier introduced retrogasserian neurectomy and cordotomy, and Cushing made outstanding contributions to surgical treatment of pain. Chippault, Jaubolay, Sicard, and Leriche developed the French school of neurosurgery and introduced the new concept of ablating the sympathetic nervous system in the management of pain. The Italian Ruggi proposed sympathectomy for visceral pain. Durante, Van Gehuchten, and de Beule of Belgium contributed authoritative experiences toward the surgical management of neuralgia. Jonnesco and Gomolu of Romania performed the first sympathectomy for angina pectoris.[21]

Radiotherapy

The discovery by Wilhelm Conrad Roentgen (Fig 1–11) on Dec. 28, 1895, of a "new kind of light"

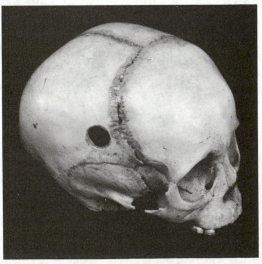

Fig 1–10.—Skull found in Peru, showing evidence of trephining. (Courtesy of the History and Philosophy of Medicine Department, University of Kansas Medical Center, Lawrence, Kansas. Reproduced by permission.)

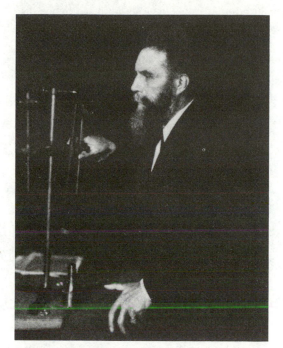

Fig 1–11.—Wilhelm Konrad Roentgen, the discoverer of x-rays. (Courtesy of the New York Academy of Medicine. Reproduced by permission.)

can be considered a great milestone in the management of pain. Soon after this discovery, roentgen rays were employed in the treatment of many conditions that were accompanied by severe and persistent pain. After the original phase of enthusiasm and the subsequent phase of pessimism had passed, roentgen therapy found its place in the management of pain.

Physical Therapy

Physical medicine made many rapid advances during the 19th century and its scope in the management of pain was enlarged.[5] The work of Edwards, Fursan, and Bernhard on light therapy, of Cavallo, Hare, Duchenne, Althouse, Testa, and D'Arsonval on electrotherapy (Fig 1–12), of Priessnitz, Winternitz, Fleury, Branch, and Baruch on hydrotherapy, of Guyot, Herschel, and Tyndall on thermotherapy, and of Graham, Weir, Mitchell, and others on mechanotherapy have contributed a great deal toward the alleviation of pain and suffering.

Perhaps the most important factors that have stood in the way of the scientific investigation of pain have been those in the human mind—religion, philosophy, and humanitarianism.

Understanding of Pain Mechanisms

For centuries religious sentiment inhibited the elucidation of the pain phenomenon, and even its control. Pain was considered a disciplinary measure for the sinners and a trial for the just. With the advent of Christianity, pain came even more definitely to be regarded as a means of enlightenment, of obtaining grace, or as a sacrament. Because bodily pain was thus regarded as a trial, a grace, and a sacrament or punishment meted out by God and it was considered "good for the soul," it was withdrawn as an object of scientific scrutiny, and any activity that tended to abolish it was inhibited.

The teachings of Aristotle, Plato, and other ancient philosophers that pain was purely an emotional process, "a passion of the soul," were accepted for 2000 years, a factor that was instrumental in delaying neurophysiologic and psychological investigations.

Soon after Johannes Müller made public his

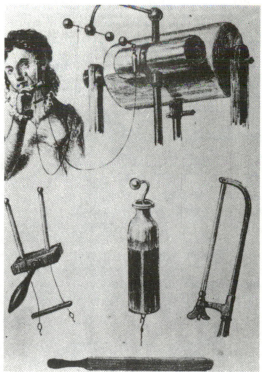

Fig 1–12.—In 1824 Charles Bew found electrotherapeutic treatment "a peculiar, and easy mode of ascertainment and cure" for tic douloureux or trigeminal neuralgia. (Courtesy of the Bakken Library of Electricity in Life. Reproduced by permission.)

theory of specific energy of nerves in the middle of the 19th century, there came into existence a new school of physiologic research composed of medical scientists who had shaken off the metaphysical shackles and had thus opened the door to the principles of scientific and experimental analysis of pain. Thus, toward the end of the 19th century there were three theories of pain: the intensive and sensory theories of the physiologists, in opposition to one another, and both opposing the emotional theory of the philosophers and psychologists. The physiologic theories were supported by the work of Goldscheider, Von Frey, Henry Head, Weir Mitchell, and other pioneers. The great bulk of work favored the sensory theory, and by the beginning of the 20th century, this had been generally accepted, even by the psychologists. Thus the traditional theory of the philosophers had been defeated.

THE TWENTIETH CENTURY

The 20th century was ushered in with many scientific advances in theories of pain. But these advances were to be dwarfed by the monumental achievements made in all phases of the pain problem during the first half of this century. The great strides made in all branches of surgery owing to better anesthesia, more liberal use of blood transfusion, and the introduction of antibiotics have made possible removal of the cause of the pain or interruption of its pathways in circumstances which previously precluded surgical intervention. The rapid development of regional analgesia has offered many newer and useful procedures in alleviating pain, e.g., continuous infusion techniques and spinal narcotics. In spite of all the achievements and in spite of the great efforts that have been made by many investigators, especially the gate control theory by Wall and Melzack, we are far from understanding pain.[22] This is due in great measure to the fact that clinical pain is only a subjective phenomenon defying objective study. It is also due to the fact that studies of the nature of pain had been almost exclusively conducted in the laboratory.

FUTURE GOALS

Presently, the resources of the anatomist, neurophysiologist, pharmacologist, and other laboratory investigators are joined with those of the clinician to solve the puzzle of pain. The united multidisciplinary effort has been richly rewarded by the discovery of the endogenous opiate system. Further work in this area is awaited with great expectations. While we await further elucidation of pain mechanisms, we must make an effort to give the various painful states an intelligent appraisal, and perhaps formulate a systematic plan for relief. This will conserve the patient's social usefulness as far as is possible. The *proper* management of pain remains the most important obligation of every physician.[23] It is hoped that this book may contribute a little toward that goal.

REFERENCES

1. Archer W.H.: The history of anesthesia, in *Proceedings of the Dental Centenary Celebration.* Baltimore, Dental Centenary Committee of the Maryland State Dental Association, 1940.
2. Allen C.W.: *Local and Regional Anesthesia.* Philadelphia, W.B. Saunders Co., 1914.
3. Macht D.I.: The history of opium and some of its preparations and alkaloids. *JAMA* 64:477, 1915.
4. Tainter M.L.: Pain. *Ann. NY Acad. Sci.* 51:3, 1948.
5. Krusen F.H.: *Physical Medicine.* Philadelphia, W.B. Saunders Co., 1941.
6. Palmer G.H. (trans.): *Homer's Odyssey.* Cambridge, Houghton, Mifflin Co., 1929.
7. Edward, Earl of Derby (trans.): *Homer's Iliad.* Philadelphia, Henry T. Coates & Co.
8. Keys T.E.: *The History of Surgical Anesthesia.* New York, Schuman's, 1945.
9. Fulton J.F., Peters C.H.: An introduction to a bibliography of the educational and scientific works of Joseph Priestley. Papers of the Bibliographical Society of America, 1936, vol. 30, p. 150.
10. Davy H.: *Researches, Chemical and Philosophical: Chiefly Concerning Nitrous Oxide, or Dephlogisticated Nitrous Air, and its Respiration.* London, J. Johnson, 1800.
11. Faraday M.: Effects of inhaling the vapors of sulphuric ether, article XVI. *Q. J. Sci. Arts Misc.* 4:158, 1818.
12. Kleiman M.: Histoire de l'anesthesia. *Anesth. Analg.* 5:122, 1939.
13. Colton G.Q.: *Anesthesia: Who Made and Developed This Great Discovery?* New York, A.G. Sherwood & Co., 1886.
14. Sertuner F.W.: Über das Morphium, eine neue Salzfähige Grundlage, und die Mekonsa ure als Hauptbestandtheil des Opiums. *Gilberts Ann. Physik.* 55:56, 1817.
15. Rynd F.: Treatment of neuralgia: Description of an instrument for the subcutaneous introduction of fluids—affections of the nerves. *Dublin Q. J. M. Sci.* 32:13, August 1945.
16. Wood A.: On a new method of treating neuralgia. *Edinburgh Med. Sci. J.* 82:265, 1855.

17. Pravaz C.G.: Sur un nouveau moyen d'operer la co-agulation du sang dans les arteres, applicable a la guerison des anevrismes. *Compt. Rend. Acad. Sci.* 36:88, 1853.

18. Spessa A.: Modo di rendere insensible una parte nella quale devesi pratticare qualche atto operatorio. *Bull. Sci. Med. (Bologna)* 11:224, 1871.

19. Koller C.: Vorlaufige Mittheilung über locale Anas-thesirung am Auge. *Klin. Monatsbl. Augenh.* 22:60, 1884.

20. Braun H.: *Die Lokal Anasthesie.* Leipsig, Verlag von Johann Ambrosius Barth, 1913.

21. Leriche R.: *Surgery of Pain.* Baltimore, Williams & Wilkins Co., 1939.

22. Melzack R., Wall P.: Pain mechanisms: A new theory. *Science* 150:971, 1965.

23. Bonica J.J.: *The Management of Pain.* Philadelphia, Lea & Febiger, 1953.

2 / Epidemiology of Pain

P. PRITHVI RAJ, M.D.

ACCURATE STATISTICS from national epidemiologic studies on the prevalence of pain and its impact on the national economy are not easy to find. However, local and regional surveys permit one to extrapolate reasonable estimates. These indicate that the cost of treating either acute or chronic pain is approximately $90 billion in the United States annually.[1] Of the 50 million accidental injuries that occur in the United States, nearly one third are associated with acute moderate to severe pain. Annually, about 400,000 accidental injuries lead to partial or permanent disability.[2] Approximately 65 million individuals in the United States suffer from chronic pain, and of these, 50 million are partially or totally disabled. In most patients with back disorders, arthritis, headache, cancer, and other chronic painful conditions, it is not primarily the underlying pathology but the pain that prevents the patient from carrying out a productive life. On the basis of these data, well over 700 million work days are lost from chronic pain, which, together with health care costs, total nearly $60 billion annually.[1]

It is important to remember the cost of human suffering, which not only produces serious physical, emotional, and affective disorders in millions of patients, but also has grave emotional and sociologic effects on members of their families. Statistics from a survey of 1,254 people across the U.S. by Lewis Harris are shown in Table 2–1.

ACUTE PAIN

It is not generally appreciated that acute pain in the postoperative period or after accidental injury or burns serves no useful purpose. If not adequately relieved, such pain can produce serious physiologic reactions that may cause significant morbidity and mortality. Similar deleterious effects may result if,

after it has served its biologic function, the severe pain of myocardial infarction, pancreatitis, or other acute visceral disorders is not alleviated. The extreme pain associated with parturition can compromise the well-being of the patient and the fetus.

Trauma

Approximately 16 million patients suffer from pain due to trauma. Acute and chronic pain from sports injuries is also becoming increasingly significant in the Western hemisphere. Fortunately, serious sports injuries are rare. In a study by Weightman and Browne, the highest injury rate occurred in contact sports like football, soccer, and rugby (4.9 per 100 participants).[3] Eleven percent of all injuries involved the head.[4] Even though in boxing indirect brain injury is produced by a blow to the chin, amateur boxing appears to be a relatively safe sport.

One of the commonest causes of serious sports injuries is skiing. Amost 500,000 persons are injured skiing each year. Approximately 225,000 fractures are due to skiing in the United States annually.

Mortality, fortunately, is rare in sports. Most deaths occur from head and cervical spine injuries and usually from severe external impact, such as being thrown from a vehicle or struck by a heavy ball or a stick.

Postoperative Pain

The incidence, intensity, and time course of postoperative pain for common procedures are not known precisely. Approximately 53 million operations are done every year in the U.S. Data based on patients' demands for analgesia suggest that among

TABLE 2–1.—EPIDEMIOLOGY OF PAIN*

Pain	Number one health complaint
Headaches	The most common pain complaint
Backaches	56%
Muscle pains	53%
Joint pains	51%
Stomach pains	46%
Menstrual pains	40%
Arthritis	Most common medical condition cited for pain
People under stress	Report more aches and pains
Working women	Have more complaints than homemakers
Doctor consulted	If the pain was felt more than six times a year in 88% of pain complainers
Pain killers prescribed	42% of patients consulted
Nonprescription drugs	Prescribed in 17% of patients
Exercises useful	In 18% of patients
People who exercise, don't smoke or drink moderately	Have less pain than their counterparts
People who exercise strenuously	Complain of more muscle pain but fewer backaches and joint pain

*Statistics from a survey of 1,254 people across the U.S. by Lewis Harris and Associates. Published in *USA Today,* October 23, 1985.

the entire postoperative population in the United States, 30% have mild pain, 30% have moderate pain, and 40% have severe pain.

Headache

One of the most common of all symptoms, headache can range from slight discomfort to excruciating pain that lasts from less than 1 hour to several days. If the headache does not recur frequently, it is considered acute pain. The prevalence of headache in the general population is about 80%–90%. Tension headache accounts for about 80% of the incidence and migrane headache for 2%–25%. Some patients have both migraine and tension headache, which appear independently in 30%–40% of the population.[5]

Waters observed that the incidence of headache declines significantly with increasing age, and is more severe in younger than in older women.[6]

Low Back Pain

Back pain occurs in 50%–80% of the population of industrial societies.[7–11] In Great Britain, 90% of all episodes of back pain remit without requiring a physician's consultation,[12] probably because most episodes of back pain are mild. In Horal's study,[8] only 3% of patients with mild low back pain sought medical attention, and even for them remission was the rule. In Fry's series,[13] 40%–50% of outpatients improved within 1 week and 90% within 8 weeks. Most of the published data are in agreement with these figures, showing 80%–90% improvement within 2 months, regardless of treatment.[8, 9, 14] Additional data indicate that recovery is rapid and complete enough that, for a given episode seen by a general practitioner, 97% of patients avoid hospitalization and 99.5% avoid back surgery.[15, 16] Furthermore, few patients suffer for a long period. In Horal's study,[8] only 2.4% of controls and 4% of sick-listed patients suffered for more than 6 months from any given episode of low back pain. Similarly, in Hult's study,[9] there was only a 4% frequency of disability of more than 6 months' duration.

At first glance, one might look at the figures and think that low back pain is not a significant problem. This is not the case. First, the general incidence of low back pain is so high that even a low percentage of persistent complainers creates a large number of chronic back pain sufferers. Second, although low back pain is characterized by a high spontaneous remission rate, it is equally characterized by a high recurrence rate. Horal noted recurrence in 90% of the patients who were sick-listed and in 67% of those who were not.[8] Other studies demonstrate a similarly high recurrence rate, in the range of 70%–80%.[7, 17] In addition, it is clear that subsequent episodes last longer and are more severe than the initial attack.[8]

There is some evidence to suggest that women may be more prone to back pain when exposed to heavy work,[18, 19] and that men may be more prone to back pain from a herniated lumbar disk.[20] However, most large studies fail to show any clear evidence that sex has a significant effect on the general frequency of back pain.[7, 8, 21, 22]

On the other hand, a significant age dependency of low back pain can be demonstrated. Data from four major studies that evaluated the frequency of back pain by decade of age may be summarized as follows: 30% of those aged 20–29 years experienced back pain, as did 51% of those aged 30–39 years, 68% of those aged 40–49 years, 73% of those aged 50–59 years, and 63% of those aged 60–69 years. In Horal's study the frequency was highest in the fifth decade of life;[8] in the studies by Hult,[9] Lawrence,[11] and Hirsch et al.[7] the frequency was highest in the sixth decade. However, the third decade is when back pain first becomes a significant problem.[8, 9]

By age 45, most people who experience back pain will have had their first episode. When the figures for age at onset are combined with the figures for peak incidence, the great majority of back pain sufferers can be placed between the ages of 25 and 55—the most productive age group.

Occupational Disability Due to Low Back Pain

There is evidence for an increase in low back symptoms in people who do heavy versus light work.[9–11, 18–21, 23–26] In a comparative study of 471 retail, light industry, and sedentary workers and 666 construction, food handling, and other heavy industry workers, the frequency of low back pain was 52% in the group that did lighter work and 64% in the heavy work group.[9] This degree of difference has been noted in many other studies.

However, if one considers only those people experiencing severe back pain, a much larger difference is noted. In Hult's study, for example, the group doing lighter work had a 6.8% incidence of severe back pain, whereas the group doing heavier work had a 10.6% incidence. This represents a 50% increase in back pain from the light to the heavy work group.

Most authors agree that the incidence of low back pain is greater in those with prolonged postural stress.[27] For example, truck and bus drivers who sit for long periods of time have a higher incidence of back pain and earlier onset.[18, 28, 29] Similarly, there is a higher incidence of back pain in miners who perform heavy work in stooped positions with poor footing.[25, 30, 31] Back pain is also more prevalent in nurses who do awkward episodic lifting.[18, 31, 32]

Occupational factors, however, are quite complex, and lifting heavy objects is not necessarily the predisposing element in back pain. Kelsey[20] was unable to demonstrate an increased risk for "disk herniation" in individuals whose jobs involved lifting, pulling, pushing, or carrying. Likewise, Rowe's industrial studies[33] did not show a preponderance of "diskogenic" back pain in heavy workers. In Hult's study,[9] the incidence of back pain and disk degeneration in weight lifters was compared with the incidence in individuals who did light and heavy work. In the older age groups, the weight lifters actually had a lower incidence of symptoms and a lower incidence of disk degeneration on x-ray.

Certain studies relate the onset of back pain to a specific accident or heavy lifting episode. In an analysis of industrial data, the percentage of individuals who recall this type of relationship is high.[23, 34, 35] In one study, over 85% of individuals with back pain related it to a specific incident.[34] In Hult's study,[9] only 30%–40% of the cases were associated with a specific accident or lifting episode. And Rowe found that trauma was rarely implicated in precipitating diskogenic backache.[33]

In the final analysis, it is not work specifically that leads to low back pain; rather, it is one's fitness to perform a certain type of work that is the significant determinant.

Manpower Costs Due to Low Back Pain

In England, more than 2% of the population are estimated to see a general practitioner each year because of back pain.[13, 36] The number of lost work days in England during a 1-year period totaled over 13,000,000. In males 75 days were lost per worker per year.[15] In Anderson's studies,[21, 37] the industrial work loss in England was approximately 18 times the overall national rate.

The rate of work loss from back pain has no less an impact on industry than the rate of hospitalization for back pain has on the health care system. In the United States in 1977, almost 400,000 people were hospitalized in short-stay hospitals for intervertebral disk displacements.[38] Interestingly, the rate of hospitalization for disk disease is 50% higher in the western United States than elsewhere in the country.[38]

As might be expected, the amount of surgery for disk prolapse is also large. In the United States in 1977, 166,000 intervertebral disks were removed surgically.[38] This figure excludes spinal fusion or other types of surgery for disorders of the lumbar spine. In the western part of the country, the rate of disk excision relative to all other operations was 50% higher than elsewhere in the country. Overall, disk excision is becoming more common in the United States. In 1973, approximately 147,000 intervertebral disks were excised, versus 166,000 in 1977.[39]

Seeing the large number of disk excisions performed, one might question how well these patients fare after surgery. Clearly, the most important indicator of success after disk excision is the percentage of pain-free patients. Though surgical management is fairly successful in eliminating the sciatic component of the pain, low back pain persists with disappointing frequency.

In a review of 3,928 previously reported cases, the average percentage of pain-free patients was 53%.[40] There was a wide range of claims, with one optimistic report showing 80% of patients free of pain following surgery. Spangford[41] showed that 60% of 2,500 patients were pain-free, although at very short follow-up. In Barr's longer follow-up,[42] only 22% of patients were free of back pain after simple disk excision. Even when he included patients who had "minor complaints," only 64% of patients could be placed in the "essentially free of back symptom" category. Hakelius,[43] in a review of patients operated on for herniated lumbar disk at the Karolinska Institute, reported that in a long-term follow-up averaging more than 7 years, only 31% of patients were free of back pain. Even if one added to the symptom-free group those patients who were improved but still had mild to moderate symptoms, the "success" rate was still only 52%. If one looks carefully at large numbers of patients who have been operated on, 50% freedom of pain is a fairly accurate measure of overall success.

It is essential to recognize what can be offered therapeutically under the best of circumstances, bearing in mind that when the circumstances are not the best, the results are substantially worse. In a recent study of Workers' Compensation patients with persistent back pain after initial surgery, the results with each successive surgery were studied. Beginning with the third operation, most patients were worse after surgery than before it.[44]

Thus, despite some optimistic reports to the contrary, it is clear that present treatment for the many patients suffering from chronic and recurrent back pain is not good. For many the appropriate treatment is uncertain; and for those who require surgery the success rate is not good. In the United States in 1971, approximately 8,000,000 people had some impairment of the back or spine, impairment being defined as a permanent defect or chronic condition causing decrease or loss of ability to perform various functions.[45] This represented almost 3.9% of the entire population.

In 1971, Haber[46] published a summary of data gathered in the Social Security Administration Study on causes of disability in the United States. Musculoskeletal conditions were at the top of the list of conditions causing disability between the ages of 18 and 64. Of the musculoskeletal conditions, impairments of the back and spine were the major cause of morbidity and disability. Even in the older age groups (45–64 years), back and spine impairments were the third leading cause of disability. Kelsey et al.[47] reviewed disability allowances granted by the Social Security Disability Board in 1973. "Displacement of the intervertebral disk" was the second most common cause of disability award for all people through the age of 49, and the third most common for the group aged 50–55 years. It must be recognized here that the term "displacement of the intervertebral disk" did not include all the remaining cases of back and spine impairments. In the 1974 nationwide National Institutes of Health Household Survey,[48] impairment of the back and spine was the third leading cause of limitation of activity and of severe disability for all ages. For individuals under 45 years of age, impairment of the back and spine was the leading cause of limitation of activity and of severe disability.

The problem seems to be on the rise. The NIH Household Survey found a 50% increase in "displaced intervertebral disk" between 1969 and 1976.[49] United States National Safety Council statistics indicate that disabling work injuries are rising faster than any other injury. This has become such an epidemic that approximately 296 of all employed individuals have a compensable back injury every year, if recurrences are included.[50]

Economic Costs of Low Back Pain

The economic dimensions of low back pain are immense: approximately $14 billion was spent on the treatment of low back pain in the United States in 1978. There is a consensus among occupational physicians that low back pain is one of the most burdensome, frequent, and problem-filled entities seen at work. The problem is enormous: by the age of 65 at least 50% of workers will be affected by low back pain. It is the leading cause of chronic disability between the ages of 19 and 45 years. In fact, low back pain is the most common complaint treated by family physicians in the United States and the 11th-ranked cause of hospitalization.

It is difficult to obtain up-to-date statistics on low back pain in the United States. According to the National Safety Council, approximately 400,000 of 590,000 cases of trunk injury resulted in low back pain in 1979.[51] Approximately 30% of all compensation claims are paid for low back pain claims. Compensation rates for low back pain in Wisconsin rose from 8% of the total case load in 1938 to 19% in 1965 and to 28% in 1978.

The injury rate yielding low back pain in light industry is approximately three to five injuries per 1,000 workers per year. In the Norton Company, which is representative of heavy industry, over 100 cases of low back pain are seen each year out of an employee population of approximately 5,000. The estimated direct and indirect costs of low back pain in this company amounted to $250,000 per year. With some 24,000 workers worldwide, the company spends close to $1 million yearly on low back pain.

Arthritis Pain

The incidence of rheumatoid arthritis in the USA is 32 per 100,000 for males and 68 per 100,000 for females. The incidence increases with age to 158 per 100,000 in the over 70 age group. It typically involves metacarpophalangeal, proximal interphalangeal, and carpal joints, elbows, knees, ankles, metatarsophalangeal joints, and temporomandibular joints. The majority of patients suffer from joint disease, pain, and stiffness during exacerbations.

Cancer Pain

Approximately 5 million people die of cancer annually in the whole world. Of these, 700,000 patients are diagnosed to have cancer in the United States, and 400,000 die of the disease. Isolated studies indicate that pain occurs in 58%–80% of hospitalized cancer patients.[7, 8] This incidence of cancer pain increases to as much as 87% in the terminal phase of the disease.

The treatment of cancer-related pain is extremely important since the advances in cancer therapy has succeeded significantly in decreasing the mortality. With longer survival time, the occurrence of cancer pain increases the incidence of chronic pain (see Chap. 20).

REFERENCES

1. Bonica J.J.: Pain research and therapy: Past and current status and future needs, in Ng L.K.Y., Bonica J.J. (eds.): *Pain, Discomfort and Humanitarian Care.* New York, Elsevier, 1980, pp. 1–46.
2. Thal E.R., Shires G.T.: Emergency assessment and management, in Giesecke A.H. (ed.): *Anesthesia for the Surgery of Trauma.* Volume 11 in *Clinical Anesthesia* series. Philadelphia, F.A. Davis Co., 1967.
3. Weightman D., Browne R.C.: Injuries in eleven selected sports. *Br. J. Sports Med.* 9:136, 1975.
4. LaCava G.: Indagine clinco stastica sulle lesioni traumatische da sport. *Minerva Med.* 1960.
5. Kunkel R.S.: Mixed headache, in Appenzeller O. (ed.): *Pathogenesis and Treatment of Headache.* Jamaica, NY, Spectrum Publications, 1976.
6. Waters W.E.: The Pontypridd headache survey. *Headache* 14:81–90, 1974.
7. Hirsch C., Jonsson B., Lewin T.: Low-back symptoms in a Swedish female population. *Clin. Orthop.* 63:171–176, 1969.
8. Horal J.: The clinical appearance of low back disorders in the City of Gothenburg, Sweden. *Acta Orthop. Scand. Suppl.* 118:8–73, 1969.
9. Hult L.: Cervical, dorsal and lumbar spinal syndromes. *Acta Orthop. Scand. Suppl.* 17:7–102, 1954.
10. Hult L.: The Munkfors Investigation. *Acta Orthop. Scand. Suppl.* 16:1–76, 1965.
11. Lawrence J.S.: Disc degeneration: Its frequency and relationship to symptoms. *Ann. Rheum. Dis.* 28:121–136, 1969.
12. Dixon A.S.J.: Diagnosis of low back pain: Sorting the complainers, in Jayson M. (ed.): *The Lumbar Spine and Back Pain.* New York, Grune & Stratton, 1976.
13. Fry J.: Back pain and soft tissue rheumatism, in *Advisory Services Colloquium Preceedings.* London, Advisory Services, Clinical and General, Ltd., 1972.
14. Dillane J.B., Fry J., Kalton G.: Acute back syndrome: A study from general practice. *Br. Med. J.* 3:82–84, 1966.
15. Benn R.T., Wood P.H.N.: Pain in the back: An attempt to estimate the size of the problem. *Rheumatol. Rehabil.* 14:121–128, 1975.
16. Wood P.: Epidemiology of low back pain, in Jayson M. (ed.): *The Lumbar Spine and Back Pain.* New York, Grune & Stratton, 1976.
17. Dehlin O., Hedenrud B., Horal J.: Back symptoms in nursing aides in a geriatric hospital. *Scand. J. Rehabil. Med.* 8:47–53, 1976.
18. Magora A.: Investigation of the relation between low back pain and occupation. *Indust. Med.* 39:31–37, 1970.
19. Nagi S.Z., Riley L.E., Newby L.G.: A social epidemiology of back pain in a general population. *J. Chron. Dis.* 26:769–779, 1973.
20. Kelsey J.L.: An epidemiological study of acute herniated lumbar intervertebral discs. *Rheumatol. Rehabil.* 14:144–153, 1975.
21. Anderson J.A.D.: Rheumatism in industry: A review. *Br. J. Indust. Med.* 28:103–121, 1971.
22. Partridge R.E.H., Anderson J.A.D., McCarthy M.A., et al.: Rheumatism in light industry. *Ann. Rheum. Dis.* 24:332–340, 1965.
23. Glover J.R.: Prevention of back pain, in Jayson M. (ed.): *The Lumbar Spine and Back Pain.* New York, Grune & Stratton, 1976.
24. Goodsell J.O.: Correlation of ruptured lumbar disc with occupation. *Clin. Orthop.* 50:225–229, 1967.
25. Lawrence J.S.: Rheumatism in coal miners. *Br. J. Indust. Med.* 12:249–261, 1955.

26. Magora A.: Investigation of the relation between low back pain and occupation. *Indust. Med.* 39:28–34, 1970.

27. Magora A.: Investigation of the relation between low back pain and occupation, three physical requirements: Sitting, standing, and weight lifting. *Indust. Med.* 41:5–9, 1972.

28. Kelsey J.L.: An epidemiological study of the relationship between occupation and acute herniated lumbar intervertebral discs. *Int. J. Epidemiol.* 4:197–205, 1975.

29. Kelsey J.L., Hardy R.J.: Driving of motor vehicles as a risk factor for acute herniated lumbar intervertebral disc. *Am. J. Epidemiol.* 102:63–73, 1975.

30. Kellgran J.H., Lawrence J.S.: Rheumatism in miners: Part II. *Br. J. Indust. Med.* 9:197–207, 1952.

31. Lawrence J.S., Aitken-Swan J.: Rheumatism in miners: Part I. Rheumatic complaints. *Br. J. Indust. Med.* 9:1–12, 1952.

32. Ferguson D.: Strain injuries in hospital employees. *Med. J. Aust.* 1:376–397, 1970.

33. Rowe M.L.: Low back pain in industry. *J. Occup. Med.* 11:161–169, 1969.

34. Kosiak M., Aurelous J.R., Hartfiel W.F.: The low back pain problem. *J. Occup. Med.* 10:288–295, 1968.

35. Troup J.D.G.: Relation of lumbar spine disorders to heavy manual work and lifting. *Lancet* 1:857–861, 1965.

36. Benn R.T., Wood P.H.N.: Statistical appendix: Digest of data on the rheumatic diseases, 4, morbidity and mortality in hospital services for rheumatism sufferers. *Ann. Rheum. Dis.* 31:522, 1972.

37. Anderson J.A.D.: Back pain in industry, in Jayson M. (ed.): *The Lumbar Spine and Back Pain.* New York, Grune & Stratton, 1976.

38. *Utilization of short-stay hospitals:* Annual summary of the United States. Vital and Health Statistics, Series 13, No. 41. Washington, D.C., U.S. Department of Health, Education and Welfare, 1977.

39. *Surgical operations in short-stay hospitals, United States.* Vital and Health Statistics, Series 13, No. 34. Washington, D.C., U.S. Department of Health, Education and Welfare, 1973.

40. Soderberg L., Sjoberg S.: On operated herniated lumbar discs. *Acta Orthop. Scand.* 31:146–152, 1961.

41. Spangford E.V.: The lumbar disc herniation: A computer-aided analysis of 2504 operations. *Acta Orthop. Scand. Suppl.* 142:1–95, 1972.

42. Barr J.S.: Low back and sciatic pain. *J. Bone Joint Surg.* 33:633–649, 1951.

43. Hakelius A.: Prognosis in sciatics. *Acta Orthop. Scand. Suppl.* 129:6–71, 1970.

44. Waddell G., Kummel E.G., Lotto W.N., et al.: Failed lumbar disk surgery following industrial injuries. *J. Bone Joint Surg.* 62:201–207, 1979.

45. *Prevalence of selected impairments, United States.* Vital and Health Statistics, Series 10, No. 99. Washington, D.C., U.S. Department of Health, Education and Welfare, 1971.

46. Haber L.D.: Disabling effects of chronic disease and impairment. *J. Chron. Dis.* 24:469–487, 1971.

47. Kelsey J.L., White A.A., Pastides H., et al.: The impact of musculoskeletal disorders on the population of the United States. *J. Bone Joint Surg.* 61:959–964, 1979.

48. *Limitation of activity due to chronic conditions, United States.* Vital and Health Statistics, Series 10, No. 111. Washington, D.C., U.S. Department of Health, Education and Welfare, 1974.

49. *Prevalence of chronic skin and musculoskeletal conditions, United States.* Vital and Health Statistics, Series 10, No. 124. Washington, D.C., U.S. Department of Health, Education and Welfare, 1976.

50. National Safety Council. *Accident Facts.* Chicago, NSC, 1976.

51. National Safety Council. *Accident Facts,* 4–24. Chicago, NSC, 1979.

3 / Organization of a Pain Clinic

FRANK MOYA, M.D.
GLORIA E. MAYNE, M.D.

THE CONCEPT OF THE pain clinic is based on the conviction that the effective management of difficult "pain" patients is possible only through the well-coordinated efforts of a group of specialists contributing their knowledge and skills to the diagnosis and solution of these patients' problems.

Patients seen in pain clinics are those for whom the routine health care system has failed.[1] They therefore demonstrate many iatrogenic problems, both medical and surgical. They present a wealth of teaching material in a unique setting, where their problems may be viewed in an interdisciplinary manner and the opinion of different specialists compared in a conference setting, without bias toward any one specialty. In a university-based pain clinic residents benefit from exposure to these patients since they exemplify the most difficult problems they will encounter in future practice. The pain clinic conference provides a forum where the activity of other specialties may be objectively assessed in a noncompetitive manner. For these reasons alone, a multidisciplinary pain clinic is essential to an integrated university medical center.

CLASSIFICATION

What is a pain clinic or center? Is it a nerve block clinic? One specialist using one or two therapeutic modalities? An acupuncture or transcutaneous electrical nerve stimulation clinic? A multidisciplinary center? A psychiatric clinic? All have been used in the management of the chronic pain patient.

A recent analysis of the American Society of Anesthesiologists' *Pain Center/Clinic Directory* revealed some interesting information regarding the organization of the 251 pain clinics listed.[2, 3] For example, over half of the clinic directors were anesthesiologists. The breakdown of directorships by specialty is as follows:

Anesthesiology	61%
Neurology/neurosurgery	11%
Psychiatry/psychology	7%
Physical medicine	4%
Orthopedics	4%
Dental	3%
Internal medicine	1%
Combinations or other	8%

In addition to these specialties, other disciplines commonly represented included physical and occupational therapy, acupuncture, social and vocational counseling, nursing, pharmacology and biofeedback, rheumatology, family practice, and oncology.

Most of the clinics surveyed were affiliated with a hospital: 44% were located in private hospitals, 30.2% in teaching units, and 5.9% in Veterans Administration hospitals. Only 15.9% were private clinics, with 3.4% listing other affiliations. Only outpatient services were offered in 14% of the units surveyed.

Regarding the size of the staff, 34% of the clinics had only one specialist and 41% had two to five specialists. Only 25% of the clinics had six or more therapeutic specialists.

The various therapeutic modalities in the clinics studied are listed below in the order of frequency.

Nerve block	87%
TENS	71%
Physical therapy	62%
Acupuncture	41.5%
Psychotherapy	41%
Behavior modification	38%

Biofeedback	37.5%
Two or fewer modalities	33%
Drug detoxification	33%
Hypnotherapy	27%
Seven or more modalities	24%
Ten or more modalities	6%

The great use of nerve blocks (87%) reflects in part the large number (61%) of anesthesiologists who are clinic directors. Regrettably, 33% of the clinics offer only one or two modalities.

In 1980 the National Institutes of Health (NIH) convened a technical review workshop of the leading pain clinic/centers in the United States. The results of that workshop are available in a monograph published by the NIH.[4]

IDEAL PAIN CLINIC

Pain clinics may be classified according to their organizational structure.[1] The ideal model is an independently budgeted, free-standing organization composed of a peer group representing different specialties, including psychology, social work, dentistry, and even law, as well as the usual medical and surgical specialties. Patient managers, selected from the physician members, act both as the clinic's liaison for the patient, the patient's family, and the referring physician, and as the medical manager who arranges the patient's course through the clinic. This course may include requisition of old records, withdrawal of medications, appointments with appropriate specialties, and various diagnostic tests. When this course is completed to the satisfaction of the individual patient's manager, the patient may be formally presented to the assembled pain clinic to request a decision concerning the most appropriate care and the possible means for implementing this advice. This conceptionally ideal organization model exists in some private-practice clinics where it has proved cost-effective, but as yet it does not appear in any academic situation.

UNIVERSITY-BASED PAIN CLINIC

The university-based multidisciplinary pain clinic must function in a self-contained world divided by medical specialty–based departments.[1] This type of clinic usually exists to meet the need of a department, a specialty training requirement, or an individual, and can exist at various administrative levels within an institution. Since it is rare that a pain clinic will operate at a level higher than that of a department, the multidisciplinary nature of the clinic and its function are usually severely compromised in the academic setting. Clinics in this situation often lack official recognition outside of their immediate department and almost never benefit from committed funds or a budget. Unfortunately, pain is not a recognized specialty, or even a subspecialty, graced with its training programs and boards. It has not yet earned its place on the academic stage.

Clinics lacking multidisciplinary support usually degrade into departmental pain clinics that emphasize the interests and specialty of the controlling department rather than the needs of the patient. This becomes a major problem for the pain clinic attempting to operate from a base within a department such as anesthesiology, neurosurgery, or physical medicine. Lack of commitment to personnel, space, and financial support on the part of the other departments involved seriously weakens the multidisciplinary nature of the clinic. Often many members of the multidisciplinary team making up the department-based clinic are professionals who have fitted in their time for the pain clinic because of personal interest without any contractual obligations. Many deals and trades must be made by the manager of the clinic to ensure the continuing unofficial participation of such professionals. Even then, the attendance of outside consultants and specialists will be irregular, not because of lack of interest, but because of conflicting commitments to their own departments. In this situation it becomes impossible to arrange a schedule binding on the members of the clinic and to ensure coverage for absences. All of this reduces the efficiency of the manager and depletes his personal energy, possibly leading to professional burnout.

Another type of university-based pain clinic is the one- or two-man, independent operation, which may be contained within a department and yet may be multidisciplinary, depending on the approach and experience of the individuals involved. This is a common form of clinic, and if patients are selected according to the resources available, a good job can be done without the administrative difficulties of managing a large group of autonomous physicians. The worst type of clinic, however, is found in this category: a specialist, either deliberately or with no malicious intent, sets up a pain clinic to justify delivering his specialty to each patient, even if it is not appropriate to that patient's needs. Unfortunately for the reputation of neurosurgery or anesthesiology, multiple surgical procedures or blocks have often been performed in this setting.

HOW TO ORGANIZE A PRIVATE PAIN CLINIC

Who?

The most important element in the success or failure of a private pain clinic is the individual responsible for its initial organization and operation. This individual may come from any of the medical disciplines, but he must have the necessary drive and determination to make it successful. A center can be multidisciplinary in its therapeutic approach, but it cannot be multidisciplinary in its administration. A successful pain clinic cannot be run by a committee.

Where?

Most private pain clinics are located in or immediately adjacent to a hospital. The advantages are obvious: proximity to the operating rooms; the availability of specialized personnel in other medical disciplines and allied health fields, of diagnostic facilities such as radiology, and of therapeutic services such as physical therapy; and the availability of critical and emergency care units.

These advantages must be weighed against the possible disadvantages found in a hospital environment, such as administrative interference; space limitations; greater cost of space, equipment, and drugs; and an unpredictable number indigent patients who must be accepted at no charge.

What?

What shall we call it—pain clinic or pain center? A facility catering primarily to private patients is best called a pain ''center.'' Private patients do not like to go to ''clinics''—except perhaps the Mayo Clinic. They associate the word ''clinic'' with charity or indigent outpatient units.

When?

When shall it be open? Clearly, an operation that can support itself financially 5 days a week is ideal, and this is certainly a goal to be desired. However, initially it may be necessary to limit the hours to 1 or 2 days per week. As the number of patients increases, the number of days can also be increased.

Commitments

A successful pain center is heavily dependent on a clear commitment of support from the hospital administration, the appropriate medical specialists and related paramedical personnel, and, above all, the medical director.

The hospital administration must provide adequate space and equipment at reasonable cost and with the least amount of administrative interference. Administrators must be convinced that a successful pain center brings not only new patients, but also new luster to the hospital.

The medical director must be able to set aside the necessary number of days per week for the center. It is not possible to schedule patients in the center subject to the vagaries of an operating room schedule. If necessary, hold the pain center open only one or two days per week—at least the patients can count on some availability. Then, little by little, as the number of patients increases, the number of days can be increased.

The organizers of the center must be prepared to absorb financial losses for at least 1 year before reaching the break-even point. Most newly organized pain centers require this much time to reach a patient volume that will make the center financially self-sustaining.

Personnel

The key person is the medical director. It is his drive and determination that will make or break the center. A large staff is not needed. Indeed, initially, a pain center can be started with just the key physician-director and one or two part-time assistants. Additional personnel can be added as required by an increased patient volume. Of course, consultative personnel should be available from all other medical and allied health disciplines, such as physical medicine and occupational therapy.

Ideally, the pain center should eventually be able to support the medical director, a full-time secretary, a nurse, a psychiatric social worker, and an acupuncturist. A part-time hypnotherapist would also be useful.

The secretary functions as an appointment secretary, receptionist, telephone operator, and billing clerk. She plays an important role in the overall smooth functioning of the center. Through careful scheduling of patients she can avoid embarrassing delays and inconvenience for everyone. By deft handling of patients over the telephone, she can save the physician time and screen out patients who obviously do not belong in the pain center. Finally, she can give the director valuable feedback regarding the patient's reaction and feelings toward the center and the therapy.

The role of the nurse can be filled by a registered nurse, a CRNA, or a medical assistant. Primarily, she functions as an assistant in the treatment room. In addition, she may instruct patients in the technique of the transcutaneous electrical nerve stimulation (TENS), exercise programs, or in the proper use of adjuvants such as heating pads, drugs, and the like.

The psychiatric social worker performs the important task of psychosocial evaluation of the patient. In addition, she provides follow-up psychosocial counseling as needed. She functions as the eyes and ears of the physician between treatments and can provide valuable feedback on the patient's progress.

The acupuncturist provides not only acupuncture but also massage and other physical therapeutic techniques.

Physical Plant and Design

The pain center can be located anywhere in the hospital. However, there are obvious advantages to keeping it relatively close to the operating room if the director is an anesthesiologist. Indeed, the recovery room has been used by some centers, especially in the early stages of a pain center's evolution. Thought should be given to the ease with which a patient can find the center, and to its proximity to the patient parking lot.

Basically, the pain center is built around the therapeutic modalities that are offered. Therefore, at the very least it should contain an office for the physician to carry out his initial consultation, and a treatment room. The office should be fully equipped, including a full-sized skeleton for patient education. The treatment room should contain all necessary drugs and equipment for nerve blocks and other therapeutic procedures performed in the center. Basic cardiopulmonary resuscitation drugs and

equipment should be immediately available. An examination table that can be quickly placed in the head-down position is also essential. The size and number of rooms needed will depend on the number of patients seen daily and the number of separate functions that will be provided.

A small quiet room will function admirably as an office for the psychiatric social worker's evaluations and follow-up counseling, as well as for the hypnotherapist on other days.

Finally, there should be a patient reception and waiting area that accommodates at least ten patients comfortably. This area should include the secretary-receptionist's work station and, preferably, a small private room for discussions with the patient regarding new appointments and professional fees. Many patients will arrive in wheelchairs or on stretchers, and all doorways, the waiting area, and traffic patterns should be designed with their special requirements in mind.

The design of the pain center should permit a neat and orderly flow of patient traffic from the reception and waiting area to the consultation office, the treatment room, and the billing clerk.

How to Start the Center

Acquiring patients, especially at the beginning, can be most difficult. However, there are various ways to stimulate interest on the part of patients and referring physicians. The most effective manner, of course, is to have one or two patients with highly successful and dramatic results. Regrettably, dramatic successes are few and far between in this field. If you are lucky enough to enjoy a great result in treating one of your early patients, then by all means bring it to the attention of your colleagues by means of informal chats in the hallway or more formal presentations at departmental meetings. Furthermore, do not discourage your patient from spreading the good news. Be sure to send a complete report on this patient to the referring physician.

Other ethical techniques that can be used to increase the number of patients include radio, television, and newspaper interviews. Because of the current great public interest in the problem of chronic pain, talks to lay groups are also a fertile field for finding patients. As soon as possible, prepare a brochure that describes in some detail what the pain center is and how it can help a patient. This is most useful for both patients and referring physicians.

THE DAILY OPERATION OF A PAIN CENTER

Making an Appointment

Although initially the pain center may not be open for patients 5 days a week, it is important that some mechanism be provided so they can make appointments to be seen. Perhaps a department secretary might function as an appointment secretary on days the pain center is closed.

Scheduling of patients should provide adequate time for each patient to receive the care necessary and appropriate for his problem. At a minimum, new patients need 1 hour for a consultation and evaluation; subsequent visits require a half-hour. Specialized procedures, such as celiac plexus or differential spinal blocks, require several hours.

All appointments should be confirmed in writing. New patients should receive a letter indicating the date, time, and precise location of the appointment. In addition, the letter should remind the patient to bring a medical summary or report from the referring physician. For the patient's convenience and information a schedule of the fees and the pain center brochure should also be enclosed. Patients coming for repeat visits are given appointment cards only to remind them of their next visit.

The Brochure

A descriptive brochure of the pain center serves as a useful guide for both the patient and referring physician.[5] Briefly and with the use of photographs, the pain center and its operation are described in some detail, including instructions on how to reach the center, how to make an appointment, what is needed for the consultation, and what to expect during the first visit. Certain patient questions should be anticipated and answered: How many visits and treatments are required? Is hospitalization necessary? What should a patient bring to the center? How much will treatment or consultation cost?

Over the years we have learned the importance of emphasizing the following points in the brochure:

1. To avoid unnecessary repetition of tests, the patient should bring or have his physician send pertinent medical records and x-ray reports.

2. The patient should prepare a one-page handwritten outline describing his pain and indicating important dates and events.

3. If possible, the patient should bring a spouse, a close friend, or a family member to the first interview.

4. The patient should bring a list of all medications he is currently taking, and a list of allergies.

A few explanatory paragraphs describing the difference between acute and chronic pain, how pain affects us, and the most common types of chronic pain problems are useful in preparing patients for the first visit. In addition, a few words indicating the different types of treatment available in the pain center are also helpful. For example:

Just as there are many different kinds of pain, so are there a variety of approaches for treating pain. These range from simple control by drugs and/or physical exercise programs to more sophisticated procedures. The latter include injections under the skin of a local anesthetic and cortisone, injections into points that trigger pain (trigger points), a variety of regional nerve blocks, injections of cortisone into the spinal canal space, acupuncture, electrical stimulation (TENS), biofeedback, hypnosis, and psychotherapy.

Mention should be made of the potential risk of adverse reactions or complications. We have found the following statements to be useful:

Just as when one is driving a car he risks having an accident, there is also the possibility of an adverse reaction or complication arising from treatment. A person may have an allergic reaction to a drug, or a complication may develop despite the most expert care. Such complications, however, are extremely rare in The Pain Center. Nevertheless, we are fully prepared for them should they occur.

Remember that chronic pain is not an emergency. Your local physician is still your primary physician. However, if you should develop a complication or reaction to a treatment received at The Pain Center, there is a member of the Department of Anesthesiology on duty 24 hours a day.

Outpatient Versus Inpatient Service

Most chronic pain problems can be treated on an outpatient basis. However, complex pain problems, surgical procedures for pain relief, continuous infusion technique, and multispecialty invasive workup necessitate treatment on an inpatient basis. In addition, a currently hospitalized patient may require pain therapy during his hospitalization. The operant conditioning units are also evolving into outpatient and inpatient centers. The structure and function of these units is detailed in Chapter 44.

The First Visit

After completing a questionnaire, the patient undergoes an office consultation and evaluation of his chronic pain problem by the director of the pain center or his associate. On the basis of this consultation, a therapeutic program is developed to help manage the problem. On rare occasions, additional medical consultations or tests may be required. Most often, however, specific treatments are recommended and started during this first visit. A psychosocial evaluation can be done as part of the first visit or no later than the second visit.

Therapeutic Techniques

Ideally, all therapeutic modalities should be available in a comprehensive pain center. Realistically, with few exceptions, this is not possible. Therefore, it is important to recognize the limitations of your particular pain center, and, if necessary, to refer your patient to another specialist or to another center to receive the appropriate therapy.

Medical Reports

The history and physical examination recorded on the patient's chart should be a relatively brief review of the facts pertinent to his pain problem. Furthermore, it must be legible so that it can be used in transferring information to third-party insurance carriers and to referring physicians or consultants. A useful final touch is a brief thank-you note to the referring physician that includes the diagnosis of the pain problem and an outline of your therapeutic game plan.

It is important to have some consistent means of following and reporting the patient's response to your therapy. One such way of evaluating therapeutic efficacy used at The Pain Center of the Mount Sinai Medical Center is shown in Table 3–1.

Fees and Payments

The patient should be made aware of your professional fee structure when he makes the first appointment. For his convenience and information, a copy

TABLE 3–1.—EVALUATION OF THERAPEUTIC EFFICACY

SUBJECT CRITERIA		
Patient	Physician	%
Excellent	Complete relief	95–100
Good	Significant improvement	70–90
Fair	Moderate improvement	40–65
Poor	Little or no improvement	<40

of your fee schedule is enclosed with the letter of confirmation. The initial consultation fee is usually commensurate with similar fees charged by other specialists in the community. Of course, there are additional charges for any treatments or tests performed.

Most patients have hospital or medical insurance. These policies vary tremendously in the coverage provided. Some pay only the hospital, some pay only the doctor, others pay both. Few policies pay the entire amount. Acupuncture, for example, is rarely covered by insurance. Because of the great variation among insurance carriers regarding reimbursement for these services, we cannot accept insurance assignment.

Direct payment by the patient should be politely requested by the billing clerk after your professional services have been rendered. An itemized receipt is then provided which can be presented by the patient to the insurance carrier for reimbursement.

A PRIVATE-PRACTICE PAIN CENTER—AN EXAMPLE

The Pain Center of the Mount Sinai Medical Center in Miami Beach, Florida, was organized in 1972 as a private-practice outpatient facility. Functionally, it is an integral part of the department of anesthesiology. It is located in the office area of the department of anesthesiology, and over the years, as The Pain Center has grown, it has cannibalized most of anesthesiology's office space. Fortunately, this does have the advantage of permitting the operation of The Pain Center and the administration of the department of anesthesiology at virtually the same time and in the same space—a highly efficient working relationship.

The Pain Center is run by a medical director assisted by two full-time physicians (including a resident in anesthesiology). These physicians are aided by a team of six assistants—two secretaries, a medical assistant, a psychosocial worker, a hypnotherapist, and an acupuncturist. Consultative personnel are immediately available from all medical disciplines, including physiotherapy.

Starting in 1972 with only a few patients a week, The Pain Center has become one of the largest private-practice outpatient facilities in the United States. The patients primarily come from the eastern half of the United States and Canada; some come from as far away as Europe and South America.

In 1982, almost 3,000 consultations and procedures to assist in the diagnosis and treatment of chronic pain problems were performed. The average age of patients was 70 years. The most common problems seen were chronic back pain (38%), herpetic neuralgia (13%), skeletal/myofascial pain (13%), headaches (9%), and cancer pain (5%). The chronic pain syndromes found most amenable to therapy are back pain, herpetic neuralgia, headaches, pancreatic cancer, and causalgia. On the other hand, the problems we find least amenable to therapy are thalamic pain syndrome, peripheral neuritis, and phantom limb pain.

Virtually all of the modern modalities of pain relief are used in the management of our patients. The most commonly used therapeutic modalities are trigger point blocks (20%), epidural or spinal steroids (18%), medical hypnosis (17%), herpetic neuralgia blocks (9%), acupuncture (9%), TENS (6%), and psychosocial counseling, used in almost all patients.

A UNIVERSITY-BASED PAIN CENTER— AN EXAMPLE

The Pain Control Center of the University of Cincinnati College of Medicine, Cincinnati, Ohio was organized in 1979 as an outpatient and inpatient facility. Functionally, it is an integral part of the department of anesthesiology. It is located in the outpatient section of the University Hospital. From its inception it has demanded a larger area every year. Presently it occupies a space of 5,000 square feet and has facilities for five examination rooms, TENS, physical therapy, behavioral medicine, and two minor surgical rooms. In addition it has space for conferences, library, billing office, consultant's offices, a reception area, and secretarial offices (Fig 3–1).

The center is directed by a medical director (anesthesiologist) with coordination provided by the pain control center manager (nurse) with the assistance of two transcriptionists, one receptionist, one secretary, and a billing manager. The pain facility includes five anesthesiologists, three clinical psychologists, two physical therapists, one dentist, four nurses, and a neurologist. A neurosurgeon and an orthopedist are on consultant staff as required.

The resident education is provided by offering three pain fellowships, every year; a junior resident rotation for 1 month; and a 6-month rotation of residents in clinical psychology. Research is coordinated by a full-time clinical research nurse.

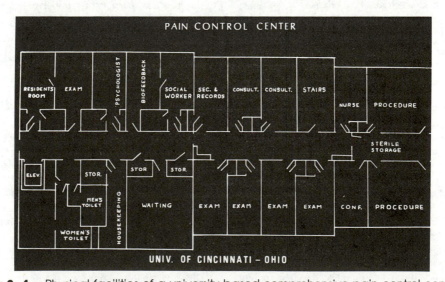

Fig 3–1.—Physical facilities of a university-based comprehensive pain control center.

The University of Cincinnati Pain Control Center is both an outpatient and inpatient facility. Approximately 5,500 patients visits are registered, with evaluation of 1,500–2,000 new patients per year. An average of ten patients are managed as inpatients every day, mainly by the resident staff. Weekly, one pain conference is attended by the multidisciplinary team and one didactic lecture is given formally for the fellows and the residents.

All modalities are provided by the center, with strengths in nerve blocks, TENS application, acupuncture, physical therapy and psychotherapy. Surgical pain-relieving procedures, like epidural stimulator placement, cordotomy, implantation of permanent epidural catheters, and pituitary adenolysis, are also provided with the assistance of the consulting neurosurgeon. The patient population treated at the center includes patients with low back pain, sympathetic pain, herpes zoster, cancer pain, paraplegia, and pain from psychosomatic causes. Drug addiction is not managed by the center.

Prolonged analgesia with continuous infusion techniques, neurolytic blocks, and intensive physical therapy is the main reason for inpatient admission. For continuous infusion the average period is about a week, and for cancer patients the stay is about 3 weeks for evaluation of spinal narcotics and permanent placement of epidural catheters.

REFERENCES

1. Black R.: Organization of multidisciplinary pain clinics. Presented at the Pain Workshop, ASA Annual Meeting, Las Vegas, 1982.
2. *Stress/Pain Manager Newsletter*. Kansas City, Missouri, May 1981.
3. American Society of Anesthesiologists: *Pain Center/Clinic Directory*. Park Ridge, Ill., ASA, 1979.
4. Ng L.K.Y. (ed.): *New Approaches to Treatment of Chronic Pain: A Review of Multidisciplinary Pain Clinics and Pain Centers*. NIDA Research Monograph 36, May 1981.
5. *A patient guide to the pain center*. Department of Anesthesiology, Mount Sinai Medical Center, Miami Beach, Fla.; Frank Moya, M.D., Director.

4 / Role of a Nurse

JENNIFER HOWELL TROTT, R.N.

EVEN THOUGH the pain experience is universal, nurses and other health care professionals have only recently begun to understand its nature and dynamics. Out of the quest for greater understanding of pain has come the development of the multidisciplinary pain control centers. As the concept of the pain control center has evolved, the role of each team member has developed and expanded.

The nurse must utilize all components of her nursing skills—assessment, planning, implementation, and evaluation—to contribute to the successful management of pain patients. In addition, excellent technical, psychosocial, and communication skills help to contribute to the plan of care formulated by the interdisciplinary pain control team. The nurse must keep in mind that, as with all chronically ill patients, she or he is involved with the family as well as the pain patient. It usually is the nurse's role to initiate family and patient teaching, to interpret and clarify, and to act as the patient's advocate. The nurse is the link between the patient/family unit and the pain management team.

Owing to development of the nursing process, nursing diagnosis, and expanded practice roles, nurses possess a unique body of knowledge and expertise to contribute to the delivery of health care. This chapter emphasizes the many ways that nurses can apply their special abilities to the discipline of pain management.

Because of their background in research and clinical practice, nurses are uniquely situated in the pain management team to coordinate pain relief modalities. As the primary coordinator of the patient's pain management, it is the nurse who makes the team's interventions work for the patient. Nurses enhance this function by developing a close relationship with the patient and family members as they implement treatment plans and provide family/patient educa-

tion. The strong bond and consequent trust fostered by the primary nurse's relationship with the patient has other important benefits. Knowing that one nurse is responsible and accountable for the patient's treatment regimen serves to reassure the patient and reduce anxiety. Such reduction in anxiety is crucial, as anxiety has been shown to increase the pain experience.

To successfully perform as primary coordinators of pain patients, nurses must have excellent assessment skills and technical ability. They will be constantly required to utilize all of the biopsychosocial and communication techniques at their disposal in order to interact effectively with both patient and family and the pain management team. The nurse becomes an advocate and interpreter, as well as implementor, educator, and monitor of the patient's progress.

With this expanded role, the clinical pain management nurse is called on to develop expertise in the following areas:

Coordination of pain assessment team
Nursing assessment and diagnosis
Individual and group patient teaching
Training patients in relaxation techniques
Use and teaching of transcutaneous electrical nerve stimulation
Coordinating patient's medications
Assisting with pain procedures (nerve block, surgery)

ADMINISTRATIVE NURSING IN THE PAIN CONTROL CENTER

The pain center nurse-administrator plans, organizes, and coordinates the implementation of nursing and other services to the patients. Although these administrative functions are not in themselves unique, their application to pain management nursing is just evolving. Heidrich[1] reported that out of 218 pain clinics surveyed in 1983, 98 did not even employ nurses. He also found that nurses saw only two thirds of patients, even though they tended to spend more than 30 minutes with each patient they saw. Nurses performed a broad range of functions, but also spent a great deal of effort on clerical matters (Table 4–1).

There are no models to utilize in structuring the nursing component of an outpatient pain center. One can now see the beginnings of structured nursing practice in pain management centers. It is hoped that formalization of models for nursing roles and functions, such as the one presented herein, will facilitate this challenging process. With nursing serving such a pivotal function in pain management, it is imperative that one adopt a consistent and unambiguous approach to this aspect of health care delivery (Figs 4–1 and 4–2).

Planning

The nurse-administrator's first task is to establish goals and priorities for nursing care. This process begins with an assessment of available personnel and resources. Because pain management is such a new field for nursing, one of the highest priorities is the education of the nursing staff. This education should include the current concepts of pain management such as the role of each individual member of the team. The nurse-administrator should work with supervisors and the pain management team to ensure that nursing goals coincide with the overall treatment goals of the center.

Once goals are clearly established, the development of staff and implementation of practice can begin. The nurse manager's role then includes over-

TABLE 4–1.—PERCENTAGE OF NURSES PERFORMING IDENTIFIED FUNCTIONS IN PAIN CONTROL CLINICS*

FUNCTION	% OF NURSES
Patient teaching	87
Illustrating procedures	74
Ordering supplies/equipment	68
VS.	50
Research	44
Completing insurance forms	21

*From Heidrich.[1] Reproduced by permission.

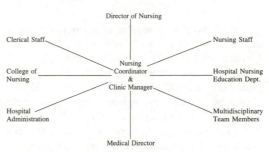

Fig 4–1.—Nursing coordinator model indicating those with whom the coordinator must interact on a daily basis. This model is used at the University of Cincinnati Pain Control Center.

seeing daily operations, collaborating with other team members, managing patient flow, facilitating staff-patient communication, and auditing the practice of the nursing staff.

Besides a broad knowledge of pain management itself, the nurse-administrator should be familiar with standard business practices utilized in the health care setting. The role of the nurse-administrator as agent and advocate of change cannot be overemphasized. The abilities to solve problems, offer innovative ideas, and supervise staff are also vital. The nurse must earn the unqualified respect of her or his professional colleagues to be successful in managing the nursing care of pain patients.

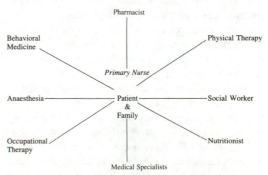

Fig 4–2.—A multidisciplinary approach indicating that the primary nurse and the patient are the focal point through which all disciplines interact. This is a practical model for clinical care wherein the nurse does not have administrative coordinating responsibilites.

Management/Administration

One of the responsibilities of the nurse-administrator is to develop a set of policies and procedures for nursing practice in a pain center. Areas that must be covered include nursing standards of care, documentation, patient instruction, admitting and discharge procedures, and record auditing. Not only are firm, consistent policies and procedures necessary for the effective operation of a clinic, they are mandatory for accreditation by the Joint Commission on Accreditation of Hospitals.

A policy/procedure manual, documentation standards, audit criteria, instruction sheet, discharge instruction sheets must be prepared for everything the nurse does in this setting. This is a large and important task since there is no nursing model of practice in pain clinics.

NURSING INTERVENTIONS

Nursing Assessment

Evaluating a patient's pain is difficult. The nurse must evaluate a patient from a physical, psychological, and social standpoint. Thorough assessment is essential. When developing this skill, the nurse must take into account her own attitudes, values, and prejudices toward pain and examine her expectations of the patient's pain tolerance and pain threshold. One must have an understanding of current knowledge about pain and its mechanisms. Johnson described the fourfold purpose of nursing pain assessment as (1) making a nursing diagnosis, (2) instituting nursing care measures or prescribed therapy, (3) helping the individual with chronic pain develop positive adaptive mechanisms, and (4) evaluating the effectiveness of interventions by determining the level of pain relief achieved.[2]

There are many assessment tools available to assist the nurse in this process. The best-known tool is the McGill Pain Assessment. This is best used on an initial assessment because it focuses on both present complaint of pain and the history of that pain. The McGill home recording card is a good tool for a follow-up assessment (Fig 4–3). The patient rates pain intensity and records the number of analgesics taken per day, the number of hours slept, and any methods of pain relief used (e.g., relaxation, guided imagery). Perhaps the most common

and quickest method of evaluating pain, whether in an acute care situation or on a follow-up visit, is to ask the patient to rate the pain on a scale from 0 to 10, where 0 represents absence of pain and 10 represents excruciating or intolerable pain. There are also simple descriptive scales and visual analogue scales available for use.

Diagnosis and Intervention

The nursing diagnosis has been defined by Durand and Prince as "a statement of a conclusion resulting from a recognition of a pattern derived from a nursing investigation of the patient."[3] For chronic pain patients, individualized goals should coincide with the overall pain center goals of increasing function or activities, decreasing pain medication, decreasing the intensity of pain, and decreasing dependence on the health care system.

Individualized patient goals should, of course, be the overall goals achievable and acceptable to the patient and the patient's family. The nurse bases interventions on specific patient priorities, current medical knowledge, the patient's level of understanding, and the nurse's own good judgment. In most pain management cases, nursing interventions focus on decreasing actual perception of pain and increasing overall patient comfort. With each visit, common effective interventions include teaching adjunct relief measures involving the patient and family in support groups, teaching about pain medications and their proper use, and just being with the patient, allowing him to express feelings and conveying acceptance of the patient as a person as well as a belief in his pain. The nurse should always remember to question patients about the methods they have used at home to relieve pain. By reinforcing noninvasive measures that have proved successful, the nurse can help the patient improve the ability to cope with future pain by relying on measures that have given relief in the past. Knowing that the nurse has the resources to deal with pain gives the patient the all-important sense of control over what is happening physically. A sense of control reduces anxiety and the patient perceives less pain.

Table 4–2 lists the accepted nursing diagnoses that are especially applicable to patients with acute or chronic pain. This list should by no means be considered exhaustive, nor should it preclude the nurse's use of good judgment and creativity in forming nursing diagnoses for individual patients. Accurate diagnoses—and interventions appropriate

McGill Home Recording Card

NAME: _____   DATE   STARTED

	Morning	Noon	Dinner	Bedtime	
M					
T					
W					
TH					
F					
SA					
SU					

PLEASE RECORD
1. Pain Intensity ∞:

    0—no pain
    1—mild
    2—discomforting
    3—distressing
    4—horrible
    5—excruciating
2. No. of Analgesics you have taken.
3. Please make note of any unusual symptoms, pains, or activities on back of card.
4. Record hours slept in morning column.

Fig 4–3.—The McGill home recording card for follow-up of a patient with pain complaints. (From Melzack R.: The McGill pain questionnaire: Major properties and scoring methods. *Pain* 1:277–299, 1975. Reproduced by permission.)

for them—are the hallmarks of effective nursing pain management.

Guided Imagery

One of the techniques a nurse may employ for chronic pain patients is guided imagery. Guided imagery denotes development of mental images that may involve any or all of the senses. The nurse must assess the individual patient's ability and readiness to attempt guided imagery before employing it.

If guided imagery seems appropriate, the nurse begins by explaining the technique to the patient. Then she or he assists the patient in exploring effective images and developing them to include the use of several senses. For example, a patient may find gardening relaxing. He is encouraged to imagine himself in a garden, while holding several fragrant flowers he can smell and touch. A recording of bird calls or bees buzzing might increase the sensation of a gardening experience. He may do the exercise with closed eyes or blindfolded to increase the use of imagination, if that provides a more satisfying experience.

Relaxation

McCaffery describes relaxation as a state of freedom from both anxiety and skeletal tension.[4] It is well known that anxiety exacerbates pain and causes the muscles to tense. Relaxation techniques can therefore be effective in the avoiding of exacerbation and reducing the amount of pain experienced. There are many methods the nurse can teach patients to use. Among them are auditory stimulation, rhythmic breathing, and counting. For these methods to be successful, the nurse must ensure that the patient is in a quiet, relaxed environment and in a comfortable position. Other methods of relaxation

TABLE 4–2.—ACCEPTED NURSING DIAGNOSES*

Comfort, alternations in: Pain
Coping, ineffective individual
Coping, ineffective family: Compromised
Coping, ineffective family: Disabling
Coping, family: Potential for growth
Diversional activity, deficit
Fear (specify)
Home maintenance management, impaired
Knowledge deficit (specify)
Noncompliance (specify)
Nutrition, alterations in: Less than body requirements
Nutrition, alterations in: More than body requirements
Nutrition, alterations in: Potential for more than body requirements
Self-concept, disturbance in
Sensory perceptual alterations
Sexual dysfunction
Sleep pattern disturbance
Spiritual distress (distress of the human spirit)
Thought processes, alterations in

*From Kim M., Montz D. (eds.): *Nursing Diagnosis*. New York, McGraw-Hill Book Co., 1981.

used commonly by psychologists and some nurses are biofeedback and hypnosis. These require specialized training and their discussion is beyond the scope of this chapter.

Distraction

Distraction is defined as the patient's transferring his focus of attention away from the painful stimulus. For example, the nurse could direct the patient to think of a favorite movie or a picture in the room. The nurse should encourage the patient to use this strategy every day during the most painful periods. The patient may find he has developed the ability to distract himself without realizing it. Watching television or taking a ride in the car can be effective distractions. The nurse should explore this technique with the patient and family because it greatly improves the patient's ability to cope with chronic pain.

Cutaneous Stimulation

As the term implies, cutaneous stimulation entails stimulating the patient's skin to relieve pain. The technique that is used most often and has been found to be very effective in pain management is transcutaneous electrical nerve stimulation. (See Chapter III.10.) Common methods of cutaneous stimulation that nurses have used for years include massage, stroking, and application of heat and cold. All are effective in reducing muscle spasm and therefore in reducing pain.

These are all techniques that nurses can teach and use on pain patients. The nurse should give a great deal of attention to helping the patient assess the effectiveness of various kinds of cutaneous stimulation, so that they may be utilized to enhance a prescribed treatment regimen.

GROUP TEACHING

Group teaching is an effective way for the nurse to communicate important information to patients, while at the same time facilitating the expression of feelings and mutual support among patients with similar problems. Patients that participate in groups feel less alone with their problems and enjoy the camaraderie in fighting the battle against pain. The topics for patient teaching groups may include cutaneous stimulation, stress management, nutrition, exercise, anxiety, medications, relaxation, and sleep. A well-prepared pain management clinical nurse can easily conduct group sessions on these topics.

Groups are most effective when kept to a maximum of 15 participants. They should meet at least once a week for 45 minutes to an hour. The nurse should plan to start new groups every 4–6 weeks to take in new patients. Many excellent texts are available for preparing nurses to utilize the art and science of group therapy and group dynamics.[5]

NURSING ASSISTANCE WITH PROCEDURES

A nurse is ideally suited to assist at nerve block procedures and at surgery for pain patients. During nerve blocks, the nurse can coordinate the preparation of the patient, assist in the explanation and signing of informed consent forms prior to block, monitor the patient during and after the block, and keep the patient emotionally stable during the procedure. If side effects appear, a nurse is ideally suited to manage them because of her expertise in drug pharmacology and intensive care training. At surgery the specialized knowledge of equipment used for such patients is helpful.

It is hoped that the nursing functions and techniques described in this chapter will serve as a model for the nursing practice of pain management, at a time when scientific nursing is just beginning to have an impact on the treatment of patients suffering from debilitating chronic pain.

The nurse has endless opportunities to develop practice in the field of pain control. These opportunities can be realized through improving assessment skill, participating in and initiating research, and communicating with other nurses about nursing roles and advances in pain management.

Pain management nursing is a specialized field. It is a stable and permanent aspect of health care delivery, and one in which nurses have a great deal to contribute. To date, the nursing approach to pain management practice has lacked consistency and definition. Nursing as a profession must take steps to standardize its position in pain management. Nursing educators, researchers, and practitioners all have a vital part in this effort. The nursing process can and must be applied to the overwhelmingly complex problem of debilitating pain if patients are to be served adequately by the entire pain management team. It is imperative that nursing define and de-

velop its own contribution to this team approach. It represents a fresh horizon for the profession, one that demands the application of the very best of nursing science, as well as the sensivity and caring spirit of nursing art.

REFERENCES

1. Heidrich G.: Survey, U.S. pain clinics 1981. Unpublished data, University of Wisconsin, Department of Anesthesiology.
2. Johnson M.: Assessment of clinical pain, in Jacox A. (ed.): *Pain: A Source Book for Nurses and Other Health Professionals.* Boston, Little, Brown & Co., 1977.
3. Durand M., Prince R.: Nursing diagnosis: Process and decision. *Nursing Forum* V(4), 1966.
4. McCaffery M.: *Nursing Management of the Patient with Pain.* Philadelphia, J.B. Lippincott Co., 1979, p. 137.
5. Turk D.C., Melchenbaum D., Genest M. (eds.): *Pain and Behavioral Medicine: A Cognitive Behavioral Perspective.* New York, Guilford Press, 1983.

5 / Role of the Physiatrist and the Physical Therapist

VICKIE M. FAIRCHILD, B.S., L.P.T.
LYNNE M. SALERNO, B.S., L.P.T.
STACY L. WEDDING, B.S., L.P.T.
ELLIOTT WEINBERG, B.S., L.P.T.

PHYSIATRIST

Physical therapy, exercises, and rehabilitation of a chronic pain patient are vital functions of any comprehensive multidisciplinary pain center. Because of his expertise in assessing disabilities in somatic functions, the physiatrist is ideally suited to plan the rehabilitation program for chronic pain patients. He can, at the initial stage of evaluation, predict the chances for full or partial recovery based on disability. This is very important to chronic pain patients, since by the time they reach the pain centers, they have also reached the end of their rope and have exhausted all other avenues of help.

In addition to the evaluation and development of a rehabilitation program for chronic pain patients, the physiatrist coordinates the treatment program with the physical therapist and occupational therapist and optimizes each mode of treatment. He participates in patient-related pain center conferences and contributes his expert knowledge toward developing an integrated program of therapy for a pain patient. His contribution to such conferences helps the other specialists develop their own therapeutic regimens. A physiatrist can and should develop education and research programs pertaining to his specialty in physical therapy pain centers. Contribution in education can be at all levels, e.g., patient, resident-fellow, other personnel in the pain center, other specialists. Research in the treatment and rehabilitation of pain patients is sorely needed. Physiatrists can play a key role in developing that research.

Unfortunately, a physiatrist is generally not interested in managing chronic pain patients. His interest normally lies in rehabilitation rather than pain control. He prefers to manage spinal cord or trauma injuries and perform diagnostic studies (e.g., electromyography) rather than be part of a multidisciplinary team to treat chronic pain patients. A physiatrist has a close relationship with neurologists and neurosurgeons in managing neurologic diseases and trauma, and with orthopedists in the rehabilitation of patients with skeletal trauma. It is not surprising, then, that only an occasional physiatrist has interest in pain control. This interest also dissipates somewhat when physiatrists realize that their best chances of success depend on working as a member of a multidisciplinary team. Presently there is heightened interest in pain control by rehabilitation centers in the United States, and the physiatrist plays a key role at such centers.

PHYSICAL THERAPIST

The role of a physical therapist in the pain center is to prevent disability and pain, restore function, promote healing, and train the chronic pain patient to cope with permanent disability. A physical therapist treats the acute pain based on specific etiology and the chronic pain based on disability and interaction with a multidisciplinary team. The elimination of pain is accomplished through noninvasive techniques such as application of heat, cryotherapy, electrical stimulation, massage, traction, mobilization, and exercises.

Utilization of appropriate technique is often initiated through evaluation. The evaluation takes into account the subjective history and objective measurements. The objective measurements consist of an evaluation of gait, posture, range of motion, joint mobility, flexibility, and muscle strength and coordination. A program is individualized for each patient after interaction with the multidisciplinary team. The progress is reported at weekly conferences, and changes in the program are made based on input by a physiatrist or the multidisciplinary team.

Group therapy sessions such as back schools and group exercises can be managed and coordinated by a physical therapist. Group physical therapy sessions are increasingly popular. The occupational therapist can take over once the pain patient has reached the stage of rehabilitation and requires further vocational training. This coordinates the smooth transition of a patient from being disabled and nonproductive to being able to lead a useful productive life even though sometimes with limited career opportunities.

6 / Role of the Anesthesiologist

P. PRITHVI RAJ, M.D.

A PAIN CLINIC or center is a functional and organizational entity that can be successfully developed at virtually any level of organization and sophistication. Basically, it is a unit in which objective means of screening and evaluating the physiologic and psychological mechanisms underlying a patient's pain problem are applied. Based on information derived from these screening tests, appropriate therapy is delineated and provided. Since objective assessment of the physiologic mechanism underlying a patient's pain is best carried out by the application of differential neural blockade, the anesthesiologist plays a key role.[1] It is his contribution that will establish the diagnosis of pathways by which pain is transmitted, and whether it has an afferent or efferent component or not. In many of the commonly encountered pain syndromes, i.e., low back pain, diskogenic pain, myofascial pain, herpes zoster and postherpetic neuralgia, reflex sympathetic dystrophy, and pain secondary to malignancy, the anesthesiologist, with his training and expertise in regional blocks, is well equipped to provide the appropriate therapy. Although the psychological aspects of pain are not his province, the anesthesiologist can, with the computerization of psychological tests, provide the necessary tests to evaluate the psychological component of the patient's pain problem. In addition, the anesthesiologist can learn some of the simpler therapeutic modalities ordinarily provided by other disciplines, such as biofeedback, physical therapy, intra-articular and intrabursal steroid injections, and so forth.

The anesthesiologist does not operate in a vacuum. Whether the pain center is at a large university medical center or at a small 50-bed hospital, the anesthesiologist is aware, or should be aware, of which specialists are able and willing to provide therapeutic measures beyond his scope. Thus, while a pain clinic may be structurally unidisciplinary (since not all disciplines are represented on a *routine* basis), the clinic becomes multidisciplinary whenever a consultant is asked to participate in the diagnosis and management of a particular pain problem. In fact, this form of "multidisciplinary" clinic, wherein one specialist guides the patient through the diagnostic and therapeutic maze and other specialists are on call to assist in specific problems, is probably the most efficient format for treating the vast majority of problems seen in a pain clinic.

The pain clinic based in a department of anesthesiology presents some unique problems. When the physician in a pain clinic admits a patient to his service or accepts responsibility for an outpatient's care, he becomes a primary care physician and has the same responsibilities as an internist, a surgeon, or any other primary care physician. This is a different approach from the one the anesthesiologist traditionally has and can result in serious conflict with the structure of an anesthesiology department. Primary care departments such as medicine and surgery have provision for directly interfacing with patients through clerks experienced in patient scheduling and have call and work schedules centered around ward patients and clinics. The anesthesiology department, on the other hand, has little experience with direct patient contact and a tight schedule that is centered around the operating room, preoperative and postoperative visits, and providing coverage for emergency cases. Because of this fundamental difference, special provision must be made for individuals working in the pain clinic so that their time commitments do not conflict with those of the department. They also need to maintain credibility and visibility among their fellow anesthesiologists, who may be unaware of, even uninterested in, their activities and protective of their own time and call obligations. The anesthesiologist heavily involved in clinical pain management may be bypassed for promotion because his heavy patient care and teaching load in the pain clinic are not taken into consideration in a service- and research-based department.

In some institutions, lack of bed space under direct control of the pain center causes inefficient management of pain patients requiring hospitalization. Admission may be required on a long-term basis for detoxification, a legitimate function of the pain clinic and one that the anesthesiologist is superbly equipped to manage. Short-term admission of patients undergoing major destructive nerve blocks for cancer pain or of patients undergoing analgesic techniques requiring chronic catheter placement or with inadvertent complications of blocks is another indication for hospitalization. Most anesthesiologists do not have admitting privileges, and beds for those purposes are ''borrowed'' from other services. The pain clinic physician must then attempt management of a patient who is on another service, under the control of interns and residents who may have no special interest in that patient's problem and often little experience in handling drug withdrawal or the complications of nerve blocks. The pain clinic physician, whom the patient has accepted as his primary physician, is now relegated to the role of a consultant whose advice may or may not be followed. The extra time and effort required in this type of invisible attending management is enormous and is another demonstration of the difficulty of pain clinic management from within an anesthesia department. These difficulties must be corrected. Anesthesiologists should have special training in pain management. Hospital privileges should include admitting privileges.

Overall, however, the expertise of the anesthesiologist is required by the multidisciplinary team in the diagnosis and therapeutic management of pain patients. Pain centers are not comprehensive enough without them.

REFERENCES

1. Black R.: The organization of multidisciplinary pain clinic. Presented before The Pain Workshop, ASA annual meeting, Las Vegas, Nevada, 1982.

7 / Role of the Neurologist and the Neurosurgeon

GERALD L. MORIARTY, M.D.
ELIZABETH BULLITT, M.D.

IT IS GENERALLY ASSUMED by specialists in neurosciences that organic pain can only be caused by abnormalities in the function of the nervous system. They take great pains to seek this abnormality by objective methods such as myelography, electromyography (EMG), or evoked somatosensory, visual, or auditory potentials prior to confirming an organic cause. Unfortunately, the incidence of pain secondary to objectively confirmable nervous system dysfunction is less than 20%. Similarly, the incidence of pain secondary to psychogenic causes is approximately 20%. It follows, then, that approximately 60% of patients have organic causes with or without psychogenic overlay. When routine diagnostic studies are conducted on such patients, they are usually negative. These patients fall into the category of those having myofascial or musculoskeletal pain. The neurologist and the neurosurgeon have difficulty in recognizing such patients as suffering from organic pain. They prefer to classify them as patients with no organic cause of pain. This is unfortunate. Thermography may be helpful in objectively confirming the myofascial causes of pain.

NEUROLOGIST

The role of the neurologist in the pain center is to perform a thorough neurologic examination, to diagnose or rule out neurogenic causes, and to predict the outcome of the neurogenic disease (if present) in a pain patient. The neurogenic causes seen in pain centers are neuropathies (diabetic, nutritional), neuralgias (tic doloroux, postherpetic neuralgia), CNS disease (multiple sclerosis, intracranial lesion,

thalamic syndrome), cancer affecting the CNS, stroke, spasticity, paraplegia, and radicular pain secondary to disk prolapse or degenerative arthritis.

It is in the realm of the neurologist to do a thorough workup on such patients by performing and evaluating the results of electrodiagnostic studies, computerized tomography, myelography, and blood chemistry studies. The neurologist plays a key role in a multidisciplinary patient conference on such patients to develop the appropriate therapeutic program.

Didactic teaching and training of residents and fellows are also essential functions of the neurologist. The teaching is directed toward obtaining and reading an EMG, myelogram, and x-ray films; training is directed toward the conduct of a proper neurologic examination.

Some neurologists have a special interest in neurophysiology. Such persons could play a key role in basic research into the mechanisms of pain. Recent advances in pain are due to such basic researches.

Experiences of a Neurologist in a University-Based Pain Center

G. Moriarty

I have the pleasure of reflecting on my experience as the neurologist consultant to a large and busy pain control center. The relationship came about during the evolution of the center when it was ready to integrate neurology into a multidisciplinary program. Prior to that, the need for a neurologic opinion was met by occasional referrals to outside consulting neurologists. The new relationship had several objectives: first, to make it simple for the pain center staff to obtain a full neurologic consultation; second, to make it possible for the neurologist to be a part of the initial therapeutic planning and continue ongoing neurologic evaluation and to care as a part of the overall management plan; and third, to provide neurologic teaching for residents and fellows in training at the pain center. This could be in the form of consultation notes, scheduled didactic conferences on topics in neurology, participation in patient care conferences, telephone discussions, or hallway consultations with a colleague.

The range of problems and the variety of patients referred to a neurologist in a pain clinic are indeed broad. The patients have in common that they hurt, and that only rarely are their neurologic problems simple. The history is usually long and involved. It may feature several illnesses, a variety of attending and consultant physicians, a colorful list of procedures and therapeutic interventions along the way, reports or rumors of medications tried and failed, a formidable bundle of photocopied medical records, and often an unmistakable tone of growing discouragement on the part of the physician who finally made the pain clinic referral.

In this center, neurology consults are seen in the center itself rather than in the consultant's office. This makes life simpler for the patients, and it allows easy communication with the referring physician in the center.

The reasons for neurologic referrals differ. Sometimes the question is what role a neurologic problem may be playing in a multifactorial, painful illness. Occasionally the underlying diagnosis needs clarification, in part because the passage of time has allowed the story to unfold. Sometimes there is a question of how much further neurologic workup should be undertaken before treatment is begun and suggestions are solicited on further treatment. Occasionally a neurologic problem may be evolving and the primary physician in the pain center needs to have its current status redefined. Often a decision as to whether a surgical procedure is called for is developed jointly with the consultant neurosurgeon.

For the consultant neurologist, the pain clinic is a veritable garden of common and unusual pathologies. Some representative of nearly every imaginable painful neurologic entity makes its appearance in a large and busy pain center. There are the muscle contraction headaches, difficult migraines, atypical facial pain syndromes. Painful neuropathies of all sorts appear; central pain syndromes related to pathology around the thalamus or within the spinal cord are not uncommon. Root and spinal cord pathologies abound. The list goes on. As expected in a referral setting as a pain center, diagnostic problems for a consultant there are frequently difficult and intriguing.

I am never left with any doubt at the end of an afternoon of consulting that the consultant has earned his fee.

But while the work is challenging, the rewards are considerable. Most patients whom the neurologist sees usually get better, and the consult is often a factor in their improvement. Most headache problems can be helped. The same is true for the painful neuropathies. Occasionally the reinvestigation of root symptoms uncovers the treatable process. And every consultant has had the thought occur as he or she drives home from work that the good accomplished that day lay less in what they did than in what they prevented from being done.

Among the chief satisfactions of the neurologist's afternoon each week in the pain center is the opportunity to participate in the clinic's educational program for residents, fellows, nurses, and psychologists. One derives satisfaction from the knowledge that his work helps physicians in other specialties be effective in their own careers. And one is reassured by seeing other physicians become excited and enthusiastic about aspects of the practice of neurology.

Finally, a pain center can be an extraordinarily fine source of patients for a neurologist with a research interest in the physiology or treatment of pain. In general, the patient population is reliable and cooperative, and they participate in a program of care that usually extends over weeks or months. When the pain clinic is located within an academic center and enjoys the multidisciplinary participation of other physicians with academic or research interests, the opportunities for collaboration become quite exciting.

Overall, for a pain center designed to provide comprehensive management of difficult pain problems, the regular in-house participation of a neurologist is an important asset, and I have always felt genuinely welcomed. For me, collaboration with the pain center offers stimulating opportunities to contribute to the care of patients, to develop an unusually close and pleasant collaborative relationship with colleagues, to contribute to the education of younger colleagues, and to cultivate research interests in an academic milieu.

NEUROSURGEON

A large number of pain patients are referred to the neurosurgeon by other physicians. Commonly they diagnose and treat radiculopathies secondary to herniated disks. In 80% of cases of disk protrusion, treatment with laminectomy and decompression is successful. However, 20% of patients experience recurring pain that increases with each operation. The neurosurgeon is frustrated in his attempts to treat such pain patients and refers them to pain centers primarily for a conservative holistic approach. The neurosurgeon also plays an essential role in treating pain due to terminal cancer, peripheral nerve injuries, cranial, and spinal cord lesions.

Technically, the neurosurgeon is trained to perform percutaneous thermocautery or cryocautery of lesions of the trigeminal ganglion, pituitary, and spinal cord (cordotomy), and permanent placement of electrodes for stimulation-produced analgesia on the spinal cord, intracranially, or on peripheral nerves.

He is a key member of the pain center team for patient education, for resident and fellow training, and for research. Community physicians usually send pain patients to the neurosurgeon. His presence helps the referral of such patients to the pain center. In return he can perform the important function of community education in chronic pain, a neglected field.

The neurosurgeon usually has adequate inpatient and academic facilities. This can provide for clinical and basic research, which can be carried out by him or his staff. He usually has enough influence in the hospital or the university to continue to provide facilities, money, and personnel to undertake research programs in pain.

The pain centers may have a neurosurgeon as the director. This may be perceived by the community as lending validity to the pain center. These centers usually are surgically oriented, with support from psychologists and physical therapists. Unfortunately, 60% of pain patients (those with pain from musculoskeletal syndromes) are not adequately treated in such centers, since evaluation and research are commonly oriented toward finding an organic basis for all pain.

Some neurosurgeons have become frustrated with the generally poor results of surgical approaches to pain patients and have in fact changed to conservative modalities, with greater success. Usually the neurosurgeon has little time to spare from a busy operating schedule and a neurosurgical clinic. This makes them poor administrators of outpatient pain centers. The neurosurgeon can be an asset to the pain center if he can evaluate pain patients for surgical indications, manage surgical patients, train fellows in neurosurgical techniques of pain relief, conduct neurophysiologic research, and provide community education on pain.

8 / Role of the Psychiatrist and the Psychologist

P. PRITHVI RAJ, M.D.

THE CHRONIC PAIN PATIENT differs from the acute pain patient in that the chronic pain patient has insignificant pathology with significant behavioral change. This behavioral change may alter a patient's personality profile, which in turn may increase the intensity of pain perceived over time. It is possible that the decrease in pain threshold may be due to alteration in central neuromodulators or neurotransmitters. A psychiatrist or a psychologist can diagnose and measure the behavioral alterations of pain patients. This gives them a key role to play in the treatment and management of chronic pain patients.

PSYCHIATRIST

The evaluation of changes in personality, mood, and other psychopathic indices can be done by the psychiatrist in the pain center. The clinical evaluation is supported by psychometric testing, including a dexamethasone suppression test. Based on this evaluation, the psychiatrist can classify the pain patient as depressed, addicted to drugs, suicidal, or malingering. He can then define and arrange the proper regimen for these patients. In an outpatient pain center, he arranges for patients needing psychiatric hospitalization for drug overdose, suicidal tendencies, or acute severe depression. If the pain center has an in-patient facility, he admits such patients directly under his care.

All chronic pain patients need adjuvant psychotherapeutic care. This may be in the form of hypnosis, biofeedback, relaxation techniques, guided imagery, operant conditions, etc. The psychiatrist helps the multidisciplinary team choose the optimum psychotherapy and evaluate its efficacy at regular intervals.

Unfortunately, not all psychiatrists are trained in managing pain patients. They gain their experience by working in the pain centers. In general, psychiatrists, who do not treat pain patients, are unaware of the modalities of pain control. This makes it difficult for the psychiatrist treating pain patients to communicate effectively with his colleagues about such patients. For instance, the psychiatrist in the pain center would encourage drug withdrawal for pain control, whereas drug use is common in routine psychiatric practice.

The psychiatrist plays a key role in specialized units that provide operant conditioning, occupational psychological therapy, and drug withdrawal programs. Psychiatrists are also important members of the pain center teams in designing therapeutic programs for routine chronic pain patients. They train residents in modes of therapy and initiate researches in specialized areas. Unfortunately, government agencies and third-party carriers are skeptical about the role of psychotherapy for chronic pain patients. This deters psychiatrists from entering the field of management of pain.

PSYCHOLOGIST

The psychologist provides day-to-day therapeutic regimens in psychotherapy. In centers where a psychiatrist is not available, the psychologist takes the psychiatrist's role and designs and evaluates programs, in addition to providing the services of hypnotherapy, biofeedback, and relaxation therapy. Drug therapy is not initiated by psychologists, but they usually recommend antidepressant medication, to the physician pain managers.

Their greatest input in the pain team is in provid-

41

ing psychometric testing, interpreting the data, and classifying the chronic pain patients to develop integrated therapeutic regimens with other members of the team. They are essential members of the operant conditioning team, offering occupational psychology and group therapy programs for stress reduction and drug withdrawal.

Unlike psychiatrists, psychologists can develop full-time careers in pain centers. This allows the development of training and research programs in pain psychology.

Many pair centers in the United States are directed by psychologists who treat pain patients. These centers believe that relieving stress, psychotherapy, and proper counseling reduce the pain sufficiently in chronic pain patients that they can cope adequately with their life. Although this is true to a certain extent, segmented single modality centers like these are not sufficient to treat difficult chronic patients such as those with low back pain, paraplegics, and cancer patients. Multimodality centers are needed for optimal care. The role of the psychiatrist and psychologist is an important one in developing that optimal care for pain patients.

9 / Role of the Orthopedist

P. PRITHVI RAJ, M.D.

IN A MULTIDISCIPLINARY pain team, an orthopedist plays a vital role in the management of pain patients. Common conditions of patients referred to pain centers include low back pain, reflex sympathetic dystrophies, cancer pain, postherpetic neuralgia, arthritis, headaches, phantom limb pain, and psychosomatic pain disorders. At many centers, low back pain, arthritis, and reflex sympathetic dystrophies account for 60%–80% of referrals.

An orthopedist has expertise in diagnosing and treating low back pain and arthritic pain secondary to the musculoskeletal causes. In addition, he can assess the functional disability of the pain patient and its prognosis, and recommend various orthopedic surgical options. The orthopedist has the facilities to admit the pain patients for workup, consultation, and treatment. Conservative methods for treating low back pain such as traction, exercise, and physical therapy (e.g., heat and massage) are routine treatment modalities for him. If he is trained to do laminectomy, he can also surgically treat herniated disks, in addition to performing other spinal surgeries. He has expertise to prescribe braces and corsets.

Chemonucleolysis is performed for the most part by the orthopedist. Since serious sequelae can occur, the experience gained by the orthopedist is essential to do such procedures.

For patients with scoliosis and back pain, the orthopedist's input is important for initial evaluation, therapeutic planning, and follow-up. Surgical intervention for such patients also falls in the province of the orpthopedist.

Patients with reflex sympathetic dystrophy usually have minor trauma to the skeleton or the myofascial tissues. The orthopedist involved with pain patients in a multidisciplinary pain center can recognize such patients early and plan an appropriate treatment. Early treatment of such patients gives the best results.

Arthritic patients may have deformities of the extremities with and without pain. These deformities are usually surgically corrected by specially trained orthopedists or by hand or plastic surgeons. In arthritic patients with pain, pain control is equally as important as selection of surgery for correcting deformities. It must be recognized that operative procedure may by itself increase the pain or result in the development of reflex sympathetic dystrophy, even though the functional disability may be improved.

Pain associated with sports injuries is now increasingly seen in the pain centers. The orthopedist is optimally suited to manage such patients. His ability to refer these patients to other members of the pain team helps to develop the optimal treatment plan.

The orthopedist improves the quality of patient care in pain centers by participating in patient conferences, resident education, and research in orthopedic-related pain syndromes. A few centers in the United States are directed by orthopedists. They usually are surgically oriented and limited to physical and occupational therapy and preliminary psychological screening. The orthopedist as a surgeon does not have enough time to devote to the pain patient. If he feels there is nothing surgical to offer, he discharges the pain patients quickly. He may not be the right specialist to administer the pain center because of lack of time and limited interest in pain patients. However, because of his broad knowledge of low back pain, arthritis, reflex sympathetic dystrophy, and sports injuries, he is an important member of the multidisciplinary pain center team.

PART II

Fundamental Considerations

10 / Basic Functions and Organization of the Nervous System

P. PRITHVI RAJ, M.D.

THE FUNCTION of the nervous system is to control the various total body activities in the conscious and the unconscious state at all times. To achieve this goal it receives literally millions of bits of information from different sensory organs and integrates them to determine the response[1] required for the preservation of life and well-being of the individual. This chapter describes the general design of the nervous system to accomplish this function.

SENSORY RECEPTORS

Most effector activities of the nervous system are initiated by information received from sensory receptors, whether these be visual, auditory, or tactile from the surface of the body.[2, 3] The sensory information can cause an immediate reaction, or its memory can be stored in the brain for minutes or years and later brought to conscious thought to help determine the reactions at some future date.

Figure 10–1 illustrates a portion of the somatic sensory system that transmits information from the sensory receptors situated on the entire surface of the body and deep structures. Information enters the nervous system through the spinal or cranial nerves and is transmitted into the spinal cord, the reticular substance of the medulla, pons, and mesencephalon, the cerebellum, the thalamus, and the somatesthetic areas of the cerebral cortex. In addition to these "primary sensory" locations, signals are also relayed to every other segment of the nervous system.[1]

Types of Sensory Receptors

There are basically five different types of sensory receptors:[4, 5]

1. *Mechanoreceptors,* which detect mechanical deformation of the receptor or of cells adjacent to the receptors.
2. *Thermoreceptors,* which detect changes in temperature, some receptors detecting cold and others warmth.
3. *Nociceptors,* which detect physical and chemical damage in the tissues.[6]
4. *Electromagnetic receptors,* which detect light on the retina of the eye.
5. *Chemoreceptors,* which detect taste in the mouth, smell in the nose, oxygen level in the arterial blood, osmolality of the body fluids, carbon dioxide concentration, and perhaps other factors that make up the chemistry of the body.[7]

Free nerve endings are found in all parts of the body. A large proportion of these detect pain. However, other free nerve endings detect crude touch, pressure, and tickle sensations, and possibly warmth and cold. Several of the more complex receptors in Figure 10–2 detect tissue deformation. These include the Merkel's disks, the tactile hairs, pacinian corpuscles, Meissner's corpuscles, Krause's corpuscles, and Ruffini's end-organs.[8] In the skin these receptors detect the tactile sensations of touch, pressure, and vibration. In the deep tissues they detect stretch, deep pressure, or any other type of tissue deformation—even the stretch of joint capsules and ligaments to determine the angulation of a joint. The Golgi tendon apparatus detects the degree of tension in tendons, and the muscle spindle detects relative changes in muscle length.

Differential Sensitivity of Receptors

Each type of receptor is highly sensitive to the one type of stimulus for which it is designed and

47

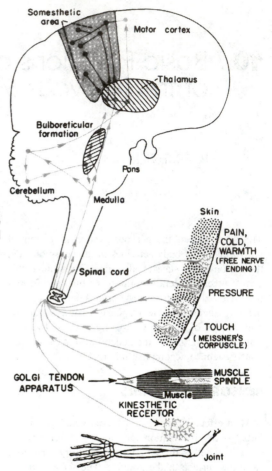

Fig 10–1.—The somatic sensory axis of the nervous system. (From Guyton.[24] Reproduced by permission.)

almost nonresponsive to normal intensities of other types of sensory stimuli.[9] For example, the rods and cones are highly responsive to light but are almost completely nonresponsive to heat, cold, pressure on the eyeballs, or chemical changes in the blood. The osmoreceptors of the supraoptic nuclei in the hypothalamus detect minute changes in the osmolality of the body fluids but have never been known to respond to sound.[10] Nociceptors in the skin are almost never stimulated by usual touch or pressure stimuli but do become highly active the moment tactile stimuli become severe enough to damage the tissues.[11]

Modality of Sensation

Each of the principal types of sensation—pain, touch, sight, sound, pressure, and temperature—represents a modality of sensation. Yet although we experience these modalities, nerve fibers transmit only impulses. How are these different nerve impulses converted to different modalities of sensation? The answer is that each nerve tract terminates at a specific point in the CNS, and the type of sensation felt when a nerve fiber is stimulated is determined by the specific area in the CNS to which the nerve fiber leads. For instance, if a pain fiber is stimulated, the person perceives pain regardless of what type of stimulus excites the fiber. This stimulus can be electricity, heat, crushing, or stimulation of the pain nerve ending by damage to the tissue cells.[12]

Adaptation of Receptors

A special characteristic of all sensory receptors is that they adapt either partially or completely to stimuli after a period of time. When a continuous sensory stimulus is applied, at first the receptors re-

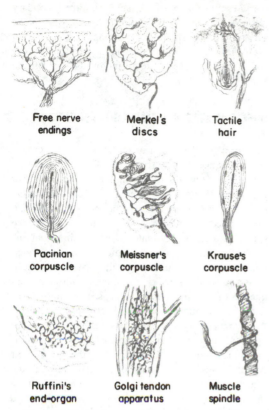

| Free nerve endings | Merkel's discs | Tactile hair |

| Pacinian corpuscle | Meissner's corpuscle | Krause's corpuscle |

| Ruffini's end-organ | Golgi tendon apparatus | Muscle spindle |

Fig 10–2.—Several types of somatic sensory nerve endings. (From Guyton.[24] Reproduced by permission.)

spond at a very high impulse rate, then progressively less rapidly, until finally many of them no longer respond at all.[13] The pacinian corpuscles adapt to extinction within a few thousandths to a few hundredths of a second, and the hair base receptors adapt to extinction within a second or more.[14] It is probable that other mechanoreceptors also adapt eventually, but some require hours or days to do so; they are therefore frequently called ''nonadapting'' receptors. The longest measured time for complete adaption of a mechanoreceptor is about 2 days for the carotid and aortic baroreceptors. Pain and chemoreceptors never adapt completely.[15]

The Nociceptors

The pain receptors in the skin and other tissues are all free nerve endings.[16] They are widespread in the superficial layers of the skin and also in certain internal tissues, such as the periosteum, the arterial walls, the joint surfaces, and the falx and tentorium of the cranial vault. Most of the other deep tissues are less extensively supplied with pain endings; nevertheless, any widespread tissue damage can summate to cause the aching type of pain in these areas.

Some nociceptors are excited only by excessive mechanical stress or mechanical damage to the tissues; these are called mechanosensitive nociceptors.[17] Others are sensitive to extremes of heat or cold and are called thermosensitive pain receptors. Still others are sensitive to various chemical substances and are called chemosensitive nociceptors. The chemicals that excite chemosensitive nociceptors include bradykinin, serotonin, histamine, potassium ions, acids, prostaglandins, acetylcholine, and proteolytic enzymes.[18] Although some nociceptors are sensitive to only one stimulus, most are sensitive to more than one stimuli.

In contrast to other sensory receptors in the body, the nociceptors adapt either poorly or not at all to continued stimulation. In fact, under certain conditions, the threshold for excitation of the nociceptors becomes progressively lower with continued stimulation. This hypersensitivity of the nociceptors is called hyperalgesia.[19]

THE MOTOR EFFECTORS

The most important ultimate role of the nervous system is control of body function. This is achieved by control or contraction of skeletal muscles, contraction of smooth muscle, and control of secretion by exocrine and endocrine glands of the body. Collectively, control of these activities is referred to as the motor function of the nervous system. The muscles and glands are effectors because they perform the functions based on commands from the nervous system. That portion of the nervous system directly concerned with transmitting signals to the muscles and glands is called the motor division of the nervous system.

Figure 10–3 illustrates the motor axis of the nervous system for controlling skeletal muscle contraction. Operating parallel to this axis is the autonomic nervous system, which controls smooth muscles and glands.[20] The skeletal muscles can be controlled at different levels of the nervous system. These include the spinal cord, the reticular substance of the medulla, pons, mesencephalon, the basal ganglia, the cerebellum, and the motor cortex. Each of these different levels plays a specific role in the control of

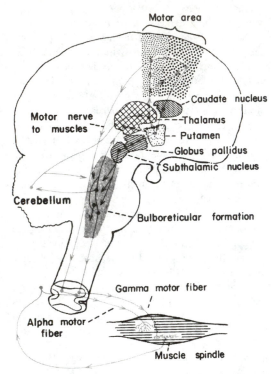

Fig 10–3.—The motor axis of the nervous system. (From Guyton.[24] Reproduced by permission.)

body movements. The lower regions are concerned primarily with automatic, instantaneous responses of the body to sensory stimuli and the higher regions with deliberate movements controlled by the thought processes of the cerebrum.[21]

INFORMATION PROCESSING

The nervous system would not be at all effective in controlling bodily functions if each bit of sensory information caused some motor reaction.[22] Therefore, a major function of the nervous system is to process incoming information in such a way that appropriate motor responses occur.[23] Indeed, more than 99% of all sensory information is discarded by the brain as irrelevant and unimportant. For instance, one is ordinarily totally unaware of the parts of the body that are in contact with clothing and/or pressure in the gluteal region while sitting.

After the important sensory information has been selected, it is channeled into proper motor regions of the brain to cause the desired responses. If a person places a hand on a hot stove, the desired pri-

mary response is to lift the hand, with the secondary response of moving the entire body away from the stove and even shouting or crying with pain. Yet even these very visible responses represent only a small fraction of the total motor system of the body.[24]

INFORMATION STORAGE—MEMORY

Only a small fraction of the sensory input causes an immediate motor response. The remainder is stored for future control of motor activities and for use in the thought processes.[25] This storage occurs mostly in the cerebral cortex, but not necessarily all of it, since the basal regions of the brain and the spinal cord can store small amounts of information.

The storage of sensory information is termed memory and is a function of the synapses.[26] Each time a particular sensory signal passes through a sequence of synapses, these synapses become facilitated in transmitting the same signal the next time. After the sensory signal has passed through the synapses many times, the synapses become so facilitated that signals generated within the brain itself can also cause transmission of impulses through the same sequence of synapses even though the sensory input has not been excited. This gives the person a perception of experiencing the original sensation, even though it is only a memory of the sensation.[27]

Once memory has been stored in the nervous system, it becomes part of the processing mechanism.[28] It helps to select the important new sensory information and to channel this information into appropriate storage areas for future use, or to motor areas for effector responses.

LEVELS OF NERVOUS SYSTEM FUNCTION

The human nervous system has inherited specific characteristics from each stage of evolutionary development. There are three major levels of the nervous system that have special functional significance: (1) the spinal cord, (2) the lower brain, and (3) the cortex.[29]

The Spinal Cord

The spinal cord of the human being still retains many functions of the multisegmental animal.[30] Sensory impulses are transmitted through the spinal nerves into each segment of the spinal cord. They can cause localized motor responses in the segment of the body from which the sensory information is received or in adjacent segments. Essentially all the spinal cord motor responses are automatic and occur almost instantaneously. They usually occur in specific patterns of response called reflexes.

Figure 10–4 illustrates two of the simpler spinal cord reflexes. To the left is the neural control of the muscle stretch reflex. If a muscle suddenly is stretched, a sensory receptor in the muscle, the muscle spindle, is stimulated and transmits nerve impulses through an afferent nerve fiber into the spinal cord. This fiber synapses directly with a motoneuron in the anterior horn of the spinal cord. The motoneuron in turn transmits impulses back to the muscle to cause the effector muscle to contract. The muscle contraction opposes the original muscle stretch. Thus, this reflex acts as a feedback mechanism to prevent a sudden change in the length of the muscle. This allows a person to maintain the body posture in desired positions despite sudden outside forces that tend to move the parts out of position.[31]

To the right in Figure 10–4 is illustrated the neural control of another reflex called the withdrawal reflex. This is a protective reflex that causes withdrawal of any part of the body from an object that causes pain,[32] e.g., if a hand is placed on a sharp object, by reflex action the hand moves away from the sharp object. This action is due to the pain signals that are transmitted to the gray matter of the spinal cord, which, after appropriate selection of information by the synapses, signal the appropriate motoneurons to cause flexion of the biceps muscle.

After the brain is removed, the spinal cord can continue to perform certain functions. For instance, an animal can under certain conditions be made to stand up. This is caused primarily by reflexes initiated from the pads of the feet. Sensory signals from the pads cause the extensor muscles of the limbs to tighten, which in turn allows the limbs to support the animal's body.

With its spinal cord transected, an animal can with its feet hanging begin walking or galloping movements with one, two, or all of its legs. This illustrates that the basic patterns for causing the limb movements of locomotion are present in the spinal cord.[33] Cord reflexes exist to cause emptying of the urinary bladder and of the rectum.

Segmental temperature reflexes are present throughout the body. Local cooling of the skin causes vasoconstriction, which helps to conserve heat in the body. Conversely, local heating of the skin causes vasodilatation, resulting in loss of heat from the body. The segmental and multisegmental reflexes of the spinal cord demonstrate that many of our moment-by-moment activities are controlled by the respective segmental levels of the spinal cord, and the brain plays only a modifying role.[34]

The Lower Brain

Most of what we call subconscious activities of the body are controlled in the lower areas of the brain, i.e., in the medulla, pons, mesencephalon, hypothalamus, thalamus, cerebellum, and basal ganglia. Subconscious control of arterial blood pres-

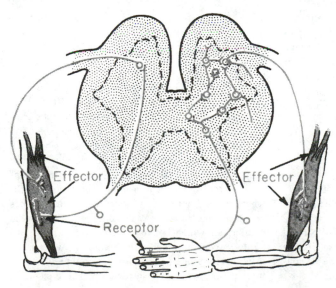

Fig 10–4.—Two spinal reflexes: *left*, muscle stretch reflex; *right*, withdrawal reflex.

sure and respiration takes place primarily in the reticular substance of the medulla and pons. Control of equilibrium is a combined function of the older portions of the cerebellum and the reticular substance of the medulla, pons, and mesencephalon. The coordinated turning movement of the head, of the entire body, and of the eyes are controlled by specific centers located in the mesencephalon, paleocerebellum, and lower basal ganglia. Feeding reflexes, such as salivation in response to taste of food and licking of the lips, are controlled by areas in the medulla, pons, mesencephalon, amygdala, and hypothalamus. And many emotional patterns, such as anger, excitement, sexual activities, reactions to pain, or reactions of pleasure, can occur in animals without a cerebral cortex.[35]

The Cortex

The cerebral cortex is primarily a vast storage area for information. Approximately three quarters of all the neuronal cell bodies of the entire nervous system are located in the cerebral cortex. It is here that most of the memories of past experiences and many of the patterns of motor responses are stored.[36] This information is ready to be called at will, to control motor functions of the body.

The cerebral cortex is an outgrowth of the lower regions of the brain, particularly of the thalamus.[37] For each area of the cerebral cortex there is a corresponding and connecting area of the thalamus, and activation of a minute portion of the thalamus activates the corresponding and much larger portion of the cerebral cortex. The thalamus can thus call forth cortical activities at will. The mesencephalon also transmits diffuse signals to the cerebral cortex, partially through the thalamus and partially through other pathways, to activate the entire cortex. This process is the state of consciousness. On the other hand, when these areas of the mesencephalon become inactive, the thalamic and cortical regions also become inactive, the process termed sleep.[38]

The Thought Processes

Some areas of the cerebral cortex are not directly concerned with either sensory or motor functions of the nervous system—for example, the prefrontal lobes and large portions of the temporal and parietal lobes. These areas are set aside for the more abstract processes of thought, but even they have direct connections with the lower regions of the brain.[39]

Large areas of the cerebral cortex can be destroyed without blocking the subconscious or even many involuntary conscious activities of the body. For instance, destruction of the somatesthetic cortex does not destroy one's ability to feel objects touching the skin, but it does destroy the ability to distinguish the shapes of objects, their character, and the precise points on the skin where the objects are touching. Thus, the cortex is not required for perception of sensation, but it does add immeasurably to the meaning of that sensation. Likewise, destruction of the prefrontal lobe does not interfere with one's ability to think, but it does destroy the ability to think in abstract terms.[40] Significantly, each time a portion of the cerebral cortex is destroyed, a vast amount of information that was stored is lost.

SYNAPSES

Information is transmitted in the CNS mainly in the form of impulses through a succession of neurons.[41] The fate of these impulses varies as information is transmitted. For example, information may be blocked in its transmission from one neuron to the next, or changed from a single impulse into repetitive impulses, or integrated with impulses from other neurons to cause highly intricate patterns of impulses in successive neurons. All these processes can be classified as synaptic functions of the neurons.[42] The synapses perform a selective action of blocking the weak signals and allowing the strong signals to continue, of amplifying selected weak signals, and of channeling the signal in different directions.[43]

The Synaptic Knob

The basic structure of the synaptic knob (presynaptic terminal) is illustrated in Figure 10–5. It is separated from the neuronal soma by a synaptic cleft having a width of 200 to 300 Angstroms. The knob has two kinds of internal structures important to the excitatory or inhibitory functions of the synapse: the synaptic vesicles and the mitochondria. The synaptic vesicles contain a transmitter substance which, when released into the synaptic cleft, either excites or inhibits the neurons by its action on the neuronal membrane, which contains either excitatory or inhibitory receptors. The mitochondria provide adenosine triphosphate (ATP), which is required to synthesize new transmitter substance.[44] The transmitter

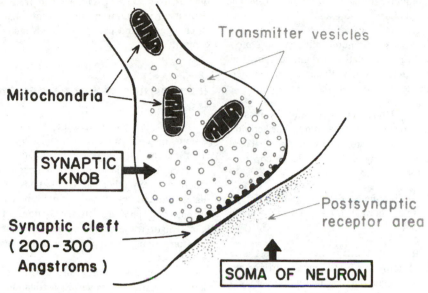

Transmitter vesicles

Mitochondria

SYNAPTIC KNOB

Synaptic cleft (200 - 300 Angstroms)

Postsynaptic receptor area

SOMA OF NEURON

Fig 10—5.—Physiologic anatomy of the synapse. (From Guyton.[24] Reproduced by permission.)

is synthesized extremely fast since the amount stored in the vesicles is sufficient for maximum activity for only a few seconds in some, to a few minutes in others.

When an action potential spreads over a presynaptic terminal, the membrane depolarization causes emptying of a small number of vesicles into the cleft; the released transmitter in turn causes an immediate change in the permeability characteristics of the postsynaptic neuronal membrane.[45] This leads to excitation or inhibition of the neuron, depending on the type of receptor substance.[46] For example, the same neuron might be excited by a synapse that releases acetylcholine but inhibited by another synapse that releases glycine. Thus, the neuronal membrane contains an excitatory receptor for acetylcholine and an inhibitory receptor for glycine. Similarly, norepinephrine released by some synapses in the CNS causes inhibition while at other synapses it causes excitation. In the first instance, the neuronal membrane contains an inhibitory receptor for norepinephrine, while in the second instance, it contains an excitatory receptor for the same transmitter.[47]

Important Transmitter Substances

There now exists good evidence for about 30 CNS transmitters.[48] The evidence confirming the presence of these transmitters includes the following: (1) the transmitter substance has been isolated from the neuronal tissue or shown to exist in specific neurons by chemical or immunologic techniques; (2) the enzymes required for synthesis of the specific transmitter have been isolated from the nervous tissue or shown to exist specifically in the synaptic knobs; (3) injection of the transmitter substance into the local neuronal areas will cause excitation or inhibition; (4) substances that prevent destruction of the transmitter will potentiate its effect on the local neurons; and (5) specific mechanisms for removing a specific transmitter after it is released have been discovered in the local tissue area. Some of the substances that fulfill many of these criteria are described below.

ACETYLCHOLINE.—Acetylcholine is secreted by neurons in many areas of the brain. Its presence has been proved beyond doubt in the striatal region of the basal ganglia and at the endings of the recurrent nerve fibers from the anterior motor neurons where they terminate on the Renshaw cell in the anterior horn of the cord. Acetylcholine is a widely used transmitter substance throughout the brain.[49] It has an excitatory effect almost everywhere, even though it is known to have inhibitory effects in some portions of the peripheral parasympathetic nervous system, for example, inhibition of the heart rate by the vagus nerves.

NOREPINEPHRINE.—Norepinephrine is secreted by many neurons, the cell bodies of which are located in the reticular formation of the brain stem and in the hypothalamus.[50] The axons of these neurons have widespread connections in the brain. In most instances they cause inhibition, although it is probable that they cause excitation in some regions. Epinephrine is secreted by fewer neurons, but in general they parallel the norepinephrine system.

DOPAMINE.—Dopamine is secreted by neurons that originate in the substantia nigra. The terminations of these neurons are mainly in the striatal region of the basal ganglia. The effect of dopamine usually is inhibition.[51]

GLYCINE.—Glycine is secreted mainly at synapses in the spinal cord. It usually acts as an inhibitory transmitter.

γ-AMINOBUTYRIC ACID (GABA).—GABA is secreted by nerve terminals in the spinal cord, the cerebellum, the basal ganglia, and many other areas. It is believed to cause inhibition.

GLUTAMIC ACID.—Glutamic acid is probably secreted by the synaptic knobs in many of the sensory pathways. It causes excitation.

SUBSTANCE P.—Substance P is released by nociceptive fiber terminals in the substantia gelatinosa of the spinal cord. In general, it causes excitation.[52]

ENKEPHALINS AND ENDORPHINS.—These are secreted by nerve terminals in the spinal cord, in the brain stem, in the thalamus, and in the hypothalamus. They act as excitatory transmitters that excite another system, which in turn inhibits the transmission of pain.[53]

SEROTONIN.—Serotonin is secreted by nuclei that originate in the median raphe of the brain stem and project to many areas, especially to the dorsal horn of the spinal cord and to the hypothalamus. It acts as an inhibitor of pain pathways in the spinal cord and is believed to modulate mood and even to cause sleep.[54]

Other substances that have been shown to have transmitter activity include peptides, amino acids, histamine, prostaglandins, and cyclic AMP.[55]

MECHANISM OF INFORMATION PROCESSING

The primary role of the nervous system is to control the body's functions. To do so, it gains infor-

mation from the environment and from within the body itself. It then transmits this information, stores it, changes it, and uses it to its advantage for body control.

Transmission of Signals and Impulses

The term information, as it applies to the nervous system, means a variety of things. For example, it could mean knowledge, or quantitative values, or the intensity of pain or light or temperature, or sensation from any other part of the body or its immediate surroundings. Thus, pain from a pinprick is information, pressure on the bottom of the feet is information, the degree of angulation of the joints is information, and a memory stored in the brain is information.

Obviously, one of the characteristics of information that must be conveyed is the quantitative intensity of the information, for instance the intensity of pain. The different gradations of intensity can be transmitted either by utilizing increasing numbers of parallel fibers or by sending more impulses along a single fiber. These two mechanisms are called respectively spatial summation and temporal summation.[24]

Spatial Summation (Multiple Fiber Summation)

Figure 10–6 illustrates the phenomenon of spatial summation, whereby increasing signal strength is transmitted by using an increasing number of fibers. Figure 10–6 shows a section of skin innervated by a large number of parallel pain nerve fibers. Each of these arborizes into hundreds of minute free nerve endings that serve as nociceptors. The entire cluster of fibers from one pain fiber frequently covers an area of skin as large as 5 cm in diameter, and this area is called the receptive field. The number of endings is large in the center of the field but becomes less and less toward the periphery. A pinprick of the skin usually stimulates endings from many different pain fibers simultaneously. But if the pinprick is in the center of the receptive field of a particular pain fiber, the degree of stimulation is far greater than if it is in the periphery of the field. Thus, a mild pinprick might stimulate only the pain fiber receiving the signal from the center of its receptive field.

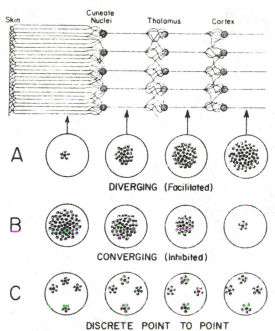

Fig 10–6.—Phenomenon of spatial summation, whereby increasing signal strength is transmitted by using an increasing number of fibers.

Temporal Summation

A second means by which signals of increasing strength are transmitted is by increasing the frequency of nerve impulses in each fiber. This is called temporal summation.

How does the brain detect the area on the body that is receiving a sensory stimulus, and how does the brain transmit impulses to individual skeletal muscles? It does this by transmitting their signals in spatial patterns through the nerve tracts. All the different nerve tracts, both in the peripheral nerves and in the fiber tracts of the CNS, are spatially organized. For instance, in the dorsal columns of the spinal cord the sensory fibers from the feet lie toward the midline, while fibers entering the dorsal columns at higher levels of the body lie progressively more toward the lateral sides. This spatial organization is maintained with precision all the way to the somatesthetic cortex.[56] Likewise, the fiber tracts within the brain and those extending into motor nerves are spatially oriented.

Processing of Signals in Neuronal Pools

The CNS contains thousands of separate neuronal pools, some of which contain very few neurons while others hold vast numbers. For instance, the entire cerebral cortex could be considered to be a single large neuronal pool. If all the surface area of the cerebral cortex were flattened out, including the surfaces of the penetrating folds, the total area of this large flat pool would be several square feet. Many separate fiber tracts enter the cerebral cortex (afferent fibers) and many others leave it (efferent fibers). Furthermore, it maintains the same quality of spatial orientation as that found in the nerve bundles. However, within this pool of neurons are large numbers of short nerve fibers by which signals spread horizontally from neuron to neuron within the pool itself.[57]

Most information is transmitted from one part of the nervous system to another through several successive neuronal pools.[58] For instance, sensory information from the skin passes first through the peripheral nerve fibers, then through second-order neurons that originate either in the spinal cord or in the cuneate and gracilis nuclei of the medulla, and finally through third-order neurons originating in the thalamus to the cerebral cortex. Such a pathway is illustrated in Figure 10–7. Recent evidence suggests that the degree of inhibition or facilitation of most neuronal pools is controlled by centrifugal nerve fibers that pass from the respective sensory areas of the cortex downward to the separate sensory relay neuronal pools. Thus, these nerve fibers help to control the faithfulness of signal transmission.

AFFERENT PAIN PATHWAYS

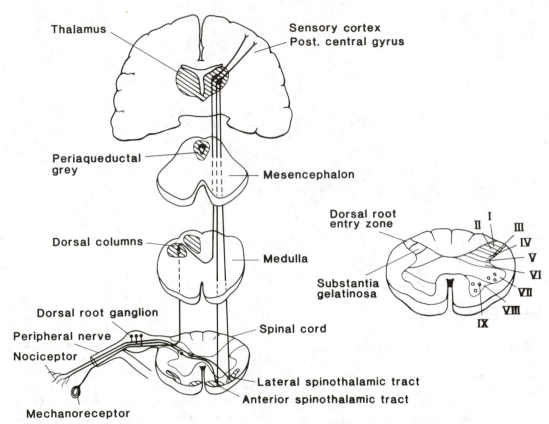

Fig 10–7.—Afferent pain pathways.

In many instances, a signal entering a pool causes a prolonged output discharge, called after-discharge, even after the incoming signal is over. After-discharge may last from a few milliseconds to many minutes. The three basic mechanisms by which after-discharge occurs are synaptic after-discharge, the parallel circuit, and the reverberatory (oscillatory) circuit.

Many neurophysiologists believe that one of the most important of all circuits in the entire nervous system is the reverberatory, or oscillatory, circuit. Such circuits are caused by positive feedback within the neuronal pool. That is, the output of a neuronal circuit feeds back to re-excite the same circuit. Consequently, once stimulated, the circuit discharges repetitively for a long time. In an animal whose spinal cord is transected in the neck, a sudden painful stimulus applied to the animal's paw will cause the flexor muscles to contract and remain contracted

a fraction of a second to more than a second after the stimulus ends. It is believed that this is caused by an after-discharge of the reverberatory type.[24]

Almost every part of the brain connects either directly or indirectly with every other part, and this creates a serious problem. If the first part excites the second, the second the third, the third the fourth, and so on until finally the signal re-excites the first part, it is clear that an excitatory signal entering any part of the brain would set off a continuous cycle of re-excitation of all parts. If this should occur, the brain would be inundated by a mass of uncontrolled reverberating signals—signals that would be transmitting no information but nevertheless would be consuming the circuits of the brain so that none of the informational signals could be transmitted. Such an effect actually occurs in widespread areas of the brain during epileptic fits.[59]

How does the CNS prevent this from happening

all the time? The answer seems to lie in two basic mechanisms that function throughout the CNS: (1) inhibitory circuits, and (2) fatigue of synapses. If the excitability of a pathway in the nervous system is too great, too many impulses are transmitted and the fatigue mechanism will automatically adjust the sensitivity of the pathway to a lower level. If the sensitivity is too low, too few impulses are transmitted, and the sensitivity of the system will automatically adjust to a higher level. Therefore, this fatigue mechanism and its recovery during rest is probably important for maintaining a proper balance among the conductivities of the respective pathways throughout the brain.

PHYSIOLOGIC CLASSIFICATION OF NERVE FIBERS

Some sensory signals must be transmitted to the CNS extremely rapidly for the information to be useful. For instance, the sensory signals that apprise the brain of the positions of the limbs during running must be transmitted extremely fast for moment-to-moment postural changes. At the other extreme, prolonged, aching pain need not be transmitted rapidly, so very slowly conducting fibers will suffice. Fortunately, nerve fibers are present in all sizes between 0.2 and 20 μ in diameter; the larger the diameter, the greater the conducting velocity. The range of conducting velocities is between 0.5 and 120 meters per second (m/sec).

In the general classification, the nerve fibers are divided into types A and C, and the type A fibers are further subdivided into alpha, beta, gamma, and delta fibers.[13]

Type A fibers are the typical myelinated fibers of spinal nerves. Type C fibers are the very small, unmyelinated nerve fibers that conduct impulses at low velocities. These constitute more than half the sensory fibers in most peripheral nerves and also all of the postganglionic autonomic fibers.

The sizes, velocities of conduction, and functions of the different nerve fiber types are given in Figure 10–8. Note that very large fibers can transmit impulses at velocities as great as 120 m/sec. On the other hand, the smallest fibers transmit impulses as slowly as 0.5 m/sec, requiring about 2 seconds to go from the big toe to the spinal cord.

Over two thirds of all the nerve fibers in peripheral nerves are type C fibers.[24] Because of their great number, they can transmit tremendous amounts of information from the surface of the

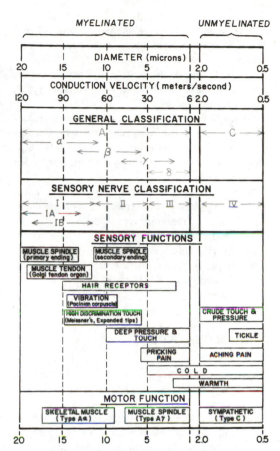

Fig 10–8.—Classification of nerve fibers, their velocity of conduction, and their functions. (From Guyton.[24] Reproduced by permission.)

body, even though their velocities of transmission are very slow. Utilization of type C fibers for transmitting this great mass of information represents an important economy of space in the nerves, for use of the larger type A fibers for transmitting all information would require peripheral nerves the size of large ropes and a spinal cord almost as large as the body itself (see Fig 10–8).

Alternate Classification

Certain recording techniques have made it possible to separate the type A-alpha fibers into two subgroups, yet these same recording techniques cannot distinguish easily between A beta and A gamma fibers. Therefore, the following classification is frequently used by neurophysiologists:

Group Ia. Fibers from the annulospiral endings of muscle spindles (average diameter about 17 μ). These are type A alpha fibers in the general classification.

Group Ib. Fibers from the Golgi tendon organs (average diameter about 16 μ; these are also type A alpha fibers).

Group II. Fibers from the discrete cutaneous tactile receptors and also from the flower-spray endings of the muscle spindles (average diameter about 8 μ; these are beta and gamma type A fibers in the other classification).

Group III. Fibers carrying temperature, crude touch, and pricking pain sensations (average diameter about 3 μ, these are type A delta fibers in the other classification).

Group IV. Unmyelinated fibers carrying pain, itch, temperature, and crude touch sensations (0.5 to 2 μ in diameter; called type C fibers in the other classification).

PAIN SENSATION

Pain is a protective mechanism for the body; it occurs whenever any tissues are being damaged, and it causes the individual to react to remove the pain stimulus. Even such simple activities as sitting for a long time on the ischia can cause tissue destruction because of lack of blood flow to the skin where the skin is compressed by the weight of the body. When the skin becomes painful as a result of the ischemia, the person shifts weight unconsciously. A person who has lost the pain sense, such as after spinal cord injury, fails to feel and therefore fails to shift weight. This eventually results in ulceration at the areas of pressure unless special measures are taken to move the person from time to time.

Pain has been classified into three different major types: pricking, burning, and aching pain.[24] Other terms used to describe different types of pain include throbbing pain, nauseous pain, cramping pain, sharp pain, and electric shock-like pain.

Pricking pain is felt when a needle is stuck into the skin or when the skin is cut with a knife. It is also often felt when a widespread area of the skin is diffusely but strongly irritated.

Burning pain, as its name implies, is the type of pain felt when the skin is burned. It can be excruciating.

Aching pain is felt not on the surface of the body, but in the deep structures. Aching pain of low intensity in widespread areas of the body can summate into a very disagreeable sensation.

What causes the differences in quality of pain sensation? The answer lies in the type of pain fiber stimulated. It is known that pricking pain results from stimulation of type A delta pain fibers, whereas burning and aching pain results from stimulation of the more primitive type C fibers.

Fast and Slow Pain Fibers

Pain signals are transmitted from the periphery to the spinal cord by small type A delta fibers at velocities between 6 and 30 m/sec and also by type C fibers at velocities between 0.5 and 2 m/sec. When the type A delta fibers are blocked without blocking the C fibers by moderate compression of the nerve trunk, the pricking type of pain disappears. On the other hand, when the type C fibers are blocked without blocking the delta fibers by low concentrations of local anesthetic, the burning and aching types of pain disappear.[16]

Because of this double system of pain innervation, a sudden onset of painful stimulus gives a "double" pain sensation: a fast pricking pain followed a second or so later by a slow burning pain. The pricking pain apprises the person very rapidly of a damaging influence and therefore plays an important role in making the person react immediately to remove himself from the stimulus. On the other hand, the slow burning sensation tends to become more and more painful over a period of time. It is this sensation that gives one the intolerable suffering of long-continued pain.

The Pricking Pain Pathway

The pricking pain pathway terminates in the ventrobasal complex in close association with the areas of termination of the tactile sensation fibers of both the dorsal-lemniscal system and the spinothalamic system (Fig 10–9). From here signals are transmitted into other areas of the thalamus and to the somatic sensory cortex, mainly to somatic area I. However, the signals to the cortex are probably important mainly for localizing the pain, not for interpreting it.

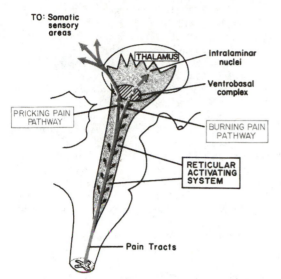

Fig 10–9.—Transmission of pain signals into the hindbrain, thalamus, and cortex via the "pricking pain" pathway and the "burning pain" pathway. (From Guyton.[24] Reproduced by permission.)

The Burning Pain Pathway

The burning and aching pain fibers terminate in the reticular area of the brain stem and in the intralaminar nuclei of the thalamus, which are themselves an upward extension of the reticular formation protruding among the thalamic nuclei. Both the reticular area of the brain stem and the intralaminar nuclei are parts of the reticular activating system.

The burning and aching pain fibers, because they excite the reticular activating system, have a very potent effect for activating essentially the entire nervous system, that is, to arouse one from sleep, to create a state of excitement, to create a sense of urgency, and to promise defense and aversion reactions designed to rid the person or animal of the painful stimulus.

The signals that are transmitted through the burning pain pathway can be localized only to very gross areas of the body.[18] Therefore, these signals are designed almost entirely for the single purpose of calling one's attention to injurious processes in the body. They create suffering that is sometimes intolerable. Their gradation of intensity is poor; instead, even weak pain signals can summate over a period of time by a process of temporal summation to cre-

ate an unbearable feeling, even though the same pain for short periods of time may be relatively mild.

Hyperalgesia

A pain pathway may become excessively excitable; this gives rise to hyperalgesia, or hypersensitivity to pain. The basic causes of hyperalgesia are (1) excessive sensitivity of the pain receptors themselves, which is called primary hyperalgesia, or (2) facilitation of sensory transmission, which is called secondary hyperalgesia.

An example of primary hyperalgesia is the extreme sensitivity of sunburned skin. Secondary hyperalgesia frequently results from lesions in the spinal cord or in the thalamus.

REFERENCES

1. Pinsker H.M., Willis W.D. Jr. (eds.): *Information Processing in the Nervous System*. New York, Raven Press, 1980.
2. Goldstein E.B.: *Sensation and Perception*. Belmont, Calif., Wadsworth Publishing Co., 1980.
3. Brown E., Deffenbacher K.: *Perception and the Senses*. New York, Oxford University Press, 1979.
4. Lynn B.: Somatosensory receptors and their CNS connections. *Annu. Rev. Physiol.* 37:105, 1975.
5. Halata Z.: *The Mechanoreceptors of the Mammalian Skin*. New York, Springer-Verlag, 1975.
6. Zimmermann M.: Neurophysiology of nociception. *Int. Rev. Physiol.* 10:179, 1976.
7. Paintal A.A. (ed.): *Morphology and Mechanisms of Chemoreceptors*. Delhi, India, Vallabhbhai Patel Chest Institute, University of Delhi, 1976.
8. Granit R.: *Receptors and Sensory Perception*. New Haven, Yale University Press, 1955.
9. Loewenstein W.R.: The generation of electric activity in a nerve ending. *Ann. NY Acad. Sci.* 81:367, 1959.
10. Gray J.A.B.: Initiation of impulses at receptors, in Magoun H.W. (ed.): *Handbook of Physiology,* section 1, vol. 1. Baltimore, Williams & Wilkins Co., 1959.
11. Perl E.R.: Sensitization of nociceptors and its relation to sensation, in Bonica J.J., Albe-Fessard D.G. (eds.): *Advances in Pain Research and Therapy.* New York, Raven Press, 1976, pp. 17–28.
12. Wilson M.E.: The neurological mechanisms of pain: A review. *Anaesthesia* 29:407, 1974.
13. McCloskey D.I.: Kinesthetic sensibility. *Physiol. Rev.* 58:763, 1978.
14. Catton W.T.: Mechanoreceptor function. *Physiol. Rev.* 50:297, 1970.
15. Bonica J.J., et al.: *Recent Advances in Pain.* Springfield, Ill., Charles C Thomas, Publisher, 1974.

16. Bonica J.J., et al. (eds.): *Proceedings of the Second World Congress on Pain*. New York, Raven Press, 1979.

17. Casey K.L.: Pain: A current view of neural mechanisms. *Am. Sci.* 61:194, 1973.

18. Bonica J.J. (ed.): *International Symposium on Pain*. New York, Raven Press, 1974.

19. Loewenstein W.R.: Excitation and inactivation in a receptor membrane. *Ann. NY Acad. Sci.* 94:510, 1961.

20. Purves D., Lichtman J.W.: Formation and maintenance of synaptic connections in autonomic ganglia. *Physiol. Rev.* 58:821, 1978.

21. Kennedy D., Davis W.J.: Organization of invertebrate motor systems, in Brookhart J.M., Mountcastle V.B. (eds.): *Handbook of Physiology*, section 1, vol. 1. Baltimore, Williams & Wilkins Co., 1977, p. 1023.

22. Wooldridge D.E.: *Sensory Processing in the Brain: An Exercise in Neuroconnective Modeling*. New York, John Wiley & Sons, Inc., 1979.

23. Schmidt R.F. (ed.): *Fundamental of Neurophysiology*. New York, Springer-Verlag, 1978.

24. Guyton A.S.: *Textbook of Medical Physiology*, ed. 6. Philadelphia, W.B. Saunders Co., 1981.

25. Freides D.: Human information processing and sensory modality: Cross-modal functions, information complexity, memory, and deficit. *Psychol. Bull.* 81:284, 1974.

26. Bennett M.V.L. (ed.): *Synaptic Transmissions and Neuronal Interaction*. New York, Raven Press, 1975.

27. Cowan W.M.: The development of the brain. *Sci. Am.* 241(3):112, 1979.

28. Asanuma H., Wilson V.J. (eds.): *Integration in the Nervous System*. New York, Igaku-Shoin, 1979.

29. Anderson H., et al.: Developmental neurobiology of invertebrates. *Annu. Rev. Neurosci.* 3:97, 1980.

30. Nichols J.C., Van Essen D.: The nervous system of the leech. *Sci. Am.* 230:38, 1974.

31. Friesen W.O., Stent G.S.: Neural circuits for generating rhythmic movements. *Annu. Rev. Biophys. Bioeng.* 7:37, 1978.

32. Hardy J.D., et al.: *Pain Sensations and Reactions*. Baltimore, Williams & Wilkins Co., 1952.

33. Szentagothai J., et al. (eds.): *Conceptual Models of Neural Organization*. Cambridge, Mass., Neurosciences Research Program, Massachusetts Institute of Technology, 1974.

34. An der Heiden U.: *Analysis of Neural Networks*. New York, Springer-Verlag, 1980.

35. Porter R. (ed.): *Studies in Neurophysiology*. New York, Cambridge University Press, 1978.

36. Bate C.M., et al.: *Development of Sensory System*. New York, Springer-Verlag, 1978.

37. Blumenthal R., et al. (eds.): *Dynamic Patterns of Brain Cell Assemblies*. Neurosciences Research Program Bulletin, vol. 12, No. 1. Cambridge, Mass., Massachusetts Institute of Technology, 1974.

38. Cowan W.M.: The development of the brain. *Sci. Am.* 241(3):112, 1979.

39. Coren S., et al.: *Sensation and Perception*. New York, Academic Press, 1979.

40. Anstis S.M., et al.: *Perception*. New York, Springer-Verlag, 1978.

41. Schmidt R.F. (ed.): *Fundamentals of Sensory Physiology*. New York, Springer-Verlag, 1978.

42. Martin A.R.: Synaptic transmission, in *MTP International Review of Science: Physiology*. Baltimore, University Park Press, 1974, vol. 3, p. 53.

43. Macagno E.R., et al.: Three-dimensional computer reconstruction of neurons and neuronal assemblies. *Annu. Rev. Biophys. Bioeng.* 8:323, 1979.

44. Cobb W.A., vanDuijn H. (eds.): *Contemporary Clinical Neurophysiology*. New York, Elsevier Scientific Publishing Co., 1978.

45. Mountcastle V.B. (eds.): *Handbook of Physiology*, section 1, vol. 1. Baltimore, Williams & Wilkins Co., 1977, p. 357.

46. Barker J.L.: Peptides: Roles in neuronal excitability. *Physiol. Rev.* 56:435, 1976.

47. Cuenod M., et al. (eds.): *Development and Chemical Specificity of Neurons*. New York, Elsevier Scientific Publishing Co., 1979.

48. Cooper J.R., et al.: *The Biochemical Basis of Neuropharmacology*. New York, Oxford University Press, 1978.

49. Ceccarelli B., Hurlbut W.P.: Vesicle hypothesis of the release of quanta of acetylcholine. *Physiol. Rev.* 60:396, 1980.

50. Gotto A.M. Jr., et al. (eds.): *Brain Peptides: A New Endocrinology*. New York, Elsevier/North-Holland, 1979.

51. Moore R.Y., Bloom F.E.: Central catecholamine neuron systems: Anatomy and physiology of the dopamine systems. *Annu. Rev. Neurosci.* 1:129, 1978.

52. Nicoll R.A., et al.: Substance P as a transmitter candidate. *Annu. Rev. Neurosci.* 3:227, 1980.

53. Snyder S.H., Childres S.R.: Opiate receptors and opioid peptides. *Annu. Rev. Neurosci.* 2:35, 1979.

54. Fields H.L., Bashbaum A.I.: Brainstem control of spinal pain-transmission neurons. *Annu. Rev. Physiol.* 40:217, 1978.

55. Bourne G.H., et al. (eds.): *Neuronal Cells and Hormones*. New York, Academic Press, 1978.

56. Somjen G.: *Sensory Coding in the Mammalian Nervous System*. New York, Appleton-Century-Crofts, 1972.

57. Kandel E.R.: Small systems of neurons. *Sci. Am.* 241(3):66, 1979.

58. Karlin A., et al. (eds.): *Neuronal Information Transfer*. New York, Academic Press, 1978.

59. Bennett T.L.: *The Sensory World: An Introduction to Sensation and Perception*. Monterey, Calif., Brooks/Cole Publishing Co., 1978.

11 / Physiology of Pain

MICHAEL BEHBEHANI, Ph.D.

THE PERCEPTION OF PAIN involves activation of sensory nociceptors, transmission through a specific set of sensory nerve fibers, and considerable integration at the spinal cord, midbrain reticular formation, and thalamic levels. This chapter considers each element of the network separately.

ACTIVATION OF NOCICEPTORS

The existence of a specific receptor for signaling noxious stimulation has only recently been established. Earlier investigators, in particular Müller, had concluded that the peripheral nerves were modality specific and that each class of fibers was responsible for transmission of one kind of sensory modality. Anatomical investigations of the skin had shown numerous types of structures, and these structures were assigned to different modalities.[1] Among these nerve endings, the small free nerve endings were designated as nociceptors. The concept of a modality-specific receptor was challenged by anatomical studies which showed that all sensation could be perceived in skin areas containing only one type of sensory end-organ.[2] In recent years, detailed physiologic experiments have reconciled these theories by providing strong evidence of specific thermal and mechanical nociceptors.[3–7] Thermal nociceptors can be excited by extreme heating (>40° C) and, to a lesser extent, by extreme cooling of the skin. They can also be excited by firm pressure. For this reason, the thermal nociceptors have been classified as polymodal receptors. These receptors have a small receptive field that, when activated, produce an increase in firing rate which is maintained for several seconds after application of the stimulus has stopped. Another property of the thermal nociceptors is that they become more sensitive after the skin has been heated. This change in sensitivity has been assumed to contribute to the hyperalgesia that develops after the skin has been burned.[8] Mechanical nociceptors are activated by extreme pressure. These have a small receptive field and, like the thermal receptors, produce a long after-discharge.

Since the stimuli that activate the nociceptors are such that, if continued, they would produce tissue damage, it has been argued that there may be a chemical intermediate between stimulus and activation of nociceptors which would make the individual aware of the danger. Several chemical agents, such as bradykinin, histamine, serotonin, and acetylcholine, can cause pain when they are injected into the skin or intra-arterially.[9, 10] Of these agents, bradykinin has been investigated most intensively.[11] Studies on perfusion of the subcutaneous space in man have shown that when an area of the skin is injured, several chemicals are released, and one of these is very similar to bradykinin. When this perfusate is injected into normal skin it produces pain. On the other hand, injection of perfusate from noninjured skin into normal skin does not produce pain.

TRANSMISSION OF PAIN THROUGH SENSORY NERVES

Numerous studies in animals and in humans have established that unmyelinated C fibers and small myelinated A delta fibers are the sensory nerve fibers that transmit pain information.[12–16] In studies by Collins et al.[12] the effect of stimulation of C and A fibers was examined in awake unanesthetized patients who were undergoing anterolateral cordotomy. In these studies, the sural nerve contralateral to the cordotomy was exposed and its distal end was cut, crushed, and fixed to a recording electrode. The proximal part of the nerve was then stimulated with a current of variable strength and frequency. When low-strength current which caused activation of the A alpha group alone was used, sensations of tap, throb, thump, touch, or flutter were perceived. As the frequency of the stimulus was increased, the sensations became more elaborate, but at no time did this type of stimulation produce the sensation of pain. When the strength of the stimulus was increased such that the activity of the A delta group of fibers could be recorded, the sensation of pain was perceived, especially at a higher frequency of stimulation. When the strength of the stimulus was increased until the activity of C fibers was predominant, the sensation of unbearable pain was elicited.

Torebjörk and Hallin[16] used a noninvasive method to stimulate and record the activity of the nerve fibers in unanesthetized human subjects. Their experiments confirmed the results obtained by Collins et al. and showed that when only the large myelinated fibers are activated, the sensation of touch or flutter is perceived. However, when the stimulus strength is increased such that A delta and C fibers are excited, pain is produced. When a low dose of local anesthetic was used to block the activity of C fibers alone, only the sensation of touch or throb, but not of pain, was elicited. On the other hand, when pressure was used to block the activity of large fibers and the conduction through C fibers was left intact, stimulation of the nerve bundle produced only the sensation of pain. In addition to these studies, there are numerous studies in cats, monkeys, and rats that indicate that conduction through C and A delta fibers is both necessary and sufficient to elicit pain.[5, 13, 17–19]

TRANSMISSION OF PAIN THROUGH THE SPINAL CORD

The information transmitted through the A delta and C fibers reaches the dorsal horn of the spinal cord and is significantly modified before it is transmitted to the brain. Anatomically, the gray matter of the spinal cord has been divided into nine laminae (Fig 11–1).[20] Physiologic studies have shown that cells in different laminae have different characteristics and that a physiologic laminar organization very similar to the anatomical laminar organization is present.[21] The functional organization of lamina I through lamina VI, which play a significant role in the transmission of pain, is discussed below.

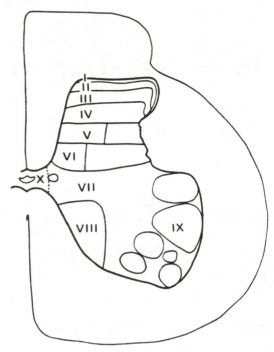

Fig 11–1.—Structure of the dorsal horn region involved in transmission of pain.

Lamina I

This thin lamina is the marginal lamina of the dorsal horn and contains loosely distributed cells. In the cat, the average size of the cells in this lamina is 8–10 μ (range, 5–25 μ). Physiologic studies on cats and monkeys[22–26] have shown that the cells in this region are predominantly excited by noxious mechanical and thermal stimulation (Fig 11–2). These cells have a high threshold and project through the anterolateral coordinate to the thalamus.

Laminae II and III

The cells in lamina II are tightly packed and small, averaging 7 μ in size. Lamina III contains tightly packed cells oriented transversely to its surface. The cells in this region are slightly larger than those in lamina II, with an average size of 9 μ. Physiologically, laminae II and III are considered to be the substantia gelatinosa (SG), although early anatomists considered lamina II alone to be the SG. Physiologic studies[27] have characterized the SG as an inhibitor pool of neurons that exerts significant

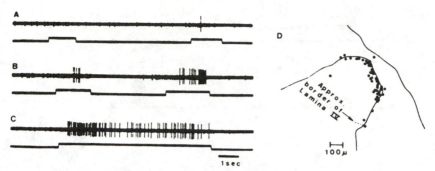

Fig 11–2.—Response of a neuron in lamina I of the cat spinal cord to stroking of the skin with a glass rod *(A)*, nonnoxious pressure *(B)*, and noxious stimulation with serrated forceps *(C)*. The location of neurons that respond to noxious mechanical or heat stimulation are shown in *(D)*. (From Willis W.D., Jr.: Physiology of dorsal horn and spinal cord pathways related to pain, in Beers R.F., Jr., Bassett E.G. (eds.): *Mechanism of Pain and Analgesic Compounds.* New York, Raven Press, 1979. Reproduced by permission.)

modulatory effects on the transmission of noxious stimuli. Cells in this region respond to touch or touch-pressure and to noxious stimulation; they have a well-defined receptive field. Most of the cells make extensive synaptic contact with other cells within these laminae and with those in lamina IV (Fig 11–3). The axons of these cells are short and only a few of them project to the thalamus through the anterolateral column.

Lamina IV

This lamina contains very large cells with diameters as large as 45 μ. The average diameter is around 15 μ. Physiologically, lamina IV cells have well-defined receptive fields. In spinal cats, the cells in this region are spontaneously active and can be excited by hair movement, touch, and nonnoxious cooling of the skin. As the intensity of the stimulation is increased, the firing rate increases in some cells, but many cells in this region fire at the same rate when stimulus intensity increases, and for this reason the cells in lamina IV are designated as small-dynamic-range cells.[21, 28]

Lamina V

The cells in this region are similar in size to those in lamina IV. In the cat, the orientation of lamina V is different from that of lamina IV and the cells tend to be oriented mediolaterally. Physiologically, the cells in lamina V have a larger receptive field than

do lamina IV cells. There is a significant difference between the response of the cell to stimulation with a light touch that is sufficient to excite the cell, whereas pressure must be applied to the peripheral field in order to increase the firing rate of the cell. In the monkey, lamina V cells respond to mechanical stimulation that ranges from light touch to noxious pressure[29–34] and to stimulation by intra-arterial injection of bradykinin (Fig 11–4).[23] The firing rate

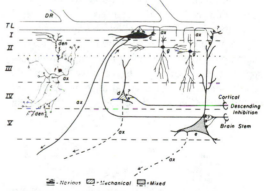

Fig 11–3.—Diagrammatic representation of the dorsal horn showing the inhibitory axosomatic connection between the substantia gelatinosa neurons *(g)* with lamina I neurons and the extent of arborization and projection of another neuron (f) in this region. (From Kerr F.W.L.: Segmental circuitry and ascending pathways of nociceptive system, in Beers R.F., Jr., Bassett E.G. (eds.): *Mechanism of Pain and Analgesic Compounds.* New York, Raven Press, 1979. Reproduced by permission.)

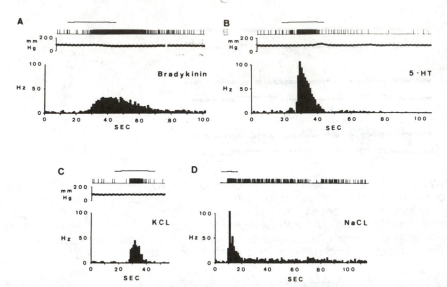

Fig 11—4.—Responses of a lamina V neuron to analgesic chemicals. Bradykinin, serotonin, KC1, and NaCl cause an increase in firing of these neurons. (From Kerr F.W.L.: Segmental circuitry and ascending pathways of the no-ciceptive system, in Beers R.F., Jr., Bassett E.G. (eds.): *Mechanism of Pain and Analgesic Compounds.* New York, Raven Press, 1979. Reproduced by permission.)

of these cells increases with the stimulus intensity; the cells respond maximally to noxious stimulation. For this reason, the cells are referred to as wide-dynamic-range cells. In addition to mechanical stimulation, cells in this region also respond specifically to noxious heat. An interesting property of lamina V cells is their adaptability. In the cat, the response of a cell fades away if repeated stimuli are applied to one region of its receptive field but the cell responds if another region of its receptive field is stimulated. Cells in this region project through the anterolateral column to the thalamus.

Lamina VI

Cells in this lamina are similar to lamina V cells in size and concentration. Physiologically, lamina VI cells respond to touch and pressure.[15, 21, 30] An important difference between lamina V and lamina VI cells is that the latter respond to joint movement, whereas lamina V cells do not. The threshold of lamina VI cells is similar to that of lamina V cells. Their receptive field is larger. Cells in this region also project through the anterolateral column to the thalamus.

GENERAL PROPERTIES OF THE DORSAL HORN

If the dorsal roots are cut between the dorsal root ganglia and their site of entry into the spinal cord, and if an electrode is placed on the proximal side of the cut rootlets, a potential called the dorsal root potential is recorded.[35, 36] This potential derives from the intrinsic activity of the dorsal horn neurons and is transmitted antidromically by electrotonic conduction. The magnitude of this potential can be changed by stimulation of different rootlets or by natural stimulation of the body at or near the area innervated by the roots. The presence of this potential led Wall and his colleague to suggest that there is a bias in the dorsal horn region that can act as a controlling mechanism.[37] Further studies on the origin of the dorsal root potential[38–43] and its effect on the transmission of the impulse through the dorsal root led Melzack and Wall to propose the gate control theory.[44] According to this theory (Fig 11–5), pain results if the firing rate in a set of neurons, designated T cells, is above a certain limit. The T cells can be excited by activities arriving in both large and small fibers whose terminals are under presynaptic control of SG cells. The SG cells are in

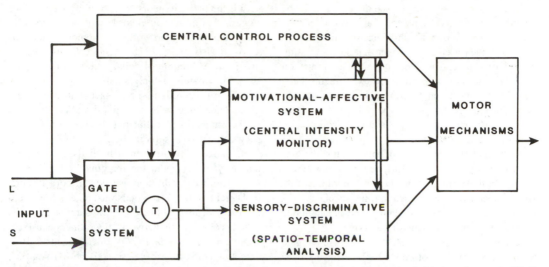

Fig 11–5.—Different neural networks and their effect (inactivation) on pain transmission through the dorsal horn, as postulated by the gate control theory of Melzach and Wall. (From Casey and Melzack.[49] Reproduced by permission.)

turn acted on by impulses arriving from small and large fibers. Small fibers cause inhibition of SG cells, whereas large fibers excite these neurons. According to this theory, when small fibers are active they cause excitation of the T cells, and by inhibiting the SG cells, they abolish the inhibitory effect of these neurons on the terminals of afferents to the T cells; therefore, the activity of the T cell rises beyond the threshold firing rate and pain results. On the other hand, when the large cells are active, they tend to increase the firing rate of the T cells. However, at the same time they excite the SG cells, which produce strong inhibitions of the terminals that synapse with the T cells and therefore prevent the afferent impulses from exciting the T cells. Thus, activity of the T cell does not increase and pain is not produced.

From the time of its proposal until the present, controversy has existed about some aspects of the gate control theory. The major point of the controversy is the interaction between large and small fibers and the presence of presynaptic inhibition.

The original hypothesis was based on studies by Wall in which a dorsal rootlet from L-6 of an unanesthetized spinal cat was cut and placed on two electrodes. One electrode was close to the spinal cord and the other on the cut end of the rootlet. When steady pressure was applied to a single toe pad, the central electrode became 150 mV negative with respect to the peripheral electrode. Since moving the joints of that leg did not alter this steady potential, they concluded that the steady dorsal root potential was due to the arrival of impulses produced by cutaneous afferents. Using stimulation of branches of a nerve bundle, they showed that the steady dorsal root potential blocked the dorsal root potential produced by nerve stimulation. Since a negative dorsal root potential indicates a depolarization of the terminals, Mendell and Wall[18] concluded that under normal physiologic conditions, there is steady depolarization of some terminals at the dorsal horn level. By adjusting stimulation conditions, they showed that when only C fibers are stimulated, only a positive dorsal root potential is obtained, and therefore they suggested that C fiber afferents hyperpolarize the terminals of large afferent cutaneous fibers. From these experiments, and based on the results of an earlier experiment by Wall[37, 45] in which he showed that the depolarization of the terminals is produced by activity in the small cells of the SG, Mendell and Wall suggested that SG cells are excited by the large fibers and inhibited by the small ones. They further suggested that the effect of C fiber activation on the effectiveness of large fibers is due to presynaptic facilitation brought about by hyperpolarization of the end terminals, whereas A fiber activation causes depolarization of the terminals through presynaptic inhibition. These suggestions have been tested by several investigators and have been supported by some experiments and contradicted by others (see review article by Nathan[47] for details).[46] In particular, experiments by Jänig and Zimmermann[48] in which intrafiber potentials were measured have shown that selective stimulation of C fibers produces depolarization at their intraspinal terminals. From these experiments Jänig and Zimmermann concluded that activation of C fibers alone does not cause hyperpolarization of the primary afferent, nor is there a postsynaptic facilitation induced by C fibers.

Additional experimental evidence against the gate control theory has been recently reported by Cervero et al.[27] In these studies (Fig 11–6), recordings from well-defined SG cells showed that these cells are excited by noxious heat application and are inhibited by brushing and squeezing of the skin.

At the time of its proposal, the T cells in the gate control theory were not defined. Experiments by a large number of investigators have provided evidence that cells in lamina V and VI can meet the criteria of T cells (for details refer to Casey and Melzack[49]). As mentioned previously, the cells in this region respond to both noxious and nonnoxious stimulation and their response increases as the stimulus strength increases.

After publication of the gate control theory, other theories dealing with transmission of pain information through the spinal cord were proposed. Among them is the balance theory, proposed by Kerr, which suggests that in the spinal cord there are nociceptive and nonnociceptive networks.[50] The nociceptive circuitry consists of small fibers, the cells in the marginal zone, the lamina I cells, and cells in the SG. According to this model, small fibers, after entry into the spinal cord, make contact with distal dendrites of the large cells in lamina I and excite them. At the same time, collaterals of the small fibers make contact with cells in the SG and excite them. These SG cells in turn establish relatively small but inhibitory contact with the marginal cells. The axons of lamina I cells then ascend the cord through the lateral column to the thalamus. The nonnociceptive network involves large fibers, lamina IV cells, and SG cells. In this network, large fibers cause activation of cells in lamina IV, designated as P or projection cells, and they also activate SG neurons, which make numerous inhibitory synapses with the lamina I cells.

In this model (Fig 11–7), activation of small fibers produces mostly an excitatory effect causing lamina I cells to fire strongly; this leads to pain. On the other hand, stimulation of large fibers leads to inhibition of lamina I cells and produces nonpainful perception. The difference between this model—the balance theory—and the gate control theory of Melzack and Wall is that the balance theory has taken

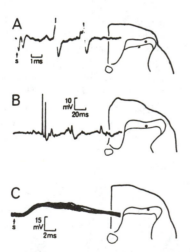
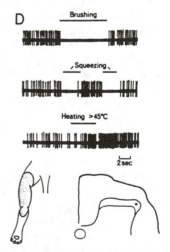

Fig 11–6.—Extracellular and intracellular recordings from substantia gelatinosa (SG) neurons. **A,** response to stimulation of the Lissauer's tract. **B,** intracellular recording from another SG neuron showing occurrence of spontaneous excitatory postsynaptic potential. **C,** EPSP produced by electrical stimulation of Lissauer's track, indicating monosynaptic connection. **D,** response of an SG neuron to brushing and nonnoxious and noxious stimulation of the skin. Note the inhibitory effect of nonnoxious stimulation and the excitatory effect of noxious stimulation on this neuron. *Insets* show location of the neurons. (From Cervero et al.[27] Reproduced by permission.)

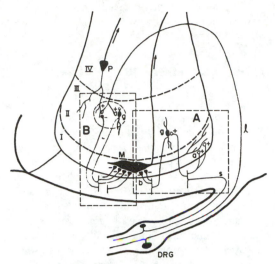

Fig 11–7.—Neural network involved in central inhibitory balance theory of pain, as proposed by Kerr. (From Kerr.[50] Reproduced by permission.)

into consideration the role of lamina 1 cells and the fact that excitation of large and small fibers produces similar responses in SG cells. There is significant evidence for the involvement of lamina I cells in pain transmission, and several studies have shown that these cells are specifically activated by noxious stimulation.[17] The hypothetical role of SG cells in Kerr's model is based on anatomical data and has not been tested physiologically.

SPINAL PATHWAYS INVOLVED IN TRANSMISSION OF PAIN

Based on anatomical results, it has been established that a dual spinothalamic system exists.[51, 52] The first part, which is laterally located and projects directly to the thalamus without relaying at any other site, sends collaterals to several regions in the reticular formation.[53, 54] Designated the neospinothalamic tract, it is phylogenetically younger and is prominently present in primate and man. The second, more medial system branches from the lateral spinothalamic tract and relays through the reticular formation. Designated the paleospinothalamic system, it is phylogenetically older than the lateral system and is present in all vertebrates.[55] Both systems are crossed and contain mostly myelinated fibers in the range of 1–7 μ, with average diameters of 4 μ. The two systems together are referred to as the an-

terolateral column. Recent studies by Mayer et al.[30] have shown that stimulation of this region of the spinal cord produces pain (Fig 11–8). In these studies, focal stimulation of the anterolateral column with pulses at a frequency of 50 Hz and a duration of 0.2 msec was used. The threshold for pain was fairly uniform and ranged from 120 to 1,000 microamp, with a median threshold of 300 microamp.

An interesting observation in these studies was the strong correlation between stimulation frequency and the production of pain sensation.[56] At a frequency of 5 Hz, no pain was elicited, whereas at 25 Hz or higher the stimulation always produced pain.

Both the lateral spinothalamic tract and the ventral spinothalamic tract are involved in pain transmission. The projections of the axons traveling in these tracts are very similar. Collaterals of these systems synapse with cells in the lateral reticular nucleus, the nucleus gigantocellularis and the nucleus paragigantocellularis in the medulla, the pontine nuclei of the subcerelus, nucleus cuneiformis, the periaqueductal gray, and the thalamic nuclei ventralis posterolateralis, medialis dorsalis, and multiformis (Fig 11–9).

Finally, there is a diffuse projection through the gray matter that is involved in the transmission of pain.[57] This system consists of short fibers that may cross and recross several times before synapsing with cells in the reticular formation. The existence

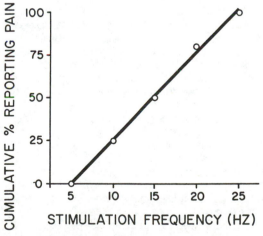

Fig 11–8.—Effect of increasing frequency of electrical stimulation of the anterolateral quadrant on pain perception in man. The ordinate is the cumulative percentage of subjects reporting pain at various stimulation frequencies. (From Mayer et al.[50] Reproduced by permission.)

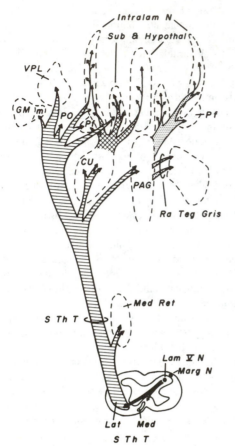

Fig 11–9.—Major components of the spinothalamic system. Note the considerable divergence of this pathway at the midbrain and thalamic levels. *CU,* cuneiformis; *Ra Teg Gris,* radiatio tegmenti grisea of uleischedal; *GM,* medical geniculate magnocellular division; *Med Ret,* medullary reticular nuclei; *PAG,* periaqueductal gray; *Pf,* parafascicular nucleus; *PO,* posterior group of nuclei of the thalamus; *S Th T,* spinothalamic tract; *VPL,* ventralis posterolateralis of thalamus; *Lat and Med.* lateral and medial spinothalamic tracts. (From Kerr F.W.L.: Segmental circuitry and ascending pathways of the nociceptive system, in Beers R.F., Jr., Bassett E.G. (eds.): *Mechanism of Pain and Analgesic Compounds.* New York, Raven Press, 1979. Reproduced by permission.)

of this pathway has been suggested in man. In the rat, it has been shown that lesion of tracts with long ascending axons, namely the anterolateral and ventral spinothalamic tracts, does not abolish the response to noxious stimulation. Therefore, a short

axon and a diffuse system that is involved in the transmission of pain through the spinal cord must exist in this species.

MEDULLARY REGIONS INVOLVED IN PAIN

As mentioned above, both the lateral and the ventral spinothalamic tracts send collaterals to the medullary and pontine reticular formation. Of major importance in the processing of pain information is the area of the nucleus gigantocellularis. This region has been extensively studied by Casey.[58, 59] In these studies, cats were trained to respond to noxious stimulation by jumping over a barrier. Later, an apparatus was implanted in the animal's head that permitted recordings from single cells as well as stimulation of this region in unanesthetized animals. As the stimulus intensity increased, the firing rate of the cells increased, and when a certain firing rate was reached, the animal jumped the barrier (Fig 11–10). Similarly, when this region was stimulated, a current intensity existed above which the animal showed escape behavior. These studies therefore indicate that an increase of cell activity in the nucleus gigantocellularis is sufficient for perception of pain.

THALAMIC NUCLEI INVOLVED IN PROCESSING OF PAIN INFORMATION

The thalamic nuclei involved in integration of pain are classified as specific and nonspecific. Specific nuclei involved in pain are the ventralis posterior lateralis (VPL) and the ventralis posterior medialis (VPM).[55, 60] The VPL receives inputs from the spinothalamic tract and the VPM receives afferents from the trigeminal sensory nuclei. Together, these nuclei have been referred to as ventrobasal nuclei.[61] Ventrobasal cells respond to noxious and nonnoxious stimuli.[7, 62–64] These cells have small and well-defined receptive fields located on the contralateral surface of the body. Based on their response, they have been classified as wide-dynamic-range cells. Because of this cellular specificity, the ventrobasal nucleus is somatotopically organized and a homunculus can be projected in this area that is in a recumbent position with the feet placed dorsolaterally, shoulders placed ventrolaterally in the VPL, and the head in the VPM.[65] Ventrobasal lesion in man has been reported to alleviate pain. However, this analgesic effect is short-lasting and

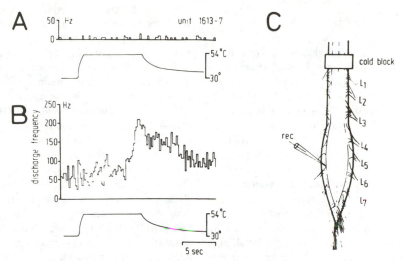

Fig 11–10.—Single unit recording from a nucleus gigantocellularis neuron in behaving cat. The firing rate of this neuron increased as the strength of cutaneous stimulation at the rate of 1 Hz was increased from below an escape-producing level to an intensity that caused escape. (From Casey.[59] Reproduced by permission.)

pain reappears within 1 year. In addition to the cells in the ventrobasal region, there are cells in the posterior nucleus of the thalamus that are excited by noxious stimulation.[66, 67] However, the majority of the cells in the posterior nucleus respond to more than one modality, and the role of this nucleus in pain is not clear.

Nonspecific Thalamic Nuclei

The center median (CM) and parafascicularis PF nuclei have been implicated in pain.[68] Electrical stimulation of these regions of the thalamus elicits feelings of anxiety that are unpleasant but not painful. There are several reports in the literature which indicate that lesion of the CM-PF causes relief of intractable pain. Anatomical studies show no direct projection from the spinothalamic tract to this region. Therefore it is believed that these intralaminar nuclei are involved in the integration of pain and nonpainful stimuli. In the monkey, it has been shown that stimulation of the nucleus giganto cellularis (NGC) causes excitation, but stimulation of the medial forebrain bundle inhibits cells in the CM-PF. Since NGC stimulation can produce pain and medial forebrain bundle (MFB) stimulation is associated with pleasure, it has been suggested that the intralaminal nuclei may be involved in motivational aspects of pain.

CORTICAL AREAS INVOLVED IN PAIN SENSIBILITY

Somatosensory areas I and II (SI, SII) and the posterior parietal areas play some role in the processing of pain.[69, 70] The somatosensory areas are located in the postcentral gyrus. The SI area is very specific and contains cells that respond to one modality of sensation. It has a receptive field on the contralateral part of the body. This area receives input from the ventrobasal nucleus to the thalamus, but very few cells in this area specifically respond to noxious stimulation. The SII area is nonspecific. Cells in this area respond to more than one modality and have receptive fields on both sides of the body. There are no cells in this area that respond specifically to pain.

In some cases, electrical stimulation of the postcentral gyrus in man produces the sensation of pain. There have been several reports that removal of the postcentral gyrus can produce elevation of the pain threshold on the contralateral side.[71, 72] However, none of these procedures has resulted in prolonged freedom from intractable pain. Another cortical area that has been shown to deal with pain is the posterior parietal area. If this area on the dominant side is lesioned, the threshold for pain does not change but pain does not produce an aversive response. This phenomenon has been called asymbolia.

DESCENDING SYSTEMS

Early investigators realized that the cells in the dorsal horn are under strong inhibitory influences from the brain.[73] Experiments by Wall[21] and later by Zimmermann (Fig 11–11) have shown that the response to noxious stimulation of cells in lamina V of the spinal cord is much more pronounced when the transmission of descending impulses from the brain is blocked by cooling the spinal cord rostral to the recording site. Several brain sites, including the pyramidal tract and the reticulospinal system, seem to be involved. In 1969, a report by Reynolds[74] started a search for the determination of one of these descending pathways. In experiments reported by Reynolds, stimulation of the periaqueductal gray area in the rat produced such strong analgesia that laparotomy could be performed without any anesthesia. These experiments were repeated by Mayer and Leibeskind,[75] Mayer and Hayes,[76] and Akil and Leibeskind[77] in the rat. Similar studies by Adams[78] and Hosobuchi et al.[79] have shown that stimulation of the periventricular gray area can cause significant and prolonged analgesia in the human. The role of monoamines in this system was examined by Akil and Leibeskind[77] and it was established that the analgesic effect of stimulation of the periaqueductal gray area, referred to as stimulus-produced analgesia, is potentiated when the concentrations of serotonin and dopamine are increased and is blocked when these monoamines are depleted. In contrast, an increase in the concentration of norepinephrine was shown to decrease stimulus-produced analgesia and depletion of norepinephrine enhanced the effect of stimulation-produced analgesia. This effect of monoamines on stimulation-produced analgesia was so similar to their effect on morphine-induced analgesia that it led Mayer and his colleagues to test the interaction between morphine- and stimulation-induced analgesia.[76] In these experiments, stimulating electrodes were placed in the periaqueductal gray area of rats and the region was stimulated over a period of 1–24 hours. It was found the prolonged stimulation of the periaqueductal gray area produces tolerance, and a cross-tolerance develops between morphine- and stimulation-produced analgesia. Later experiments showed that, like morphine-induced analgesia, stimulation-produced analgesia is blocked by the morphine antagonist, naloxone.[30, 80] The mechanism of the production of stimulation-produced analgesia was examined by Leibeskind and Mayer[81] and Carstens et al.,[82] and it was shown that stimulation of the periaqueductal gray area causes a decrease in response to noxious stimulation of cells in the lamina V of the spinal cord. Since

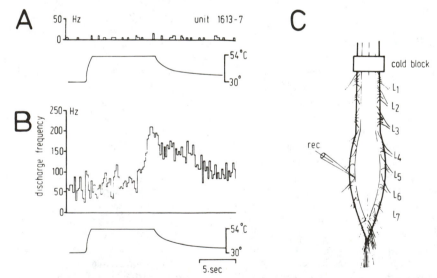

Fig 11–11.—Effect of reversable blockage of descending influence on a dorsal horn neuron response to radiant heat stimulation of the skin. **A,** response before; **B,** response after blocking. The transmission of impulses through the rostral parts of the spinal cord by cooling as shown in **C.** (From Zimmerman M., Handmerker H.O.: Advances in *Neurology*, Vol 4. New York, Raven Press, 1974. Reproduced by permission.)

there are very few direct projections from the periaqueductal gray area to the spinal cord, it was clear that analgesia produced by stimulation of the periaqueductal gray area must involve other brain regions. Since morphine-induced analgesia involved serotonergic pathways and since raphe nuclei contain the highest concentration of serotonin, Proudfit and Anderson[83] examined the effect of lesioning of the medullary raphe nuclei. They showed that the analgesia produced by morphine and by stimulation of the peri aqueductal gray area is abolished when the nucleus raphe magnus is lesioned. To determine the spinal pathways that mediate morphine- and stimulus-induced analgesia, Basbaum et al. lesioned several known tracts in the spinal cord and showed that both morphine-induced analgesia and stimulation-produced analgesia are blocked when the dorsolateral funiculus is destroyed.[84, 85] Later, using retrograde transport of horseradish peroxidase, it was shown that the major source of dorsolateral funiculus axons is the cells in the nucleus raphe magnus and its surrounding area.[86-88] Efferent projection of the nucleus raphe magnus was examined by injection of radiolabeled leucine, and it was found that the cells in this region project mainly to cells in laminae I and V of the dorsal horn.[89] The ascending laminar projection of the nucleus raphe magnus includes the periaqueductal gray, the intralaminar thalamic nuclei, and several sites in the hypothalamus.[90] The afferent projection to the nucleus raphe magnus has been examined in several studies and includes the periaqueductal gray area, the nucleus cuneiformis, and the medullary gigantocellularis nucleus.[91] A strong interaction between the periaqueductal gray and the nucleus raphe magnus has been found in physiologic experiments in cats and rats. Pomeroy and Behbehani have shown that electrical stimulation of the nucleus raphe magnus leads to excitation of nucleus raphe magnus neurons. Behbehani and Fields[92] showed that injection of glutamic acid into the periaqueductal gray area leads to excitation of nucleus raphe magnus neurons and produces analgesia (Fig 11–12). Since glutamic acid only excites cell bodies, these studies prove that activation of the cell bodies and not the axon of passage is the source of nucleus raphe magnus excitation by the periaqueductal gray area. In the same studies, they showed that localized lesions of the nucleus raphe magnus block the analgesic effect of glutamate injected into the periaqueductal gray area.

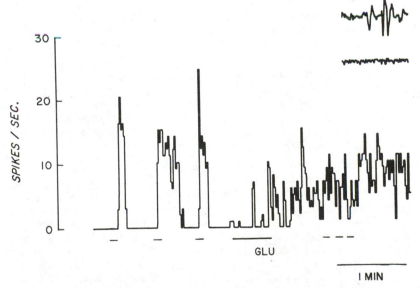

Fig 11–12.—Response of a nucleus raphe magnus neuron to injection of glutamic acid into the periaqueductal gray in the rat. This cell responded to noxious stimulation (indicated by *bars*) of left and right pain and tail by excitation. Glutamic acid injection caused an increase in the firing rate of this cell and decreased its response to noxious stimulation. Simultaneous EMG recording shows withdrawal response before *(top inset)* and its inhibition after *(botton inset)* injection of glutamic acid. (From Behbehani and Fields.[92] Reproduced by permission.)

Fields and Anderson have shown that stimulation of the periaqueductal gray area in the cat also causes excitation of nucleus raphe magnus neurons.[93]

In addition to electrical and glutamate-induced excitation of the periaqueductal gray area, it has been shown that injection of morphine and neurotensin into the periaqueductal gray also produces excitation of nucleus raphe magnus neurons and analgesia.[94, 95] These studies therefore indicate that the analgesic effect of periaqueductal gray stimulation is mediated through activation of the nucleus raphe magnus region. Stimulation of the nucleus raphe magnus has been shown to inhibit the cells in laminae I and V of the spinal cord,[96–98] and its analgesic effect can be abolished by naloxone.[99] Since these cells are the origin of the spinalothalamic tract,[100] the analgesic effect of nucleus raphe magnus stimulation is therefore due to inhibition of these neurons. Also, since there is a significant projection from the nucleus raphe magnus to the substantia gelatinosa, the nucleus raphe magnus region must be involved in modulation of pain by altering the activities of these neurons.

TRANSMITTERS INVOLVED IN PAIN

Anatomical studies have shown that there is a high concentration of substance P–containing terminals in the dorsal horn region (Fig 11–13).[101] Substance P is a peptide that has an excitatory effect in most areas of the spinal cord and the brain. Physiologic studies have shown that iontophoretically applied substance P excites laminae I and V of the spinal cord.[102–104] In behavioral experiments, Yaksh et al. showed that depletion of substance P produces strong analgesia.[105] Since after rhizotomy, the concentration of substance P drastically decreases,[106] it is believed that the primary afferents involved in nociception excite dorsal horn neuron by release of substance P. In the spinal cord there is a high concentration of enkephalinergic neurons and terminals.[101] Iontophoresis of enkephalin in this area produces strong inhibition, which is reversed by naloxone.[107] Since the concentration of enkephalin or the number of enkephalinergic neurons does not decrease following rhizotomy or lesion of the spinal cord rostral to the measurement site, it is believed that enkephalinergic neurons are interneurons that are activated by descending systems. It has been suggested that enkephalin neurons make presynaptic connections with the dorsal root afferents and inhibit them. In addition to substance P and enkephalin, serotonin and norepinephrine are also involved in

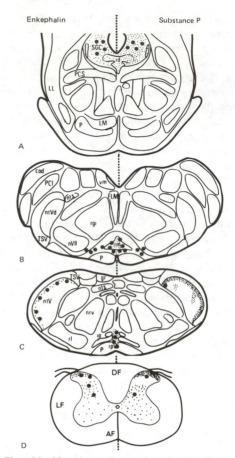

Fig 11–13.—Location of enkephalin-positive *(left side)* and substance P–positive *(right side)* cell bodies *(asterisks)* and nerve terminals *(dots)* in the lower brain stem and spinal cord. *AF,* anterior funiculus; *cod,* nucleus cochlearis dorsalis; *DF,* dorsal funiculus; *FLM,* fasciculus longitudinalis medialis; *gr,* nucleus gracilis; *io,* nucleus olivaris inferior; *LF,* lateral funiculus; *LL,* lemniscus lateralis; *LM,* lemniscus medialis; *nrv,* nucleus reticularis medullae oblongatae pars ventralis; *nts,* nucleus tractus solitarii; *ntV,* nucleus tractus spinalis nervi trigemini (spinal trigeminal nucleus); *ntVd,* nucleus tractus spinalis nervi trigemini pars dorsomedialis; *nVII,* nucleus originis nervi facialis; *P,* tractus corticospinalis; *PCI,* pedunculus cerebellaris inferior; *PCS,* pedunculus cerebellaris superior; *rd,* nucleus raphe dorsalis; *rgi,* nucleus reticularis gigantocellularis; *rl,* nucleus reticularis lateralis; *rm,* nucleus raphe magnus; *rp,* nucleus raphe pallidus; *SGC,* substantia grisea centralis; *TSV,* tractus spinalis nervi trigemini; *vm,* nucleus vestibularis medialis. The nomenclature as well as the cross sections of the lower brain stem are according to Palkovits and Jacobowitz.[101]

the processing of pain information in the spinal cord.[108–111] Iontophoretic application of 5-hydroxy-tryptamine (5-HT) can cause inhibition or excitation of dorsal horn neurons. In intact animals, 5-HT causes excitation of a majority of neurons, but in animals with spinal lesions the majority of cells are inhibited by 5-HT. The mechanism for this change in the reaction to 5-HT is not clear at this time. In intact animals, it has been shown that stimulation of the periaqueductal gray area increases 5-HT concentration. However, it is not clear which cells are involved in the release of 5-HT, nor their exact location in the spinal cord known. Injection of labeled 5-HT into the fourth ventricle leads to an accumulation of labeled 5-HT in the dorsal horn gelatinosa and marginal laminae and there is a strong overlap between the projection from the nucleus raphe magnus and the serotonin-containing terminals.[96] Similarly, the concentration of norepinephrine in the spinal cord increases when the periaqueductal gray area is stimulated for several seconds. Since intrathecal injection of norepinephrine into the spinal cord produces analgesia, it is possible that norepinephrine is an inhibitory transmitter in the spinal cord. The origin of the norepinephrine-containing terminals in the spinal cord is not clear. However, Behbehani and Pert have shown that lesioning of noradrenergic nuclei in the brain stem (A1 nuclei of Dahlstrom and Fuxe[112]) does not abolish the analgesic effect of periaqueductal gray stimulation.

The transmitters that activate the reticular and thalamic neurons involved in pain are not known. The role of substance P, acetylcholine, norepinephrine, and glutamic acid in the reticular formation and in particular in the nucleus raphe magnus has been studied. However, the exact role of these transmitters in transmission of pain is yet to be established.[113–115] Thalamic nuclei also respond to the above transmitter, but their pharmacology has not been as extensively studied as in the dorsal horn cells (Fig 11–14).

Since enkephalins are analgesics and a definite enkephalinergic pathway exists,[116] their effect in the pain system has been extensively studied.[107] It has been shown that the majority of the cells in the central pain pathway are inhibited by enkephalins.[117] Nevertheless, the natural mechanism through which enkephalins are released is not known. Several manipulations, such as acupuncture,[118] stress, and placebos, which produce analgesia are mediated through the release of enkephalin because their effect is totally or partially blocked by naloxone, but the mechanism through which those processes cause

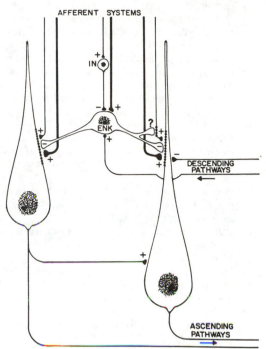

Fig 11–14.—A network that accounts for activation of enkephalin interneuron by descending systems which produce inhibition of the dorsal horn neuron by noxious stimulation. (From Zieglgansberger.[107] Reproduced by permission.)

the release of enkephalin remains a challenge for future studies.

REFERENCES

1. Müller J.: Von den Ergentumlichkeiten der einzelnen Nerve, in Kobling L. (ed.): *Handbuch der Physiologie des Menschen.* Coblenz, Holscher, 1844, pp. 667–682.
2. Weddel G., Palmer E., Paillie W.: Nerve endings in mammalian skin. *Biol. Re.* 30:159–195, 1955.
3. Duclaus R., Kenshalo D.R.: The temperature sensitivity of the type I slowly adapting mechanoreceptor in cats and monkeys. *J. Physiol. (London)* 224:647–664, 1972.
4. Iggo A.: Activation of cutaneous nociceptors and their actions on dorsal horn neurons. *Adv. Neurol.* 4:1–9, 1974.
5. Iggo A.: Cutaneous heat and cold receptors with slow conducting C fibers. *Q. J. Exp. Physiol.* 44:362–370, 1959.
6. Iggo A.: Cutaneous mechanoreceptors with afferent C fibers. *J. Physiol.* 152:337, 1960.
7. Ishizima B., Yoshimasu N., Fukushima T., et al.: Nociceptive neurons in human thalamus. *Confina Neurologica* 37:99–106, 1975.

8. LaMotte R.H., Thalhammer J.G., Torebjörk H.E., et al.: Peripheral neural mechanisms of cutaneous hyperalgesia following mild injury by heat. *J. Neurosci.* 2:765–781, 1982.

9. Collier H.J.J., Schneider C.: Nociceptive response to prostaglandins and analgesic actions of aspirin and morphine. *Nature New Biol.* 236:141–143, 1972.

10. Keele C.A., Armstrong D.: *Substances Producing Pain and Itch*. London, Edward Arnold Lt., 1964.

11. Lim R.K.S., Krauthamer G., Guzman F., et al.: Central nervous activity associated with pain evoked by bradykinin and its alteration by morphine and aspirin. *Proc. Natl. Acad. Sci. USA* 63:705–712, 1969.

12. Collins W.F., Nulsen F.E., Randt C.T.: Relation of peripheral nerve fiber size and sensation in man. *Arch. Neurol.* 3:381, 1960.

13. Hallin R.G., Torebjörk H.E.: Activity in unmyelinated nerve fibers in man. *Adv. Neurol.* 4:19–27, 1974.

14. Hensel H., Iggo A., Witt I.: A quantitative study of sensitive cutaneous thermoreceptors with C afferent fibres. *J. Physiol. (London)* 153:113–126, 1960.

15. Meyer R.A., Campbell J.N.: Evidence for two distinct classes of unmyelinated nociceptive afferents in monkey. *Brain Res.* 224:149–152, 1981.

16. Torebjörk H.E., Hallin R.C.: Perceptual changes accompanying controlled preferential blocking of A and C fibre: Responses in intact human skin nerve. *Exp. Brain Res.* 16:321–332, 1973.

17. Burgess P.R., Perl E.R.: Myelinated afferent fibers responding specifically to noxious stimulation of the skin. *J. Physiol. (London)* 190:541–562, 1967.

18. Mendell L., Wall P.D.: Presynaptic hyperpolarization: A role for fine afferent fibers. *J. Physiol. (London)* 172:274–294, 1964.

19. Pert E.R.: Myelinated afferent fibers innervating the primate skin and their response to noxious stimuli. *J. Physiol. (London)* 197:593–615, 1968.

20. Rexed B.: The cytoarchitectonic organization of the spinal cord in the cat. *J. Comp. Neurol.* 23:259–281, 1954.

21. Wall P.D.: The laminar organization of dorsal horn and effects of descending impulses. *J. Physiol. (London)* 188:403–423, 1967.

22. Applebaum A.E., Beall J.E., Foreman R.D., et al.: Organization and receptive fields of primate spinothalamic tract neurons. *J. Neurophysiol.* 38:572–586, 1975.

23. Besson J.M., Consellor C., Hamann K.F., et al.: Modification of dorsal horn cell activities in the spinal cord after intra-arterial injection of bradykinin. *J. Physiol. (London)* 221:189–205, 1972.

24. Besson P., Perl E.R.: Response of cutaneous sensory units with unmyelinated fibers to noxious stimuli. *J. Neurophysiol.* 32:1025–1043, 1969.

25. Brown A.G., Franz D.N.: Responses of spinocervical tract neurons to natural stimulation of identified cutaneous receptors. *Exp. Brain Res.* 7:231–249, 1969.

26. Christensen B.N., Perl E.R.: Spinal neurons specifically excited by noxious or thermal stimuli: Marginal zone of the dorsal horn. *J. Neurophysiol.* 33:293–307, 1970.

27. Cervero F., Molony V., Iggo A.: Extracellular and intracellular recording from neurons in the substantia gelatinosa Rolandi. *Brain Res.* 136:565–569, 1977.

28. Gregor M., Zimmermann M.: Characteristics of spinal neurons responding to cutaneous myelinated and unmyelinated fibres. *J. Physiol. (London)* 221:555–576, 1972.

29. Fields H.L., Clanton C.H., Anderson S.D.: Somatosensory properties of spinoreticular neurons in the cat. *Brain Res.* 120:49–66, 1977.

30. Mayer D.J., Price D.D., Becker D.P.: Neurophysiological characterization of the anterolateral spinal cord neurons contributing to pain perception in man. *Pain* 1:51–58, 1975.

31. Price D.D., Mayer D.J.: Neurophysiological characteristics of anterolateral quadrant neurons subserving pain in M. mulatta. *Pain* 1:59–72, 1975.

32. Price D.D., Hull C.D., Buchwald N.A.: Intracellular response of dorsal horn cells to sural nerve A- and C-fiber stimuli. *Exp. Neurol.* 33:291–309, 1971.

33. Trevino D.L., Maunz R.A., Bryan R.N., et al.: Localization of the cells of origin of the spinothalamic tract in lumbar enlargement of cat. *Exp. Neurol.* 34:64–77, 1972.

34. Randic M., Yu H.H. Effects of 5-hydroxytryptamine and bradykinin in cat dorsal horn neurons activated by noxious stimuli. *Brain Res.* 111:197–203, 1976.

35. Barron D.H., Matthews B.H.C.: Intermittent conduction in the spinal cord. *J. Physiol. (London)* 85:73–103, 1935.

36. Barron D.H., Matthews B.H.C.: The interpretation of potential changes in the spinal cord. *J. Physiol. (London)* 92:276–321, 1938.

37. Wall P.D.: The origin of a spinal cord slow potential. *J. Physiol. (London)* 164:508–526, 1962.

38. Burke R.E., Rudomin P., Vyklicky L., et al.: Primary afferent depolarization and flexion reflexes produced by radiant heat stimulation of the skin. *J. Physiol. (London)* 213:185–214, 1971.

39. Dawson G.D., Merrill E.G., Wall P.D.: Dorsal root potentials produced by stimulation of fine afferents. *Science* 167:1385–1387, 1970.

40. Eccles J.C., Krenjevic K.: Potential changes recorded inside primary afferent fibres within the spinal cord. *J. Physiol (London)* 149:25–213, 1959.

41. Eccles J.C., Schmidt R.F., Willis W.D.: Depolarization of the central terminals of cutaneous afferent fibres. *J. Neurophysiol.* 26:646–661, 1963.

42. Hodge D.J.: Potential changes inside afferent terminals secondary to stimulation of large and small diameter peripheral nerve fibres. *J. Neurophysiol.* 35:30–43, 1972.

43. Schmidt R.F., Trautwein W., Zimmermann M.: Dorsal root potentials evoked by natural stimulation of cutaneous afferents. *Nature (London)* 212:522–523, 1965.

44. Melzack R., Wall P.D.: Pain mechanism: A new theory. *Science* 150:971–979, 1965.

45. Wall P.D.: Presynaptic control of impulses at the first central synapse in cutaneous pathway. *Prog. Brain Res.* 12:92–115, 1964.

46. Franz D.N., Iggo A.: Dorsal root potentials and ventral root reflexes evoked by nonmyelinated fibers. *Science* 162:1140–1142, 1968.

47. Nathan P.W.: The gate-control theory of pain: A critical review. *Brain* 99:123–158, 1968.

48. Jänig W., Zimmermann M.: Presynaptic depolarization by myelinated afferent fibers evoked by stimulation of cutaneous C fibers. *J. Physiol. (London)* 214:29–50, 1971.

49. Casey K.L., Melzack R.: Neural mechanisms of pain: A conceptual model, in Way E., Leon G. (eds.): *New Concepts in Pain and Its Clinical Management.* Philadelphia, F.A. Davis Co., 1967, pp. 13–31.

50. Kerr F.W.L.: Pain: A central inhibitory balance theory. *Mayo Clin. Proc.* 50:685–670, 1975.

51. Noordenbos N., Wall P.D.: Diverse sensory functions with almost totally divided spinal cord: A case of spinal cord transection with preservation of part of one anterolateral quadrant. *Pain* 2:185–195, 1976.

52. Kerr F.W.L.: Neuroanatomical substrates of nociception in the spinal cord. *Pain* 1:325–356, 1975.

53. Castiglioni A.J., Gallaway M.C., Coulter J.D.: Origin of brainstem connections to spinal cord in monkey. *J. Comp. Neurol.* 178:328–346, 1977.

54. Denny-Brown D., Kirk E.J., Yanagisawa N.: The tract of Lissaur in relation to sensory transmission in the dorsal horn of spinal cord in the macaque monkey. *J. Comp. Neurol.* 151:175–200, 1973.

55. Bowsher D.: The termination of secondary somatosensory neurons within the thalamus of Macaca mulatta: An experimental degeneration study. *J. Comp. Neurol.* 117:213–227, 1961.

56. Kerr F.W.L.: The ventral spinothalamic tract and other ascending systems of the ventral funiculus of the spinal cord. *J. Comp. Neurol.* 159:335–355, 1975.

57. Basbaum A.I.: Conduction of the effects of noxious stimulation by short-fiber multisynaptic systems of the spinal cord in the rat. *Exp. Neurol.* 40:699–716, 1973.

58. Casey K.L.: Responses of bulboreticular units to somatic stimuli eliciting escape behavior in the cat. *Int. J. Neurosci.* 2:15–28, 1971.

59. Casey K.L.: Escape elicited by bulboreticular stimulation in the cat. *Int. J. Neurosci.* 2:29–34, 1971.

60. Casey K.L.: Unit analysis of nociceptive mechanisms in the thalamus of the awake squirrel monkey. *J. Neurophysiol.* 29:727–750, 1966.

61. Poggio G.F., Mountcastle V.B.: The functional properties of ventrobasal thalamic neurons studied in unanesthetized monkeys. *J. Neurophysiol.* 26:775–806, 1963.

62. Hellon R.F., Mitchell D.: Characteristics of neurons in the ventrobasal thalamus of the rat which respond to noxious stimulation of the tail. *J. Physiol. (London)* 250:29P–30P, 1975.

63. Kenshalo D.R. Jr., Giesler G.J., Leonard R.B., et al.: Responses of neurons in primate ventral posterior lateral nucleus to noxious stimuli. *J. Neurophysiol.* 43:1594–1614, 1980.

64. Krauthamer G., McGuinness C., Gottseman L.: Unit responses in the ventrobasal thalamus (UPL) of the cat to bradykinin injected into somatic and visceral arteries. *Brain Res. Bull.* 2:229–306, 1977.

65. Andersen P., Eccles J.C., Sears T.A.: The ventrobasal complex of the thalamus: Types of cells, their responses and their functional organization. *J. Physiol.* 174:370–399, 1964.

66. Curry M.J.: The exteroceptive properties of neurons in the somatic part of the posterior group (PO). *Brain Res.* 44:439–462, 1972.

67. Guilhaud G., Caille D., Besson J.M., et al.: Single unit activities in ventral posterior and posterior group thalamic nuclei during nociceptive and non-nociceptive stimulation in the cat. *Arch. Ital. Biol.* 115:38–56, 1977.

68. Albe-Fessard D., Kruger L.: Duality of unit discharges from cat centrum medianum in response to natural and electrical stimulation. *J. Neurophysiol.* 25:3–20, 1962.

69. Erickson T.C., Bleckmenn W.J., Woolsey C.N.: Observations on the postcentral gyrus in relation to pain. *Trans. Am. Neurol. Assoc.* 77:57–59, 1952.

70. Whitsel B.L., Roppalo J.R., Werner G.: Cortical information processing of stimulus motion on primate skin. *J. Neurophysiol.* 35:691–717, 1972.

71. Horrax G.: Experience with cortical excisions for the relief of intractable pain in the extremities. *Surgery* 20:593–602, 1946.

72. Stone T.T.: Phantom limb pain and central pain: Relief by ablation of portion of posterior central cerebral convolution. *Arch. Neurol. Psychiatry* 63:739–748, 1950.

73. Hagbarth K.E., Kerr D.I.B.: Central influences on spinal afferent conduction. *J. Neurophysiol.* 17:295–307, 1954.

74. Reynolds D.V.: Surgery in the rat during electrical analgesia induced by focal brain stimulation. *Science* 164:444–445, 1969.

75. Mayer D.J., Liebeskind J.C.: Pain reduction by focal electrical stimulation of the brain: An anatomical and behavioral analysis. *Brain Res.* 68:73–93, 1974.

76. Mayer D.J., Hayes R.L.: Stimulation produced analgesia: Development of tolerance and cross tolerance to morphine. *Science* 188:941–943, 1975.

77. Akil H., Liebeskind J.C.: Monoaminergic mecha-

nisms of stimulation produced analgesia. *Brain Res.* 94:279–296, 1975.

78. Adams J.E.: Naloxone reversal of analgesia produced by brain stimulation in human. *Pain* 2:161–166, 1976.

79. Hosobuchi Y., Adams J.E., Linchitz R.: Pain relief by electrical stimulation of the central gray matter in human and its reversal by naloxone. *Science* 197:183–186, 1977.

80. Pert A., Walter M.: Comparison between reversal of morphine and electrical stimulation induced analgesia in the rat mesencephalon. *Life Sci.* 19:1023–1032, 1976.

81. Liebeskind J.C., Mayer D.J.: Somatosensory evoked responses in mesencephalic central gray matter of the rat. *Brain Res.* 27:133–151, 1971.

82. Carstens E., Yokota T., Zimmermann M.: Inhibition of spinal neuronal responses to noxious skin heating by stimulation of mesencephalic periaqueductal gray in the cat. *J. Neurophysiol.* 42:558–568, 1979.

83. Proudfit H.K., Anderson E.G.: Morphine analgesia blocked by raphe magnus lesion. *Brain Res.* 98:612–618, 1975.

84. Basbaum A.I., Marley N.J.E., O'Keefe J., et al.: Reversal of morphine and stimulus-produced analgesia by subtotal spinal cord lesion. *Pain* 3:43–56, 1977.

85. Hayes R.L., Price D.D., Bennett G.J., et al.: Differential effects of spinal cord lesions on narcotic and non-narcotic suppression of nociceptive reflexes: Further evidence for the physiologic multiplicity of pain modulation. *Brain Res.* 155:91–101, 1978.

86. Basbaum A.I., Clanton C.H., Fields H.L.: Opiate and stimulus-produced analgesia: Functional anatomy of a medullospinal pathway. *Proc. Natl. Acad. Sci. USA* 73:4685–4688, 1976.

87. Basbaum A.I., Fields H.L.: The origin of descending pathways in the dorsolateral funiculus of the spinal cord of the cat and rat: Further studies on the anatomy of pain modulation. *J. Comp. Neurol.* 187:513–532, 1979.

88. Leichnetz G.R., Watkins L., Griffin G., et al.: The projections from nucleus raphe magnus and other brain stem nuclei to the spinal cord in the rat: A study using the HRP blue reaction. *Neurosci. Lett.* 8:119–124, 1978.

89. Abols I.A., Basbaum A.I.: Afferent connections of the rostral medula of the cat: A neural substrate for midbrain-medullary interactions in the modulation of pain. *J. Comp. Neurol.* 201:285–297, 1981.

90. Basbaum A.I., Clanton C.H., Fields H.L.: Ascending projections of nucleus raphe magnus in the cat: An autoradiographic study. *Anat. Rec.* 184:354, 1976.

91. Gallagher D.W., Pert A.: Afferents to brainstem nuclei (brainstem raphe, n. reticularis pontic caudalis and n. gigantocellularis) in the rat demonstrated by microiontophoretically applied horseradish peroxidase. *Brain Res.* 144:257–275, 1978.

92. Behbehani M.M., Fields H.L.: Evidence that an excitatory connection between the periaqueductal gray and the nucleus raphe magnus mediates stimualtion produced analgesia. *Brain Res.* 170:85–93, 1979.

93. Fields H.L., Anderson S.D.: Evidence that raphe-spinal neurons mediate opiate and midbrain stimulation-produced analgesia. *Pain* 5:333–350, 1979.

94. Behbehani M.M., Pomeroy S.L.: Effect of morphine injected in their periaqueductal gray on the activity of single units in nucleus raphe magnus of the rat. *Brain Res.* 149:266–269, 1978.

95. Behbehani M.M., Pert A.: Behavioral and neurophysiological evidence for involvement of nucleus raphe magnus in analgesia produced by neurotensin. *Neurosci.* 2:806, 1982.

96. Fields H.L., Basbaum A.I.: Brainstem control of spinal pain transmission neurons. *Annu. Rev. Physiol.* 40:193–221, 1978.

97. Fields H.L., Basbaum A.I., Clanton C.H., et al.: Nucleus raphe magnus inhibition of spinal cord dorsal horn neurons. *Brain Res.* 126:441–454, 1977.

98. Giesler G.J. Jr., Gerhard K.D., Yezieroski R.P., et al.: Postsynaptic inhibition of primate spinothalamic neurons by stimulation in nucleus raphe magnus. *Brain Res.* 204:184–188, 1981.

99. Oliveras J.L., Hosobuchi Y., Redjemi F., et al.: Opiate antagonist, naloxone, strongly reduces analgesia induced by stimulation of raphe nucleus (centralis inferior). *Brain Res.* 120:221–229, 1977.

100. Willis W.D., Trevino D.L., Coutler J.D., et al.: Responses of primate spinothalamic tract neurons to natural stimulation of hind limb. *J. Neurophysiol.* 37:358–372, 1974.

101. Hökfelt T., Jung L., Dahl A., et al.: Immunohistochemical analysis of peptide pathways possibly related to pain and analgesia: Enkephalin and substance P. *Proc. Natl. Acad. Sci. USA* 74:3081–3085, 1977.

102. Hayes A.G., Tyers M.B.: Effect of capsaicin in nociceptive heat, pressure and chemical thresholds and on substance P levels in the rat. *Brain Res.* 189:561–564, 1980.

103. Henry J.L.: Effects of substance P on functionally identified units in cat spinal cord. *Brain Res.* 113:439–451, 1976.

104. Randić M., and Miletić V.: Effect of substance P in cat dorsal horn neurons activated by noxious stimuli. *Brain Res.* 128:164–169, 1977.

105. Yaksh T.L., Farb D.H., Leeman S.E., et al.: Intrathecal capsaicin depletes substance P in the rat spinal cord and produces prolonged thermal analgesia. *Science* 206:481–483, 1979.

106. Jessel T.M., Iversen L.L., Cuello A.C.: Capsaicin-induced depletion of substance P from primary sensory neurons. *Brain Res.* 152:183–188, 1978.

107. Zieglgansberger W.: An enkephalinergic gating system involved in nociception, in Casta E., Trabucch M. (eds.): *Neural Peptides and Neuronal Communication*. New York, Raven Press, 1980, pp. 425–434.

108. Carstino E., Fraunhoffer M., Zimmermann M.: Serotonergic mediation of descending inhibition from midbrain periaqueductal gray but not reticular formation of spinal nociceptive transmission in the cat. *Pain* 10:149–167, 1981.

109. Yaksh T.L., Tya G.M.: Microinjection of morphine into the periaqueductal gray evokes the release of serotonin from spinal cord. *Brain Res.* 171:176–181, 1979.

110. Yaksh T.L.: Direct evidence that spinal serotonin and noradrenaline terminals mediate the spinal antinociceptide effects of morphine in periaqueductal gray. *Brain Res.* 160:180–185, 1979.

111. Zemlan F.P., Corrigan S.A., Paeff D.W.: Noradrenergic and serotonergic mediation of spinal analgesia mechanisms. *Eur. J. Pharmacol.* 61:111–124, 1980.

112. Dahlstrom A., Fuxe K.: Evidence for the existence of monoamine neurons in the central nervous system. *Acta Physiol. Scand. Suppl.* 2470:1–30, 1967.

113. Behbehani M.M., Pomeroy S.L., Mack C.E.: Interaction between central gray and nucleus raphe magnus: Role of norepinephrine. *Brain Res. Bull.* 6:361–364, 1981.

114. Behbehani M.M.: The role of acetylcholine in the function of nucleus raphe magnus and in the interaction of this nucleus with the periaqueductal gray. *Brain Res.*, in press.

115. Pomeroy S.L., Behbehani M.M.: Response of nucleus raphe magnus neurons to iontophoretically applied substance P in rats. *Brain Res.* 202:464–468, 1980.

116. Pert C.B., Kuhar M.J., Snyder S.H.: Opiate receptor: Autoradiographic localization in rat brain. *Proc. Natl. Acad. Sci. USA* 73:3729–3733, 1976.

117. Duggan A.W., Hall J.G., Headley P.M.: Morphine, enkephalin and the substantia gelatinosa. *Nature* 264:456–458, 1976.

118. Mayer D.J., Price D.D., Rafizi A.: Antagonism of acupuncture analgesia in man by the narcotic naloxone. *Brain Res.* 121:368–372, 1977.

12 / Neurologic Examination

P. PRITHVI RAJ, M.D.

THE IMPORTANCE of the history and the neurologic examination in the diagnosis of pain of neurogenic origin cannot be overemphasized. The purpose of the neurologic evaluation is to determine whether there is an organic lesion causing pain.

THE HISTORY

Every examination must be preceded by an accurate history. A skillfully taken history, with careful analysis and interpretation of the chief complaints and the course of the illness, frequently indicates the probable diagnosis even before physical, neurologic, and laboratory examinations are performed. The history should be recorded clearly and concisely in a logical, well-organized manner. It can never be sufficiently complete, and no symptom may be unanalyzed.

The history should be obtained from the patient if at all possible. The patient should be encouraged to give a detailed account of the illness in his or her own words. The physician should intervene only to exclude obviously irrelevant material, to obtain amplification on statements that seem to be vague or incomplete, or to lead the patient into areas from which useful information may be obtained. Rarely, however, is the patient's spontaneous narrative complete enough to make the diagnosis certain, and it is usually necessary to augment the account by means of leading questions regarding specific details.

Young children and sedated or confused patients obviously are unable to give a suitable history. Those who are in severe pain may not be able to give a satisfactory history for themselves. Consequently, it may be necessary on some occasions to corroborate or supplement the history given by the patient with one given by a relative or friend, or it may be necessary to obtain the entire history from someone else. Members of the family may also be able to give important information about changes in behavior, of which the patient may not be aware.

A history or an examination that is directed exclusively toward the nervous system is incomplete. It may seem irrelevant at times to follow the history of the present illness with a detailed medical history, but neurologic manifestations or complications are frequently the first clinical evidence of serious systemic diseases. First, the patient's general health prior to the onset of the present illness is recorded. Then a history of past illnesses, operations, and accidents or injuries is obtained, with the date, nature, and sequelae of each period of incapacitation. The patient is also questioned about any susceptibility to disease and any reactions to illness, operations, and injuries. The past medical history is followed by the marital history, occupational history, family history, and information about the patient's interests, habits, contacts, and other social, economic, and adjustment factors that may have influenced the patient's life and may have been important in bringing on the present painful condition.

PHYSICAL EXAMINATION

The general appearance of the patient may yield important information. Manifestations of acute or chronic illness should be sought, and special note should be made of signs of fever, pain, or distress; evidence of loss of weight, emaciation, or cachexia; the appearance of physical strength or weakness; the general motor behavior and any irregular or unusual attitudes, outstanding mannerisms, bizarre activities, restlessness, and an increase or decrease in motor activity; the relative position of the trunk, head, and extremities; and the posture and attitude in standing, walking, sitting, or lying down. The degree of cooperation; the appearance of apathy, lethargy, and fatigue; the presence of alertness or nervous tension; and the promptness or delay in responses should be recorded. Note should be made of any outstanding abnormalities in development or structure, such as gigantism, dwarfism, gross deformities, amputations, contractures, unusual conformations, or disproportion between parts of the body.

The vital signs, i.e., temperature, pulse and respiratory rates, and blood pressure, should be recorded in every instance. The head should be examined by inspection, palpation, percussion, and auscultation (noting the presence of bruits); the neck and spine by inspection (both at rest and on movement), palpation, and percussion.

To complete the physical study of the patient, various laboratory examinations and related diagnostic procedures are necessary.

The Sensory System

Abnormalities of sensation may be characterized by an increase in, impairment of, or loss of feeling. An increase in sensation is usually manifested by pain, the severity of which depends on the tissues affected, the duration, extent, and quality of the stimulus, the personality of the individual, and his or her powers of discrimination. Perversions of sensation take the form of paresthesias, dysesthesias, and phantom sensations. Impairment and loss of feeling result from a lessening of the acuity of the sense organs, a decrease in the conductivity of the fibers or tracts, or a dysfunction of higher centers with a consequent decrease in powers of recognition or of perception.[1]

The sensory examination is an attempt to discover any loss of or decrease or increase in one or all types of sensation, dissociation of sensation with loss of one type but not of others, loss in ability to recognize differences in degrees of sensation, misinterpretations or perversions of sensation, and areas of localized tenderness or hyperesthesia. More than one of these may occur simultaneously.[2]

To determine whether the patient has had changes in sensation or is experiencing spontaneous sensations of an abnormal type, the examiner should inquire whether the patient has any pain, paresthesias, or loss of feeling, and whether the patient has experienced such phenomena as numbness, burning, pressure, distension, tingling, pruritus, feelings of weight or constriction, girdle sensations, percep-

tions of absence of portions of the body, or "phantom limb" manifestations.

It is advisable, to investigate the sensory system early in the course of the neurologic examination. Although a simple procedure, it must be painstakingly performed and the findings evaluated with great care. The results depend largely on subjective responses, but occasionally objective manifestations such as withdrawal of the part stimulated or wincing may aid in the delineation of areas of sensory change. The results of the sensory examination may at times seem unreliable and confusing, and under such circumstances conclusions must be drawn with care. It may be necessary to postpone the sensory investigation if the patient has become fatigued or to repeat the test on consecutive days if consistent and satisfactory results are to be obtained. In fact, the examination should always be repeated at least once to confirm the findings. If the patient notices no subjective changes in sensation, the examiner can rapidly test the entire body, bearing in mind the major sensory nerve and segmental supply to the face, trunk, and extremities. The changes demonstrated are marked on the chart (Figure 12–1). It is helpful in appraisal if areas of change in different sensory qualities, such as pain, touch, and temperature, are indicated individually on the chart.

Sensations may be classified into various categories. For the routine neurologic examination, the major sensory modalities to be tested are the *exteroceptive sensations, the proprioceptive sensations,* and the so-called *combined sensations,* in which cerebral sensory functions play an important part.

Exteroceptive Sensations

The exteroceptive sensations are those that arise from or originate in sense organs in the skin or mucous membranes and respond to external agents and changes in the environment. They may also be designated as superficial sensations. There are three major types: (1) pain, (2) temperature, and (3) touch.[3, 4]

EXAMINATION OF SUPERFICIAL PAIN SENSATION.—Many different procedures for testing superficial pain sensation have been described. Perhaps the simplest method, one as reliable as any, is the use of a common pin. Algesimeters and other apparatus for quantitative testing are sometimes recommended, but their use actually adds little information to the clinical examination. The pin should be a sharp one, so that with minimal pressure it is

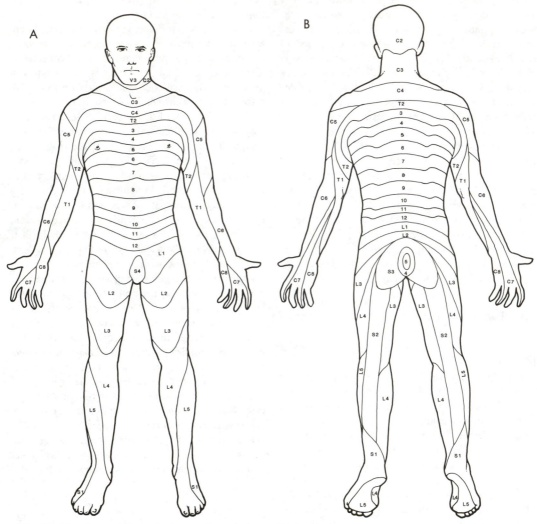

Fig 12—1.—A and **B,** anterior and posterior dermatomes of the body. (From Baker A.B., Baker L.H.: *Clinical Neurology.* Vol. 1. New York, Harper & Row, 1983. Reproduced by permission.)

possible to elicit a sensation of sharpness and pain. The patient is best examined with his or her eyes closed. Alternate stimulations should be made with the head and point of the pin, and the patient should be instructed to indicate whether the pain is "sharp" or "dull." The patient should also be asked whether there is any difference in the intensity of the stimulus in different areas. This mode of examination, if carried out in a painstaking manner, may be more satisfactory than one that involves the use of complicated instruments.[5] Very slight changes can sometimes be demonstrated by asking a cooperative patient to indicate the changes in sensation when a nearly vertical

pin point is stroked or drawn lightly over the skin in such a manner that the subject does not notice disagreeable pain.

The latent time in the response to stimulation is eliminated and the delineation is most accurate if the examiner proceeds from areas of lesser sensitivity to those of greater sensitivity, rather than the reverse. If there is hyperalgesia, for example, the examiner should proceed from the normal to the hyperalgesic area. If the stimuli are applied in too close proximity and if they follow each other too quickly, there may be summation of impulses; on the other hand, if conduction is delayed the patient's response may refer to a previous stimulation. Algesia and algesthesia are the terms used to indicate pain sensibility. In recording the response to pain stimulation, alganesthesia and analgesia designate areas insensitive to pain; hypalgesia, those areas having decreased sensitivity; and hyperalgesia, those showing increased sensitivity.

EXAMINATION OF TEMPERATURE SENSATION.—Temperature sensations are tested by the use of glass or metal tubes containing either cracked ice or hot water. A beam of light that does not indent the skin and stimulates a restricted area is also valuable in testing heat sensation. For quantitative evaluation one may use a thermophore, which is kept at a constant temperature by means of a rheostat, or an electric thermometer or thermopile. The patient is asked to respond by saying "hot" or "cold." For testing cold the stimuli should be from 41° to 50° F (5°–10° C); for testing warmth, from 104° to 113° F (40°–45° C). Temperatures much lower or higher than these elicit responses of pain rather than of temperature. In almost every instance the absence of one variety of temperature sensation is accompanied by the absence of the other, although there may be cases in which one is involved while the other remains partially intact. The cutaneous distribution of the absence of heat sensation is usually larger than that of absence of cold sensation.[6] Changes in temperature sensibility are recorded by the terms thermanesthesia, thermhypesthesia, and thermhyperesthesia, modified by the adjective hot or cold.

EXAMINATION OF TACTILE SENSATION.—Various means are available for evaluating tactile sensations. General tactile sensibility is tested by the use of a light stimulus such as a camel's hair brush, a wisp of cotton, a feather, a piece of tissue paper, or even a very light touch with the fingertip. Touch is tested along with pain when the examiner alternately stimulates the patient with the point and head of a pin. Stroking of the hairs is also a delicate means of testing this type of sensation. For a very detailed examination, as in experimental investigations, Frey hairs or an esthesiometer in which the stimulating element is a thin nylon wire may be used. The stimulus should be so slight that no pressure is exerted on subcutaneous tissues. Allowance must be made for thicker skin on the palms and soles and for especially sensitive skin in the fossae. The examiner asks the patient to say "now" or "yes" when the stimulus is felt, or, better still, to point to the area stimulated.[7]

Similar stimuli may be used for evaluating discriminatory tactile sensation, but this is best tested on the hairless, or glabrous, skin, and movement of hairs must be avoided. In addition, discriminatory sensation is examined by determining the patient's ability to accurately localize tactile stimuli and by investigating two-point discrimination. Localization is most acute on the palmar surfaces of the fingers, especially the thumb and index fingers. Two-point, or spatial, discrimination may be considered both a delicate tactile modality and a more complex sensation requiring cerebral interpretation.

Anesthesia, hypesthesia, and hyperesthesia are the terms that designate changes in tactile sensation; unfortunately, these terms also denote changes in all types of sensation. Thigmanesthesia denotes loss of light touch. Loss of sensation on stimulation or movement of the hairs is known as trichoanesthesia. Loss of tactile localization may be designated by the term topoanesthesia.

EVALUATION OF EXTEROCEPTIVE SENSATIONS.—In delineating and recording changes in superficial sensations, differentiation between changes due to lesions of the peripheral nerves, of

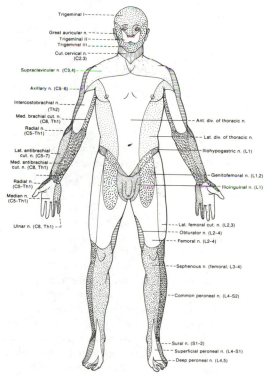

Fig 12–2.—Cutaneous distribution of the peripheral nerves on the anterior aspect of the body. (From Baker A.B., Baker L.H.: *Clinical Neurology.* Vol. 1. New York, Harper & Row, 1983. Reproduced by permission.)

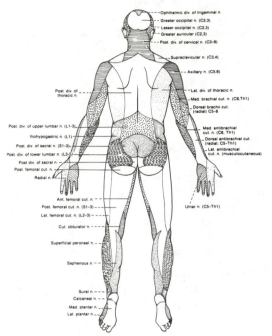

Fig 12–3.—Cutaneous distribution of the peripheral nerves on the posterior aspect of the body. (From Baker A.B., Baker L.H.: *Clinical Neurology.* Vol. 1. New York, Harper & Row, 1983. Reproduced by permission.)

the nerve roots, and of the cerebrospinal axis is important.

Peripheral Nerve Lesions.—In peripheral nerve lesions the areas of anesthesia, hypesthesia, or hyperesthesia correspond to the areas of sensory distribution of specific nerves (Figs 12–2 and 12–3). All types of sensation, including the proprioceptive, are altered within the distribution of the affected nerve or nerves. There is, however, an individual variation in the areas supplied by the peripheral nerves, so the resulting change differs with each patient. There are also areas of algesic overlap, especially for pain and temperature sensations; for light touch, this algesic overlap is less widespread. The demonstrable area of anesthesia in a lesion of a specific nerve is usually smaller than the cutaneous area that the nerve supplies. Consequently, with careful testing the examiner may demonstrate first an area of slightly hypalgesia, with loss of ability to distinguish slight differences in pain and thermal stimuli; then an area of marked hypalgesia and hypesthesia, within which, however, coarse tactile stimuli may be identified; and finally, an area of complete anesthesia and analgesia. In the

nerves supplying the face and body, there is usually a certain amount of "crossing" at the midline, more on the body than on the face. Therefore, an organic anesthesia almost always ends before the midline is reached.

Lesions of the Nerve Roots.—In lesions confined to the nerve roots there are areas of anesthesia, hypesthesia, analgesia, or hypalgesia limited to the segmental distribution of these roots. All types of sensation are affected. Instead of sensory loss there may be hyperesthesia and radicular or girdle pains in the same distribution. The skin areas innervated by specific segments of the spinal cord or their roots or dorsal root ganglions are called dermatomes.[8, 9]

The segmental innervation of the extremities is somewhat complex, in part owing to the migration of the limb buds during evolution. As a result, the fourth and fifth cervical dermatomes approximate the first and second thoracic on the upper chest, and the first and second lumbar dermatomes are close to the sacral dermatomes on the inner aspect of the thigh near the genitalia (see Fig 12–1).

Lesions of the Cerebrospinal Axis.—In lesions of the brain stem and spinal cord, or the cerebrospinal axis, the anesthesia follows the segmental rather than the peripheral distribution. The level of involvement can be localized accurately if the following is recalled: the interaural or vortex-mental line forms the border between the areas supplied by the trigeminal nerve and the second cervical segment; the fifth and sixth cervical segments supply the radial side of the arm, forearm, and hand; the eighth cervical and first thoracic segments supply the ulnar side of the forearm and hand; the fourth thoracic segment supplies the nipple level; the tenth thoracic segment supplies the umbilicus; the twelfth thoracic and first lumbar segments supply the groin; the first three lumbar segments supply the anterior aspect of the thigh; the fourth and fifth lumbar segments supply the anterior aspect of the leg; the first and second sacral segments supply the sole of the foot and posterior aspect of the leg and thigh; and the fourth and fifth sacral segments supply the perianal region.

In hysteria (conversion reaction), there are changes in sensory perception that do not correspond to organic nerve distribution and that may be influenced by suggestion. As a consequence, anesthesia extending exactly to the midline or even beyond it and other changes that do not correspond to peripheral nerve, root, or segmental supply, such as the so-called glove and stocking types of anesthesia, are often indicative of hysterical change. The borders of the anesthetic areas are sharply defined, but they may vary from examination to examination. It may be noted, however, that in spite of marked anesthesia these individuals can identify objects placed in their hands and can perform skilled movements and fine acts for which cutaneous sensations are indispensable. In addition, they may retain postural sensation even though all other sensations are lost. There may be a midline change for the sense of vibration over the bony areas, such as the skull or sternum, making it obvious that the condition does not have an organic basis.

Proprioceptive Sensations

The proprioceptive sensations are those that arise from the deeper tissues of the body, principally from the muscles, ligaments, bones, tendons, and joints. Kinesthesia is the sensation by which muscular motion, weight, and position are perceived. Bathyesthesia is deep sensibility, or that from the parts of the body below the surface, such as the muscles and joints. Myesthesia is muscle sensation, or the sensibility of impressions coming from the muscles.

SENSES OF MOTION AND POSITION.—The sense of motion, also known as the kinetic sense or the sensation of active or passive movement, consists of an awareness of motion in various portions of the body. The sense of position or of posture consists of an awareness of the position of the body or its parts in space. Some observers use the term arthresthesia to designate the perception of joint movement and position and statognosis to indicate the awareness of postures.

By passively moving the subject's digits the examiner can determine the subject's appreciation of movement and recognition of direction, force, and range of movement as well as ability to judge the position of the digits in space. The normal individual should be able to appreciate movement of one or two degrees at the interphalangeal joints and even less movement at more proximal joints. With minimal involvement the first loss is the sense of position of the digits; then the sense of motion is lost. As the pathologic process becomes more extensive, these senses may be lost for an entire extremity or, at times, for the entire body. In the foot, these sensations are lost in the small toes before they disappear in the great toe; in the hand, involvement of the little finger may precede involvement of the ring, middle, index finger, or thumb.

In testing, the completely relaxed digits should be grasped laterally with as little pressure as possible and passively moved. The examiner's fingers should be applied parallel to the plane of movement to eliminate variations in pressure. The digit being tested should be separated from other digits so that there may be no clues from contact. The patient should be instructed not to attempt active movement of the digit, as such an attempt may provide a clue to its position. If the senses of motion and position are lost in the digits, larger portions of the body, such as the leg and forearm, should be examined.

Sensations of motion and position may also be tested by placing the fingers of one of the patient's hands in a certain position while the eyes are closed, then asking the patient to describe the position or to imitate it with the other hand. The hands may be held outstretched; with loss of position sense, one hand may waver or droop. One of the outstretched hands is passively raised or lowered while the eyes are closed, and the patient is asked to place the other hand at the same level. The foot may be passively moved while the patient's eyes are closed, and the patient asked to point to the great toe or the heel. When performed with the eyes closed, certain tests for ataxia, such as the finger-to-nose test and the heel-to-knee-to-toe test, are effective in demonstrating the senses of motion and position. The senses of motion and position are also evaluated by observing the station and gait. A patient with significantly disturbed sensations of movement and of position in the lower extremities is not aware of the position of the feet or of the posture of the body. The Romberg sign is positive when the patient is able to stand with feet together and eyes open but sways or falls when the eyes are closed. Sensations of motion and position contribute to the recognition of shape, size, and weight. Their absence may be manifested not only by recognizable changes in sensory acuity but also by difficulties with coordination, known as sensory ataxia.

SENSE OF VIBRATION.—The ability to perceive the presence of vibration when an oscillating tuning fork is placed over certain bony prominences is termed pallesthesia.[10, 11] A tuning fork at 128 Hz (C^0) is most frequently used, although some authorities believe that a fork of 256 Hz (C^1) may bring out finer changes in the vibration threshold. Sensation is tested on the great toe, medial and lateral malleoli of the ankle, tibia, anterior-superior iliac spine, sacrum, spinous processes of the vertebrae, sternum, clavicle, styloid processes of the radius and ulna, and fingers. Not only the intensity but also the duration is noted. It should be emphasized that both the intensity and duration depend to a large extent on the force with which the fork is struck and the interval between the time it is set in motion and the time of application. Hence, all observations are relative.[12] Quantitative tests for vibration have been described in which an electrically stimulated oscillating rod or vibrating applicator (pallesthesiometer) is used; because the pallesthesiometer may vary in amplitude or vibration or intensity but generally not in frequency, the threshold of perception of vibratory sensibility can be determined quantitatively.[13, 14]

For adequate testing, the tuning fork is placed in maximum vibration and held on the great toe or over the lateral medial malleolus until the patient no longer feels it vibrate. The examiner then notes whether the vibration can still be felt at the wrist or over the sternum of clavicle. Better still, the patient's perception of vibration can be compared with the examiner's own perception. Loss of vibratory sense is referred to as pallanesthesia.

PRESSURE SENSATION.—Pressure sense is tested by firm touch on the skin with the finger or a blunt object and by pressure on the subcutaneous structures, such as the muscle masses, the tendons, and the nerves themselves, either by using a blunt object or by squeezing the tissues between the fingers. Both the appreciation and the localization of pressure are tested. For quantitative testing one may use the Head pressure esthesiometer or the piesimeter, an instrument in which the differentiation in focal pressure is estimated in grams. The term piesesthesia means pressure sensibility, and baresthesia is sometimes used to signify the sensibility for pressure or weight; this must be differentiated from barognosis (the appreciation, recognition, and differentiation of weight). Deep pain sensibility is tested by strong pressure applied over the muscle masses, tendons, and nerves.

DEEP PAIN SENSATION (PRESSURE PAIN).—Deep pain is more diffuse and less well localized than is superficial pain. Deep pain sense is tested by squeezing the muscles or tendons, by pressure on those nerves that lie close to the surface, or by pressure on the testicles or the eyeballs. Before the loss of deep pain sense, there is a delayed response to painful stimulation for both superficial and deep pain. Abadie's sign in tabes dorsalis is the insensibility of the Achilles tendon to pressure, and Biernacki's sign is the absence of pain on pressure on the ulnar nerve. Tenderness should not be considered as increased acuity for deep pain. Tinel's sign is a tingling sensation in the distal end of an extremity on pressure over the site of a divided nerve; it points to beginning regeneration of the nerve.

Combined Sensations: Cerebral Sensory Functions

The term combined sensation has been used to describe those varieties of sensation that require the utilization of more than one faculty for recognition. They are not mere combinations of sensation, however; in every instance a cortical component is necessary for the final perception. The resulting manifestations are perceptual and discriminative functions rather than the simple appreciation of the stimulation of primary sensory endings.

The faculty of perceiving and understanding the form and nature of objects by touch and of identifying and recognizing them is termed stereognosis. Loss of this ability is termed astereognosis or tactile agnosia. Astereognosis can be diagnosed only if cutaneous and proprioceptive sensations are present; if these are significantly impaired, the primary impulses cannot reach consciousness for interpretation.

The recognition of weight or the ability to differentiate between weights is termed barognosis; loss of this ability is known as baragnosis. It is tested by the use of objects of similar size and shape but of different weights, which may be appraised by holding them in the hand, either unsupported or resting on a table; unsupported is preferable. It is essential that the senses of motion and position be intact.

Recognition of texture is a special variety of stereognosis in which the patient is asked to identify similarities and differences, but it can probably be considered a specific type of combined sensation. It is tested by asking the subject to differentiate between cotton, silk, and wool, or between wood, glass, and metal.

Two-point or spatial discrimination is the ability to differentiate between stimulation by one and stimulation by two points. A Weber's compass or a calibrated two-point esthesiometer is used, and the patient is stimulated by either a single point or the simultaneous application of two points. The minimum distance between the two points when they are felt separately is noted. The distance varies considerably in different parts of the body. Two points can be differentiated from one at a distance of 1 mm on the tip of the tongue, at 2 to 4 mm on the fingertips, at 4 to 6 mm on the dorsum of the fingers, at 8 to 12 mm on the palm, and at 20 to 30 mm on the dorsum of the hand. Greater distances are necessary for differentiation on the forearm, upper arm, torso, thigh, and leg. The findings on the two sides of the body must always be compared. Two-point discrimination is sometimes considered a variety of critical tactile sensibility that is carried through the dorsal funiculi; Head[2] placed it in the epicritic system. Clinically, however, it has been found that loss of two-point discrimination with preservation of tactile sensation results from lesions of the parietal lobe.

The Cranial Nerves

The cranial nerves should be examined individually and in consecutive order.

Olfactory Nerve

The olfactory nerve is a sensory nerve with but one function, that of smell; it is tested by the use of nonirritating, aromatic substances.[15] Each nostril is examined individually while the other is occluded. The ability to smell should be determined by having the patient inhale forcibly, or sniff, the test materials through each nostril, and then comparing the results from the two sides. Probably the most satisfactory test substances are freshly ground coffee, tobacco, vanilla, and volatile oils such as benzaldehyde (bitter almond oil), oil of cloves, and oil of lemon. The use of a package of cigarettes or a tube of toothpaste from a patient's bedside stand may be of value in carrying out a rough, qualitative test.

Loss of the sense of smell is known as anosmia. Intranasal conditions may seriously interfere with the sense of smell, and there may be an individual variation in smell efficiency. The perception of the presence of an odor, even without the ability to identify and name the test substance, is sufficient evidence to rule out anosmia. Unilateral loss of smell is much more significant than bilateral anosmia, which may be caused by sinusitis, colds, and heavy smoking.[16, 17]

Optic and Ocular Nerves

The major function of the optic nerve is tested by examination of the various manifestations of the visual sense: quantity (acuity) of vision, range (fields) of vision, and special components of vision, such as color vision and day and night blindness. Finally, the optic nerve and the retina are examined by means of an ophthalmoscope.

In examining the function of ocular nerves (the oculomotor, trochlear, and abducens nerves) and the cervical sympathetic fibers to the intraocular structures, it is necessary to consider individually the pupils, the eyelids, the extraocular movements, and the position of the eyeball within the orbit. Details on the examination of the optic and ocular nerves are found in standard textbooks.

Trigeminal Nerve

The trigeminal (or fifth cranial) nerve is a mixed nerve, i.e., it carries both motor and sensory fibers. It is the largest of the cranial nerves and, because of connections with the third, fourth, sixth, seventh, ninth, and tenth cranial nerves and with the sympathetic nervous system, one of the most complex.

MOTOR FUNCTIONS.—The principal motor functions of the trigeminal nerve are examined by testing the motor power of the muscles of mastication. In disturbances of function of the motor division of the nerve, there is ipsilateral paresis or paralysis of the masticatory muscles. There is weakness or loss of power in motions of the mandible. The jaw is deflected toward the side of the involved nerve, and the patient is unable to deviate it toward the nonparalyzed side. In bilateral paresis the jaw droops, owing to the pull of gravity, and all muscle power is lost.

The function of the muscles of mastication may be tested by carrying out the following procedures:

1. The patient clenches the jaw while the examiner palpates the contraction of the masseter and temporalis muscles on each side; if there is either weakness or paralysis on one side, contraction is absent or defective.

2. The patient opens the mouth. Owing to the action of the pterygoids, especially the external pterygoids, which draw forward the condyle of the mandible and protrude the jaw, paralysis of the muscles of mastication is evidenced by deviation of the jaw to the side of the paralyzed muscles. Deviation is appraised by noting the relationship between the upper and lower incisor teeth. By placing a ruler or pencil in a vertical position in front of the nose, the examiner may be able to tell whether there is a deviation of the mandible. In paralysis of the facial nerve there may be an apparent deviation of the jaw owing to weakness of the muscles of facial expression.

3. The patient moves the jaw from side to side against resistance; with paralysis of the fifth nerve

on one side the patient is able to move the jaw to the paralyzed side but not to the nonparalyzed side.

4. The patient protrudes and retracts the jaw, and any tendency toward deviation is noted.

5. The patient bites on a tongue depressor with the molar teeth, and the depth of the tooth marks on the two sides is noted and compared. If the tongue blade can be pulled out while the patient is biting on it, there is a weakness of the muscles of mastication.

6. The jaw reflex is tested.

7. The tone, volume, and contour of the muscles of mastication are noted, and a check is made for fasciculations. If there is atrophy of these muscles, concavities above and below the zygoma are visible or palpable.

The other muscles supplied by the fifth nerve cannot be examined adequately, but, if possible, their function should be evaluated. With paralysis of the mylohyoid and anterior belly of the digastric, flabbiness or flaccidity of the floor of the mouth may be apparent on palpation. With paralysis of the tensor veli palatini, the uvula may be slightly tilted to the affected side, and the palatal arch on that side may appear broader and lower than normal. The levator veli palatini, however, is more important than the tensor veli palatini in elevation of the soft palate, and paresis of the tensor is masked if the muscles supplied by the tenth nerve are intact. Paralysis of the tensor tympani is not apparent objectively, but the patient may complain of difficulty in hearing high tones and of dysacusis for high tones.

SENSORY FUNCTIONS.—In testing sensation in the distribution of the trigeminal nerve, both skin and mucous membrane sensations are considered. The various exteroceptive functions (superficial pain, hot, cold, and light touch sensations) are examined individually, and changes in them are charted. The cornea, conjunctiva, nostrils, gums, tongue, and insides of the cheeks are also examined.

Lesions of the sensory portion of the nerve alter or destroy sensibility in the distribution of the affected portion. An attempt should be made to differentiate between sensory changes of peripheral origin, i.e., those resulting from lesions of one or more of the primary divisions of the nerve, and changes in the segmental distribution that follow lesions of the cerebrospinal axis. With the latter there may also be dissociation of sensations. Areas of tenderness and "trigger" or "dolorogenic" zones should be sought, and it is important to test for sensory extinction on the face. In differentiating or-

ganic from hysteric anesthesias of the face, it must be recalled that there is less crossing at the midline on the face than elsewhere on the body and that the skin over the angle of the jaw is not supplied by the fifth nerve but by the second or third cervical nerve through the great auricular nerve.

Proprioceptive sensations carried by the trigeminal nerve cannot be adequately tested.

REFLEXES.—The trigeminal nerve participates in many reflex responses. Since it is the principal sensory nerve of the face, in most instances the afferent portion of the reflex arc is carried through the nerve; in some of the responses, however, it conveys the efferent portions of the arc as well.

Mandibular Reflex.—To elicit the reflex the examiner's index finger is placed over the middle of the patient's chin, holding the mouth slightly opened. Then the finger is tapped with the reflex hammer. The response is a contraction of the masseter and temporalis muscles, which causes a sudden closing of the mouth. The chin itself may be tapped, or the examiner may lace a tongue blade over the lower incisor teeth and tap the protruding end. A unilateral response may sometimes be elicited by tapping the angle of the jaw or by placing a tongue blade over the lower molar teeth and tapping the protruding end. The afferent impulses for this reflex are carried through the sensory portion of the trigeminal nerve, and the efferent impulses are carried through its motor portion; the reflex center is in the pons.[18]

Corneal Reflex.—To elicit the corneal reflex, the examiner touches the cornea lightly with a wisp of cotton, a piece of string, or a hair. It is best to moisten the cotton to avoid irritating the cornea. The patient should turn the eye to the side away from the examiner, who should approach from the side to eliminate the blink or visual-palpebral reflex. Both the upper and lower portions of the cornea should be tested. In response to this stimulus there is a blinking or closing of the ipsilateral eye, i.e., the direct corneal reflex, as well as a closing of the opposite eye, i.e., the consensual corneal reflex. The afferent portion of the reflex arc is mediated by the ophthalmic division of the trigeminal nerve, whereas the efferent or motor response is a function of the facial nerve, which conveys the impulse to the orbicularis oculi. The reflex center is in the pons.[19]

When corneal anesthesia is the result of a unilateral trigeminal sensory lesion, stimulation fails to produce either the direct response on the affected side or the consensual response on the opposite side. Stimulation on the unaffected side elicits both responses, however. With a seventh nerve lesion and paralysis of the orbicularis oculi, the direct response is absent on that side but the contralateral consensual reflex is maintained; when the opposite cornea is stimulated, the direct response is present but the consensual reflex is absent. On occasion, the bulbar conjunctiva is stimulated rather than the cornea, the conjunctival reflex: this may be absent in normal individuals, especially those with a high threshold for pain, and is often absent in hysteria. It is much less significant clinically than the corneal reflex.

Loss of the corneal reflex is an early sign of trigeminal nerve involvement and indicates interruption of the sensory impulses carried through the ophthalmic division. The response decreases with lowering of consciousness, and the reflex is widely used as an index of the depth of anesthesia and of coma. Occasionally it is absent when there are lesions of the opposite cerebral hemisphere.[20]

Facial Nerve

Predominantly a motor nerve, the facial nerve innervates the muscles of facial expression. In addition, it carries parasympathetic secretory fibers to the salivary and lacrimal glands and to the mucous membranes of the oral and nasal cavities. It also conveys various types of sensation, including exteroceptive sensation from the region of the ear drum, taste sensation from the anterior two thirds of the tongue, general visceral sensation from the salivary glands and mucosa of the nose and pharynx, and proprioceptive sensations from the muscles it supplies. Anatomically, the motor division of the nerve is separated from the portion that carries sensation and parasympathetic fibers; this latter part is frequently referred to as the nervus intermedius.

MOTOR FUNCTIONS.—Testing of motor functions involves the examination of the facial expression muscles. First the face is inspected, mobility of facial expression observed, and any asymmetry or abnormality of the facial muscles noted. A one-sided appearance while the patient is talking or smiling, inequality of the palpebral fissures, infrequent or asymmetric blinking, smoothness of the face and absence of normal wrinkling, or increased wrinkling may all give clues to facial nerve involvement. It should be noted whether the abnormality is more marked during emotional stress or during voluntary effort.

The patient is asked to contract various muscles individually and in unison. The patient is asked to frown, wrinkle the forehead, raise the eyebrows, and corrugate the brow; to close the eyes, both singly and bilaterally, first lightly then tightly, and then against the examiner's resistance; to draw back the angles of the mouth, show the teeth, grimace, blow out the cheeks, purse the lips, whistle, and retract the chin muscles. Retraction of the angles of the mouth is noted both on voluntary effort and on smiling, and voluntary and emotional responses of all muscles are compared. Function of the platysma muscle is tested by having the patient open the mouth and pull down the corners against resistance or bite the teeth together firmly. The tone of the muscles of facial expression is noted, and a check is made for atrophy and fasciculations. The presence of abnormal movements such as oral facial dyskinesias, tremors, spasms, tics, grimacing, and athetoid, myoclonic, and choreiform movements should be recorded. Immobility of the face should be appraised.

The functions of the stylohyoid muscle and the posterior belly of the digastric muscle cannot be adequately tested. If they are paralyzed, however, there may be some weakness of deglutition with regurgitation of food. Weakness of the stapedius muscle may cause hyperacusis, especially for low tones.

REFLEXES.—There are several reflexes connected with the facial nerve, and they should be tested.[21]

Orbicularis Oculi Reflex.—Percussion at the outer aspect of the supraorbital ridge, over the glabella, or around the margin of the orbit, or a sudden stretching of the orbicularis muscle is followed by a reflex contraction of this muscle with resulting closing of the eye.[22] The response is usually bilateral. This is a deep muscle-stretch reflex, and the corneal reflex may be considered its superficial counterpart. The afferent portion of the arc may be carried through both the facial nerve (as proprioceptive impulses) and the trigeminal nerve; the efferent impulses pass through the facial nerve. The reflex center is in the pons. The strength of response varies in individuals, but the reflex is diminished to absent with nuclear and peripheral lesions of the facial nerve and is absent in coma. It is preserved or exaggerated in supranuclear varieties of facial palsy and in pyramidal lesions above the nucleus of the seventh nerve. In cases of extrapyramidal disease, the response is also exaggerated and may continue with repeated stimuli, whereas in the normal individual it disappears after a few stimulations; this persistent response is sometimes referred to as Myerson's sign.

Palpebral-Oculogyric Reflex.—A turning upward of the eyeballs when the eyes are closed or when an attempt is made to close the eyes is known as the palpebral-oculogyric reflex. This response is exaggerated in peripheral varieties of facial palsy (Bell's phenomenon).

Chvostek's Sign.—Chvostek's sign is a spasm (tetanic, cramplike contraction) of the ipsilateral facial muscles that appears when the exit area of the facial nerve anterior to the ear is tapped. Its presence indicates hyperirritability of the nerve. An important sign in tetany, it is also observed in other conditions in which there is increased reflex irritability.

SENSORY FUNCTIONS.—The sensory functions of the facial nerve cannot be adequately examined. The exteroceptive innervation supplies a relatively inaccessible area, i.e., the external auditory canal and tympanic membrane. These areas also receive exteroceptive innervation from other nerves, and the areas of distribution overlap. Deep, general visceral, and proprioceptive sensations cannot be evaluated. As a result, the sensory examination of the seventh nerve is limited to the testing of taste.

Taste is tested by using four common flavors: solutions of sugar, sodium chloride, acetic acid, and quinine are most frequently utilized. It is important when testing the patient's sense of taste to examine the anterior and posterior portions of each half of the tongue individually. The tongue should be protruded during the entire test; the patient should not be allowed to speak during the examination. For an accurate test, the words sweet, salty, sour, and bitter are written on a piece of paper. The various test substances are then placed on the portion of the tongue that is being tested, and the subject is asked to point to the word that signifies the taste perceived. The test substances may be placed on the tongue either by using a cotton applicator that has been dipped into the solution or by the use of a pipette. The mouth should be rinsed with water between tests. Bitter substances should be tested last because they leave the most aftertaste.

Loss and diminution of taste are called, respectively, ageusia and hypogeusia. Perversions or abnormal perceptions of taste are called parageusias.

There is marked individual variation in taste. Complete ageusia is rare unless there is also loss of smell. Age, wasting diseases, coating of the tongue, and excessive smoking diminish the power of taste. If there is loss of taste, the possibility of disease of the tongue should be eliminated first.

PARALYSIS OF FACIAL NERVE.—In a peripheral facial paralysis, or prosopoplegia, there is flaccid paralysis of all the muscles of facial expression on the involved side, and the paralysis is usually complete.[23] There is loss of function of the frontalis, corrugator, and orbicularis oculi muscles, the nasal muscles, the muscles of the mouth, and the platysma, together with paralysis of the stylohyoid, the posterior belly of the digastricus, the auricular muscles, and, in certain instances, the stapedius. The affected side of the face is smooth, the eyebrow droops, the eye cannot be closed, and the angle of the mouth may be depressed. When the patient attempts to close the eye on the involved side, the eyeball turns upward until the cornea is hidden. Known as Bell's phenomenon, this is a synkinesis of central origin in which the levator palpebrae superioris, the superior rectus, and the inferior oblique muscles participate. It is an exaggeration of the palpebral-oculogyric reflex.

Certain confirmatory signs of facial paresis may be elicited when the peripheral paralysis is not complete. The patient, for instance, may be able to close the eye on the involved side but be unable to close it against the resistance of the examiner's fingers. The examiner may find it easier to open this eye against the patient's resistance than to open the eye on the normal side. If the lids are passively opened and then allowed to close, the normal lid closes quickly, whereas on the involved side the closing is retarded and incomplete. The patient should be asked to close each eye individually. Inability to close the eye on the involved side without simultaneously closing its mate may indicate a facial weakness or may be the only residual of a facial palsy.

To test for the Dutemps and Cestan sign (levator sign), the patient is asked to look down and then to close the eyes slowly. The sign is present if the upper lid on the paralyzed side moves slightly upward, elevated by the levator palbebrae superioris because its function is no longer counteracted by the orbicularis. To test for the Negro sign the patient is asked to look up; the eyeball on the paralyzed side deviates outward and goes higher, owing to overaction of the superior rectus and inferior oblique muscles.

The platysma sign of Babinski is a failure of the

platysma to contract on the involved side when the mouth is opened. The corneal reflexes, both direct and consensual, are absent on the involved side, a result of impairment of the motor portion of the reflex arc. The consensual reflex remains on the sound side when the cornea on the involved side is touched.

A minimal facial paresis on one side must be differentiated from a facial contracture on the opposite side; if the latter is present, the normal side appears to be the weaker. It must also be differentiated from developmental asymmetry and facial hemiatrophy. Unequal palpebral fissures because of ptosis on one side may suggest the presence of a facial weakness on the opposite side. Measurement of nerve conduction time and electromyography often aid in differential diagnosis and in evaluation of prognosis.

FACIAL PARALYSIS OF CENTRAL ORIGIN.—With a central, or supranuclear, facial palsy, there is paresis of the lower portion of the face with relative sparing of the upper portion. The paresis is rarely complete, and it is always contralateral to the pathologic lesion.

The central variety may be called a paresis of the lower face, whereas the peripheral variety is a paralysis of the entire face. Differentiation between the two is rarely difficult.

Acoustic Nerve

The eighth cranial (acoustic or auditory) nerve is composed of two fiber systems blended into a single nerve trunk. These are the cochlear nerve, or the nerve of hearing, and the vestibular nerve, which subserves equilibration, coordination, and orientation in space. They originate in separate peripheral receptors and have distinct central connections. They differ so greatly both in anatomical relationships and in their respective functions that they should be considered separate nerves.

EXAMINATION OF COCHLEAR NERVE: HEARING TESTS.—Hearing is tested in a variety of ways. The patient's ability to understand soft and loud tones and low and high pitches is noted. Signs of deafness, such as a tendency to turn the head in listening, lip reading, or speaking with a loud voice, may give valuable information. If there is any history or difficulty in hearing or if the hearing is to be tested, the external auditory canal should be examined with an otoscope to eliminate any wax, pus, blood, foreign bodies, or exudate from the area and to determine whether the tympanic membrane is intact. The mastoid region should be examined for swelling and tenderness.

To test hearing, the examiner may first note the distance from each ear at which the subject is able to hear either the whispered or the spoken voice. Despite the inaccuracy of the voice test, it may be more valuable from a practical point of view to test acuity for the spoken voice than to measure hearing accurately in terms of intensity or decibels. If properly performed, the voice test can be useful and reliable.[24]

Hearing is further tested by noting the patient's ability to perceive the noise made when the examiner rubs thumb and index finger together in front of the external auditory meatus; for more critical testing, a watch is used. Each ear is tested while the other is occluded. The watch is first held outside the range of hearing of the ear being tested and is then brought toward the ear until the patient is first able to hear it. The distance from the ear is noted, and the examiner compares the patient's acuity hearing with his or her own. The high-pitched sound of a watch makes this test impractical for patients with nerve deafness and for elderly individuals, however. The Politzer acoumeter, an instrument that gives a clicking sound similar to that of a watch but louder, may be used if the patient is unable to hear a watch.

The use of a tuning fork also gives specific information. The patient's hearing can be compared with that of the examiner, and the relative auditory acuity on each side can be noted. Air conduction is tested by placing a tuning fork in front of the external auditory meatus; bone conduction, by placing it on the mastoid process. Both the intensity or quantity of the sound and the duration are noted.

The Rinne test is used to compare the patient's air conduction and bone conduction.[25] The vibrating tuning fork is placed firmly against the mastoid process, and the patient is asked to indicate when it is no longer heard. It is then placed in front of the external auditory meatus, and the period of time during which it is heard there is noted. In the normal individual, or when the Rinne test is positive, the tuning fork is heard twice as long by air conduction as it is by bone.

The Weber test is carried out by placing a vibrating tuning fork over the forehead or the vertex of the skull. In the normal individual the sound is heard in both ears, i.e., it is not lateralized. If one ear is occluded, the sound is heard more loudly on that side. In conductive deafness the sound is lateralized to the involved side and the Weber test is said to be positive. In sensorineural deafness the sound is heard by the uninvolved ear and the Weber test is said to be negative.

Glossopharyngeal Nerve

The glossopharyngeal and vagus nerves are intimately associated with each other and are similar in function. Both have motor and autonomic branches with nuclei of origin in the medulla. Both conduct exteroceptive sensation, as well as general and special visceral sensation, to similar or identical fiber tracts in the brain stem. The two nerves leave the skull together and course through the neck in a similar manner, and in many instances they supply the same structures. The two are frequently affected by the same disease process, and often it may be difficult to differentiate involvement of one from that of the other.

The various functions of the ninth nerve are difficult to test, principally because the areas of distribution are also supplied by other more important nerves. In addition, many of the structures it supplies are inaccessible.

The motor supply of the ninth nerve probably goes only to the stylopharyngeus muscle. The only objective manifestation of a motor lesion of the ninth nerve may be a slight unilateral lowering of the palatal arch at rest, although the two sides elevate equally well when an effort is made.[26]

The autonomic functions of the glossopharyngeal nerve can be evaluated by noting the function of the parotid gland. If highly seasoned food is placed on the tongue, a copious flow of saliva may be seen to issue from Stensen's duct. This may be called salivary reflex. The salivameter has been developed for the quantitative testing of salivary secretion.

Only certain sensory functions of the glossopharyngeal nerve can be tested.[27] The areas to which branches of this nerve supply exteroceptive sensation are the posterior portion of the tympanic membrane and the posterior wall of the external auditory meatus. These regions, which are also supplied by the fifth, seventh, and tenth cranial nerves, are inaccessible to clinical testing. The glossopharyngeal nerve supplies the special visceral sensation of taste to the posterior third of the tongue. Possibly with the vagus, it also supplies special visceral sensation to the epiglottis, the region of the arytenoid cartilage, the hard and soft palates, the anterior pillars, and the posterior pharyngeal wall. This function may be tested in a manner similar to that described

earlier for the testing of taste, but examination by the use of a galvanic current is more satisfactory.

The function of the glossopharyngeal nerve that is most available to clinical testing is that concerned with general visceral sensation. This can be tested best in the throat and on the base of the tongue. The ninth nerve carries "common sensation" from the mucous membrane in the regions of the tonsils, the fauces, the opening of the eustachian tubes, the lateral and posterior surfaces and a narrow rim along the inferior margin of the soft palate, the uvula, the posterior third of the dorsum of the tongue, the glossoepiglottic and pharyngoepiglottic folds, and the lingual surface of the epiglottis. One branch supplies the mucous membrane of the side of the tongue halfway to the tip. These areas are examined in the same manner as sensation is tested elsewhere.

Elicitation of the pharyngeal and palatal reflexes is an important part of the examination of the glossopharyngeal nerve. The pharyngeal or gag reflex is elicited by applying a stimulus, such as a tongue blade or a cotton applicator, to the posterior pharyngeal wall, tonsillar region, faucial pillars, or even the base of the tongue. If the reflex is present, the pharyngeal musculature is elevated and constricted, and the tongue is retracted. This reflex is used physiologically to initiate deglutition. The afferent impulses of the reflex arc are carried through the glossopharyngeal nerve, whereas the efferent element is conducted through the vagus nerve. The reflex center is in the medulla.

The palatal or uvular reflex is tested by stimulating the lateral and inferior surfaces of the uvula or soft palate with a tongue blade or a cotton applicator. Elevation of the soft palate and retraction of the uvula result. If the stimulus is directed toward one side of the soft palate, there is greater elevation on that side, together with ipsilateral deviation. The center for this reflex is also in the medulla. The motor portion of the reflex arc is carried through the vagus (and possibly the glossopharyngeal) nerve; the sensory component is carried through the glossopharyngeal (and possibly the vagus) nerve. The trigeminal nerve, however, also supplies a part of the soft palate; for this reason, the palatal reflex may be retained with ninth nerve lesions.

Both of these reflexes are lost with interruption of either the afferent or the efferent pathway. They are sometimes absent without pathologic significance but are most likely to be missing with lesions of the glossopharyngeal nerve. It is most significant if their absence is unilateral.

Vagus Nerve

In spite of its great size, many functions, and importance in regulation of vital functions, the vagus nerve can be clinically tested only with difficulty. Present means for its examination are inadequate.

EXAMINATION OF MOTOR FUNCTIONS.—The motor branches of the vagus nerve, which supply the soft palate, pharynx, and larynx, are more available to clinical testing than are most of the other branches of the nerve.[26]

Soft Palate

In examining the soft palate, the physician observes the position of the soft palate and uvula at rest and the position and movements during quiet breathing or on phonation. Any congenital asymmetry or the surgical removal of the uvual is noted, the palatal reflex is tested, and the character of the voice and the ability to swallow are appraised. Special attention should be paid to dysarthria and to dysphagia for liquids or solids.

With a unilateral vagus paralysis the findings include a weakness of the soft palate, unilateral lowering and flattening of the palatal arch, and deviation of the median raphe to the normal side. On phonation, the uvula is retracted to the nonparalyzed side. The normally functioning tensor veli palatini, which is innervated by the trigeminal nerve, may prevent marked drooping of the palate. The palatal reflex is lost on the involved side, owing to interruption of the motor rather than the sensory pathways. There usually is little difficulty with articulation or deglutition, although in acute unilateral lesions there may be a "nasal" quality to the speech, dysphagia (more marked for liquids than for solids), and some regurgitation of fluids into the nose on swallowing. These problems are usually transient, however.

With bilateral vagus paralysis the palate cannot be elevated on phonation, although it may not droop markedly. The palatal reflex is absent ilaterally. Because the nasal cavity is not closed from the oral cavity, speech has a characteristic nasal quality. There is special difficulty with palatal and gutteral sounds such as k, q, and ch. The sound b becomes m, d becomes n, and k becomes ng. There may be marked dysphagia, especially for liquids, and fluids may be regurgitated into the nose on attempts to swallow.

Pharynx

The functions of the pharyngeal muscles are examined by noting their contraction on phonation, by observing the elevation of the larynx on swallowing, by testing the pharyngeal reflex, and by noting the character of the patient's speech and his or her ability to swallow liquids and solids. If the superior constrictor is not functioning, Vernet's "rideau phenomenon" or a "curtain movement" of the pharyngeal wall toward the nonparalyzed side may be observed at the beginning of phonation. Normally, the larynx is elevated on swallowing; with paralysis of the middle and inferior constrictors this either does not occur or occurs only once or twice rather than repeatedly. The pharyngeal reflex is absent on one side with unilateral lesions, on both with bilateral lesions.

With paresis of the pharynx there may be some dysarthria, but this is usually minimal unless there is associated involvement of the soft palate or the larynx. Coughing may be impaired, and there may be loss of the cough reflex. There may also be difficulty in swallowing, especially in swallowing solid foods. Dysphagia, however, is marked only with acute unilateral or bilateral lesions.

Larynx

In the examination of the larynx the character and quality of the voice, any change of articulation, difficulty with respiration, and impairment of coughing are noted. A mirror examination of the larynx or a direct laryngoscopic examination should be carried out if there is hoarseness that is not readily explained by an acute inflammatory process, if there is dysarthria, or if there are any suggestions of vagus nerve involvement. Normally, the vocal cords are abducted on inspiration and adducted on phonation and coughing. In addition, there is reflex adduction on irritation of the larynx. In examining the larynx the physician notes the appearance and position of the vocal cords at rest, their movements during phonation and inspiration, and their response on coughing and irritation. Sensation of the upper larynx, a function of the internal branch of the superior laryngeal nerve, may also be tested. With paralysis of the laryngeal musculature there is often difficulty in speaking, but occasionally there is almost complete involvement of the larynx on one side without an appreciable effect on the voice.

EXAMINATION OF AUTONOMIC FUNCTIONS.—Since the vagus nerve is the inhibitor of the heart, paralysis causes tachycardia whereas stimulation causes bradycardia. The heart rate and, to a certain extent, the respiratory rate may be slowed slightly by pressure on the eyeball or by painful stimulation of the skin on the side of the neck. This is called the oculocardiac reflex or Aschner's ocular phenomenon. The afferent portion of the reflex arc is carried through the trigeminal nerve and the efferent portion is carried through the vagus nerve. The reflex is inconstant, unstandardized, and influenced by emotion. Usually the pulse is not slowed more than five to eight beats per minute, and it may be necessary to test the response during electrocardiography in order to be certain of the results. The oculocardiac reflex is an index of vagal hyperirritability; it is absent with vagus paralysis.

Vagus nerve paralysis may also cause depression, acceleration, or irregularity of the respiratory rate and alterations of gastrointestinal function. The other autonomic functions of the vagus nerve cannot be tested by the oculocardiac reflex.

EXAMINATION OF SENSORY FUNCTIONS.—The sensory elements of the vagus nerve cannot be adequately tested.[27] The exteroceptive branches supply the tympanic membrane, part of the external acoustic meatus, and part of the pinna. These areas are inherently difficult to examine; furthermore, they are also supplied by the fifth, seventh, and ninth cranial nerves. Sensation to the meninges, taste in the region of the epiglottis, and general visceral afferent supply cannot be adequately tested. It is possible that the vagus nerve carries some sensation from the posterior pharyngeal wall, but anesthesia of the pharynx in isolated vagus nerve lesions is rare.

EXAMINATION OF REFLEXES.—The vagus nerve plays a part in many autonomic or visceral reflexes, and loss of these reflexes may follow a lesion of the tenth nerve.

Vomiting Reflex.—Exaggeration of the palatal and pharyngeal reflexes may cause the retching, vomiting, or regurgitation reflex, also carried through the ninth and tenth nerves. Excessive stimulation or hyperirritability of these nerves may initiate reverse peristalsis in the esophagus and stomach, resulting in forceful ejection of material from the stomach. The vomiting reflex may be also produced by stimulation of the wall of the lower pharynx, the esophagus, the stomach, the duodenum, or the lower gastrointestinal tract. Vomiting may also be precipitated by stimulation of the internal ear (vestibular portion of the eighth nerve). Phenomena such as salivation, nausea, hyperhidrosis, and pallor may be associated with vomiting, owing to stimulation of vasomotor and secretory centers.

Swallowing Reflex.—Stimulation of the pharyngeal wall or back of the tongue initiates swallowing movements. Food is moved into the esophagus by the action of the tongue, palatine arches, soft palate, and pharynx. The presence of the bolus of food acts as a stimulus for deglutition.

Cough Reflex.—Stimulation of the mucous membrane of the pharynx, larynx, trachea, or bronchial tree elicits a cough response. Stimulation of the tympanic membrane or external auditory canal also elicits this response.

Nasal (Sneeze) Reflex.—A violent expulsion of air through the nose and mouth occurs in response to stimulation of the nasal mucous membrane. The reflex response is similar to that in coughing; however, because in the nasal reflex the faucial pillars contract and the soft palate descends, the air is directed chiefly through the nose.

Sucking Reflex.—Stimulation of the lips results in a series of sucking movements that involve the lips, tongue, and jaw. The response is elicited by bringing some object, such as a nipple to the lips. This reflex is largely a striated muscle response, but it is probably of autonomic origin. Normally present immediately after birth, it is lost after infancy. Like the snout reflex, it is present in adults with certain types of diffuse brain disease or severe cerebral degenerations. Under some circumstances testing for the orbicularis oris reflex causes not only puckering or protrusion of the lips but also sucking and even tasting, chewing, and swallowing movements. This exaggerated response is also known as the Alz, mastication, or "wolfing" reflex. When present, the reflex may be elicited by lightly touching, stroking, or tapping the lips, stroking the tongue, or stimulating the palate.

Hiccup (Singultus).—The hiccup is a sudden reflex contraction of the diaphragm that causes a forceful inspiration. There is an associated laryngeal spasm with sudden arrest of inspiration by closure of the glottis, which produces the peculiar inspiratory sound. The phenomenon usually results from irritation of the stomach wall or of the diaphragm. The phrenic nerves are the important pathways, but the vagus nerve may also play a part through both its sensory and motor functions.

Yawning.—Yawning is deep, prolonged inspiration, usually involuntary, through the open mouth; it is often accompanied by stretching movements of the neck and body.[28] Under most circumstances it is a complex respiratory reflex that occurs during fatigue and sleepiness, usually in response to chemical stimulation. Yawning may be a symptom of encephalitis or brain stem or cerebral disorders; it may also be brought on by suggestion and boredom.

Carotid Sinus Reflex.—Stimulation of the carotid sinus or of the carotid body by digital pressure at the bifurcation of the common carotid artery (either unilateral or bilateral) causes reflex stimulation of the vagus nerves and of the cerebral centers governing vegetative functions. The afferent impulses are carried through the carotid branch of the glossopharyngeal nerve to the medulla; the efferent impulses, through the vagus and sympathetic nerves. In certain susceptible individuals, often those with an appreciable amount of arteriosclerosis, stimulation of either the carotid sinus or body causes slowing of the heart rate, decrease in cardiac output, fall in blood pressure, and peripheral vasodilatation.[29] In pathologic states, pressure at the bifurcation of the common carotid artery or stimulation of the carotid body may produce vertigo, pallor, loss of consciousness, and occasionally convulsions. If hyperactivity of this reflex is suspected, it should be tested with caution—only unilateral stimulation should be used.

Spinal Accessory Nerve

The eleventh nerve is entirely motor in function. The accessory portion functions with the glossopharyngeal and vagus nerves and cannot be distinguished from them. It is in reality an integral part of the vagus. The spinal portion of the nerve supplies two important muscles: the sternocleidomastoid and the upper portion of the trapezius. The former muscle is innervated almost entirely by the eleventh nerve, although it may be supplied by a few fibers from the anterior divisions of the second and third cervical nerves. The amount of innervation to the trapezius varies with the individual, but only the upper part is supplied by the accessory nerve; the lower part is innervated by the third and fourth cervical nerves.

The function of the sternocleidomastoid muscle is appraised by inspection and palpation as the patient rotates the head against resistance. The contraction of the muscle can be seen and felt. With unilateral paresis there may be little change in the position of the head in the resting state, and rotation and flexion can be carried out fairly well by the other cervical muscles. A weakness of rotation can be observed, however, if the examiner places a hand against one side of the patient's chin and asks the patient to counteract this resistance.

With complete unilateral paralysis the occiput cannot be pulled toward the paralyzed side, and as a result the face is turned toward that side by the contralateral muscle and cannot be turned toward the normal side. If the chin is bent down against resistance, there is further deviation of the face toward the paralyzed side. The paralyzed muscle is flat and does not contract, so that it no longer stands out or becomes tense when attempts are made to turn the head toward the opposite shoulder or to flex the neck against resistance. There may be contracture of the contralateral normally functioning muscle.

The two sternocleidomastoid muscles can be examined simultaneously by having the patient flex the neck while the examiner exerts pressure under the chin or against the forehead, or by having the patient turn the head from side to side. If both are paralyzed, anteroflexion of the neck is difficult, and the head assumes an extended position.

In addition to testing the motor power of the sternocleidomastoids, the examiner should note their tone, volume, and contour. With nuclear or infranuclear lesions there may be atrophy, and fasciculations may be seen in the former. The sternocleidomastoid reflex may be elicited by tapping the muscle at its clavicular origin. Normally there is a prompt contraction. The reflex is innervated by the accessory and upper cervical nerves; when these nerves are diseased, the reflex is lost.

The function of the trapezius muscle is tested by having the patient shrug and retract the shoulders against resistance. The movements may be observed, and the contraction may be seen and palpated. Muscle power should be compared on the two sides. With unilateral paralysis of the trapezius the shoulder cannot be elevated and retracted, the head cannot be tilted toward that side, and the arm cannot be elevated above the horizontal. In addition, there is a tendency for the upper portion of the scapula to fall laterally, while the inferior angle of the scapula is drawn inward. The outline of the neck is changed; there is a depression or drooping of the shoulder contour, and the levator scapulae becomes subcutaneous. The paralyzed muscle becomes atrophic and fasciculations may be seen. There may be contracture of the normal muscle.

The two trapezius muscles can be examined simultaneously by having the patient extend the neck against resistance. When both muscles are paralyzed, there is weakness of extension of the neck, and the head may fall forward. The patient is unable to raise the chin, and the shoulders appear to be square as a result of atrophy of both trapezius muscles.

With bilateral paralysis of the spinal accessory nerves the ability to rotate the neck is diminished. The head may fall either backward or forward, depending on whether the sternocleidomastoids or the trapezii are the more involved. Since other cervical muscles, e.g., the scaleni, splenii capitis, and longi colli, are also important in rotation, deviation, flexion, and extension of the head and neck, complete paralysis of the neck muscles never occurs in lesions of the spinal accessory nerve.

Hyperkinetic manifestations with tonic or clonic spasm of the muscles supplied by the accessory nerve are encountered more frequently than paralytic phenomena. The involvement is most marked in the sternocleidomastoid muscles, but the trapezius and other muscles of the neck may also be affected. The muscular contractions cause a turning or deviation of the head or neck, known as wryneck or torticollis.

Hypoglossal Nerve

The examination of the hypoglossal nerve consists of an evaluation of the motor functions of the tongue. Motor power is tested; the position of the tongue on protrusion and at rest, as well as the strength and rapidity of movement in all directions are noted; weakness, paralysis, atrophy, and abnormal movements are observed.

The position of the tongue at rest in the mouth is first noted. The patient is then asked to protrude it; to move it in and out, from side to side, and upward and downward, both slowly and rapidly; and to press it against each cheek while the strength of this pressure is tested by the examiner's finger placed on the outside of the cheek. The patient may also be asked to curl the tongue upward and downward and to elevate the lateral margins.

If there is unilateral paralysis or paresis of the tongue muscles, the organ deviates toward the involved side on protrusion.

Motor System

The examination of motor functions involves not only the determination of muscle power but also an evaluation of tone and bulk, a study of coordination and gait, an observation of abnormalities of movement, and, on occasion, special electrical and chemical tests.

During the examination of motor functions the patient should be warm and comfortable. The posture and build, muscular development and bulk, active and passive movements, and any deformities and skeletal abnormalities should be noted. The character of the spontaneous active movement should be observed, as well as any abnormal movements. The two sides of the body should always be compared, and any asymmetries noted. Before testing motor power, it is helpful to inquire about handedness.

Motor Strength and Power

In an examination for strength and power active motility is especially important. In general, this is tested in two ways: by having the patient carry out movements against the examiner's resistance and by having the patient resist the examiner's active attempts to move fixed parts. On occasion, however, movements that are carried out without resistance or even with assistance may have to be tested. For example, it may be necessary to observe muscle strength when the parts are supported in water. Passive movements may also be tested to ascertain range or limitation of motion.

Adequate knowledge of the function of the individual muscles is essential.[30, 31] In addition to the action of isolated muscles or groups of muscles in simple or complex acts, the peripheral nerve and segmental innervation of each important muscle must be known in order to distinguish peripheral nerve and plexus lesions from those that involve segmental structures.

The examiner should determine whether power has been retained or whether there is complete paralysis, paresis, barely perceptible movement with or without assistance, movement against gravity, or various degrees of sustained power, either spontaneous or against resistance. The part of the body to be examined is placed in a position that permits the muscle to act directly and at the same time inhibits as far as possible the action of muscles of similar function. The proximal portion of a limb must be fixed when the movements of the distal portion are being tested; for instance, the humerus should be fixed when pronation is tested so that the patient does not use the shoulder to compensate for a weakness in pronation. Spasm and contracture may limit range of motion and simulate paresis.

It is important to palpate the muscles as well as to observe their contraction, especially when there is a decrease in power. Even the futile effort to move a muscle may be accompanied by a synergistic contraction of neighboring or antagonistic muscles which may be palpable but not visible. Paresis may be mistaken for paralysis if the movement takes place in an unfavorable attitude, as, for instance, in overcoming the effect of gravity. In the presence of weakness, the biceps and triceps muscles can contract more easily if the elbow is raised outward to the height of the shoulder so that the forearm can be moved in the horizontal plane. The extensors of the wrist can act better when the arm is hanging at the side than when it is raised to the horizontal. Grip may appear weak in a radial palsy if it is tested while the hand is hanging down, but if the wrist is passively extended, the flexors of the fingers contract.

It is usually possible to evaluate muscle strength and power sufficiently well by observation and palpation, without recourse to special instruments. The subjective impression of the investigator is usually sufficient. On occasion and for special purposes, a dynamometer or myosthenometer may be used, especially when exact quantitative measurements are desired.

Muscle function may be graded in various ways. The following classification is acceptable:

0. There is no muscle contraction.

1. There is a flicker, or trace, of contraction without actual movement, or contraction may be palpated in the absence of apparent movement. There is minimal or no motion of joints (0%–10% of normal movement).

2. The muscle moves the part through a partial arc of movement with gravity eliminated (11%–25% of normal movement).

3. The muscle completes the whole arc of movement against gravity (26%–50% of normal movement).

4. The muscle completes the whole arc of movement against gravity, together with variable amounts of resistance (51%–75% of normal movement).

5. The muscle completes the whole arc of movement against gravity and maximum amounts of resistance several times without signs of fatigue; this is normal muscular power (76%–100% of normal movement).

S. Spasm of muscle occurs.

C. Contraction of muscle occurs.

Since there is a marked individual variation in muscle strength, a diffuse deficiency in strength of moderate degree usually is of little significance. The presence of local muscle weakness or paralysis is of importance, however, and such changes have definite diagnostic value in peripheral and central nervous system lesions. If weakness is found, it should be determined whether the weakness involves a specific muscle or various muscles supplied by a certain segment of the spinal cord, whether it involves a specific movement for which more than one muscle is used, or whether it involves an entire extremity.

Diffuse weakness may be found in such conditions as the myopathies and myositis. In myasthenia gravis there is a decrease in endurance and an increase in fatigability; the weakness improves after rest. Diffuse weakness may also be the result of poor muscular development or inadequate muscular training, or it may be found in chronically ill patients. The weakness of elderly persons is an exaggeration of the normal aging process as it affects skeletal muscles.[30, 31]

The motor examination may have to be modified in various disease states, in confused and stuporous patients, and in infants and young children. Often, only a rough estimate of function can be made. In the presence of coma, assessment of motor function may have to be limited to observation of spontaneous movements, the position of the extremities, asymmetries of voluntary movement on the two sides, or withdrawal of a part in response to painful stimulation. In infants, also, motor function may have to be tested largely by observing spontaneous movements and noting the position of the body parts when the infant is prone, supine, seated, or upright. Resistance to passive movement and response to reflex testing give indirect evidence of muscle strength.

Detailed testing should be directed at individual muscles as well as movements involving groups of muscles. Strength and power should be carefully observed and impairment or loss of function noted. Testing of the muscle supplied by those cranial nerves which have motor functions has already been described. In the examination of the motor system the testing should include appraisal of movements and muscles of the neck, shoulder girdles and upper extremities, thorax and abdomen, trunk, and hip girdles and lower extremities.

Muscle Tone

The evaluation of tone is entirely a matter of judgment and can be learned only by experience.

The most important criterion in the examination of tone is the resistance of muscles to passive manipulation when they are relaxed and voluntary control is absent. In the testing of tone passive, not active, movement is normally examined, and the degree of tension present on passive stretching of muscles is noted, as well as extensibility and range of motion.

Changes in tone are more readily detected in the muscles of the extremities than in those of the trunk. When an individual extremity is tested, the patient is asked to "give the extremity to the examiner" and to relax completely, avoiding all tension. The part is moved passively, first slowly through a complete range of motion, then at varying speeds. The examiner may shake the forearm to and fro and note the excursions of the patient's voluntarily relaxed hand. The resistance to movement and the power to maintain postures against external forces are noted, both on slow and rapid motion and on partial and full range of motion. Tone may also be tested by raising the head, arms, or legs of the recumbent patient and then allowing them to drop; by noting the pendulousness of the legs when the limbs of the seated patient are raised and allowed to drop; by observing the range of motion of the arms after shaking the patient's shoulders; and by noting the range of movement of a part in response to a slight blow. The distribution of any abnormality in tone and the movements or muscles involved, as well as the type and degree of change, should be recorded.

Abnormalities of Muscle Tone

Abnormalities of tone may occur in the presence of disease of any portion of the motor system.

Hypotonicity, or flaccidity, is characterized by a decrease in or loss of normal tone. The muscle lies inert and is flaccid and flabby, or soft to palpation. The joints involved offer no resistance to passive flexion or extension, even when such movement is carried out rapidly. The excursion of the joints may be normal, but it is usually increased; there is absence of a "checking" action on extremes of passive motion. Involved limbs do not steadily maintain positions into which they are brought either actively or passively. If such an extremity is lifted and allowed to drop, it falls with a flail-like motion. A slight blow causes it to sway through an excessive excursion. In the Babinski tonus test there is an exaggerated flexibility of the forearm against the upper arm; passive flexion of the forearm against the upper arm while the latter is extended at the shoulder reveals a decrease in tone followed by an increase in flexibility and mobility so that the elbow can be bent to a more acute angle than normal. The muscle stretch reflexes are usually decreased or absent. Such a change is found with disease of the anterior horn cells, peripheral nerves, myoneural junction, or muscle tissue itself. It may also be found if there is interference with proprioceptive pathways.

Hypertonicity is usually caused by lesions central to the anterior horn cells, most frequently from involvement of the extrapyramidal or pyramidal systems, with loss of those impulses that normally inhibit one.[22, 32, 33]

Extrapyramidal rigidity, which occurs in lesions of the basal ganglia and their connections, is a state of fairly steady muscular tension that is equal in degree in opposing muscle groups. In the extremities it may involve both flexor and extensor muscles. There is resistance to passive movement in all directions, throughout the entire range of motion, and it is continuous from the beginning to the end of the movement. It is sometimes referred to as waxy or "lead pipe" resistance.

Spasticity is a state of slight to severe muscular tension or contraction in response to passive stretching. Passive movement of the extremity may be carried out with comparative freedom if it is done slowly, but tension appears as soon as rapid or forceful movement is attempted; "blocking" limits further movement. Passive movement may also be carried out with little resistance through a limited range of motion, but extremes of movement, such as complete flexion or extension, likewise result in blocking and limitation of further movement. There may be an elastic, springlike resistance to stretching at the beginning of movement, especially if the part is moved abruptly. At a certain point after the initial resistance, the muscle relaxes. This waxing and waning of resistance is sometimes referred to as a "clasp knife" phenomenon. In the Babinski tonus test there is reduced flexibility of the forearm against the upper arm; passive flexion of the forearm against the upper arm while the latter is extended results in decreased mobility, and the forearm cannot be flexed beyond an obtuse angle.[34]

Conditions That Affect Muscle Tone

Diseases of the pyramidal system (or pyramidal and related systems) cause a spastic paralysis that is often characterized by sustained contraction of specific groups of muscles. In hemiplegia of cerebral origin, for instance, the spasticity is most marked in the flexor muscles of the upper and extensor muscles of the lower extremity. This causes postural flexion of the arm and extension of the leg; as a result, the extremities are held in a characteristic position. The arm is adducted and flexed at the shoulder, the forearm is flexed at the elbow, and the wrist and fingers are flexed. There may be forced grasping. The lower extremity is extended at the hip, knee, and ankle, and there is inversion with plantar flexion of the foot. Marked spasm of the adductors of the thigh may be present. Passive resistance to extension is greater than that to flexion in the upper extremities; passive resistance to flexion is greater than that to extension in the lower extremities. Occasionally, however, with relatively complete spinal cord lesions the lower extremities may be in flexion rather than extension, resulting in paraplegia in flexion. This occurs when the spinal cord lesion is so extensive that the vestibulospinal and other extrapyramidal pathways, as well as the pyramidal tracts, are affected.

Catatonic rigidity is similar to extrapyramidal rigidity but may be accompanied by bizarre posturing and mannerisms. Decerebrate rigidity is characterized by marked rigidity and sustained contraction of all the extensor (antigravity) muscles. Reflex rigidity, or spasm of skeletal muscle, is a response to sensory irritation, usually to pain. It is a state of sustained involuntary contraction accompanied by muscle shortening. The contracted muscles, which are raised, are firm and resistant on palpation.

In myotonia there is a generalized increase in muscle tone with persistence of contraction and delay in relaxation. In tetany there are tonic muscle spasms, and there is hyperirritability of the muscular and nervous systems to all stimuli. In tetanus there is a generalized increase in muscle tone which may affect the face and jaw muscles, abdominal and spinal muscles, and extremities. In the stiff-man syndrome there are painful tonic muscular spasms with progressive rigidity of the muscles of the neck, trunk, and proximal parts of the extremities.

Muscle Volume and Contour

Muscle volume and contour are examined and atrophy or hypertrophy appraised by inspection, palpation, and measurement.

The general muscular development and the size of the individual muscles and muscle groups are appraised. Symmetric parts of the two sides of the body should be compared and the muscular landmarks carefully scrutinized. Any flattening, hollowing, or bulging of the muscle masses should be investigated. The muscles of the face, shoulder and pelvic girdles, and distal parts of the extremities should be especially noted. The palmar surfaces of the hands, the thenar and hypothenar eminences, and the interosseous muscles should be examined specifically.

The muscle masses should also be carefully palpated and their volume, contour, and consistency noted. In order to determine the degree of atrophy or of hypertrophy, measurements may be essential. A tape measure, calipers, or an oncometer may be used. The size of the individual muscles and the circumference and size of the extremities are measured and compared, and the distribution of changes is noted.

Coordination

Many special tests are used in evaluating coordination, but often careful observation of the patient during the examination as a whole may provide a great deal of information. The way in which the patient lies down, sits, stands, and walks should be observed.[35] Performance while dressing and undressing should be noted, as should tremors and hyperkinesias. The patient may be asked to carry out simple acts such as writing his or her name, using simple tools, drinking a glass of water, and tracing lines with a light pen while no support is given at the elbow. Tests for coordination may be divided into those concerned with equilibratory and nonequilibratory functions.

EQUILIBRATORY COORDINATION.—Equilibratory coordination, or cordination of the body as a whole, is noted in the examination of posture, or station, and gait. The patient may first be observed in the lying or seated position; only gross disturbances of coordination are apparent in these positions. There may be oscillations or unsteadiness of the body, and the patient may be unable to fix properly and coordinate the spinal, trunk, pelvic, and shoulder muscles. The patient may lack the ability to maintain a steady seated position and may sway or fall if seated without support. There may be nodding movements of the head.

It is usually in the standing position, however, that the moderate disturbances of equilibratory coordination first become apparent. The patient is asked to stand with the eyes open and then with them closed. The position of the body as a whole and that of the feet, shoulders, and head should be noted, as should tremors, swaying, and lurching.

Difficulty with balance may be accentuated if the patient stands with the feet in a tandem relationship, i.e., with one heel directly in front of the opposite toes, especially if he or she attempts to follow movements with the eyes, not the head. The patient may be given a light push, first toward one side and then toward the other, and then may be asked to stand on one foot at a time while the other leg is fixed at the knee. In all these tests, sensory ataxia can be differentiated from the cerebellar type because in sensory ataxia the difficulty is accentuated when the eyes are closed (the positive Romberg test). Unilateral cerebellar or vestibular disease can be differentiated from vermis involvement by laterality of unsteadiness.

Coordination of the body as a whole may also be tested by asking the patient to rise from a lying to a seated position and then to an erect one without using the hands; to bend forward, flex the trunk, touch the floor with the hands, and then resume the erect position; to bend the head and trunk as far backward as possible; and to bend from side to side. In rising from the supine position the patient may fail to press on the lower extremities, thus raising the legs, especially the one on the involved side, instead of lifting the trunk forward. In rising from a seated position the patient may fail to flex the thighs and pull the knees and trunk forward, and accordingly will be unable to secure or maintain balance. In bending forward the patient may be unable to coordinate the functions of the spinal, pelvic, and lower extremity muscles to maintain balance. In bending backward the patient may fail to flex the knees to prevent falling. In bending from side to side there may be more difficulty with balance on the involved side and a tendency to fall toward that side.

Gait is tested by having the patient walk forward and backward with the eyes open and then closed, follow a straight line, or walk tandem. Any swaying, staggering, or deviation should be noted. Disturbances of function that are moderately evident in testing station may become more marked in the examination of gait.

NONEQUILIBRATORY COORDINATION.—In testing nonequilibratory coordination the examiner is concerned with the patient's ability to carry out discrete, often relatively fine, intentional movements with the extremities.

In the finger-nose-finger test the patient touches the tip of the index finger to the nose, then touches the tip of the examiner's finger, and again touches the tip of his or her own nose. The examiner's finger is moved about during the test, and the patient touches it when it is held in various positions. The examiner may withdraw the finger slowly, noting the patient's ability to follow it accurately while making repeated efforts to touch it.

In the finger-to-finger test the patient is asked to abduct the arms to the horizontal and then bring in the tips of the index fingers through a wide circle to approximate them exactly in the midline. This is done slowly and rapidly and with the eyes open and closed.

The usual test for dysdiadochokinesia is carried out by having the patient alternately pronate and supinate the hands, either outstretched or with the elbows fixed to the sides. Any movement, however, that is concerned with reciprocal innervation and alternate action of agonists and antagonists can be used. The movements are performed as rapidly as possible. The patient may be asked to open and close the fists alternately, tap on a table with the fingers, pat the knees with the palms and dorsa of the hands alternately, or touch the tip of the thumb repetitively to the tip of each finger rapidly and in sequence.[36] The lower extremities may be tested by having the patient rapidly flex the ankle or rapidly flex and extend the toes. Rate, rhythm, accuracy, and smoothness of movements are noted.

The check movements of antagonistic muscles, the ability to contract the antagonists immediately after relaxation of the agonists, and the brake mechanism after the sudden release of a resistance opposing a strong voluntary movement are all evaluated in the Holmes rebound test. The patient is asked to flex the arm at the shoulder and forearm at the elbow and to clench the fist firmly. The elbow may be supported on a table, or it may be held close to the body with no support. The examiner pulls on the wrist against resistance and then suddenly releases it. In the normal individual, the contraction of the biceps and other flexors of the forearm is followed almost immediately by contraction of the triceps, the tendency toward flexion is checked by the rapid action of the antagonists, and the movement of the limb is arrested. In contrast, when the strongly flexed extremity of a patient with cerebellar disease is suddenly released, the individual is unable to stop the contraction of the flexors and follow it immediately by contraction of the triceps. There is loss of the "checking factor," and as a consequence, the hand flies up to the shoulder or mouth, often with considerable violence.

Station and Gait

STATION.—To test station, the patient is asked to stand with the feet closely approximated, first with the eyes open and then with the eyes closed. Any unsteadiness, swaying, deviation, or tremor should be noted. Station may be further evaluated by having the patient stand on one foot at a time, on the toes and then on the heels, and in a tandem position with one heel in front of the toes of the other foot; these tests should be made both with the eyes open and with them closed. The patient may be given a slight push to see if it causes a fall to one side, forward, or backward. Additional tests include having the patient hop on one foot, mark time, rise from a supine or seated position, stoop and resume the erect position, or bend forward, backward, and to each side.

GAIT.—The gait is also tested with the patient's eyes open and closed, and the patient should be asked to walk not only forward but also backward, sideward, and around a chair. Other tests involve walking on the toes and then on the heels; following a line on the floor; walking tandem; walking in a sideward direction and overstepping or crossing one foot over the other in doing so; walking forward and turning rapidly; walking forward and backward repeatedly six to eight steps with the eyes closed; walking slowly, then rapidly, then running; climbing stairs. The patient may be asked to rise abruptly from a chair, stand erect, walk, stop suddenly, and turn quickly on command (Fournier test).

Various abnormalities of gait are of diagnostic importance in neurologic diseases. Some of them may even be considered pathognomonic of certain disease processes.

Gait of Weakness.—Chronic illness of prolonged duration and even acute illness of short duration may cause an abnormality of locomotion. It is characterized mainly by unsteadiness and the desire for support. The patient may stagger and sway from side to side and may anxiously reach for a chair or even a wall for support.

Gait of Sensory Ataxia.—Interruption of the proprioceptive pathways in the spinal cord is the most frequent cause of the gait of sensory ataxia. The patient is no longer aware of the position of the lower extremities in space, or even of the position of the body as a whole, if visual impulses are not correlated with proprioceptive ones. Locomotion may not be conspicuously abnormal when the patient walks with the eyes open. If there is any marked involvement, however, it will be noted that the gait is irregular and jerky even with the eyes open and that the patient walks with a broad base, throwing out the feet and coming down first on the heel and then on the toes with a slapping sound or "double tap." The phase of progression is lengthened because more time is needed to execute the muscular movements required to place the feet on the floor. The patient watches the feet and keeps the eyes on the floor while walking. When the eyes are closed, the feet seem to shoot out, the staggering and unsteadiness increase, and the patient may be unable to walk.

Gait of Cerebellar Ataxia.—Caused by involvement of the coordinating mechanisms in the cerebellum and its connecting systems, the gait of cerebellar ataxia is present when the eyes are open or closed. It is a staggering, unsteady, irregular, lurching, titubating, wide-based gait. While the patient is walking, tremors and oscillatory movements of the entire body may be noted. The difficulty may be referred to as a "drunken gait"; it is also seen in alcoholic intoxication, drug intoxication, and similar states. The swaying and deviation are toward the affected side when disease is localized to one cerebellar hemisphere or its connections.

Gait of Spastic Hemiplegia.—Any lesion that interrupts the pyramidal innervation to one half of the body causes the gait of spastic hemiplegia. When walking, the patient holds the arm tightly to the side, rigid and flexed, and does not swing it in a normal fashion. The arm can be extended only with difficulty. The leg is held stiffly in extension and flexed with difficulty (Figure 2); consequently, the patient drags or shuffles the foot and scrapes the toes. With each step the patient may tilt the pelvis upward on the involved side to aid in lifting the toe off the floor and may swing the entire extremity around in a semicircle from the hip, or circumduct it. The phase of support is shortened because of weakness, and the phase of progression is lengthened because of spasticity and slowing of movement.

Gait of Spastic Paraplegia.—The gait of spastic paraplegia is encountered in congenital spastic paraplegia, congenital spastic diplegia, cerebral spastic infantile paralysis (Little's disease), and related conditions. There is spastic paresis of both lower extremities, with less marked involvement of the upper extremities. Usually, in addition to the extensor deformity of the lower limbs with equinus position of the feet and shortening of the Achilles tendons, there is pronounced obturator or adductor spasm. As a result, the patient walks with a bilateral stiff, shuffling gait, dragging the legs and scraping the toes. There is also adduction of the thighs, so the knees may cross with each step; this produces the scissors type of gait. The steps are short and slow, and the feet seem to stick to the floor. Swaying and staggering may suggest an element of ataxia, but there is usually no true loss of coordination.

Parkinsonian Gait.—In the various extrapyramidal syndromes, especially Parkinson's disease and related conditions, there is an abnormality of gait characterized by rigidity, bradykinesia, and loss of associated movements. The gait is slow, rigid, and shuffling; the patient is stooped and walks with small, mincing steps. There may be propulsion and festination. The patient may have difficulty initiating the act of locomotion.

Steppage Gait.—The steppage gait appears in association with a foot drop and is caused by weakness or paralysis of dorsiflexion of the foot and/or the toes. The patient either drags the foot in walking or, in attempting to compensate for the foot drop, lifts the foot as high as possible to keep the toes from scraping the floor. Thus there is an exaggerated flexion at the hip and knee; the foot is thrown out, and the toe flops down before either the heel or the ball of the foot strikes the floor, making a characteristic sound. The phase of support is shortened. The patient is unable to stand on the heels, and when he or she stands with the foot projecting over the edge of a step, the forefoot drops.

Dystrophic Gait.—The dystrophic gait is seen in the various myopathies in which there is weakness of the hip girdle muscles. It is most characteristic of muscular dystrophy but may also be present with myositis and allied disorders. The patient stands and walks with a pronounced lordosis. In walking there is a marked waddling element because of difficulty in fixing the pelvis. The patient walks with a broad base and shows an exaggerated rotation of the pelvis, rolling or throwing the hips from side to side with every step to shift the weight of the body. This compensatory lateral movement of the pelvis is due in a large part to weakness of the gluteal muscles.

Hysterical Gaits.—Individuals with hysteria or other abnormalities in the psychomotor sphere may show various derangements of station and gait. Such a patient may be unable either to stand or to walk despite the absence of paralysis. Results of tests for power, tone, or coordination may be normal if carried out while the patient is lying down. The gait is nondescript and bizarre, and it may vary from the normal in a way that does not conform to any specific organic disease pattern. It is often irregular and changeable, with elements of ataxia, spasticity, and other types of abnormality. There may be suggestions of monoplegia, hemiplegia, or paraplegia, yet the limbs can be used in an emergency. The abnormality may be unilateral or bilateral. In anxiety states there may be marked tremulousness of the extremities while the patient is standing or walking.

The Reflexes

The reflexes are significant for many reasons. Changes in their intensity and character may be among the earliest and most delicate indications for disturbance in CNS function. Furthermore, testing of the reflexes is more objective than many other procedures of the neurologic examination. The attention, cooperation, and intelligence of the patient are not as important in the testing of the reflexes as they are in other portions of the neurologic examination, and the reflexes can usually be adequately evaluated even when the other tests cannot be carried out, i.e., in infants and children, in confused individuals, in those of low intelligence, and in stuporous and comatose patients. The integrity of the motor and sensory systems can sometimes be appraised more adequately by examining the reflexes than by a detailed investigation of these systems.

Not all the reflexes can be tested in the routine neurologic examination, however, and many have no clinical importance. The majority of those that are important are muscular responses, and the muscle involved rather than the point of stimulation is the important factor.[37, 38]

When a muscle is passively stretched, its fibers react by resisting the stretch and entering into a state of increased and sustained tension, or contraction. In reflex response, either direct or indirect stimulation of any muscle results first in a lengthening reaction; then the proprioceptive impulses carried to the nervous system from sensory organs within the muscle itself call forth an increase in tension, and a shortening reaction or contraction follows. A sudden stimulus, such as a brief, sharp impact, is followed by an immediate response with a pull exerted longitudinally through the muscle. The reflex excitation is decreased by inhibiting impulses from higher centers. If these inhibiting influences are removed, there is an increase in reflex activity. Some muscles react more strongly than others; for example, the extensor muscles of the thigh and leg, which are important in standing and walking, react more promptly and strongly than do the flexor muscles.

Reflexes may be categorized into the following groups: (1) muscle-stretch reflexes, (2) superficial reflexes, (3) pyramidal tract responses, (4) reflexes of spinal automatism, (5) postural and righting reflexes, (6) associated movements, and (7) miscellaneous neurologic signs, including those of extrapyramidal dysfunction, meningeal irritation, tetany, and frontal lobe release. Conditioned or acquired reflexes are those in which, as the result of certain experiences, a specific response may be called forth by an indifferent stimulus; they depend on the integrity of the cerebral cortex, are developed through training and association, and cannot be considered with the other reflexes.

Muscle-Stretch Reflexes

The muscle-stretch reflexes are those that are elicited in response to a stimulus applied to either tendons or periosteum, or occasionally to bones, joints, fasciae, or aponeurotic structures. They are often called deep tendon or periosteal reflexes. Because the stimulus is mediated through the deeper sense organs, e.g., the neuromuscular and neurotendinous spindles, they may be referred to as proprioceptive reflexes. They are all, however, muscle-stretch reflexes and are produced by indirect stimulation of muscles and their response to a sudden stretch imposed on them.

The muscle-stretch reflexes are best tested by using a soft rubber percussion hammer. The activity or briskness of the response depends largely on the tone in the muscles. For an accurate determination of the reflexes, the examiner should feel the contraction by placing one hand over the muscle that responds. When the reflexes are tested, the patient should be relaxed and as comfortable as possible. The position of the extremities should be symmetric. The mechanical stimulus should be a quick, direct one, but no greater than necessary.

The examiner should note the degree of activity of the reflexes, which is estimated by the speed and vigor of the response, range of movement, and length of contraction. Reflexes may be classified as normal, sluggish, diminished, absent, exaggerated, and markedly hyperactive. For the purposes of clinical note-taking, some neurologists grade them as follows: 0, absent; +, present but diminished; + +, normal; + + +, increased but not necessarily to a pathologic degree; + + + +, markedly hyperactive, often with associated clonus. It is important to note the equality of the response on the two sides, and unequal reflexes may be as significant as either increased or absent reflexes. As far as possible, the deep reflexes should be named by the muscles involved rather than by the site of stimulation or the nerves involved.

Muscle-Stretch Reflexes of the Upper Extremities

The biceps, triceps, brachioradialis, and finger flexor reflexes are the most important muscle-stretch reflexes of the upper extremities. The biceps, triceps, and brachioradialis reflexes should be obtained without difficulty in normal individuals. The finger reflex is a little difficult for the inexperienced examiner to elicit, but it is present in most normal persons. Wartenberg[38] considered it one of the most important reflexes in the upper extremity. Other reflexes of the upper extremities may be elicited only to a slight extent in normal persons. If they are conspicuous, the presence of general reflex exaggeration can be assumed.

BICEPS REFLEX.—The arm is held in a relaxed position, with the forearm midway between flexion and extension and in slight pronation. This position is obtained most satisfactorily if the patient's elbow is resting in the examiner's hand. The examiner places his or her thumb over the biceps tendon and taps the thumb with a reflex hammer (Fig 12–4). The response is a contraction of the biceps muscle with flexion of the forearm on the arm, often accompanied by supination. If the reflex is exaggerated, the reflexogenic zone is increased, and the reflex may even be obtained by tapping the clavicle. Also, with exaggeration of this reflex there may be associated flexion of the wrist and fingers and adduction of the thumb. The sensory supply of this reflex is through the midcervical nerves, and the motor supply is through the musculocutaneous nerve (fifth and sixth cervical segments).

TRICEPS REFLEX.—The triceps reflex is elicited by tapping the triceps tendon just above its insertion on the lolecranon process of the ulna. The arm is held midway between flexion and extension, and it may rest on the examiner's hand or on the patient's thigh. The response is a contraction of the triceps muscle, with extension of the forearm on the arm. The sensory and motor innervations are through the radial nerve (sixth through eighth cranial segments). The so-called paradoxic triceps reflex consists of a flexion of the forearm following stimulation at the olecranon. This response appears when the arc of the triceps reflex is damaged, as, for example, in lesions of the seventh and eighth cervical segments; in such cases the stimulus calls forth a flexion response, unopposed by the triceps muscle (Fig 12–5).

BRACHIORADIALIS (RADIAL PERIOSTEAL OR SUPINATOR) REFLEX.—If the styloid process of

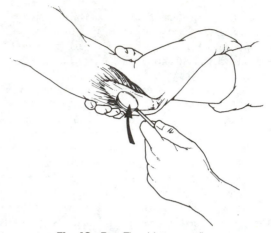

Fig 12–5.—The triceps reflex.

the radius is tapped while the forearm is in semiflexion and semipronation, the forearm flexes on the arm and supinates. The latter response is more marked if the forearm has been extended and pronated, but there is less flexion. If the reflex is exaggerated, there is associated flexion of the wrist and fingers with adduction of the forearm. The principal muscle involved is the brachioradialis. The innervation of this reflex is through the radial nerve (fifth and sixth cervical segments). In the presence of pyramidal tract involvement or other conditions causing reflex hyperactivity and involvement of the fifth cervical segment or its neuroaxes, there may be contraction of the flexors of the hand and fingers, without flexion and supination of the forearm. This is termed inversion of the radial reflex (Fig 12–6).

PRONATOR REFLEX.—If either the styloid process or the posteroinferior surface of the ulna is tapped while the forearm is in semiflexion and the wrist is in semipronation, there is pronation of the forearm, often with adduction of the wrist. There may also be flexion of the wrist and fingers. The same response may be obtained by stimulating the palmar surface of the lower aspect of the radius, causing brief supination that is followed by pronation. The major muscles participating are the pronators teres and quadratus.

Muscle-Stretch Reflexes of the Lower Extremities

PATELLAR (QUADRICEPS) REFLEX.—The patellar reflex, or the knee jerk, is characterized by contraction of the quadriceps femoris muscle, re-

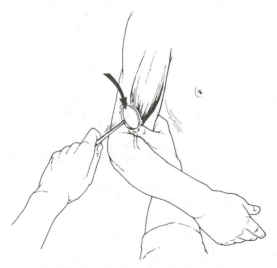

Fig 12–4.—Testing the biceps reflex.

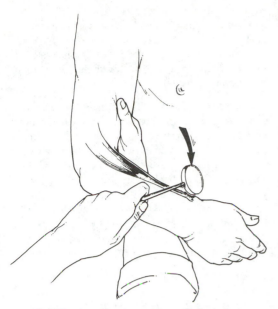

Fig 12–6.—The brachioradialis reflex.

sulting in an extension of the leg on the thigh, in response to a stimulus directed toward the patellar tendon. A sharp blow on the tendon draws down the patella and stretches the quadriceps muscle. This is followed by contraction of the muscle. If the reflex irritability is high, the contraction is abrupt and strong and the amplitude of the movement is large (Fig 12–7).

The reflex is best tested with the patient seated in a chair with the feet resting on the floor. The examiner places one hand over the quadriceps femoris muscle in order to feel the contraction and with the other hand taps the patellar tendon, or ligamentum patellae, just below the patella. If the patient is lying in bed, the examiner should partially flex the knee by placing one hand beneath it; it is advisable to lift both knees and to have the heels resting lightly on the bed. Many examiners test the patellar reflex by having the patient sit on the edge of a table with the legs hanging over the edge in such a manner that the feet do not touch the floor or by having the patient sit with one leg crossed over the other and tapping the patellar tendon of the superior leg.

If the patellar reflex is exaggerated, there may be not only extension of the leg but also adduction of the thigh. Occasionally, both extensor response and adduction may be bilateral. The response may also be obtained, if the reflex is exaggerated, by stimulating the tendon of the quadriceps femoris muscle just above the patella; this is known as the suprapatellar or epipatellar reflex. The tendon can be tapped directly, or, with the patient recumbent, the examiner can place the index finger on the tendon and tap the finger or push down on the tendon. Contraction of the quadriceps muscle causes a brisk upward movement of the tendon, together with extension of the leg. Patellar clonus may be elicited in marked exaggeration of the patellar reflex. Absence of the patellar reflex is known as Westphal's sign; this has been described as one of the cardinal signs of tabes dorsalis. The patellar reflex is innervated by the femoral nerve (second through fourth lumbar segments).

ADDUCTOR (TIBIOADDUCTOR) REFLEX.—With the thigh in slight adduction, the medial epicondyle of the femur is tapped in the vicinity of the

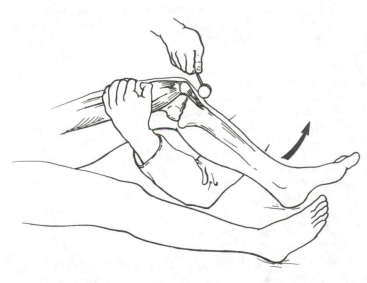

Fig 12–7.—Position to elicit the patella reflex in a supine position.

adductor tubercle, or the medial condyle of the tibia may be stimulated. The response is a contraction of the adductor muscles of the thigh with inward movement of the extremity. If the reflex is exaggerated, there may be crossed or bilateral adduction. The innervation of this reflex is through the obturator nerve (second through fourth lumbar segments). When the reflexes are exaggerated, an adductor response can also be elicited by tapping the spinous processes of the sacral or lumbar vertebrae while the patient is seated or by tapping the crest or superior spines of the ilium.

INTERNAL HAMSTRING (SEMITENDINOSUS AND SEMIMEMBRANOSUS, OR POSTERIOR TIBIOFEMORAL) REFLEX.—Stimulating the tendons of the semitendinosus and semimembranosus muscles just above their insertions on the posterior and medial surfaces and medial condyle of the tibia elicits the internal hamstring reflex. This is best done with the patient in the recumbent position, the leg abducted and partly externally rotated and the knee slightly flexed. The examiner's fingers are placed over the lower portions of the muscles and their tendons on the medial aspect of the leg just below the knee, and the fingers are tapped with the reflex hammer. The response is an increased flexion of the leg on the thigh, with slight internal rotation of the leg. This reflex is supplied through the tibial portion of the sciatic nerve (fourth lumbar through second sacral segments).

EXTERNAL HAMSTRING (BICEPS FEMORIS OR POSTERIOR PERONEOFEMORAL) REFLEX.—Elicited by stimulating the tendon of the biceps femoris muscle just above its insertion on the lateral side of the head of the fibula and the lateral condyle of the tibia, the external hamstring reflex is tested with the patient either recumbent or lying on the opposite side. With the patient's leg in moderate flexion at the knee, the examiner places the fingers over the tendon of the biceps femoris muscle on the lateral aspect of the leg just below the knee and taps the fingers. The response is a contraction of the muscle, resulting in flexion of the leg on the thigh and moderate external rotation of the leg. The reflex may also be elicited by tapping the head of the fibula; this is known as the fibular reflex. The nerve supply for the long head of the biceps is through the tibial portion of the sciatic nerve, but the short head of the biceps is supplied by the common peroneal portion of the sciatic nerve (fifth lumbar through second or third sacral segments).

TENSOR FASCIAE LATAE REFLEX.—The tensor fasciae latae reflex is tested by tapping over the tensor fasciae latae muscle at its origin near the anterosuperior iliac spine while the patient is in the recumbent position. The response consists of slight abduction of the thigh. The reflex is innervated by the superior gluteal nerve (fourth lumbar through first sacral segments).

GLUTEAL REFLEX.—Tapping the lower border of the sacrum or the posterior aspect of the ilium near the origin of the gluteus maximus muscle is followed by a contraction of this muscle with extension of the thigh. The reflex is best tested with the patient in a recumbent position but with his or her weight on the opposite side so that there is moderate flexion of the ipsilateral thigh. It may also be elicited with the patient in the prone position. The reflex is innervated by the inferior gluteal nerve (fourth lumbar through second sacral segments).

ACHILLES (TRICEPS SURAE) REFLEX.—Also called the ankle jerk, the Achilles reflex is obtained by tapping the Achilles tendon just above its insertion on the posterior surface of the calcaneus. Contraction of the posterior crural (gastrocnemius, soleus, and plantaris) muscles follows, with resulting plantar flexion of the foot at the ankle. If the patient is seated or is lying in bed, the thigh should be moderately abducted and rotated externally, the knee flexed, and the foot in moderate inversion; the examiner should place one hand under the foot to produce moderate dorsiflexion at the ankle. If the reflex is obtained with difficulty, the patient should press the foot against the examiner's hand in order to tense the tendon. If it cannot be elicited in this manner, the patient should kneel on a chair, preferably on a soft surface, with the feet projecting at right angles. The reflex may also be obtained while the patient is lying prone with the feet in moderate dorsiflexion (Fig 12–8).

If the Achilles tendon reflex is exaggerated, it may be elicited by tapping the sole of the foot, the medioplantar reflex, or by tapping the anterior aspect of the ankle, the paradoxic ankle reflex. In more marked exaggeration, spontaneous clonus may be obtained when the tendon is tapped, or it may be possible to elicit transient or sustained ankle clonus. The Achilles tendon reflex is innervated by the tibial nerve (first and second sacral segments, and possibly by the fifth lumbar segment).

Diminution or Absence of the Muscle-Stretch Reflexes

If there is hypoactivity of the reflexes, i.e., if the response is sluggish and/or the range of response is

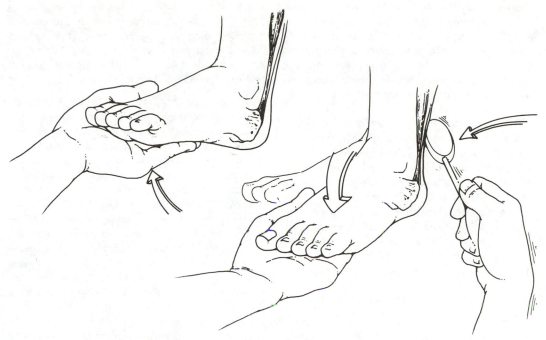

Fig 12–8.—Testing the achilles tendon reflex.

diminished, an increased intensity of the stimulus or repeated blows may be necessary to elicit them. A single stimulus may be subliminal. If muscle-stretch reflexes are not obtained, even with reinforcement, they are considered to be absent.

Diminution of the reflexes usually results from an interference with the conduction of the impulse through the reflex arc, and absence indicates a break in the reflex arc. Such changes may be associated with dysfunction of the receptor, afferent pathway, intercalcated neuron, motor unit, efferent pathway, or effector apparatus.

The muscle-stretch reflexes may also be either diminished or absent in various other conditions. Whereas they may be exaggerated in the early stages of coma, they are absent in deep coma, narcosis, deep sedation, and often in deep sleep. These reflexes are characteristically lost with nerve block, nerve root block, and caudal and spinal anesthesia. In asthenic states, hypothyroidism, and severe toxemias resulting from drug intoxication or infectious disease the muscle-stretch reflexes are diminished and often lost. They may be either diminished or lost in the presence of increased intracranial pressure, especially with posterior fossa tumors, or exhaustion following extreme exertion. They are also absent in spinal shock and in Adie's syndrome.

In paraplegia in flexion it may not be possible to obtain the muscle-stretch extensor reflexes because of spasm of the antagonist, or flexor muscles. In addition, the flexor reflexes are hyperactive.

The reflexes may appear to be absent in neurologic disorders in which there is marked spasticity with contractures and in diseases of the joints characterized by inflammation, contractures, and ankylosis. Here their absence is apparent rather than real, since motility of the joint is lacking or moving the joint causes pain.

Hyperactivity of the Muscle-Stretch Reflexes

Hyperactivity of the muscle-stretch reflexes is characterized by a decrease in the reflex threshold, increase in the speed of response (decrease in latent period), exaggeration of vigor and range of movement, prolongation of muscular contraction, and extension of the reflexogenic zone (zone of provocation). A minimal stimulus may evoke the reflex, and reflexes that are not normally obtained may be elicited with ease. There may be a wide zone of areas for effective stimulation in the neighboring bones and joints, and application of the stimulus to structures at some distance from the usual site may cause the response. The response may involve adjacent or even contralateral muscles, and the contraction of one muscle may be accompanied by contraction of others; e.g., extension of the leg may be accompanied by adduction of the thigh, or there may be bilateral extension of the legs. One stimulus may be followed by repeated contractions and relaxations, owing to repeated volleys of discharges, so clonus may be obtained. The muscle-stretch reflexes are exaggerated in association with an increase in the tone of the contracting muscles.[39]

The muscle-stretch reflexes are increased with lesions of the pyramidal system (in the accepted clinical sense of this term). They are normally under partial inhibition by higher centers, not only the pyramidal cortex but also extrapyramidal centers and suppressor areas in the brain stem reticular formation. When this inhibiting effect is removed, there is an overresponse and the reflexes are exaggerated.

The muscle-stretch reflexes are also exaggerated in the early stages of coma and anesthesia, as well as in tetany, tetanus, and strychnine poisoning. Cold and exercise may increase the reflex response, although extreme exercise may be followed by areflexia.

Superficial Reflexes

The superficial reflexes are those that are elicited in response to the application of a stimulus to either the skin or mucous membrane. These reflexes are not muscle-stretch reflexes but are skin-muscle responses. Inasmuch as the stimulus is a superficial one, they are sometimes known as exteroceptive reflexes, but probably the deep pressure, or proprioceptive, endings are also stimulated. These reflexes respond more slowly to the stimulus than do the muscle-stretch reflexes, their latent period is more prolonged, and they fatigue more easily.

SUPERFICIAL ABDOMINAL REFLEXES.—Gentle stroking of the skin of the abdomen or scratching it with a blunt object is followed by homolateral contraction of the abdominal muscles and retraction of deviation of the linea alba and umbilicus toward the area stimulated. This reflex should be tested with the patient recumbent and the abdominal wall thoroughly relaxed. The arms should be at the sides and the head down to avoid tension of the abdominal musculature. Sometimes the reflex is obtained most satisfactorily at the end of expiration. A blunt point such as a wooden applicator or a broken tongue blade is a satisfactory stimulus, although a pin may be used if applied lightly. If the object is too blunt there may be no response, and a painful stimulus may call forth a defense reaction. Too firm a stimulus may elicit the abdominal muscle reflex. The abdominal reflexes have been subdivided as follows (Fig 12–9):

1. Epigastric Reflex.—A stimulus directed from the tip of the sternum toward the umbilicus or from the breast or costal margin diagonally toward the umbilicus is followed by a contraction of the upper abdominal muscles with a dimpling and draw-

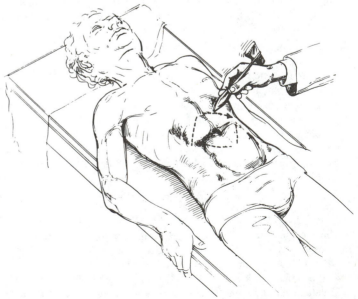

Fig 12–9.—Testing the superficial abdominal reflexes. (From Hoppenfield S.: *Physical Examination of the Spine and Extremities.* New York, Appleton-Century-Crofts, 1976. Reproduced by permission.)

ing in of these muscles. Usually there is no retraction of the umbilicus. This reflex is innervated by the intercostal nerves from the fifth through the seventh thoracic segments.

2. Upper Abdominal or Supraumbilical Reflex.—The upper abdominal reflex is elicited by stimulating the skin of the upper abdominal quadrants, usually in a diagnonal fashion downward and outward from the tip of the sternum or in a horizontal fashion starting externally and going medially. There is a contraction of the abdominal musculature and a diagonal deviation of the umbilicus upward and outward toward the side of the stimulus. This reflex is innervated by the intercostal nerves from the seventh through the ninth thoracic segments.

3. Middle Abdominal or Umbilical Reflex.—Stimulation of the skin of the abdomen at the level of the umbilicus either by a horizontal stimulus, starting externally and proceeding medially, or by a vertical stimulus along the lateral abdominal wall at the level of the umbilicus is followed by a lateral deviation of the linea alba and umbilicus. This reflex is innervated by the intercostal nerves from the ninth through the eleventh thoracic segments.

4. Lower Abdominal, Infraumbilical, or Suprapubic Reflex.—The lower abdominal reflex is elicited by stimulating the skin of the lower abdominal quadrants either diagonally in an upward and outward direction from the region of the symphysis pubis or horizontally, starting externally and proceeding medially. The abdominal muscles contract and the umbilicus deviates diagonally toward the site of stimulation. This reflex is innervated by the lower intercostal, iliohypogastric, and ilioinguinal nerves (eleventh and twelfth thoracic and upper lumbar segments). Bechterew's hypogastric reflex consists of a contraction of the lower abdominal muscles in response to stroking the skin on the inner surface of the homolateral thigh.

The superficial abdominal reflexes may be difficult to obtain or evaluate in ticklish individuals. They may be absent in acute abdominal conditions (Rosenbach's sign), obesity, abdominal distention, or bladder distention. It may be impossible to obtain them in individuals with relaxed abdominal walls, such as elderly people and women who have borne children. These reflexes may be absent on one side due to the presence of an old abdominal incision. Their absence is not significant under these circumstances, but their absence in young individuals, especially in muscular men, is definitely pathologic.

If there is diminution of the reflex response, the reflex may fatigue easily: it may be elicited once or twice and then disappear. If the reflex is diminished or absent, the lower abdominal reflex is usually affected first. In unilateral abdominal paralysis the abdominal reflexes may be inverted, with deviation of the umbilicus to the opposite side.

Cremasteric reflex.—Stroking the skin on the upper, inner aspect of the thigh, from above downward, with a blunt point, or pricking or pinching the skin in this area elicits the cremasteric reflex. The response consists of a contraction of the cremasteric muscle, with homolateral elevation of the testicle. The reflex may be absent in elderly males, in individuals who have a hydrocele or varicocele, and in those who have had orchitis or epididymitis. The innervation is through the first and second lumbar segments (ilioinguinal and genitofemoral nerves). This reflex is not to be confused with the scrotal reflex, a visceral reflex that is characterized by a slow, vermicular contraction of the dartos muscle on applying a cold object to the scrotum or on stroking the perineum (Fig 12–10).

Plantar reflex.—Stroking the plantar surface of the foot from the heel forward is normally followed by plantar flexion of the toes. This reflex is innervated by the tibial nerve (fourth lumbar through first or second sacral segments). This flex-

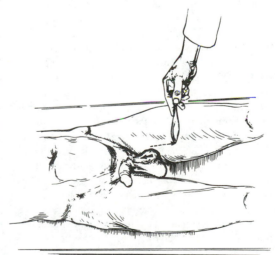

Fig 12–10.—The cremasteric reflex. (From Hoppenfield S.: *Physical Examination of the Spine and Extremities.* New York, Appleton-Century-Crofts, 1976. Reproduced by permission.)

ion response is the normal one after the first 12–18 months of life, but, like the palmar reflex, it is more significant in its pathologic variation—the Babinski sign.[40, 41] The normal response may be difficult to obtain in individuals with plantar callosities, and in ticklish persons there may be a voluntary withdrawal with flexion of the hip and knee. In every normal individual there is a certain amount of plantar flexion of the toes on stimulation of the sole of the foot. If the short flexors of the toes are paralyzed, there may be an extensor response.

SUPERFICIAL ANAL REFLEX.—The cutaneous (superficial) anal reflex consists of a contraction of the external sphincter in response to stroking or pricking the skin or mucous membrane in the perianal region. This reflex is innervated by the inferior hemorrhoidal nerve (second through fourth or fifth sacral segments).

Diminution or Absence of the Superficial Reflexes

The superficial reflexes, like the muscle-stretch reflexes, are either diminished or absent when the continuity of the reflex arc—afferent nerve, motor center, efferent nerve—is disturbed. The superficial reflexes, especially the abdominal and cremasteric reflexes, have a special significance, however, if their absence is associated with an exaggeration of the muscle-stretch reflexes (dissociation of reflexes) or if they are absent when there are signs of pyramidal tract involvement.[42–44] In addition to a spinal reflex arc, the superficial reflexes have a superimposed cortical pathway. Impulses ascend to the parietal areas of the brain, where they connect with the motor centers in the pyramidal or the premotor areas. Efferent impulses then descend either in the pyramidal pathways or in intimate association with them. As a consequence, an interruption of the reflex arc at a higher level or a lesion anywhere along the pyramidal pathway usually causes either diminution or absence of the superficial reflexes. The change is on the side of the body contralateral to the lesion if the lesion is above the pyramidal decussation, homolateral if below.

The abdominal reflexes are absent in deep sleep, surgical anesthesia, and coma, as well as in the presence of violent emotions such as fear. Absent in the newborn, they appear after about 6–12 months, at about the time the plantar response begins to assume the normal pattern. Apparent abdominal reflexes, which are elicited in about one third of the infants examined, differ from the normal adult response in that the reaction is diffuse and is often associated with movements of the legs. It must always be borne in mind that both the abdominal and the cremasteric reflexes may be absent in physiologic states not resulting from nervous system disease.

HOFFMANN AND TROMNER SIGNS AND FLEXOR REFLEXES OF THE FINGERS AND HAND.—To elicit the Hoffmann sign, the examiner supports the patient's hand, dorsiflexed at the wrist, so that it is completely relaxed and the fingers are partially flexed. The middle finger is partially extended and either its middle or distal phalanx is grasped firmly between the examiner's index and middle fingers. With a sharp flick of the thumb, the examiner nips or snaps the nail of the patient's middle finger, causing a forcible increased flexion of this finger followed by sudden release. If the Hoffmann sign is present, this is followed by flexion and adduction of the thumb and flexion of the index finger, and sometimes flexion of the other fingers as well. The sign is said to be incomplete if only the thumb or only the index finger responds.

Responses in the Lower Extremities

RESPONSES CHARACTERIZED BY DORSIFLEXION OF THE TOES.—In the normal individual stimulation of the plantar surface of the foot is followed by plantar flexion of the toes, the small toes flexing more than the great toe. The response is usually a fairly rapid one. This is the normal plantar reflex, and superficial reflex innervated by the fourth lumbar through the first or second sacral segments of the spinal cord by means of the tibial nerve (Fig 12–11, A and B).

In disease of the pyramidal system there is an inversion of the normal reflex, the Babinski sign, consisting of dorsiflexion of the toes, especially of the great toe, together with a separation or fanning of the toes. The two essential manifestations were described separately by Babinski as the *phenomene des orteils* (the dorsiflexion of the toes) and the *signe de l'éventail* (the fanning). In addition, especially if the response is marked, there is dorsiflexion at the ankle, with flexion at the knee and hip, and possibly slight abduction of the thigh. These associated movements are brought about by contraction of the anterior tibial, hamstring, tensor fasciae latae, and related muscles. They are a part of the spinal defense reflex mechanism. The contraction of the

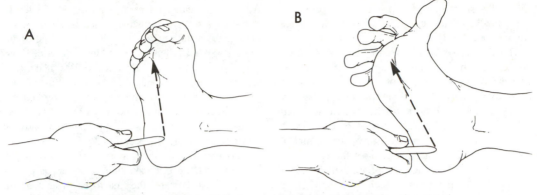

Fig 12–11.—a, Babinski test—normal. **b,** Babinski test—abnormal.

tensor fasciae latae is often referred to as Brissaud's reflex. The dorsiflexion of the toes may be the only visible effect, but the contraction of the thigh and leg muscles is always present and can be detected by palpation.[45–47]

The Babinski sign is elicited by stimulating the plantar surface of foot with a blunt point, preferably a matchstick, a toothpick, a wooden applicator, or a broken tongue blade. Some examiners prefer to use the thumbnail or a pin. The stimulus is directed from the heel toward the ball of the foot and toes and is stopped at the metatarsophalangeal joints. It should be a threshold stimulus, as light as possible. Tickling, which may cause voluntary withdrawal, and pain, which may bring about a reversal to flexion as a nociceptive response, should be avoided. Both the inner and the outer aspects of the sole of the foot should be stimulated. If the response is difficult to obtain, it may be elicited more easily by stimulating the lateral aspect of the sole. The stimulus may also be applied along the metatarsal pad from the little to the great toe. The sign is obtained with less difficulty if the patient is in the recumbent position with the hips and knees in extension and the heels resting on the bed; however, it may be obtained if the patient is seated with the hips flexed, the knee moderately extended, and the patient's foot held either in the examiner's hand or on the examiner's knee. The response may sometimes be reinforced by rotating the patient's head to the opposite side. It may be inhibited when the foot is cold and increased when the foot is warm. It may be abolished by flexion of the knee, and in 50% of cases it is abolished by placing an Esmarch bandage around the leg.

The characteristic response is one of slow, tonic dorsiflexion of the great toe and the small toes with fanning, or separation, of the toes. The phenomenon may show itself in formes frustes, which are also significant. For instance, there may be no response whatever to plantar stimulation, or either dorsiflexion or fanning may occur separately. There may be flexion of the hip with no movement of the toes. If there is paralysis of the dorsiflexors, there may be no Babinski sign even though one is expected. These variations and incomplete responses are sometimes referred to as equivocal Babinski signs. They are all significant, and the examiner should describe the response rather than make an arbitrary statement that the Babinski sign is either present or absent.[6, 48–50]

The response to plantar stimulation may be difficult to evaluate, especially if the plantar surface of the foot is overly sensitive. In individuals with plantar hyperesthesia, frequently encountered in the peripheral neuritides, there may be reflex withdrawal that interferes with the response. Under such circumstances, it may be necessary to hold the foot at the ankle.

When the reflex is pronounced, there may be either contralateral or bilateral responses, with an increase in the reflexogenic zone so that the phenomenon may be obtained by stimulation of other than the usual sites. Occasionally, in the presence of extensive disease, there may be a spontaneous Babinski sign or manipulation of the foot or leg, or the toes may be held in a constant dorsiflexion and fanning position.

False responses, or pseudo-Babinski signs, may occur in the absence of pyramidal tract disease. The voluntary withdrawal in overly sensitive individuals, the responses in plantar hyperesthesia, and the reactions from too strong a stimulus may give the appearance of a Babinski sign. In athetosis and chorea there may be a false response due to the hyperkinesia. If the short flexors of the toes are paralyzed, there may be apparent dorsiflexion following plantar stimulation.

The Babinski sign has been called the most important sign in clinical neurology. If definitely present, it is always evidence of organic disease. The dorsiflexion reaction is the normal one in the newborn, and the response to plantar stimulation gradually assumes its normal form at 6 to 18 or 24 months of age. The development of the normal response probably coincides, as does the appearance of the abdominal reflexes, with the myelinization of the pyramidal pathways, which is incomplete at birth.

The Babinski sign may also be obtained in states of unconsciousness. It is sometimes present in profound sleep, deep anesthesia, profound narcosis, drug and alcohol intoxication, insulin and hypoglycemic shock, the postconvulsive state of epilepsy, coma due to hyperglycemia and uremia, posttraumatic states, and other conditions in which there is complete loss of consciousness. The Babinski sign may be obtained in normal individuals following injection of scopolamine in sufficiently large doses, and a latent Babinski phenomenon may be brought out following the injection of a smaller amount. The injection of physostigmine in physiologic doses may abolish a Babinski response, and a unilateral response is sometimes abolished by simultaneous bilateral stimulation.

There are many other pyramidal tract responses in the lower extremities that are characterized by dorsiflexion of the toes. In fact, there are so many modifications that they cannot all be listed. Some merely indicate an increase in the reflexogenic zone; others, however, are important because they can be elicited in patients in whom, for some reason, the plantar surface of the foot cannot be stimulated. The important modifications include the Oppenheim sign, which is elicited by applying heavy pressure with the thumb and index finger to the anterior surface of the tibia, mainly on its medial aspect, and stroking down from the infrapatellar region to the ankle; the response is a slow one and usually occurs toward the end of stimulation. The Gordon sign is obtained by squeezing or applying deep pressure to the calf muscles. The Schaefer sign is produced by deep pressure on the Achilles tendon. The Chaddock sign is elicited by stimulating the lateral aspect of the foot with a blunt point; the stimulation is applied under and around the external malleolus in a circular direction. In recent years, Gonda[51] and Allen[52] have independently described a sign that is elicited by forceful downward stretching or snapping of the distal phalanx of either the second or the fourth toe, and Allen and Cleckley[53] described one that is produced by a sharp upward flick of the second toe or by pressure applied to the ball of the toe. The examiner may flex the toe slowly, press on the nail, and twist the toe and hold it for a few seconds. These responses cannot be elicited as frequently as the Babinski sign, but occasionally it is possible to elicit one or more of them when the Babinski cannot be obtained. The Babinski sign, however, is probably the most delicate, the first to be evident in the presence of disease, and the one that occurs most frequently. The Chaddock sign is next in frequency. It may be worth trying two maneuvers simultaneously, such as the one described by Babinski and that described by Oppenheim, to bring out a latent dorsiflexion response.

RESPONSES CHARACTERIZED BY PLANTAR FLEXION OF THE TOES.—In the newborn infant there is a grasp reflex in the foot as well as in the hand, and tonic flexion and adduction of the toes may occur in response to a light pressure on the plantar surface of the foot, especially its distal portion. Normally, this disappears by the end of the first year, but it may persist with abnormalities of development or reappear with disease of the opposite frontal lobe.

In addition to the superficial plantar reflex, there is a plantar muscle reflex that consists of flexion of the toes in response to sudden stretching. This is barely, if at all, perceptible in normal persons but is present with reflex hyperactivity and, therefore, with pyramidal tract lesions.

There are several manifestations or exaggerations of the plantar muscle reflex. The Rossolimo sign is elicited by tapping the ball of the foot, percussing the plantar surface of the great toe, tapping or stroking the balls of the toes, or giving a quick, lifting snap to the tips of the toes. The test should be carried out while the patient is lying in the recumbent position with the leg extended. The Mendel-Bechterew or dorsocuboidal sign is elicited by tapping or stroking the outer aspect of the dorsum of the foot in the region of the cuboid bone, or over the fourth and fifth metatarsals. This is also known as the tarsophalangeal reflex. Following both of these maneuvers there is only slight dorsiflexion of the toes or no movement whatever in the normal individual. In the presence of pyramidal tract disease, however, there is a quick plantar flexion of the toes, especially of the smaller ones.

Plantar flexion of the toes may be elicited occasionally by application of the stimulus to other portions of the foot or ankle. Bechterew found that percussion of the middle of the sole or of the heel was followed by a plantar flexion response. In the medioplantar reflex of Guillain and Barré and the heel reflex of Weingrow there is plantar flexion with fanning of the toes when the midplantar region of the foot or the base of the heel is tapped. The antagonistic anterior tibial reflex of Piotrowski is characterized by plantar flexion of the ankle and sometimes of the toes when the belly of the anterior tibial muscle is tapped. Tapping the anterior aspect of the ankle joint produces the paradoxic ankle reflex, consisting of plantar flexion of the foot. Some of these responses correspond to accessory methods of eliciting the Achilles tendon reflex and may indicate a spread of the reflexogenic zone. Although they are found in pyramidal tract lesions, their presence may indicate merely a functional hyperirritability of the reflexes. These reflexes probably have less diagnostic value than the Rossolimo and Mendel-Bechterew signs.

Reflexes of Spinal Automatism

Like the pyramidal tract signs, the spinal defense reflexes, or the reflexes of spinal automatism, become manifest when the inhibiting action of the higher centers has been removed. These reflexes, while present only in pathologic states in human beings and higher animals, are phylogenetically and ontogenetically related to responses seen in lower forms. They are clinical homologues of reflexes seen in "spinal" and decerebrate animals.

FLEXION SPINAL DEFENSE REFLEX.—In a manner of speaking, the flexion spinal defense reflex (Babinski), also known as the pathologic shortening reflex, the reflex of spinal automatism (Marie), reflex flexor synergy, the withdrawal reflex, and the *réflexe* or *phenomene des raccourcisseurs,* is an exaggeration of the Babinski sign. If the Babinski sign is marked, there is a spread of the reflexogenic zone so that the response may be obtained not only by stimulation of the plantar surface of the foot but also by stimulation of the dorsum of the foot and the anterior surface of the tibia, or by a painful stimulus to any part of the foot, toes, or leg. Also, if the

response is marked and is due to a spinal lesion that is transverse or partially transverse, it is obtained not only on the side stimulated but also on the contralateral side.

With lesions of the spinal cord, especially if they are transverse or nearly transverse, stimulation below the level of the lesion calls forth the flexion spinal defense reflex, with flexion at the hip and knee, dorsiflexion at the ankle, and usually dorsiflexion of the great toe and dorsiflexion and fanning of the small toes. If the response is a bilateral one, there is also a crossed flexor reflex. It may be evoked by any type of stimulus, but it is most frequently produced by a painful or nociceptive stimulus. Pricking, scratching, or pinching the skin on the dorsal aspect of the foot or ankle, hot or cold stimuli, deep pressure, squeezing the toes, or extreme flexion of the toes or foot (Marie-Foix sign) may initiate the response. At times it may be brought on by moving the foot, testing the reflexes, touching the skin lightly, or even by the weight of bedclothes. It may be elicited by stimulation of either cutaneous or proprioceptive endings, or by stimuli from the viscera (e.g., distention of the bladder) at any site below the level of the lesion. The upper border of the reflexogenic zone usually corresponds to the lower limit of the spinal lesion and thus may be important in localization. Sometimes a more painful stimulus is needed to elicit the response near the level of the lesion than to elicit it farther down. It is important to bear in mind, however, that a painful stimulus above the level of the lesion may cause voluntary movements of the upper part of the body, which may be followed by a reflex response of the lower portion; this may constitute a false withdrawal reflex.

Various modifications of the flexion spinal defense reflex may be obtained. The most important of these are described below.

RIDDOCH'S MASS REFLEX.—The flexion spinal defense reflex may be accompanied in certain instances by muscular contractions of the abdominal wall, by dorsiflexion of the toes and feet, by flexion of the knees and hips, by evacuation of the bladder and bowels, and by sweating, reflex erythema, and pilomotor responses below the level of the lesion. Seen in relatively complete transverse spinal lesions after the period of spinal shock has passed, it is an indication of grave spinal injury. The reflexogenic zone may be extended to the bladder, and the entire reflex complex may be precipitated by distention of the bladder. Priapism and even ejaculation may be a part of the response. The mass reflex may at times be utilized in therapy in the reductation of bladder function.[54]

CROSSED EXTENSOR REFLEX.—Stimulation of the foot or leg on one side may cause flexion of that extremity with an extension response in the other leg. This is the crossed extensor reflex, or *phenomene d'allongement croise,* sometimes known as Philippson's reflex. It is indicative of a partial or incomplete spinal lesion.

Paraplegia in Flexion

In certain cases of transverse involvement of the spinal cord, the frequently repeated and easily elicited flexion defense reflexes result in involuntary flexor spasms which occur with increasing frequency. The process terminates eventually in a fixed flexion reflex, with a permanent state of flexion of the hips and knees and dorsiflexion of the ankles and toes. The exaggeration of the flexion reflex holds the limbs in a position of flexion for longer and longer intervals until they can no longer be actively or even passively extended. The legs may be completely flexed so that the knees press firmly against the abdominal wall. This is known as paraplegia in flexion. The slightest stimulus, even the weight of clothes or bedclothes or the sudden uncovering of the legs, may elicit the flexion response until finally a permanent flexion occurs. Even after the development of a fixed flexion reflex, any additional stimulus may aggravate the degree of flexion. Secondary contractures may develop at the joints. Such flexion indicates a relatively complete spinal lesion with interruption of all descending impulses, extrapyramidal (vestibulospinal) as well as pyramidal.

This flexion position of the lower extremities is in contradistinction to the extension position that occurs with pyramidal lesions in the cerebrum or the corticospinal pathway above its decussation. In these lesions, while the upper extremity is usually in a position of flexion, the lower extremity is more likely to be in a position of extension, with more marked paralysis of the flexor muscles.

Paraplegia in Extension

Paraplegia with extensor rigidity usually results from supraspinal lesions or from incomplete spinal lesions. There is increased tone of both extensor and flexor muscles, but the spasticity predominates in the extensors. Hyperactivity of the extensor reflexes (patellar and Achilles muscle-stretch reflexes) results, and clonus may be obtained. There is tonic extensor spasm of the lower limbs, with the legs in adduction and slight internal rotation. This syndrome probably is the result of predominant involvement of the pyramidal pathways without associated dysfunction of the extrapyramidal efferent tracts. Nevertheless, it has been observed in patients with complete transverse myelitis.

Miscellaneous Neurologic Signs

Miscellaneous neurologic signs, some of them reflexes, some closely related to defense and postural reflex mechanisms, and others more varied in nature, are elicited in certain diseases of the nervous system.

SIGNS OF MENINGEAL IRRITATION.—Signs of irritation of the meninges are most frequently elicited in association with inflammatory involvement of the meningeal tissues. However, they may also be present secondary to the presence of foreign material in the subarachnoid space, as in the case of a subarachnoid hemorrhage, or they may be associated with increased CSF pressure, as in aseptic meningitis and meningism.[55]

Nuchal (cervical) rigidity.—Nuchal rigidity is probably the most widely recognized and frequently encountered sign of meningeal irritation, and the diagnosis of meningitis is rarely made in its absence. It is characterized by stiffness of the neck and resistance to passive movement, with pain and spasm on attempts at motion. There is resistance to passive flexion, and the chin cannot be placed on the chest; there may be resistance to hyperextension and to rotatory movements as well. The rigidity may vary from slight resistance to flexion to complete resistance to all movements. It particularly affects the extensor musculature (Fig 12–12).

Kernig's Sign.—With the patient recumbent, the examiner flexes the patient's thigh to a right angle and then attempts to extend the leg on the thigh.[56] This passive extension at the knee is accompanied not only by pain and resistance, due to spasm of the hamstring muscles, but also by limitation of extension. Full extension of the leg is impossible if the hip is in flexion. According to some

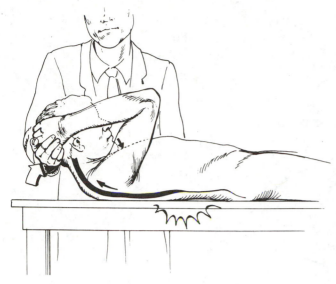

Fig 12–12.—The test for meningeal irritation. There is resistance to passive flexion and the chin cannot be placed on the chest. Pain is produced in the back. (From Hoppenfield S.: *Physical Examination of the Spine and Extremities.* New York, Appleton-Century-Crofts, 1976. Reproduced by permission.)

definitions, Kernig's sign is positive if the leg cannot be extended on the knee to over 135° while the thigh is in flexion. To elicit Lasègue's sign, which is similar, attempts are made to flex the thigh at the hip while the leg is held in extension. This, when positive, is also accompanied by pain in the sciatic notch and resistance to movement. Both Kernig's and Lasègue's signs are positive in meningitis, probably due to stretching of and tension on the irritated nerve roots and meninges, but both are also positive in sciatica and in irritation of the lumbosacral nerve roots or plexus due to a ruptured intervertebral disk or other causes. In the latter conditions, however, they are usually unilateral, while in meningitis they are bilateral.[56]

Lasègue's Sign.—Flexion of the thigh at the hip while the leg is extended at the knee causes stretching of the sciatic nerve. This is the Lasègue maneuver, often called the straight-leg-raising test. Such stretching may be done as an active process if the patient bends forward while the legs are extended at the knees. As a dianostic neurologic test it is done by passively flexing the hip of the supine patient while holding the leg in extension at the knee. The patient does not experience radiating pain when this maneuver is carried out if there is disease of the hip joint, but with either disease or irritation of the sciatic nerve, or of the nerve roots that enter into it, there is pain in the sciatic nerve. This is the positive Lasègue sign. The procedure is similar to that used in eliciting the Kernig sign, in which the thigh is

flexed at the hip and then an attempt made to extend the leg at the knee. Both, when positive, indicate irritation of the meninges or of the lower lumbosacral nerve roots (Fig 12–13).

The examiner should note both the angle of flexion of the hip at which pain occurs and the amount and site of the pain experienced by the patient. The pain may be felt as a tight sensation or as actual pain in the lumbar or sacral region, gluteal region, posterior aspect of the thigh, or the popliteal space, or sometimes in the opposite limb. The test is most positive if the maneuver reproduces the patient's subjective pain. Pain produced by flexion of less than 40° is indicative of movement of an affected nerve root against a protruded disk; if pain does not occur until flexion has been carried to 70°–80°, it may be assumed that there is an abnormally sensitive nerve root but not necessarily a demonstrable lesion of the root or protruded disk. Evidence of sciatic nerve or nerve root irritation can also be elicited by conducting the examination while the patient is seated with the thighs at a right angle to the hips. The leg is then passively extended at the knee until pain is produced. It is generally believed, however, that the supine position is preferable to the seated position for carrying out these maneuvers.

To test for the buckling sign the straight-leg test is carried out as described, i.e., by passively flexing the hip while the knee is extended until the knee begins to flex or buckle.

Various modifications of the Lasègue test give additional information. The pain may be more se-

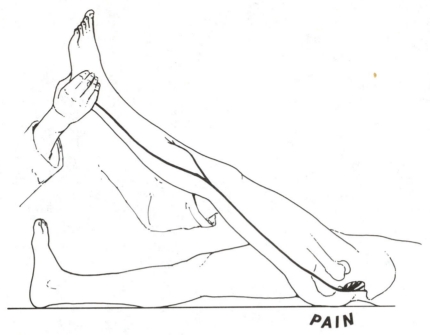

PAIN

Fig 12–13.—Straight leg raising test (Lasègue's sign).

vere, or elicited sooner, if the test is carried out with the thigh and leg in a position of adduction and internal rotation (Bonnet's sign). Dorsiflexion of the foot (Bragard's sign) or of the great toe (Sicard's sign) while the examination is being performed increases stretching of the tibial portion of the sciatic nerve and aggravates the pain. The examiner may flex the patient's hip until the first manifestations of pain are noted and then flex either the toe or foot. Sometimes the pain is brought on while the patient is supine, with the thighs and legs extended, merely by dorsiflexion of the foot or great toe. This aggravation of pain by passive dorsiflexion of the foot is sometimes called Gower's sign (Fig 12–14). All the modifications of the Lasègue maneuver in which either the foot or the great toe is dorsiflexed may be called nerve stretching tests; the term Spurling's sign is also used.

In some patients with low back pain with lumbosacral radiation, flexion of the nonpainful thigh while the knee is extended causes an exacerbation of pain on the affected side. This has been called the crossed straight-leg-raising test, and some observers believe it is pathognomonic of disk herniation.

Trousseau's Sign.—Compression of the arm by squeezing or constricting it with the hand or by means of a tourniquet or sphygmomanometer cuff is followed by paresthesias of the fingers and then of the hand and forearm, then by twitching of the fingers, and finally by cramping and contraction of the muscles of the fingers and hand with the thumb strongly adducted and the fingers stiffened and slightly flexed at the metacarpophalangeal joints and clustered about the thumb—the so-called accoucheur's hand. There may be a latent period of 0.5–4 minutes. Similar pressure around the leg of thigh may be followed by spasm of the foot and toe muscles. A modification of this is carried out in the von Bonsdorff technique in which a pneumatic cuff is placed over the arm and is kept moderately inflated for about 10 minutes. It is then removed and the patient is told to hyperventilate. Typical tetanic spasm occurs much earlier in the previously ischemic arm than in the other arm.

Nerve Pressure Signs.—Tension on the sciatic nerve is increased when the tibial nerve is pressed in the popliteal space. The Lasègue maneuver is carried out to the angle where pain is first noted, and then the knee is flexed about 20°. Following this the hip is further flexed to a degree just short of that causing pain, and firm pressure is applied in the popliteal space over the tibial nerve. When the test is positive, this causes sharp pain in the lumbar re-

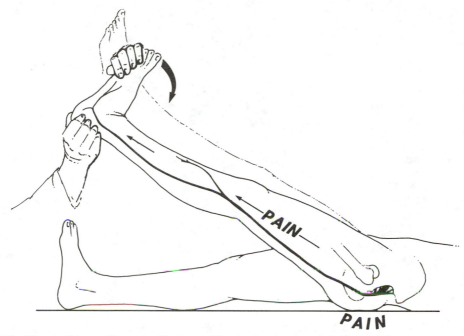

Fig 12–14.—In this position, dorsiflexion of the foot causes pain in the sciatic nerve distribution (Gower's sign).

gion, affected buttock, or along the course of the sciatic nerve. This test may also be carried out with the patient seated on a table. The affected leg is extended passively at the knee to the point at which pain is reproduced. It is then flexed slightly, and pressure is applied in the popliteal space, which in cases of sciatic nerve or nerve root irritation causes pain.

O'Connell's Test.—In this test, the Lasègue maneuver is first carried out on the sound limb, and the angle of flexion and site of pain are recorded; the pain may be on the opposite side (Fajersztajn's sign). Then the test is carried out on the affected limb, and the angle and site of pain are again noted. Then both thighs are flexed simultaneously while extension is maintained at the knee. The angle of flexion permitted when the thighs are flexed simultaneously may be greater than that allowed when the affected limb is flexed alone or when either is flexed separately. Finally, once both thighs have been flexed to an angle just short of that which produces pain, the sound limb is lowered to the bed; this may result in a marked exacerbation of pain, sometimes associated with paresthesias.

Reverse Straight-Leg-Raising Test.—With the patient lying prone, the knee is flexed to its maxi-

mum. The normal individual should complain of quadriceps tightness. With disk disease there is pain in the back or in the sciatic nerve distribution on the side of the lesion.

Viets and Naffziger Tests.—Increase of the intracranial or intraspinal pressure exaggerates radicular pain in patients with space-occupying lesions pressing on the nerve roots. The pressure may be increased temporarily by coughing, sneezing, and straining, and by digital compression of the jugular veins. Pressure should be maintained until the patient complains of a feeling of fullness in the head, and the test should not be considered negative until venous return has been impeded for at least 2 minutes. Jugular compression can also be carried out with a sphygmomanometer cuff, maintaining a pressure of 40 mm Hg for 10 minutes (Naffziger test) (Fig 12–15). The patient may be in either the recumbent or upright position. In a patient with a ruptured intervertebral disk there is radicular pain in the distribution of the affected nerve roots following jugular compression. The pain is similar to that which follows coughing and straining, and the Viets and Naffziger tests are rarely positive in patients whose pain is not aggravated by coughing and straining. Occasionally the pain may be noticed on

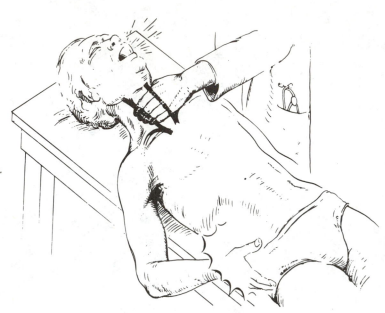

Fig 12–15.—The Naffziger test increases intrathecal pressure. (From Hoppenfield S.: *Physical Examination of the Spine and Extremities.* New York, Appleton-Century-Crofts, 1976. Reproduced by permission.)

the release of the pressure. A similar aggravation of the pain may sometimes be brought about merely by having the patient perform the Valsalva maneuver.

Patrick's Sign.—Patrick's sign consists of pain in the hip when the heel or the external malleolus of the painful extremity is placed on the opposite knee and the thigh is pressed downward. The pain thus occurs on simultaneous flexion, abduction, external rotation, and extension of the involved hip. It may be noted that the knee on the affected side is kept elevated when the maneuver is carried out and cannot be pressed toward the bed. Patrick's sign is positive in hip joint disease but is usually absent in sciatic nerve involvement (Fig 12–16).

Ely's Sign.—Ely's sign is probably indicative of contracture of the fascia lata. With the patient prone on the examining table, the examiner flexes the leg on the thigh, bringing the heel toward the buttock. In a positive test, the pelvis rises from the table during such flexion and the thigh is abducted.

Autonomic Nervous System

The examination of the autonomic nervous system yields important information in neurologic disease. Certain of the procedures used are routine ones and should be carried out in every neurologic appraisal, but others are special tests used only under certain circumstances.[57, 58]

General Observation of the Patient

The following are the aspects of the physical examination to which special emphasis should be given.

ENDOCRINE STATUS.—Evidence of endocrine imbalance, such as dwarfism, gigantism, acromegaly, cretinism, and other signs of dysfunction of the pituitary, pineal, thyroid, adrenal, and sexual glands may be related to disease of the autonomic nervous system. The degree of physical development, including sexual maturity and evidence of senescence, is also important.

REGULATION OF VITAL PROCESSES.—The body temperature, as well as the temperature of the extremities and of isolated portions of the body, should be noted. Blood pressure should be taken in both arms with the patient recumbent, seated, and standing; the pulse rate and regularity, as well as the respiratory rate and rhythm, should be noted. Either vertigo or faintness with changes of position may be significant.

SKIN AND MUCOUS MEMBRANES.—Important evidence of autonomic dysfunction may be found in the skin and mucous membranes. There may be changes in color, such as pallor, erythema, flushing, or cyanosis. Color changes with alteration of position may be valuable diagnostic criteria. Variations in texture, consistency, and appearance of the skin

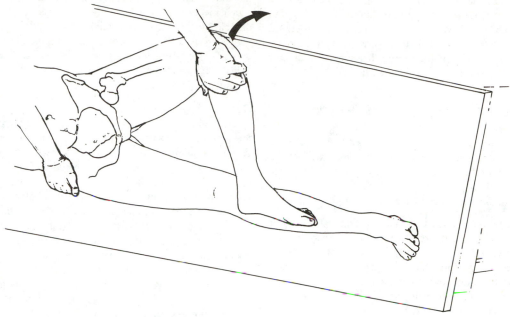

Fig 12–16.—The Patrick or Fabere test.

that are diagnostically significant include glossiness, hardness, thickening, wasting, scaling, seborrhea, looseness or tightness, oiliness, and moisture or dryness. Urticaria, generalized or localized edema, angioneuritic edema, hemiedema, trophedema, myxedema, dermographia, herpetic lesions, vesicles, bullae, perforating ulcers, and decubiti should be noted.

PERSPIRATION.—Disease of the autonomic nervous system may be characterized by any of the following: excessive perspiration, decreased perspiration, anhidrosis, and localized changes in sweating.

HAIR AND NAILS.—Hypertrichosis, hypotrichosis, abnormal distribution of hair, localized loss of hair (alopecia), abnormal brittleness, color change, and localized or premature graying of the hair may be significant. Important abnormalities of the nails include brittleness, striations, fissuring, and cyanosis.

EXTREMITIES.—The examiner should note the development, color, and temperature of the extremities as a whole, the character and pulsation of the arteries, and the influence of changes in position.

SALIVATION AND LACRIMATION.—The secretory responses of the salivary and lacrimal glands to physical and psychic stimulation may give information about autonomic nervous system dysfunction.

FAT METABOLISM.—Conditions such as obesity, wasting, lipodystrophy, and adiposis dolorosa are seen in autonomic dysfunction. The localization of wasting and the bodily distribution of the adipose tissue should be noted.

BONES AND JOINTS.—Changes in bone structure and arthropathies of various types may result from diseases of the autonomic nervous system.

EVIDENCE OF LOCALIZED INVOLVEMENT.—The presence of specific and focal changes, such as Horner's syndrome, gives evidence of focal alteration in the autonomic nervous system.

Autonomic Nervous System Reflexes

Many reflexes that are important to the neurologic examination are essentially responses of the autonomic nervous system. Some of these may be classified as mucous membrane and orificial reflexes, others as true visceral reflexes. Because all are smooth muscle and glandular responses, the reaction is a slower one than that which takes place in striated muscle reflexes. In many instances, however, the smooth muscle response is accompanied by contraction of striated muscle.

The autonomic nervous system reflexes that involve the cranial nerves, e.g., the lacrimal, salivary, sneeze, sucking, cough, vomiting, and carotid sinus reflexes, were included in the discussions of the individual nerves. Pupillary reflexes are discussed elsewhere in this volume. There are other reflexes, largely of autonomic origin, that should be elicited in the neurologic examination, however.

Special Tests of Autonomic Function

In addition to the general observation of the patient and the elicitation of the autonomic nervous system reflexes, there are many special tests and examinations that may be important in evaluating the autonomic nervous system.

SWEATING TEST.—The sweating test is easy to carry out, and the results may be observed over the surface of the entire body. The chronologic appearance of perspiration and quantitative differences may be noted, and photographs may be made at any stage of sweat development.[59, 60] Various methods of color determinations of sweating are available. Cobalt blue papers that turn pink when moist can be laid over the areas to be tested; iodine in oil can be painted on the skin and the painted areas dusted with a starch powder that turns a bluish black in the presence of iodine and moisture; the skin can be painted with a solution of ferric chloride and then dusted with tannic acid powder that turns black in the presence of iron and moisture. A more convenient method consists of dusting the skin with 1,4-dihydroxyanthraquinone 2,6-disulfonic acid [Quinizarin Compound (Burroughs Wellcome)]; this is a grayish violet when dry but becomes a deep purple when moistened. The moisture on the skin may also be evaluated by palpation or measured with a hygrometer;[61] it is often possible to see the droplets of sweat on the skin, especially on the papillar ridges of the fingers, with the use of the plus-20 lens of the ophthalmoscope.[62]

Various diaphoretic procedures may be used. Thermoregulatory or heat sweating is produced by the use of external heat after the ingestion of hot fluids and acetylsalicylic acid. Large electric bakers or cradles are placed over the patient, the open ends covered with woolen blankets. An electric heat cabinet may be used. Emotional sweating is produced centrally and corresponds to the spontaneous hyperhidrosis of normal persons. It may be elicited by emotional stimuli, intellectual strain, or painful cutaneous sensation. Emotional sweating differs in distribution from thermoregulatory sweating in that it is more localized. The response also varies with the individual. Drug sweating is produced by the subcutaneous injection of 5 mg of pilocarpine hydrochloride. It acts peripherally, stimulating the glands innervated by postganglionic cholinergic fibers. The response to drugs is more variable than that to heat, and the resulting perspiration may be irregular and spotty.

PILOMOTOR RESPONSE.—Stimulation of the sympathetic nerves causes contraction of the arrectores pilorum muscles, resulting in erection of the cutaneous hairs; this phenomenon is known as cutis anserina, or "goose flesh." Piloerection may be provoked by gentle stroking of the skin, tickling, scratching with a pin, or the application of cold. Ice, cotton soaked in alcohol or ether, or a methyl chloride spray may be used. Piloerection is elicited best at the nape of the neck, in the axillas, on the abdominal wall, and at the upper border of the trapezius muscle. The patient should be in a warm room, since cold influences the response. It may be helpful to warm the body before the application of a cold stimulus. Emotional stimuli may also provoke piloerection.

The reaction appears slowly, after a latent period of 4–5 seconds, is complete or at its maximum in 7–10 seconds, and lasts 15–20 seconds. Piloerection first occurs at the site of stimulation and then spreads slowly and widely. If a massive stimulus is used, such as chilling the neck with ice, pinching the skin in the cervical region or at the upper border of the trapezius muscle, tickling or scratching the axilla, or applying cold to the axilla or the abdominal wall, there is a descending response which takes about half a minute to become manifest and lasts 1–2 minutes. This is seen best on the trunk and the extensor surfaces of the extremities. Symmetric parts of the body should be observed. If one side of the body is stimulated, the response is ipsilateral, but if the midline is stimulated, the response is bilateral.

VASOMOTOR RESPONSE.—Vasodilation causes flushing of the skin, and vasoconstriction is followed by pallor. When the sympathetic division of the autonomic system is interrupted, vasoconstriction is prevented so that temporary vasodilation and flushing result. The pallor that follows slight pressure on the skin disappears more quickly in the involved than in the normal areas. The test may be carried out by warming the surface of the body with towels wrung out of very hot water. If there are transverse spinal lesions, vasodilation occurs, with flushing, redness, and an increase in skin temperature below the level of the lesion. The vasodilation is most marked at the upper level of the vasoparalytic lesion, and there may be a distinct zone of hyperemia on the skin corresponding to the upper limit of the sensory zone of hyperalgesia. The hyperalgesic and hyperemic areas indicate the level of root involvement and the uppermost point of the spinal cord lesion. If warming of the skin is followed by sudden chilling of the skin with towels wrung out of ice water, there is a decrease in the vasoconstrictor response to cold below the level of a spinal lesion. As is true in the case of the pilomotor response, the vasomotor test depends on a number of factors and affords only limited and indirect information; it is difficult to evaluate and provides less reliable information than the sweating test.

REFLEX ERYTHEMA.—Stimulation of the skin by stroking it with a blunt point is followed by focal vasodilation. Localized flushing develops, and often a wheal or welt is produced. This response is assumed to depend on the axon reflex and the liberation of histamine. A three-phase reaction has been described, similar to the responses that follow histamine administration. First, there is a local red reaction, or the production of a red line along the site of pressure. This is followed in about half a minute by a spreading flush, or flare, which may be present for a distance of about 3 cm on each side of the scratch. In susceptible individuals, the area of the flare then becomes elevated, with the development of a wheal, often with a broad white line in its center; the red area may be bordered by a white zone. The vasoconstricting effect of the sympathetic division interferes with this response, and the reaction is increased when the sympathetic influence is diminished. Exaggeration of reflex erythema is called dermographia.

HISTAMINE FLARE.—The intracutaneous injection of 0.1 mg of phosphate histamine causes a localized red reaction followed by the development of a flare and a wheal; this is similar to the response produced by stroking the skin with a blunt point.[63, 64]

SKIN TEMPERATURE STUDIES.—The vasomotor tonus is reflected in the surface temperature of the body, and interruption of the sympathetic division with resulting vasodilation is followed by a rise in temperature; stimulation of the sympathetics with consequent vasoconstriction is accompanied by a fall in temperature. Quantitative skin temperature determinations can be made and are more accurate and more objective than the observation of flushing and pallor. Not only is it possible to evaluate the continuity of the sympathetic pathways by such determinations made in the resting state, but also valuable additional information may be obtained by noting the response to peripheral nerve and sympathetic block, spinal and general anesthesia, warming or cooling of different portions of the body, foreign protein injections, and the use of autonomic blocking agents.

DETERMINATION OF SKIN RESISTANCE.—Although affected to a certain extent by local factors, the resistance of the skin to passage of an electric current through the body is influenced largely by the activity of the sweat glands. It is known that section of a peripheral nerve is followed by a great and permanent increase in the resistance of the portion of skin supplied by that nerve to the passage of a minute, imperceptible current, whereas stimulation of a peripheral nerve is followed by a decrease in skin resistance. The autonomic component of the nerve is the important factor in this resistance, since areas deprived of autonomic supply show a greatly increased resistance even though other components of the peripheral nerves are intact. The change seems to be correlated with the function of the sweat glands, since the resistance is low if the sweat glands are active and high if they are inactive. The changes compare closely with those in sweating. Vasodilation may also play a part in skin resistance changes.

Skin resistance is measured by means of a dermometer, an instrument that is an essential part of the polygraph. Various types of instruments have been used.[65–67]

CAPILLARY MICROSCOPY.—When a beam of light is focused on either a fingernail or an area of skin on which a drop of cedar oil has been applied, the capillary loops become visible through the low-power objective of the microscope. During vasoconstriction, clumps of stagnant erythrocytes can be seen within the capillaries; during vasodilation, the red blood cells shoot through the vessels so rapidly they are visible only as a rapid flicker. Furthermore, if there is spasm, changes in the size and shape of the capillary loops may be seen, together with tortuosity and loss of normal hairpin-shaped forms.

PLETHYSMOGRAPHIC STUDIES.—Arteriocapillary tension can be measured and the expansile pulsation of an extremity determined at any desired level by means of an oscillometer or a plethysmograph. Such studies make it possible to estimate the arterial pulsation of an extremity and differentiate between vasospasm and arterial obstruction.

Suspected Hysteria and Malingering

In the evaluation of every patient who has symptoms of nervous system dysfunction it is essential to differentiate between those manifestations that are organic in origin and those that are psychogenic in origin. Furthermore, if nonorganic changes are present, it is essential to distinguish between those that are consciously induced or feigned (malingering) and those that are unconsciously motivated (hysterical).

Psychogenic manifestations may closely resemble organic ones, and the differentiation between the two may present diagnostic difficulties. Furthermore, organic and nonorganic disease may exist simultaneously. If the patient is seen only during malingering or hysterical attacks, the entire illness may appear to have a psychogenic origin and the organic factors may be overlooked.

There is no special routine for the neurologic examination to detect hysteria and malingering. The complete routine for the neurologic appraisal must be carried out in every case.[68–73]

In taking the history, the examiner should attempt to differentiate between organic and nonorganic factors; this applies not only to the symptoms that are directly referable to the nervous system but also to somatic symptoms in general. The history of previous adjustment to the environment, the home situation, employment, and emotional stresses and strains has great significance. Such information should be obtained not only from the patient but also from relatives and friends. The history of the present episode should include the details of the precipitating experience (trauma, emotional strain, mental shock) and of the evolution of the symptoms following their first appearance. If there was an accident, the details should be obtained. It is important to know how the injury occurred, whether witnesses were present, and if the accident was reported. The examiner should attempt to determine whether there was any loss of consciousness, whether the patient was able to move or walk after the injury, and whether medical treatment was given immediately. It is often desirable to have the patient reenact the injury and compare present muscle power with that before the accident.

In the neurologic examination it must be borne in mind that the manifestations which do not fit into the organic pattern may be of psychic origin. In the sensory examination, for instance, hysterical and malingering changes never correspond accurately to peripheral nerve, root, or spinal segmental distribution.

REFERENCES

1. Adrian E.D.: *The Basis of Sensation: The Action of the Sense Organs.* London, Christopher's, 1928.
2. Head H.: Six clinical lectures on the diagnostic value of sensory changes in diseases of the nervous system. *Clin. J.* 40:337, 358, 375, 390, 408, 1912; 42:23, 1913.
3. Sinclair D.: *Cutaneous Sensation.* London, Oxford University Press, 1967.
4. Weddell, G., Miller S.: Cutaneous sensation. *Annu. Rev. Physiol.* 24:199, 1962.
5. Dyck P.J., O'Nrien P.C., Bushek W., et al.: Clinical versus quantitative evaluation of cutaneous sensation. *Arch. Neurol.* 33:651, 1966.
6. Nathan P.W., Rice R.C.: The localization of warm stimuli. *Neurology* 16:533, 1956.
7. Halnan C.R.E., Wright G.H.: Tactile localization. *Brain* 83:677, 1960.
8. Foerster O.: The dermatomes in man. *Brain* 56:1, 1933.
9. Keegan J.J., Garrett F.D.: The segmental distribution of the cutaneous nerves in the limbs of man. *Anat. Rec.* 102:409, 1948.
10. Goff, G.D., Rosner B.S., Detre T., et al.: Vibration perception in normal man and medical patients. *J. Neurol. Neurosurg. Psychiatry* 28:503, 1965.
11. Plumb C.S., Meigs J.W.: Human vibration perception: I. Vibration perception at different ages (normal ranges). *Arch. Gen. Psychiatry* 4:611, 1961.
12. Toomey J.A., Kopecny L., Mickey S.: Measurement of sensation: I. Vibratory sensation. *Arch. Neurol. Psychiatry* 61:663, 1949.
13. Calne D.B., Pallis C.A.: Vibratory sense: A critical review. *Brain* 89:723, 1966.
14. Steiness I.: Vibratory perception in normal subjects: A biothesiometric study. *Acta Med. Scand.* 158:315, 1957.
15. Bedichek R.: *The Sense of Smell.* New York, Doubleday, 1960.
16. Schneider R.A.: The sense of smell in man: Its physiologic basis. *N. Engl. J. Med.* 277:299, 1967.
17. Sumner D.: On testing the sense of smell. *Lancet* 2:895, 1962.
18. McIntyre A.K., Robinson R.G.: Pathway for jaw-jerk in man. *Brain* 82:468, 1959.
19. Magladery J.W., Teasdall R.D.: Corneal reflexes: An electromyographic study in man. *Arch. Neurol.* 5:265, 1961.
20. Rose R.T.: Corneal reflex in hemispheric disease. *J. Neurol. Neurosurg. Psychiatry* 35:877, 1972.

21. Weingrow S.M.: Facial reflexes. *Arch. Pediatr.* 59:234, 1933.

22. Rushworth G.: Spasticity and rigidity: An experimental study and review. *J. Neurol. Neurosurg. Psychiatry* 23:99, 1960.

23. Drachman D.A.: Bell's palsy: A neurological point of view. *Arch. Otolaryngol.* 89:173, 1969.

24. von Bekesy E.: *Experiments in Hearing,* Wever E.G. (trans.-ed.). New York, McGraw-Hill Book Co., 1960.

25. Crowley H., Kaufman R.S.: The Rinne tuning fork test. *Arch. Otolaryngol.* 84:406, 1966.

26. Edwards H.: Neurological disease of the pharynx and larynx. *Practitioner* 211:729, 1973.

27. Bosma J., Grossman R., Kavanagh J.: Impairment of somesthetic perception and motor function in the oral and pharyngeal area. *Neurology* 17:649, 1967.

28. Montagu A.: On yawning. *JAMA* 182:732, 1962.

29. Engel G.L.: On the existence of a cerebral type of carotid sinus syncope. *Neurology* 5:565, 1950.

30. Adams R.D.: *Diseases of Muscles: A Study in Pathology,* ed. 4. Hagerstown, Md., Harper & Row, 1975.

31. Walton J.N. (ed.): *Diseases of Voluntary Muscle,* ed. 3. Edinburgh, Churchill Livingstone, 1974.

32. Penry J.K., Hoefnagel D., van den Noort S., et al.: Muscle spasm and abnormal postures resulting from damage to interneurones in spinal cord. *Arch. Neurol.* 3:500, 1960.

33. Thomas J.F.: Muscle tone, spasticity, rigidity. *J. Nerv. Ment. Dis.* 132:505, 1961.

34. Landau W.M.: Spasticity: The fable of the neurological demon and the Emperor's new therapy. *Arch. Neurol.* 31:217, 1974.

35. Kremer M.: Sitting, standing, and walking. *Br. Med. J.* 2:63, 121, 1958.

36. Fisher C.M.: A simple test of coordination in the fingers. *Neurology* 10:745, 1960.

37. Bronisch F.W.: *The Clinically Important Reflexes.* New York, Grune & Stratton, 1952.

38. Wartenberg R.: *The Examination of Reflexes: A Simplification.* Chicago, Year Book Medical Publishers, Inc., 1945.

39. Bergman P.S., Hirschberg G.G., Nathanson M.: Measurement of quadriceps reflex in spastic paralysis. *Neurology* 5:542, 1955.

40. Fiorentino M.R.: *Reflex Testing Methods for Evaluating C.N.S. Development.* Springfield, Ill., Charles C Thomas, Publisher, 1963.

41. Grimby I.: Normal plantar response: Integration of flexor and extensor reflex components. *J. Neurol. Neurosurg. Psychiatry* 26:39, 1963.

42. Arieff A.J., Tigay E.L., Pyzik S.: Superficial and deep reflexes in spinal cord injuries. *Neurology* 8:933, 1958.

43. Lehoczky T., Fodors T.: Clinical significance of dissociation of abdominal reflex. *Neurology* 3:453, 1953.

44. Magladery J.W., Teasdall R.D., French I.H., et al.: Cutaneous reflex changes in development and aging. *Arch. Neurol.* 3:1, 1960.

45. Babinski J.: Sur le reflexe cutane plantaire dans certaines affections organizues du systeme nerveux central. *CR Soc. Biol. (Paris)* 3:207, 1896.

46. Landau W.M., Clare M.H.: The plantar reflex in man: With special reference to some conditions where the extensor response is unexpectedly absent. *Brain* 82:321, 1959.

47. Walshe F.: The Babinski plantar response: Its forms and its physiological and pathologic significance. *Brain* 70:529, 1956.

48. Brain R., Wilkinson M.: Observations on the extensor plantar reflex and its relationship to the functions of the pyramidal tract: With special reference to (1) the plantar reflex in infancy, (2) the crossed extensor plantar reflex, and (3) extension of the great toe as an associated movement. *Brain* 82:257, 1959.

49. Landau W.M.: Clinical definition of the extensor plantar response. *N. Engl. J. Med.* 295:1149, 1975.

50. Szapiro M.: The Babinski sign. *J. Neurol. Neurosurg. Psychiatry* 23:262, 1960.

51. Gonda V.E.: A new tendon stretch reflex: Its significance in lesion of the pyramidal tract. *Arch. Neurol. Psychiatry* 48:531, 1942.

52. Allen I.M.: Application of stretch reflex of identification of lesion of upper motor neurone. *NZ Med. J.* 44:237, 1945.

53. Allen I., Cleckley H.: A new pyramidal sign of great frequency. *J. Nerv. Ment. Dis.* 97:146, 1943.

54. Head H., Riddoch G.: The automatic bladder, excessive sweating and some other reflex conditions in gross injuries of the spinal cord. *Brain* 40:188, 1917.

55. O'Connell J.E.A.: The clinical signs of meningeal irritation. *Brain* 69:9, 1946.

56. Wartenberg R.: The signs of Brudzinski and Kernig. *J. Pediatr.* 37:679, 1950.

57. Appenzeller O.: *The Autonomic Nervous System: An Introduction to Basic and Clinical Concepts,* ed. 2. Amsterdam, North-Holland, 1976.

58. Pick J.: *The Autonomic Nervous System: Morphological, Comparative, Clinical and Surgical Aspects.* Philadelphia, J.B. Lippincott Co., 1970.

59. Guttman L.: Topographic studies of disturbances of sweat secretion after complete lesions of peripheral nerves. *J. Neurol. Neurosurg. Psychiatry* 3:197, 1940.

60. List C.F., Peet M.M.: Sweat secretion in man: I. Sweating responses in normal persons. *Arch. Neurol. Psychiatry* 39:1228, 1938.

61. Bullard R.W.: Continuous recording of sweating rate by resistance hygrometry. *J. Appl. Physiol.* 17:735, 1962.

62. Kahn E.A.: Direct observation of sweating in peripheral nerve lesions: Its use as a simple diagnostic test. *Surg. Gynecol. Obstet.* 92:22, 1951.

63. Loeser L.H.: The cutaneous histamine reaction as a test of peripheral nerve function. *JAMA* 110:2136, 1938.

64. Tonick B., Beck W.C.: The histamine flare in the

evaluation of peripheral nerve lesions. *War Med.* 8:386, 1945.

65. Jasper H., Robb P.: Studies of electrical skin resistance in peripheral nerve lesions. *J. Neurosurg.* 2:261, 1945.

66. Redlich F.C.: Organic and hysterical anesthesia: A method of differential diagnosis with the aid of the galvanic skin response. *Am. J. Psychiatry* 102:218, 1945.

67. Richter C.P., Woodruff B.G.: Lumbar sympathetic dermatomes in man: Determined by the electrical skin resistance method. *J. Neurophysiol.* 8:323, 1945.

68. Chodoff F.: The diagnosis of hysteria. *Am. J. Psychiatry* 131:1073, 1974.

69. DeJong R.N.: *The Neurologic Examination: Incorporating the Fundamentals of Neuroanatomy and Neurophysiology,* ed. 4. Hagerstown, Md., Harper & Row, 1979, pp. 721–739.

70. Slater E.: Diagnosis of "hysteria." *Br. Med. J.* 1:1395, 1965.

71. Walshe F.: Diagnosis of hysteria. *Br. Med. J.* 2:1451, 1965.

72. Woodruff R.A. Jr., Clayton P.J., Guze S.B.: Hysteria: Studies of diagnosis, outcome, and prevalence. *JAMA* 215:425, 1971.

73. Woolsey R.M.: Hysteria: 1875 to 1975. *Dis. Nerv. Syst.* 37:379, 1976.

13 / Evaluation of the Patient With the Complaint of Pain

RICHARD G. BLACK, M.D.

THE SIMPLE ACT of presenting a complaint of pain to his physician increases the patient's risk of receiving poor care and the physician's chance of doing harm. The very nature of a pain complaint directs attention away from the patient and toward the site of the pain and its presentation. No need is felt to further investigate the patient as a whole or suspect other problems not as easily disclosed as a physical pain problem. Because the complaint of pain, usually meaning nociception or physical hurt, is so common and has been experienced by all mankind, both the patient and the physician feel comfortable dealing with it. Pain is therefore a ''safe'' expression of ''disease'' or suffering for the patient since it is completely acceptable as a significant problem at face value. The physician readily accepts the suggestion of a simple physical problem with understandable relief that this patient does not have time-consuming psychological, job, or marital problems to be heard. Many patients with pain complaints, however, already have or do develop secondary problems that can present significant difficulties in management. In spite of its high incidence and usually successful management, the expression of pain as a persisting complaint remains poorly understood and therefore frequently mismanaged.

Acute pain and chronic pain are two distinctly different disease states sharing only the expression of pain. Both physician's and patient's past experiences with acute pain are frequently carried over into the area of chronic pain, with bad results. When patients with long-standing complaints of headache, low back pain, vague abdominal discomfort, or myofascial problems are treated in the same manner as patients with acute pain problems related to significant pathology, the response is often unpredictable. The usual drugs or operative procedures known to be successful for the acute problem are applied for chronic pain and only transiently help the patient, who often becomes worse. Both the patient and physician become desperate, seeking stronger medications and even mutilating operations, until they regard each other as incompetent or psychologically disturbed. Referral is made to other specialists until the patient, in his rounds from physician to physician, is blamed totally for his problems, and becomes firmly labeled with the regrettable terms of ''crock'' or ''crazy.''

The physician is as much a victim of this situation as the patient. The highly specialized nature of his training has narrowed his view of the patient's problem and eliminated all consideration except physical disease, biochemical disorders, or extreme psychological problems. In the case of the specialist, this tunnel vision may become even more extreme and be directed at one particular organ system or therapeutic approach. The adage ''When the only tool you have is a hammer, everything looks like a nail'' may seem appropriate in describing the response of some specialists to the complaint of pain. The hammer may take the form of surgery, nerve block, prescription pad, acupuncture, or some other modality of therapy, which have in common only financial support from third-party carriers.

The successful management of a patient with chronic intractable pain requires that a correct and specific diagnosis be made, leading to formulation and execution of an appropriate plan for therapy. A correct diagnosis is particularly difficult to make in patients with the chronic pain syndrome, since these individuals often present with an established diagnosis or label which, when critically examined, will be found inappropriate, outdated, or dangerously useless. Often this label is a mere description of an initiating disease entity which may have little or no relation to the patient's current problem. A preexisting problem, such as disk disease, may be used to explain the pain from a myofascial problem or hamstring contractures. Unless a correct diagnosis is made, inappropriate therapy will result. A correct diagnosis will lead to appropriate therapy. It is the meaning of "diagnosis" that is important in this statement and especially important when treating the patient with the chronic pain syndrome.[8] A diagnosis must include all of the factors affecting the suffering of the patient. These include any physical, psychological, and socioeconomic problems. These factors are more likely to be ignored the more definitive the prevailing diagnosis and the more specialized the training of the physician.

This lack of understanding of the suffering, expressed as pain by the patient with support from his family, can seriously affect the outcome of his care and the quality of his life. The word pain, or its equivalents, may have many meanings ranging from fear, to an annoying sensation, to extreme nociception such as that which may accompany invasion of bone or nerve by tumor.[1] The words used may be the same, the sensation invisible, and the display of suffering completely unrelated to the intensity of the nociceptive sensation. A patient's expression of his suffering as pain may hide his underlying unexpressed feelings of depression, anxiety, fear, or inability to tolerate a specific social situation. Failure of the health care professional, relatives, and friends to acknowledge factors other than severe nociception as being important in the problem will lead to escalating use of heavy analgesic medications and multiple surgical attacks on the pain pathways. Meanwhile, the meaning of the patient's cry for help is kept hidden. As if by common agreement, fear of dying, of further suffering, and of losing control remains unexpressed in our society.[2]

Consideration must be given to the definition of the word pain. These range from "Pain is an experience, whether physical or mental which the patient dislikes," by C. S. Lewis,[3] to R. A. Sternbach's relativistic definition: "Pain is an abstract concept which an observer may use to describe: (1) a personal, private sense of hurt; (2) a harmful stimulus which signals current or impending tissue damage; (3) a pattern of responses which operate to protect the organism from harm."[4] An acceptable working definition of pain is "an unpleasant experience which we primarily associate with tissue damage or describe in terms of tissue damage, or both."[5] This definition, proposed by H. Merskey, combines subjective experience, an apparent physical pain generator, and the response by which an outside observer would agree one was in pain. Melzack and Torgerson have suggested that pain might be described in terms of several sensory and affective dimensions. They have made a substantial contribution concerning the language used to describe pain.[6] The concept of pain as suffering with components of hurt, anxiety, and depression has also been developed in an attempt to assign clinically useful descriptors to the complaint of pain.[7]

Injury-associated pain accompanying job loss or pain related to a life-threatening disease has another important component. These pains constantly remind the patient of his condition and increase his anxiety over imagined fates, all worse than reality. The involuntary increase in muscle tension and the increased attentiveness to body sensations maintain the problem through the development of myofascial problems and increased anxiety. When the patient has been diagnosed as having a malignancy, even though it may be cured or inactive, the situation is worse. Emphasis is now given to the patient's imagined painful death. Even normal subpainful sensations become associated in the mind with cancer and result in suffering that is nonresponsive to the usual analgesics and only poorly responsive to convincing statistics of cures and long life expectancies.

In order to comprehend the real meaning of a patient's complaint of pain, attention must be directed to the components of his problem and to understanding the nature of his pain and how it might differ from the complaint of pain usually seen in a medical practice. In addition to evaluating the amount of nociception present, the physician must attempt to ascertain whether it is acute or chronic in nature. Acute pain is most commonly seen, most responsive to therapy, and may be the most severe in nature. Responding differently is chronic pain, meaning chronic nociception, which differs from acute pain in that (1) chronic pain no longer serves a protective or warning function but has become an end onto itself; (2) the pain is low grade in nature and appropriate to some definable, often diffuse, inflammatory or neuritic process; (3) the patient's condition is remarkably stable, becoming neither better nor worse over the years with the therapies attempted; and (4) the patient has made a functional adaptation to his condition, managing in some way to lead a life-style as normal as possible under the circumstances. Chronic pain, meaning chronic nociception, must not be confused with the syndrome of chronic pain, a stable, severe, psychosocial maladaption to life.[8] There are many sufferers of chronic nociception such as paraplegics, arthritics, and some individuals with malignancies who lead reasonably normal, functional lives. In contrast are the depressed, dependent victims of the chronic pain syndrome with their poor premorbid adjustment, high incidence of medication dependency, and disturbed social functioning.

Many patients have a presentation characteristic enough to constitute an entity, the chronic pain syndrome.[8] Its presence is characterized by a significant deviation from peer group normality in the patient's life-style and in his relations with others. Of note is failure to show any progressive improvement, while at the same time rarely becoming worse. There are intractable, often multiple pain complaints, many of which are inappropriate to existing physical problems or illnesses. A history of multiple physician contacts with many nonproductive diagnostic procedures is usually elicited. Irritating to the examiner is the patient's excessive preoccupation with his complaints, which are strongly reinforced by his family and friends. All sufferers of the chronic pain syndrome have a responsive audience for their suffering and in a most skillful manner play to that audience to obtain immediate gains. Features of depression, anxiety, and neuroticism are present.[8–10] Strong dependency needs are characteristic, and child abuse is often disclosed in the family history. The victim of this syndrome has no realistic plans for the future or practice with any therapy requiring time or active participation on his part. Care must be taken to differentiate these pain patients from individuals with sociopathic and psychopathic traits who may mimic the pain patient but, in contrast, have deliberate manipulative gains as their goal. This latter class of patients requires psychiatric management and have no place in a pain center.

In its later stages, the chronic pain syndrome is accompanied by excessive use of short-acting medications, particularly analgesics but also the benzodiazepines and hypnotics. It is the chronic long-term use of such medications that produces a toxic alteration of CNS function resembling an organic brain syndrome. This further confuses the diagnostic picture and makes it impossible for the victim of this disease to have any insight into his problem, with or without outside help.[10–12] These patients, in their confused state, often present so strongly and with such sympathetic support from family and friends that surgery directed at pain relief or further prescriptions for these same drugs may seem most appropriate, even expedient, to the unwary physician,

who by now wishes he were rid of the patient. This medication problem and the obsession with disease are often seen in a more acute form in the cancer patient and his family unit.

Disabling secondary problems soon follow establishment of the chronic pain syndrome and almost predictably occur in the cancer victim as well. Despair at the seemingly useless and endless nature of the suffering leads to increased anxiety and depression. Concern over loss of income, work, and social contacts combines with the patient's own failing physical abilities to increase anxiety. There is also fear of failing mental abilities secondary to the central effects of the analgesics and other medications taken. These same factors add to the depression already present. The use of narcotic and synthetic analgesics, as well as the benzodiazepines, directly causes depression through central neuropharmacologic effects, magnifying any depression already present.[12] Sleep patterns are altered by the presence of pain and the use of short-acting analgesics on an ''as-needed'' basis.[8] The use of hypnotics on a regular basis alters the percentage of time spent in each of the individual stages that are part of the regular physiologic sleep pattern. This imbalance results in an abnormal and unrestful sleep period which significantly decreases the feeling of well-being. The effect is similar to the jet lag experienced by travelers who cross many time zones. When this primary disturbance of the circadian rhythm has established itself, progressive physical and mental deterioration inevitably follows. Particularly terrible are the long lonely night hours spent thinking of one's fate, and the beginning of each new day in a state of exhaustion.

Since pain is an acceptable affliction in our society and one especially worthy of sympathy, environmental rewards in the guise of attention by well-meaning friends and family act to keep the individual in his role as the patient, or ill person.[5, 12] This interaction nurtures the helper while increasing illness behavior in the patient. The patient, having received and still receiving the special benefits of being ill, is placed in the difficult position of being unable to justify acting well again.[13] In addition, activities recognized as beneficial to self-image, such as driving a car, working, and socializing, that might make the individual feel worthwhile and a functional member of his family or society, are taken away by well-meaning friends. By doing this, these friends unintentionally increase the duration and severity of the illness while making themselves feel better.

This is especially apparent in the cancer patient who, because of the forebidding nature of his disease, receives considerable sympathy and attention. Soon well-meaning friends and relatives systematically take away those everyday activities which identify the individual as an independent autonomous human being. First, the patient is given rides from place to place. Then help, or actual interference, with housework and chores follows, and finally there is a premature taking over of all body functions before they are physiologically lost. Careful examination of the situation from a behavioral viewpoint shows that the patient is being accelerated through the normal course of his illness. All semblance of well behavior is suppressed and the role of the invalid encouraged. By assuming the role of helper, family and friends become legitimately bound to the patient and his illness and are therefore free to verbalize their feelings and participate in events centered around the patient. These actions are useful coping mechanisms for family and friends but may be disastrous for the patient.[14, 15]

Both patient and family must make difficult, sometimes impossible changes to break out of this vicious self-propagating cycle of illness behavior. Both the helper and the helped must decrease, modify, or stop altogether such behaviors or actions which have given immediate reward or enjoyment, and they must start to do some new things, often difficult and undesired, for which the negative consequences of failure are remote and not previously experienced, and the positive rewards equally distant.[13]

The pain patient in his desperate search for relief from his suffering is exposed to a high risk of iatrogenic complications at the hands of well-meaning physicians. These physicians are not malicious but are practicing according to the experience gained from years of training and practice. A considerable part of their experience with pain is with the acute variety. They are poorly trained, if indeed trained at all in the chronic management of suffering made up of physical hurt and severe psychological stress. In transferring their experience with management of acute pain to the suffering of the chronic pain patient, less than optimum care is often delivered. Abuse of short-acting analgesic medications is responsible for the majority of unsatisfactory results obtained in attempting to treat low-intensity chronic pain with analgesics and surgical measures, including destructive interventions on the nerve pathways. Many physicians versed in the valuable effects of short-acting analgesics in acute pain will mistakenly apply the same therapeutic regimens to the patient with chronic ongoing pain problems, even those secondary to malignancies, and ultimately make the patient much worse. This is analogous to treating diabetes, a chronic disease, with regular or short-acting insulin. The management, while possible, would be less than satisfactory.

As noted with the chronic pain syndrome, the long-term use of short-acting analgesics on an as-needed basis results in escalation of their use, psychological depression from their effects on CNS neurotransmitters, and a resulting increase in the intensity of pain reported by the patient.[11] Nonanalgesic drugs such as tranquilizers, hypnotics, and muscle relaxants also have cumulative toxic side effects and play as important a role in this problem as do analgesics.[11, 12] Confusion of cognitive functions can result from continued long-term use of prescription and over-the-counter drugs and may result in a clinical state similar to an organic brain syndrome. This problem is commonly ignored by many examining physicians, even though it contributes significantly to misdiagnosis and inappropriate therapy. Chronic pain patients who are chronic users of analgesic medications report less pain after these medications are discontinued and time is allowed for detoxification.[8, 16] This applies equally well to the patient with the diagnosis of a malignancy. So important, and sometimes subtle or even occult, is this problem that *a basic principle in the management of pain patients is that whenever excessive or chronic use of medication is even suspected, it must be withdrawn before a meaningful diagnostic evaluation can be attempted.* While this may not be reasonable in a patient with significant nociception, such as from bone metastases, equally satisfactory conditions for a meaningful diagnostic evaluation can be obtained if the blood level of the analgesic medication is kept constant, either by oral use of an effective long-acting agent on a time contingency basis or else by continuous intravenous infusion of an analgesic agent. Sensations secondary to cyclically changing blood levels of analgesics administered on an as-needed basis can create demands for medication which are often presented as pain complaints. The constant blood level of analgesic obtained by either of the two techniques will separate these pain complaints from pain complaints related to nociceptive input.

With the time-contingency use of long-acting analgesic medications, it is possible to achieve a balance between the steady or continuous component of nociceptive input and the blood level of analgesia, with almost negligible side effects from cerebral cortical intoxication. With as-needed or even regular use of short-acting agents, lasting usually 2–3 hours but given on a q4h basis, larger doses are necessary to achieve a reasonable duration of action. Intervals of administration are kept longer than the duration of the desired analgesic effect in order to avoid respiratory depression. This will ultimately result in behavior changes and dependency needs associated with administration of medication rather than level of nociception. These occur, as noted, related to the sensations produced by rapidly changing blood levels of drug and anticipation of return of pain.

A DIAGNOSTIC APPROACH TO THE PATIENT WITH CHRONIC PAIN

The patient with a persisting complaint of pain who has already made the rounds of many physicians and clinics without relief must be considered a proved failure of the health care delivery system. A new approach is therefore necessary for the successful management of this type of patient. Any new approach should be based on increased one-to-one patient-physician contact and a diagnostic scheme that systematically examines all possible contributing factors, even those not presently considered a part of medical and surgical practice.

Whereas such patients represent only a relatively small percentage of all patients, they do consume a disproportionately large percentage of the available health care services. The system they have interacted with was designed to make efficient use of both physicians and facilities to permit more patients to be treated in less time and at a lower cost. Unfortunately, inherent in this efficiency is a reduction in physician-patient contact time as various activities requiring patient contact are delegated to assistants. The patients who fail this system—those with the more obscure problems such as multisystem disease, psychological overlay, or dependency needs—apparently do not respond to this type of efficient approach and begin seeing other physicians in their quest for help. This help-seeking behavior becomes more desperate, yet more stereotyped, and nonproductive. Direct access to specialists is easily obtained with the resulting management becoming more and more technical, as the elusive psychological and sociologic factors constituting the ''art of medicine'' are ignored. Unfortunately, these patients require, even demand, more time than the average patient, and many physicians are understand-

ably reluctant to spend the required time with the patient. Indeed, if there is any single factor that will ensure success in the management of these patients, it is the amount of time spent by the physician in meaningful contact with the patient and his family. Unfortunately, few physicians realize that these patients will eventually take the time from the physician in one way or another and that it is really more efficient to give it under controlled conditions. More time should be scheduled for meeting with this type of patient and the appointment should be made for the end of the day when the interview may be allowed to run over without disrupting the clinic.

Many physicians have wondered why certain patients have not responded, or do not continue to respond, to surgical or medical interventions that have already proved successful in other patients with acute complaints. An explanation for this is that the physician's training has caused him to focus on physical factors and to ignore the difference between acute and chronic pain. Evaluation of social and psychological factors is time-consuming and little attention is paid to it except in a last desperate attempt to solve the patient's problem by referral to a psychiatrist who is not able to manage the patient's many and by now very real physical problems. Thus, social and economic factors are almost never considered early enough in the patient's management, which leads to development of the chronic pain syndrome in that patient.

Since the patient with chronic pain already has an intimate relation with the health care system through multiple, often simultaneous physician contacts, it is often but erroneously assumed that somewhere by someone this patient is receiving comprehensive care, complete physical evaluations, coordinated medication management, and whatever necessary psychological support. This is often not the case. Many patients, not just pain patients, receive fractionated care from multiple physicians. Some even assume that an annual visit to a specialist, say for renal disease, constitutes their complete yearly checkup, with the result many do not even have a family physician. In spite of the voluminous records accompanying chronic pain patients, these patients may have not received a thorough examination of the site of their pain or a comprehensive pain history. It behooves the physician managing these patients to begin anew with a detailed history, functional inquiry, and physical examination. For each of these areas there is specialized information to be sought when the patient complains of pain.

Unlike the routine patient, for whom it is generally enough to attend to the acute physical problem, the patient with a complaint of persisting pain must be assessed simultaneously for physical, mental, and environmental factors.[7] It is essential that the patient, his family, the physician, and the nursing staff understand that these items are interrelated. The patient's active cooperation in evaluation of each of these factors is just as important for him as is his active participation in his own self-care. Participation of the spouse and other involved family members is also necessary, since the family may be the determining factor in reinforcing the need for illness behavior by the patient and in maintaining the patient's status as an invalid. A family unit that will not readily agree to such an encompassing diagnostic and therapeutic plan will probably not achieve the desired reversal of the patient's invalidism and dependency. Without this change family relations will remain superficial, and close bonding of family members, if it ever existed, will be lost.

In the history, consideration must be given to the state of the patient prior to the onset of his pain problem. If this was normal, a return to normality can be expected. If, however, the patient has been health care dependent with a long history of health care–seeking behavior at times of stress in his life, it is usually unrealistic to expect improvement beyond his previous best level of functioning. Similarly, a positive history of addictive behavior, whether to medications, tobacco, alcohol, or illicit drugs, is a bad prognosticator. These findings do not suggest that therapeutic management should not be attempted but that the goals, the final outcome of that management, must be realistic for that patient. It is, however, characteristic of patients with the chronic pain syndrome that they expect to be physically much better than they ever have been, and that they look forward not to improvement, but a pain-free life with no problems.

Important prognostic factors are listed in Table 13–1. Some of the premorbid factors have been considered above. If the nociceptive component is present, significant, and responsive to treatment, improvement can be expected. However, if nociception is minimal or even imaginary, or if there is somatizing depression or pain dependency, then little

can be expected from use of analgesics or surgical attacks on the pain pathways of the sensory nervous system.

The resources of the individual are important in planning for the future of the patient following therapy. Laborers with grade school educations and no marketable skills are most difficult to rehabilitate. It is even difficult to find alternatives for their pain behavior, which may be both face-saving and productive of an adequate guaranteed income. Planned retirement with medical justification but not carrying a limit on desired physical activity may be an acceptable and honorable way out for these individuals trapped in a high technology society. The professional person with an education and other individuals with marketable skills have a higher probability of good functional recovery. Hobbies, realistic plans for retirement or alternate work, and outside interests are also favorable prognosticators. If this latter kind of patient does not make good progress, his underlying organic condition and psychological factors should be most carefully reassessed.

Most unfortunate of the diagnostic labels applied to patients is that of cancer. Histologically proved and appropriately treated, it now becomes an explanation for every ache or discomfort and an excuse for the early use of strong narcotic analgesics, all too frequently on an as-needed basis.[17] Foley estimates that approximately 30% of the pain syndromes that occur in cancer patients have no relationship to the underlying cancer or cancer therapy.[18] Complaints that actually represent the patient's expressions of fear, depression, and anxiety are regarded as strong nociceptive responses and treated by the early use of strong analgesics. At this time these only confuse the patient's thinking and increase morbidity, through lack of activity, constipation, and nausea. Lack of activity by itself leads to painful myofascial problems, contractures, and dystrophies related to the autonomic nervous system. These patients would do much better if treated with appropriate psychotropic drugs, sympathy, and a scheduled exercise or activity regimen. Less suffering would result for the patient and his family.

Cancer is typically a silent disease, with most patients not expressing their suffering as a complaint of pain until made aware of their diagnosis.[19] Only an exact diagnosis of the cause of their suffering, be it nociception, anxiety, or depression, will permit an understanding of the cause of the patient's pain complaint, and only with this exact diagnosis can appropriate therapy be instituted. As noted in Table 13–2, premorbid and nociceptive factors are impor-

TABLE 13–1.—MANAGING SUFFERING IN CHRONIC PAIN

PREMORBID	NOCICEPTION	RESOURCES
Good	Present	Strong
Bad	Absent	Weak

TABLE 13–2.—MANAGING SUFFERING IN CANCER

PREMORBID	NOCICEPTION	RESOURCES	PROGNOSIS
Good	Present	Strong	Good
Bad	Absent	Weak	Bad

tant in evaluating the outcome of management, just as in the chronic pain patient. While resources are important, the prognosis of how much useful life expectancy remains is more important. If time is short, more aggressive attacks on the nervous system and heavy use of analgesics may be appropriate. With a favorable prognosis or long life expectancy, these therapies may ultimately lead to the disasters of drug dependency and reinforced illness behavior.

The history of the patient's pain complaint should be elicited in a manner that will leave in the mind of the examiner a clear picture of the time course and anatomical progression of the pain problem since its onset. Detailed interest in the patient's problem, shown by the examiner in obtaining this history, will help reestablish the patient's confidence in physicians and begin establishing a new patient-physician relationship. During the time required to obtain this information the examiner has an opportunity to observe the patient's body mechanics and mood changes while the patient is distracted in recalling past details of this problem. His past interactions with his peer group, employers, and physicians should also be inspected for any indications of sociopathic or other disturbed patterns of behavior. A good starting point is to inquire when the current pain complaint was first felt. The type of onset, gradual or sudden, should be noted. If it is motion-related, the patient should be asked to demonstrate the position he was in and the action he was performing when the pain first occurred. Was the patient able to continue his activities that day or was he immediately crippled? If the injury was job-related, what were the interpersonal relations in the work setting at the time as interpreted by the patient? Injuries may anticipate loss of a job or represent acting out of interpersonal relations.

The immediate management of the injury and its effect should be noted. Further therapy should be documented with details as to indication, effect on the pain problem, and effect on social economic status. It must always be very carefully determined if the pain following surgery or any therapy was the same as the pain before the procedure. Many times iatrogenic problems have been introduced by inappropriate or unnecessary procedures.

The intensity of the pain at its various stages is important. Daily variations may give clues to arthritic processes, characterized by early morning stiffness, and inflammatory traumatic processes, which are made worse by activity and improved with rest. The changes in the pain complaint between work days and weekends may point to unrecognized stresses in the home or work situation. Information of this type is best collected in advance. The patient should be instructed to keep a daily diary in which he records his hourly activity, medication use, and some measure of the intensity of pain. This should be kept on an hourly basis for several weeks prior to the next physician contact. If the patient is unwilling to participate to this extent in his care it is unlikely that he will benefit from anything else the physician might do for him.

The presence of the spouse or other most significant individual from the patient's peer group during the interview is so helpful as to be essential. Often other distinctly different versions of various incidents may be revealed, especially concerning the use of medications and alcohol, and the setting presents an ideal opportunity to judge the quality of the relationship between the couple. The presence of parents or children is not recommended since, in most cases, their relation to the patient is not at a peer level except perhaps for a mature daughter managing an elderly mother or mother-in-law in her home.

Often a careful, accurate description of the character of the pain and its location is enough to identify the pathophysiologic mechanisms involved. This description should be evoked at the same time that a physical examination of area involved is done. The patient is requested to indicate the area of the pain and describe its apparent size and depth. Localized discrete pains are generally somatic in nature, in contrast to visceral, autonomic, or vascular problems. The depth of pain may indicate myofascial, bone, or nerve entrapment problems, and the relation of the primary pain site and its radiation pattern to dermatomes often indicates nerve root–related problems. The character of the pain is documented next. Descriptors such as those published by Melzack may be suggested to the patient, who may have difficulty describing a sensation for which he has no words.[6] With experience, the examiner will realize that certain pain descriptors fit very closely with known pathophysiologic states. The immediate time course of the pain, whether steady, throbbing, or intermittent is noted. Pains of a throbbing character should be checked for a relation to the pulse.

Factors affecting the pain should be systematically documented in three categories: those increasing the pain, those not affecting the pain, and those decreasing the pain. In addition to factors volunteered by the patient, specific questions should be directed at factors that the examiner thinks might be related to or might confirm any suspected pathology. It is convenient to arrange these findings in a table so that patterns characteristic of certain conditions become apparent.

In addition to the above points, a complete orthopedic and neurologic examination must be done. This should include a full range of motion measurements, thermography, and electromyography, when indicated. If, after all the examinations have been done and the results of tests reported, no apparent cause of the patient's complaint can be identified, a careful reevaluation of the diagnostic process used

is in order. Errors of omission are common. While at first thought these might imply the missed rectal examination, or the lack of flexion-extension films and examination for long tract signs in a neck evaluation, etc., the more common error in dealing with chronic pain is some factor unfamiliar to the physician or specialist. The usual reason is a simple lack of time to spend with the patient and his family to understand and acknowledge the effect of these factors on his problems.

A diagnostic approach that has proved most useful entails grouping the patient's complaint into various components which are then individually evaluated.[7] These components are then combined to form a pain profile for that individual patient at that particular time. This may be done for both acute pain (Fig 13–1) and for chronic pain (Fig 13–2). The highest peaks in this profile are considered the major problem areas and are treated first in the course of the patient's management. This will bring about the greatest improvement in the shortest time.

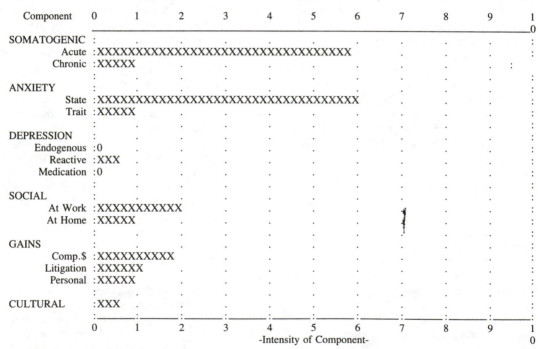

Fig 13–1.—Computer-generated graph demonstrates the magnitude of each of the components of suffering in a patient with a complaint of short-term acute pain. This form of presentation may be used to direct treatment at those factors contributing most to the patient's disease. In this example, treatment of the nociceptive component alone with analgesics, immobilization, or even appropriate surgery would be expected to have the greatest effect. The anxiety state is also a significant component and should improve as the acute pain resolves.

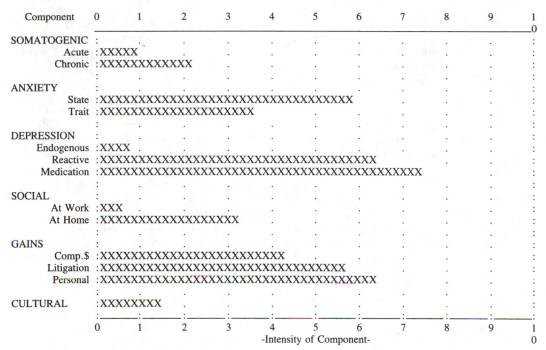

```
Component    0    1    2    3    4    5    6    7    8    9    1
                                                              0
SOMATOGENIC :    .    .    .    .    .    .    .    .    .    :
       Acute :XXXXX    .    .    .    .    .    .    .    .    :
     Chronic :XXXXXXXXXXX    .    .    .    .    .    .    .    :
             :    .    .    .    .    .    .    .    .    .    :
ANXIETY      :    .    .    .    .    .    .    .    .    .    :
       State :XXXXXXXXXXXXXXXXXXXXXXXXXXXXXXXXXXX    .    .    :
       Trait :XXXXXXXXXXXXXXXXXXXXX    .    .    .    .    .    :
DEPRESSION   :    .    .    .    .    .    .    .    .    .    :
  Endogenous :XXXX .    .    .    .    .    .    .    .    .    :
    Reactive :XXXXXXXXXXXXXXXXXXXXXXXXXXXXXXXXXXXXXXX    .    :
  Medication :XXXXXXXXXXXXXXXXXXXXXXXXXXXXXXXXXXXXXXXXXXXXX  :
             :    .    .    .    .    .    .    .    .    .    :
SOCIAL       :    .    .    .    .    .    .    .    .    .    :
     At Work :XXX .    .    .    .    .    .    .    .    .    :
     At Home :XXXXXXXXXXXXXXXXX    .    .    .    .    .    .    :
             :    .    .    .    .    .    .    .    .    .    :
GAINS        :    .    .    .    .    .    .    .    .    .    :
     Comp.$  :XXXXXXXXXXXXXXXXXXXXXXXXXX    .    .    .    .    :
  Litigation :XXXXXXXXXXXXXXXXXXXXXXXXXXXXXXX    .    .    .    :
    Personal :XXXXXXXXXXXXXXXXXXXXXXXXXXXXXXXXXXXX    .    .    :
CULTURAL     :XXXXXXXX    .    .    .    .    .    .    .    .    :
             :____:____:____:____:____:____:____:____:____:____:
             0    1    2    3    4    5    6    7    8    9    1
                           -Intensity of Component-           0
```

Fig 13–2.—Computer-generated graph demonstrates the magnitude of each of the components of suffering in a patient with the chronic pain syndrome. Treatment of the nociceptive component alone with analgesics or surgery would probably make little difference to the patient's overall suffering. Depression, both reactive and secondary, has developed into a significant problem. The medication-related depression is iatrogenic, related to narcotic and benzodiazepine use.

The components found to be most useful are as follows:

Somatogenic—This refers to the physical hurt or nociceptive component of the pain problem. It may result from irritation of nerve or periosteal tendon insertions, presence of inflammation, obstructed viscera, or effects of a reflex sympathetic dystrophy. This component is further divided into:

Sa—an acute component generally adequately managed with the usual measures of immobilization, surgery, and analgesic medications. If at all possible, the source of the nociception should be treated rather than symptoms.

Sc—a chronic component difficult to manage with medications or procedures on the nervous system but usually responsive to a well-kept exercise, range of motion, and activity program. In some cases constantly maintained appropriate blood levels of long-acting analgesics are useful, as is TENS.

Anxiety—This refers to the patient's anxiety state at the time of diagnosis. It may be a major component in the suffering of cancer patients who have been technically "cured," when a friend or family member succumbs to a similar malignancy. Two components may be considered:

As—anxiety state, related to the patient's overall situation. It may involve concern over support and raising of children, loss of income, or other issues peripheral to the disease itself.

At—anxiety trait, or the individual's natural tendency to be anxious. It will be apparent in a well-taken chronological history.

Depression—This refers to the patient's degree of depression at the time of diagnosis. Suicidal ideation should be sought out if the depressive component is high or is starting to improve. It is further divided into:

De—endogenous depression, a not uncommon and often misdiagnosed problem.

Dr—reactive depression, which may represent an appropriate and normal response to a bad situation.

Dm—depression secondary to use of medications, an exogenous chemical depression common with the extended use narcotic analgesics, benzodiazepines, and hypnotics.

Social—This factor refers to stress resulting from the patient's social situation. It is divided into two problem areas, the home and the place of work. Signs secondary to the presence of illness, changes in physical appearance, disability resulting from illness, or the need to wear braces or stimulators may have profound effects on the patient's ability to accept himself or be accepted by others. Pain may be employed as an acceptable excuse in avoiding exposure to stressful social situations.

Sw—problems at work.

Sh—problems at home.

Gains—This factor refers to gains received by the patient from his pain behavior. It is divided into areas of:

Gc—gains from financial compensation.

Gl—gains anticipated or realized from litigation. Both of these gains are characteristic of the chronic pain patient. They may exist only in the patient's hopes and are often unrealistically exaggerated.

Gp—personal gains from family and friends. The patient has become the center of attention and may unconsciously or deliberately employ his suffering to maintain his power to manipulate others. Chronic pain patients often have few other social skills, so care must be taken to retrain these individuals in their social skills before eliminating their personal gains.

Cultural—This refers to modifying factors peculiar to the individual patient's culture. In "multigeneration" cohesive families, illness, even impending death, may be accepted in an appropriate and supportive manner with much support for the dying family member. This attitude may unfortunately result in too much support for a chronically but not terminally ill family member. In contrast, in some cultures illness may be abhorrent and its victim isolated. Cancer is considered a contagious disease by some. In such homes the patient may be isolated from spouse and children at a time of greatest need.

This approach heightens the health care professional's awareness of the various components contributing to the patient's suffering. Especially emphasized is the important distinction between acute and chronic pain and the many psychosocial influences present. While it is possible by directed questioning, careful physical examination, simple psychological testing, and the assistance of a social worker to establish a reasonably correct formal profile for the patient, this is not always necessary or desirable. Once the concept is accepted, with attention directed to the various parameters, a bedside estimate of the pain profile is often enough. Therapy should then be directed where it will be most effective and least harmful.

REFERENCES

1. Loeser J.D., Black R.G.: A taxonomy of pain. *Pain* 1:81–84, 1975.
2. Cassel E.J.: The nature of suffering and the goals of medicine. *N. Engl. J. Med.* 306(3):639–645, 1982.
3. Lewis C.S.: *The Problem of Pain.* New York, MacMillan, 1973.
4. Sternbach R.A.: Strategies and tactics in the treatment of patients with pain, in *Pain and Suffering: Selected Aspects.* Springfield, Ill., Charles C Thomas, Publisher, 1970, pp. 176–185.
5. Merskey H.: *Psychology Aspects of Pain Relief: Relief of Intractable Pain.* Amsterdam, Excerpta Medica, 1971, pp. 90–115.
6. Melzack R., Torgerson W.S.: On the language of pain. *Anesthesiology* 34:50–59, 1971.
7. Black R.G., Chapman, C.R.: The SAD index for clinical assessment of pain, in Bonica J.J., Albe-Fessard D. (eds.): *Advances in Pain Research and Therapy.* New York, Raven Press, 1976, vol. 1, pp. 301–306.
8. Black R.G.: The chronic pain syndrome. *Surg. Clin. North Am.* 55(4):999–1011, 1975.
9. Sternbach R.A.: *Pain and Depression: Somatic Manifestations of Depressive Disorders.* Amsterdam, Excerpta Medica, 1974, pp. 107–119.
10. Sternbach R.A.: *Pain Patients: Traits and Treatment.* New York, Academic Press, 1974.
11. Black R.G.: *Use and Misuse of Medications in Chronic Pain Management.* Walter Reed Pain Symposium, 1979, in press.
12. Hendler H.N.: The psychopharmacology of chronic pain, in *Diagnosis and Medical Management of Chronic Pain.* New York, Raven Press, 1979, chap. 24.

13. Fordyce W.E.: *Behavior Methods for Chronic Pain and Illness*. St. Louis, C.V. Mosby Co., 1976.

14. Fordyce W.E.: The office management of chronic pain. *Minn. Med.* 57:185–188, 1974.

15. Fordyce W.E.: Treating chronic pain by contingency management. *Adv. Neurol.* 4:83–589, 1974.

16. Swerdlow M.: The pain clinic. *Br. J. Clin. Pract.* 26:403, 1972.

17. Woodford J.M., Fielding J.R.: Pain and cancer. *J. Psychosom. Res.* 14:365–370, 1970.

18. Foley K.M.: Pain syndromes in patients with cancer, in Bonica J.J., et al. (eds.): *Advances in Pain Research and Therapy*. New York, Raven Press, 1979, vol. 2.

19. Bonica J.J.: *The Management of Pain*. Philadelphia, Lea & Febiger, 1953.

14 / A Psychosomatic Approach to the Diagnosis of Chronic Pain

THOMAS OXMAN, M.D.

THE BIOMEDICAL MODEL of disease is a diagnostic obstacle to managing the chronic pain patient. It assumes that symptoms or illness are deviations from the norm of measurable, biologic variables.[1] When such deviation is not measurable, health professionals may be tempted mistakenly to diagnose functional (psychogenic) pain rather than organic pain.

Patterns of pain cannot be understood in purely physiologic terms. Pain is a subjective experience that signals actual or perceived injury, and the meaning of the injury plays a primary role in determining the severity of the pain response. Ninety years ago, Marshall[2] and Strong[3] proposed that suffering consisted of an initial sensation and a reaction to the sensation. In an impressive test of this hypothesis, Beecher[4] compared 150 civilians undergoing elective surgery with 150 soldiers wounded in battle. He found there was no relationship between the extent of a wound and the pain experienced. Only 32% of the military casualties requested narcotics, compared to 83% of the civilian group. The primary factor accounting for this difference was the psychological state of the soliders; they had just been relieved of the even greater pain of weeks of uninterrupted shell fire. An analogous finding was made by Peterson et al.[5] in a study of antacids and gastric ulcer. When measured by endoscopy, more ulcers were healed by antacids than placebos; however, there was no correlation of patient symptom report with healing or decrease in ulcer size. These examples suggest that whatever the immediate pathologic cause of the pain, psychological and social expectations are always involved.

The best framework for approaching management of chronic pain patients is a biopsychosocial model as proposed by psychosomatic medicine. The writings of Hippocrates demonstrate the Greeks' belief in the interaction of psychological and social factors with somatic factors: lower socioeconomic groups were reported to have more somatic complaints.[6] Although the word ''psychosomatic'' is of Greek origin, its modern scientific use is a 19th century German invention. The work of Freud and psychoanalysis is most often associated with the term psychosomatic as a symbolic conversion of psychological conflict into a somatic symptom. Nevertheless, Pavlov, Cannon, and Wolff broadened the concept to include careful empirical studies of the physiologic processes mediating a variety of psychosocial stresses.[7, 8] More recently Lipowski has attempted to clarify psychosomatic medicine as a discipline. In his view,[7, 9] psychosomatic medicine is a scientific discipline concerned with the interaction of biologic, psychological, and social variables that determine health and illness. Psychosomatic medicine is also a comprehensive or holistic approach to prevention, diagnosis, management, and rehabilitation. It is most closely associated with the clinical teaching and research activity of consultation-liaison psychiatry. Psychosomatic medicine is not the study of putative psychogenic causes of somatic disorders. The concept of a psychogenesis of somatic disorders is obsolete and has been replaced by the concept of multicausality of all physical and mental disorders.

Within this broad framework, psychosomatic medicine consists of several overlapping, useful approaches to assessing and managing the psychosocial aspects of chronic pain: operant conditioning; cognitive behavioral psychology; psychoanalysis (psychodynamics); and psychiatry.

OPERANT CONDITIONING

Behavioral psychology, which developed from Pavlov and learning theory, focuses on events preceding and following symptoms in order to change the symptoms; etiology is relatively unimportant.[9] Rather than seeking the identity of physical or psychological stimuli for pain behavior responses, operant conditioning looks at environmental antecedents and the consequences of pain behavior that reinforce pain. The investigative approach changes from "what causes the pain" to "what happens when the patient hurts and what happens when he does not." After observable positive and negative consequences in the patient's environment are identified, appropriate modification of those consequences is attempted. Common positive reinforcers of any pain behavior, regardless of etiology, are attention, rest, time out from stress, medication, and compensation. On the other hand, negative reinforcement commonly comes from chronic avoidance of postures or activities that only acutely resulted in pain. The positive and negative reinforcement of communicating pain occurs to some extent in all chronic pain patients and is usually not psychopathologic.

Behavioral psychology using operant conditioning is a different approach to disease than is the biomedical model or psychiatry. For example the medically trained psychiatrist employs eclectic neuropharmacologic, psychodynamic, and social theories of disease to devise hypotheses of etiology and treatment. Because of the identifiable methodologic approach of learning theory, some behaviorists view psychosomatic medicine as a broad area of interest rather than a discipline.[10] Nevertheless, the development of cognitive psychology and cognitive behavior therapy has resulted in a wider interdisciplinary collaboration of psychology, and psychiatry.

COGNITIVE BEHAVIOR THEORY

Cognitive behavior theory and therapy are based on the thesis that an individual's affect and behavior are largely determined by his subjective appraisal of events.[11-13] The cognitive approach differs from learning theory in that it emphasizes the patient's verbal or conscious attitudes and assumptions as well as observable behaviors. Although several psychoanalysts contributed important concepts to cognitive therapy,[14] cognitive therapy differs from the psychodynamic approach by not dealing with unconscious symbolic meanings.[11-13] Beecher's comparison of the difference in narcotic use between soldiers and civilians is an excellent example of cognitive theory.[4]

Cognitive behavioral psychology and consultation-liaison psychiatry have both promoted a theory of coping and adaptation that is relevant to chronic pain. Lipowski,[15] Moos and Tsu,[16] and others[17-19] have combined cognitive behavioral theory and crisis theory[20, 21] into a model of coping and adaptation. Crisis theory is concerned with how people deal with either disaster or major life transitions. Accordingly, it has both a threatening, negative component and a growth-promoting, positive aspect. In reference to the crisis of physical illness, Lipowski[15] has defined coping as "all cognitive and motor activities which a sick person employs to preserve his bodily and psychic integrity, to recover reversibly impaired function and compensate to the limit for any irreversible impairment . . . [which] may be evaluated as adaptive or maladaptive."

Moos and Tsu[16] have described seven major adaptive tasks of serious illness such as chronic pain: (1) dealing with pain and incapacitation, (2) dealing with the hospital (clinic) environment and special treatment procedures, (3) developing adequate relationships with professional staff, (4) preserving a reasonable emotional balance, (5) preserving a satisfactory self-image, (6) preserving relationships with family and friends, and (7) preparing for an uncertain future.

The adaptive or maladaptive manner in which any individual copes with these tasks is influenced by the meaning of the pain to the individual and the coping skills available to him. Both the meaning of pain and coping skills are determined by interaction with preexisting conditions which include personality style, stage of life, family style, and socioeconomic environment. For example, a person's cultural background influences his expression of pain. Families with strong and active Italian or Jewish heritage encourage the expression of pain while those with a strong and active Irish heritage encourage stoic acceptance of pain.[22, 23]

The stage of a person's life cycle[20, 24] should also be considered in understanding the meaning of the pain. For example, an adolescent already struggling with the body changes of puberty may have more difficulty with a physically deforming pain source than would a married middle-aged man. Similarly, a person's current life situation is an additional factor that influences the meaning of pain. A happy marriage, high job satisfaction, and a stable economic situation are factors that should promote adaptive coping.

Based on these factors and the particular cause of the pain, the meaning of the pain can be experienced as a challenge, an enemy, a punishment, a weakness, a relief, a leverage, an irreparable loss, or a virtue.[15]

PSYCHODYNAMICS

With the exception of a few specific psychiatric illnesses discussed below, pain is rarely initiated or maintained by psychological factors alone. Nevertheless, the description of personality structure derived from psychoanalysis is helpful in understanding a coping and adaptation model of illness and in working with pain patients. Psychologically normal persons have different personality styles that influence the way they perceive and respond to any stressful situation such as pain.

Normal personality styles can be classified in several different fashions. Kahana and Bibring,[25] for example, describe seven *normal* personality structures: (1) the dependent, (2) the orderly, controlled, (3) the dramatizing, emotional, captivating, (4) the self-sacrificing, (5) the guarded, querulous, (6) the superior feeling, and (7) the uninvolved, aloof. The stress of pain will exacerbate any of these personality structures. Recognizing these normal response styles sometimes guides the physician in planning and communicating diagnosis and treatment plans. For example, the dependent person requires warm support balanced with firm limits on undue reliance on the physician. The controlled person who habitually tries to order events in an attempt to master them will insist on detailed explanations and instructions. It is helpful to repeatedly offer such a patient just what he seeks. The dramatizing patient may present his symptoms in an attention-seeking manner and may be uninterested in explanations. It is usually helpful to respond to this type of patient by appreciating his courage and letting him express his fears while providing support with less detailed treatment explanations. The guarded person who is normally somewhat mistrustful may blame others, including his doctors, for his pain and suffering. With the guarded patient it is helpful to be scrupulously open and honest and to avoid vagueness or evasions.

At some point every clinician who treats chronic pain patients is likely to encounter some in whom psychological factors are actually the primary cause of intractable pain: psychogenic pain. Patients with psychogenic pain are described as having a long-standing ''pain-prone'' personality.[26, 27] This profile has been eloquently described by George Engel.[26] In this type of patient the psychodynamic approach again provides a useful theoretical model.

From earliest life human relations are related to pain and pain relief. Pain is one stimulus for crying, a signal that usually brings relief and comforting by the parent. Thus, crying often becomes the stimulus for obtaining comfort, with little correlation to the severity of the peripheral injury or source of pain. Pain is also early associated with punishment and thus guilt. According to Engel, this is often the crucial dynamic of the intractable pain-prone patient: pain becomes a welcomed expiation for guilt; pain is more bearable than guilt, and accordingly a relatively preferred state. The psychogenic pain patient will then experience himself as long-suffering and abused. Engel has described several family dynamics that can lead to this experience: (1) parents who were physically or verbally abusive, (2) a physically abusive alcoholic father and a submissive mother, (3) a parent who showed affection only by remorse after punishing the child, (4) cold distant parents who responded affectionately only when the child was sick, (5) a parent or close relation who suffered illness for which the child was made to feel responsible, either by family remarks or the child's own aggressive acts or fantasies toward the relative, and (6) a child who deflected and suffered aggression directed from one parent to the other. These background factors are usually revealed by the patient if asked.

The study of psychodynamics has also contributed to our understanding of the concept of ''compensation neurosis.'' In observing the dynamics of disability in compensation cases, Hirschfeld and Behan[28] described the concept of a predisposing dependent personality style. Paradoxically, it is extremely difficult for the disability-prone patient to acknowledge and seek help or fulfillment of dependency needs. At some point soon before an accident, tension and stress increase and are accompanied by a sense of disappointment, frustration, and lack of being appreciated. When an injury occurs in someone with these two conditions, the distress and sense of impairment become understandable and acceptable, the result of an external event that could happen to anybody. Prior to this, many may have performed excessively beyond average expectations as if atoning for guilt. When pain occurs they are able to become helpless sufferers, finally express long-denied needs, and be dependent and passive as the pain replaces work for atonement. As summarized by Weinstein, "the accident transforms an unacceptable emotional disability into an acceptable physical disability. With social and financial reinforcement, disability becomes a permanent way of life."[29]

Patients with a pain-prone personality or compensation neurosis are a heterogeneous group with a wide spectrum of severity. As described, these conditions are not considered specific psychiatric disorders. It must be emphasized that compensation neurosis does not entail malingering for financial gain. More important, the majority of patients with chronic pain do not have a pain-prone personality. Nevertheless, a precise diagnosis is important because the treatment of such patients is difficult and cure is unlikely. These patients are not good candidates for psychotherapy. Their pain symptom is a strong adaptive response and they are characteristically unable to recognize and talk about their conflicts. They are frustrating to physicians because they do not get better and, despite even obvious psychological conflicts, often refuse psychiatric referral.

PSYCHIATRIC DISORDERS

There are several psychiatric disorders associated with pain that will be encountered at one time or another: depression, somatoform disorders; anxiety disorders; factitious illness; schizophrenia; paranoia; and organic brain syndromes, especially dementia.

Primary and secondary depression are by far the commonest psychiatric disorders encountered. Patients with primary depressive illness often present to the primary care physician with a somatic complaint such as pain.[30] More common for the pain specialist is depression secondary to chronic pain.[31] This may be due to the psychological effect of suffering and/or changes in the serotonergic and noradrenergic neurotransmitter systems in common to both pain and depression. In either case, the pain specialist should ask all patients about the eight principal symptoms of depression (Table 14–1). Seventy percent of patients with four or five of these eight symptoms which have lasted longer than 2 weeks will respond to antidepressant drug treatment.[32] Early recognition is important to alleviate suffering and hasten recovery.

Somatoform disorders are a new classification in

TABLE 14–1.—DIAGNOSIS OF MAJOR DEPRESSIVE DISORDER

Two-week history of five or more of the following:

1. Depressed mood (sadness; crying; hopelessness; helplessness; guilt; low self-esteem; boredom)
2. Sleep disturbance (less total sleep, longer sleep latency, early A.M. awakening, midcycle awakening; less stage IV sleep, shorter REM latency)
3. Fatigue, loss of energy
4. Agitation or retardation (apprehension, dread, tension, somatization, panic)
5. Loss of interest in usually stimulating activities (job, hobbies, social, sexual)
6. Suicidal or death thoughts
7. Poor appetite or weight change; clothes fit differently
8. Decreased concentration or confused thinking

the *Diagnostic and Statistical Manual,* 3d edition *(DSM-III),* of the American Psychiatric Association.[33] Somatoform disorders include older concepts such as hysteria, conversion, hypochondriasis, and the pain-prone personality. However, unlike the older nebulous and stigmatizing terms, somatoform disorders now have specific definitions (Table 14–2). The underlying principles of these disorders are:

1. Physical symptoms that suggest a physical disorder.

2. No demonstrable organic findings or known physiolgic mechanisms.

3. Evidence of or presumption that the symptoms are associated with psychological factors.

4. Symptoms are *not* voluntarily controlled.

The prevalence of somatoform disorders varies from 0.2% to 7%, depending on the population studied and the method of diagnosis.[34] Prevalance at the higher range may be expected in the practice of a pain specialist. In 50% of patients with somatization, the presenting complaint is pain.[35]

There are several important reasons for diagnosing these disorders and for using the *DSM-III* criteria. First, physicians making the diagnosis of psychogenic pain should be aware there is a risk that patients thought to have psychogenic pain may have an unrecognized somatic disease that could explain the symptoms. This was the case in 47 of 277 patients (17%) given the diagnosis of conversion reaction in five follow-up studies compiled by Lazare.[36] Similarly, patients with organic disease can have conversion symptoms. It is not enough to "rule out organic disease." The physician also must establish the presence of psychosocial stress or conflict. A history of previous conversion reactions is also helpful. If there is evidence to make the diag-

TABLE 14–2.—DSM-III CRITERIA FOR SOMATOFORM DISORDERS

SOMATIZATION DISORDER

A. Physical symptoms
   Duration of several years
   Onset before age 30
B. Take medications other than aspirin, or change life-style, or see doctor for 14 (females) or 12 (males) of the following symptoms without substantial physical or laboratory findings:
   Difficulty swallowing
   Voice loss
   Double vision
   Blurred vision
   Blindness
   Fainting
   Memory loss
   Seizures
   Trouble walking
   Weakness, paralysis
   Urinary retention
   Abdominal pain
   Nausea
   Vomiting (not pregnant)
   Bloating, gas
   Multiple food intolerances
   Diarrhea
   Very painful menstruation
   Very irregular menstruation
   Increased bleeding with menstruation
   Excess vomiting with pregnancy
   Sexual indifference
   Lack pleasure with intercourse
   Pain with intercourse
   Back pain
   Joint pain
   Extremity pain
   Nonintercourse genital pain
   Pain with urination
   Other pain, except headache
   Shortness of breath
   Palpitations
   Chest pain
   Dizziness

PSYCHOGENIC PAIN

A. Severe and prolonged pain is predominant complaint
B. Pain is inconsistent with neuroanatomy or pain is much greater than pathophysiology
C. Psychological etiology:
   Onset with stimulus of conflict or need, or
   Pain allows avoiding noxious activity, or
   Pain gains environmental support not otherwise available
D. No other psychiatric disease
   Not tension headache

CONVERSION DISORDER

A. Loss or alteration in physical function suggests physical disorder
B. Evidence of psychological etiology:
   Onset with stimulus of conflict or need, or
   Avoid noxious activity, or
   Gain environmental support not otherwise available
C. Not under voluntary control
D. After physical examination and laboratory tests, no known organic explanation
E. Symptoms not limited to pain or sexual dysfunction

HYPOCHONDRIASIS

A. Preoccupation with having serious illness
   Unrealistic intepretation of physical signs/symptoms
B. Thorough physical exam negative for serious illness
C. Persists despite medical reassurance

nosis of somatization disorder by *DSM-III* criteria, it is unlikely that any other explanation for the symptom will develop.

Another important reason for using specific diagnostic criteria for psychiatric illness is that somatoform, depressive, and anxiety disorders may coexist or their symptoms may overlap. Somatic complaints such as fatigue, backache, or headache are often the initial symptoms of depression or anxiety. Conversely, patients with somatization disorder may develop depression or anxiety. Since the treatment for these three types of disorders differs, it is important to diagnose them appropriately.

Factitious illness and malingering are two other mental conditions that may present to the pain specialist and require specific diagnosis. Unlike somatoform disorders, both factitious illness and malingering entail conscious production of the symptom. In factitious illness there is no obvious gain from the symptom other than to be in the patient role. This bizarre situation is often entitled the Munchausen syndrome and is characterized by sustained, multiple hospitalizations. The patient with factitious illness will often have extensive medical knowledge and present a dramatic but vague history. Such individuals may inflict self-injury or undergo painful medical procedures even if dangerous. Although they are aware of their behavior, it has a compulsive, driven quality. Malingering is differentiated from factitious illness by the obvious secondary gain, such as money or shelter. It is not considered a mental disorder.

SPECIFIC METHODS OF PSYCHOSOMATIC INVESTIGATION

Clinical Interview

Each of the behavioral disciplines (psychiatry, psychodynamics, behaviorism, and cognitive psychology) lends itself to particular types of questions and observations that elicit psychosocial factors in chronic pain. These factors are useful in understanding the meaning of the pain in each patient's situation in order to plan the most specific type of treatment. By themselves, none of the four disciplines is comprehensive enough to help in the evaluation and treatment of a majority of pain patients. Because psychsomatic medicine and consultation-liaison psychiatry incorporate aspects of all four disciplines, a

psychosomatic approach is the most comprehensive for evaluation of the pain patient. Using a psychosomatic approach, biologic, psychological, and social factors can be ordered by priority for treatment with one or more of the appropriate disciplines. Ideally a consultation-liaison psychiatrist (proficient in general psychiatry, psychopharmacology, and cognitive psychology) and a clinical psychologist (proficient in cognitive behavior therapy, relaxation training, and recognition of depressive disorders) should be available to the pain specialist.

Figure 14–1 reviews and illustrates the major components of a psychosomatic approach to the evaluation of pain. The information in this model is useful to assess the degree of potential for an adaptive, positive outcome and for planning the major emphasis of treatment. Most of the necessary information can normally be obtained in standard history and clinical interview with the patient and family members. Referral to a mental health professional is not necessarily indicated if the clinician is willing to conceptualize and organize the clinical data using such a model.

The mental status examination is an essential part

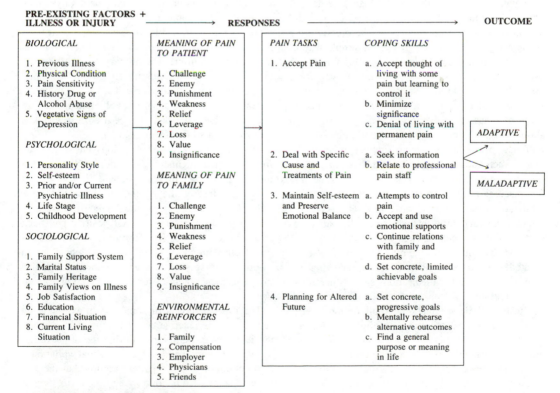

Fig 14–1.—A psychosomatic approach for the evaluation of chronic pain. (Adapted from Lipowski[15, 17] and Moos and Tsu.[16])

of the medical history and examination. Major depressive illness, delirium, and somatoform disorders are the psychiatric disorders most likely to be encountered. Special care should be taken to elicit a history of the eight signs of depression listed in Table 14–1. At least 10% of chronic pain patients have a treatable depressive illness.[31] Somatic complaints, including pain, are also frequently the presenting complaint of depressive illness in primary care.[30, 35] Since most patients are seen by other physicians before referral to pain specialists, undiagnosed depressive illness is less common in referred patients. Nevertheless, the pain specialist should always be aware of possible depression. Furthermore, susceptible individuals living with chronic pain can develop depressive illness. Distinguishing endogenous from reactive depression is less important than evaluating the eight signs of depression. The examiner should use persistent questioning when the initial response is negative. For example, rather than just asking "How do you sleep," it is useful to ask for additional details: "What time do you go to bed? How long does it take you to fall asleep? How many times do you wake up at night? How long does it take you to fall back to sleep? What time do you get up? How tired are you upon arising? How would you have answered these questions before suffering chronic pain?" Serial weights are a simple way to evaluate appetite and food intake. Questions such as, "Does food taste good to you? Do you force yourself to eat? Do you eat when you are nervous? Do your clothes fit differently?" are more specific ways of assessing appetite changes. The physician should also periodically ask about hopelessness, thoughts of giving up, and suicidal thoughts or plans. Such questioning does not induce suicide and has great preventive value because it opens the way for discussion, appropriate pharmacotherapy, hospitalization, and/or psychiatric referral. Decreased interest and concentration are assessed by patient report as well as checking cognitive function.

Some assessment of cognitive function is also indicated, especially in elderly patients receiving one or more psychotropic medications such as narcotics, antidepressants, or benzodiazepines. Quick screening tests include orientation, recall of three unrelated words after 3 minutes, and digit span forward and backward. A person who is not mentally retarded and cannot repeat a series of five digits forward and three digits in reverse should be presumed to have an organic brain syndrome (e.g., delirium or dementia) until proved otherwise. Reduction of medications and/or further investigation is indicated.

Table 14–3 lists several questions useful for eliciting psychosocial factors that lead to amplified pain sensations or are indicative of a somatoform disorder (somatization disorder, psychogenic pain, or hypochondriasis). This line of questioning generally assumes that the pain symptom is not feigned or voluntary (malingering or factitious illness). Such knowledge is not always easy to come by. Generally, malingerers will not submit to painful procedures in order to obtain their obvious goal, their symptoms are not presented in the context of emotional conflict, and they obtain no pain relief from suggestion, hypnosis, or intravenous barbiturates. Patients with a factitious disorder will often have: (1) a history of numerous hospitalizations, frequently in multiple cities; (2) extensive knowledge of medical terms and hospital routines; (3) a history of substance abuse; and (4) a psychological connection to the medical profession (e.g., a grudge, an important family member who is a physician, prior employment in the medical field).

If the pain specialist judges a pain symptom to be involuntary and excessive in relation to known somatic disease, then amplification of pain can be viewed on a continuum between a neurophysiologic personality trait and a somatoform disorder. The more questions in Table 14–3 that are clearly answered in the affirmative, the more likely it is that the patient is suffering a primary somatoform disorder rather than secondarily amplifying a primary pain complaint. In either case, the physician-patient interaction will be of primary therapeutic consequence. Table 14–2 can also be used as a checklist to diagnose a somatoform disorder.

In addition to gathering biopsychosocial data from the medical history, questioning for environmental reinforcers of pain behavior is useful. Following Fordyce et al.,[37–39] the series of questions in Table 14–4 helps to assess the degree of the reactive component to pain and to elicit positive and negative pain reinforcers. It is fruitful to ask these questions both with and without family members present in order to assess the degree of reinforcement they give and their potential for change with simple education.

The time pattern is of some use in assessing the severity of the reactive component of pain. Usually the intensity of pain varies during the day with activity, distraction, and mood. Seasonal variation is also common. When a patient reports that the pain never changes from hour to hour, day to day, or season to season, that nothing helps and it is only getting worse, then the clinician should consider

TABLE 14–3.—QUESTIONS FOR IDENTIFYING PSYCHOSOCIAL CONDITIONS LEADING TO AMPLIFIED PAIN SENSATIONS

CHILDHOOD EXPERIENCES

1. Did the patient grow up with a parent who had chronic illness that affected family life?
2. Did the patient grow up with sick siblings who received special attention?
3. Did the family discourage or encourage the expression of affect (anger, crying) other than when ill?
4. Does the patient feel he had an unhappy childhood or was there a history of abuse by (verbal, physical, sexual) or alcoholism in the parents?
5. Did the patient see the doctor frequently or was he sickly?

MEANING OF THE PAIN

6. What worries the patient most about the pain?
7. Are there important persons in the patient's life who may have suffered a similar pain or illness?
8. Are there any recent losses, gains, defeats, or successes occurring near the onset of the pain? Any changes at home or work?
9. Does the onset of the pain coincide with any important anniversaries?
10. Does the patient wonder why this is happening to him? Does he come up with reasons, particularly associated with guilt? Are guilty feelings a prominent aspect of the patient's life experience?

QUESTIONS SUGGESTIVE OF SOMATOFORM DISORDERS

11. Does the pain allow the patient to avoid some noxious activity?
12. Does the patient gain support not otherwise available from the environment?
13. Is the pain symptom involuntary?
14. Is the pain inconsistent with known neuroanatomy or in excess of the illness or injury?
15. Does the patient have a chronic history of numerous unexplained physical symptoms, beginning before age 30, for which the patient frequently visited one or more physicians?
16. Is it difficult to get the patient to talk about anything other than his medical status?
17. Is the patient absolutely convinced he is ill and emotions play no role at all?
18. Does the patient report negative therapeutic responses and disparage prior physicians?
19. Is it hard for the patient to believe the physician when he says the *cause* of the pain is nothing serious to worry about? Does the patient often worry that he has a serious (life-threatening) illness?
20. If a disease is brought to the attention of the patient (by radio, television, newspapers, other people), does he worry that he has it?

that psychological factors may be far more important than somatic factors. Sometimes this line of questioning elicits responses of uniqueness such as "this must be the worst pain you've had to treat" or "nobody has ever experienced such a pain."

TABLE 14–4.—PAIN INTERVIEW: ENVIRONMENTAL REINFORCERS

1. *Time Pattern*
   a. Sleep: Does the pain awake you from sleep? How often? Does falling asleep alleviate the pain?
   b. Calendar: Do changes in the seasons affect your pain?
   c. Trend: What is the overall trend of your pain (better, worse, same, varies)?
2. *Pain Behavior:* How would I know if you were in pain? How does your family know? What is their response? How do friends know? How do co-workers, employers know? What are their responses?
3. *Pain Activators:* Which activities bring on or exacerbate pain, according to the patient? What is the value of these activities to the patient? Which activities induce or exacerbate pain according to the family? What do they perceive the value of these activities to be? Does the patient push himself to his limits frequently? How does he take his medications, as needed or fixed schedule? Does tension increase pain?
4. *Pain Diminishers:* Which activities decrease pain, according to the patient and/or family? What is the value of these activities to the patient? Is patient aware of relaxation reducing pain?
5. *Changes in Routines:* What changes in patient activity have occurred (e.g., job loss, hobbies increase)? What changes in family life have occurred (e.g., wife must return to work, decreased fighting)?

This sense of singularity is another sign of an important psychological component and should initiate search for features of the pain-prone personality.

Questions regarding pain behavior, pain activators, and pain diminishers are useful in assessing positive and negative reinforcers of pain behavior. Guarding and "overreacting" may be learned responses that continue only because they earlier successfully avoided the punishment of activities which used to but no longer would cause pain. A patient may also reveal his pain more to those who give attention, such as family or physicians, rather than to employers, or vice versa. If a patient displays more grimacing or pain complaints in the presence of family or when particular family members are mentioned, interpersonal relations may be an important psychological factor. If family members are to change their reinforcement, they will be aided by knowing the first signs a patient uses to convey his pain.

Activities that induce pain can include specific physical activity such as lifting or vacuuming. Stress or conflict with specific people or agencies can also induce pain. Psychological factors or malingering may be operative if low value activities (such as an unpleasant job) induce pain but high value activities with equivalent physical exertion (such as hobbies or sports) do not. Pleasant or positive reinforcers of pain behavior include rest, drugs, compensation, and removal from stress. Changes in routines are important in assessing the impact on the family. Spouses who must reluctantly return to work are an indication for early family involvement in therapy. Marriages with preexisting conflicts may result in divorce at this point. A genuinely supportive and accepting family bodes a more favorable prognosis.

Planning cognitive therapy is aided by assessing which coping skills are indicated and how well they are employed. In conjunction with the adaptive tasks of illness, Moos and Tsu also delineated seven types of coping skills.[16] As shown in Table 14–3, these types can be consolidated and specifically applied to chronic pain. The first group consists of a continuum of emotional and cognitive acceptance of pain. This can range from a constructive minimization to delusional denial. The time course of the pain is important in assessing the use of this group of skills. Early in an illness causing pain, such as a myocardial infarction or a burn, it may be protective for the patient to suppress the seriousness and chronicity of pain. Later in an illness such as cancer or irreparable herniated disks, it can be pathologic and dangerous. The second set of skills includes relating to professional staff and seeking relevant information and using it appropriately. For example, someone with migraine headache might seek a physician who would appropriately explain the complex pathophysiology and the potential roles of stress and diet. The individual would then use this information to modify his life-style without excessively constricting his life. Other types of pain information include learning specific procedures such as operating a transcutaneous electrical nerve stimulator, a proper exercise program, recordkeeping, and the appropriate use of medication. The third group of coping skills includes requesting reassurance and emotional support. A patient with chronic pain frequently becomes frustrated and loses self-esteem. It is necessary for the pain patient to be able to discuss and display feelings with family and professionals rather than withdrawing. This group of skills also includes setting and attempting concrete, limited goals. Achievement of goals boosts self-esteem and setting a series of smaller goals allows for increased chances of success compared to a larger goal. Careful planning can center on gradually increasing exercise tolerance, initial return to part time work, and a gradual increase in socialization.

Stepwise, concrete planning helps prevent disappointments and setbacks. The fourth group of skills, rehearsing alternative outcomes, overlaps with the third group and is indicated when irreversible life changes are required. When it is clear that permanent damage and pain will prevent return to certain jobs or activities, it is beneficial to imagine and anticipate the disappointment and necessary changes. In conjunction with recalling prior successful adaptation, mental rehearsal can increase rehabilitation success. This group of coping skills can incorporate finding a general purpose or meaning in life. A renewed purpose may come from increased religious activity or devotion to family. A meaning for life can palliate the pain resulting from losses and encourage one to do one's best in a difficult situation.

To illustrate many of the types of analyses discussed above, the following case history is outlined in Figure 14–2 according to a psychosomatic approach for chronic pain evaluation.

A 36-year-old married man was referred to the University of Cincinnati Pain Control Center for chronic left upper extremity pain following traumatic amputation of three fingers on his left hand. His hand was caught in a lawn mower while working as a groundskeeper 5 years prior to his initial evaluation at the Pain Control Center. He had been hospitalized six times for surgical repair and skin grafting. His left hand demonstrated evidence of advanced reflex sympathetic dystrophy. He was hostile toward and suspicious of the Pain Control Center staff, resulting in his leaving the hospital before completion of a continuous brachial plexus infusion of marcaine. He had taken acetaminophen and codeine (120 mg) every 4–6 hours for 3 years, but complained that nothing really gave him relief of pain. He believed the pain was not only getting worse but actually, like a poison, spreading up his arm to eventually kill him. He displayed obvious physical discomfort on any procedures or examinations. He reported side effects to numerous medications, including antidepressants, even at low doses. He had not suffered or complained of major somatic symptoms prior to his injury.

He had been treated for depression once prior to the injury. At the time of psychosomatic evaluation, he reported marked depression with crying, sadness, helplessness, insomnia, anorexia, and passive suicidal ideation. Despite living with the pain for 5 years, he still believed something could be done to eliminate it totally, but the doctors were not telling him what it was.

The patient had been employed on his job only 3 months prior to his accident. He refused to release the employer from liability and the employer had

PRE-EXISTING FACTORS + INJURY
(Left hand caught in lawn mower at work)

RESPONSE

BIOLOGICAL

1. Amputation of fingers and scarring of skin grafts
2. High pain sensitivity
3. Narcotic abuse
4. Right handed

PSYCHOLOGICAL

1. Guarded, querulous, and hostile personality style
2. Low self-esteem from narcotics, job failures and body image
3. Treated for depression during divorce prior to injury
4. Fatherhood

SOCIOLOGICAL

1. Comes from family of nine children with history of psychiatric treatment
2. Brother died of cancer, age 36, on excess drugs
3. Mother ill with diabetes and arteriosclerotic vascular disease but also with somatization
4. Unemployed on disability, facing bankruptcy
5. Living in small trailer with pregnant wife, two children from first marriage, one child from second marriage
6. Some college education but only one in family to do so

↔

MEANING OF PAIN TO PATIENT

1. Enemy-conscious meaning
2. Weakness as a man-unconscious meaning
3. Relief from job failures-unconscious meaning

MEANING OF PAIN TO FAMILY

1. Weakness in patient
2. Loss of income

ENVIRONMENTAL REINFORCERS

Positive:
 1. Narcotics
 2. Compensation
Negative:
 3. No possible increase in disability payments despite inflation

↔

PAIN TASKS

1. Does not accept

2. Is not dealing with specific illness and therapy
3. Is not maintaining self-esteem and emotional balance
4. Is not planning for an altered future

COPING SKILLS

—Is using denial, wants total relief

—Does not trust physicians, will not stay in hospital

—Depressed
—Physical fights with wife

—Unrealistic general goal of immediate, high paying job
—No specific concrete goals
—Does use care of all his children as his general purpose in life

Fig 14–2.—Example of a psychosomatic analysis of a chronic pain patient.

refused to give him alternative employment following his accident. He was given total, permanent disability payments by the state as a result of his injury. He met his second wife while hospitalized following his injury. After they were married he obtained custody of two children from his first marriage because his ex-wife abandoned them. He and his second wife had a 2-year-old son, and she was pregnant again. She had to return to work full time yet still prepare dinner and help clean house. The patient did what he could around the house; however, his wife had little tolerance for his pain complaints and disability. She accused him of being a drug abuser and they had physical fights on occasion. They lived in a three-room trailer. Despite her salary and his disability payments they were considering bankruptcy proceedings to meet the demands of their creditors.

Elicitation of the patient's family history revealed that he was the third of nine children. His father died of cancer at age 55. His brother died of cancer at age 36, accompanied by prolonged drug abuse. His mother had been a chronic somatizer but also suffered from end-stage vascular complications of diabetes. His family ridiculed him for being the only one of his siblings with any college eduction yet failing to maintain any job for more than 1 year.

As can be gathered from this brief history, the patient presented with a poor prognosis and few psychosocial assets. Nevertheless, by arranging the multiple factors using a biopsychosocial and coping model (see Fig 14–2), three advantages were gained. First, the overwhelming number of factors were made more understandable by organizing them. Second, the organization made it easier to understand the patient's situation and decrease negative feelings toward him. Third, it became easier to set priorities of treatment. The first priority was establishing a trusting relationship, because of the negative effects of his guarded personality style. Although narcotic abuse and his desire for total pain relief were major problems, to confront them immediately without trust seemed fruitless. Immediate involvement with the wife also was indicated because of the physical abuse and the conflicting meanings of the pain to the couple. Two self-esteem bolstering factors that were identified for future exploration were his desire for education and the pride he took in fatherhood.

This example and the psychosomatic approach in general both make use of all four of the behavioral sciences discussed. A behavioral modification analysis was considered in assessing social and family reinforcement for pain behavior. A cognitive approach was of importance in understanding and planning modification of the meaning of the pain to the patient and the coping skills he was currently employing to deal with the meaning. A psychodynamic approach was necessary in recognizing both the effects of personality style and also the difference between the conscious and unconscious meanings of the pain. A psychiatric approach was required to diagnose depressive illness and narcotic abuse. This combined psychosomatic approach resulted in appropriate treatment, as evidenced by the outcome: 16 months after initial evaluation, the patient was trusting the staff of the Pain Control Center, showing no hostility, had discontinued all narcotics, was taking antidepressants, had improved communication with his wife, and was beginning a new job with an acknowledgment of the possibility of failing but the need to keep trying.

REFERENCES

1. Engel G.L.: The need for a new medical model: A challenge for biomedicine. *Science* 196:129–136, 1977.
2. Marshall H.R.: *Pain, Pleasure, and Aesthetic.* London, Macmillan Publishing Co., 1894, p. 30.
3. Strong C.A.: The psychology of pain. *Psychol. Rev.* 2:329–347, 1895.
4. Beecher H.K.: Relationship of significance of wound to pain experienced. *JAMA* 161:1609–1613, 1956.
5. Peterson W.L., Sturdevant A.L., Frank L.H.D., et al.: Healing of duodenal ulcer with an antacid regimen. *N. Engl. J. Med.* 297:341–345, 1977.
6. Lowy F.H.: Management of the persistent somatizer, in Lipowski Z.J., Lipsitt D.R., Whybrow P.C. (eds.): *Psychosomatic Medicine: Current Trends and Clinical Applications.* New York, Oxford University Press, 1977, pp. 510–522.
7. Lipowski Z.J.: Review of consultation psychiatry and psychosomatic medicine: I. General Principles. *Psychosom. Med.* 29:153–171, 1967.
8. Lipowski Z.J.: Psychosomatic medicine in the seventies: An overview. *Am. J. Psychiatry* 134:233–244, 1977.
9. Lipowski Z.J., Morgan C.D.: Psychosomatic and behavioral medicine and liaison psychiatry: New trends in research and clinical applications, in Manschreck (ed.): *Psychiatric Medicine Update: Mass. General Hospital Reviews for Physicians.* New York, Elsevier, 1979, pp. 3–22.
10. Pomerleau O.F., Brady J.P.: Introduction: The scope and promise of behavioral medicine, in Pomerleau O.F., Brady J.P. (eds.): *Behavioral Medicine: Theory and Practice.* Baltimore, Williams & Wilkins Co., 1979, pp. xi–xxvi.
11. Lazarus R.S.: *Psychological Stress and the Coping Process.* New York, McGraw-Hill Book Co., 1966.
12. Lazarus R.S.: Psychological stress and coping in adaptation and illness. *Int. J. Psychiatry Med.* 5:321–333, 1977.
13. Turk O.C.: Cognitive behavioral techniques in the management of pain, in Foreyt J.P., Rathjin D.P. (eds.): *Cognitive Behavior Therapy: Research and Applications.* New York, Plenum Press, 1978, pp. 199–232.
14. Beck A.T., Rush A.J., Shaw B.F., et al.: *Cognitive Therapy of Depression.* New York, Guilford Press, 1979, pp. 1–33, 61–86.
15. Lipowski Z.J.: Physical illness, the individual, and the coping process. *Psychiatry Med.* 1:90–102, 1970.
16. Moos R.H., Tsu V.D.: The crisis of physical illness: An overview, in Moos R.H. (ed.): *Coping with Physical Illness.* New York, Plenum Medical Book Co., 1977, pp. 3–21.

17. Lipowski Z.J.: Psychosocial aspects of disease. *Ann. Intern. Med.* 71:1197–1206, 1969.
18. Mechanic D.: Illness behavior, social adaptation, and the management of illness. *J. Nerv. Ment. Dis.* 165:79–87, 1977.
19. Coelho G.V. (ed.): *Coping and Adaptation: A Behavioral Sciences Bibliography.* Chevy Chase, Md., National Institute of Mental Health, 1969.
20. Erikson E.H.: *Childhood and Society,* ed. 2. New York, W.W. Norton, 1963.
21. Caplan G.: *Principles of Preventative Psychiatry.* New York, Basic Books, 1964.
22. Sternbach R.A.: Psychophysiology of pain. *Int. J. Psychiatry Med.* 6:63–73, 1975.
23. Zola I.K.: Culture and symptoms: An analysis of patients' presenting complaints. *Am. Soc. Rev.* 31:615–620, 1966.
24. Levinson O.J.: *The Seasons of a Man's Life.* New York, Ballantine Books, 1978.
25. Kahana R.J., Bibring G.L.: *Psychiatry and Medical Practice in a General Hospital.* New York, International University Press, 1964, pp. 108–123.
26. Engel G.L.: "Psychogenic" pain and the pain-prone patient. *Am. J. Med.* 26:899–918, 1959.
27. Blumer D., Heilbronn M.: The pain-prone disorder: A clinical and psychological profile. *Psychosomatics* 22:395–402, 1981.
28. Hirschfeld A.H., Behan R.C.: The accident process: III. Disability: acceptable and unacceptable. *JAMA* 197:85–89, 1966.
29. Weinstein M.R.: The concept of the disability process. *Psychosomatics* 19:94–97, 1978.
30. Cadoret R.J., Widmer R.B., Troughton E.P.: Somatic complaints: Harbinger of depression in primary care. *J. Affective Disord.* 2:61–70, 1980.
31. Pilowski I., Chapman C.R., Bonica J.J.: Pain, depression, and illness behavior in a pain clinic population. *Pain* 4:183–192, 1977.
32. Cassem N.H.: Depression, in Hackett T.P., Cassem N.H. (eds.): *Massachusetts General Hospital Handbook of General Hospital Psychiatry.* St. Louis, C.V. Mosby Co., 1978, pp. 209–225.
33. American Psychiatric Association: *Diagnostic and Statistical Manual,* ed. 3. Washington, D.C., American Psychiatric Association, 1980.
34. Coryell W.: Diagnosis specific mortality: Primary unipolar depression and Briquet's syndrome (somatization disorder). *Arch. Gen. Psychiatry* 38:939–942, 1981.
35. Kenyon F.E.: Hypochondriacal states. *Br. J. Psychiatry* 129:1–14, 1976.
36. Lazare A.: Hysteria, in Hackett T.P., Cassem N.H. (eds.): *Massachusetts General Hospital Handbook of General Hospital Psychiatry.* St. Louis, C.V. Mosby Co., 1978, pp. 117–140.
37. Fordyce W.E., Fowler R.S., Lehmann J.F., et al.: Operant conditioning in the treatment of chronic pain. *Arch. Phys. Med. Rehabil.* 54:399–408, 1973.
38. Fordyce W.E.: Pain viewed as learned behavior. *Adv. Neurol.* 4:415–422, 1974.
39. Fordyce W.E.: Treating chronic pain by contingency management. *Adv. Neurol.* 4:583–589, 1974.

15 / Investigations

15A / Electromyography

SARJIT SINGH, M.D.
LALIGAM N. SEKHAR, M.D.

THE HISTORY of electrodiagnosis can be traced to Erb,[1] who studied electrical reaction of muscle on a completely denervated muscle. Piper,[2] using a string galvanometer, recorded voluntary muscle contractions in the forearm flexor of a man. However, clinical electromyography (EMG) was introduced by Denny-Brown and Pennybaker[3] using bipolar needle electrodes for recording motor unit action potentials. In the 1950s, with the introduction of measurement of motor nerve conduction velocities[4, 5] and subsequently sensory nerve conduction velocities,[6] interest reverted to the study of peripheral nerve and spinal cord disorders.

The introduction of digital computers for extracting small biogenic signals from ''noise'' and for carrying out very complete statistical analysis has made electrodiagnostic procedures more rewarding in the clinical evaluation of peripheral nerve, muscle, and spinal cord disorders. In addition to conventional methods of recording motor and sensory conduction velocities, and EMG studies, it is important to study two late responses, the F response and the H response.

In the last decade, introduction of short-latency, somatosensory evoked potential (SSEP) studies made it possible to evaluate central conduction pathways, thus improving the diagnostic workup of patients with peripheral nerve and spinal cord lesions.

Electrodiagnostic methods can be very useful in evaluating the cause of painful disorders, particularly those due to radicular and peripheral nerve–related processes. In this chapter, particular atten-

tion will be paid to EMG, motor conduction studies, and sensory conduction studies. Evoked potential recording and other sophisticated studies such as the F response and the H response are mentioned briefly.

The study of electrical activity of contracting muscle provides information concerning the structure and function of motor units. The nerve fibers that supply the muscle are extensions of anterior horn cells and give off terminal branches that supply a large number of muscle fibers. The nerve cell and the muscle fibers it supplies are called the motor unit. When the fibers of a motor unit are activated, the muscle fibers contract and their action potentials summate so that a relatively large complex potential, known as the motor unit action potential, can be recorded. EMG is a technique by which the action potentials of contracting muscle fibers and a motor unit are recorded and displayed.

EMG APPARATUS AND TECHNIQUE

A capacitor-coupled amplifier and a cathode ray oscilloscope are the basic instruments. Electrical changes recorded by the electrodes represent voltages from a few microvolts to more than 10 mV, and these must be amplified before they can be displayed for analysis. In clinical practice, the ear can identify certain EMG features more readily than the eye, so it is of value to have an auditory record of potential changes amplified through a loudspeaker. Permanent records may be made directly with a camera, or the data may be stored on magnetic tape.

In clinical practice, muscle action potentials are usually recorded by extracellular electrodes placed in close proximity to the muscle fibers. There are several varieties of recording electrodes in common use. When large volumes of muscles are to be sampled, small metal disk electrodes may be used. The most commonly used electrodes are the concentric or coaxial type of needle electrode. Such electrodes are satisfactory for most purposes and they record activity within a few cubic millimeters with good reliability.

Sterilization of needle electrodes by heat, gas, or liquid germicide reduces the risk of infection.

The electrode is inserted through the skin and into the muscle with the limb relaxed. During insertion, the presence or absence of excessive insertion activity is recorded. A search is then made in different parts of the relaxed muscle for spontaneous electrical activity. After the patient contracts the muscle voluntarily, the motor unit potentials during different grades of voluntary contraction are observed with the electrode at different sites within the muscle (Fig 15A–1).

Normally, resting muscle is electrically silent. If the recording needle electrode is placed near the motor end-plate, potentials can be recorded from the normal resting muscle ("end-plate noise"); these potentials consist mainly of miniature end-plate potentials (MEPPs) and must be distinguished from fibrillation potentials.

ABNORMAL FINDINGS ON EMG

Insertional Activity

When the needle is inserted into the muscle, there is usually a brief burst of action potentials (Fig 15A–2) which ceases when the needle is stable. Increased insertional activity is seen in all forms of denervation as well as in polymyositis.

Fibrillation Potentials

These are small potentials, most commonly 0.5–2 msec in duration and having an amplitude of 30–100 mV (Fig 15A–3). Fibrillation is the contraction of a single muscle fiber and appears when the muscle fiber has lost its nerve supply. Fibrillation potentials may be seen in certain primary muscle diseases such as polymositis or occasionally in dystrophy. Fibrillation potentials recorded in patients with peripheral nerve or spinal root injuries suggest denervation and will continue until the muscle fiber is reinnervated.

Positive Sharp Waves

These potentials are larger than fibrillation potentials and consist initially of a positive spike followed by a slow change of potential in a negative direction

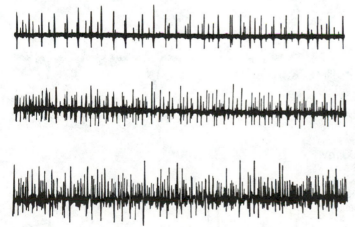

Fig 15A–1.—Interference patterns. *Top,* the pattern recorded from a single motor unit. With increased effort, the frequency of the discharge increases and additional units are recruited *(middle* and *bottom).*

$\overline{}$1mV

200 msec   +

$\longmapsto$

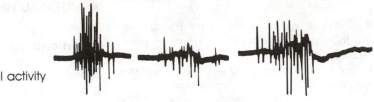

Fig 15A–2.—Insertional activity in normal muscle.

1mV

100msec +

(see Fig 15A–3). The total duration may be greater than 10 msec. These positive sharp waves probably arise from the fiber that has been damaged by the recording needle electrode.

Fasciculations

Fasciculations are spontaneous contractions of a group of muscle fibers or of motor units large enough to produce visible contractions of muscle without involving movement at the joint. Fasciculations may occur in healthy subjects and in patients with conditions affecting the lower motor neuron and irritation of the nerve roots. They are of much more significance when they occur in slowly advancing destructive disease of the anterior horn cells, such as amyotrophic lateral sclerosis and progressive spinal muscular atrophy (see Fig 15A–

3,B). They are seen often in early stages of poliomyelitis. They are also seen in compressive anterior nerve root lesions secondary to herniation of the nucleus pulposus and spondylosis.

Diseases such as polymyositis, muscular dystrophy, and other myopathies reduce the population of fibers per motor unit and thereby produce a potential of lower voltage and shorter duration. Diseases that reduce the population of functional motor neurons or of axons within the peripheral nerve decrease the number of motor units that can be recruited in affected muscle.

MOTOR NERVE CONDUCTION STUDIES

Techniques are now available for percutaneous stimulation of peripheral nerve and for recording

A

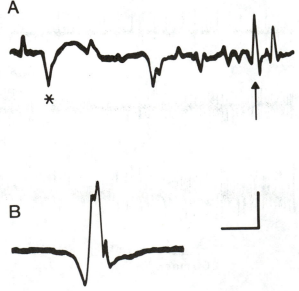

Fig 15A–3.—Fibrillations and positive sharp waves. **A,** the recording from a denervated muscle. The activity is spontaneous, and no interference pattern could be produced by voluntary effort. Fibrillations *(arrow)* are 1–2 msec in duration and 50–200 mV in amplitude. A positive sharp wave (mainly positive) is indicated by the *asterisk.* **B,** fasciculation recorded from a patient with amyotrophic lateral sclerosis.

*

B

muscle action potentials when a motor nerve is stimulated and nerve action potentials when a sensory nerve is stimulated. The study of sensory and motor nerve conduction velocities provide is useful in the recognition and accurate localization of peripheral nerve pathology, including the peripheral nerve entrapments. The motor nerve is stimulated at two points along its course and the evoked potentials from the muscle it supplies are recorded. The nerve conduction velocity is calculated by dividing the distance in centimeters between the two points by the time difference in milliseconds between the proximal and distal latencies (Fig 15A–4).

Nerve conduction velocities in a normal subject vary from a minimum of 40–45 meters per second (m/sec) to a maximum of 70–90 m/sec, depending on which nerve is studied. Values are lower in infants, reaching the adult range by the age of 2–4 years (Table 15A–1).

Apparatus

In nerve conduction measurements, the potential detected from the muscle or the nerves is evoked by nerve stimulation. Rectangular pulse generators are the most common type of stimulators used because the amplitude and duration of rectangular pulses can be easily changed and measured. The stimulator is capable of delivering voltages up to 150 V in amplitude at a duration of 0.1–3 msec with a variable frequency. The evoked potentials in the muscle can be recorded either with a concentric needle or with a surface electrode.

The commonly used electrode in motor nerve conduction studies is the surface electrode, consisting of a small disk about 1 cm in diameter made of stainless steel or silver that is covered with electrode jelly and applied to the skin. In usual practice, two electrodes are used, one applied over the belly of the muscle and the other over the tendon. Evoked sensory potentials are recorded with ring or disk electrodes. Needle electrodes have been used for sensory nerve conduction studies; this increases the amplitude of potentials.

Technique

Motor nerve conduction velocity measurement entails stimulating a nerve at one point and recording the response either at the muscle or at some distance along the nerve. The former applies to motor nerve and the latter to sensory nerve conduction studies. Motor nerve conduction studies can be carried out on nerves accessible to stimulation. In the

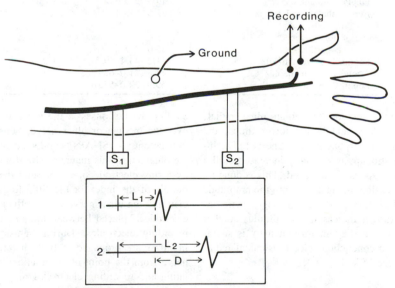

Fig 15A–4.—Determination of motor conduction velocity. The median nerve is stimulated at two points, S_1 and S_2. The distal latency (L) is the time from application of the stimulus to the onset of the action potential. It represents the time taken for conduction over the distance A_1 and through the neuromuscular junction. The motor conduction velocity is given by the equation $\frac{L_2 - L_1}{D}$.

TABLE 15A–1.—Normal Motor Conduction Velocity
and Distal Latency

SEGMENT	VELOCITY (Meters/sec)	LATENCY (msec)
Ulnar nerve		
Axilla–wrist	60.0 (56.0–62.7)	2.8 (2.3–3.4)
Axilla–elbow	63.4 (SD 5.3)	
Elbow–wrist	56.4 (SD 4.8)	2.6 (2.0–3.4)
Axilla–wrist	59.4 (SD 4.1)	
Median nerve		
Axilla–antecubital fossa	7.1 (60.3–86.4)	3.3 (2.8–4.2)
Antecubital fossa–wrist	60.1 (54.3–65.0)	
Axilla–wrist	64.3 (59.8–70.4)	
Axilla–elbow	67.9 (SD 7.7)	
Elbow–wrist	57.0 (SD 5.0)	3.9 (SD 0.4)
Radial nerve		
Erb's point–above elbow	72.0 (56–93)	
Above elbow–distal forearm	61.6 (48–75)	
Elbow–forearm	62.0 (SD 5.1)	2.4 (SD 0.5)
Suprascapular nerve		
Erb's point–supraspinatus		2.6 ± 0.3
Erb's point–infraspinatus		3.4 + 0.4
Femoral nerve		
Above inguinal ligament–vastus Medialis		6.1–8.4
Below inguinal ligament–vastus Medialis		5.5–7.5
Below inguinal ligament–rectus Femoris		5.5 ± 0.5
Peroneal nerve		
Fibula head–ankle	49.5 ± 5.6	5.1 (SD 0.5)
Across fibular head–tib. anterior	62.6 ± 3.4	
Posterior tibial nerve		
In thigh–gastrocnemius	56.0 ± 5.6	
Popliteal–above malleolus	51.2 (43.4–59.5)	2.1–5.6
Above–below malleolus	44.8 (21.0–67.0)	
Popliteal–medial malleolus	49.9 (37.0–57.0)	

upper limbs, these include the median, ulnar, radial, and axillary nerves, and in the lower limbs, the sciatic, femoral, tibial, and peroneal nerves. The intensity of the stimulus is gradually increased until a supramaximal response is achieved. This is done by gradually increasing the intensity until the amplitude of the muscle action potential no longer increases and then by further increasing the stimulus another 25% to ensure that the stimulus intensity is supramaximal. Motor conduction velocity is calculated as shown in Figure 15A–4.

SENSORY CONDUCTION

Sensory conduction studies are carried out by stimulating the digital nerves on the fingers and re-cording the responses at the wrist, elbow, or axilla over the median or ulnar nerve. Sensory nerve action potentials (SNAPs) conducted orthodromically are obtained in this manner. The stimulus is applied by a ring electrode placed around the base and the middle of the index or the little finger for the median and the ulnar nerves, respectively. The ground electrode is placed between the stimulating and the recording electrodes. During sensory stimulation, impulses are propaged in both directions along the nerve from the point of stimulation, and the stimulating and recording electrodes may be reversed to obtain antidromic conduction. Orthodromic conduction denotes impulse propagation along an axon in a normal direction for sensory fibers. This corresponds to impulse traveling from distal to proximal. Antidromic conduction refers to impulse propagation in a direction opposite to normal, i.e., from proximal to distal in the case of sensory conduction. Median and ulnar nerves are stimulated at the wrist and the responses are recorded with a ring electrode placed around the index finger or the little finger, respectively. Both sensory and motor fibers are stimulated, but only antidromically conducted sensory action potentials are recorded at the digit. With antidromic examination, usually a higher amplitude response is obtained.

In the lower limbs, sensory conduction studies can be carried out on peroneal, sural, saphenous, and posterior tibial nerves. Sensory conduction studies have considerably improved with the use of electronic signal averaging.

Techniques are now available by which small signals can be superimposed and better evaluated with electronic averaging. Body temperature and age of the patient considerably affect the conduction velocities. Both sensory and conduction velocities decrease with lower limb temperature. In infants,

young children, and adolescents, the conduction velocity is slower than in adults (Table 15A–2).

REFLEXES AND EVOKED POTENTIALS

H Reflex

The H reflex is the electrical analogue of the tendon jerk, the electrical stimulus being applied to the afferent fibers of the muscle spindles rather than the nerve endings themselves. In the lower limb, it is elicited by stimulation of the popliteal nerve and recorded from the gastrocnemius soleus muscle. It can also be recorded in the upper limbs of normal infants.[7] The blink reflex obtained in the face by stimulating the ophthalmic branch of the trigeminal nerve and recording the reflex contraction of the oculus orbicularis muscle can also provide information about the function of both nerves.[8]

TABLE 15A–2.—NORMAL SENSORY CONDUCTION VALUES

NERVE	CONDUCTION VELOCITY (Meters/sec)	LATENCY (msec)
Median nerve		
Digits II and III–wrist		
(orthodromal)	58.6 (SD 4.7)	3.0 (SD 0.25)
(antidromal)	57.4 (SD 3.8)	3.2 (SD 0.25)
Wrist–digit I	48.0 (SD 4.5)	
Wrist–Digits II and III	57.0 (SD 4.1)	
Ulnar nerve		
Digits IV and IV–wrist		
(orthodromal)	56.7 (SD 4.2)	3.0 (SD 0.2)
(antidromal)	54.9 (SD 3.9)	3.2 (SD 0.3)
Digit V–wrist (orthodromal)	51.9 (SD 5.6)	2.8 ± 0.2
Digit IV–wrist	54.8 (SD 4.9)	3.0 ± 0.2
Radial nerve		
Forearm–thumb	58.1 (50–68)	2.6 (2.0–3.3)
Thumb–wrist	58.0 (SD 6.0)	
Femoral nerve		
Saphenous, orthodromic antidromic	54.8 ± 1.9	
	49.6 ± 6.2	
Peroneal nerve		
Medial dorsal cutaneous, antidromic	51.2 ± 5.7	
Posterior tibial nerve		
Medial plantar nerve, orthodromic	36.6 ± 7.9	
Lateral plantar nerve, orthodromic	31.7 ± 4.4	
Sural nerve		
Antidromic from midcalf to lat. malleolus	46.2 ± 3.3	

F Response

When motor nerves are stimulated, action potentials travel orthodromically as well as antidromically. The antidromic impulses are capable of firing the motor neurons in the spinal cord, and this response can be recorded distally in the musculature. F responses were initially observed in the small muscles of the foot by Magladery and McDougal.[9] F responses can be distinguished from H responses. When a series of such responses are recorded, F responses are enhanced by supramaximal stimulation, whereas increasing the stimulus intensity inhibits H responses. F responses can be recorded from all muscles (although more they are prominent in antigravity muscles), while H reflexes are limited to antigravity muscles.

The conduction velocity of the proximal segments of the nerve can be measured by using the F response. Such determination can particularly aid in diseases where proximal, focal pathology may be seen, such as the Guillain-Barré syndrome, carcinoma, and rheumatoid arthritis, and in the evaluation of radiculopathies.[10]

Evoked Potentials

The availability of computerized signal averaging has made possible the extraction of the responses evoked at the cortex (after peripheral sensory stimulation) from the background electroencephalographic activity. Such evoked responses can be elicited after peripheral cutaneous (somatosensory evoked potential, or SSEP), visual (visual evoked potential, or VEP), trigeminal (trigeminal evoked response, or TER), or auditory (auditory evoked response, or AEP) stimulation by recording over the appropriate cortical area. In each type of evoked response, different positive and negative peaks with short or long latency can be distinguished. The neural generators for many of these peaks have been identified. The methodology and interpretation of these studies will not be discussed here in detail.

In the extremities, evoked potentials are typically elicited by median or tibial nerve stimulation. However, essentially any segmental cutaneous nerve can be stimulated to obtain SSEPs. This makes it possible to evaluate lesions of the peripheral nerves or roots which cannot be easily studied by SNAP or other methods. Thus, stimulation of the fifth finger can be used to study the eighth cervical root, and stimulation of the lateral femoral cutaneous nerve can be used to evaluate a patient with neuralgia parasthetica. The trigeminal evoked potential can be used in studying a patient with facial pain.[11-15]

ROLE OF ELECTRODIAGNOSTIC STUDIES IN CLINICAL DIAGNOSIS

Localized Processes

Localized peripheral nerve and radicular problems are a common cause of pain, and electrodiagnostic studies are very useful in their diagnosis. Such localized processes are of two types: entrapment neuropathies, which cause compression of the nerves in a fibrous or a bony tunnel; and neuropathies that result from injuries to the nerve due to trauma following operations, or due to scar entrapment. In such nerve lesions, pressure applied briefly may cause only a transient conduction blockade, but prolonged pressure or severe trauma causes wallerian degeneration distal to the injury. Intermediate grades of injury may result in segmental demyelination and may compromise the intraneural vasculature, which in turn may accentuate the lesion. The presence of fine, unmyelinated regenerating axons, and the formation of artificial synapses between the injured or regenerating axons (ephaptic transmission), have been implicated in the production of pain due to such lesions. Persons with systemic disorders such as diabetes, and lupus erythematosus may be predisposed to the development of such localized lesions. These lesions will be considered in the order of the nerves involved.

Median Nerve (Fig 15A–5)

CARPAL TUNNEL SYNDROME.—Carpal tunnel syndrome is caused by compression of the nerve in the tunnel between the transverse carpal ligament and the bones of the wrist. Because the space is also occupied by the tendons of the fingers, a variety of disorders may give rise to this syndrome. These include tenosynovitis, rheumatoid arthritis, rubella immunization, diabetes mellitus, gout, amyloidosis, myxedema, acromegaly, multiple myeloma, pregnancy, and mucopoly saccharidosis. The symptoms usually consist of pain and numbness. The pain caused may be felt only in the fingers, in the entire hand, or even in the forearm and arm. In cases where the pain extends proximally, there may be an

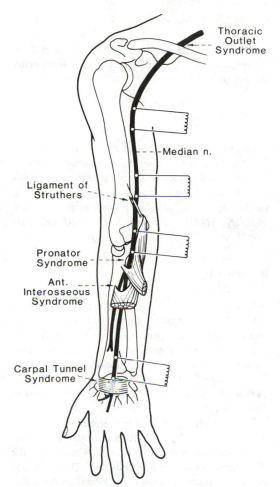

Fig 15A–5.—Sites of entrapment of the median nerve.

associated radiculopathy, which is a predisposing factor to distal nerve compression. In advanced cases, atrophy of the thenar muscles is present. Tinel's sign may be elicited by tapping the nerve at the wrist. Phalen's sign (reproduction of the symptoms by flexion of the wrist) may also be elicited.

ELECTRODIAGNOSIS.—Changes of sensory conduction precede motor conduction across the wrist. Since the SNAP study is performed between the fingers and the wrist, it does not have the same localizing value as motor studies. Prolongation of distal motor latency, in combination with normal motor velocity in the forearm segment of the nerve, is diagnostic. In advanced cases, however, retrograde axonal degeneration may cause the slowing of conduction in the forearm. EMG changes in the thenar muscles occur late in the disease.

PRONATOR TERES SYNDROME.—Entrapment of the median nerve may occur as it passes between the heads of the pronator teres or under the edge of the flexor digitorum sublimis. Symptoms may mimic carpal tunnel syndrome, but weakness of muscles proximal to the wrist and Tinel's sign over the entrapped point are distinguishing features. Phalen's sign is absent. Electrodiagnostically, there is no slowing of distal motor latency, and there may be slowing of motor conduction in the forearm segment. The diagnosis is established by EMG when it demonstrates denervation of median innervated muscles in the forearm with sparing of the pronator teres.

ANTERIOR INTEROSSEOUS SYNDROME.—This is due to entrapment of the anterior interosseous branch of the median nerve, with motor changes restricted to the flexor pollicis longus, flexor digitorum profundus to the second finger, and the pronator quadratus. Pain is uncommon with this syndrome but may occur occasionally.

OTHER ENTRAPMENT LESIONS.—Other entrapment lesions of the median nerve include compression caused by the lacertus fibrosus, which is a fascial band connecting the biceps tendon to the flexor carpi radialis, and compression caused by the ligament of Struthers, or a supracondylar spur just above the elbow.

Ulnar Nerve (Fig 15A–6)

AT THE ELBOW.—Ulnar neuropathy at the elbow is a common and a well-recognized entity. It may be due to recurrent trauma to the nerve behind the medial epicondyle, entrapment of the nerve in the cubital tunnel as it passes through the heads of the flexor carpi ulnaris, or entrapment of the nerve as it passes through the medial intermuscular septum. Pain is common and often involves the hand, forearm, and elbow. It may occasionally extend more proximally. Trophic changes may be prominent in some patients. Weakness and wasting of the small muscles of the hand and a sensory deficit in the ulnar distribution are present in advanced cases.

ELECTRODIAGNOSTIC STUDIES.—Motor conduction velocity can be measured across the elbow; a delay localizes the lesion to the elbow. The procedure must be standardized because values are affected by the position of the elbow and by an interstimulus distance less than 10 cm. SNAP studies,

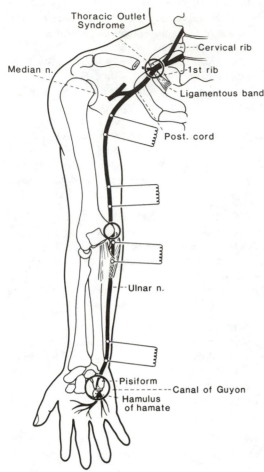

Fig 15A–6.—Sites of entrapment of the ulnar nerve.

unless performed segmentally, do not localize the lesion. However, abnormal SNAP studies may correlate with a poorer prognosis. EMG abnormalities may be noted in the flexor carpi ulnaris, first dorsal interosseous, adductor pollicis, and hypothenar muscles.

AT THE CANAL OF GUYON.—Entrapment of the nerve may occur in the canal of Guyon as the nerve passes between the hook of the hamate and the pisiform bone. This lesion may or may not be associated with pain or sensory abnormalities, since the superficial palmar cutaneous branch separates as the nerve enters the canal. Electromyographically, changes occur in the adductor pollicis and the first dorsal interosseous muscles, while some or all of the hypothenar muscles are spared.

Other Ulnar Nerve Lesions

Other ulnar nerve lesions may be caused by trauma, catheterization of the brachial artery, or by the use of crutches.

Radial Nerve

Lesions of the radial nerve rarely cause pain and therefore will not be considered in detail. Injury to the superficial branch of the radial nerve may, however, be associated with pain in the dorsal wrist and hand area, in association with Tinel's sign at the site of injury. SNAP studies can demonstrate such a lesion.

Brachial Plexus

Brachial plexus lesions are a common cause of pain. Most commonly, they are associated with trauma caused by a penetrating wound, local pressure, or traction. Injuries may be associated with fractures and dislocations of the humerus, clavicle fractures, birth trauma, or operations. The other causes of brachial plexus lesions are summarized in Table 15A–3.

The thoracic outlet syndrome is an unusual cause of lower brachial plexus involvement. More common lesions such as those of the C-8 root or of the ulnar nerve should be ruled out first. The syndrome consists of arterial, venous, and neural entities. The four most important causes are listed in Table 15A–3.

The clinical diagnosis of a lesion at the level of the brachial plexus is based on careful sensory and

TABLE 15A–3.—LESIONS OF THE
BRACHIAL PLEXUS

Traumatic: Penetrating and missile wounds; traction injuries; injuries associated with fractures and dislocations; birth injuries; iatrogenic (intraoperative) traction and laceration; hematoma after axillary artery catheterization; crutch-induced lesions

Brachial neuritis: Sporadic; related to sera or vaccines; familiar recurrent variety

Radiation-induced neuropathy

Cancer-related breast carcinoma; Hodgkin's disease, lymphomas

Drug-related; heroin addiction

Thoracic outlet syndrome: Cervical rib; scalesus anticus syndrome; costoclavicular syndrome; hyperabduction syndrome motor examination and knowledge of the anatomy (Fig 15A–7). It is important to distinguish preganglionic lesions, which have a poorer prognosis, from postganglionic lesions. An intact triple response to histamine or cold stimulation, the presence of Horner's sign, and the presence of meningoceles on myelography indicate a preganglionic lesion. Occasionally, however, a meningocele may be associated with an intact anterior or posterior root. The presence of Tinel's sign at Erb's point that migrates distally indicates a postganglionic lesion.

ELECTRODIAGNOSTIC STUDIES.—Electrodiagnostic studies include EMG of muscles, SNAP response, motor conduction and latency measured by stimulation at Erb's point, and the F response. Sparing of the paraspinal muscles on EMG indicates a lesion close to the root, probably a preganglionic lesion. The presence of an intact SNAP in the absence of a cortical evoked response also indicates a preganglionic lesion. Conduction studies of the distal segments from Erb's point may reveal a low or absent motor or sensory response, depending on the degree of axonal degeneration. In the thoracic outlet syndrome, needle electromyography usually does not reveal abnormal spontaneous activity, but motor unit potentials may be polyphasic and giant, and recruitment patterns may be decreased. Conduction studies (of the ulnar nerve) have been reported to show motor slowing across the outlet, or abnormal SNAPs.

Femoral Nerve

Femoral neuropathy is an uncommon cause of pain. Such neuropathy may be caused by pelvic or hip fractures, avulsion of the iliac muscle, pelvic or abdominal operations, and difficult delivery. Abdominal aortic aneurysms and hemorrhage into the psoas muscle may also occasionally involve the femoral nerve. The saphenous branch of the femoral nerve may be involved by entrapment or traumatic lesions, and patients may present with a painful neuropathy.[16]

Electrically, the femoral nerve may be studied by EMG of the innervated muscles and by motor conduction velocity measurements after stimulation of the nerve above and below the inguinal ligament. Saphenous nerve conduction studies (by stimulating the nerve above the medial malleolus and recording at the inguinal ligament) and evoked cortical potential studies after stimulation of the saphenous nerve are also useful in studying lesions of the saphenous and femoral nerves.

Sciatic Nerve and Lumbosacral Plexus (Fig 15A–8)

Proximal lesions of the sciatic nerve and the lumbosacral plexus are usually associated with trauma. Hip fractures and pelvic fractures are the most fre-

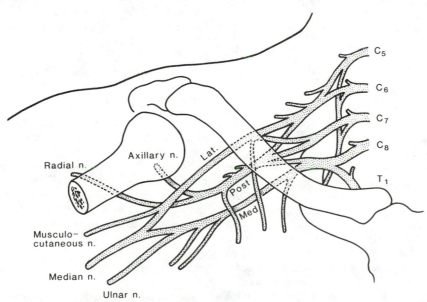

Fig 15A–7.—The brachial plexus and its branches.

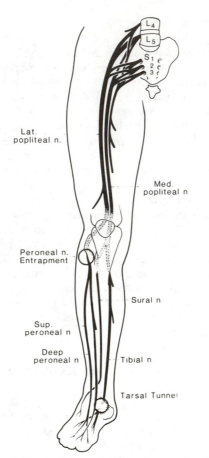

Fig 15A—8.—The sciatic nerve and entrapment sites.

quent causes. The lumbosacral plexus can be also affected by retroperitoneal hemorrhage into the psoas muscle. Lesions of the sciatic nerve in the gluteal area can also be caused by injection injuries, hip operations, hematomas, and vaginal operations. In the thigh, lesions of the sciatic nerve are uncommon and are usually caused by fractures or penetrating injuries.

The peroneal division of the sciatic nerve is more frequently involved than the tibial division. This has been explained by Sunderland as being due to the larger size and smaller number of funiculi in this nerve, and due to the relative fixation of the nerve at the fibular head. The peroneal nerve is most frequently involved as it passes around the neck of the fibula, due to fractures, prolonged sitting in a cross-legged position, or ganglion cysts of the superior tibiofibular joint. The etiology may not be evident in some patients.

The tibial division of the sciatic nerve may also be injured by traumatic lesions, but injuries of this nerve in the thigh are almost always associated with peroneal nerve lesions. The tarsal tunnel syndrome results from entrapment of this nerve underneath the flexor retinaculum at the ankle. The pain due to this syndrome occurs in the medial aspect of the foot, but may extend into the calf. Sensory abnormalities are present in the plantar aspect of the foot but spare the heel since the medial calcaneal nerve exits above the flexor retinaculum. Motor weakness involves the intrinsic foot muscles.

ELECTRODIAGNOSTIC STUDIES.—The lumbosacral plexus and the sciatic nerve and its branches can be studied by needle EMG, motor nerve conduction, SNAP studies, tibial H responses, and the tibial and peroneal F responses.

The proximal sciatic nerve may be studied by sampling the hamstring muscles, the short head of the biceps femoris being supplied by the peroneal division and all others by the tibial division. Motor conduction studies have been performed using a deep needle electrode near the gluteal fold. The sensory conduction has been measured by stimulating the three medial toes and by using needle electrodes to record from the nerve. The proximal sciatic portion has been studied without the use of deep needle electrodes by using the tibial H response and the tibial and peroneal F responses.

The tibial and peroneal nerves are studied by motor conduction and SNAP measurements. Motor conduction studies are performed by stimulating at the knee and ankle while recording from the distal musculature. The tibial segment crossing the tarsal tunnel is studied by stimulation above and below the tarsal ligament. Orthodromic SNAP studies of the superficial peroneal, sural, and medial plantar nerves have been performed.

LATERAL FEMORAL CUTANEOUS NERVE.—The lateral femoral cutaneous nerve can become entrapped at its point of passage through the attachment inguinal ligament, resulting in a painful dysesthetic syndrome. Predisposing conditions include obesity, pregnancy, anomalous course of the nerve, and wearing a corset. The SNAP of this nerve can be measured, but it is technically difficult.

Cranial Nerves

Electrodiagnostic studies may be quite useful in the diagnosis of pain syndromes relating to the cranial nerves, particularly the trigeminal nerve. While the diagnosis of classic trigeminal neuralgia is quite easily made on the basis of the history, the diagnosis of other facial and dental pain syndromes (atypical trigeminal neuralgia, trigeminal neuropathy, and atypical facial pain syndromes) may be difficult. Trigeminal somatosensory evoked potentials following gum stimulation are often abnormal in these syndromes and may have a value in predicting response to operative treatment such as microvascular decompression, or glycerol rhizotomy.[12-15] EMGs from the masseter and temporalis muscles can be recorded and may indicate the presence and the site of lesion of the nerve.

In patients with accessory nerve palsy, shoulder and neck pain may be a prominent symptom, and an accurate diagnosis can be made by the clinical examination, in conjunction with EMG studies of the trapezius and sternomastoid muscles.

Radiculopathy

Isolated root pathology is a common cause of pain and may be caused by fractures, disk herniation (Fig 15A–9), chronic degenerative arthritis, tumors, and Guillain-Barré syndrome. The clinical localization to root involvement depends on the pattern of motor and sensory abnormalities (on the basis of well-known dermatomal and myotomal charts), as well as the accentuation of symptoms by maneuvers that stretch the roots (such as those eliciting Lasèque's sign) or that cause an increase in intraspinal pressure (such as the Valsalva maneuver).

Electrically, EMG abnormalities are most useful in studying root pathology. The muscles may exhibit abnormal spontaneous activity such as fibrillation potentials, positive sharp waves, and bizarre high-frequency responses. Localized polyphasic motor unit potentials may be the only finding in a large number of patients. Involvement of paraspinal muscles indicates a lesion of the roots or anterior horn cells. Recently the H reflex has been used to study lesions of the S-1 root, and F waves were used to study the proximal conduction responses after stimulation of the median, ulnar, posterior tibial, and peroneal nerves. Rockswold et al. have introduced a catheter into the bladder, stimulated the bladder wall, and studied EMG activity in the anal sphincter. The response was thought to be a reflex arc passing through the pelvic nerves, the cauda equina, entering through the sacral cord, and exiting through the pudendal nerves. This technique can be

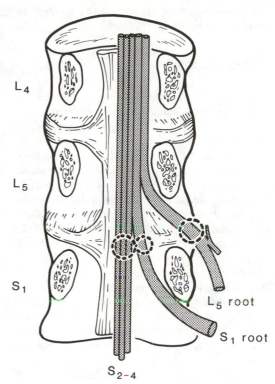

Fig 15A–9.—Disk herniation causing radiculopathy.

useful in studying lesions of the cauda equina.[17] Finally, it must be remembered that electrodiagnostic studies, particularly EMG, may be entirely normal in patients with radiculopathy.

Diffuse Processes

Among diffuse processes causing pain syndromes, polyradiculopathies and polyneuropathies are the most important.

Polyradiculopathy

Many polyneuropathies involve the proximal aspect of the neuron and technically should be termed polyradiculoneuropathy. Examples include the Guillain-Barré syndrome, diabetic neuropathy, and carcinomatous or inflammatory meningitis. Polyradiculopathy may be distinguished from polyneuropathy on EMG by the presence of changes in the paraspinal muscles. On conduction studies, conduction over the proximal segments can be measured by using F responses and H reflexes.

Polyneuropathy

Peripheral polyneuropathies are manifested by motor, sensory, and autonomic signs and symptoms. They may be bilateral and symmetric, or asymmetric. Pain and dysesthesia are common accompaniments of polyneuropathies, and electrodiagnostic studies are an essential element in their diagnosis. Electrodiagnostic studies can reveal the presence or absence of polyneuropathy, the distribution of the lesions, and whether the neuropathy is of a myelin or an axonal type.

Demyelinating processes occur in Dejerine-Sottas disease, Refsum's disease, diabetes, and the Guillain-Barré syndrome. They are characterized by slow conduction values and are usually associated with increased temporal dispersion and decreased amplitude of the evoked responses. SNAP abnormalities usually precede the motor changes, and the lower extremities are involved more often than the upper.

Axonal degeneration is seen in alcoholic polyneuropathy amyloidosis, Friedreich's ataxia, and porphyria. Electrical studies reveal abnormal spontaneous activity on EMG, while the remaining axons conduct at nearly normal velocity. The evoked motor response may be decreased in amplitude. However, many diseases may have a mixture of axonal and myelin degeneration.

Polymyositis

Although diffuse bilateral muscle weakness is the cardinal clinical symptom of polymyositis, tenderness and pain of the involved muscles are present in about half the cases. About 50% of cases of polymyositis are associated with a skin lesion and are termed dermatomyositis. The etiology of this condition is usually a collagen disease or carcinoma. Parasitic infestation with *Trichinella spiralis* or with Toxoplasma gondii can also produce a painful generalized myositis.

In polymyositis, multiple abnormalities are usually present on EMG examination. There is a prolonged insertional activity. Fibrillation potentials, trains of positive sharp waves, and bizarre high-frequency potentials are seen. The motor unit potentials are decreased in amplitude and duration, and

the interference pattern is increased. A certain degree of neuromuscular blockade may be demonstrable in some patients on repetitive stimulation. However, unlike the polyneuropathies, the motor and sensory conduction velocities are normal in polymyositis.

CONCLUSION

Pain is a highly subjective phenomenon, often difficult to separate from accompanying psychological problems. When the cause of a patient's pain is not diagnosed, he is often branded as a "crazy person." The electrodiagnostic studies described in this chapter can be very useful in preventing this dilemma. They also provide information to the physician and the surgeon about the location and extent of the lesion. After appropriate treatment, they can be useful in the follow-up of painful disorders.

REFERENCES

1. Erb W.: *Handbook of Electrotherapeutics.* New York, W. Wood, 1883.
2. Piper H.: *Elektrophysiologie menschlicher Muskeln.* Berlin, 1912.
3. Denny-Brown D., Pennybaker J.B.: Fibrillation and fasciculation in voluntary muscle. *Brain* 61:311, 1938.
4. Hodes R., Larrabee M.G., German W.: The human electromyogram in response to nerve stimulation and conduction velocity of motor axons: Studies on normal and on injured nerves. *Arch. Neurol. Psychiatry* 60:340, 1948.
5. Simpson J.A.: Electrical signs in the diagnosis of carpal tunnel and related syndromes. *J. Neurol. Neurosurg. Psychiatry* 19:275–280, 1956.
6. Gilliatt R.W., Sears T.A.: Sensory nerve action potentials in patients with peripheral nerve lesions. *J. Neurol. Neurosurg. Psychiatry* 21:109, 1958.
7. Thomas J.E., Lambert E.H.: Ulnar nerve conduction. *J. Appl. Physiol.* 15:1, 1960.
8. Kimura J., Powers J.M., Van Allen M.W.: Reflex response of orbicularis oculi muscle to supraorbital nerve stimulation: Study in normal subjects and in peripheral facial paresis. *Arch. Neurol.* 21:193, 1969.
9. Magladery J.W., McDougal D.B.: Electrophysiological studies of nerve and reflex activity in normal man: I. Identification of certain reflexes in the electromyogram and the conduction velocity of peripheral nerve fibers. *Bull. Johns Hopkins Hosp.* 86:265–290, 1950.
10. Young R.R., Shahani B.T.: Clinical value and limitations of F-wave determination. *Muscle Nerve* 1:248–249, 1978.
11. Eisen A.A.: *The somatosensory evoked potential,*

minimonograph No. 19. American Association of Electromyography and Electrodiagnosis, 1982, p. 16.

12. Bennett, M.N., Janetta P.J.: Evoked potentials in trigeminal neuralgia. *Neurosurgery* 13:242–247, 1983.

13. Bennett M.H., Lunsford L.D.: Percutaneous retrogasserian glycerol injection for tic douloureux: Part II. Results and implications of trigeminal evoked potential studies. *Neurosurgery,* in press.

14. Buettner U.W., Petruch F., Scheglmann K., et al.: Diagnostic significance of cortical somatosensory evoked potentials following trigeminal nerve stimulation, in Courjon J., Mauguiere F., Rveol M. (eds.): *Clinical Applications of Evoked Potentials in Neurology.* New York, Raven Press, 1982, pp. 339–345.

15. Stohr M., Petruch F., Scheglmann K.: Somatosensory evoked potentials following trigeminal nerve stimulation in trigeminal neuralgia. *Ann. Neurol.* 9:63–66, 1981.

16. Sekhar L.N., Alemo-Hammad S.: *Saphenous Neuropathy and Subsartorial Canal Syndrome.* Submitted for publication.

17. Rockswold G.L., et al.: Electrophysiological technique for evaluating lesions of the conus medullaris and the cauda equina. *J. Neurosurg.* 45:321, 1976.

15B / Radiography

P. PRITHVI RAJ, M.D.

THE LARGE NUMBER of diagnostic modalities available for the evaluation of chronic pain attests to the fact that objective confirmation of subjective pain is difficult to achieve in the majority of patients. This section reviews the various radiologic techniques available for diagnosis.

The available radiologic procedures fall into three categories, based on the expertise of the radiologist and the availability of equipment. Although availability and experience may ultimately alter the order of use, presently the commonest radiographic techniques for the diagnosis of chronic pain pathology are plain radiography, myelography, and bone scans. These techniques may be used singly or in combination. According to Berg,[1] supplemental procedures include epidural venography, computerized tomography, angiography, and arthrography. Epidurography and diskography are less commonly used, controversial procedures.

PLAIN RADIOGRAPHY

The standard anteroposterior (AP), lateral, and oblique projections are the ones most commonly used in screening the cervical, thoracic, and lumbosacral spine and various joints of the body. Spot films coned to the area of pathology (e.g., angled AP and oblique views of the sacroiliac joints) may supplement the standard views, if clinically indicated.

Readily diagnosed by these studies are cases of ankylosing spondylitis with bamboo spine appearance, spondylolisthesis, a defect of the pars interarticularis, disk space narrowing, sclerosis of adjoining end-plates, fractures, anomalies, osteophytes, osteolytic neoplasms, scoliosis, abnormalities of joints, calcification, arthritis, and derangements of the joints (Figs 15B–1 through 15B–4).

Standard plain radiography may be supplemented by complex motion tomography to improve assessment of interosseous lesions or anatomical alignment of fractures.

Unfortunately there are limitations to these studies. Limitations include significant radiation exposure, increased pain during the study (the patient must be in an uncomfortable difficult position), poor detail of the region under study, and absence of soft tissue for radiographic detail.[2–7]

RADIONUCLIDE SCANS

Radionuclide bone scans are more sensitive in detecting early bone lesions than are plain radiographs. This is because 50% distraction of the cancellous bone is needed before a lytic process is radiographically apparent. Bone scan is the first study choice in almost all cases of metastatic disease (Fig 15B–5) and in most cases of suspected primary neoplasm. Early inflammatory conditions and Paget's disease are easily detected on bone scans.

MYELOGRAPHY

Myelography has been performed since 1919, when Dandy introduced air contrast into the spinal canal.[8, 9] Shortly thereafter, Mixter and Barr used the technique to investigate intervertebral disk protrusion and nerve root irritation.[10] In 1944, iophendylate (Pantopaque) was introduced into the subarachnoid space, and until recently myelography was most often performed with this agent (Figs 15B–6 and 15B–7).

Various water-soluble agents have been tried over the years, including methiodal sodium (Abrodil), meglumine iothalamate (Conray meglumine), and meglumine iocarnate (Dimer-X). Because of neurotoxicity, these agents have been discarded. Since 1978, metrizamide (Amipaque) has all but replaced Pantopaque for lumbar myelography (Fig 15B–8).

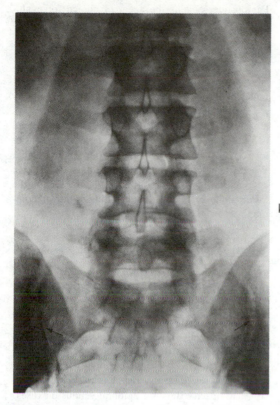

Fig 15B–1.—Plain radiograph showing ankylosing spondylitis in the sacroiliac joints.

Fig 15B–2.—Plain radiograph showing severe degenerative arthritis of the lumbar spine at L4–L5 and L5–L1 levels.

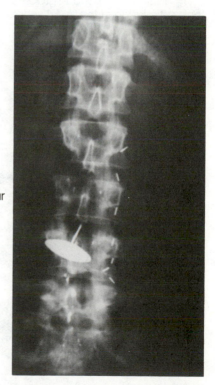

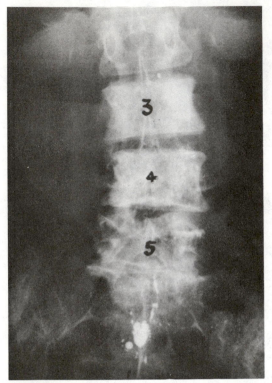

Fig 15B–3.—Plain radiograph showing osteoblastic lesion of the L3–L4 vertebrae due to prostatic cancer with metastases.

Pantopaque remains the agent of choice for evaluating spinal block, for posttherapeutic follow-up studies, for evaluating obese patients, and in cases where there are contraindications to metrizamide. The reader is referred to Sachett and Strother's excellent work on the techniques of using metrizamide.[11]

Myelography with Pantopaque clearly shows large extradural defects. The more laterally located or subtle lesions on the nerve root sleeve are easier to visualize with the less viscous metrizamide. When myelographic studies are done, one must keep in mind that disk protrusion may be seen in the asymptomatic patient.[4] This finding is not uncommon.

SUPPLEMENTAL STUDIES

Epidural Venography

The object of this technique is to reveal the status of veins lying against the posterior longitudinal ligament in various states of chronic pain (e.g., after disk protrusion) (Fig 15B–9). Initially it was performed by interosseous injection of spinous processes to opacify Batson's epidural venous plexuses. Fortunately this painful technique was discarded in favor of the technique described by Gargano et al. in which the ascending lumbar and radicular veins are selectively catheterized via the femoral vein.[12]

Fig 15B–4.—Plain radiographs showing Sudek's atrophy of the left foot (bottom).

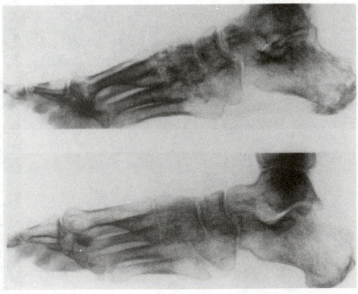

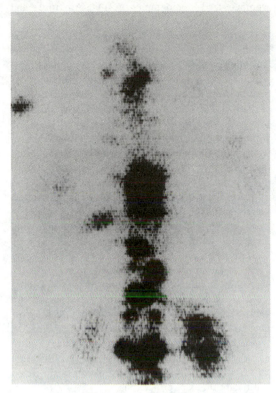

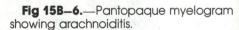

Fig 15B–5.—Radionuclide ^{99m}Tc-DP scan. Note increased radioactivity in multiple areas, indicating prostatic metastases. (From Stanton-Hicks M., Boas R.A.: *Chronic Low Back Pain.* New York, Raven Press, 1982. Reproduced by permission.)

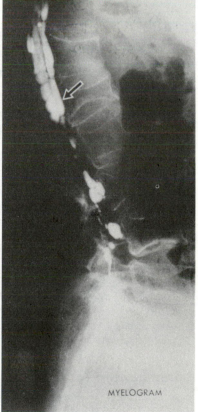

Fig 15B–6.—Pantopaque myelogram showing arachnoiditis.

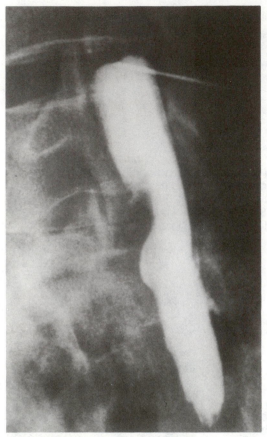

Fig 15B–7.—Pantopaque myelogram showing disk prolapse.

Epidural venography has been reported to be comparable in accuracy to metrizamide myelography.[13] The low false negative rate of venography[1] indicates the high confidence level that may be sustained following a normal study.

Epidural venography is indicated when myelography is normal or equivocal (especially with a wide lumbosacral epidural space or short caudal sac), there is a strong clinical evidence of L5–S1 disk protrusion, or the patient refuses myelography or myelography is contraindicated. Epidural venography is contraindicated in patients with iodine hypersensitivity, in patients who have had previous laminectomy at that level, or no facilities are available for interpretation of the studies.

Computerized Tomography

The most recent and undoubtedly the most important advances in the diagnostic armamentarium is computerized tomography (CT). Ambrose and Hounsfield developed it as a clinically usable tool in 1973 for head scanning.[14, 15] As newer generation scanners became available, fast, high-resolution scanning and thin overlapping sections have provided the clinician with a noninvasive method of examining the CNS and surrounding structures (Fig 15B–10). The ability to vary the window width allows all structures from dense bone to fat to be examined individually or together. The multiplanar reconstruction capability allows sagittal, coronal, and more recently three-dimensional visualization from the initial axial section.[16]

The CT has been used equally well in children as in adults. It is indicated in infection, abscesses, space-occupying lesions, and metastases involving bone, soft tissues, and organs.

Herniated disk visualization by CT scan may prove to be one of its most valuable uses (Fig 15B–11). Arachnoiditis with distortion of the subarachnoid pouch is easily shown by the CT scan and can be differentiated from facet hypertrophy, callus formation from fusion, or recurrent disk.

Evaluation of fracture and massive injuries have been remarkably improved with CT. The limitation of CT in trauma is the poor evaluation of the vertical height on axial projections.

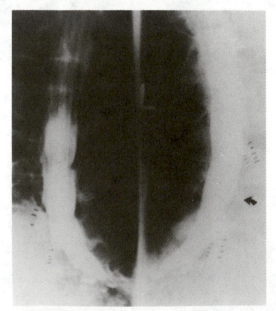

Fig 15B–8.—Metrizamide myelogram showing right L5 nerve root sleeve cutoff. (From Stanton-Hicks M., Boas R.A.: *Chronic Low Back Pain.* New York, Raven Press, 1982. Reproduced by permission.)

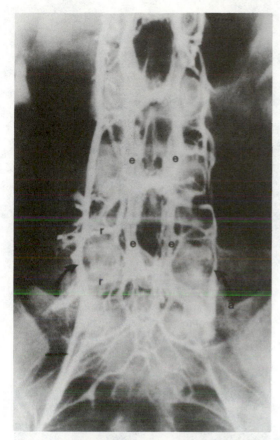

Fig 15B–9.—Normal epidural venogram. a, ascending lumbar veins; r, radicular venous branches; e, symmetric filling. (From Stanton-Hicks M., Boas R.A.: *Chronic Low Back Pain.* New York, Raven Press, 1982. Reproduced by permission.)

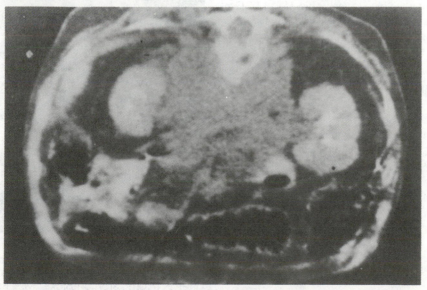

Fig 15B–10.—CT scan of midabdomen showing extensive pancreatic tumor with displacement of the kidney and invasion of the vertebral body. (From Stanton-Hicks M., Boas R.A.: *Chronic Low Back Pain.* New York, Raven Press, 1982. Reproduced by permission.)

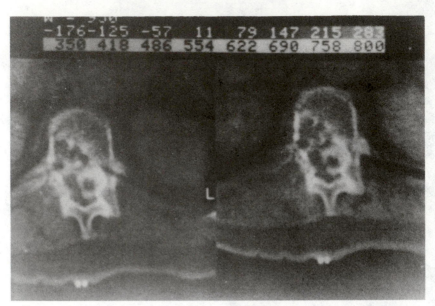

Fig 15B–11.—*Left,* normal CT scan of lumbar region. *Right,* CT scan of lumbar region showing disk prolapse. (From Stanton-Hicks M., Boas R.A.: *Chronic Low Back Pain.* New York, Raven Press, 1982. Reproduced by permission.)

Angiography

The introduction of intra-arterial contrast by selective catheterization of a regional artery has a limited application for chronic pain. It is primarily used for arteriovenous malformations and aneurysms, and for indicating the blood supply (Fig 15B–12). Generally, angiography is a final definitive study coupled with possible therapy via embolization of arteriovenous malformations or tumors.

Arthrography

Static and cinearthrography following injection of contrast material into a joint reveals additional pathologic information that supplements findings on plain radiography (Fig 15B–13). Arthrography is useful when tears or other abnormalities in cartilage of a joint are suspected.

CONTROVERSIAL STUDIES

Epidurography and Discography

Sanford and Doub introduced air into the epidural space in 1941.[17] Injection of contrast to improve vi-

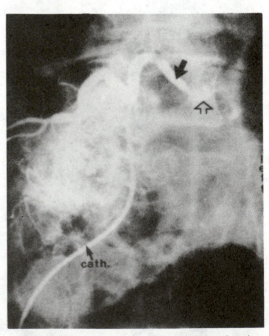

Fig 15B–12.—Lateral angiogram of spine showing filling of hemangioblastoma. Contrast was injected into the right subclavian artery. (From Stanton-Hicks M., Boas R.A.: *Chronic Low Back Pain.* New York, Raven Press, 1982. Reproduced by permission.)

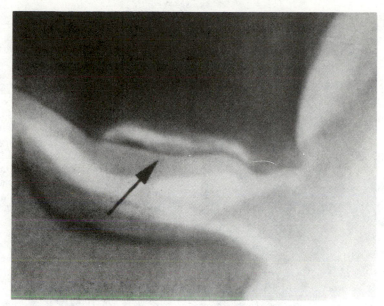

Fig 15B–13.—Arthrogram with contrast material of the right knee joint with osteochondrosis issecans in the medial femoral condyle.

sualization of the epidural space and nerve root sleeve to delineate the pressure change from disk protrusion was first reported in 1963.[18] Its use is suggested when myelography is equivocal or normal, especially when the L5–S1 epidural space is wide (Fig 15B–14). Gupta correlated epidurograms with clinical and operative findings in 255 patients with spinal disorders.[19] In most cases, the caudal approach was used to facilitate the study of the sacral canal. The dispersion of the solution in the epidural space was directly proportional to the speed of injection. When 80 ml of contrast material was used, the cervical space was visualized without tilting the table. Contrast material dispersal was symmetric in 88.2% of cases and was not related to the direction of the tip of the needle. There was a negative correlation between epidurographic findings and surgical findings in 10% of patients. Gupta found epidurography useful for repeated visualization of the epidural space following surgery for spinal compression.

Some adverse reactions can occur on epidurography. In Gupta's study, 56% of patients complained of severe backache and 82 of 90 patients with prolapsed disk complained of sciatica. The pain lasted for 10 minutes and did not require treatment. Water-soluble agents such as meglumine iothalamate can produce CNS toxicity. Patients may experience muscle twitchings, difficulty breathing, and clonic

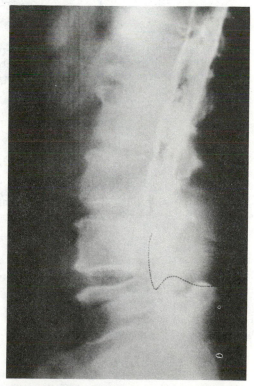

Fig 15B–14.—Epidurogram in the lumbar region showing normal epidural space.

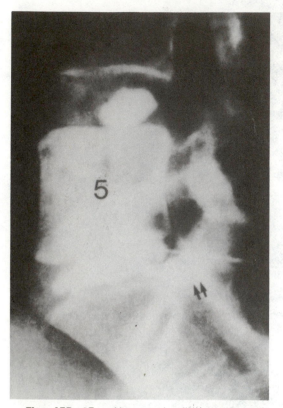

Fig 15B–15.—Abnormal diskogram with posterior extravasation of the dye following posterolateral disk injection. (From Stanton-Hicks M., Boas R.A.: *Chronic Low Back Pain.* New York, Raven Press, 1982. Reproduced by permission.)

convulsions. The treatments for such cases is intravenous diazepam with barbiturates for 24–48 hours. Usually patients recover fully after this period. Metrizamide has been shown to be the least toxic agent to the CNS and is now routinely recommended for epidurograms.

Diskography is performed by percutaneously injecting contrast material in the intervertebral disk.[20] Indications for its use are the same as for epidurography, although it has also been used as the primary radiographic study for disk disease (Fig 15B–15). Despite numerous studies, diskography remains controversial and is not widely used as a diagnostic tool.

REFERENCES

1. Berg D.J.: The radiologic evaluation of back pain, in Stanton-Hicks M., Boas R. (eds.): *Chronic Low Back Pain.* New York, Raven Press, 1982.
2. Fridenberg Z.B., Shoemaker R.C.: The results of nonoperative treatment of ruptured lumbar discs. *Am. J. Surg.* 88:933–935, 1954.
3. Fullenlove T.M., Williams A.J.: Comparative roentgen findings in symptomatic and asymptomatic backs. *Radiology* 68:572–574, 1957.
4. MacNab I.: Negative disc explorations. *J. Bone Joint Surg.* 53A:891–903, 1971.
5. McRae D.: Asymptomatic intervertebral disc protrusion. *Acta Radiol.* 46:9027, 1955.
6. Spengler D.M., Freeman C.W.: Patient selection for lumbar discectomy. *Spine* 4:129–134, 1979.
7. Splithoff C.A.: Lumbosacral junction: Roentgenographic comparison of the patients with and without backaches. *JAMA* 152:1610–1613, 1953.
8. Dandy W.E.: Roentgenography of the brain after the injection of air into the spinal canal. *Ann. Surg.* 70:397–403, 1979.
9. Dandy W.E.: Ventriculography following the injection of air into the cerebral ventricles. *Ann. Surg.* 68:5–11, 1941.
10. Mixter W.J., Barr J.S.: Rupture of the intervertebral disc with involvement of the spinal canal. *N. Engl. J. Med.* 112:210, 1934.
11. Sachett J.F., Strother C.M.: *New Techniques in Myelography.* New York, Harper & Row Publishers, Inc., 1980.
12. Gargano F.P., Meyer J.D., Sheldon J.J.: Transfemoral ascending lumbar catheterization of the epidural veins in lumbar disc disease: Clinical application and results in the diagnosis of the herniated intervertebral disc of the lumbar spine. *Radiology* 111:329–336, 1974.
13. Van Damme W., Hessels G., Verhelst M., et al.: Relative efficacy of clinical examination, electromyography, plain film radiography, myelography and lumbar phlebography in the diagnosis of low back pain and sciatica. *Neuroradiology* 18:109–118, 1979.
14. Ambrose J.: Computerized transverse scanning (tomography): Part 2. Clinical application. *Br. J. Radiol.* 46:1023–1047, 1973.
15. Hounsfield G.N.: Computerized transverse axial scanning (tomography): Part 1. Description of system. *Br. J. Radiol.* 46:1012–1022, 1973.
16. Glenn W.V. Jr., Rhodes M.L., Altschuler E.M., et al.: Multiplanar display computerized body tomography application in the lumbar spine. *Spine* 4:382–392, 1979.
17. Sanford H., Doub H.P.: Epidurography, a method of roentgenologic visualization of protruded intervertebral discs. *Radiology* 36:712–716, 1941.
18. Luyendijk W.: Canalography, roentgenological examination of the peridural space in the lumbosacral part of the vertebral canal. *J. Belge Radiol.* 46:236–253, 1963.
19. Gupta R.C.: *Epidurography: A Diagnostic Aid in Spinal Lesions.* Allahabad, India, Bhargava & Co., 1978.
20. Lindblom K.: Diagnostic puncture of intervertebral discs in sciatica. *Acta Orthop. Scand.* 17:231–239, 1948.

15C / Thermography

P. SEBASTIAN THOMAS, M.D.
HOWARD L. ZAUDER, M.D., PH.D.

THERMOGRAPHY is a noninvasive procedure that images the temperature distribution of the body surface. Although the technique involves neither radiation nor other risk to the patient, it is more sensitive in detecting the distribution of pain than are many of the currently employed methods. In contrast to conventional radiographic examinations, CT scans, and myelography, which demonstrate only anatomical lesions, thermography shows functional changes in circulation consequent on damage to nerves, ligaments, muscles, or joints.

Two types of thermographic equipment are currently available: (1) infrared thermography, or telethermography, and (2) liquid crystal thermography, or contact thermography

BASIS

Infrared Thermography

Thermography is based on the phenomenon that any object not at absolute zero temperature emits infrared (IR) radiation invisible to man. The spectrum ranges from 0 to 9 meters, visible to some birds, to nearly 1 meter, where it blends into the band of radio waves. The properties of different wavelengths of IR radiation vary widely. Some wavelengths are useful in biochemical analysis, some in crime analysis, some in cooking, and some were once popular in deep-heat therapy in physical medicine.

Electronic or telethermography consists of a camera similar to a television camera that detects IR radiation produced by the body surface. The object is scanned by fast rotating mirrors and its heat emission is projected to a IR radiation sensor.[1] The IR emission is converted to electrical signals and displayed on a black-and-white or color monitor similar to a conventional television receiver. The mid-temperature level of the thermal image is adjusted so that maximum information is gained.

Liquid Crystal Thermography

Contact thermography utilizes cholesterol crystals that change color with changes in surface temperature. The proper range of liquid crystals applied to the body provides a color map of temperature distribution.

Crystals may be painted or sprayed on the skin; however, the use of a flexible material impregnated with crystals is more efficient. The Flexi-Therm system consists of a series of inflatable transparent boxes about 11×14 inches in size; each box has one flexible thermosensitive side, which is applied to the body. Since each box provides a limited temperature-color scale consisting of five colors, the proper box must be selected for each portion of the body. Initially, the proper box is selected by trial and error. The same box should be used for contralateral parts to allow comparison.

Liquid crystal thermography (LCT), or contact thermography, is less expensive than electronic thermographic modes and yields quantitative absolute temperature images. The scale, however, is nonlinear. LCT requires minimum space and the equipment is ready to use without preparation. LCT is therefore most useful when the patient load is not great and the technique is used only occasionally. Electronic thermography requires a supply of liquid nitrogen and a room large enough to frame the body in the picture.

LCT is used in our facility in two different modes. When a full-body thermogram is required the patient is scheduled for the test, which takes about 1 hour. The disrobed patient is cooled for about 15 minutes in a draft-free room at 21° C (65° F). This emphasizes the differences in heat distribution. The thermogram is usually recorded with a Polaroid camera, and the films are kept with patient records.

Thermography should include not only that part of the body in which pathology is suspected but also the contralateral part for assessment of asymmetry. In addition, relevant dermatomes must be examined if segmental involvement is to be detected.[1]

Standardization of thermographic evaluation includes standardization of the environment as well as of the views and their interpretation. Since only one aspect of one portion of the body can be visualized on thermography at any one time, multiple standard views are necessary. Upper body standard thermography includes views of the neck, upper back, the lateral portion of the shoulders and arms, posterior oblique shoulder views, and the dorsal and volar aspects of the forearms and hands. In this manner, all dermatomes can be evaluated. Lower body thermographic views include the lower back and buttocks, the posterior and anterior thighs, the knees and legs, the lateral aspects of the legs, as well as vicus of the "walking" position from each side. The dorsum of feet and the heels and soles are then imaged with lower midtemperature level settings. The thermogram is usually repeated at 10-minute intervals to determine if thermographic changes are constant or transient. Repetition of imaging is particularly important for medicolegal documentation.

The full thermogram is read and evaluated with total knowledge of the patient's subjective complaints at the time of the examination. The films can then be read in a manner analogous to an x-ray film by a knowledgeable person who is familiar with the pictures of different pathologic conditions (e.g., disk disease, root involvement, trigger points). Examination of the patient by the interpreter of the thermogram is not required.

We use another kind of thermogram, the immediate or short thermogram. This is obtained as part of the patient's examination and is usually limited to the involved areas. The immediate or short thermographic examination can be done without precooling the patient. If radicular involvement is suspected, thermography is extended to include relevant views of the extremities. Immediate thermography, then, becomes an extension of the physical examination. Because it renders immediate results, this mode allows correlation of the thermographic findings with the results of physical examination.

Thermography shows temperature distribution in the superficial layer of the skin only. IR radiation detection reaches only 1 mm in depth. However, often deep tissue pathology including metastases to the bone can be detailed on thermography. Reflex mechanisms are probably involved.

The first step in evaluation of a thermogram is assessment of asymmetry; a side-to-side difference of 1° C involving 25% of the evaluated area is considered abnormal.[2] Some physiologic asymmetries, however, are normal: the dominant arm and shoulder may be 1° C warmer than the contralateral side.

Distortion of physiologic temperature distribution patterns (e.g., the warmer diamond in the lumbosacral area, the tadpole in the upper back) indicates pathology. A change in physiologic temperature gradients (proximal-distal in limbs, radioulnar in digits) is abnormal.[3]

Changes in thermal distribution are identified as corresponding to a dermatome or to an area supplied by a peripheral nerve or by an artery. Varicose veins show up as hot serpent-like structures or as small hot spots. Larger hot spots (about 10 mm in diameter) have been described over trigger points and tender areas.

Acute pain usually appears as hot areas, while chronic pain usually appears as an area of decreased temperature. Inflammation appears as hot areas. Deep tissue pathology may be conveyed to the surface by circulation. Muscle spasm or contraction can be detected by increased heat in skin overlying the active muscle. Artifacts are not unusual on thermograms. One frequent artifact is produced by skin folds, which conserve heat by decreased cooling and show up as hot streaks. A Polaroid picture or slide taken of the patient's back and neck helps to identify skin folds and to correlate them with hot areas on the thermogram. Once the thermograms have been interpreted, the results are correlated with the patient's complaints, including a "pain picture," and with clinical and other investigative findings.

CLINICAL APPLICATIONS

The clinical applications of thermography are myriad. It has been used in a variety of disorders, including bone and joint disorders, fractures, burns, grafts, infection, myofascial pain syndrome, musculoskeletal disorders, neurovascular compression, reflex sympathetic dystrophy, soft tissue injury, sprains, stroke, thoracic outlet syndrome, tumors, vascular disease, and wound healing. The purpose of this section is to discuss the usefulness of thermography in the diagnosis and treatment of pain syndromes.

Low Back Pain

Foremost among its uses is the diagnosis and treatment of low back pain syndromes. Pochaczevsky[4] compared IR and LCT thermograms and found that the findings of both correlated. He used LCT in the evaluation of spinal root syndromes. His data indicate that LCT compared favorably with EMG and myelographic findings in these patients, suggesting the usefulness of LCT as a diagnostic aid complementing EMG and myelography.

In spinal nerve root irritation, there are always changes along the affected dermatone, owing to the sympathetic hyperactivity at the affected nerve root. Thermography, therefore, is useful in documenting treatment in patients with nerve root irritation. In 20 patients undergoing epidural steroid injections for low back syndrome with signs of radiculopathy, Thomas et al.[5] studied the thermographic changes immediately before and after the block and 3 weeks after cessation of all epidural steroid blocks. All patients had positive thermograms before a block. A 1.5° C temperature difference between the extremities was considered abnormal. The thermogram was found to be normal in 17 of 20 patients who reported pain relief, indicating absence of radiculopathy (Figs 15C–1 through 15C–3, Plate 1). Thermography therefore can be used to document treatment results. It can also be used in place of visual analogue as a measure of the intensity of pain and as an indicator of the efficacy of epidural steroid injections for low back pain syndrome.

Psychogenic Pain

Hendler and co-workers tried to differentiate psychogenic pain and malingering from true organic pain syndromes.[6] They evaluated 224 patients who were diagnosed as having psychogenic pain by the referring physicians. In a 14-month period, it was found that 43 (19%) had abnormal thermograms of the extremities where the patients were complaining of pain. A temperature difference of 1° C between the extremities was considered abnormal. Hendler et al. attributed the abnormal thermograms to reflex sympathetic dystrophy, nerve root irritations, or facet syndrome. They concluded that thermography is useful for validating the complaint of pain in the absence of the EMG or nerve conduction velocity studies and other investigatory findings.

Industrial accident victims and patients on compensation usually have a secondary gain in having pain. Even in a structured pain clinic, it is sometimes difficult to discriminate between organic and psychogenic reasons for pain. Routine thermography provides valuable data on the organic causes of pain. Since there are no false negatives in medical thermography, it is a useful tool for screening of malingering and psychogenic pain.

Reflex Sympathetic Dystrophy

Reflex sympathetic dystrophy is a pain syndrome that is often overlooked, misdiagnosed, or recognized too late. The interruption of sympathetic nervous system, if performed early, can provide immediate pain relief and resolution of the physiopathologic process. In the early stages of reflex sympathetic dystrophy, physical laboratory and x-ray studies often yield negative results and the problem requires the clinical skills of most physicians. Thermography may confirm an organic cause of pain and allow quantification of the severity of the disorder.

CASE 1.—A 20-year-old man with a history of trauma to the hand presented for treatment. The extremity was put in cast for 4 weeks. Following removal of the cast, patient reported burning pain of the hand, and by the time of admission to the pain clinic he had a decrease in temperature of the hand and evidence of hyperpathia and hair loss with smooth and shiny skin. A diagnosis of reflex sympathetic dystrophy was made and documented by the LCT, as illustrated in Figures 15C–4 (Plate 1) and 15C–5 (Plate 2). The diagnosis correlated well with the complaint of pain and the clinical finding of hyperpathia along the whole hand.

Vascular Lesions

CASE 2.—A 63-year-old woman was admitted to the hospital with the diagnosis of rheumatoid vasculitis of over 20 years' duration and with gangrene of the tips of the left index, middle, and ring fingers. Prior to this admission, she had undergone multiple surgical procedures for repair of joint deformities. Her current therapy consisted of prednisone, 60 mg/day, and d-penicillamine, 125 mg/day, which produced only marginal resolution of the gangrene.

Physical examination revealed severe joint deformities. Splinter hemorrhages of both hands were present, with gangrene evident on the 2d, 3d, and 4th fingertips on the left hand. A 7° C temperature difference distal to the left proximal interphalangeal joints was present, and these fingers were extremely tender to touch.

Because of the poor response to medical therapy, a sympathetic stellate ganglion block was performed using 7 ml of 0.25% bupivacaine (Marcaine). LCT was performed prior to (Fig 15C–6, Plate 2) and immediately following the procedure (Fig 15C–7, Plate 2). The efficacy of the block is indicated by the postblock thermogram, which demonstrated a rise in temperature of the affected fingers, indicating increased blood flow. The patient's pain was significantly decreased. She subsequently underwent two additional sympathetic blocks after discharge, and her progress was evaluated and documented using thermography (Fig 15C–8, Plate 2). Subsequently the patient had complete resolution of symptoms.

Myofascial Pain Syndrome and Trigger Points

Myofascial pain syndromes constitute a group of disorders characterized by very sensitive small areas in the muscles or ligaments. Trigger points have a specific and typical area of referred pain. The treatment of trigger points includes ultrasound and deep kneading massage, but the best therapy is trigger point injection with local anesthetics. Trigger points can be accurately located by thermography.[7]

CASE 3.—A 38-year-old man, otherwise healthy, was referred to the pain clinic following extensive workup for pain in the upper back and left shoulder. Demonstration of trigger on thermography facilitated locating the areas for injection therapy (Figs 15C–9 and 15C–10, Plate 3).

REFERENCES

1. Wexler C.E.: *An Overview of Liquid Crystal and Electric Lumbar Thoracic and Cervical Thermography.* Tarzana, Calif., Thermographic Services, Inc., 1981.
2. Uematsu S. (ed.): *Medical Thermography: Theory and Clinical Applications.* Los Angeles, Brentwood Publishing Co., 1976.
3. Pochaczevsky R.: Liquid crystal thermography of the spine and extremities. *J. Neurosurg.* 56:386–395, 1982.
4. Pochaczevsky R.: Contact thermography of spinal root compression syndromes. *Am. J. Neuroradiol.* 3:243–250, 1982.
5. Thomas P.S., Chen L., Yuan H.A., et al.: Liquid crystal thermography: A noninvasive technique to document treatment results in patients with low back syndrome. Read before the IVth World Congress of Pain, Seattle, Washington, September 1984.
6. Hendler N., Uematsu S., Long D.: Thermographic validation of physical complaints in "psychogenic pain" patients. *Psychosomatics* 23–3:283–287, 1982.
7. Fischer A.A.: Thermography and pain. Read before the annual meeting of the American Academy of Physical Medicine and Rehabilitation, San Diego, 1981.

15D / Differential Nerve Block Studies

P. PRITHVI RAJ, M.D.
SOMAYAJI RAMAMURTHY, M.D.

IN A PATIENT with intractable and chronic pain, one must investigate, as much as possible, the origin and physiology of that pain before initiating therapy. The knowledge derived from studying the pain mechanisms can prevent serious sequelae to therapy (e.g., surgery) and allows one to predict which modalities will be helpful in treating such complex chronic pain. One investigative study that examines pain pathways and the central and peripheral components of pain is the differential nerve block study. It can be performed on any mixed nerve containing A alpha, beta, delta and C fibers and at any site, such as brachial and lumbosacral plexuses, major peripheral nerves, and in subarachnoid and epidural regions.

The technique of differential nerve block is based on the work of Gasser and Erlanger, who demonstrated that stimulating a mixed peripheral nerve produces a compound action potential that changes with the varying distances of the stimulating electrode.[1] At a suitable distance, A alpha, beta, and delta fibers can be separated. Based on these data, peripheral nerve fibers were classified into A, B, and C fibers (Table 15D–1). Different local anesthetics and concentrations have selective sensitivities for A alpha and delta and C fibers.[2] A delta fibers carry sharp pain, while dull burning pain is transported by C fibers. Preganglionic autonomic fibers (B fibers) are most susceptible to local anesthetic agents, followed by C fibers and then A delta fibers.[3, 4]

TECHNIQUE OF DIFFERENTIAL SPINAL BLOCK

Antegrade Spinal Block

The differential spinal block is a pharmacologic approach to differentially blocking sympathetic and somatic fibers. It is applicable to patients who have pain in the lower extremities, low back, lower abdomen, or pelvis.

The patient is informed that local anesthetic drugs of different concentration are injected into the spinal fluid. The possibility of post-spinal tap headache is explained. Written informed consent is then obtained. It is helpful to tell the patient that one of the four different solutions used may relieve the pain, or in some instances none of them may relieve the pain.

Preparation

Procaine is the most commonly used drug. It is available in 10% concentration for spinal use. Four 10-ml syringes, numbered 1 through 4, are used. Nine ml of 0.9% saline without preservative is taken up in a 10-ml syringe and 1 ml of 10% procaine is added and mixed well to obtain the 1% solution. Five ml of the 1% solution is aspirated into syringe No. 4, 2.5 ml is aspirated into syringe No. 3, and 2.5 ml of saline is added to make 0.5% solution; 2.5 ml of 1% solution is diluted to a volume of 10 ml with 0.9% saline in syringe No. 2 to give 0.25% solution; and 5 ml of 0.9% saline is drawn into syringe No. 1.

The patient must have pain at the time of this test; otherwise it must be postponed. Patients should be advised not to take an analgesic the morning of the test.

An intravenous infusion is started and the patient is positioned with the painful side on the table. The painful area is marked, and a painful maneuver is done to reproduce the pain, (e.g., palpation, movment of the limb).

After the patient is prepared and draped, the subarachnoid space is entered with a 25-gauge, 3½-inch needle at the L3–4 interspace. Free flow is con-

TABLE 15D–1.—GENERAL CLASSIFICATION OF MIXED PERIPHERAL NERVE FIBERS

FIBER	DIAMETER (μ)	CONDUCTION VELOCITY (M/SEC)	FUNCTION	
			Sensory	Motor
A fibers	2–20	6–120	Muscle tendon and spindle	Skeletal muscle and spindle control
Alpha	10–20	60–120	Vibration	
Beta	5–15	30–80	Deep pressure touch	
Gamma	3–7	10–50		
Delta	2–5	6–30	Pricking pain; cold, warmth	
C fibers	0.5–2	0.5–2	Crude touch, pressure, tickle, aching pain, cold, warmth	Sympathetic

firmed in all quadrants. The blood pressure is checked, and sensation is checked with a pinprick. The temperature of the painful area is recorded with a cutaneous probe. A placebo solution is injected after the patient has been told that one of the drugs is being injected. Five minutes later blood pressure, sensation, and temperature are evaluated. If there is pain relief, it is checked by repeating the aggravating maneuvers. If the pain relief lasts for 20 minutes, the needle is removed and the duration of placebo response noted.

If there is no pain relief or the pain reappears within 20 minutes, 5 ml of 0.25% procaine (syringe No. 2) is injected.

If there is evidence of sympathetic block with complete pain relief without loss of pinprick sensation, a sympathetic mechanism is confirmed. This patient is a candidate for further sympathetic blocks.

If there is partial pain relief, the degree of pain relief is noted. If there is no evidence of sympathetic block, or if there is no pain relief despite the sympathetic block, 5 ml of 0.5% (No. 3 syringe) is injected and the pinprick sensation is checked.

If there is no pain relief despite loss of pinprick sensation, or if there is no sensory loss, 1% solution (syringe No. 4) is injected to obtain motor block. Occasionally 1 ml of 5% procaine may be necessary to achieve complete motor block. The needle is removed and the patient is turned supine. Blood pressure, sensation, temperature, and motor block are evaluated. If there is pain relief despite complete sensory loss over the affected area and motor block, the cause of pain is proximal to the site of block. It is not possible to distinguish between psychogenic pain, malingering encephalation, or a CNS lesion. But the most important conclusion reached is that a peripheral procedure such as surgery or nerve block is unlikely to be successful. Further unnecessary surgery can be avoided. Techniques such as hypnosis, behavior modification, and antidepressants may

be of value. Procaine takes approximately 1 hour to wear off.

This procedure can be done on an outpatient basis.

Retrograde Spinal Block

For a standard differential spinal block the patient must lie on the side, with a needle in the back, sometimes up to one hour. This can be avoided with a continuous catheter technique, which also increases the incidence of post-spinal tap headache. Also, end points with each solution sometimes are not clearly delineated.

A retrograde differential spinal block avoids the above drawbacks. The spinal tap and the placebo injection are performed as in the standard technique. If plaebo does not relieve the pain, 2 ml of 5% procaine, which is prepared by mixing 1 ml of 10% procaine for spinal with 1 ml of CSF (sp. gr 1015) or 1 ml of normal saline, is injected. The patient is turned supine after the needle is removed. Because 5% proacine in CSF is hyperbaric, the position of the patient is adjusted to achieve a block at the T-10 or T-6 level. After sensory and complete motor block is established, pain relief is evaluated. If the patient has no pain relief despite complete sensory and motor block, the etiology is proximal to the site of block (i.e., spinal roots). Peripheral procedures such as surgery and nerve blocks will not be helpful.

If pain is relieved, it is due to a sympathetic or a somatic mechanism. After waiting approximately an hour for the block to wear off, the pain relief is evaluated. If pain is relieved despite the reappearance by sensation, the mechanism is likely to be sympathetic, since the pain relief outlasts the duration of the block. Also, sympathetic block is likely to outlast sensory block because the concentration

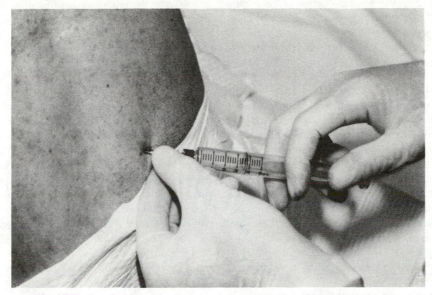

Fig 15D–1.—Epidural technique in progress for differential studies.

necessary to block the B fibers is exceeded for a longer period.

If the pain comes back at the same time that sensation reappears, a somatic mechanism is diagnosed.

Xylocaine may be used in patients allergic to ester compounds.

In many patients, sympathetic and somatic mechanisms coexist in varying proportions. Sympathetic blocks relieve that component (e.g., burning pain), but the somatic mechanism must be treated separately.

Differential Epidural Block

Some physicians prefer differential blocking with an epidural technique to prevent post-spinal tap

TABLE 15D–2.—RETROGRADE DIFFERENTIAL EPIDURAL BLOCK*

TIME (Min)	BP (mm Hg)	PULSE (Beats/Min)	SUBJECTIVE FEELINGS	MOTOR POWER LEG	MOTOR POWER KNEE BEND	MOTOR POWER TOES	SENSATION ON PINPRICK	TEMP. (° F) R LEG	TEMP. (° F) L LEG
Control	116/65	72	Pain and discomfort in back, L hip, and L thigh	X	X	X	X	86	88
0	120/76	76		X	X	X	X	86	88
10	112/70	72	Feeling of warmth, some pain				to t-9	89	93
20	120/60	72	No pain				to T-6	92	94
60	120/60	72	No pain	X	X	X	to T-9	96	96
70	120/60	72	Some return of pain	X	X	X	X	90	92
80	120/60	72	Return of pain to preblock level	X	X	X	X	88	89

*The results of a differential epidural block (20 ml of 3% 2-chloroprocaine injected into epidural space at zero minute) in a 45-year-old man with pain in the low back, left hip, and left thigh and a history of four surgical procedures in the lumbar area. Findings showed that the pain was transmitted via A delta and C fibers. Following the investigative differential blocking, the relief obtained by a series of sympathetic blocks was not enough. Stimulation by percutaneously inserted epidural electrodes gave the patient 70% pain relief. Note that blood pressure and pulse were stable during the differential study. Hypotension may make the test unreliable.

headache and also to have the option of inserting a catheter.[5, 6] This allows the patient to be in a comfortable position for evaluation. Both antegrade and retrograde evaluations have been done.[6] In the retrograde method, 20 ml of a 3% solution of 2-chloroprocaine is injected via an epidural needle or after an epidural catheter is placed (Fig 15D–1). This volume is needed to ensure that all the lumbosacral nerve roots in the epidural space will be bathed. In patients suspected of having epidural fibrosis or other occlusive pathology, spreading of the local anesthetic in the epidural space is a problem. This can be corrected by inserting a catheter and adding enough of the drug in 5-ml increments until the lumbosacral plexus distribution is adequately blocked. One can then evaluate-the-pain pathways as the patient is recovering from the block. Tables 15D–2 through 15D–4 show the results of retrograde differential epidural block in three different pain syndromes.

2-Chloroprocaine is chosen because of its rapid onset of action and rapid disappearance. Rapid onset permits quick determination of the height and intensity of the block; psychogenic pain can be differentiated from sympathetic or somatic pain at this stage. Rapid disappearance permits assessment of C, A delta, and A alpha fiber function within 1 hour. Usually only one dose (20 ml) of 2-chloroprocaine is required for retrograde assessment in the lumbar region. Rapid elimination of 2-chloroprocaine by plasma cholinesterase facilitates the patient's return to normal physiologic status. This is necessary if the procedure is to be done on an outpatient basis.

DIFFERENTIAL BRACHIAL OR LUMBOSACRAL PLEXUS BLOCK

Differential blocking of these plexuses can be done to delineate the pain mechanisms. The volume of the local anesthetic should be the same as that used for surgical anesthesia (see Table 15D–2). The site of blocking should be such that all branches of the plexuses are blocked above the suspected peripheral pathology (e.g., interscalene approach for Pancoast tumor pain and lumbar approach for groin pain). A catheter should be placed for repeated injections. It is best to start with a lesser concentration of the local anesthetic and inject a greater concentration every 30 minutes if the pain is not relieved. One can start initially with 40 ml of saline for evaluation of placebo effect. If there is no pain relief, 40 ml of 0.25% lidocaine is injected at 30 minutes, followed by 40 ml of 0.5% lidocaine and 1% lidocaine at succeeding 30-minute intervals. Vital signs are monitored throughout the procedure and the test is continued only if they are stable at the time of repeated injection.

One can try retrograde evaluation of plexus block after injecting 40 ml of 1.5% lidocaine at one time, just as in the retrograde differential spinal or epidural block. However, there are no data in the literature to show which technique is better (Table 15D–5).

TABLE 15D–3.—RETROGRADE DIFFERENTIAL EPIDURAL BLOCK*

| TIME (Min) | BP (mm Hg) | PULSE (Beats/Min) | SUBJECTIVE FEELINGS | MOTOR POWER | | | SENSATION ON PINPRICK | TEMP. (° F) | |
				LEG	KNEE BEND	TOES		R LEG	L LEG
Control	134/84	60	Burning pain in left fool					91	86
0	148/80	64	Burning pain in left foot	X	X	X	X	90	86
10	120/80	88	75% pain relief	25%	X	X	T-10	95	90
20	114/82	76	Total pain relief				T-8	95	92
60	140/96	64	Total pain relief	X	X	X	T-12	95	92
70	140/96	64	Total pain relief	X	X	X	X	94	92
80	138/94	64	Total pain relief	X	X	X	X	92	90

*The results of a differential epidural block (20 ml of 3% 2-chloroprocaine) in a 22-year-old man with pain in the left foot. At first evaluation at the pain control center patient gave the history of motor vehicle accident 6 months previously. He sustained a medial malleolar fracture at the ankle which was surgically corrected and put in a cast. The fracture healed normally, but the patient complained of burning pain in his left foot, especially after weight-bearing. A diagnosis of reflex sympathetic dystrophy of the left leg was made and retrograde differential epidural block was done to confirm the diagnosis. Findings seen above show that total relief of pain was obtained by blocking the C fibers only. A delta and A alpha nerve fibers did not transmit the nociceptive impulses. A series of six lumbar sympathetic blocks (left) were done at 2-week intervals with adjuvant physical therapy. The patient recovered completely.

TABLE 15D–4.—RETROGRADE DIFFERENTIAL EPIDURAL BLOCK*

| TIME (Min) | BP (mm Hg) | PULSE Beats/Min | SUBJECTIVE FEELINGS | OBJECTIVE FINDINGS | | | | TEMP. (° F) | |
| | | | | MOTOR POWER | | | SENSATION ON PINPRICK | | |
				LEG	KNEE BEND	TOES		R LEG	L LEG
Control	106/88	100	Severe pain in abdominal region	X	X	X	X	88	91
0	110/70	128	Pain in same abdominal region	X	X	X	X	88	91
10	110/70	100	Pain—same	25%	X	X	T-10	86	90
20	106/88	92	Pain—same			75%	T-4	94	92
60	118/70	92	Pain—same	X	X	X	T-10	90	91
70	120/70	92	Pain—same	X	X	X	X	89.5	90
80	120/70	92	Pain—same	X	X	X	X	88.5	90

*The results of a differential epidural block (20 ml of 3% 2-chloroprocaine injected into epidural L2–3 space at time zero) in a 24-year-old woman with chronic abdominal pain. Prior to admission to the pain control center the patient had a diagnosis of chronic pancreatitis for 12 months. During her previous workup and treatment, she had cholecystectomy and multiple ERCP. She became dependent of narcotics and in the interim found it difficult to wean her off the drugs. At initial pain evaluation, it was unclear whether her pain was visceral, somatic, or central. First, a celiac plexus block was carried out which intensified her pain. Second, a retrograde differential epidural block was done to diagnose peripheral vs. central pain. The findings given in the table show clearly that the pain was central in origin since total motor, sensory, and sympathetic nerve fiber loss of function did not change her perception of pain. Her subsequent treatment consisted of behavioral therapy and a drug withdrawal program, with moderate success.

TABLE 15D–5.—DOSAGE OF LOCAL ANESTHETICS FOR DIFFERENTIAL STUDIES

| AGENTS | TECHNIQUES | | | | | |
| | SPINAL | | EPIDURAL | | BRACHIAL PLEXUS | |
	ANTEGRADE VC*	RETROGRADE VC	ANTEGRADE VC	RETROGRADE VC	ANTEGRADE VC	RETROGRADE VC
Procaine	5 ml saline 5 ml 0.25% 5 ml 0.5% 5 ml 1.0% (in some cases may need 2 ml of 5%)	2 ml 5%	5 ml cervical 10 ml thoracic 20 ml lumbar 30 ml caudal			
Lidocaine	—	2 ml 5%	saline 0.25% 0.5% 1.0% 2.0%	2%	40 ml saline 40 ml 0.25% 40 ml 0.5% 40 ml 1.0%	40 ml 1.5%
2-chloroprocaine	—		3%		saline 40 ml 1% 40 ml 2% 40 ml 3%	40 ml 3.0%

*VC, volume concentration.

REFERENCES

1. Gasser H.S., Erlanger J.: Role of fiber size in establishment of nerve block by pressure or cocaine. *Am. J. Physiol.* 88:581–591, 1929.
2. Nathan P.W., Sears T.A.: Some factors concerned in differential nerve block by local anesthetics. *J. Physiol. (London)* 157:565–580, 1961.
3. Gentry, W.D., Newman M.C., Goldner J.L., et al.: Relation between graduated spinal block technique and MMPI for diagnosis and prognosis of chronic low back pain. *Spine* 2:210–213, 1977.
4. McCollum D.E., Stephen C.R.: Use of graduated spinal anesthesia in the differential diagnosis of pain of the back and lower extremities. *South Med. J.* 57:410, 1964.
5. Raj P.P.: Sympathetic pain mechanisms and management. Read before the second annual meeting of the American Society of Anesthesiologists, Hollywood, Fla., March 10–11, 1977.
6. Raj P.P.: Case history 2: Nesacaine for retrograde differential epidural blocking: Nesacaine (Chloroprocaine hydrochloride), in *Case Studies in Obstetrical and Surgical Regional Anesthesia*. New York, Pennwalt Corp., 1979, pp. 8–12.

15E / Psychological Testing and the Dexamethasone Suppression Test

THOMAS OXMAN, M.D.

PSYCHOLOGICAL TESTING

RESEARCH ON psychological testing of pain patients has proceeded along three basic themes: description of the chronic pain patient, discrimination between so-called functional and organic pain, and prediction of outcome. With respect to all three themes, the Minnesota Multiphasic Personality Inventory (MMPI) has been the most popular psychometric instrument.[1] The MMPI is a self-administered test consisting of 566 true-false questions. It can usually be completed in less than 2 hours and then scored by hand or computer. The MMPI gives scores for hypochondriasis (Hs), depression (D), hysteria (Hy), psychopathic deviate (Pd), masculinity-femininity (Mf), paranoia (Pa), psychasthenia (Pt), schizophrenia (Sc), hypomania (Ma), social introversion (Si), and four scales that measure reliability and consistency of responses (L, F, K, Lb).

Use of the MMPI for description and discrimination of pain patients is controversial. Many studies in chronic pain patients show elevations in the three scales Hs, D, and Hy, the "neurotic triad." For treatment planning of specific disorders the clinical labels for the MMPI scales have become less meaningful as psychiatric diagnostic criteria have become more specific in *DSM-III*. This is especially true for depressive illness, anxiety disorders, and somatoform disorders. Various scale configurations as well as absolute scores have been suggested to separate psychogenic from somatic pain patients. However, as discussed by Sternbach,[2] several of these "functional" patterns are also found in "organic" patients with many chronic diseases such as arthritis or multiple sclerosis. In addition, some studies suggest that the presence of psychological disturbance leads to a different style of pain expression regardless of the presence or absence of obvious organic evidence.[3] The authors of those reports that show statistical differences between a functional and organic group caution that there is a great degree of overlap.[4] It is also possible that a physician's belief as to whether a patient's pain is organic or not may influence the patient's self-perception; reported studies have not controlled for this possibility. When patients in these studies are diagnosed as having functional pain, there are no universal criteria, and usually no consideration of the poorly understood myofascial pain syndromes that do not show up on laboratory or radiologic examination.[5] In view of this evidence, several authors have cast doubt not only on the validity of testing for discrimination of functional from organic pain, but also on the existence of the dichotomy between functional and or organic pain[1, 2, 6, 7]

Correlations of outcome with MMPI profiles appear somewhat more promising.[1, 2, 4, 8] MMPI studies of subjects with low back pain have predicted better outcome with lower pretreatment Hs, D, and Hy scores.[1, 4, 8] Sternbach[2] has retrospectively described two MMPI configurations associated with good outcome and two with poor outcome. The former he has termed the "reactive depression" and the "somatization reaction" profiles and the latter the "hypochondriacal" and the "manipulative reaction" profiles. These patterns need cross-validation by others as well as correlation with clinical interview. The practical significance for psychological testing appears to lie in the prediction of successful treatment. The danger of this predictive use of psychological testing is that it may lead the pain specialist to refuse treatment to potentially "unsuccessful" patients rather than to postpone serious procedures in such patients. Continuing research is necessary, and successful interpretation of the MMPI results requires extensive clinical experience by a psychologist. The results of the MMPI should not be taken out of context of the patient's history and the clinical interview, and thus should not be the sole determinant of treatment plans.

TESTS SPECIFIC FOR PAIN ASSESSMENT

As discussed in other parts of this book, pain has several dimensions, including intensity, duration, emotion, and meaning. Any psychological test useful in clinical management of pain should assess several of these dimensions. Probably the most widely used test of this type is the McGill Pain Questionnaire (MPQ).[9] This test consists of 78 pain adjectives divided into 20 categories. The categories are in turn separated into three major dimensions: sensory, affective, and evaluative. Patients are asked to select not more than one appropriate word from each category. Several different methods of scoring are possible, some of which require sophisticated statistical analysis. Research has suggested validity of the three dimensions.[10] The MPQ can be used to measure the impact of various treatments over time. It has also been suggested as an unobtrusive method of obtaining emotional information from those chronic pain patients who are "hypervi-

gilant to any implication of psychogenicity of their pain."[11] As with the MMPI, however, until further empirical research correlates these three MPQ dimensions with physiologic and clinical mechanisms, their descriptive names remain somewhat arbitrary and should not be used without a clinical interview for planning treatment.

The concept of the MPQ has also been combined with psychophysical pain rating procedures which derive from sensory decision theory.[12] This promising work is still more applicable to experimental pain than clinical pain and is not yet practical for routine use.

DEPRESSION AND THE DEXAMETHASONE SUPPRESSION TEST

The report of depression and particularly its associated signs (Fig 15E–1) is not uncommon in patients with pain. Usually the diagnosis of a depressive illness that will be responsive to antidepressants

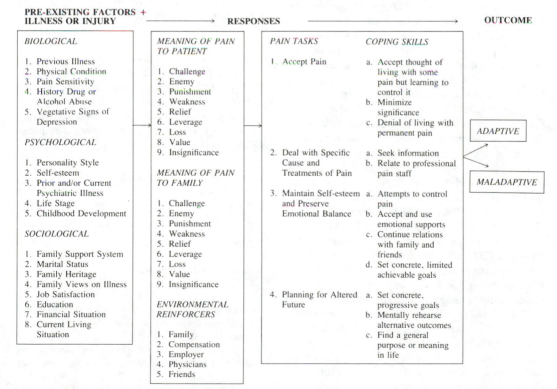

| PRE-EXISTING FACTORS + ILLNESS OR INJURY | | RESPONSES | | OUTCOME |

BIOLOGICAL	MEANING OF PAIN TO PATIENT	PAIN TASKS	COPING SKILLS	
1. Previous Illness		1. Accept Pain	a. Accept thought of living with some pain but learning to control it	
2. Physical Condition	1. Challenge			
3. Pain Sensitivity	2. Enemy			
4. History Drug or Alcohol Abuse	3. Punishment		b. Minimize significance	
5. Vegetative Signs of Depression	4. Weakness		c. Denial of living with permanent pain	ADAPTIVE
	5. Relief			
	6. Leverage			
PSYCHOLOGICAL	7. Loss			
	8. Value	2. Deal with Specific Cause and Treatments of Pain	a. Seek information	
1. Personality Style	9. Insignificance		b. Relate to professional pain staff	MALADAPTIVE
2. Self-esteem				
3. Prior and/or Current Psychiatric Illness	MEANING OF PAIN TO FAMILY			
4. Life Stage		3. Maintain Self-esteem and Preserve Emotional Balance	a. Attempts to control pain	
5. Childhood Development	1. Challenge		b. Accept and use emotional supports	
	2. Enemy			
SOCIOLOGICAL	3. Punishment		c. Continue relations with family and friends	
	4. Weakness			
1. Family Support System	5. Relief			
2. Marital Status	6. Leverage		d. Set concrete, limited achievable goals	
3. Family Heritage	7. Loss			
4. Family Views on Illness	8. Value			
5. Job Satisfaction	9. Insignificance	4. Planning for Altered Future	a. Set concrete, progressive goals	
6. Education				
7. Financial Situation	ENVIRONMENTAL REINFORCERS		b. Mentally rehearse alternative outcomes	
8. Current Living Situation				
	1. Family		c. Find a general purpose or meaning in life	
	2. Compensation			
	3. Employer			
	4. Physicians			
	5. Friends			

Fig 15E–1.—A psychosomatic approach for the evaluation of chronic pain. (Adapted from Lipowski Z.J.: *Ann. Intern. Med.* 71:1197, 1969; Lipowski Z.J.: *Psychiatr. Med.* 1:90, 1970; Moos R.H., Tsu V.D.: In Moos R.H. (ed.): Coping With Physical Illness, New York, Plenum Press, 1977.

can be made by detailed questioning about the eight signs of depression. A depression-specific screening questionnaire may be of use to alert the physician to take extra time in eliciting the right signs of depression. The Zung Self-Rating Depression Scale (SDS) or the Symptom Check List-90 (SCL-90) are two recommended screening devices.[13, 14] Sometimes, however, the severity of the pain complaint and the organic pathology make it difficult to diagnose depressive illness. The dexamethasone suppression test (DST) is receiving increasing attention as a biologic marker for depressive illness in difficult diagnostic situations. Research has linked dysfunction of the hypothalamic-pituitary-adrenal axis with depressive illness, possibly through a common neurotransmitter dysfunction. Classically, the DST has been used as a screening test for Cushing's disease. Several studies have now applied the DST to depressive illness and pain.[15, 16]

The usual method for a DST includes predexamethasone and postdexamethasone blood cortisol sampling. The number of samples and the dose of dexamethasone used are quite variable. Normal plasma cortisol demonstrates a diurnal variation up to 25 μ/100 ml in the early morning and up to 8 μ/100 ml around midnight. Bearing in mind the lack of consensus over the method of choice and the cost to and comfort of the patient, we recommend an 8 A.M and 11 P.M. pretest blood cortisol sample followed by 1 mg of dexamethasone at 11 P.M., and then 8 A.M. and 4 P.M. samples the following day. For outpatients who have transportation difficulties, the next best alternative would be to have the patient take 1 mg of dexamethasone at 11 P.M. at home and come to the office for an 8 A.M. and/or 4 P.M. sample. Failure to adequately suppress plasma cortisol below 5 μ/100 ml at 8 A.M. or 4 P.M. is consistent with depressive illness, as is a predexamethasone 8 A.M. cortisol level greater than 25 μ/100 ml and an 11 P.M. plasma cortisol greater than 8 μ/100 ml. An abnormal DST will occur in up to 50% of patients with depressive illness.[15, 17] False positive results may be obtained in the presence of Cushing's syndrome, other primary endocrine illnesses, ectopic ACTH-producing tumors, renovascular hypertension, chronic renal failure requiring hemodialysis, alcohol withdrawal, protein-calorie malnutrition, obesity, and chronic use of diphenylhydantoin or barbiturates. False negative results occur with chronic corticosteroid therapy.

The following case describes the usefulness of the DST.

A 32-year-old married woman with a 2-year history of chronic left knee pain and leg pain following an automobile accident presented for treatment. She had a fractured patella, several ruptured ligaments, and a history of four operations. She was able to continue working part time as a computer operator but became increasingly despondent over her inability to pursue her athletic hobbies. She was placed on 100 mg of amitriptyline daily at bedtime for sleep and possible depression. When she presented to the pain control center for treatment, she complained of occasional crying spells, thoughts of not wanting to continue living in chronic pain, and insomnia marked by trouble falling asleep and midcycle awakening. Amitriptyline was increased to 225 mg nightly with some improvement in sleep but no change in mood or pain. On admission to the hospital for continuous epidural infusion, the DST revealed a pretest 8 A.M. cortisol value of 20 μ/100 ml, and 8 A.M. and 4 P.M. postdexamethasone cortisol levels of 25 μ/100 ml and 15 μ/100 ml. Amitriptyline was discontinued because of side effects, but the DST results, in conjunction with the patient's depressed affect and insomnia, suggested she had an inadequately treated depression. Desipramine was prescribed at a dose of 200 mg. nightly, and after 2 weeks she noted significant improvement in affect and sleep.

The DST may also be used in assessing how long to maintain a person on antidepressants. As many as 50% of patients can relapse within 6 months of clinical recovery from depressive illness. Antidepressant therapy should probably be continued in patients whose DST does not show a normal response despite clinical improvement.

REFERENCES

1. Strassberg D.S., Reimherr F., Ward M., et al.: The MMPI and chronic pain. *J. Consult. Clin. Psychol.* 49:220-226, 1981.
2. Sternbach R.: *Pain Patients: Traits and Treatments.* New York, Academic Press, 1974.
3. McCreary C., Turner J., Dawson E.: Principal dimensions of the pain experience and psychological disturbance in chronic low back pain patients. *Pain* 11:85-92, 1981.
4. McCreary C., Turner J., Dawson E.: Differences between functional versus organic low back pain patients. *Pain* 4:73-78, 1977.
5. Raj P.P., McLennan J.E., Phero J.C.: Assessment and management of planning of chronic low back pain, in Hicks M.S., Boas R. (eds.): *Chronic Low Back Pain.* New York, Raven Press, 1982, pp. 71-99.
6. Hackett T.P.: The pain patient: Evaluation and treat-

ment, in Hackett T.P., Cassem N.H. (eds.): *Massachusetts General Hospital Handbook of General Hospital Psychiatry*. St. Louis, C.V. Mosby Co., 1978, pp. 41–63.

7. Freeman C., Calson D., Louks J.: The use of the M.M.P.I. with low back pain patients. *J. Clin. Psychol*. 32:294–298, 1976.

8. Hendler N., Viernstein M., Gucer P., et al.: A preoperative screening test for chronic back pain patients. *Psychosomatics* 20:801–808, 1979.

9. Melzack R.: The McGill pain questionnaire: Major properties and scoring methods. *Pain* 1:277–299, 1975.

10. Kremer E., Atkinson J.H.: Pain measurement: Construct validity of the affective dimension of the McGill pain questionnaire with chronic benign pain patients. *Pain* 11:93–100, 1981.

11. Morgan C., Kremer E., Gaylor M.: The behavioral medicine unit: a new facility. *Compr. Psychiatry* 20:79–89, 1979.

12. Gracely R.H., Dubner R.: Pain assessment in humans: A reply to Hall. *Pain* 11:109–120, 1981.

13. Hedlund J.L., Viewweg B.W.: The Zung self-rating depression scale: A comprehensive review. *J. Operat. Psychiatry* 10:51–64, 1979.

14. Derogatis L.R., Rickels K., Rock A.F.: The SCL-90 and the MMPI: A step in the validation of a new self report scale. *Br. J. Psychiatry* 128:280–289, 1976.

15. Kalin N.H., Risch S.C., Janowsky D.S., et al.: Use of the dexamethasone suppression test in clinical psychiatry. *J. Clin. Psychopharmacol*. 1:64–69, 1981.

16. Carroll B.J., Feinberg M., Greeden J.F., et al.: A specific laboratory test for the diagnosis of melancholia. *Arch. Gen. Psychiatry* 38: 15–22, 1981.

17. France R.D., Krishan K.R., Houpt J.L., et al.: Differentiation of depression from chronic pain with the dexamethasone suppression test and DSM-III. *Am. J. Psychiatry* 141:1577–1579, 1984.

16 / Pain Syndromes and Rationale for Management

16A / Neurogenic Pain

STEPHEN E. ABRAM, M.D.

MATT J. LIKAVEC, M.D.

AFTER COMPLETION of the history, physical examination, and other investigative procedures, an acute or a chronic pain syndrome can be categorized into one of five groups: neurogenic musculoskeletal, sympathetic somatic, visceral, or psychogenic. Some patients, however, present with a combination of neurologic and myofascial pain, neurologic and skeletal pain, musculoskeletal pain, or musculo-sympathogenic pains. Most usually exhibit psychogenic pain behavior (Fig 16A–1). How can one develop a management applicable to all these complex syndromes? The answer might be found by looking at the physiologic and psychological changes that occur as a result of the anatomical pathologies.

Any pain reaching consciousness must involve the nervous system by transmission of nociceptive pathways through the spinal cord and thalamus to the primary pain cortex and limbic (interpretive) cortex. However, the term "neural pain" should be limited to situations where the pain originates from the nerve tissue itself, be it in CNS or in the peripheral nervous system. Common examples of pain of neurogenic origin involving the CNS are thalamic syndrome, brain and spinal cord tumors, and multiple sclerosis; examples of pain involving the peripheral nervous system are various radiculopathies, postherpetic neuralgias, trigeminal neuralgia, and diabetic neuropathy. Pain of CNS origin is discussed in chapter 16E. Peripheral neurogenic pain is discussed in this chapter under the headings of rad-

iculopathy, peripheral neuralgia, and peripheral neuropathy.

RADICULOPATHY

Pain that follows the distribution pattern of a single dermatome is usually the result of a pathologic process involving a nerve root close to its emergence from the spinal column (Figs 16A–2 and 16A–3). Pain is often "shooting" or "electric" in nature, but other qualities, such as burning, throbbing, or aching, may be described. Weakness of muscles supplied by that segment and loss of sensation within the dermatome are commonly seen. Maneuvers that place tension on the affected root reproduce the pain.

Acute pain results from irritation and inflammation of the nerve root, frequently because of prolonged mechanical compression by herniated disk material, osteophytes, or tumor.[1] Chemical radiculitis may result from degenerating glycoprotein material from the herniated nucleus puloposus.[2] Neural swelling, ischemia, and eventually, loss of neural elements and fibrosis occur, leading to chronic pain resistant to most types of therapy.[3]

Injection of corticosteroid preparations into the epidural space adjacent to the irritated nerve root produces lasting relief for the majority of patients with relatively acute radicular pain.[4] Early treatment of the inflammatory response with local steroids

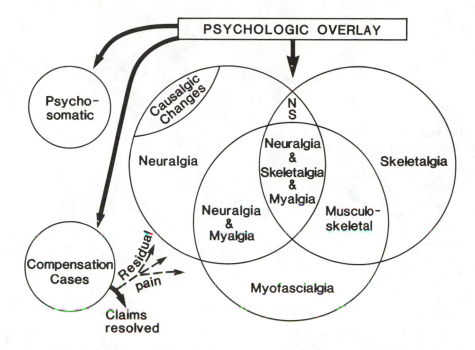

NS = NEUROSKELETAL PAIN, e.g. facet syndrome, spondylolesthesis

Fig 16A–1.—Etiologies of chronic pain. The "pure" category is rare and is seen as the acute manifestation of chronic pain. As pain becomes chronic, complex syndromes evolve and require multimodality therapeutic management. (From Raj P.P., McLennan J.E., Phero J.C.: Assessment and management of planning of chronic low back pain, in Hicks M.S., Boas R. (eds.): *Chronic Low Back Pain.* New York, Raven Press, 1982. Reproduced by permission.)

probably prevents some of the irreversible changes that occur with chronic inflammation.

PERIPHERAL NEURALGIA

Severe pain and marked cutaneous hypersensitivity may result from many types of peripheral nerve pathology. Trauma, including crushing injury, laceration, avulsion, and compression, may cause degeneration of sensory axons. During and often after regeneration, the cutaneous areas supplied by the nerve remain hyperpathic.

Toxic and metabolic neuropathies, such as those caused by diabetes, alcoholism, and certain drugs, may produce constant neuralgic pain and dysesthesias. Herpes zoster causes similar symptoms in addition to the cutaneous rash. Some types of neuralgic pains such as tic douloureux are episodic. Nerve function is normal at times, but severe, lancinating pain occurs suddenly and transiently, often initiated by a stimulus to a trigger area within the distribution zone of the nerve. The sympathetic nervous system is important in the pathophysiology of some neuralgias. The toxic and metabolic neuropathies may improve with sympathetic blocks, and there is at least anecdotal evidence that sympathetic blocks performed during the acute phase of herpes zoster decrease the incidence of postherpetic neuralgia.

In mixed nerves, the larger fibers are more susceptible to certain types of insult, particularly ischemia. Following such injuries there may be loss of many large afferent fibers with preservation of most of the small fibers that subserve nociceptive functions. Either through changes in the function of the peripheral nerve or through a dorsal horn "gating" mechanism,[5] touch, pressure, and proprioceptive

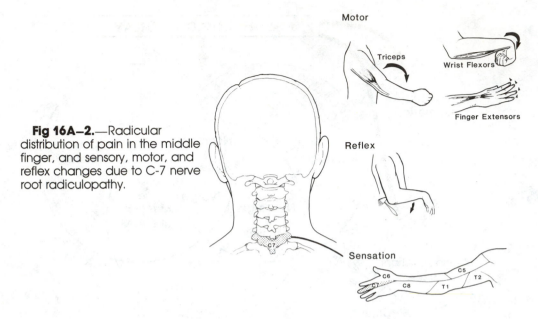

Fig 16A–2.—Radicular distribution of pain in the middle finger, and sensory, motor, and reflex changes due to C-7 nerve root radiculopathy.

stimuli, which are normally transmitted by large afferent fibers, evoke pain.

Several types of treatment may be helpful in controlling neuralgic pain. Some anticonvulsants, such as diphenylhydantoin and carbamazepine, are often effective in the episodic type of neuralgias such as tic douloureux. Sympathetic blocks or peripheral nerve blocks with local anesthetic or anesthetic-steroid mixtures may be helpful for constant neuralgic pain and hyperpathia. Transcutaneous electrical stimulation is occasionally of benefit in such cases.

Trigeminal Neuralgia

Trigeminal neuralgia is not really a disease but a manifestation of underlying disordered physiology. Even though trigeminal neuralgia has various etiologies, it presents with a consistent clinical syndrome. This clinical syndrome is manifested by the classic features of (1) Painful paroxysms. These are described as lightning, shooting, or lancinating pains. They last anywhere from a few seconds to a couple of minutes at most. (2) Pain provoked by obvious stimuli. The stimulus can be as slight as touching the side of the face, eating, a breeze blowing across the face, brushing the teeth, or any other insignificant type of mechanical stimulus. (3) Pain confined to the trigeminal nerve zone. This is classically in division V_2 or V_3. The pain does not

spread out to shoot down the neck or up over the head, nor does it leave the distribution of the trigeminal nerve zone. (4) Pain referred to only one side of the midline. (5) No hypesthesia or hypalgesia on neurologic examination. (6) Long episodes of pain-free intervals lasting minutes, hours, days, or months.[6–8]

As is obvious from these criteria, trigeminal neuralgia is a presenting symptom complex. There are all kinds of facial pains that should not be confused with trigeminal neuralgia. Also, trigeminal neuralgia is not synonymous with any long-lasting chronic facial pain. True trigeminal neuralgia should fulfill the above six criteria.

There is also the syndrome of "atypical trigeminal neuralgia," which bears a superficial resemblance to true trigeminal neuralgia. The differences lie in the fact that atypical trigeminal neuralgia often is associated with constant burning, aching pain, with severe exacerbations based on the background of pain. There may or may not be trigger points in trigeminal neuralgia. There is often hyperactive autonomic dysfunction in atypical trigeminal neuralgia, and there may be hypesthesia or hypalgesia detected more frequently in the atypical facial pain.[9] Also, atypical facial pain does not respond to the usual medical treatment for trigeminal neuralgia.

The clinical differences between atypical trigeminal neuralgia and trigeminal neuralgia are brought out to emphasize that the statistics on painful afflic-

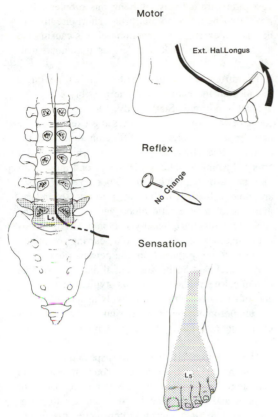

Motor

Ext. Hal.Longus

Reflex

No Change

Sensation

L₅

Fig 16A–3.—Radicular distribution of pain in the lateral aspect of the foot, and sensory, motor, and reflex changes due to S-1 nerve root radiculopathy.

tion of the face characteristic of *true* trigeminal neuralgia apply only to this state. Treatment modalities commonly applied to true trigeminal neuralgia have had only mixed results with the atypical facial pains.

The signs and symptoms of trigeminal neuralgia are basically defined by its criteria. Facial pain that fulfills the six listed criteria qualifies as trigeminal neuralgia. There are some things to add, however, concerning this clinical state. At times trigeminal neuralgia can be so debilitating that people refuse to eat, if mastication brings on the pain. Large weight losses are not uncommon in this disease entity. Some patients become recluses because of their fear of going outside and exposing even part of their face to stimulation by something as quiet as a wisp of air. Dental hygiene often deteriorates because of the patient's inability to maintain proper mouth care.

The physician may notice that these patients talk with only one side of their mouth and look as if they have partial paralysis of one side of their face; these protective mannerisms have developed out of fear of initiating a painful attack. In examining women with the disease, one often finds makeup not applied to one part of the face because of the fear of inciting an incident.[7]

The pain of trigeminal neuralgia is severe. Afflicted persons describe the pain as worse than that of a kidney stone. I have had one patient tell me that he would live with kidney stone pain again rather than go through recurrent attacks of trigeminal neuralgia. Among the mysteries of the clinical complex of trigeminal neuralgia which make physicians sometimes reticent to make the diagnosis or doubt the veracity of the patient's word is that the symptoms sometimes abate. As included in the six criteria, there may be long periods of no symptoms. This means that not only will the patient not have the attacks of pain, but pressure or stimulation on the previous trigger point will be without effect.

There is another source of clinical confusion because the trigger zones often associated with the mouth and teeth, the disease may be unrecognized for years, or patients may seek other treatment after multiple dental, surgical, or orthodontic procedures. All of these may appear successful for a short time, but later the same pain recurs. Because of the inconsistency of the symptoms and the episodes of remission, a patient might have had a number of unnecessary surgical procedures.

There are few statistics of interest in true trigeminal neuralgia. The disorder is more common in women than in men—about 60% of the patients are women. The disease usually occurs in the fifth and sixth decades of life.[10] This is an important clinical point, for if the disease seems to present at an earlier age, one should consider a demyelinating process or an associated tumor. The pain usually involves the second and third division of the trigeminal nerve. The first division is involved in less than 5% of cases.[11]

Etiology and Pathology

Consistent pathologic changes take place in the trigeminal ganglia that are more marked in people with trigeminal neuralgia. These degenerative changes are thought to be the anatomical basis for the altered neuronal function. These microscopic changes, documented by light and electron microscopy, are characterized by intact ganglion cells with some vacuolization, degenerative hypermyelinization, segmental myelinization with denuding of the axis cylinders, and axonal thickenings and tortuosity.[12] These consistent anatomical findings in persons with trigeminal neuralgia should lay to rest any idea that the ganglia are normal in trigeminal neuralgia.

From reviewing the literature, it appears that there are a number of possible etiologies which can cause this pathologic description and which are associated with the symptoms of trigeminal neuralgia. Among the two most common etiologies for this pathologic picture associated with trigeminal neuralgia are mechanical deformation of the nerve root entry zone, and demyelinating illness.

In line with recent contributions in the literature it appears that a number of mechanical factors can be the cause of the classic syndrome of trigeminal neuralgia. These appear to cause some sort of mechanical deformation at the nerve root entry zone. The nerve root entry zone is that area of the nerve of the cranial nerve where it enters the brain stem. Studies indicate that any sort of pressure applied at the nerve root entry zone of the fifth cranial nerve can be the cause of the classic syndrome of trigeminal neuralgia.[13] The most common cause of this mechanical distortion appears to be distortion of the entry zone by branches of ectatic atherosclerotic branches of the superior cerebellar artery. Other ectatic and aberrant arteries have been described as causing pressure in that area and to be associated with classic trigeminal neuralgia.[14] Mechanical distortion of nerve root entries by small tumors, arteriovenous malformations, cysts, and even venous structures has been described, and such distortion in turn has been associated with classic trigeminal neuralgia.

The other major cause of trigeminal neuralgia appears to be demyelinization from multiple sclerosis. Trigeminal neuralgia is a well-known symptom complex that is associated with multiple sclerosis. It seems that demyelinating plaque in the nerve root entry zone or even in the pons itself can evolve into a clinical picture of trigeminal neuralgia.[15]

Even with some knowledge of mechanical factors and demyelinization and pathologic changes, we still do not know how these aberrations of pathology, and what we believe are the primary etiologies, can cause the abnormal neurophysiologic events that manifest as trigeminal neuralgia. A number of investigators are actively studying this problem. It is not clear whether abnormal firing, short circuits, abnormal reflex arcs, or something else is causing the aberrant impulses that manifest as trigeminal neuralgia.[11]

The differential diagnosis of trigeminal neuralgia includes all the entities that can possibly cause this clinical syndrome. Statistically, the most common cause of the syndrome is a pressure exerted on the nerve root entry zone of the fifth cranial nerve in the posterior fossa by a loop of the superior cerebellar artery.[14] Multiple sclerosis is the second most common cause of the syndrome. Other possible causes are tumors (benign, malignant, primary, secondary, metastatic, etc.), ectatic blood vessels (besides the superior cerebellar), aneurysms, and arteriovenous malformations, cysts, arachnoid scarring, or indentation from bony spurs from the petrous ridge.[7]

Also included in the differential diagnosis of true trigeminal neuralgia are various atypical facial pains and other facial syndromes involving pathology of the temporomandibular joint, sinuses, orbit and orbital contents, gums, teeth, and other oral structures.

The workup of a patient with suspected trigeminal neuralgia includes not only a thorough physical and neurologic examination, but also an examination of the oral and facial contents. With respect to radiologic workup, it is currently considered mandatory to obtain CT scans of the brain, with and without contrast. Radiologic evaluation of the orbits and sinuses and mouth is also indicated if there is any question as to the underlying etiology of a tic-like pain.

Treatment

Treatment of trigeminal neuralgia entails four basic approaches: (1) medication, (2) injection of nerve branches and trigger points, (3) percutaneous radiofrequency trigeminal rhizotomy, and (4) open surgical procedures.

The medical treatment of trigeminal neuralgia entails the use of three drugs: diphenylhydantoin, mephenesin, and carbamazepine. Diphenylhydantoin has been used for years in the treatment of trigeminal neuralgia. It is tolerated well, usually with minimal side effects. However, because of toxicity in some patients, and because its efficacy seems to fall off with time and control of pain appears to be incomplete, it is not used as often as it once was. In our experience, only about 15%–20% of patients with tics appear to derive sustained relief of symptoms with diphenylhydantoin. The dosage of this medication is 300–600 mg/day.[16]

Mephenesin has been shown to be effective in the treatment of trigeminal neuralgia. We have very little experience with the use of this drug.[17]

Carbamazepine (Tegretol) has an excellent track record in the treatment of tic pain. Relief of tic pain occurs in more than 60% of patients and appears to be sustained in quite a few for an extended period of time. The problem with the drug is its toxic effects, which may include leukopenia and liver damage. For this reason, Tegretol is started at low dosages, 200 mg twice a day, and blood counts and LFTs are checked at intervals. Because of toxic reactions the Tegretol may have to be stopped.[8, 18]

The second method of treating trigeminal neuralgia is by injection of the trigger points or involved branch of the trigeminal nerve with a local anesthetic and alcohol. The rationale for this treatment is as follows: (1) It allows patients to experience the kind of numbness they would have following radiofrequency rhizotomy and decide whether they could live with it. (2) It allows the rare debilitated patients a period of oral intake so that they can become better operative risks. (3) In the unusual case of ''atypical'' facial pain it is of help in deciding whether a patient definitely has a tic-like pain or not. Procaine has been injected into the superior or-

bital or manidublar branch of the nerve to see how people like it.[7] For more permanent blocks, alcohol is used.

The third treatment of trigeminal neuralgia is percutaneous rhizotomy. It is believed that partial destruction of the sensory pathway for the impulses of the trigeminal neuralgia will interrupt the pain. Percutaneous rhizotomy is carried out with needle electrocoagulation of the percutaneous route. Temperature coagulation is used to destroy A delta and C fibers, which carry painful stimuli, yet maintain function of the A fibers.[7] The results depend on the differences in myelination and fiber diameter: patients maintain touch perception yet have analgesia.

An insulated needle is placed through the cheek into the foramen ovale under radiographic control (Fig 16A–4). Needle localization is confirmed anatomically by radiography and physiologically by the feeling of dysesthesias in the appropriate nerve root. After needle placement is confirmed, a radiofrequency current is used in a controlled, graded manner to thermally injure the trigeminal ganglion and rootlets in order to create an area of analgesia.[19] The advantage of this technique is that it can be done on almost any patient with minimal, short-term, reversible anesthesia (e.g., IV pentothal). This includes elderly patients and those who are severely debilitated. Because of the physiologic and anatomical localization and testing, the physician can be fairly certain what areas are involved. And a

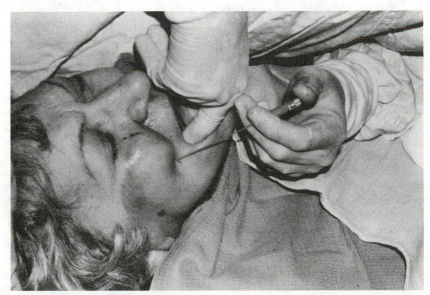

Fig 16A–4.—Needle insertion for radiofrequency percutaneous rhizotomy of trigeminal ganglion in a patient with trigeminal neuralgia. (Courtesy of James Phero, D.M.D.)

graded lesion can be created that can be enlarged or increased in the future. There is nothing in this technique that prevents the physician from repeating it a second or third time.[7, 18]

The disadvantages of the radiofrequency techniques are its side effects. The first major side effect is the sensory deprivation, which some people find intolerable; they would rather have the pain than the dysesthetic numbness. A small number of patients end up with diplopia because of the technique. Other patients have reported some facial weakness and some difficulty chewing properly. V_1 lesions have a slight incidence of keratitis. A small percentage of patients end up with herpes keratitis in the area of the lesion. The most terrible side effect and complication of this technique is anesthesia dolorosa, or painful anesthesia involving the area of the lesion. The pain is severe and debilitating and responds poorly to any treatment. Extreme measures such as lobotomy or mesencephalotomy have been attempted in the past in order to take care of this painful complication. Fortunately anesthesia dolorosa occurs in a very small percentage of patients who undergo percutaneous rhizotomy. Approximately 93% of patients who undergo the procedure have good results, and their condition is improved.[2, 16, 18]

Finally, percutaneous trigeminal rhizotomy is indeed a destructive procedure, and pain specialists, by and large, abhor the idea of creating lesions to control pain.

The fourth method of controlling trigeminal neuralgia is open surgery. Three procedures are available: extradural sensory root section through a temporal craniotomy, posterior fossa microvascular decompression of the trigeminal nerve, and posterior fossa microvascular decompression of the trigeminal nerve with partial sensory root section.

Extradural sensory root section was the standard procedure for years and has been used by such giants as Frazier, Grant, and Cushing. The procedure is carried out through a subtemporal approach extradurally on the side affected by trigeminal neuralgia. After subtemporal dissection to the area of the foramen ovale, the rootlets constituting the sensory roots of V_2 and V_3 are sectioned. The operative mortality from this procedure is low, but facial weakness occurs in as many as 7%–10% of patients.[21] One should always remember that the procedure is an open surgical procedure as well as a destructive ablative one.

The second major operative procedure involves the posterior fossa approach to the trigeminal nerve.

The idea behind this operation is that most trigeminal neuralgia is caused by vascular compression of the nerve root entry zone of the trigeminal nerve by a branch of the superior cerebellar artery. Hence a posterior fossa approach is used with microscopic magnification to approach cranial nerve. Upon approaching it the surgeon will find an indentation of the trigeminal nerve root entry zone by a branch of the superior cerebellar artery. By discretely dissecting the arachnoid free, this branch of the superior cerebellar artery can be dissected free from the trigeminal nerve and a small padding used to make sure that the vessel does not go back and imprint on the nerve.[15, 22]

This procedure, too, is an open procedure, and elderly and debilitated patients are not candidates for it. In addition, it has all the complications associated with an open surgical procedure.

Nevertheless, the advantages of microvascular decompression are numerous. Most important, it is not an ablative or destructive procedure, so patients will have normal facial sensation postoperatively. Second, it allows thorough exploration of the area of pathology. Small tumors, cysts, veins, and other pathology can be identified and handled as necessary. Third, anesthesia dolorosa does not occur afterward.[23]

The results of open microvascular decompression are indeed excellent and appear to be as good as those of percutaneous radiofrequency rhizotomy, with good results being reported more than 90% of patients in most series.[19, 20, 23]

The third operative procedure that is considered for trigeminal neuralgia is a posterior fossa approach with microvascular decompression and a partial sensory nerve root section. The idea is that not only is the underlying pathology taken care of by decompressing the nerve root entry zone, but results in the few remaining failures could be enhanced by partial root section.[24] Too few of these procedures have been done in a large series to analyze how patients do, compared with patients who had the two more standard procedures, the percutaneous radiofrequency rhizotomy of an open microvascular decompression. However, one must question whether having the best of both worlds is worth buying the complications of both worlds.

At present trigeminal neuralgia appears to be one treated medically first, with Tegretol, and after Tegretol fails, an operative procedure is considered. The choice of this operative procedure, in our opinion, is percutaneous radiofrequency rhizotomy or an open posterior fossa microvascular decompression.

A thorough discussion with the patient and the surgeons involved will help one make the decision. See Loeser[6] for an excellent approach.

PERIPHERAL NEUROPATHY

Peripheral neuropathy includes any primary disorder of peripheral motor, sensory, or autonomic neurons. The clinical signs are muscle weakness, varying degrees of atrophy, and sensory and autonomic dysfunction.

Among neuropathies, nerve entrapment, leprosy, and diabetes mellitus are probably the most common worldwide. The precise cause of many neuropathies is unknown, and their diagnosis depends on their association with other diseases such as diabetes mellitus, carcinoma, or uremia.

Compression and Entrapment Syndromes

The peripheral nerve trunks of the extremities are particularly prone to compression and entrapment. The three most common entrapment neuropathies are carpal tunnel syndrome, tardy ulnar palsy, and tardy common peroneal nerve palsy.

Carpal Tunnel Syndrome

In this syndrome, the median nerve as it passes through the carpal tunnel is compressed by a ganglion, a degenerative joint, or an inflamed, thickened synovium caused by rheumatoid arthritis or similar disorders. Carpal tunnel syndrome usually affects women. Pricking pain and numbness are most prominent in the thumb, the thenar aspect of the palm, and first three digits, especially at night. Relief by shaking the hand is characteristic. Aching discomfort may extend up to the arm. Atrophy of the thenar muscles is a late sign. In many cases it is possible to reproduce the painful numbness by holding the wrist in extreme flexion (Phalen's sign, Fig 16A–5). Tingling may also occur when the skin is percussed over the carpal tunnel (Tinel's sign, Fig 16A–6).

Nerve conduction studies confirm the syndrome. The latency is usually prolonged. Treatment is directed toward prevention of activities that aggravate the syndrome, or release of compression and entrapment by percutaneous steroid injections or surgery.

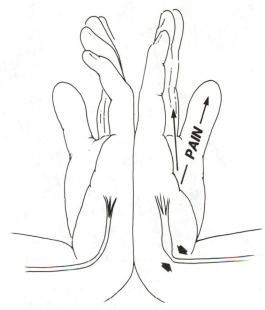

Fig 16A–5.—Phalen's sign.

Stellate ganglion blocks have also been helpful in reducing the burning discomfort associated with this syndrome.

Meralgia Paresthetica

Obese patients who wear tight corsets or clothes and patients with a pendulous abdomen may develop superficial paresthesia and burning discomfort in the distribution of the lateral cutaneous nerve of the thigh. It is due to compression of the nerve as it passes beneath the inguinal ligament. Nerve blocks of the lateral femoral cutaneous nerve or a lumbar sympathetic block is indicated for severe burning pain. Wearing loose clothes and weight loss are good methods by which pain relief can be maintained.

Neuropathy Associated With Diabetes Mellitus

The frequency of diabetic neuropathy ranges from 5% to 60% and increases with age and the duration of diabetes. It seems unlikely that a single mechanism underlies the various types of diabetic neuropathy. Nerve damage from ischemia to distal lower limbs is one mechanism and responsible for one variety; compression may be responsible for another.

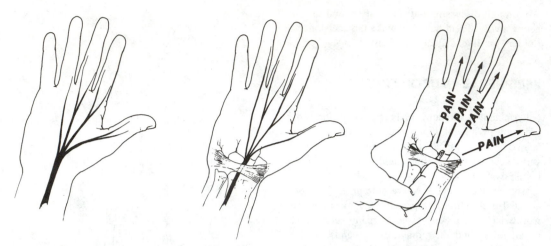

Fig 16A–6.—Tinel's sign, and neuropathy of the carpal tunnel syndrome. *Left,* median nerve. *Middle,* compression of the median nerve in the carpal tunnel. *Right,* Tinel's sign.

The pathology may be a diffuse microangiopathy of endoneural capillaries with ischemia. Alternative explanations include immunologic or biochemical derangements (e.g., insulin deficiency, phospholipid deficiency). A period of severe weight loss may often precede the development of diabetic polyneuropathy or diabetic amyotrophy. Diabetic amyotrophy involves proximal portions of the peripheral nerves, commonly lumbar roots and plexuses. Pain in this condition is centered in the thigh and extends to the medial side of the leg, followed by the onset of muscle weakness and atrophy. Recovery from this condition may require months or years. Until that time, pain is controlled by epidural and sympathetic blocks, as needed, followed by exercises and stabilization of diabetes with increased protein intake in the diet.

REFERENCES

1. Howe J.F.: A neurophysiologic basis for the radicular pain of nerve root compression, in Bonica J.J. (ed.) *Advances in Pain Research and Therapy.* New York, Raven Press, vol. 3, 1979, pp. 647–657.
2. Marshall L.L., Trethewice E.R., Curtain C.C.: Chemical radiculitis. *Clin. Orthop.* 29:61–67, 1977.
3. Murphy R.W.: Nerve roots and spinal nerves in degenerative disc disease. *Clin. Orthop* 60:46–60, 1977.
4. Pace B.L.: Psychophysiology of pain: Diagnostic and therapeutic implications. *J. Fam. Pract.* 5:553–557, 1977.
5. Melzack R., Wall P.D.: Pain mechanisms: A new theory. *Science* 150:971–979, 1965.
6. Loeser J.D.: What to do about tic douloureux. *JAMA* 239:1153–1155, 1978.
7. White J.C., Sweet W.H., Thomas C.C.: *Pain of the Neurosurgeon: A Forty Year Experience.* Springfield, Ill., Charles C Thomas, Publisher, 1969, chaps. 5, 8, and 9.
8. Voorhies R., Patterson, R.H.: State of the art: Management of trigeminal neuralgia (tic douloureux). *JAMA* 245:2521–2523, 1981.
9. Yonas H., Jannetta P.J.: Neurinoma of the trigeminal root and atypical trigeminal neuralgia: Their commonality. *Neurosurgery,* 6:273–277, 1980.
10. Harris W.: An analysis of 1433 cases of paroxysmal trigeminal neuralgia (trigeminal tic) and the end results of gasserian alcohol injection. *Brain* 63:209–224, 1940.
11. Tytus J.S.: General considerations, medical therapy, and minor operative procedures for trigeminal neuralgia, in Youmans J.R. (ed.): *Neurological Surgery.* Philadelphia, W.B. Saunders Co., 1982, pp. 3534–3546.
12. Kruger L.: Structural aspects of trigeminal neuralgia: A summary of current findings and concepts. *J. Neurosurg.* 26:109–190, 1967.
13. Kerr F.W.L.: Etiology of trigeminal neuralgia. *Arch. Neurol.* 89:15–25, 1963.
14. Janetta P.J.: Trigeminal neuralgia and hemifacial spasm: Etiology and definitive treatment. *Trans. Am. Neurol. Assoc.,* 100:89–91, 1965.
15. Lazar M.L., Kirkpatrick J.B.: Trigeminal neuralgia and multiple sclerosis: Demonstration of the plague in an operative case. *Neurosurgery* 5:711–717, 1979.
16. Braham J., Saia A.: Phenytoin in the treatment of trigeminal and other neuralgias. *Lancet* 2:892–893, 1960.
17. King R.B.: The medical control of tic douloureux: Preliminary report on the effect of mephenesin on facial pain. *J. Neurosurg.* 15:290–298, 1958.
18. Dalessio D.J.: Treatment of trigeminal neuralgia, editorial. *JAMA* 245:2519–2520, 1981.

19. Tew J.M.: Treatment of trigeminal neuralgia by percutaneous rhizotomy, in Youmans J.R. (ed.): *Neurological Surgery*. Philadelpha, W.B. Saunders Co., 1982, vol. 6, p. 3564–3579.
20. Tew J.M.: Treatment of trigeminal neuralgia: Viewpoint. *Neurosurgery* 4:93, 1979.
21. Tytus J.S.: Treatment of trigeminal neuralgia by through temporal craniotomy, in Youmans J.R. (ed.): *Neurological Surgery*. Philadelphia, W.B. Saunders Co., 1982, vol. 6, pp. 3580–3585.
22. Janetta P.J.: Treatment of trigeminal neuralgia by microoperative decompression, in Youmans J.R. (ed.): *Neurological Surgery*. Philadelphia, W.B. Saunders Co., 1982, vol. 6, pp. 3589–3603.
23. Janetta P.J.: Treatment of trigeminal neuralgia: Viewpoint. *Neurosurgery* 4:93, 1979.
24. Swanson S.E., Farhaat S.M.: Neurovascular decompression with selective partial rhizotomy of the trigeminal nerve for tic douloureux. *Surg. Neurol.* 18:3–6, 1982.

16B / Musculoskeletal Pain

STEPHEN E. ABRAM, M.D.
P. PRITHVI RAJ, M.D.

MYOFASCIAL PAIN may be due to one or more of the following causes: reflex muscle spasm, ischemia of the myofascial structures, decreased nutrition, fatigue of the muscle due to excessive use, and muscle injury. In most instances the mechanism of pain involves an interference with oxidative processes in the muscle caused by a decrease in the supply of oxygen, enzymes, and other nutrients necessary for muscle metabolism.

When fatigue follows overexertion, pain and soreness are experienced hours or days later. These may result from increases in cellular metabolites and water that stimulate nociceptive nerve endings. Once the painful state is produced, it can be perpetuated by feedback cycles from myofascial trigger points.[1] Muscle spasm is associated with pain and tenderness of the affected muscle. The pain is constant and diffuse. When the group of muscles is activated by motion, sharp stabbing pain may be experienced. Trigger points that are extremely sensitive to touch and pressure are anatomically located in the muscles. Analgesics and muscle relaxants have no effect on these muscle spasms, and the patient becomes restless, irritable, tense, and fatigued. This in turn aggravates the muscle spasm, and a vicious cycle ensues.

Pain of myofascial origin can be caused by various conditions. These include postural disturbances, degenerative lesions, and inflammation.

The skeletal pain may arise from pathology of the bone, periosteum, ligaments, or joints. There are many systemic diseases, e.g., rheumatoid arthritis, that involve those structures. Metastatic tumors frequently involve bone at multiple sites and cause pain by periosteal pressure. Benign skeletal pain as part of low back or cervical pain may result from diffuse or focal spondylitic changes in the spine that narrow the spinal canal. Facet joint bony changes, pseudarthroses, nonunion of fractures, spondylolysis, and spondylolisthesis are all common causes of skeletal pain (Figs 16B–1 through 16B–3).

INFLAMMATORY DISORDERS

Inflammation of joints, tendons, and other somatic structures is an extremely common and troublesome source of chronic pain. The inflammatory process may be primary, as in rheumatoid or psoriatic arthritis, or it may be secondary to joint degeneration, as in osteoarthritis. Much of the pain is related to the inflammatory process itself, with the consequent release of prostaglandins and other substances that activate or sensitize nociceptors.[2] However, other pain mechanisms may become important. Myofascial trigger points are frequently found in arthritis patients, and neurogenic mechanisms may develop as a result of joint overgrowth and spurring with resultant neural compression or irritation (Fig 16B–4).

Therapy is generally directed toward reduction of inflammation. Aspirin and other nonsteroidal antiinflammatory drugs reduce pain at least partly through inhibition of prostaglandin synthesis.[3] Occasionally corticosteroids may be injected into affected joints or bursae or around inflamed tendons or ligaments. Such therapy should not be done repeatedly, as weakening of tendons may occur, and joint deterioration may result from loss of the inflammatory response and pain which normally occur when joints are overstressed. Transcutaneous electrical stimulation is sometimes useful. Treatment of associated myofascial and neuralgic pain should be undertaken as soon as it becomes evident.

192

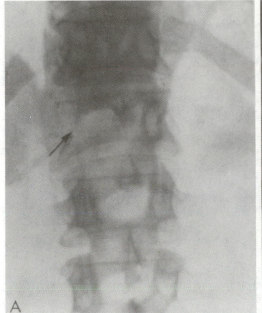 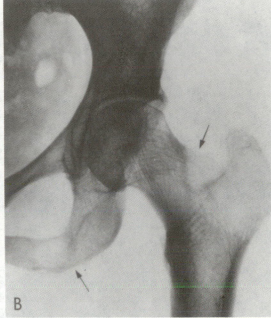

Fig 16B–1.—Metastatic tumor of the vertebral spine. **A,** AP view of the thoracolumbar region of a 53-year-old man. Note osteolytic lesion on the right of the body of the 12th thoracic vertebra and on the 12th rib. Lesion represented metastasis of a hypernephroma. **B,** AP view of the left hip joint of a 34-year-old woman. Note cherry-sized osteolytic lesion in the horizontal ramus of the pubis and an egg-sized osteolytic lesion in the great trochanter. The diagnosis of secondary hypernephroma was confirmed histologically. (From Matzen P.F., Fleissner H.K.: *Orthopedic Roentgen Atlas.* New York, Grune & Stratton, 1970. Reproduced by permission.)

RHEUMATOID ARTHRITIS

Rheumatoid arthritis is a systemic disease of unknown cause.[4] The frequency of extra-articular manifestations justifies the concept of rheumatoid disease, but in the majority of patients clinical and pathologic findings and disability are the result of chronic inflammation of synovial membranes. There is striking heterogeneity among patients regarding mode of onset, pattern of joint involvement, frequency of extra-articular manifestations, and clinical course. There is a tendency for symmetric involvement of hands, wrists, and feet. Spontaneous remissions and exacerbations are characteristic. About 10%–20% of patients have complete remissions, whereas the remainder experience sustained fluctuating activity. Joint injury results from formation of chronic granulation tissue (pannus), the product of proliferative and exudative synovitis; this is capable of altering articular and periarticular structures.

Incidence and Epidemiology

The frequency of rheumatoid arthritis, based on limited population surveys in Europe and North America, is in the range of 1%–3%.[5] It is two to three times more common in females. Onset is most frequent in the fourth and fifth decades of life, but it may occur at any age. There are no consistent trends relating prevalence to geography, climate, or culture. An increased frequency of a histocompatibility antigen (HLA-DW4) has been observed in rheumatoid arthritis subjects.

Pathology

The pathologic elements of chronic synovitis include exudation, cellular infiltration, and the proliferation of granulation tissue.[6] Although polymorphonuclear leukocytes predominate in synovial

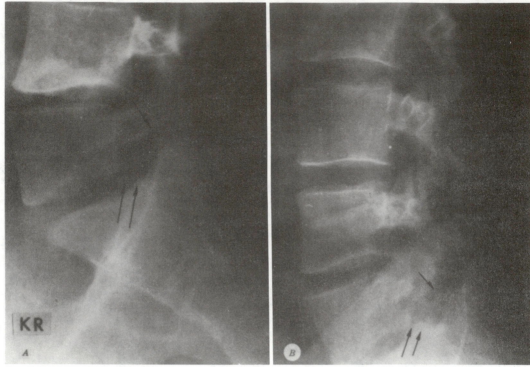

Fig 16B–2.—Roentgenograms of identical twins with spondylolisthesis of L5-S1. **A,** lateral roentgenogram of lumbosacral area of twin who had progressive back pain requiring spinal fusion. **B,** lateral roentgenogram of second twin, who never had any back symptoms. (From McCarty D.J.: *Arthritis and Allied Conditions,* ed. 9. Philadelphia, Lea & Febiger, 1979. Reproduced by permission.)

fluid, the principal infiltrating cells in synovial membranes are lymphocytes. Multinucleated giant cells may be seen.

The role of inflammation in the production of articular, periarticular, and extra-articular injury is evident. A variety of lysosomal enzymes, neutral proteases, and synovial collagenases are capable of hydrolyzing constituents of connective tissue, and the role of such enzymes in the induction of tissue injury seems explicit.

Immunologic Features

Synovial tissue in rheumatoid arthritis often displays histologic features characteristic of lymphoid organs, with prominent collections of lymphocytes and plasma cells, sometimes in the form of germinal centers.[7] Immunoglobulin synthesis has been demonstrated in rheumatoid synovial tissue by immunohistologic and tissue culture studies. There is evidence for a role of immune complexes in the induction of inflammation.

Rheumatoid Factors

Rheumatoid factors are autoantibodies reactive with the Fc portion of IgG. Anti-globulin activities are associated with the three major classes of immunoglobulins (IgM, IgG, and IgA), but, because of the enhanced agglutinating property of IgM antibodies, standard tests measure predominantly IgM Rheumatoid factors. Rheumatoid factors form soluble complexes with their antigen (IgG).[8, 9] The complexes of IgM rheumatoid factor with IgG have a sedimentation coefficient of approximately 22S, whereas the complexes formed with IgG rheumatoid factors are very heterogeneous, sedimenting in the "intermediate" range between IgG and IgM.

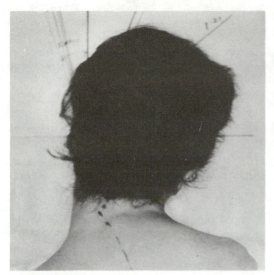

Fig 16B–3.—Myofascial pain in the neck and shoulder.

Infectious Agents

A number of clinical and pathologic features of rheumatoid arthritis are mimicked by animal models of disease where microbial causes are explicit, in particular chronic arthritis in swine induced by species of *Mycoplasma* and by *Erysipelothrix insidiosa*.

Clinical Manifestations

MODE OF ONSET.—Usually rheumatoid arthritis has an insidious onset, often beginning with poorly localized arching and stiffness. These early symptoms may be attributed to ''grippe,'' and the subsequent evolution of frank synovitis may be sufficiently slow that the patient does not seek medical attention for many weeks. A variety of precipitating factors have been entertained (trauma, environmental change, infections, and psychological stress), but none of these is constant in the antecedent history. Most patients manifest symmetric polyarthritis early in the course of the disease, but a significant number (approximately one third) have inflammation limited to one or two joints.

SYMPTOMS.—Pain, the dominant symptom, corresponds to the pattern and intensity of joint involvement, whereas stiffness is more generalized and is characteristically maximal after periods of physical inactivity. Morning stiffness is an almost

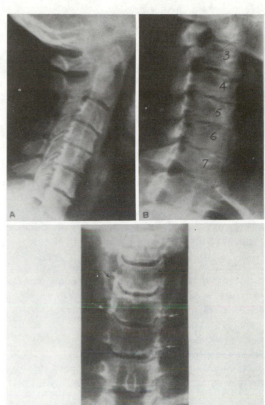

Fig 16B–4.—Cervical arthritis with narrow cervical canal. Lateral **(A)**, oblique **(B)**, and anteroposterior **(C)** views of the cervical spine show hypertrophic changes with marked spur formation at the margins of the lateral interbody joints. (From McCarty D.J.: *Arthritis and Allied Conditions*, ed. 9. Philadelphia, Lea & Febiger, 1979. Reproduced by permission.)

invariable feature; its intensity and duration can guide one in the assessment of disease activity.

The majority of patients experience constitutional symptoms such as weakness, increased fatigability, and diminished appetite. Temperature elevation in excess of 38° C is uncommon. Many patients complain of coldness and hypesthesias and paresthesias in the hands and feet (in the absence of signs of nerve entrapment).

Physical Signs

The physical signs of rheumatoid arthritis vary enormously according to anatomical patterns, severity, and stage of disease. The "classic" articular and extra-articular expressions are features of chronic rheumatoid arthritis.

GENERAL EXAMINATION.—Observations of gait and performance of simple tasks, such as removal of clothing, may reveal evidence of stiffness or specific anatomical patterns of disease. Many, but not all, patients appear chronically ill and undernourished. Dependent edema not attributable to other causes is an infrequent but significant feature. Easy bruising and increased fragility of skin are common in patients with chronic disease. Nodules are most commonly found in subcutaneous tissue. Nodules are characteristically localized over points of pressure of friction, most commonly the extensor surfaces of the proximal forearms (Fig 16B–5).

SKELETAL MANIFESTATIONS.—The invariable signs of swelling, tenderness, and pain on motion in early cases may seem poorly localized to joints. A common mode of onset, with symmetric involvement of the distal upper extremities, is diffuse swelling of the hands and wrists. Warmth is usually evident, especially over the large joints such as the knee, but skin erythema is infrequent. Swelling reflects varying degrees of synovial thickening and

proliferation and increased volume of synovial fluid. From palpation and ballottement, the examiner can usually estimate the relative roles of effusion and synovial proliferation.

Muscle atrophy of the affected extremities may be evident within weeks of onset of rheumatoid arthritis. Whether this relates to primary myopathic change or disuse is moot, but rarely an overt myopathy, indistinguishable from polymyositis, may be a feature of the disease.

EXTRA-ARTICULAR MANIFESTATIONS.—Many of the features of rheumatoid arthritis that are associated with diffuse vasculitis were mentioned in the section on pathology. The clinical expressions of vasculitis (neuropathy, chronic skin ulcers, digital gangrene, and, rarely, visceral arteritis) and the clinical patterns associated with disseminated granulomas are invariably features of chronic "classic" disease and are rarely encountered in patients who lack the rheumatoid factor.

There are usually no problems in interpretation of neurologic signs related to peripheral neuropathy, nerve entrapment (median nerve involvement at the wrist is common), and radiculopathy. In contrast, the insidious progression of muscle weakness secondary to myelopathy from C1–C2 subluxation can

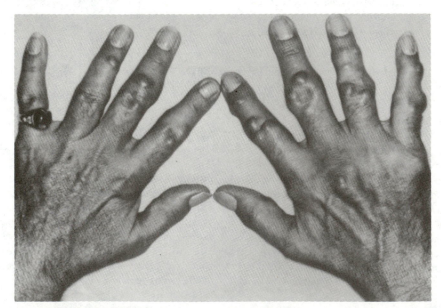

Fig 16B–5.—Rheumatic arthritis of the upper extremity: "rheumatoid nodulosis." These multiple rheumatoid nodules and palindromic rheumatism in a diabetic man were thought at first to be gouty arthritis. A diabetologist thought these were xanthomas. His grip strength was nearly normal and he felt generally well. (From McCarty D.J.: *Arthritis and Allied Conditions,* ed. 9. Philadelphia, Lea & Febiger, 1979. Reproduced by permission.)

mistakenly be attributed to "arthritis" and associated constitutional symptoms.

Clinical Course and Prognosis[4]

Statistics regarding the natural history of rheumatoid arthritis are based on studies in large rheumatic disease units where patients are not representative of the entire population of rheumatoid arthritics, i.e., they tend to have more severe and sustained disease. Patients with more remitting patterns of disease are less apt to be entered into prognostic studies. However, even the published figures allow one to present a reasonably optimistic outlook to the patient. After 10–15 years of disease, over 50% of patients remain fully employed and only about 10% are completely incapacitated. About 10%–20% of patients have virtually complete remission; the course followed by the remainder is extremely varied. The average patient with episodic exacerbations and partial remissions will experience gradual progression of deformity and disability. The minority, with sustained disease activity and only slight remissions, may become completely disabled within a few years of onset. The features associated with a poor prognosis, in a statistical sense, are (1) classic pattern of disease (symmetric polyarthritis with subcutaneous nodules and high titers of rheumatoid factor), (2) sustained disease of more than 1 year's duration, (3) onset before age 30, and (4) extra-articular manifestations of rheumatoid arthritis.

Roentgenographic Findings

Osteoporosis, especially in juxta-articular locations, may be evident within weeks of the onset of disease. Loss of articular cartilage, shown by reduction in the apparent "joint space," and bone erosions are rarely evident before several months of sustained disease. Subluxations, dislocations, and bony ankylosis, if they occur, are still later phenomena. Diffuse osteoporosis is common with chronic disease and is heightened by adrenocorticosteroid therapy (Fig 16B–6).

Laboratory Findings

Mild anemia, similar to that associated with chronic infection, is common in rheumatoid arthritis. Anemia is usually normocytic and normochronic, but if there is accompanying iron deficiency, the erythrocytes may be slightly hypochronic and microcytic. Leukocytosis, eosinophilia, and thrombocytosis are occasional laboratory features.

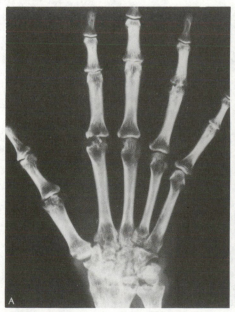 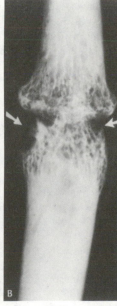

Fig 16B–6.—X-ray films of the hand in rheumatoid arthritis. **A,** typical radiographic changes of moderately advanced rheumatoid arthritis with periarticular demineralization, cartilage narrowing, erosive disease showing a proximal distribution, and sparing of the distal interphalangeal joints. **B,** magnificaiton of fourth proximal interphalangeal joint demonstrates fusiform soft tissue swelling and extensive erosion of the head of the proximal phalanx. (From McCarty D.J.: *Arthritis and Allied Conditions,* ed. 9. Philadelphia, Lea & Febiger, 1979. Reproduced by permission.)

The erythrocyte sedimentation rate (ESR) is increased above the normal range is virtually all patients with active rheumatoid arthritis. There are a variety of other acute-phase reactants in the serum which reflect inflammatory activity, but none of them matches the simplicity of the ESR or exceed its sensitivity.

Rheumatoid synovial fluid is usually turbid with reduced viscosity, increased protein content, and a slight reduction of glucose levels relative to the blood. Leukocyte counts (predominantly polymorphonuclear cells) vary between a few thousand to more than 50,000 cells per cubic millimeter. Cells containing inclusions are common, but these may be seen in other types of exudative synovitis.

There are no tests that are specific for rheumatoid arthritis, although the term rheumatoid factors has been applied to autoantibodies reactive with IgG. A variety of test systems are available, but more laboratories utilize the latex fixation test, in which polystyrene latex particles coated with IgG are agglutinated by rheumatoid factors. Less commonly applied systems include the bentonite flocculation test and a variety of hemagglutination tests employing erythrocytes coated with immunoglobulins. The latex fixation test result is positive (1:80 titer or higher) in approximately 70% of rheumatoid subjects. Although test results are positive in less than 5% of healthy control subjects, the rheumatoid factor is associated with other connective tissue syndromes, liver disease, and a variety of infectious diseases such as bacterial endocarditis, tuberculosis, syphilis, and leprosy. The frequency of positive test results for rheumatoid factor in the general population increases with age.

Differential Diagnosis

Differential considerations are numerous and vary according to the pattern of disease.[5] There is seldom confusion in identifying classic rheumatoid arthritis, but symmetric involvement of hand and wrist joints can be a feature of other syndromes. Differentiation is more difficult and complex in patients with early acute polyarthritis or in those with arthritis limited to one or a few joints.

The most common form of chronic arthropathy, degenerative joint disease, is usually quite distinct from rheumatoid arthritis. Minimal inflammatory signs, absence of constitutional symptoms, ESR determinations in the range of normal, and the char-

acteristic radiographic findings usually serve to identify degenerative joint disease.

Gout and chondrocalcinosis may mimic chronic rheumatoid arthritis. The most definitive basis for their identification is polarized light microscopy of synovial fluid.

Other connective tissue syndromes such as systemic lupus erythematosus (SLE) and progressive systemic sclerosis are infrequently associated with chronic deforming joint change. Their differentiation from rheumatoid arthritis is based on characteristic multisystemic patterns of disease. Certain serologic features of SLE, especially hypocomplementemia and the antibodies to native deoxyribonucleic acid, are rare in rheumatoid arthritis.

The majority of patients with arthritis and psoriasis are indistinguishable from patients in the spectrum of rheumatoid arthritis. The designation psoriatic arthritis as a separate entity is in part arbitrary, but certain clinical and laboratory features of psoriatic arthritis aid in its differentiation from rheumatoid arthritis.

Management

In the management of rheumatoid arthritis, the physician should keep the following facts in mind: (1) in most patients the disease is chronic; (2) spontaneous remissions occur in almost all patients; (3) the majority of subjects can continue to lead active lives with varying degrees of restrictions; and (4) complications of drug therapy, most notably adrenocorticosteroids, can cause greater morbidity than the underlying disease.

The patient and the doctor must be educated not to expect or seek a short-term solution. The physician can present a reasonably optimistic prognosis, based on knowledge of the natural history of rheumatoid arthritis, and can assure the patient that there are conservative means of ameliorating symptoms and minimizing disability.

Weight reduction in obese patients should have high priority. If the diet is well balanced, there are no indications for vitamin supplementation. The anemia of rheumatoid arthritis does not respond to hematinic therapy except to the extent that iron deficiency may be a complicating feature.

Psychological depression is a common consequence of chronic rheumatoid arthritis. From the physician, the patient needs sympathetic understanding of his problems and a willingness to help solve them. When depression is severe, these efforts may be facilitated by the use of antidepressive medication. If anxiety, restlessness, and insomnia are complicating features, the use of mild sedatives or tranquilizers may be indicated.

A basic program that is applicable to all patients includes (1) rest, (2) employment of salicylates for the relief of pain and suppression of inflammation, and (3) maintenance of joint function by physical measures. Some but not all patients will be candidates for medicinal therapy other than salicylates and/or orthopedic surgical procedures.

Physical Measures

The choice of various heat modalities (warm pool, tank, bath, shower, diathermy, or ultrasound) depends primarily on the areas affected and the availability of services. Diathermy and ultrasound treatments are contraindicated in patients with mental implants. A warm pool permitting exercise under water is optimal for the patient with very severe symptoms, but for most individuals a hot bath or shower will suffice. Morning stiffness and pain will be minimized by ingestion of salicylates followed by a hot bath.

The goals of an exercise program are (1) maintenance of motion of affected joints, and (2) prevention of muscle atrophy. Both of these can be achieved without submitting inflamed joints to the task of work. An active exercise program for the lower extremities can maintain motion and strength without heavy weight-bearing, allowing the right combination of rest and exercise. The rate of progression from gentle passive exercises, required for the most symptomatic patient, to a more active program will vary according to the pattern of involvement and the response to therapy. In order that the patient avoid assuming a passive dependent role, it is crucial that emphasis be placed on what he or she can do independent of supervision.

Other Antirheumatic Therapy

For the patient whose response to salicylate therapy has not been adequate, several other anti-inflammatory agents can be employed. These include indomethacin, phenylbutazone (and oxyphenbutone), antimalarial drugs (chloroquine and hydroxychloroquine), gold compounds, and several compounds (propionic acid derivatives and tolmetin) marketed in the United States after 1975.[10, 11] The adrenocorticosteroid drugs are the most potent anti-inflammatory medications available, but their value, for reasons stated below, is limited. Unfortunately all medications employed for the treatment of rheumatoid arthritis, except gold compounds, have in common the property of promoting peptic ulceration.

Codeine and related analgesics may be required on a temporary basis, but their chronic use should be discouraged.

Intra-articular Adrenocorticosteroid Therapy

Several adrenocorticosteroid preparations suitable for intra-articular therapy will temporarily suppress signs and symptoms of synovitis. This mode of therapy is helpful for a patient whose disability relates primarily to disease in one or two joints. With rigorous antiseptic technique, the risk of infection is low. If there is any question of antecedent infection at the time of arthrocentesis, intra-articular steroids should not be administered.

Orthopedic Surgery

Orthopedic surgeons are playing an increasingly important role in the management of rheumatoid arthritis. The value of reconstructive surgery in the rehabilitation of selected subjects is well established. Techniques of arthroplasty and prosthetic joint replacement have improved dramatically during the past decade. The rationale for synovectomy is sound, i.e., the removal of chronic pannus and its destructive potential, but proof of its efficacy is lacking. Disease frequently recurs in regenerated synovium, but the intensity of recurrent inflammation tends to be less. On the basis of current experience, synovectomy is probably warranted for patients with sustained (several months or more) proliferative synovitis affecting knee, hand, and wrist joints.

DEGENERATIVE JOINT DISEASE (OSTEOARTHRITIS)

Early degeneration of articular cartilage probably begins in all subjects by the end of the second decade of life.[12] In the pathologic sense, degenerative joint disease is a normal response to aging. If the incidence of degenerative joint disease is estimated by minimal roentgenographic criteria, approximately 90% of the population are affected by age 40. Although only a small proportion of those with abnormal roentgenograms are symptomatic, degenerative joint disease is the most common cause of chronic disability.

Degenerative joint disease is sometimes classified as primary or secondary. The latter denotes the acceleration or augmentation of wear by abnormal stresses associated with injuries, obesity, and mechanical joint disturbances. Primary degenerative joint disease, in which there is no abnormal wear or forces, is probably influenced by one or more biochemical abnormalities that impair cartilage metabolism.

ing and fibrillations. Abrasion of fibrillated cartilage results in progressive loss of cartilaginous surfaces and exposure of subchondral bone.

Subsequent to ulcerations of cartilage, new bone formation occurs at the margin of articular cartilage. These marginal osteophytes appear on roentgenograms as characteristic spurs. Other osseous changes include cysts of varying size beneath the joint surface and remodeling of subchondral bone (Fig 16B–7).

Changes in synovial membranes, including fibrosis, hypertrophy, and occasionally synovitis, appear to be secondary to events affecting articular cartilage. Rarely, the pathologic features of inflammation mimic those of rheumatoid arthritis.

Pathology[13]

The earliest lesions of degenerative joint disease are microscopic alterations of articular cartilage. These include diminution of metachromatic material, decreased numbers of chondrocytes, fatty degeneration, alteration of collagen fibrils, and surface irregularities. Later morphological changes include localized softening of the cartilage with surface flak-

Etiology and Pathogenesis

In response to injury, the metabolic activity of chondrocytes increases, but their capacity to replicate and form new matrix is limited.[13] Secondary degenerative joint disease occurs when the forces of wear and tear exceed the restricted capacity for repair. When degenerative joint disease develops, frequently in familial patterns, in the absence of ab-

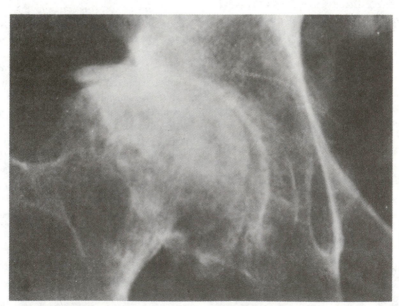

Fig 16B–7.—Osteoarthritis of the hip. There is advanced osteoarthritis with superolateral migration, extensive marginal osteophytosis, and remodeling of the femoral head and acetabular roof. (From McCarty D.J.: *Arthritis and Allied Conditions*, ed. 9. Philadelphia, Lea & Febiger, 1979. Reproduced by permission.)

normal stresses, it is presumed that accelerated degeneration results from one or more biochemical abnormalities affecting cartilage metabolism.[14] Chemical studies of degenerative cartilage have revealed several abnormalities: decreased water and chondromucoprotein contents and alterations in the profile of glycosaminoglycans. Some of these changes could be mediated by the action of lysosomal hydrolases, but the nature of the presumed biochemical defect in degenerative cartilage remains unknown.

Clinical Patterns of Degenerative Joint Disease[12]

Pain is the dominant symptom of degenerative joint disease but, as noted earlier, disease that is roentgenographically moderate to severe may be asymptomatic. Pain is aggravated by joint motion or weight-bearing. Transient stiffness after periods of inactivity is common. Loss of articular cartilage and osseous hypertrophy result in bony enlargement and malignant of joints and crepitation on motion. Mild tenderness to palpation and effusions are common, but other inflammatory signs are usually absent.

The Hand

Heberden's nodes are bony protuberances at the dorsal margins of the distal interphalangeal joints (Fig 16B–8). Early Heberden's nodes have a soft cystic consistency and may be associated with prominent inflammatory signs. The chronic stage of Heberden's nodes, characterized by bony enlargement and angular deformities, is usually minimally symptomatic. Heredity and sex are prominently involved in the development of Heberden's nodes. They are much more common in women. On the basis of family studies, it has been postulated that a single autosomal gene is involved which is dominant in females and recessive in males.

Patients with Heberden's nodes frequently show degenerative changes in other joints of the hands. The misinterpretation of proximal interphalangeal joint involvement (Bouchard's nodes) as rheumatoid arthritis is a common error. Metacarpophalangeal joint involvement is rare. Pain on the radial side of the wrist caused by degenerative disease in the first carpometacarpal joint is a frequent manifestation.

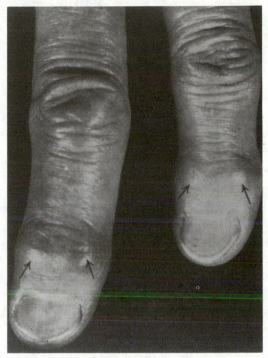

Fig 16B–8.—Heberden's nodes affecting index and middle fingers. (From McCarty D.J.: *Arthritis and Allied Conditions*, ed. 9. Philadelphia, Lea & Febiger, 1979. Reproduced by permission.)

Coxarthrosis (Malum Coxae Senilis)

Symptoms of primary degenerative hip disease usually appear in the later decades of life, but in as many as half of cases there is evidence of antecedent hip disease such as congenital dysplasia, slipped capital femoral epiphysis, or Legg-Calvé-Perthes disease. In addition, a variety of acquired disorders such as rheumatoid arthritis and avascular necrosis of the femoral head may lead to degenerative hip disease. Groin pain on motion or weight-bearing is the dominant symptom, and this is often referred to the medial aspect of the thigh or knee. Over a period of months to a few years, the majority of patients become seriously disabled because of pain and restricted motion.

Degenerative Disease of the Knee

Involvement of the knees is the most common source of major disability in degenerative joint disease. Although mild synovitis and effusion may be present, joint enlargement primarily reflects bone proliferation. Crepitation on motion is a consistent finding. Degenerative changes are usually more prominent in the medial compartment of the knee, leading to varus deformity.

Vertebral Degenerative Joint Disease, Including Herniated Disk Syndromes

Two sets of articulations are present at all levels of the spinal column: the intervertebral disks and the posterior zygapophyseal joints. In addition to these, the cervical spine (between C-2 and C-7) has articulations between the lateral aspects of adjacent vertebral bodies, usually referred to as the joints of Luschka. Degenerative changes in the joints of Luschka are the most common cause of pain in the cervical area.[15] At lumbar levels, degeneration and herniation of the nucleus pulposus of the intervertebral disks are usually the bases for symptoms (Fig 16B–9).

CERVICAL SPINE.—The close proximity of cervical nerve roots to the joints of Luschka makes them vulnerable to irritation or compression from any derangement in or about the joints.[15] Since the greatest amount of stress in the cervical spine occurs at C4–C5 and C5–C6 levels, degenerative changes in the intervertebral disks and the joints of Luschka are most common there. Osteophytic spurs at the margins of the joints of Luschka may impinge on nerve roots as they leave the intervertebral foramina. The pattern of pain and neurologic findings varies according to the level involved: pain is frequently in the supraclavicular and upper trapezius regions but can be referred to the occiput and more distal upper extremity. Discomfort is aggravated by motion of the neck, particularly rotation and lateral bending (Fig 16B–10).

If there is degeneration of the intervertebral disks in the cervical spine, the joints of Luschka provide a barrier against lateral herniation of the nucleus pulposus. The protrusion and subsequent osteophytic reaction may therefore encroach directly on the spinal cord rather than on the nerve roots. The progression of the resulting cervical myelopathy may be insidious and painless.

LUMBAR SPINE.—Symptoms of degenerative disease of the lumbar spine are nearly always attributable to involvement of intervertebral disks.[16] Protrusion or extrusion of degenerated disks is directed

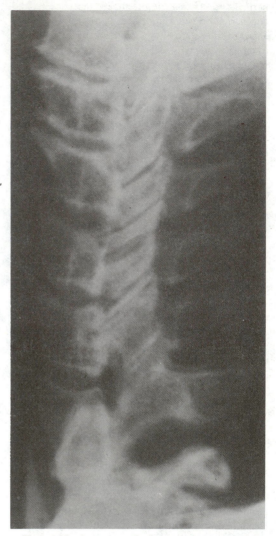

Fig 16B–9.—Moderately advanced degenerative disk disease involving the mid and lower cervical regions with narrowing, osteophytosis, and subchondral sclerosis. Minor degenerative changes are also present in lower apophyseal joints. (From McCarty D.J.: *Arthritis and Allied Conditions,* ed. 9. Philadelphia, Lea & Febiger, 1979. Reproduced by permission.)

posterolaterally, impinging on nerve roots or the cauda equina. Although any of the lumbar disks can herniate, this most commonly occurs at L4–L5 and L5–S1. Patients with herniated lumbar disks frequently have a history of mild or recurrent backache prior to development of more acute discomfort. Pain radiates distally into one or the other lower extremity and is aggravated by spinal movement, partic-

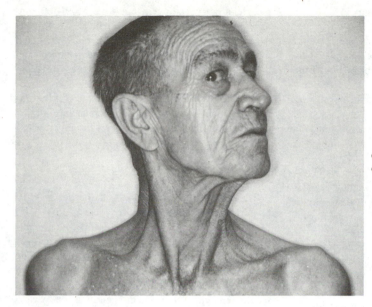

Fig 16B–10.—Torticollis in a man with degenerative arthritis of the cervical spine.

ularly bending to the side of the pain. There is usually marked paravertebral tenderness and aggravation of pain by straight leg raising. Loss of suppression of the ankle jerk and sensory deficit in the lateral border and sole of the foot and toes suggest L5–S1 root compression. No reflex change, a sensory deficit in the lateral leg and mediodorsal aspect of the foot, and weakness of the toe extensors suggest L4–L5 root compression.

Laboratory Findings

There are no specific laboratory abnormalities of degenerative joint disease. The ESR is usually normal. The synovial sedimentation rate is usually normal. Synovial fluid is clear and exhibits high viscosity and normal mucin clotting. Leukocyte counts in synovial fluid vary, in the range of 200–2,000/cu mm. Fragments of cartilage are frequently identified in the fluid.

Roentgenographic Features

Osteophyte formation at the margins of affected joints is the basis for the most striking roentgenographic feature of degenerative joint disease, but earlier and more common findings, resulting from destruction of articular cartilage, are narrowing of the interosseous joint space and subchondral bone sclerosis. Radiolucent cysts, varying in size from a few millimeters to several centimeters, may be seen in periarticular bone.

Degeneration of cervical and lumbar disks results in interspace narrowing. Exostoses at the margins of vertebral bodies may coalesce with adjacent osteophytes, causing fusion at one or more levels. Roentgenographic documentation of intervertebral herniation is best observed on anteroposterior and lateral roentgenograms. For visualization of osteophytes encroaching on foramina, especially important in the cervical spine, oblique projections are required.

Differential Diagnosis

In their typical expressions, degenerative joint disease and rheumatoid arthritis are easily distinguished. The latter is usually associated with evidence of systemic disease, prominent signs of joint inflammation, and the characteristic symmetric pattern of disease affecting the hands and wrists. When a patient presents with signs of mild inflammation in one or two weight-bearing joints of the lower extremities, the differentiation between these two syndromes is more difficult. In that setting a normal ESR, a negative rheumatoid factor test result, and minimal abnormalities in the synovial fluid support the diagnosis of degenerative joint disease. No test singly or in combination can be viewed as diagnostic; even the roentgenographic demonstration of marginal osteophytes may be a secondary change in rheumatoid arthritis. In the most experienced hands, there is a small percentage of patients in whom the diagnosis remains indeterminate.

A common diagnostic error is the interpretation of degenerative changes in proximal interphalangeal joints of the hands as evidence of rheumatoid arthritis. The deformities that characterize Heberden's and Bouchard's nodes may be marked, but this pattern of degenerative joint disease is not associated with prominent signs of inflammation, and the metacarpophalangeal joints and wrist joints are rarely or never affected.

Important aspects of differential diagnosis involve the recognition of syndromes in which secondary development of degenerative joint disease may occur. These include hemochromatosis, neuropathy, chondrocalcinosis, alcaptonuria, hypermobility of joints (including the Ehlers-Danlos syndrome), mechanical derangements of joints, and a variety of metabolic disorders that affect the support of articular cartilage by subchondral bone.

There should never be confusion in the differentiation of degenerative joint disease of the vertebral column from ankylosing spondylitis. Patients with the latter are almost invariably young men, and the roentgenographic features are distinct from those associated with degenerative joint disease.

Treatment

The management of degenerative joint disease is highly varied, depending on anatomical patterns and the degree of joint deformity. An optimistic forecast is appropriate for most individuals. Patients should understand that disability can be minimized even though there is no specific remedy. The common statement that "nothing can be done for your kind of arthritis" is false.

Drugs

No medication has been shown to retard the development or progression of degenerative joint disease. The requirement for analgesic drugs is varied; many patients have so little pain that they require no medicinal therapy. Aspirin in moderate dosage is usually helpful for the patient with pain. Sustained salicylate therapy is superior to intermittent or erratic dosage. A common problem in degenerative joint disease, regardless of anatomical location, is the occurrence of intermittent episodes of increased pain which tend to subside spontaneously. For these recurrent episodes, phenylbutazone (100–300 mg/day) or indomethacin may be beneficial. Continuous use of drugs other than salicylates is rarely indicated in degenerative joint disease. Some patients with disabling hip pain, however, experience sufficient relief of symptoms with phenylbutazone or indomethacin to warrant maintenance therapy. It is common practice to prescribe muscle relaxants for the pain and muscle spasm of vertebral disease.

Physical Measures

There are two general goals in the design of a physical medicine program for degenerative joint disease: minimizing the forces of work and weight-bearing that apply to affected joints, and maintenance of normal joint alignment and motion. The patient with hip or knee disease should be instructed to avoid unnecessary walking or stair climbing. This recommendation is not inconsistent with the performance of an exercise program (in non-weight-bearing attitude) which can maintain muscle power and joint motion. Quadriceps isometric exercise for degenerative joint disease of the knees is particularly important. There is a powerful rationale for weight reduction for the obese patient with involvement of the spine or lower extremities. The use of a cane or a crutch can reduce forces of weight-bearing applied to a symptomatic hip or knee by as much as 50%. In selected patients with an unstable knee, fitting of a brace may be beneficial.

Certain physical measures are selectively relevant to degenerative joint disease of the spine. Patients need to learn to live with the altered mechanics of their spine. With cervical involvement, hyperextension and hyperflexion should be avoided. The patient should sleep supine with no more than one pillow. Most, but not all, patients with cervical radicular pain will be helped by intermittent traction. If this is beneficial, there are inexpensive devices for applying intermittent cervical traction at home. When symptoms are acute, wearing a cervical collar will restrict movement and minimize pain.

The patient with symptomatic degenerative disease of the lumbar spine should sleep on a hard mattress and avoid bending and lifting activities. A program of graded postural exercises is important when pain has subsided. External support provided by a lumbosacral corset will frequently minimize mild chronic symptoms. When lumbar disk herniation results in severe pain or nerve deficit, hospitalization is usually indicated. The majority of such patients will experience a remission of symptoms within a 2- to 3-week period. Consideration of surgical therapy is appropriate for those patients who fail to respond to conservative management.

Surgical Management

The main anatomical areas affected by degenerative joint disease that are amenable to orthopedic surgical therapy are the hip, the knee, and the vertebral column. Several surgical procedures are appropriate for the patient with debilitating hip pain. These include arthrodesis (if the disease is unilateral), mold arthroplasty, osteotomy, and total joint replacement. In most centers, the last is the preferred procedure. Operative procedures for the knee with degenerative joint disease include debridement, osteotomy, and a variety of prosthetic arthroplasties. If there is reasonable preservation of motion and stability of the malaligned knee, tibial or femoral osteotomy is frequently beneficial. When there is a serious disability attributable to malalignment and instability of the knee, one or another prosthetic procedure may be indicated. However, the successes, to date, of knee joint replacement have not been as predictable as have comparable procedures for the hip.

Virtually all orthopedic surgeons agree that surgical procedures for degenerative disease of the spine are appropriate only after there has been a systematic and sustained trial of conservative management. If radicular pain is relentless or if there are increasing neurologic deficits from nerve root involvement or myelopathy, surgical correction is warranted.

ANKYLOSING SPONDYLITIS[17, 18]

In ankylosing spondylitis (also known as Marie-Strumpell spondylitis, von Bechterew's syndrome, and rheumatoid spondylitis), there is prominent involvement of spinal articulations, sacroiliac joints, and paravertebral soft tissues. Because one third to one half of patients with ankylosing spondylitis manifest synovitis in peripheral joints (especially hips and shoulders), the syndrome was formerly viewed as a variant of rheumatoid arthritis. However, several features of ankylosing spondylitis are distinct from those of rheumatoid arthritis: (1) prominent ligamentous calcification and ossification with a tendency to bony ankylosis; (2) male preponderance; (3) impressive evidence of genetic transmission in selected kindreds; (4) symptomatic benefit with medications, notably phenylbutazone and indomethacin, that are minimally effective in rheumatoid arthritis; (5) absence of rheumatoid factor and rheumatoid nodules; and (6) the association of certain extra-articular manifestations such as iridocyclitis and aortitis.

Etiology

The cause of ankylosing spondylitis is unknown. The disease has been found to be 30 times more prevalent among the relatives of spondylitic patients than among relatives of controls. The striking association of ankylosing spondylitis with the histocompatibility antigen HLA-B27 has provided insight into the genetic transmission of the syndrome and, additionally, has helped define a group of spondylitic disorders. This category includes Reiter's syndrome, a subset of juvenile rheumatoid arthritis, psoriatic spondylitis, and inflammatory bowel disease that exhibits spinal involvement. The manner in which this histocompatibility antigen influences pathogenesis is unknown. Infectious causes have long been suspected but never established.

Incidence and Prevalence

Ankylosing spondylitis is a common cause of back pain in young men. The male-to-female ratio is approximately 8:1. In an English survey, the incidence of ankylosing spondylitis was 1 in 2,000 among the population at large.

Pathology

On the basis of symptoms and early radiographic findings, the disease appears to begin in the sacroiliac joints, with subsequent involvement of zygapophyseal and costovertebral articulations, interspinous ligaments, and paravertebral tissues. The characteristic immobility of the spinal column results from bony ankylosis of zygapophyseal joints and ossification of paravertebral structures. Syndesmophytes, the bony bridges which unite adjacent vertebral bodies, form in the outer lamellae of the anulus fibrosus and adjacent connective tissue fibers. The pathologic character of synovial inflammation is not distinct from that of rheumatoid arthritis.

Clinical Manifestations

In the majority of cases the onset of ankylosing spondylitis, usually in the second or third decade of life, is insidious. The initial symptoms are usually low back pain and stiffness; rarely, the first symptoms may relate to involvement of hip, shoulder, or peripheral joints. Symptoms may be sufficiently mild that the patient seeks no medical attention for months. At the other extreme, there may be debilitating pain at the outset, associated with fever, severe fatigue, and weight loss. In most patients, however, constitutional symptoms are not prominent. Pain and stiffness, which are maximal after periods of inactivity, often interrupt sleep in the early morning hours. Radicular and sciatic patterns of pain are common. The pattern and rate of spinal ankylosis are varied. The majority of patients experience gradual cephalad progression of spinal immobility, but the disease may remain confined to the sacroiliac joints and lumbar segments (Fig 16B–11). The development of the poker-back type of spinal deformity usually evolves gradually over a period of 10 years or more. The majority of patients remain fully employed. Hip involvement, the most common cause of occupational disability, is now amenable to prosthetic surgery.

Physical signs are limited in the early stages of disease. Sacroiliac joint involvement may be evident from palpation of these joints or from orthopedic maneuvers which produce sacroiliac joint movement. Paravertebral muscle spasm and tenderness are common. Physical signs associated with the chronic phase of ankylosing spondylitis relate primarily to spinal immobility. The most accurate estimate of lumbar flexion is accomplished by comparing midline measurements from the sacrum to T-12 in flexion and extension. The normal difference in these two measurements is approximately 3 inches. The presence and progression of costovertebral joint involvement can be documented by measurements of chest expansion.

The most important extra-articular manifestations of ankylosing spondylitis are iridocyclitis, occurring in approximately one quarter of patients, and aortitis. The frequency of aortic insufficiency has been as high as 4% in some series. Cardiac conduction disturbances, most frequently first degree AV block, occur in about 10% of cases. Cauda equina involvement, a rare but significant complication of longstanding spondylitis, is manifest as urinary or rectal sphincter incompetence and pain and sensory loss in the sacral distribution.

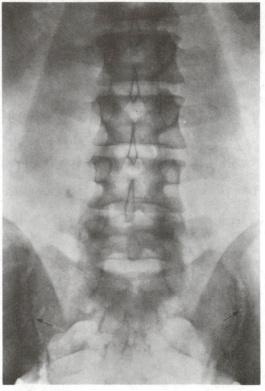

Fig 16B–11.—Ankylosing spondylitis. AP view of the lumbar spine and sacrum of a 27-year-old man shows undulating outline of the sacroiliac joints, more pronounced on the right than on the left. (From Matzen P.F., Fleissner H.K.: *Orthopedic Roentgen Atlas.* New York, Grune & Stratton, 1970. Reproduced by permission.)

Roentgenographic Findings

Characteristic roentgenographic findings of ankylosing spondylitis involve the following structures: sacroiliac joints, zygapophyseal articulations, vertebral bodies, and paravertebral soft tissues. Changes in the sacroiliac joints are the earliest and most consistent findings. The margins of subchondral bone are blurred, followed by subchondral sclerosis and bony erosions. Progressive narrowing of the interosseous joint space and sacroiliac fusion develop slowly over a period of years. Sclerotic and erosive changes in zygapophyseal and costovertebral articulations are common but less readily demonstrated by x-ray. Calcification and ossification of the anulus fibrosus and adjacent paravertebral ligaments give rise to the characteristic syndesmophytes that gradually bridge adjacent vertebral bodies. In advanced cases this results in the so-called bamboo spine (Fig 16B–12). In addition to sacroiliac joints, other cartilaginous articulations such as the symphysis pubis and sternomanubrial joints may be involved. There is a tendency for ossification of ligaments and tendon insertions.

Diagnosis

Ankylosing spondylitis should be suspected in anyone, particularly a young male, with persistent or recurrent low back pain and stiffness or recurrent sciatic pain. Although associated phenomena such as elevation of the ESR, thoracic girdle pain, arthritis in the lower limbs, and iridocyclitis will enhance the suspicion, early diagnosis should not be ex-

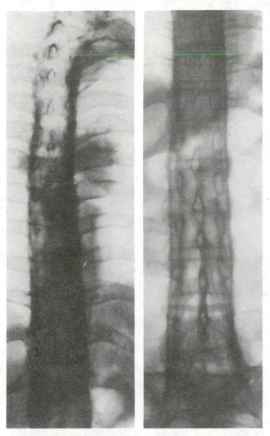

Fig 16B–12.—Bamboo spine. AP and lateral views of the cervical spine of a 42-year-old patient with Bechterew's disease show almost complete ankylosis. Only the joints of the atlas are still incompletely fused. (From Matzen P.F., Fleissner H.K.: *Orthopedic Roentgen Atlas*. New York, Grune & Stratton, 1970. Reproduced by permission.)

cluded on the basis of normal roentgenograms, because several months or, rarely, a few years may elapse before the development of roentgenographic changes. Although degenerative joint disease can result in back pain and loss of spinal motion, this is a problem of later decades of life, and the roentgenographic features are distinct from ankylosing spondylitis. Joint disease identical to ankylosing spondylitis can be a feature of ulcerative colitis, regional enteritis, Reiter's syndrome, and psoriasis.

Treatment

The highest-priority goal in the management of ankylosing spondylitis is the maintenance of a functional posture. It is doubtful that any medication will prevent ankylosis of those spinal segments involved, but the suppression of pain and inflammation is essential before an appropriate physical medicine program can be instituted.

Indomethacin and phenylbutazone are usually more effective than other anti-rheumatic agents in the control of pain and stiffness, but an initial trial of salicylate therapy (3.6–4.5 gm/day) is recommended. For those patients who do not experience sufficient relief of symptoms with salicylates, indomethacin, 100–150 mg/day, or phenylbutazone, 100–300 mg/day, is indicated. With control of symptoms, the dose of either indomethacin or phenylbutazone should be gradually reduced to the lowest level that will maintain improvement. Systemic adrenocorticosteroid therapy may be required for the control of iridocyclitis. Although roentgen therapy, directed at areas of involvement, is effective in control of symptoms, this mode of treatment is not recommended because of the demonstration of chromosomal injury and an observed incidence of leukemia that is ten times greater in patients so treated than in the general population.

For the management of ankylosing spondylitis, emphasis should be given to the institution and maintenance of an exercise program. In order that flexion deformity of the spine be avoided, the patient should sleep on a firm mattress, preferably without a pillow. There should be a twice-daily performance of exercise directed at the maintenance of erect posture, strengthening of paraspinal muscles, and promotion of chest cage motion. A hot bath or shower will often facilitate exercise activity. If physical medicine measures fail to check the progression of flexion deformity, back splints or braces may be tried. In carefully selected individuals with advanced flexion deformity, spinal osteotomy can improve posture, but this is associated with a significant risk of neurologic complications. For the patient with severe hip involvement, the most frequent cause of major disability, prosthetic hip replacement offers dramatic relief.

REFERENCES

1. Bonica J.J.: General considerations of musculoskeletal pain, in Bonica J.J. (ed.): *The Management of Pain.* Philadelphia, Lea & Febiger, 1953.
2. Terenius L.: Biochemical mediators in pain. *Triangle* 20:19–26, 1981.
3. Vane J.R.: The mode of action of aspirin-like drugs. *Agents Actions* 8:430–431, 1978.
4. Duthie J.R.R., et al.: Course and prognosis in rheumatoid arthritis. *Ann. Rheum. Dis.* 23:193, 1964.
5. Short C.L., Bauer W., Reynolds W.E.: *Rheumatoid Arthritis.* Cambridge, Harvard University Press, 1957.
6. Hollingsworth J.W.: *Local and Systemic Complications of Rheumatoid Arthritis.* Philadelphia, W.B. Saunders Co., 1968.
7. Zvaifler N.J.: the immunopathology of joint inflammation in rheumatoid arthritis. *Adv. Immunol.* 16:265–336, 1973.
8. Winchester R.J., Agnello V., Kunkel H.G.: Gamma globulin complexes in synovial fluids of patients with rheumatoid arthritis: Partial characterization and relationship to lowered complement levels. *Clin. Exp. Immunol.* 6:689, 1970.
9. Ruddy S., Austen K.F.: The complement system in rheumatoid synovitis: I. An analysis of complement activities rheumatoid synovial fluids. *Arthritis Rheum.* 13:713, 1970.
10. Freyberg R.H., Ziff M., Baum J.: Gold therapy for reheumatoid arthritis, in Hollander J.L., McCarty D.J. Jr. (eds.): *Arthritis and Allied Conditions,* ed. 8. Philadelphia, Lea & Febiger, 1972.
11. Cooperating Clinics Committee of the American Rheumatism Association: A controlled trial of cyclophosphamide in rheumatoid arthritis. *N. Engl. J. Med.* 283:883, 1970.
12. Sokoloff L.: *The Biology of Degenerative Joint Disease.* Chicago, University of Chicago Press, 1969.
13. Mankin H.J.: Biochemical and metabolic aspects of osteoarthritis. *Orthop. Clin. North Am.* 2:19, 1971.
14. Kellgren J.H., Lawrence J.S., Bier F.: Genetic factors in generalized osteoarthritis. *Ann. Rheum. Dis.* 22:237, 1969.
15. Friedenberg Z.B., Miller W.T.: Degnerative disc disease of the cervical spine. *J. Bone Joint Surg.* 45A:1171, 1963.
16. Armstrong J.R.: *Lumbar Disc Lesions.* ed. 3. Baltimore, Williams & Wilkins Co., 1965.
17. Gilliand B.E., Mannik M.: Ankylosing spondylitis, in *Harrison's Principles of Internal Medicine,* ed. 10. New York, McGraw-Hill Book Co., 1983.
18. Calabro J.J.: Diagnosis of low back pain, in Stanton-Hicks M., Boas R. (eds.): *Chronic Low Back Pain.* New York, Raven Press, 1982.

16C / Sympathetic Pain

STEPHEN E. ABRAM, M.D.

SOMATIC REGION

Sympathetic pain in the somatic region is due to overactivity of the peripheral sympathetic nervous system involving the somatic structures (Fig 16C–1). The two common syndromes in which this pain appears are causalgia and reflex sympathetic dystrophy.[1, 2] True causalgia follows partial injury to a major nerve trunk such as the sciatic nerve or its large branches. Reflex sympathetic dystrophy is much more common and may occur following the minor trauma to neural structures that accompanies fractures or soft tissue injuries. Reflex sympathetic dystrophy is also not unusual as a iatrogenic complication of surgical or neurolytic therapy. Clinical characteristics include burning, poorly localized pain, often with a stabbing component, hyperesthesia, and vasomotor and sudomotor alterations leading to trophic changes that themselves may provide noxious afferent stimuli to perpetuate the syndrome.

Mechanism

The pathophysiology of these conditions may be based, at least partially, on reflex sympathetic hyperactivity with resultant hypoperfusion, release of algesic chemicals, such as prostaglandins or bradykinin, and increased sensitivity of nociceptors.[3] Increased spontaneous and evoked firing rates in afferent nerve fibers or in cells in the spinal cord may also play a role.

Mechanisms of Causalgia and Reflex Sympathetic Dystrophy

During the early phases of injury the pain is due to damage to A delta and C fibers. They promptly develop hypersensitivity to circulating norepineph-rine, pressure, and movement. These fibers then fire spontaneously, which causes the typical pain of sympathetic origin. Shortly afterward, small neuromas form which sprout small myelinated and unmyelinated fibers.[4] These normally silent fibers can generate, even in the absence of stimulation, an ongoing barrage of impulses that traverse the afferent fibers to the spinal cord (Fig 16C–2). These basic physiologic processes can be solely responsible for initiating and sustaining the burning pain of causalgia during its early phase.

This peripheral pathophysiology causes lesser inhibition or facilitation in dorsal horn and other parts of the CNS. Initially the effect is reversible with effective therapy. On the other hand, if somatic sympathetic pain does not improve spontaneously, the abnormal function in the CNS becomes self-sustaining and independent of the abnormal peripheral input. The important clinical implication is that adequate therapy with sympathetic blocks or surgical sympathectomy produces permanent relief in the early course of the disease but fails to do so in the later stages.

Peripheral Vascular Disease

Somatic sympathetic pain can be caused by peripheral vascular disease. In many peripheral vascular diseases there is increased sympathetically induced vasoconstriction, ischemia, tissue damage, pain, and trophic changes which can be wholly or partially reversed by sympathetic interruption. The somatic sympathetic pain can be produced by acute vascular disorders in which sudden and severe circulatory insufficiency of the limb develops, e.g., trauma, embolism, thrombosis, or chemical irritation. The local lesion initiates reflex spasm of the collateral vessels. If not relieved early by adequate therapy, including sympatholytic blocks, the reflex vasospasm leads to thrombosis and may terminate

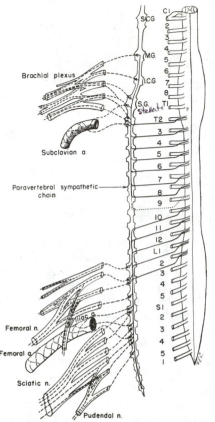

Fig 16C–1.—Anatomy of the peripheral sympathetic nervous system. Preganglionic fibers originate from the spinal cord from T2–L2. Sympathetic ganglia are shown as interconnected with each other in a sympathetic chain. Formation of stellate ganglion *(S.G.)*, inferior cervical ganglion *(I.C.G.)*, middle cervical ganglion *(M.G.)*, and superior cervical ganglion *(S.C.G.)* is identified. The postganglionic fibers traversing the somatic structures via nerves and vessels are identified. (From Bonica J.J.: *Clinical Applications of Diagnostic and Therapeutic Nerve Blocks*. Springfield, Ill., Charles C Thomas, 1959, p. 146. Reproduced by permission.)

in gangrene or chronic vasospastic disorders. Common examples of chronic vasospastic disorders caused by reflex vasospasm are Raynaud's phenomenon or disease, thromboangiitis obliterans (Buerger's disease), and arteriosclerosis obliterans.[5]

There are a number of other less important disorders of the extremities in which sympathetic hyperactivity contributes to the pathophysiology and

which can be benefited by sympathetic interruption.[6] These include hyperhydrosis, acute bursitis, tendinitis, tenosynovitis, and other traumatic and infectious disorders, including acute herpes zoster.

Rationale for Management

Repeated local anesthetic blocks of the sympathetic chain usually produce prompt, permanent relief of symptoms in reflex sympathetic dystrophy. Such treatment benefits some patients with causalgia, but the majority require sympathectomy for permanent relief. In both syndromes, persistent pain and permanent disability are likely if appropriate therapy is not carried out early.

Several other conditions may respond to interruption of sympathetic activity, including atypical facial pain, certain neuropathies, Raynaud's disease, hyperhydrosis, and the chronic pain and vasoconstriction seen after frostbite.

VISCERAL REGION

In general, the viscera have sensory receptors for no other sensation besides pain. Pain in the visceral tissues is usually diffuse, rather ill-defined, and frequently referred to distant points.[7] This pain is transmitted by afferent autonomic nerve fibers.

One of the most important differences between somatic pain and visceral pain is that highly localized damage to the viscera rarely causes pain. For instance, a surgeon can cut the gut entirely in two in a patient who is awake without causing significant pain. On the other hand, any stimulus that causes diffuse stimulation of nociceptive nerve endings in the viscus causes extremely severe pain. For instance, ischemia caused by occlusion of the blood supply to a large area of gut stimulates many diffuse nociceptive fibers at the same time and can result in extreme pain.[7]

Causes of Visceral Pain

Any stimulus that excites nociceptive nerve endings in diffuse areas of the viscera causes visceral pain. Such stimuli include ischemia of visceral tissue, chemical damage to the surfaces of the viscera, spasm of the smooth muscle in a hollow viscus, distention of a hollow viscus, and stretching of the ligaments.

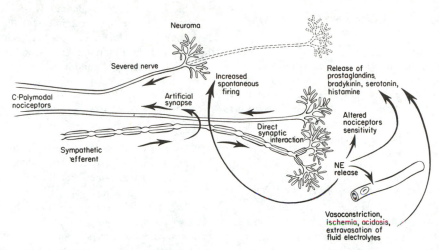

Fig 16C–2.—Some proposed mechanisms of interaction between sympathetic efferent and nociceptive afferent fibers in causalgia.[4]

Essentially all the true visceral pain originating in the thoracic and abdominal cavities is transmitted through afferent nerve fibers that run in the sympathetic nerves.[8] These are small unmyelinated type C fibers and therefore can transmit only burning and aching types of pain.

ISCHEMIA.—Ischemia causes visceral pain in exactly the same way that it causes pain in other tissues, presumably because of the formation of acidic metabolic end-products or tissue degenerative products, such as bradykinin and proteolytic enzymes, that stimulate the pain nerve endings.[9, 10]

CHEMICAL STIMULI.—On occasion, damaging substances leak from the gastrointestinal tract into the peritoneal cavity. For instance, proteolytic acidic gastric juice often leaks through a ruptured gastric or duodenal ulcer. This juice causes widespread digestion of the visceral peritoneum, thus stimulating extremely broad areas of pain fibers. The pain is usually extremely severe.

SPASM OF A HOLLOW VISCUS.—Spasm of the gut, the gallbladder, a bile duct, the ureter, or any other hollow viscus can cause pain in exactly the same way that spasm of skeletal muscle causes pain.[11] This possibly results from mechanical stimulation of the pain endings. Another possible cause is diminished blood flow to the muscle combined with increased metabolic need of the muscle for nutrients. Thus, relative ischemia could develop, which causes severe pain.

Often, pain from a spastic viscus occurs in the form of cramps, the pain increasing to a high degree of severity and then subsiding, the cycle renewing itself rhythmically once every few minutes. The rhythmic cycles result from rhythmic contraction of smooth muscle. For instance, each time a peristaltic wave travels along an overly excitable spastic gut, a cramp occurs. The cramping type of pain frequently occurs in gastroenteritis, constipation, menstruation, parturition, gallbladder disease, or ureteral obstruction.

OVERDISTENTION OF A HOLLOW VISCUS.— Extreme overfilling of a hollow viscus also results in pain, presumably because the tissues themselves are overstretched. However, overdistention can also collapse the blood vessels that encircle the viscus or that pass into its wall, thus perhaps promoting ischemic pain.

Insensitive Viscera

A few visceral areas are almost entirely insensitive to pain of any type. These include the parenchyma of the liver and the alveoli of the lungs. Yet the liver capsule is extremely sensitive to both direct trauma and stretch, and the bile ducts are also sensitive to pain. In the lungs, even though the alveoli are insensitive, the bronchi and the parietal pleura are both very sensitive to pain.

"Parietal" Pain Caused By Visceral Damage

In addition to true visceral pain, some pain sensations are also transmitted from the viscera through nerve fibers that innervate the parietal peritoneum, pleura, or pericardium.[12] The parietal surfaces of the visceral cavities are supplied mainly by spinal nerve fibers (somatic) that penetrate from the superficial distribution to deeper viscera.

Characteristics of Parietal Visceral Pain

When a disease affects a viscus, it often spreads to the parietal wall of the visceral cavity. This wall, like the skin, is extensively innervated by the spinal nerves, not by the afferent visceral sympathetic nerves. The innervating spinal nerves include the "fast" delta fibers. Therefore, pain from the parietal wall of the visceral cavity is frequently very sharp and piercing in quality, although it can also have burning and aching qualities as well if the pain stimulus is diffuse. For example, a knife incision through the parietal peritoneum is very painful, even though a smaller cut through the visceral peritoneum or through a gut is not painful.

Localization of Visceral Pain

Pain from the different viscera is frequently difficult to localize. First, the brain does not know from firsthand experience that the different organs exist, and therefore any pain that originates internally can be localized only generally. Second, sensations from the abdomen and thorax are transmitted by two separate pathways to the CNS—the true visceral pathways and the parietal pathway. The true visceral pain is transmitted via afferent fibers of the autonomic nervous system. The CNS refers this sensation to surface areas of the body often far from the painful organ. On the other hand, parietal sensations are conducted directly from the parietal peri-

TABLE 16C–1.—VISCERAL PAIN PATHWAY AND SITE OF NERVE BLOCK

STRUCTURE OF VISCERA	NOCICEPTIVE PATHWAY	SITE OF NERVE BLOCK FOR PAIN RELIEF
HEAD AND NECK Meninges, blood vessels, glands	Cranial Nerves VI, VII, IX	T1–T2 preganglionic fibers *or* cervical ganglia *or* appropriate cranial nerves
CHEST Heart	Middle and inferior cervical cardiac and thoracic cardiac nerves	T1–T5 Preganglionic fibers *or* cervicothoracic (T5) sympathetic ganglion
Lung	Via sympathetic nerves Parietal pleura:	T1–T8 sympathetic ganglion
Esophagus Thoracic aorta	Intercostal nerves Phrenic nerves Brachial plexus	

ABDOMEN
  Stomach
  Pancreas
  Liver, gallbladder
  Small intestines
  Cecum, ascending,
    and one half of
    transverse colon
	Splanchnic nerves	Celiac ganglion
		Splanchnic nerves

Left half of transverse colon, descending colon, and rectum	Nervi erigentes	Mesenteric ganglion *or* left T11, T12 sympathetic ganglion *or* S2–S4 somatic afferents
Kidney, ureter, upper bladder	Sympathetic nerves	T10–L2 preganglionic sympathetic fibers or T11–L1 sympathetic ganglion
Uterus and cervix	Sympathetic nerves	T6–L2 preganglionic fibers *or* T10–L1 sympathetic ganglion

Lower bladder—
  urethra, testes
  prostate
	Nervi erigentes and pelvic plexus	T10–L1 sympathetic preganglionic fibers *or* S2–S4 afferent somatic fibers

toneum, pleura, or pericardium and are usually localized directly over the painful area.

The True Visceral Pathway for Transmission of Pain

Most of the internal organs of the body are supplied by unmyelinated C fibers that traverse the visceral sympathetic nerves into the spinal cord and thence up the anterolateral spinothalamic tract along with the pain fibers from the somatic structures. A few visceral pain fibers—those from the distal portion of the colon, from the rectum, and from the bladder—enter the spinal cord through the sacral parasympathetic nerves, and some enter the CNS through various cranial nerves (see Fig 16C–1). These include fibers in the glossopharyngeal and vagus nerves which transmit pain from the pharynx, trachea, and upper esophagus. Some fibers from the surfaces of the diaphragm as well as from the lower esophagus are also carried in the phrenic nerves (Table 16C–1).

The position in the spinal cord to which visceral afferent fibers pass from each organ depends on the segment of the body from which the organ developed embryologically. The heart originated in the neck and upper thorax; consequently, the heart's visceral pain fibers enter the cord all the way from C-3 down to T-5. The stomach had its origin approximately from the seventh to the ninth thoracic segments of the embryo, and consequently the visceral afferents from the stomach enter the spinal cord between these levels. The gallbladder had its origin almost entirely in the ninth thoracic segment, so that the visceral afferents from the gallbladder enter the spinal cord at T-9.

Because the visceral afferent pain fibers are responsible for transmitting referred pain from the viscera, the location of the referred pain on the surface of the body is in the dermatome of the segment from which the visceral organ was originally derived in the embryo. Some of the areas of referred pain on the surface of the body are shown in Figure 16C–3.

The Parietal Pathway for Transmission of Abdominal and Thoracic Pain

A second set of pain fibers penetrates inward from the spinal nerves to innervate the parietal peritoneum, parietal pleura, and parietal pericardium. Retroperitoneal visceral organs and perhaps portions

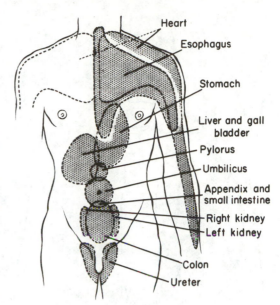

Fig 16C–3.—Pain referred to the surface of the body from the viscera. (From Guyton.[8] Reproduced by permission.)

of the mesentery are also innervated to some extent by parietal pain fibers. The kidney, for instance, is supplied by both visceral and parietal fibers.

Pain from the viscera is frequently localized to two surface areas of the body at the same time because of the dual pathways for transmission of pain. Figure 16C–4 illustrates dual transmission of pain from an inflamed appendix. Impulses pass from the appendix through the sympathetic visceral pain fibers into the sympathetic chain and then into the spinal cord at approximately T-10 to T-11; this pain is referred to an area around the umbilicus and is of the aching, cramping type. On the other hand, pain impulses also often originate in the parietal peritoneum where the inflamed appendix touches the abdominal wall, and these impulses pass through the spinal nerves into the spinal cord at a level of approximately L-1 or L-2. This pain is localized directly over the irritated peritoneum in the right lower quadrant of the abdomen and is of the sharp type.

Rationale for Management of Visceral Pain

Chemical or surgical interruption of the peripheral sympathetic nervous system has produced prolonged and sometimes permanent relief of visceral pain.

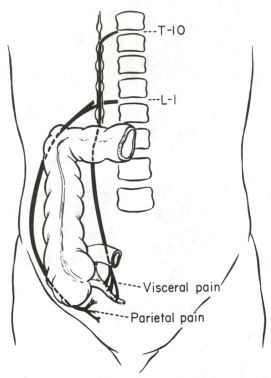

Fig 16C–4.—Visceral and parietal pathways of appendicitis. Note that the visceral pain pathway enters the spinal cord in the sympathetic fibers at the T10 level, whereas the parietal pain enters the somatic pain pathway at L1. (From Guyton.[8] Reproduced by permission.)

Pain in the visceral structures of the head, neck, and thoracic region can be relieved by stellate or thoracic sympathetic chain interruption. Pain of the upper abdominal viscera can be relieved by the celiac plexus block, whereas pain of the lower abdominal and pelvic viscera can be relieved by lumbar sympathetic blocks. Drugs like analgesics and antispasmotics for chronic visceral pain have not been efficacious in the long run. They may be useful as an adjunct and for short, acute episodes of pain. While physical methods like transcutaneous electrical nerve stimulation have not been helpful, acupuncture may alleviate visceral pain and is worth a try. Biofeedback, hypnotherapy, and relaxation therapy have their advocates and are successful in selected cases.

REFERENCES

1. Mitchell S.W., Morehouse G.R., Keen W.W.: *Gunshot Wounds and Other Injuries of Nerves.* Philadelphia, J.B. Lippincott Co., 1964.

2. Bonica J.J.: Causalgia and other reflex sympathetic dystrophies, in Bonica, J.J., Liebeskind J.C., Albe-Fessard D. (eds.): *Advances in Pain Research and Therapy.* New York, Raven Press, 1979, vol. 3, pp. 141–166.

3. Zimmerman M.: Peripheral and central nervous mechanisms of nociception, pain and pain therapy: Facts and hypotheses, in Bonica J.J., et al. (eds.): *Advances in Pain Research and Therapy.* New York, Raven Press, 1979, vol. 3, pp. 3–32.

4. Wall P.D., Gutnick M.: Ongoing activity in peripheral nerves: The physiology and pharmacology of impulses originating from a neuroma. *Exp. Neurol.* 43:580–593, 1974.

5. Bonica J.J.: *Sympathetic Nerve Blocks From Pain: Diagnosis and Therapy.* Vol. 1: *Fundamental Considerations and Clinical Applications.* Winthrop Breon Laboratories, 1984.

6. Dan K., Tanakak H., Kamihara Y.: Herpetic pain and T-cell subpopulation, in Bonica J.J., Liebeskind J.C., Albe-Fessard D. (eds.): *Advances in Pain Research and Therapy.* New York, Raven Press, 1979, vol. 3.

7. Cervero F.: Deep and visceral pain, in Kosterlitz H.W., Terenius L.Y. (eds.): *Pain and Society.* Weinheim, Verlag Chemie, 1980, pp. 263–282.

8. Guyton A.C.: Visceral pain. Somatic Sensation: Pain, visceral pain, headache and thermal sensations, in Guyton A.C. (ed.): *Textbook of Medical Physiology.* Philadelphia, W.B. Saunders Co., 1981, pp. 611–625.

9. Baker D.G., Coleridge H.M., Coleridge J.C.G., et al.: Search for a cardiac nociceptor: Stimulation by bradykinin of sympathetic afferent nerve endings in the heart of the cat. *J. Physiol.* 306:519–536, 1980.

10. Foreman R.D., Ohata C.A.: Effects of coronary artery occlusion on thoracic spinal neurones receiving viscerosomatic inputs. *Am. J. Physiol.* 238:H667–H674, 1980.

11. Cervero F.: Afferent activity evoked by natural stimulation of the biliary system in the ferret. *Pain* 13:137–151, 1982.

12. Morrison J.F.B.: The afferent innervation of the gastro-intestinal tract, in Brooks F.P., Evers P.W. (eds.).: *Nerves and the Gut.* New York, CBS Inc., 1977, pp. 297–326.

ADDITIONAL READINGS

1. Carstens E., Yokota T.: Viscerosomatic convergence and responses to intestinal distension of neurones at the junction of midbrain and posterior thalamus in the cat. *Exp. Neurol.* 70:392–402, 1980.

2. Hancock H.B., Foreman R.D., Willis W.D.: Convergence of visceral and cutaneous input onto spinothalamic tract cells in the thoracic spinal cord of the cat. *Exp. Neurol.* 47:240–248, 1975.

3. Leck B.F.: Abdominal and pelvic visceral receptors. *Br. Med. Bull.* 33:163–168, 1977.

4. Widdicombe J.G.: Enteroceptors, in Hubbard J.I. (ed.): *The Peripheral Nervous System.* New York, Plenum Press, 1974, pp. 455–485.

16D / Psychogenic Mechanisms

STEPHEN E. ABRAM, M.D.

ALTHOUGH certain pain problems are initiated by psychogenic factors, some physical mechanisms may be activated, resulting in stimulation of nociceptors or neuronal pools in the CNS. The resulting perception of pain is as real as the perception of pain induced by physical injury. The release of biogenic amines may lead to headaches and other pain problems. Involuntary increases in motor nerve activity produce chronically increased muscle tone and the genesis of myofascial pain syndromes. Elevated sympathetic activity may alter peripheral nociceptor activity. Alterations in intrinsic pain control mechanisms may lead to decreased pain threshold or tolerance.

Several psychological factors are thought to be important in the pathogenesis of psychogenic pain. These are described below.

DEPRESSION

Psychological depression frequently accompanies chronic somatogenic pain, and relieving the pain often alleviates the depression.[1] It has been postulated that both pain and depression are influenced by levels and turnover rates of certain brain amines, particularly serotonin. Drugs which increase availability of these amines, such as certain tricyclic antidepressants and serotonin precursors, such as L-tryptophan, can ameliorate depression and diminish pain perception.[2] On the other hand, depression may be the underlying element behind pain complaints. The pain may arise after a disease, injury, or medical treatment, but the disease or injury only serves as the trigger for pain behaviors and complaints.[3] Vigorous attention to the somatic aspects of pain complaints may destroy the patient's mechanism of compensation, allowing the depression to break through, with potentially serious consequences.

SOCIAL AND VOCATIONAL FACTORS

Pain is not only a socially acceptable complaint, it may also, in many instances, be financially compensable. It is not surprising, therefore, that headache, backache, or neck or shoulder pain become defenses against situations which the patient finds intolerable.[4] Unpleasant personal relationships and tedious, unrewarding work situations may be escaped through intractable pain. Financial rewards through the Workmen's Compensation Act and publicly funded disability programs provide incentives for perpetuating pain complaints.

Painful injuries that prevent the family breadwinner from working may result in the nonworking spouse having to earn a living. The reversal of roles may be tolerable only through continued pain complaints, thus justifying the former breadwinner's ongoing inability to fulfill that role. Thus, previously somatogenic mechanisms may become psychogenic.

LEARNING PROCESSES

Even when obvious secondary gain factors are absent, learning through reinforcement of certain behavioral responses may take place in patients with chronic pain, leading to "operant pain" problems.[5] Pain medications prescribed on an as-needed basis may act as direct reinforcers if the patient finds the sedative and analgesic effect of the drug pleasant. He exhibits behavior (complaining of pain, asking for medication) which is reinforced by the dispensing of the medication. Such behavior may persist long after nociceptive input ceases. Likewise, attention from physicians or a spouse may reinforce certain pain behavior.

Indirect reinforcement of pain behaviors occurs when the behavior leads to avoidance of an aversive or unpleasant consequence. Lying in bed avoids not

215

only discomfort associated with physical activity, but other aversive events, such as an unpleasant job or threatening social interactions.

Punishment of activity or "well behavior" may also be involved in the learning process. Supportive family members may admonish the patient for attempting to increase his physical activity.

MANAGEMENT

Recognition and appropriate treatment of depression are essential when it is the underlying cause of pain complaints. Such patients must be distinguished from those with depression secondary to long-standing somatogenic pain problems.

When operant pain mechanisms are responsible for much of a patient's disability, treatment consists of changing the illness behavior reinforcers in an effort to extinguish those responses which are causing continued disability. Family members and other physicians must be instructed to stop rewarding medication-seeking, inactivity, and verbal pain complaints and to actively reinforce increased physical activity and social interaction. Fordyce[5] outlines six objectives: (1) an increase in activity level, (2) a reduction of pain behaviors evocative of protective action by others, (3) a reduction in pain-related medication use, (4) a restoration of "well behaviors," e.g., social skills, interpersonal activities, (5) modification of reinforcing contingencies in the patient's immediate environment, and (6) a reduction in health care utilization.

Despite the development of new psychological treatment methods, there remains a group of patients who do not respond to psychological or medical treatment efforts. Such patients are often disruptive of treatment programs in which they are enrolled. Swanson et al.[6] has outlined some of the common characteristics of such patients, which include a complicated medical and surgical history, a psychiatric history indicating a traumatic childhood and adolescence, accident proneness, very long pain duration with impaired ability to work, repeated treatment failures, denial of psychiatric factors, analgesic and sedative dependency, and evidence of psychopathology on psychological tests. It is important to recognize such patients and to attempt to minimize the drain on medical resources which they represent, as any diagnostic or therapeutic intervention is bound to be fruitless.

REFERENCES

1. Sternbach R.A.: Psychological factors in pain, in Bonica J.J., Albe-Fessard D. (eds.): *Advances in Pain Research and Therapy*. New York, Raven Press, 1976, vol. 1, pp. 293–299.
2. Ward N.G., Bloom V.L., Friedel R.O.: The effectiveness of tricyclic antidepressants in the treatment of co-existing pain and depression. *Pain* 7:331–341, 1979.
3. Menges L.J.: Chronic pain patients: Some psychological aspects, in Lipton S., Miles J. (eds.): *Persistent Pain: Modern Methods of Treatment*. London, Academic Press, 1981, pp. 87–98.
4. Pace B.L.: Psychophysiology of pain: Diagnostic and therapeutic implications. *J. Fam. Pract.* 5:553–557, 1977.
5. Fordyce W.E.: Leaving processes in pain, in Sternbach R.A. (ed.): *The Psychology of Pain*. New York, Raven Press, 1978, pp. 49–72.
6. Swanson D.W., Swenson W.W., Maruta T., et al.: The dissatisfied patient with chronic pain. *Pain* 4:367–378, 1978.

16E / Central Pain

MATT J. LIKAVEC, M.D.

CENTRAL PAIN has been defined in various ways. Some people mean by central pain a diffuse and severe pain that is usually continuous in nature, with periods of increasing severity. Hyperpathia is frequently found in the general region where the pain is felt. This definition can be fulfilled by any number of lesions that affect the CNS. Spinal pain, for example, would be considered a form of central pain. This pain is normally referred to the area innervated by the nerves involved in the central lesion.

In its more classic description, central pain denotes the pain of the thalamic lesion, as described by Dejerine and Roussy.[1] The features of this syndrome are described very well in White and Sweet's original monograph.[2] The central pain of thalamic lesions has the following seven characteristics: (1) a spontaneous and constant character which may have aching, boring, gnawing, burning, icy, crushing, or other unpleasant components; (2) different or more pain is superimposed on the constant character, and there may be spontaneous paroxysms that are sometimes evoked by external stimuli; (3) the threshold for appreciation of pinprick may be elevated; (4) pain is usually referred over a wide area that may or may not include the spot stimulated; (5) touch, cold, heat, and pinprick may all evoke the same diffuse and unpleasant sensation that is much more disagreeable than pain evoked from the normal side; (6) there is often an abnormally long period between the onset of the effective stimulant and the sensations which last afterward; and (7) the pain long outlasts the stimulus, which may be quite brief.[2]

On reviewing the literature, it is apparent that pain with the above seven classic features for a thalamic lesion has often been evoked by lesions not only in the brain, but in the spinal cord, the brain stem, and the cerebral hemispheres. It is of note that Foerster in 1927 hypothesized corticofugal pathways for inhibiting pain impulses because of the existence and clinical presentation of the central pain.[3] This was long before the existence of endorphin demonstrated and the descending endorphin system described in the 1960s and 1970s. Our discussion will be confined to lesions of the thalamus.

ETIOLOGIES OF CENTRAL PAIN

The most common cause of central pain of the thalamic nature is a cerebrovascular accident. Usually a small CVA is manifested by hemianesthesia and some hemiparesis contralateral to the lesion. Over a period of weeks to months the hemianesthesia gradually dissipates and is replaced by a particularly disagreeable sensation that has become known as central pain. Among the other causes of "central pain on a thalamic basis" have been reported tumors (both glial and otherwise), arteriovenous malformations, trauma, scars, repeated ischemic insults, resolving blood clots, and emboli.[4] This list of lesions gives us an excellent idea that the thalamic central pain center is not one of specific etiology, but rather one of disordered physiology from the disruption of normal anatomical pathways.

The anatomical area involved by this lesion obviously lies in the thalamus. The question is whether it is specific thalamic nuclei that are disturbed or whether the disturbance is in the inputs and outputs. Interruption of axons from the cortex very seldom produces a central thalamic pain type of syndrome. Some of our present understanding of the disease state derives from empirical observations having to do with endorphins, and corticofugal pathways which being treated empirically with some results better than in the past.[5] Presently, central pain is thought to be related to altered synapses or imbalances located in the area of the ventral posterior thalamus, according to White and Sweet.[6]

APPROACH TO PATIENTS WITH CENTRAL PAIN

As with a great number of painful states, the human organism learns to adapt with time. Most patients who develop a central pain–like symptom complex will, after months, have some clinical improvement, so they are not left on terribly addicting drugs and do function. This observation is brought out because one would like to restrain the surgeon from doing anything uncorrectable on these patients. The results of surgical procedures on the CNS are irreversible, and if the symptom complex is going to improve over time, with some temporizing measures, it is best to stay the hand of the surgeon.

Once the consideration has been made for a central pain syndrome, a thorough history and physical examination must be completed. Based on the information derived, one is often able to come up with some etiology. For example, someone with diffuse arteriosclerotic cardiovascular disease is more likely to have thalamic syndrome on the basis of a small CVA. There is more hemianesthesia and hemiparesis associated with this than would be expected with a small infarct. If the symptom complex follows trauma, one must consider the possibility of either a traumatic lesion or an associated blood clot causing the problem. Therefore, once the physical examination and history are completed and there is a well-documented neurologic examination on the chart, the next step is neuroradiologic evaluation. The neuroradiologic evaluation includes a CT scan as a minimum. If the CT scan suggests that further pathology exists or that the pathology cannot be explained readily, or if there is a concern about a vascular abnormality, an angiogram should be obtained. The reason for this aggressive approach in the evaluation of a patient with central pain is the possibility of finding a treatable lesion, perhaps a cyst or an arteriovenous malformation.[7]

Once a treatable CNS lesion has been ruled out, the next step is to make the patient more comfortable. Because of the severe hyperpathic nature of the patient's discomfort, narcotics are of little help and have a high addictive potential. We suggest trying either Dilantin or Tegretol as the first measure in the hope of influencing the pattern of neuronal discharge. Unfortunately, this works infrequently. If this proves to be without success, we next proceed to a cocktail of Elavil and Prolixin. The goal of this drug therapy is to try to make the patient more comfortable, while the central pain state becomes more manageable on its own.

There is some evidence that the β-endorphin system has something to do with the transmission of central pain.[8, 9] With this in mind, we sometimes increase the Elavil to levels that begin to cause side effects.

It is also important to remember that other pathology in the involved areas of altered sensibility can aggravate the pain state. An example is severe arthritis involving one knee or one hip, when that side of the body is involved in the central pain syndrome. Therefore, one should not forget to treat associated pathologic conditions in the area. Because of the severe pain state, it is important that patients have physical therapy so that the areas of altered sensibility do not end up with frozen joints. Along with physical therapy, adequate rest and a reasonable diet are suggested. These all sound like the usual platitudes that doctors tell patients when there is nothing to do, but the fact remains that if the whole organism is doing well, areas of altered sensibility will not be as troublesome.

Operative Approaches

The operative approach to central thalamic pain continues to be troublesome, although there are a number of new findings. Various peripheral procedures have met with only minimal results. Although there is a well-described case by Frazier et al. in which various peripheral procedures relieved the pain,[10] such is a rarity.

Sympathetic blocks, sympathectomy, and various brachial plexus nerve blocks have all proved to be of minimal success.[11] Central pain in the spinal cord has occasionally been alleviated by central procedures. Nonetheless, these procedures have not proved helpful for thalamic pain. Trigeminal tractotomy in other lesions, at least in the brain stem, has also met with only mixed results.[5, 11]

Perhaps the most exciting area in pain research, and the most exciting prospect for the treatment of central pain, lies in manipulation of the β-endorphin system. Good results in the treatment of thalamic pain syndromes have been achieved with stimulation of the periventricular gray and with stimulation of the internal capsule. In an excellent article, Adams et al. described four patients with thalamic pain syndrome in whom good results were achieved with internal capsule stimulation.[4] They and other investigators point out that stimulation either of the periaqueductal gray or of the posterior region of the internal capsule gives pain relief. Because stimulation of the internal capsule appears to give more paresthesia, the stimulation may be slightly better for deafferented pain.[12, 13] Stimulation of the periventricular gray, on the other hand, seems to give rise to an increase of β-endorphins in the cerebrospinal fluid (CSF). It appears that at least some of this pain relief is due to the β-endorphin system because the administration of naloxone will block the relief.[5, 14]

Unfortunately, stimulation of brain areas is not widely available. A number of groups are actively exploring this technique and following their patients closely. The reasons are as follows: (1) the procedure requires a delicate stereotactic placement into specific anatomical structures of the CNS; (2) ethical issues may be raised about people with ''stimulators in the brain'' in terms of changing their personalities or affecting their behavior; and (3) this area is still highly experimental, with little practical experience. More data need to be accumulated before widespread use of these techniques can be encouraged.[15]

In summary, for the unfortunate patient with thalamic pain, one tries to do the following: (1) optimize the organism; (2) try various nonaddicting drugs in order to help the patient with the painful syndrome; (3) delay surgical therapy for at least 3–6 months in the hope that this syndrome will gradually abate, as it does in most cases; (4) avoid ablative procedures that have shown to have very poor results; and (5) if all else fails, attempt stereotactic placement of an electrode into the CNS in the hope that stimulation can affect some relief.

PATHOLOGIC INTRACRANIAL PAIN

In reality, all pain is pathologic. Functional, happy, and productive existence as we know it is pain free. Pain prevents us from being our most productive selves. However, pain of itself is seldom the pathology; it is merely a manifestation of some underlying pathology. Pain acts as a warning to the organism that something is wrong. From a strictly evolutionary viewpoint, it is a useful development. When pain does become apparent the human being will do one of three things: (1) try to alleviate the pain, (2) restrict the activity that brings on the pain, and (3) seek advice for relieving the underlying pathologic process.

This section considers intracranial pain secondary to obvious intracranial pathology (e.g., a tumor, trauma, vascular pathology).

Neither tumor cells nor glial scar tissue nor abnormal blood vessels have fine pain-sensitive nerve endings, so these in and of themselves cannot cause pain. Also, most clinicians are aware that some large processes inside the head cause no pain, whereas some very small pathologic processes can cause much pain. This brings us face to face with the fundamental fact of nervous system pathology. It is not only what is affected by the pathologic process but where it is affected that gives a nervous system lesion the ability to delineate symptoms.

Intracranial pain follows certain pathways. Based on these pathways and the tissue endings are involved, certain clinical syndromes emerge. From these clinical syndromes we can determine exactly what the process is and how to go manage the syndrome.

The pain of intracranial disease is referred to certain areas based on the anatomical distribution of the nerves that innervate the head. The trigeminal, glossopharyngeal, vagal, and first three cervical nerves are the nerves most involved in the transmission of pain from intracranial structures. The supratentorial anterior and middle fossae are innervated by the sensory nerve findings from the fifth cranial nerve. The posterior fossa and the infratentorial structures are innervated partly by cervical nerves C-1, C-2, and C-3, and partly by cranial nerves IX and X. Further understanding of pain syndromes builds on this anatomy.

Next, we must consider what the pain-sensitive structures are in the head. First, the skin, subcutaneous tissue, muscle, arteries, and periosteum of the skull are all pain sensitive. Second, the structures around the eye, the ear, and the nasal cavities are pain sensitive. Third, intracranial venous sinuses and tributaries and large veins have pain endings in them. Fourth, parts of the dura at the base of the brain and arteries within the dura mater and the pia-arachnoid appear to have some pain sensitive fibers. And fifth, the trigeminal nerve, the glossopharyngeal nerve, the vagus nerve, and the first three cervical nerves are pain-sensitive structures.

Therefore, the way to approach pain syndromes is (1) to know what the innervation is, (2) to realize what pain-sensitive structures are involved, and (3) using knowledge innervation and pain-sensitive structures, to come up with certain clinical syndromes that indicate roughly the anatomical location of the lesion.

Finally, processes in the supratentorial compartment often localize pain to the orbital or frontal region. A posterior fossa lesion often results in headache in the occipital-nuchal region. Some posterior fossa or tentorial lesions or lesions in the occipital area of the supratentoral fossa give deferred pain to the ear or to the back of the neck. Usually the location of the pain from an anatomically and pathologically localized lesion is homolateral. However, this is not always the case. Several references are available for a more complete discussion of the anatomy and findings mentioned briefly here.[5, 16–20]

The problem comes down to the fact that the symptom of headache is universal. At some time during a normal life span, probably everyone has a headache. Fortunately most of the time the headache is not associated with any neuropathologic process, but is simply part of the human condition. One should also remember that there are a number of clinical syndromes, characterized by recurrent headache, in which no definable neuropathologic process is involved—at least no gross lesion like a brain tumor, aneurysm, or arteriovenous malformation. The understanding of these headaches has been growing over the years. Some are related to neurochemistry problems. Some are related to the increased sensitivity of various vascular receptors in the head. Some headaches are caused by diffuse collagen disease. Some headaches are idiopathic. Among the principal varieties of headache that are chronic and recurrent and are often not associated with other problems are migraine, cluster headaches, tension headaches, psychiatric headaches, cough and exertional headaches, occipital neuralgia, and the headaches associated with various and sundry medical diseases, such as the headaches associated with hypertension, carotidynia, Costen's syndrome, Toloso-Hunt syndrome, retropharyngeal neuralgia, postherpetic neuralgia, acrocyanotic headaches, arteries, and "atypical facial pain." All of these conditions are associated with chronic recurrent headaches.[19–21]

The best means of determining whether patients with headache have significant intracranial pathology is a good neurologic examination and a good history. What the physician is looking for is definitive evidence that a discrete anatomical area of the CNS that is involved, or physical findings that can be ascribed to a discrete CNS area. A suspicious finding might be a field defect on vision testing, or an inability to read on the neurologic examination, or some other obvious weakness. It is when the history or the physical examination points to a CNS anatomical location that the index of suspicion is highest for CNS pathology. Unfortunately, we must rely on neurologic symptoms because there doesn't appear to be anything pathognomic or diagnostic about the pain of a tumor or often the pain of a vascular lesion. The best caveat is that if it doesn't

all add up in the history, pay extreme attention to the physical examination. Of course, there will be times when neither the history nor the physical examination will help localize the problem. When this occurs, our recommendation is to proceed with a diagnostic radiographic workup rather than curse the darkness.

After completion of the history and physical, the diagnostic workup for someone with a headache that does not fall into a classic diagnostic syndrome begins with CT scans of the head, with and without contrast. The CT scan should not only be directed toward the intracranial contents, but should also be through the orbits and the sinuses when indicated. In approximately 90% of cases of diagnosable, anatomically localized pathology, the CT scan will be diagnostic. One shortcoming to the diagnostic abilities of the CT scan has to do with vascular pathology.

With vascular pathology (e.g., aneurysm, arteriovenous malformation, or some other vascular malformation), the CT scan will often not pick it up unless it reaches a certain critical size. Therefore, if there is clinical suspicion of a vascular pathology, either a vascular malformation or an aneurysm, or if there is vascular occlusion, a complete cerebrovascular radiographic workup is mandatory. At present, this workup entails selective cerebral angiography. In the future, with improvement in diagnostic and radiographic techniques, digital subtraction angiography (DSA) may have a place in the continued workup of someone thought to have vascular pathology.

On completion of the CT scan and the vascular workup, if one is still left without an etiology, the next step is a lumbar puncture. The purposes of the lumbar puncture are as follows: first, it gives the examiner the opportunity to measure the intracranial pressure; and second it allows one to measure the various constituents of the CSF, including cells, glucose, and protein, and yields specimens for VDRL, culture studies for bacteria, fungi, myocobacteria, and other chemical evaluations.

The next step in the diagnostic workup of a patient with headache includes radiologic studies. If there is referred pain from the temporomandibular joint, films of this area are indicated. If the pain can be localized to a particular area of the head, films of that area should be obtained. The second shortcoming of the CT scan is its diagnostic accuracy in the evaluation of certain bony areas. The reason is the summation of densities, which the computer does automatically. This is especially true for lesions at the base of the brain. MRI scanning is proving increasingly helpful for these lesions.

After the completion of CT studies, lumbar puncture, and radiographic studies, 99% of the diagnosable intracranial pathologic conditions will have been identified. The remaining 1% must be dealt with on a follow-up basis with continued evaluations. With time, and by following the patient, one may be able to discern a pathology that was not evident.

Headache After Head Trauma

Immediately after significant head trauma, the victim, if he is awake, is entitled to a headache. The reason is quite simple: direct irritation of the nerve endings involving the face, scalp, periosteum, or dura can quite easily cause someone pain. This intracranial pain is usually self-evident and is treated with evaluation of the appropriate CNS insult, therapy of that, and suppression of the pain if the patient is awake.

If the patient who is wide awake after an insult begins to complain bitterly of increasing intracranial pain, this can be cardinal feature of a developing blood clot, with intracranial shifts and/or herniation. This complaint is best evaluated by a neurosurgeon.

In a second group are patients who, after a head injury, complain of constant or throbbing headaches, and on workup and evaluation the size of the ventricular system is found to be increased. The intracranial pressure is elevated slightly. Compensation of this increased intracranial pressure by drainage of the CSF, either by lumbar puncture or by shunting, relieves the pressure and pain. The type of headache appears to be merely that associated with hydrocephalus and possibly plateau waves.[20, 23, 25]

In a third group of patients with posttraumatic headache are those with delayed headache. Patients with minimal objective findings after head trauma may complain bitterly of nagging, aching headaches weeks or months later. These people invariably appear to constitute a litigious population. In large series of head trauma victims, the patients with mild head injuries and scores on the Glasgow coma scale of 13–15 when evaluated in the emergency room make up a large proportion of those with headaches later on. This has been described by a number of investigators as the postconcussive syndrome.[26, 27] In most cases the syndrome subsides over the next weeks to months. In a small number of patients the headache picture does not subside and appears to be constant and aggravating. Our only recommendations are first, to make sure that any intracranial pathology is ruled out, and second, to treat the patient on a protocol designed not to addict him. This would mean trying the patient on something like Elavil and increasing endogenous endorphin production in the hope of relieving pain, or perhaps a trial of propranolol to decrease vascular reactivity. It is only by trying these nonaddicting therapeutic measures that we can treat these people without them becoming analgesic abusers.

Vascular Headaches

The true vascular headache can be one of four types. The first type is associated with an acute bleeding episode. Bleeding might be from an aneurysm or AVM, but a small jet of blood pours into the subarachnoid space and stops abruptly. If it does not stop abruptly, the patient dies. When it does stop abruptly and the patient is not knocked to the ground or made comatose, the patient will complain of the acute onset of the worst headache of his life.[20] With this history, the diagnostic workup is not too difficult. A problem arises in managing hyperhistrionic patients who get a bad tension headache and complain of the worst headache of their lives. Unfortunately, these patients will be forced to undergo diagnostic workups, including CT scans and lumbar punctures, to rule out the possibility of subarachnoid hemorrhage. However, it is better to consider this course than to disregard the symptoms and miss the patient with a treatable subarachnoid hemorrhage.

The second type of vascular headache is one associated with a growing vascular lesion, either an aneurysm or an AVM. This is usually caused by irritation of the surrounding meninges or stretching of the blood vessels and is more the throbbing, pounding type of headache that is often localizable to one spot. An aneurysm stretching or pushing on dura will cause a headache referred to a certain part of the head, depending on the innervation of the area of dura that is irritated.[27] It is sometimes helpful if the patient with such a throbbing headache develops a third nerve or other sort of localizable neurologic deficit, which would be a clue that something is going wrong. When in doubt, we proceed with the workup outlined earlier.

The third type of headache associated with vascular pathology is the vascular headache of thrombosis. Certain patients with intracranial thrombosis of the internal carotid artery complain bitterly of an aching or throbbing headache located behind the eyes.[28] Unfortunately, this is neither pathognomonic nor diagnostic. However, it does show that because of the thrombotic process, something is going on in the adventitial layers of the involved blood vessel, and this will cause the pain syndrome.

The fourth type of headache associated with vascular disease is the headache related to the migraine syndrome. It is thought that migraine headache comes from dilation of the arteries of the cortical surface and in the meninges, and that the dilation and increased flow and stretching of these vascular structures cause the increasing headache. The situation is much more complicated than our brief description implies, with serotonergic and adrenergic neurochemistries involved in the pathophysiology of migraine. However, it is the fourth type of vascular headache, and when it falls in line with clear clinical symptoms, the diagnosis is not difficult to make and the treatment is fairly obvious.[20, 29]

The Pain of Tumor

The first type of tumor pain is that associated with increased intracranial pressure. This can be either from hydrocephalus of an obstructing lesion or because the mass has reached a critical size. The pain associated with hydrocephalus can be either occipital or bifrontal. It is sometimes described as intermittent, sometimes as constant in nature. The key is the consideration of intracranial pathology, not necessarily a specific description of the headache. The headache associated with a mass reaching a critical size can be due to two causes. The first cause is a shift of intracranial contents, with consequent irritation of the compromised dura, meninges, and blood vessels. The second cause is possible dural irritation from the mass reaching such a size that it irritates the nerve endings and the dura in the blood vessels in the area. The last type of headache associated with tumor is diffuse headache. This has no specific characteristic and seems to vary from patient to patient, according to intracranial tumor pathology. The headaches may be constant, intermittent, throbbing, pounding, sharp, dull, aching, irritating, lancinating, etc. A key feature is that the patient perceives this headache as distinctly different from any other headache he has ever had. The difference in onset should suggest workup for a tumor.[18-20, 27]

The following approach is suggested for diagnosing intracranial pain. First, a good history and physical examination may delineate a clinical syndrome that is recognizable and at times treatable, or a neurologic deficit, or an anatomically localized area of irritation that would lead one to think of intracranial pathology. On completion of this step, if there is no answer available, neuroradiologic and continued diagnostic workup are indicated. Only if vascular pathology is suspected should angiography be done, because of its associated risks. If the diagnosis is still not evident, I attempt various nonaddicting therapies, including tricyclic antidepressants, beta blockers, biofeedback, TENS, some muscle relaxants, and the judicious use of narcotics. A stratified approach, such as the one described, should help the examiner rule out intracranial pathology and diagnose the cranial pathology of a treatable syndrome. Such an approach also minimizes the tendency of the American patient with intracranial pain to medicate himself into oblivion.

REFERENCES

1. Dejerine J., Roussy G.: Le syndrome thalamique. *Rev Neurol.* 14:521–532, 1906.
2. White J.C., Sweet W.H.: *Pain: Its Mechanisms and Neurosurgical Control.* Springfield, Ill., Charles C Thomas, Publisher, 1955.
3. Foerster O.: *Die Leitungsbahnen des schmerage Fühls und die chirurgische Behandlung der Schmerzzustande.* Berlin, Urban & Schwarzenberg, 1974.
4. Adams J.E., Hosobuchi Y., Fields H.L.: Stimulation of the internal capsule for relief of chronic pain. *J. Neurosurg.* 41:740–744, 1974.
5. Hosobuchi Y., Rossier J., Bloom F.E., et al.: Stimulation of human periaqueductal gray for pain relief increases immunoreactive β-endorphin in ventricular fluid. *Science* 203:279–281, 1979.
6. White J.C., Sweet W.H., Thomas C.C.: *Pain and the Neurosurgeon: A Forty-Year Experience.* Springfield, Ill., Charles C Thomas, Publisher, 1969, chapters 5, 8, and 9.
7. Mayo Clinic: *Clinical Examinations in Neurology,* ed. 5. Philadelphia, W.B. Saunders Co., 1981.
8. Ignelzi R.J., Hampton Atkinson J.: Pain and its modulation: Part 1. Afferent mechanisms. *Neurosurgery* 6:577–583, 1980.
9. Ignelzi R.J., Hampton Atkinson J.: Pain and its modulation: Part 2. Efferent mechanisms. *Neurosurgery* 6:584–590, 1980.
10. Frazier C.H., Lewy F.H., Rowe S.N.: The origin and mechanisms of paroxysmal neurologic pain and the surgical treatment of central pain. *Brain* 60:44–51, 1937.
11. Long D.M.: Surgical therapy of chronic pain. *Neurosurgery* 6:273–277, 1980.

12. Richardson D.E., Akil H.: Pain reduction by electrical brain stimulation in man: Part 1: Acute administration in periaqueductal periventricular sites. *J. Neurosurg.* 47:178–183, 1977.

13. Richardson D.E., Akil H.: Pain reduction by electrical brain stimulation in man: Part 2. Chronic self-administration in the periventricular grey matter. *J. Neurosurg.* 47:184–194, 1977.

14. Akil H., Mayer D.J., Liebeskind J.C.: Antagonism of stimulation provided analgesia by naloxone, a narcotic antagonist. *Science* 191:961–962, 1976.

15. Sweet W.H.: Intracerebral electrical stimulation for the relief of chronic pain, in Youmans J.R. (ed.): *Neurological Surgery.* Philadelphia, W.B. Saunders Co., 1982, vol. VI, chap. 136.

16. King R.B., Young R.F.: Cephalic pain, in Youmans J.R. (ed.): *Neurological Surgery.* Philadelphia, W.B. Saunders Co., 1982, vol. VI, chap. 118.

17. Ray B.S., Wolff H.G.: Experimental studies of headache. *Arch. Surg.,* 41:813–856, 1940.

18. Northfield D.W.C.: Some observations on headache. *Brain.* 61:133–162, 1938.

19. Adams R.D., Victor M.: *Principles of Neurology,* ed. 2. New York, McGraw-Hill Book Co., 1981.

20. Reskin N.H., Appenzeller O.: *Headache.* Philadelphia, W.B. Saunders Co., 1980.

21. Menkes J.H.: *Textbook of child neurology,* ed. 2. Philadelphia, Lea & Febiger, 1980, chap. 11.

22. Weinstein M., Modic M.T., Paulicek W.A.: Intravenous digital subtraction angiography of the head and neck, in Weiss M. (ed.): *Clinical Neurosurgery.* Baltimore, Md., Williams & Wilkins, Co., 1982, vol. 29, chap. 28.

23. Ommaya A.K., Gennavelli T.A.: Cerebral concussion and traumatic unconsciousness, *Brain* 97:633–654, 1974.

24. Langfitt T., Weinstein J.D., Kasses N.F.: Cerebral vasomotor paralysis produced by intracranial hypertension. *Neurology* 15:622–641, 1965.

25. Epstein F., Martin A.E., Walk A.: Chronic headache in the shunt-dependent adolescent with nearly normal ventricular volume: Diagnosis and treatment. *Neurosurgery* 3:351–355, 1978.

26. Rimel R.W., Giordan B., Barth J.T., et al.: Disability caused by minor head injury. *Nuerosurgery* 9:221–228, 1981.

27. Mackenzie I.: The clinical presentation of cerebral angioma. *Brain* 76:184–214, 1953.

28. Ratcheson R.A.: Clinical diagnosis of atherosclerotic carotid artery disease. *Clin. Neurosurg.* 129:464–481, 1982.

29. Carrol J.D.: Migraine: General management. *Br. Med. J.* 2:756-757, 1971.

16F / Pain Secondary to Paraplegia or Quadriplegia

MATT J. LIKAVEC, M.D.

AMONG THE MOST emotionally taxing people to deal with in the setting of chronic pain are patients who have pain on top of paraplegia or quadriplegia. These patients are usually intact mentally but are extremely damaged from their spinal cord lesion. The physician wants to be able to do something for their pain because he is unable to do anything for their basic spinal lesions. And yet these patients present with some of the most bizarre and unusual painful complaints, including pain in parts of the body that don't feel and spasms in parts of the body that don't move. In many of the interactions, the unspoken theme is that if something is done for the pain, the patient "knows" his function will improve.

The only way to deal with these patients successfully and fairly is the same way one deals with other pain patients—directly, with compassion, and with honesty.

Fortunately, only about 15%–20% of patients with severe spinal cord injury have severe disabling pain.[1, 2] On questioning, the majority of paraplegic patients report various aches and pains they appear able to live with. Nevertheless, the pain from spinal cord injury can be quite severe and debilitating.

ETIOLOGY

The etiology of spinal cord pain is not completely known. Obviously the primary lesion, with interruption of nervous continuity at the level of insult, sets the scene for subsequent pain. However, why do only 15% of these patients subsequently have disabling pain? The answer appears not to lie in pathology of the cord, which is usually hemorrhagic necrosis at the site of the lesion. Furthermore, much of the pain of spinal cord lesions cannot be traced to the injured spinal cord segment but emanates from the surrounding bony, ligamentous, and muscular structures. Bony instability at the site of injury can be very painful.[5] Also, improper positioning

and therapy of limbs and joints innervated above the level of a lesion can cause considerable pain.[6]

The empirical fact does remain, in any analysis of severe pain attributed to the spinal cord itself in spinal cord injury, the level of the cord just proximal to the lesion is the critical area in the genesis of the pain. This fact becomes apparent on review of all therapies involved in manipulating the nervous system distal to the level of the insult. Therapy aimed at the nervous system distal to the level of the insult shows uniformly poor results.[7]

A number of hypotheses have been proposed to explain the physiologic basis for the anatomical location of the "spinal" pain in these debilitated patients. One line of reasoning links the pain from the traumatized spinal cord to hyperactivity of spinal neurons, i.e., almost an epilepsy of the spinal neurons.[8] It is suggested that the inhibitory influences of the spinal neurons just above the level of the spinal insult have been interrupted and the neurons are now firing abnormally in a new neuronal milieu, which causes pain.

A second line of reasoning raises the possibility of collateral pathways that bypass the level of injury of the spinal cord in carrying the pain impulses cephalad. One possible explanation for this would be an anatomical location outside the spinal cord.[6]

A third line of reasoning implicates disruption of normal circuits, with previously suppressed impulses becoming painful. This may explain why especially partial conus lesions have the highest tendency to become painful afterward.[9]

RATIONAL MANAGEMENT APPROACH

Any therapy for spinal pain must take into account the possible influence of outside factors. Only in the context of the *total* patient can a rational approach be designed and a successful management scheme executed.

Workup

An approach to spinal pain starts with a thorough history and physical examination. The history should cover the onset of the pain, aggravating factors, alleviating factors, duration of pain, location of pain, possible relief by medications, and the other kinds of criteria that are reviewed in all pain states. Next, the physician must go into the emotional and psychological background of the patient. A recent loss may be making a previously tolerable pain state now unbearable. In line with this approach, the physician must inquire into topics like employment, rehabilitation potential and direction, sexuality, a problem with meeting financial needs, or just an unrealistic view (either positive or negative) of the patient's compromised state.[6]

After the history is completed a thorough physical examination must be done. The examination must not only document what the patient's deficits are, but must also investigate hyperpathic zones, loss of mobility in joints above and below the lesion, and the presence decubiti, sore spots, and other problems. The physical examination findings must be checked against earlier examinations that the patient has had. A rise in one or two segments of anesthesia may be the harbinger of a posttraumatic syringomyelia, which can also bring on a painful state. This examination may be difficult to do because of the loss of mobility and various dysesthic areas, but it must be done completely and repeated at intervals during the treatment program.[6]

After the history and the physical examination are completed, attention is directed toward the laboratory and radiologic evaluation. Not only must the usual blood, electrolytes, and hepatic indices be checked, but the urine must be cultured, and also any sores or decubiti. Liver disease, a urinary tract infection, an infected decubitus, and other nonspinal pathologies are all well-known provocateurs of spinal pain.

The radiographic workup proceeds with plain x-ray films of the involved spinal area and any areas of referred pain. This is to check for spinal stability, possible vertebral collapse, the presence of foreign bodies, and other bony pathology. Before any surgical procedure is contemplated, good judgment dictates that the radiographic workup include a CT scan (with contrast in the subarachnoid space) of the involved spinal area, and also a myelogram if any doubt remains about local pathology after the CT study.

On unusual occasions electromyograms (EMGs) and nerve conduction studies have been helpful in documenting progressive anterior horn cell dropout, but by and large they have not proved necessary.

Treatment

Once the above workup is completed and the findings have been analyzed, the possibility of any "extrinsic" lesion should have been ruled out. Entities or states that can be uncovered by the workup just described include depression, psychological maladjustment, syringomyelia, spinal instability, vertebral collapse, retained foreign body, urinary tract infection, spastic or atonic bladder, decubitus, and so forth.

With the exclusion of extrinsic treatable inciting factors for spinal pain, we are left with three approaches to the problem: pharmaceutical, anesthetic, and surgical.

The practice of starting the paralyzed patient on low doses of narcotics and titrating for the problem is to be condemned. A possibly chronic, fluctuating, lifelong painful state can rarely be handled safely with long-term narcotics because of their highly addictive potential.

In my experience, diphenylhydantoin and carbamazepine have seldom been of any help, although I have had one patient each who responded to each drug. Nonsteroidal anti-inflammatory drugs have rarely touched the spinal pain. Tricyclic antidepressants alone or in combination with other drugs have been of some help in painful states.[5] I have had a number of patients who have responded to these agents (perhaps because of their endorphin effects) and have become more comfortable, although none of the patients has become pain free. I attempt drug therapy first because the anesthetic and surgical therapies are ablative and irreversible.

For patients who do not respond to drug therapy, the next option is anesthesia. Sympathetic and epidural blocks with local anesthetics have been tried in the hope of predicting whether more permanent chemical blocks will prove helpful. This approach has not proved helpful.[5] The experience of Sir Ludwig Guttman in the British Isles suggests that a subarachnoid phenol block around and above the level of the injury and a segment or two higher may be successful.[5] The problem with this therapy is threefold: first, difficulty of the technique and nonspecificity of the lesion; second, compromise of bowel and bladder function in incomplete lesions; and third, the inability to use the technique above the lower thoracic area because of potential compromise of respiratory control centers in the cervical cord.

Present surgical options include a number of standard procedures from the past as well as some promising procedures for the future. Among the standard surgical therapies are open cordotomy, percutaneous cordotomy, and cordectomy. Localized rhizotomies, lysis of adhesions, and sympathectomy have all had their proponents in the past but have not proved to be of sustained benefit.

Open cordotomy has been the surgical therapy with the longest follow-up for the treatment of spinal pain. White and Sweet in their classic monograph point out some of the limitations and caveats for this procedure. Included in their warnings were the necessity of doing bilateral anterolateral open procedures, the necessity of doing the procedure at slightly different spinal cord levels, and the necessity of creating the cordotomy at a high enough level. The drawbacks to this procedure are first, it is an open operation, and second, although the results are good, they are not uniformly successful. One can expect good results about 90% of the time.[10]

Percutaneous cordotomy came into its own with the 1960s. There are some reasonable results with it. The advantages of the procedure are the ability to do it on the awake patient, the ability to stage the operation, the ability to gauge the lesion with stimulation techniques, and the ability to repeat it if necessary. Morbidity and mortality from the procedure are minimal. There is difficulty however with higher spinal cord lesions for anterior cordotomy to be efficacious. The other disadvantage is the caveat that percutaneous cordotomies should not be done bilaterally high in the neck because of the risk of inducing Ondine's curse. Results of the procedure are usually good, but recurrences and painful dysesthetic states have occurred.[5, 11]

Cordectomy is the ultimate surgical procedure for spinal pain and must involve the area just proximal to the damaged segment to be successful. However, cordectomy is limited to the lower spinal cord and is an open, major surgical procedure, with its risks. The other problems associated with cordectomy are that it will make any partial lesion into a complete one, and many patients have a great deal of difficulty facing the prospect of ''cutting'' their spinal cords, even with their pain. This procedure seems to take away any minimal lingering subconscious hope of regaining function.[9]

Nashold and his colleagues have recently suggested dorsal root entry zone lesions at the level of the spinal cord insult and one level above.[2] Review of their data suggests that the surgical procedure might work better for more peripheral lesions involving the cauda equina or peripheral nerves.[12] Nonetheless, their work should be followed closely.

The placement of epidural stimulators may be considered in patients with spinal cord pain.[5] However, there is often associated scarring and unusual anatomy (e.g., from gunshot wounds) that make the placement technically very difficult. In our hands, the epidural stimulators have not proved helpful.

One major line of research that may lead to some practical developments for this state involves techniques that have arisen from research on endorphins. The possibility of thalamic or central gray area stimulation has not been explored much in these spinal patients but is a consideration.[13, 14] Also the local continuous pump infusion of minimal doses of narcotics might be helpful in these patients.[15]

SUMMARY

Patients with pain following spinal cord injury are among the most difficult of pain patients to manage. Fortunately, there are a number of avenues that can be explored in helping them with their pain problem, and a number of procedures can be attempted that have good statistical possibilities of success. Unfortunately, the physicians that treat paraplegic or quadriplegic patients with pain cannot give them back spinal cord function and sometimes may further damage the nervous system.

REFERENCES

1. Kahn E.A., Peet M.M., The technique of anterolateral cordotomy. *J. Neurosurg.* 5:276–283, 1948.
2. Nashold B.S., Bullit E.: Dorsal root entry zone lesions to control center pain in paraplegics. *Neurosurgery* 55:414–419, 1981.
3. Freeman L.W., Heimburger R.F.: Surgical relief of pain in paraplegic patients. *Arch. Surg.* 55:433–440, 1947.
4. Tinsley M. Compound injuries of the spinal cord. *J. Neurosurg.* 3:306–309, 1946.
5. Long D.M.: Neurological surgery, in Youmans J.R. (ed.): *Pain of Spinal Origin.* Philadelphia, W.B. Saunders Co., 1982, vol. VI, chap. 126.
6. Guttman L.: *Spinal Cord Injuries: Comprehensive Management and Research.* Oxford, England, Blackwell Scientific Publications, 1976.
7. Long D.M.: Surgical therapy of chronic pain. *Neurosurgery* 6:317–328, 1980.

8. Loeser J.D., Ward A.A., White L.E.: Chronic Deafferentation of Human Spinal Cord Neurons. *J. Neurosurg.* 29:48–50, 1968.

9. Druckman R., Lende R.: Central Pain of Spinal Cord Origin. *Neurology* 15:518–522, 1965.

10. White J.C., Sweet W.H.: *Pain: Its Mechanisms and Neurosurgical Control.* Springfield, Ill., Charles C Thomas, Publisher, 1955.

11. Rosomoff H.L.: Bilateral Percutaneous Cervical Radiofrequency Cordotomy. *J. Neurosurg.* 31:41–46, 1969.

12. Nashold Jr., Blaine S. and Ostdahl R.H.: Dorsal Root Entry Zone Lesions for Pain Relief. *J. Neurosurg.* 51:p. 59–69, 1979.

13. Meyerson B.A., Boethius J., Carlsson A.M.: Percutaneous central gray stimulation for cancer pain. *Appl. Neurophysiol.* 41:57–65, 1978.

14. Hosobuchi Y., Rossier J., Bloom F.E., Guillemin R.: Stimulation of Human Periaqueductal Gray for Pain Relief Increases Immunoreactive β-Endorphin in Ventricular Fluid. *Science* 203:279–281, 1979.

15. Onofrio B.M., Yaksh T.L., and Arnold P.G., Continuous Low-Dose Intrathecal Morphine Administration in the Treatment of Chronic Pain of Malignant Origin. *Mayo Clinic Proc.* 56:516–520, 1981.

PART **III**

Pain in Specific Situations

17 / Postoperative Pain

MICHAEL STANTON-HICKS, M.D.

IT IS AN INDICTMENT of modern medicine that such an apparently simple problem as relief of postoperative pain remains largely unsolved.[11] Such is the present state of affairs regarding our inability to successfully and consistently manage the pain of surgery.

While no one would question the success of modern anesthesia and analgesia to provide optimal conditions for surgery with a minimum of discomfort and disturbance for the patient, it is apparent that the standard methods of pain management fall short of providing satisfactory analgesia.[8] Presently, postoperative pain is treated by oral and parenteral administration of nonnarcotic and narcotic analgesics. Mather has pointed out that even though many new potent analgesic drugs have been introduced to clinical practice in the last 50 years, their inability to provide adequate pain relief is due not to their lack of potency, but rather to iatrogenic circumstances.[25] These are:

1. The orders are poorly written. They are frequently inappropriate with regard to the type and severity of pain.

2. The orders are not explicit and are open to misinterpretation by the nursing staff, such that suboptimal doses are frequently administered.

3. There is a frequent failure to understand that patients differ in their analgesic requirements.

Obviously, if oral or parenteral drugs are to achieve their analgesic effects, an adequate plasma concentration of the drug must be attained to equilibrate with receptors involved in the production of analgesia. A knowledge of pharmacokinetics of the analgesics is necessary to understand the factors that are responsible for the uptake, distribution and excretion of such drugs.[25]

Since in all but the mildest of postoperative pain, narcotics are the agent of choice, the following discussion focuses on these drugs. Studies show that blood drug concentrations following parenteral administration are totally unpredictable. This in turn produces a varying quality of analgesia. However, with the advent of intensive care units allowing close monitoring, the intravenous (IV) route is now increasingly utilized.[5, 6, 32] With the IV technique, some of the barriers responsible for uneven drug absorption are removed. It is simpler to titrate a dose that will safely and quickly achieve a desired analgesic effect.

An extension of this idea is the predetermined intermittent or continuous IV administration of narcotics based on a dosage schedule that has been calculated according to pharmacokinetic principles.[18] Following a loading dose of analgesic agent, the subsequent dosage schedule is calculated to obtain a rate that will maintain optimal analgesia under similar circumstances. Unfortunately, such standard conditions are not routinely obtained in clinical practice. Nevertheless, compared with oral or intramuscular routes of administration, this technique achieves infinitely better analgesia.

A recent innovation and an extension of the same principles governing IV administration of narcotics for analgesia is the use of mechanical devices that allow the patient to administer a predetermined dose of a particular agent.[18, 40] Such devices can be programmed to allow repetitive increments of drug to be self-administered, while limits can be set that will prevent toxic amounts from being delivered. In addition, computer technology has enabled ''fail-safe'' alarms to be built into these machines. The main disadvantages of such systems are the high cost of the apparatus and the small group of selected patients that would benefit from this technique.[19]

TECHNIQUES OF ANALGESIA

Drugs

Oral Administration

INDICATIONS.—Common indications for the oral administration of drugs for analgesia are minor surgery, ambulatory surgery, endoscopic procedures, and for the manipulations and reapplication of plaster casts.

DRUGS.—The nonnarcotic drugs customarily used for the above indications are aspirin and paracetamol; the narcotic drugs are pentazocine, codeine, and meperidine.

DOSAGE.—Pentazocine (tablet form) is given in a dosage of 25–100 mg q3h. For children aged 6–12 years, the dosage is 25 mg q3h. Codeine phosphate (tablet form) is given in a dosage of 10–60 mg q4h. In children, the dosage is 3 mg/kg q4h. Meperidine (tablet form) is given in a dosage of 150 mg q4h.

COMMENT.—The side effects of codeine and meperidine are common to all narcotic analgesics, with sedation, euphoria, nausea, vomiting, and respiratory depression usually being dose related. Pentazocine may produce hallucinations. Pentazocine or codeine can be used for mild to moderate pain, while meperidine should be reserved for more severe pain.

Because of the variability of absorption with oral administration, it is useful to anticipate postoperative pain by giving a small dose of narcotic IV within the last 15 minutes of the surgical procedure. In this way, severe pain is alleviated in the time it takes for the orally administered dose of narcotic to become effective. In addition, because the effects of the two narcotics would be additive, a smaller dose of oral medication will suffice. However, it must be remembered that because of factors that affect the uptake of these drugs, it may be necessary to administer a second dose of analgesic if the pain has not been relieved adequately after 90 minutes. The second dose should be half the original dose.

Intramuscular Injection

DRUGS.—Pentazocine, codeine, meperidine, morphine, and buprenorphine are the narcotic drugs commonly given by intramuscular injection for the control of postoperative pain.

DOSAGE.—The dosages of these drugs are as follows: pentazocine, 30–60 mg q3h (in children, 0.5–1 mg/kg q3h); codeine, 25–30 mg q3h; meperidine, 25–200 mg q3h (in children aged 6–12 years, 0.2 mg/kg); morphine, 5–20 mg q4h (in children aged 6–12 years, 0.2 mg/kg); buprenorphine, 300–600 μg q4h.

Intravenous Injection

DRUGS.—Morphine, meperidine, fentanyl, and methadone are the narcotic drugs that may be given by IV infusion for the control of postoperative pain.

DOSAGE.—Usually, the dosage of narcotics given by IV injection is "titrated," i.e., given in small amounts until the desired level of analgesia is achieved. It is preferable to use small boluses of any agent so that the systemic effects can be readily observed while unwanted side effects such as nausea and respiratory depression can be held to a minimum. This, in fact, is the basis for the continuous IV infusion of narcotics. Only small differences in the pharmacokinetic properties of meperidine, fentanyl, morphine, and methadone occur in most healthy patients. Following IV administration, the redistribution of drugs from blood occurs, firstly, to highly perfused tissues like brain, kidney, liver and heart to the less well perfused tissues like muscle and skin, and ultimately to fat which is the least well perfused tissue in which drugs like meperidine, fentanyl and methadone have such a high affinity.[23] The half life of this redistribution phase for each of these opiates is somewhere between one and 30 minutes, depending on whether arterial or venous blood concentrations are measured, and the number of components or sub-phases into which one may wish to resolve this entire phase. Elimination of the drug is much slower than redistribution, meperidine, morphine, and fentanyl having typically slow elimination half lives of around 2–6 hours, while methadone is as long as 30 hours.[24] Because of the pharmacokinetic variability reported for opiates, and the fact that there seems to be no convincing evidence of a direct correlation between weight and dose for effect, bolus injections will of necessity yield varying blood concentrations and, consequently, varying levels of analgesia. More important to successful analgesia would appear to be the altered perfusion rates to various regions in the body. Such regional differences occur in conditions such as cirrhosis, or viral hepatitis, postoperatively after the influence of anesthetic drugs, and under circumstances of the co-administration of particular drugs having enzyme inducing properties. If one bypasses the absorption phase through use of an intravenous infusion, invariably the analgesic response will be related to the variability of steady state concentrations. These, in turn, are controlled solely by systemic clearance which is dependent on the hepatic enzymes, i.e., extraction ratio and blood flow. IV infusion, by bypassing the absorption phase, is no more than the titration of a patient's analgesic response to repeated tiny doses of opiates.

Intravenous Infusion

DRUGS.—Narcotics commonly given by IV infusion for the control of postoperative pain are morphine, meperidine, fentanyl, buprenorphine, and methadone.

GENERAL PRINCIPLES.—The agonist narcotics, morphine, meperidine, and fentanyl, and the synthetic agonist/antagonist narcotics, of which buprenorphine is an example, seem to share similar pharmacokinetic characteristics, whereas methadone is quite different.[4]

After IV infusion, the redistribution phase of the first four agents is fast, i.e., the half-life of the narcotic in this phase is less than 30 minutes. However, the elimination phase of the drug takes longer (2-6 hours). The half-life of methadone is extremely slow, and the drug takes 30 or more hours to be eliminated.[20]

Because of the rapid redistribution phase, a loading dose of the agent must be given so that analgesia is provided before the steady-state blood level of drug is reached that will ensure continued adequate relief of pain. Continuous IV infusion, by removing the peaks and troughs in blood narcotic concentrations, helps maintain a constant ratio between the drug input or infusion rate and the drug output or total body clearance, once an equilibrium (steady state) between the blood and tissue concentration has been reached.

The following are examples of dosages that have been determined for meperidine, fentanyl, and morphine in patients who have undergone major abdominal surgery: meperidine, 25 mg/hr; fentanyl, 0.045 mg/hr; and morphine, 2.5 mg/hr. Little clinical data are yet available for buprenorphine, although its pharmacokinetic characteristics are very similar to the foregoing narcotic agonists, in which case one might expect an infusion rate that would be determined by its relative potency and of a similar order.

Methadone, on the other hand, has a low clearance and a long half-life. After redistribution, the plasma concentration will drop slowly, i.e., if a dose of 15-20 mg is given IV, it will take at least 12-24 hours before analgetic levels subside. It would therefore be inappropriate to use such an agent for continuous IV infusion. However, such characteristics would be very desirable in an analgesic agent because no complicated IV devices or extra nursing attention would be required. Unfortunately, any untoward side effects would also decline slowly in a parallel with the slow drug clearance.

Transcutaneous Electrical Nerve Stimulation

Based on the gate control mechanism proposed by Wall and Melzack, in which selective stimulation of large-diameter cutaneous afferent pathways inhibits pain, electrical devices that percutaneously stimulate such fibers have been developed for the management of chronic pain.[22] Such nerve stimulators have been used to determine the suitability of certain patients for the implantation of dorsal column stimulators for controlling certain chronic pain syndromes. Following the prognostic use of these units, skin analgesia was often observed and the potential application to other types of pain relief was recognized.

Essentially such electrical units are battery powered and provide a square wave stimulus which may be biphasic. The frequency can be altered, although for stimulation of large afferent fibers, a frequency of 100–150 at a current flow of 20–25 mamps is most effective. The duration of each pulse is 250–400 msec.

Various types of electrodes have been developed for use with these stimulators and vary from small patch electrodes to strips that can be placed on either side of a wound. For large paramedian or median abdominal incisions, electrodes in long strips are best to use. They must be sterile and should be placed close to the skin margins and so must be included in the wound dressing.

When small patch electrodes are used, the patients can be encouraged to experiment with different positions to find one that will produce optimal pain relief.

How often one should use the stimulator varies from individual to individual and with the severity of pain. A useful routine with which to commence is to apply the current for 20–30 min at 4-hr intervals. This sequence seems very successful in reducing the pain in some 70% of individuals after abdominal surgery. Following upper abdominal surgery, the stimulator can be used to enable the patient to tolerate chest physical therapy.

COMMENT.—Transcutaneous electrical nerve stimulation (TENS) as a means of inhibiting the acute pain of injury is certainly not as effective as nerve blocks, but when used after abdominal surgery it is almost as effective as parenteral narcotics and does not induce the undesirable side effects of respiratory depression, nausea, vomiting, and urinary retention. Several randomized studies have shown that the analgesia provided is better than placebo effect. This was confirmed when the patients conclusively demonstrated the placebo effect with nerve stimulators that had their batteries removed. What is still lacking, however, is a good randomized controlled study of the cardiovascular effects and of the effects on stress hormones when this form of analgesia is compared with another standard form of pain relief.

Although the pain relief using TENS remains incomplete, the concurrent administration of small doses of parenteral opiates will provide the additional analgesia needed to achieve almost complete relief of pain without the side effects often associated with the exclusive use of parenteral narcotics. Some early reports of postoperative TENS claimed a reduction in the frequency of postoperative ileus and pulmonary atelectasis.[27] Subsequent studies, however, have not confirmed these earlier observations. The main disadvantage of TENS is the management of the electrodes which, for their integrity and continued function, require excellent skin contact. Any movements, sweating, secretions, and disconnection of the cables, particularly to those electrodes that are included in the dressing, can interfere with the continuity of analgesia; nevertheless, TENS is a practical alternative form of pain relief.

Nerve Blocks

Intercostal Blocks

The use of intercostal blocks for postoperative pain management has been under emphasized, and as a consequence their application has been under utilized. Intercostal block is perhaps the easiest of all nerve blocks to perform because of the proximity of the nerve to its principal landmark, the rib.[9, 26] Although the procedure carries the potential hazard of pneumothorax, this complication can be avoided by understanding the local anatomy and using an impeccable technique.

Most of the pain from abdominal surgery arises from the parietal peritoneum and the incision. Intercostal nerve blocks can therefore provide adequate analgesia and the relief from muscle spasm within the territory of innervation. In the chest, intercostal blocks can be used to provide analgesia after rib resection and thoracotomy.[13, 14]

ANATOMY.—The intercostal nerves are the anterior primary rami of the thoracic spinal outflow. There are 11 nerves and one subcostal nerve under the 12th rib. With slight variation, most intercostal nerves, after their formations from their respective spinal nerve roots, pass directly to the adjacent rib and divide into a main nerve, which travels with its intercostal artery and vein in the subcostal groove, and a collateral intercostal nerve, which travels in parallel with the main nerve but in the lower margin of the intercostal space (Fig 17–1). The collateral nerve, when present, travels in the same tissue plane between the inner and innermost intercostal muscles. The main nerve is both sensory and motor throughout its distribution, whereas the collateral nerve is purely motor in its supply.

In the midaxillary line the main intercostal nerve gives off a perforating branch that divides superficial to the muscle into anterior and posterior branches, which supply the skin over the lateral part of the chest and abdomen. The main intercostal nerve in the upper six intercostal spaces passes anteriorly and ends as the interior cutaneous branch, which perforates the muscle to supply the skin over the anterior chest and parietal pleura. The lower six nerves supply the skin over the abdomen and the parietal peritoneum and abdominal muscles.

PHYSIOLOGIC EFFECTS.—Block of an intercostal nerve proximal to its perforating branch will pro-

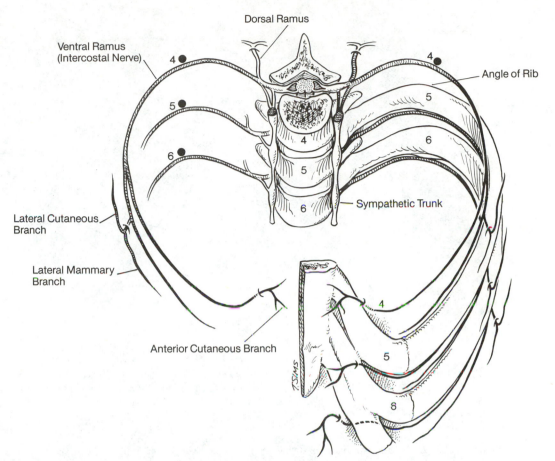

Fig 17–1.—Anatomy of the intercostal nerve and its distribution with its branches along the ribs. (From Raj P.P. [ed.]: *Handbook* *of Regional Anesthesia.* New York, Churchill Livingstone, Inc., 1985. Reproduced by permission.)

duce analgesia in its dermatome with only slight overlap in the adjacent spaces, and paralysis of the muscles it supplies. For most abdominal wounds, block of the lower five to six nerves is required bilaterally, although for a muscle-splitting incision or subcostal incision, block of intercostal nerves on the right side will generally provide satisfactory analgesia without the need for a bilateral block.

Technique.—The patient may be in the prone position, if it is feasible, or turned on his or her side. For an effective block of each intercostal nerve, the injection must be made proximal to the origin of the lateral perforating branch. The 12th rib is identified and the overlying skin is fixed with the second and third fingers of the left hand. A 20-gauge short bevel needle is introduced until it con-

tacts the rib. The skin and needle together are drawn caudad as the tip is "walked" over the surface of the rib until it reaches the inferior edge, at which point it is advanced no more than 3 mm (Fig 17–2). At this depth, the tip should have traversed the inner intercostal muscle and should be lying in the space between the inner and innermost intercostal muscles. After prior aspiration, 2–3 ml of local anesthetic solution are injected in each intercostal space. Usually ten intercostal blocks will provide satisfactory abdominal analgesia unless, as already explained, a limited unilateral block will suffice for a unilateral wound site.

An alternative to multiple intercostal injection sites has recently been redescribed by Murphy and takes note of the anatomy of the intercostales intimi and subcostales muscles whose fibers traverse more

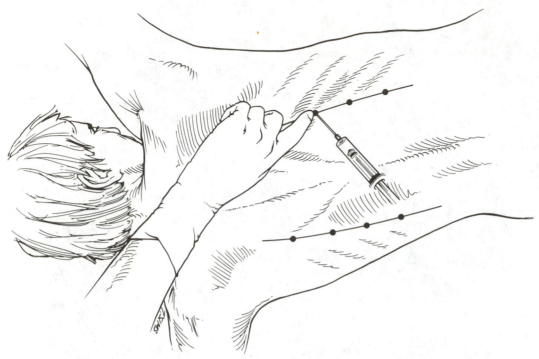

Fig 17–2.—Technique of intercostal block at the angles of the ribs. Note the palpation of the inferior edge of the rib and penetration of the needle below it. (From Raj P.P. [ed.]: *Handbook of Regional Anesthesia.* New York, Churchill Livingstone, Inc., 1985. Reproduced by permission.)

than one intercostal space.[29] The former muscles are disposed as a sheath within the lateral wall of the thorax, while the subcostales muscles lie in the paravertebral gutter. These two muscles and the sterno-costalis muscle comprise a group, the transversus thoracis group of muscles, which form the innermost boundary of the intercostal space. A consequence of this anatomy is that when sufficient local anesthetic solution is introduced in one intercostal space, it will flow proximally, and then spread superiorly and inferiorly to reach other intercostal nerves. It is a simple matter to take advantage of this anatomy by placing an epidural catheter through an 18-gauge thinwall Tuohy needle directed proximally in the intercostal space. This can then be used to provide analgesia over a series of intercostal nerves for as long as required.

Thoracotomy presents a different situation in that the surgeon can very simply apply the local anesthetic under direct vision from within the thoracic cavity. For a thoracotomy wound it is generally necessary to block four to five nerves at the level of the thoracotomy and one or two intercostal nerves at the drainage tube site. Even though the drainage tube itself may irritate the pleura at sites distant from the blocked nerves, the pain relief provided is still better than no relief at all.

METHODS AND AGENTS.—Two principal methods of intercostal nerve block are available for alleviating postoperative pain: a local anesthetic block with the long-acting amide local anesthetic bupivacaine or etidocaine, or a cryoblock, utilizing a cryoprobe under direct vision to freeze the nerves.

Bupivacaine 0.5% or etidocaine 1%, both with epinephrine 5 μg/ml, will each produce excellent analgesia for 12–18 hours. Cryoanalgesia, when correctly applied, can provide analgesia for several weeks.

The significant advantages of nerve block over centrally acting opiate analgesics are the avoidance of central depression and the provision of almost complete pain relief, facts which make chest physical therapy simple while allowing patients voluntarily to clear their own pulmonary secretions more easily. Lung function is therefore improved, and in many cases patients with compromised lung function who would normally require mechanical ventilation are spared this imposition with its inevitable morbidity. The principal disadvantages of intercostal nerve block are the fact that several injections must be made each time the analgesia is reinforced, theoretically increasing the risk of pneumothorax, and toxicity of local anesthetic injections must always be considered, particularly when 10 or more ribs are injected. It should be noted that highest peak blood local anesthetic levels are obtained following intercostal block.[1]

The principal advantage of cryoanalgesia over local anesthetic intercostal blocks is the extensive duration achieved.[20] The disadvantage is the fact that the technique is not available in every institution, in addition to which it requires practice, more time to produce an effective neuroblock, and cooperation with the surgeon. In institutions where a large number of thoracic operations are performed, this form of analgesia is certainly a practical feasibility, whereas for itinerant thoracic surgery, a local anesthetic block is a simpler and equally effective solution, the only real disadvantage being its relatively short duration of action. However, if advantage is taken of the catheter technique, servicing the catheter becomes a simple matter.[2]

The technique of intercostal block is simple and, with practice, ten blocks performed bilaterally require no longer than 2–3 minutes for their performance.

Epidural Block

Epidural analgesic agents, when used for postoperative pain, may be administered by intermittent injection or as a continuous infusion (Fig 17–3). While the intermittent method is certainly the most popular, continuous infusion technique carries a slightly better overall quality of analgesia.[30] For intermittent epidural analgesia to be successful, close medical or nursing support is necessary to insure reinjection of the epidural catheter as soon as the patient commences to experience pain, otherwise tachyphylaxis will develop rapidly, making subsequent use of the technique all the more difficult to sustain.

A particular advantage of the intermittent injection technique is that the overall total dose of local anesthetic is much lower than that which is required for a continuous infusion.

TECHNIQUE OF INTERMITTENT INJECTION.—The provision of postoperative epidural analgesia often follows use of the technique as a component or whole of the surgical anesthetic, in which case the puncture site is always made at the center of the particular spinal segments that subserve the operation site. In this way, the most economical dose of local anesthetic that will provide analgesia can be employed.[3] It is difficult to give a predictable rule of thumb in determining the dose requirements for postoperative analgesia, but a volume about two-thirds of that used for surgical anesthesia will provide satisfactory dermatomal spread of analgesia.

Through trial and error, some adjustments may be required, and should tachyphylaxis develop, it will be necessary to increase the volume in order to maintain the same extent of analgesia. The limiting factor in each case is the total dose of anesthetic, because it would obviously be undesirable to use a higher concentration in the lumbar region due to the potential motor block which could ensue.

To prevent or delay the onset of tachyphylaxis, the interval between the onset of pain and reinjection should be kept to a minimum and the catheter should be placed in the center of the spinal segments relaying the nociceptive input.[4] The initial dose must be kept as small as possible and a long-acting local anesthetic must be chosen.

Provision of the epidural service is the most difficult aspect to achieve unless nursing staff members are trained in its complete management.[34] As is the case with the parenteral administration of narcotic analgesics, nurses should be able to assume responsibility for the reinjection of epidural catheters whenever pain recurs. Under such circumstances, the development of tachyphylaxis is delayed, the duration of analgesia is optimal, and doses of local anesthetic can be kept to a minimum. There is little experimental or clinical evidence that changing from one agent to another will preempt or reverse tachyphylaxis once it has developed.

TECHNIQUE OF CONTINUOUS INFUSION.—Considerable experience has been gained in the last 20 years in the use of continuous epidural infusions.[7, 12, 17, 37] The simplest method is to make up a sterile solution of local anesthetic in a bottle or plastic bag which can then be attached to the epidural catheter by an IV infusion set (Fig 17–4). The method is comparatively safe because the solution is weak and the high resistance offered by the epidural catheter prevents any inadvertent sudden infusion of local anesthetic. Such dilute solutions of

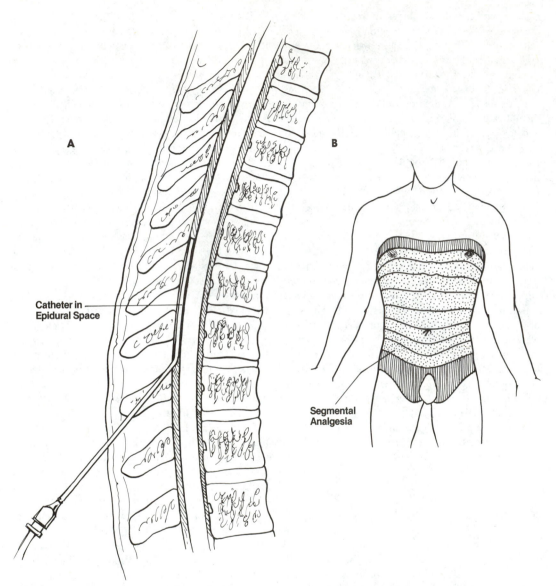

A

Catheter in
Epidural Space

B

Segmental
Analgesia

Fig 17–3.—A, placement of epidural catheter for intermittent or continuous infusion. **B,** segmental analgesia provided by thoracic epidural block. (From Raj P.P. [ed.]: *Handbook of Regional Anesthesia.* New York, Churchill Livingstone, Inc., 1985. Reproduced by permission.)

local anesthetic can also be given by volumetric infusion pumps. With experience, the dose can be predetermined. The dose will vary with the severity of pain, the number of dermatomes requiring analgesia, and the onset of tolerance. Such infusion systems assume a steady state in pharmacokinetic terms, a fact which does not pertain clinically.[41] It may therefore be necessary, when the analgesic level recedes, to administer a bolus injection in order to reestablish the block to its former extent. Another disadvantage of continuous infusion systems is that a much larger overall dose is required to maintain effective analgesia.[42] One way around this is to use an intermittent infusion device which mimics the intermittent or "timed dose" that is given manually. Such pumps can be set to give a bolus dose at predetermined intervals of time. Again, the overall dose of local anesthetic will be greater than that

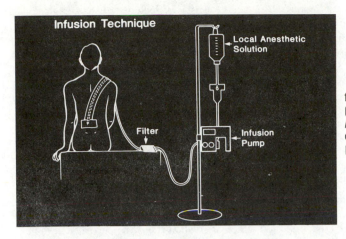

Fig 17—4.—Arrangement used for continuous epidural analgesia. (From Raj P.P. [ed.]: *Handbook of Regional Anesthesia.* New York, Churchill Livingstone, Inc., 1985. Reproduced by permission.)

which would be used if personnel were employed in the response to pain, but the onset of tachyphylaxis will also be delayed. The "human factor" in responding to a complaint of pain is removed by such devices but the total dose is still much less than would be the case if a continuous infusion were used. This author has found the following protocol for continuous infusion to be effective in most cases of postoperative abdominal and prosthetic hip surgical pain. When epidural analgesia has been used for the surgical procedure, it is normal practice to wait for the onset of pain and then to administer a dose 7–10 ml of 0.25% bupivacaine. One hour after the administration of this dose, a continuous infusion of 0.125% bupivacaine is commenced at a rate of 10 ml/hr for abdominal surgery and 5 ml/hr for hip surgery. Generally speaking, the local anesthetic blood levels reflected will be no greater than 0.5 µg/ml. This rate of infusion is generally sufficient to keep most patients free of pain during the first 48 hours. Occasionally, some discomfort will break through the analgesia provided, in which case it may be necessary to give an additional bolus injection of 0.25% bupivacaine. The reader is also referred to Chapter 36 in this volume for a more extensive description of this technique and some of its associated problems.

MAINTENANCE OF INDWELLING CATHETERS.—If the epidural catheter has been securely fixed at the time of insertion and an appropriate dressing applied, it will usually continue to function well for the duration of most postoperative pain applications. It is not necessary to "bury" the catheter beneath the skin as a means of stabilizing its entry site, a procedure often undertaken for chronic pain treatment. Normally, a simple sterile technique with appropriate dressing and adequate fixation with tape will suffice. An "Op site"® can be used in those cases where incontinence or other external source of fluid contamination is possible. Whether one routes the catheter along the back to a site on the nape of the neck or brings it around the flank to an anterolateral position on the abdomen will generally be determined by such factors as wound site and obesity of the patient. Most infections that occur in the epidural space are not due to external contamination but rather have as their source an endogenous infection elsewhere in the body. However, the use of a bacterial filter does reduce the risk of particulate contamination. Glass particles are often shed by the ampule each time one is opened. Such particles have been associated with the formation of a sterile granuloma. However, such sequelae are extremely rare, judging from the paucity of reports in the literature.

DRUGS USED FOR CONTINUOUS EPIDURAL BLOCK.—Only long-acting local anesthetics, e.g., bupivacaine and etidocaine hydrochloride, should be employed for continuous epidural block in the control of postoperative pain. Recently intraspinal opiates have been introduced as an alternative to local anesthetics. While there appear to be many advantages in the use of opiates, such as the absence of autonomic effects, avoidance of hypotension, longer duration, and reduced toxicity, other kinds of side effects such as profound respiratory depression are possible, and although dose related, they may be quite unpredictable in given patients.[15]

Because opiate administration does not produce an autonomic block, loss of this modality in the postoperative period may be undesirable in patients who have undergone vascular surgery or other patients who, because of their obesity, are at serious risk for thromboembolic phenomena. In other words, autonomic block, although possibly associated with hypotension, is therapeutically advantageous and hence commends the use of local anesthetic over narcotics alone for most cases.[39] This fact has prompted the combination of local anesthetics and narcotics by several observers.[28, 42] Müller et al. using a number of combinations of bupivacaine and etidocaine with opioid agonists and the newer synthetic agonist/antagonist opioids have enjoyed considerable success. They found that not only did this combination provide very satisfactory postoperative analgesia of a greater duration than that which could be obtained through the use of local anesthetic alone, it provided, in addition, the benefits of sympathetic block, inhibition of the stress response and maintenance of bowel motility. Another important attribute of the sympathetic block is the preservation of blood supply to anastomotic junctions in the gut after bowel surgery. Very stable hemodynamic conditions prevailed during the course of this analgesia which was administered both by intermittent injections and continuous infusions. Another benefit from the combined usage of opioid and local anesthetic is the much smaller dose of either agent needed to achieve a desired effect than would be necessary if either were to be used alone.

Miscellaneous Techniques

DEXTRAN AND LOCAL ANESTHETICS.—Since Loder used a combination of lidocaine and high molecular weight dextran (150,000) for the use of extending the duration of intercostal blocks in association with post-thoracotomy analgesic treatments,[21] investigators have tried to identify the mechanism by which such substances could prolong the action of local anesthetics. Both in vivo and in vitro studies have tended to produce conflicting data either supporting a longer duration or action or refuting such an effect. The mechanisms that have been postulated are the pH of the solution, the absorptive effect of the dextran molecules, and the osmotic effect, a fact which is related to the size of the molecule.

Most recently, a randomized double blind study by Simpson et al. was able to show that a combination of high molecular weight dextran (110,000) together with epinephrine 1:200,000 prolonged the action of 0.5% bupivacaine for a mean duration of

8.8 hours. This is a doubling of the duration that one would generally expect from a solution of bupivacaine and epinephrine when used for this procedure.

When carrying out the technique of field block for inguinal herniorrhaphy, it is important to deposit at least 20 ml of solution 1 cm medial to the anterior superior iliac spine in a series of fan-wise injections each of which must penetrate the deep fascia overlying the external oblique muscle in order to block the ilioinguinal and iliohypogastric nerves. From the same site, 15 ml of solution should be used to block the internal inguinal ring to anesthetize the visceral fibers on the hernial sac and the genitofemoral nerve which pierces the deep fascia at this point. A further 20–25 cc of solution should be deposited at the external inguinal ring down to the pubic tubercle and superiorly along the rectus sheath and superficial to the skin in order to block not only the sensory L_1 fibers which cross the midline from the other side, but also the terminals S_2, S_3, and S_4 branches which enter at the external ring. Successful block for surgery and postoperative analgesia of the inguinal canal is assured when larger volumes, namely, 60–80 ml of a dilute local anesthetic solution rather than a lesser volume of more concentrated local anesthetic solution is employed.

PERFUSION OF SURGICAL WOUNDS.—The perfusion of surgical wounds with local anesthetic solutions has been carried out for many years with varying degrees of success. A recent study has shown that if a wound such as cholecystectomy is perfused with a solution of either saline or bupivacaine over a period of 48 hours, the analgesic requirement is reduced by 70%. It seems that rather than attributing a placebo effect to the saline, it may well be that by removal of humoral substances the genesis of postoperative pain is significantly lessened. Interestingly, no significant restoration of the vital capacity towards preoperative values occurred with either solutions, results which are in agreement with other investigators who have compared similar respiratory parameters under the influence of epidural block or parenteral narcotic administration.

Such a simple technique which was not associated with toxicity, infection, or impaired wound healing, and which can be administered merely through a regular surgical drain tube must commend its use at least to those patients in whom narcotic administration may be contraindicated, or as an adjunctive technique for such surgical procedures as cholecystectomy. An administration protocol of 0.5% bupivacaine administered every four hours has been shown to provide satisfactory analgesia for a total period of 48 hours.

CONTINUOUS BRACHIAL PLEXUS ANALGESIA.—The value of continuous brachial plexus analgesia for postoperative pain has been grossly underestimated.[34] Major trauma of the upper extremity with dismemberment, repeated plastic surgical procedures and major vascular and nerve injury repair are all primary indications for the use of continuous brachial plexus analgesia.

Apart from providing useful postoperative analgesia, the advantage of sympathetic blockade being maintained for several days is difficult to refute. Many studies have shown the benefits of continuous sympathectomy on graft survival.

TECHNIQUE.—A catheter may be placed into the brachial plexus sheath at the level of the interscalene space, infraclavicular region, or it can be placed in the axillary sheath from an axillary approach to the plexus. When using the over-the-needle cannula technique, at least a 2½-inch needle must be chosen, otherwise the cannula will become dislodged. One manufacturer has made available a special cannula-over-needle and catheter set for continuous plexus anesthesia (Plexifix)®* which enables the operator to enter the axillary sheath either in the axilla or from a supraclavicular approach following which the catheter may be introduced through the cannula for a distance of several centimeters, thus enabling the catheter to be fixed to the skin at a distance from the site of insertion. The most effective way of identifying the axillary sheath, particularly when using the specially designed short bevel needle, is the loss of resistance technique using a syringe filled with local anesthetic. The combined "click" and loss-of-resistance as the needle tip penetrates the sheath will ensure identification of this tissue plane. If after entry, difficulty in inserting the catheter is experienced, the cannula and catheter should be withdrawn and a new attempt at identifying the space should be made. Because 0.375%–0.5% bupivacaine has such a long duration of action, it is generally not necessary to use a continuous infusion technique. The lower concentration should be used whenever no motor block is desired and epinephrine 5 μg/ml should always be added to the solution unless otherwise contraindicated.

---

*Burron/Braun, Bethlehem, Pennsylvania.

INSUFFLATION BLOCK.—Good analgesia and the prevention of pelvic cramps after tubal ligation can be achieved by spraying local anesthetic on the fallopian tubes under direct vision through the suction port of the laparoscope at the end of the procedure. Ten cc of 0.25% bupivacaine with epinephrine 5 μg/ml sprayed onto each fallopian tube will achieve analgesia, preventing cramps for 6–24 hours. While the intensity of pain is low, it still requires the use of either nonnarcotic or narcotic analgesics in most patients during the first 6–24 hours. This technique which can be performed at the end of surgery is simple to do and requires only a matter of minutes for its completion.[36]

ANALGESIA FOR AUGMENTATION MAMMOPLASTY.—Augmentation mammoplasty is often done as an outpatient procedure under either general or regional anesthesia. When a field block employing 0.375% bupivacaine with epinephrine 2.5 μg/ml of the perforating branches of the intercostal nerves is employed, postoperative analgesia is often sufficient to obviate the need for any analgesics at all. Likewise, when a thoracic epidural at T_1-T_4 is employed with 0.5% bupivacaine, analgesia in the postoperative period is similar to that achieved by field block.

NONCONVENTIONAL POSTOPERATIVE ANALGESIA IN CHILDREN.—Inpatient or outpatient surgical procedures on the perineum and lower limbs in children are often associated with a stormy and combative early recovery phase. While it is normal to employ a general anesthetic technique, it is a simple matter, in addition, to perform a single-shot caudal anesthetic with 0.25% bupivacaine.[33] The dose can be calculated from the following formula: 0.1 ml/spinal segment/year or 0.5 ml/kg.

The only potential problem with postoperative caudal analgesia is a delay in micturition in some children, although this is not sufficiently problematic to preclude use of the technique for postoperative analgesia.

A special indication for the use of transcutaneous electrical nerve stimulation for postoperative pain after thoracic surgery in children has recently been described.[17] The impairment of respirations following operations to correct the congenital abnormality of pectus excavatum or carinatum, poses a challenge for adequate pain control in the postoperative period. Normally, very large doses of parenteral narcotics are required with their potential for severe respiratory depression and further hampering a return to normal pulmonary function. Intercostal blocks are out of the question because of the extremely high blood levels that would result from the number of intercostal spaces needing to be blocked. Thoracic epidural analgesia would be ideal, however, only a few anesthesiologists would have the training and skill to perform this procedure.

The technique requires that two electrodes be placed parallel to the incision before a sterile dressing is applied. With the patient still under anesthesia, the electrodes are connected to an output device and the current raised until slight muscle movement is detected. The output is then decreased until this disappears after which this setting is maintained during the postoperative period. The degree of analgesia achieved by this method can reduce the morphine requirements from as little as 3 mg during the first postoperative day to no narcotics at all during the postoperative course. Although only two patients were described in the foregoing communication, the results are so good as to suggest that this technique may be quite successful for this particular surgical procedure.

Drugs and Dosages for Nerve Blocks

The two long-acting agents, bupivacaine and etidocaine hydrochloride, are employed for postoperative pain control.

Etidocaine 1% or bupivacaine 0.5% are the most suitable concentrations to use for intercostal blocks. These solutions will provide the maximum duration of action while still remaining within a safe nontoxic range, even when as many as ten intercostal nerves are to be blocked.

For thoracic epidural analgesia, where motor block is of little consequence, etidocaine 0.5%–0.7% can be used. For analgesia in the lumbar or caudal epidural regions, bupivacaine is the agent of choice for postoperative pain relief. The optimal concentration is 0.25%–0.5%. These concentrations are suitable for intermittent techniques.

Considerable disagreement exists as to the optimum strength of local anesthetics for epidural infusion techniques. There is agreement, however, with regard to the range of dosage for bupivacaine and etidocaine (Table 17–1).

Drugs and Dosages for Intraspinal Narcotics

The clinical use of epidural narcotics, while still controversial, is increasing. The decision to use epidural narcotics over local anesthetics will rest on an intelligent evaluation of the pharmacologic result required in each case. When the decision to use epidural opioids has been made, the current choice of drugs is limited to three opioids: morphine, meperidine, and fentanyl. Most experience has been gained with morphine, the dose of which for satisfactory pain relief after abdominal surgery has varied from 3 to 10 mg. While it is difficult to reconcile any specific dose with the reports of clinical respiratory depression, the dosage range of epidural opioids shown in Table 17–2 is not likely to be associated with life-threatening respiratory depression. Having said this, however, the potential for life-threatening respiratory depression still remains.[15] This may arise from the summation effect of a previously administered sedative and/or narcotic, or as a result of the subsequent administration of such drugs being superimposed on the actions of the intraspinal opioid. It could also arise as a result of the dural penetration by the epidural catheter causing a relative overdose of narcotics in the subarachnoid space. It might arise as a result of the combined increase of intrathoracic and intra-abdominal pressures during coughing or straining, having the effect of redirecting epidural venous flow into the basivertebral system and tending to flush a high concen-

TABLE 17–1.—LOCAL
INFUSION CHARACTERISTICS

SITE	DRUG (%)	RATE (mg/hr)	PEAK PLASMA LEVEL (μg/ml)
Thoracic Bupivacaine	0.125–0.25	12–20	0.6
Etidocaine	0.5–0.7	15–30	—
Lumbar Bupivacaine	0.125–0.25	22–30	1.2

TABLE 17–2.—TYPICAL DOSAGE SCHEME
FOR EPIDURAL NARCOTICS

DRUG	RANGE
Morphine	0.5–5.0 mg
Hydromorphone	0.5–1 mg
Buprenorphine	0.3 mg
Methadone	1 mg
Meperidine	50 mg
Fentanyl	50–100 mcg
Fentanyl infusion	100–200 mcg bolus; 66 mcg/hr.

tration of opioids to the midbrain centers. Finally, it might also be an idiosyncratic reaction in a given patient. It should be noted that respiratory depression is referred to as early and late, the early depression representing the systemic vascular uptake of narcotics with the late depression being a manifestation of the rostrad movement of narcotic via the cerebrospinal fluid or internal vertebral venous plexus. The range there has varied from 0.75 hours to 13 hours. Generally it can be said that those drugs like morphine which are highly hydrophilic and highly ionized will tend to be associated with late respiratory depression, whereas drugs like fentanyl and meperidine which are highly lipid soluble and highly ionized are more likely to be associated with early respiratory depression if at all. Personal experience with morphine during the past four years would suggest that a dose of 4 mg in 5–6 ml of saline will provide good postoperative analgesia in most adults for a variety of thoracic, abdominal, pelvic, and orthopedic surgery of the hip and lower limbs. As an alternative to saline, 0.25% bupivacaine may be substituted. This dose will provide satisfactory analgesia in about 85% of patients. Respiratory depression requiring treatment has not been seen using this dose. With a drug such as morphine which is highly hydrophilic, nursing the patient in a semi-Fowler position will increase the safety of the procedure by impeding rostral spread of the narcotic. The mean duration of analgesia using morphine is 16 hours. It would appear in the light of studies undertaken during the past five years that the lipophilic drugs such as meperidine and fentanyl appear to have the best efficacy/safety ratio and, in addition, to have a lower incidence of minor side effects (pruritis, nausea, vomiting, and urinary retention), although strict comparative studies have still not been undertaken.[10] In addition, the peridural route offers singular advantages because of the ability to titrate dose requirements and the ease with which repeated doses or an infusion can be used. For these reasons, a long-acting hydrophilic drug like morphine really has no advantage over the other narcotics when used for epidural analgesia in postoperative pain because personnel are still required to monitor the respiratory status and to oversee each dose and the operation of infusion pumps. A typical dosage scheme for fentanyl infusion is shown in Table 17–2.

Mention has already been made of combining opioids and local anesthetic solutions. Müller et al. have found that combining a dose of morphine, 0.05 mg/kg BW, with bupivacaine, 10 ml 0.25%, will provide a mean duration of analgesia of 20 hours + 4.6 hours. If, however, it is desired to maintain the sympathetic block throughout the analgesic period, the local anesthetic must be injected in a volume which has been shown to provide adequate dermatomal analgesia for the surgical procedure every 5–6 hours.

A recent innovation and embodiment of the same principles employed with patient controlled intravenous narcotic therapy is the self administration of epidural meperidine for postoperative pain. Similar wide variations in the individual analgetic requirements were observed as have been noted with the intravenous demand analgesia technique.[44] Using a highly lipid soluble drug, this technique might offer an alternative to either intermittent or infusion techniques in providing satisfactory postoperative analgesia. By allowing the patient to respond to his own pain, important pharmacodynamic aspects of opioid action are addressed and perhaps a best efficacy/safety ratio for spinal opioid administration will be achieved. Much work, however, still needs to be done in this area before its complete safety and utility are realized.

Rawal and Wattwil have shown that a naloxone infusion of 5 µg/kg/hr will partially reverse the respiratory depression of a 4-mg epidural dose of morphine as detected by depression of the CO_2 response.[31] If this dose is doubled to 10 µg/kg/hr, any depression as measured by these means is prevented. Also, the side effects of nausea, pruritus, and urinary retention are attenuated without any degradation of the sensory analgesia.

Therefore, it seems that a dose of morphine has been found which can provide analgesia without incurring the risks of respiratory depression. Furthermore, the use of highly lipid soluble opioids like fentanyl and meperidine given by infusion further reduce the risk of late respiratory depression. The combination of a narcotic and local anesthetic can achieve a lower dose of either drug, thereby reducing even further the possibility of toxicity being manifested. Having said this, however, when using epidural opioids for postoperative pain, it is desirable in the light of conventional experience to have such patients either in an area of high surveillance (postoperative ward) or to have some form of apnea monitor attached to the patient whenever he is returned to a semiprivate or private room.

REFERENCES

1. Braid D.P., Scott D.B.: The systemic absorption of local anesthetic drugs. *Brit. J. Anesth.* 37:394, 1965.

2. Bromage, P.R.: *Epidural Analgesia*. Philadelphia, W.B. Saunders Co., 1978, pp. 100–105.

3. Buckley P., Simpson R.: Relief of pain following upper abdominal operations by thoracic epidural block with etidocaine. *Acta Anesth. Scand.* (Suppl.) 60:76–79, 1975.

4. Bullingham R.E.S., McQuay H.J., Moore A., et al.: Bupivacaine kinetics. *Clin. Pharm. Ther.* 38:667–672, 1980.

5. Check W.A.: Results are better when patients control their own analgesia. *J.A.M.A.* 247:945–947, 1982.

6. Church J.J.: Continuous narcotic infusions for relief of postoperative pain. *Br. Med. J.* 1:977–979, 1979.

7. Cleland J.G.P.: Continuous peridural and caudal analgesia in surgery and early ambulation. *Northwest Med. J.* 48:26, 1948.

8. Cohen F.L.: Postoperative surgical pain relief: Patient's status and nurses medication choice. *Pain* 9:265–274, 1980.

9. Cronin K.D., Davies M.J.: Intercostal block for postoperative pain relief. *Anesth. Int. Care* 4:459–461, 1976.

10. Cousins M.J., Mather L.E.: Intrathecal and epidural opioids. *Anesthesiology* 61:276–310, 1984.

11. Postoperative Pain, editorial *Br. Med. J.* 2:517–518, 1978.

12. Evans K.R.L., Carrie L.E.S.: Continuous epidural infusion of bupivacaine in labour: A simple method. *Anesthesia* 34:310–315, 1979.

13. Faust R.A., Nauss L.A.: Post-thoracotomy intercostal block: Comparison of its effects on pulmonary function with those of intramuscular meperidine. *Anesth. Analg. Curr. Res.* 55:542, 1976.

14. Galway J.E., Caves P.K., Dundee J.W.: Effect of intercostal blockade during operation on lung function and the relief of pain following thoracotomy. *Br. J. Anesth.* 47:730–735, 1975.

15. Glynn C.J., Mather L.E., Cousins M.J., et al.: Spinal narcotics and respiratory depression. *Lancet* 2:356–357, 1979.

16. Green R., Dawkins C.J.M.: Postoperative analgesia: The use of continuous drip epidural block. *Anesthesia* 21:372, 1966.

17. Hinkle A.J., Koka B.V.: Transcutaneous electrical stimulation for pain control after thoracic surgery in children. *Reg. Anesthes.* 8:163–165, 1983.

18. Hull C.J., Sibbald A.: Control of postoperative pain by interactive demand analgesia. *Br. J. Anesth.* 53:385–391, 1981.

19. Hull C.J.: Opioid infusions for the management of postoperative pain, in Smith G., Covino B.G. (eds.): *Acute Pain*. London, Butterworth, 1985, pp. 155–279.

20. Lloyd J.W., Barnard J.D.W., Glynn C.J.: Cryoanalgesia: A new approach to pain relief. *Lancet* 2:932, 1976.

21. Loder R.E.: A local anaesthetic solution with longer action. *Lancet* 2:346, 1960.

22. Long D.M.: Electrical stimulation for the control of pain. *Arch. Surg.* 112:884, 1977.

23. Mather L.E., Tucker G.T., Pfug A.E., et al.: Meperidine kinetics in man: Intravenous injection in surgical patients and volunteers. *Clin. Pharm. Ther.* 47:21–30, 1975.

24. Mather L.E.: Determination of drug action. *Anaesth. Int. Care* 8:233–247, 1980.

25. Mather L.E.: Pharmacokinetics and pharmacodynamic factors influencing the choice, dose and route of administration of opiates for acute pain, in Bullingham R. (ed.): *Clinics in Anaesthesiology*. London, W.B. Saunders Co., 1983.

26. Moore D.C., Bridenbaugh L.D.: Intercostal nerve block in 4333 patients: Indications, technique and complications. *Anaesth. Analg. Curr. Res.* 41:1, 1962.

27. Nelson G.D., Printy A.L.: Electrical surface stimulation for control of acute postoperative pain and prevention of ileus. *Surgical Forum* 24:447, 1973.

28. Müller H., Borner U., Gips H., et al.: Intraoperative peridurale Opiatanalgesie, in Wust H., Stanton-Hicks M., Zindler M. (eds.): *Neue Aspekte in der Regionalanaesthesie*, vol. 3. *Anaesthesiology and Intensive Care Medicine*. Heidelberg, Springer Verlag, 1984, pp. 152–163.

29. Murphy D.F.: Continuous intercostal nerve blockade. An anatomical study to elucidate its mode of action. *Br. J. Anaes.* 56:627–30, 1984.

30. Raj P.P., Denson D., Finnsson R.: Prolonged epidural analgesia: Intermittent or continuous, in Meyer J., Nolte H. (eds.): *Die kontinuierliche Periduralanaesthesie*. Stuttgart, Georg Thieme Verlag, 1983, pp 26–37.

31. Rawal N., Wattwil M.: Respiratory depression following epidural morphine. An experimental and clinical study. *Anesth. Analg.* 63:8–14, 1984.

32. Rutter P.C., Murphy F., Dudley H.A.F.: Morphine: Controlled trial of different methods of administration for postoperative pain relief. *Br. Med. J.* 1:12–13, 1980.

33. Schulte-Steinberg O., Rahlfs V.W.: Caudal anaesthesia in children and spread of 1 percent lignocaine: A statistical study. *Br. J. Anaesth.* 42:1093, 1970.

34. Selander D.: Catheter technique in axillary plexus block. *Acta Anaesth. Scand.* 21:324–329, 1977.

35. Simpson P.J., Hughes D.R., Long D.H.: Prolonged local analgesia for inguinal herniorrhaphy with bupivacaine and dextran. *Ann. R. Coll. Surg. Eng.* 64:243–246, 1982.

36. Burney R.G., Soni V.: Intraperitoneal local anesthetics for tubal ligation. *Regional Anesthesia* 7:74, 1982.

37. Spoerel W.J., Thomas A., Gerula G.R.: Continuous epidural analgesia: Experience with mechanical injection devices. *Canad. Anaesth. Soc. J.* 17:37, 1970.

38. Stanton-Hicks, M.: Continuous epidural anaesthesia: advantages and disadvantages, in Van Kleef J.W., Burm A.G.L., Spierdijk J. (eds): *Current Concepts in*

Regional Anaesthesia. The Hague, Martinus Nijhoff, 1984, pp. 226–236.

39. Stanton-Hicks M.: Spinal opiate analgesia (subarachnoid and epidural): Clinical aspects, in Scott D.B., McClure J. Mc., Wildsmith J.A.W., Sodertalje, I.C.M. (eds.): *Regional Anaesthesia.* Vienna, I.C.M., 1985, pp. 140–146.

40. Tamsen A., Hartvig P., Dahlstrom B., et al.: Endorphans and on-demand pain relief. *Lancet* 1:769–780, 1980.

41. Tucker G.T., Mather L.E.: Pharmacokinetics of local anaesthetic agents. *Br. J. Anaesth.* 47:213–224, 1975.

42. Tucker G.T., Cooper S., Littlewood D., et al.: Observed and predicted accumulation of local anaesthetic agents during continuous extradural anaesthesia. *Br. J. Anaesth.* 49:237–241, 1977.

43. Van Steenberge A.: Peridural anaesthesia in caesarian section, in Van Kleef J.W., Burm A.G.L., Spierdijk J. (eds): *Current Concepts in Regional Anaesthesia.* The Hague, Martinus Nijhoff, 1984, pp. 123–129.

44. Zaren B., Hartwig P., Tamsen A.: Patient-controlled analgesic therapy with epidural pethidine for postoperative pain relief, in Wust H., Stanton-Hicks M., Zindler M. (eds.): *Neue Aspekte in der Regionalanaesthesie,* vol. 3, *Anaesthesiology and Intensive Care Medicine.* Heidelberg, Springer-Verlag, pp. 173–176, 1984.

18 / Pain Relief in Obstetrics

J. STEPHEN NAULTY, M.D.
SANJAY DATTA, M.D.
GERALD OSTHEIMER, M.D.

MOST WOMEN experience parturition as a painful process, and some form of analgesia is employed in an overwhelming number of parturients. The reported percentage of patients requiring analgesia ranges from 60% to 99% of all parturients, depending on the population studied and the setting of delivery.[1, 2] Since there are approximately 4 million births per year in the United States alone,[3] the discomfort produced by uterine contractions, cervical dilation, and fetal descent undoubtedly represents the most common painful condition treated by anesthesiologists. However, obstetric analgesia differs in many important respects from other pain conditions. The most obvious difference is that *two* patients are affected simultaneously by the treatment of labor pain, and occasionally techniques that provide comfort for the mother can be harmful to the fetus. In addition, the pregnant woman has a significantly altered physiology and different responses to anesthetic maneuvers than a nonpregnant woman. Preexisting disease processes may be altered by pregnancy, and other disease processes are unique to pregnancy, such as toxemia of pregnancy, peripartum cardiomyopathy, and obstetric complications, which can profoundly affect the anesthetic management of the parturient. This chapter discusses (1) the changes that occur in maternal physiology during parturition, (2) various methods of pain control in obstetrics, and (3) analgesic techniques that are used in the high-risk parturient.

THE PAIN OF PARTURITION

Childbirth is described by most women as a painful process.[4] Labor pain is a subjective sensory ex-

perience initiated by stretching of the cervix, distention of the lower uterine segment, and ischemia of uterine muscle fibers with accumulation of metabolites. Nerve impulses stimulated by these factors travel from the uterus and birth canal via two major pathways, as described below.

UTERINE AND CERVICAL PAIN.—The efferent nerve fibers from the uterus and cervix are somatic sensory fibers that travel with the sympathetic nervous supply to the uterus. These fibers pass through the paracervical tissue along the uterine artery and then through the inferior, middle, and superior hypogastric plexuses to the sympathetic chain. The impulses then enter the spinal cord through the 10th, 11th, and 12th thoracic nerves (Fig 18–1).

PERINEAL PAIN.—Impulses arising from the vagina, vulva, and perineum travel a different pathway. Sensory innervation of the area is through the pudendal nerve, which enters the CNS at the second, third, and fourth sacral nerves.

On entering the CNS, these impulses undergo modulation in the posterior horn of the spinal cord and descend to the brain stem through the ipsilateral and contralateral spinothalamic tracts. In the brain stem, the impulses stimulate the reticular formation and tegmental tract, and then continue upward to the ventral posterolateral nucleus of the thalamus. From there, fibers project to the sensory cortex for localization and discrimination of pain. It is important to note that nerve fibers also *arise* from the medulla, thalamus, and cortex and project to the dorsal horn of the spinal cord. There they participate in the modulation of pain impulses entering the spinal cord and create a feedback loop whereby labor pain may provide analgesia for itself (Fig 18–2).

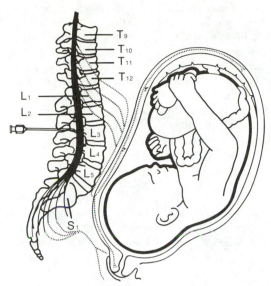

Fig 18–1.—Pain pathways during parturition. (From Ostheimer G. (ed.): *Manual of Obstetric Anesthesia.* New York, Churchill Livingstone, 1984. Reproduced by permission.)

There are also projections to the prefrontal cortex and the limbic system which stimulate the motivational and affective components of pain. It is these motivational-affective components that can be modulated by psychological factors such as attention, suggestion, anxiety, expectations, and prior conditioning.

Labor Pain

The normal pattern of the pain of parturition, then, can be predicted from the above information. During the first stage of labor, increasing uterine contractions lead to progressive uterine muscle ischemia, cervical dilation, and distention of the lower uterine segment. This leads to a progressive increase in painful sensation, which is felt mainly in the distribution of the 10th, 11th, and 12th thoracic dermatomes. The most severe labor pain usually occurs during the acceleration phase of labor, when cervical dilation and the strength of uterine contractions reach their maximum.

In the second phase of labor and during delivery, stretching of the tissues of the vagina and perineum is added to the pain of uterine contractions. These sensations are mainly felt in and referred to the distribution of the second, third, and fourth sacral dermatomes.

Reflex Effects of Labor Pain

Nerve impulses that arise from the process of parturition produce not only the subjective sensation of

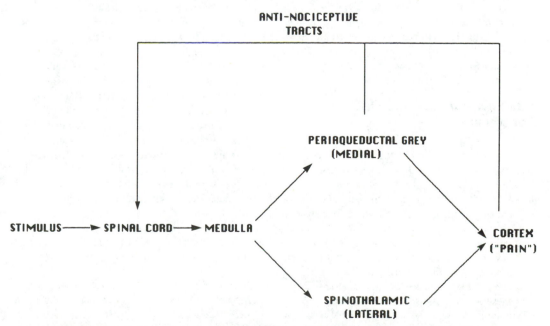

Fig 18–2.—Pain pathways in labor. Note feedback loop for antinociception.

pain, but also a number of physiologic changes in the maternal-fetal unit that may be of considerable significance. The most profound changes are observable in the cardiovascular, respiratory, musculoskeletal, endocrine, and central nervous systems.

CARDIOVASCULAR.—The process of parturition stimulates the sympathetic nervous system and produces increases in cardiac preload and afterload; the combination of these factors produces an increase in cardiac output by as much as 60% during labor.[5] Tachycardia, hypertension, and arrhythmias may occur. Uterine blood vessels have been shown to be particularly sensitive to sympathetic tone, and Shnider et al. have demonstrated that experimentally produced pain can reduce uterine blood flow in pregnant ewes by release of endogenous catecholamines.[6] In addition, newborns of mothers that have received *no* analgesia have been found to have higher concentrations of lactate and lower pH blood levels at birth.[7]

RESPIRATORY.—Hyperventilation is a common response to painful stimulation. Arterial carbon dioxide is severely reduced in some patients during labor. The resulting respiratory alkalosis may produce fetal hypoxia by shifting the maternal oxyhemoglobin dissociation curve to the left,[8] leading to decreased oxygen release at the placenta.[9]

MUSCULOSKELETAL.—Maternal skeletal muscle expulsive efforts (''bearing down'') may become an uncontrollable urge as a result of labor pain. Obstetric anesthesia has been shown to control these reflexes and decrease the metabolic acidosis that may result from excessive muscular efforts.[10]

Administration of Obstetric Anesthesia

Properly administered obstetric analgesia not only reduces the psychological or subjective component of pain but also may be beneficial in preventing undesirable reflex effects in some patients. For example, patients with severe mitral valve regurgitation may develop cardiac decompensation and congestive heart failure as a result of the severe cardiovascular stresses (i.e., increased preload, afterload, and cardiac output) produced during labor. Properly administered obstetric analgesia or anesthesia will prevent these adverse effects from developing.

Numerous methods of pain relief have been employed in obstetric practice. The selection of any given technique depends on the stage of labor, maternal condition, fetal condition, and experience of the anesthesiologist and obstetric team.

Pain of the first stage of labor may be relieved in many ways. Paracervical, paravertebral, epidural, and spinal anesthetics may be used to prevent noxious impulses from entering or ascending the spinal cord. The sensation of pain may be also blocked by systemic or intraspinal analgesia with narcotics or by inhalation analgesia with N_2O, trichloroethylene, or methoxyflurane. Finally, the motivational-affective component of pain may be alleviated with psychological methods, hypnosis, or acupuncture.

These techniques may be continued in the second stage of labor. In addition, the pudendal nerve may be blocked to relieve perineal pain. All of these techniques are currently used in obstetric anesthesia practice and are discussed at greater length in the following section.

CURRENT OBSTETRIC ANESTHETIC PRACTICE

Obstetric anesthesia has traditionally been a stepchild of many anesthesia departments. Because of unpredictable and widely fluctuating manpower requirements, many anesthesia departments cannot or will not provide 24-hour obstetric anesthesia coverage. The American Society of Anesthesiologists (ASA) viewed this as an undesirable development and in 1978 published a position paper which stated that parturients were entitled to the same level of anesthetic care as elective surgical patients.[11] Ideally a full-time anesthesiologist should be available, as should modern equipment for administering anesthetics and monitoring the parturient. In 1970 the American College of Obstetricians and Gynecologists conducted a survey which revealed that in only 37% of hospitals were personnel specifically trained in anesthesia administering obstetric anesthetics,[12] and a similar study in 1980 showed only slight progress, with approximately 50% of hospitals providing adequate anesthetic coverage in the obstetric suite.[13] It is hoped that the growing interest in regional anesthetic techniques, pain control, and perinatal medicine will ''spill over'' into obstetric anesthesia and produce an improvement in this chronic staffing problem.

In another survey, anesthesia was deemed directly responsible for 8% of 950 maternal deaths in the United States.[14] More than two thirds of these deaths were judged to have been preventable. Similar results have been obtained in Great Britain,[15] with the most common cause of anesthetic mishap in the obstetric suite being unfamiliarity with the pathophysiology of obstetric disease and the use of unfamiliar techniques in the parturient. The practitioner who wishes to provide adequate care for the parturient should have an easy familiarity with the techniques commonly used in obstetric anesthesia and should practice these techniques regularly. For example, if obstetric epidural anesthesia is administered only a few times a year for special cases, the technique will be considerably less familiar than on a busy obstetric service where thousands of women are administered such anesthetics every year. Bonica has stated, "In case there is a choice between poorly administered anesthesia and no anesthesia, the latter should be selected."[16] This is no less true today. However, many of the techniques that will be described as typical of obstetric anesthesia have considerable utility in the operating room environment and can (and should) be "practiced" in the operating room, in a premedicated, cooperative patient, before they are attempted on the frequently noncooperative obstetric patient who is in severe, acute pain.

Obstetric Anesthesia Without Drugs

Psychoanalgesia

Psychoanalgesia is a term that encompasses a number of techniques designed to minimize the noxious effects of the pain of parturition. These techniques include natural childbirth, described by Dick-Read in 1944,[17] Jacobsen's physiologic relaxation technique,[18] and the Lamaze[19] and Bradley[20] techniques. Modern psychoanalgesic techniques combine a number of these approaches. They emphasize antenatal preparation and education to allay many of the anxieties associated with parturition: relaxation techniques to minimize the contribution of skeletal muscle spasm due to labor pain, and the development of conditioned responses to uterine contractions to distract the parturient from the sensation of pain. These techniques do not make childbirth painless (despite the claims of some of their proponents), but instead may convert a painful experience to a controllable, positive experience. Psychoanalgesic techniques have proved to be very useful and generally adequate for delivery in about 20%–30% of parturients.[21] When combined with other analgesic methods, psychoanalgesia may be effective in a larger percentage of the population.

Psychoanalgesia, however, is not without risk. The breathing techniques of psychoanalgesia are designed to minimize hyperventilation, but some parturients do develop severe hyperventilation, with maternal arterial carbon dioxide tensions as low as 12–15 mm Hg. Carbon dioxide tensions in this extremely low range will displace the maternal oxyhemoglobin dissociation curve to the left and interfere with placental oxygen exchange. Saling and Ligidas in 1969 reported that neonates of hyperventilating parturients were more acidotic than neonates of a control group that did not hyperventilate.[22] These adverse effects can be prevented with adequate obstetric analgesia. For example, Zador and Nillson in 1974 found that fetal acid-base balance during prolonged labor was better maintained if women received epidural anesthesia than if they received no analgesia or small doses of systemic narcotic drugs.[23]

In addition, psychoanalgesic techniques require a high level of personal concentration and are not entirely reliable. Some enthusiasts of psychoanalgesic techniques promote them as being applicable to all deliveries. Therefore, a woman who experiences severe pain during parturition and who wishes further anesthesia may feel she has failed. When one is interviewing a parturient prior to initiating an analgesic technique, it is important to stress that not all patients find psychoanalgesia techniques adequate and that further anesthetic intervention is *not* uncommon.

Hypnosis

Another method of disrupting the motivational-affective element of the pain of parturition is via hypnotic suggestion. It is possible to provide adequate maternal analgesia with hypnosis in highly suggestible patients. However, there appears to be little effect on the reflex effects of labor pain.[24] The effect of hypnotic analgesia on the neonate is poorly documented, with most authors merely assuming that no neonatal effects should be present. Preparation of the patient for hypnotic analgesia requires a large number of conditioning sessions prior to delivery. During these sessions the parturient is taught to produce analgesia of some part of the body (typically an arm or leg) and is then conditioned to transfer this analgesia to the abdomen and perineum to provide pain relief during labor and delivery. A successful series of conditioning sessions allows the parturient to perform this maneuver during labor without the hypnotist actually being present. The hypnotic state has been reported to shorten labor[25] and the acid-base status of the neonate is apparently improved, at birth and in the hour following, over what is seen in patients who received either no analgesia or other forms of analgesia.

Notwithstanding these advantages, hypnoanalgesia is only rarely employed in obstetric practice today. Lack of use of this technique probably arises from the relative paucity of skilled practitioners and from the economic and staffing problems of obstetric units in general. In addition, Wahl[26] reported a high incidence of psychological complications ranging from anxiety to frank psychosis following hypnosis for obstetric analgesia. This is certainly an area where further investigation should be carried out.

Acupuncture

Because acupuncture and its variant, transcutaneous electrical nerve stimulation (TENS), appear to be completely safe for the mother and newborn, their use for relief of labor pain has been investigated. Wallis et al.[27] have reported that 19 of the 21 patients in their study described adequate analgesia when the traditional acupuncture points were used for vaginal hysterectomy and dysmenorrhea. However, the investigators judged that none of the subjects had adequate analgesia. Several authors[28, 29] have investigated TENS during labor, with a variety of electrode sites. "Success" rates varying from 3% to 20% of patients reporting adequate analgesia have been achieved in the above series, but these percentages are less than those generally reported for psychoanalgesic techniques. It must be concluded that while acupuncture and TENS are useful in many painful states, their role in obstetric analgesia is extremely limited.

Obstetric Analgesia Using Drugs

Labor pain that is not adequately controlled by nondrug techniques will require additional analgesic intervention. These techniques include the intramuscular (IM), intravenous (IV), or inhalation administration of sedative or analgesic drugs, or the perineural application of local anesthetics or narcotics.

Techniques of IV or IM Medication

The systemic administration of sedatives, tranquilizers, and narcotics to the parturient is probably the most popular method of achieving obstetric analgesia today. In the past, large doses of these drugs were employed to create a "twilight sleep." An increasing realization of the adverse effects of excessive medication on both mother and fetus has led to a reduction in dosage of these drugs. In addition, better understanding of maternal uptake, distribution, and placental transfer of drugs has led to a more rational and safer selection of methods of administration and timing of these drugs in labor.

In current practice, small doses of minimally depressant drugs are administered IV early in labor, which produces a minimum amount of placental transfer of these medications and hence a minimally depressed neonate.

The major groups of drugs employed today are the sedative-tranquilizers, the narcotic analgesics, and the dissociative anesthetics.

SEDATIVE-TRANQUILIZERS.—These drugs are administered to the parturient to diminish the adverse motivational-affective component of labor pain. Examples include barbiturates, phenothiazines, and benzodiazepines.

Barbiturates.—Secobarbital (Seconal) and pentobarbital (Nembutal) have been employed in obstetrics. Because of their prolonged effects, their principal use today is in the early latent phase of labor when delivery is not likely to occur before 12–24 hours. Barbiturates have been described to have an "antianalgesic effect"[30] and may convert a minimally uncomfortable, controlled patient into a hyperventilating, confused, and unmanageable one. For this reason, they are rarely used today.

Phenothiazines.—Promethazine (Phenergan) and propiomazine (Largon) are the drugs in this class commonly employed in obstetrics. Hydroxyzine (Vistaril), although not a phenothiazine, has similar properties. These drugs are useful for relieving anxiety, and hence modify the response to painful stimulation. They are less likely than the barbiturates to cause "antianalgesia" or to potentiate the actions of the narcotic analgesics. In addition, they are useful in controlling nausea and vomiting, which may be severe enough in some parturients to produce maternal dehydration. In the recommended dosages (promethazine, 50 mg; propiomazine, 20 mg; hydroxyzine, 50–100 mg), these drugs appear to have minimal depressant effects on both mother and fetus.[31]

Benzodiazepines.—Diazepam (Valium) is one of the most widely prescribed drugs in the world, and it is not surprising that it has been employed as an anxiolytic agent in obstetrics. Its use is controversial but it is capable of reducing maternal anxiety, decreasing narcotic dosage, and antagonizing the convulsions associated with local anesthetic toxicity or eclampsia. When used in small doses (2.5–10 mg IV), diazepam appears to be without significant adverse fetal or neonatal effects.[32]

NARCOTICS

Narcotics, one of the earliest means of pain relief in obstetrics, are today still the most commonly employed form of analgesia in obstetrics. Indeed, with the recent developments in narcotic pharmacology, they are also one of the most exciting areas in obstetric analgesic research. This section discusses the basic pharmacology of the narcotic drugs, pertinent aspects of their *perinatal* pharmacology, methods of narcotic administration, the selection of narcotic drugs useful in obstetrics, and the indications for and contraindications to their use.

Narcotic Pharmacology

Opiate Receptors

The narcotic analgesics act by stimulating an opiate receptor that is found in many locations throughout the CNS. These drugs act by binding to the receptor and altering its conformation.[33] More than one type of opiate receptor exists,[34] each with particular drug affinities and responses, just as there are many kinds of adrenoreceptors. Thus, to adequately describe the pharmacology of a narcotic drug, we must describe what type of opiate receptors it affects (receptor specificity) and in what way it affects these receptors (agonist-antagonist activity).

RECEPTOR SPECIFICITY.—At this time, the exact nature and specificity of opiate receptors have not been elucidated. In general, it may be said that the preponderant opiate receptors in the brain are the so-called mu receptors, which seem to mediate the central analgesic effects of these drugs, as well as respiratory depression.[35] Examples of mu-stimulating narcotic drugs are morphine, meperidine, and fentanyl. Kappa and delta receptors are found predominantly in the spinal cord and, when stimulated, seem to produce spinal analgesia.[36] They also seem to be responsible for the sedative and dysphoric reactions seen with narcotics that stimulate these receptors, such as pentazocine. Other opiate receptors have been characterized that are found primarily in smooth muscle, called sigma receptors. However, it must be remembered that the specificity of these receptors is far from absolute, and the classification is based on the relative binding of various drugs. Thus, a drug that is described as a mu-stimulating drug, such as morphine, merely binds most strongly to mu receptors and is perfectly capable of producing some effect at other receptor sites.

AGONIST-ANTAGONIST ACTIVITY.—The alteration in conformation of an opiate receptor produced by the application of a narcotic drug is capable of altering neural transmission, probably at synaptic junctions. Drugs that bind the receptor and cause this change in neural (pain) sensitivity (analgesia) are called *agonists*. Examples of such drugs are morphine, alphaprodine, meperidine, and fentanyl. In another class are the narcotic drugs that bind to the receptor (in most cases very avidly) but do not seem to cause the conformational change in the receptor that produces analgesia. Because of their high affinity for the receptor, these drugs are capable of displacing the agonist drugs from the receptor and "reversing" their effects, and therefore are known as narcotic *antagonists* (e.g., naloxone, naltrexone). Yet a third interaction with the receptor is possible. Some drugs have a high affinity for the receptor and therefore displace the pure antagonist drugs from the receptor in a competitive manner. Unlike the pure antagonists, however, these drugs are capable of producing some analgesic effect themselves and therefore are called *agonist-antagonist* drugs. Examples of this class are levallorphan, pentazocine, nalbuphine, and butorphanol. These drugs are typically kappa receptor agonists and mu receptor antagonists, and it is tempting to view this receptor specificity as the explanation for their peculiar actions.[37]

Peripartum Pharmacology

When narcotics are used in obstetrics, they are used to relieve labor pain, but with the additional requirement that no adverse effects be produced in either mother or baby. All narcotic drugs readily cross the placental barrier and can exert neonatal effects in normal doses. In order to achieve maternal analgesic without neonatal depression, the method of administration, selection of the appropriate drug, and selection of the appropriate patient are all important variables to be considered.

Method of Administration

Many methods of administration have been used in obstetrics in an attempt to minimize the amount of the drug administered to the mother that reaches the baby.

IM ADMINISTRATION.—IM administration of drugs is easy to perform but leads to uneven analgesia, late respiratory depression, and profound neonatal effects if not properly timed.[38] For these reasons, many centers have abandoned this method.

IV ADMINISTRATION.—This method is frequently used to provide analgesia in labor. The effects of an IV injection of narcotic are more predictable, making timing of doses easier. However, achieving a steady blood level of narcotic sufficient to provide analgesia is difficult, and the parturient frequently suffers either underdosage or overdosage. Continuous IV infusion of short-acting narcotics (e.g., alfentanyl) or self-administration of IV narcotics may overcome this limitation.[39, 40]

INTRATHECAL ADMINISTRATION.—Application of narcotic drugs in the immediate vicinity of the spinal cord (e.g., intraspinal or peridural injections) produces high concentrations of drug in the posterior horn of the spinal cord and can produce analgesia, at least in postoperative patients.[41] The utility of this approach has been difficult to demonstrate in labor, probably because an inappropriate drug (morphine) is the one most extensively studied. It appears that morphine must be injected into the subarachnoid space to provide reliable pain relief during labor, and this method of administration has been associated with an unacceptably high incidence of side effects.[42] Epidural administration of a more lipid-soluble, dura-penetrating drug (e.g., fentanyl) shows promise,[43] as does the use of agonist-antagonist (kappa receptor) drugs, such as butorphanol and nalbuphine.[44] At present, this is an experimental technique and should not be applied indiscriminantly to laboring patients.

Drug Selection

An ideal narcotic for perinatal use would provide good analgesia, no maternal respiratory depression, no other maternal side effects (nausea, pruritus, dysphoria), no neonatal effects (short- or long-term), and no adverse effects on maternal-infant interactions.

Obviously, at present no such drug or technique can provide these ideal effects. The drugs that most closely approach this goal are the agonist-antagonist drugs, such as butorphanol and nalbuphine.[45]

Patient Selection

Narcotic drugs can only provide analgesia. They do not take the place of major regional anesthetic techniques when these are indicated. They should not be used when it is necessary to prevent deleterious effects arising from the reflex responses to labor pain, as is desirable in patients with severe cardiac disease. They are at present most useful in primiparas in early labor, as adjuncts when inserting major regional anesthetics in uncontrollable patients, and in multiparas with relatively short, predictable labors with minimal pain. When used intrathecally, they are useful only in the first stage of labor, and they do not provide adequate analgesia for operative obstetric procedures.[46]

In summary, narcotic analgesics have had a major role in reducing the discomfort of labor and may play an even larger role if improved methods of administration and more suitable drugs can be found.

GENERAL ANALGESIA AND ANESTHESIA

The further extension of the concept of systemic medication for the relief of labor pain is general analgesia and anesthesia. General *analgesia* entails the administration of subanesthetic concentrations of inhalation agents (nitrous oxide, methoxyflurane, trichloroethylene) that provide analgesia roughly equivalent to that achieved by narcotic analgesics. The goal of general analgesia is for the patient to remain awake and cooperative, and to maintain protective laryngeal reflexes during administration of the inhalation agent. General *anesthesia* further extends the scope of inhalation analgesia and provides a profound analgesia, amnesia, hypnosis, and muscle relaxation.

Various types of general anesthesia and analgesia are available, using a wide variety of drugs. The techniques commonly applied to obstetrics include intermittent inhalation analgesia, dissociative general anesthesia (ketamine), and a general endotracheal anesthesia supplemented with neuromuscular blockers.

Intermittent Inhalation Analgesia

This technique, first used by Simpson in 1847, entails inhalation by the parturient of subanesthetic concentrations of inhalation agents. This technique may have an advantage over narcotics because of the rapid onset and reversibility of the analgesia produced.

The technique is simple in concept: the parturient self-administers an anesthetic agent from an inhaler device during the time of contractions. However, this apparent simplicity is a major hazard of the technique since the staffing of many obstetric units may lead to inadequate observation of the parturient, and this danger is great because the physiology of the pregnant state predisposes to overdosage with inhalation anesthesia. The functional residual capacity of the lungs is reduced and alveolar ventilation is increased, which, combined with the reduced anesthetic requirements in pregnancy, leads to a rapid induction of the unconscious, *anesthetized* state, rather than the analgesic state desired. Thus, the major risk of inhalation analgesia is inadvertent, unobserved overdosage, with loss of consciousness and protective laryngeal reflexes. Maternal regurgitation, vomiting, and aspiration may then occur, leading to airway obstruction, asphyxia, and aspiration pneumonitis. If the parturient is *carefully* observed, however, the risk of overdosage may be minimized, and inhalation analgesia might be self-administered reasonably safely in special circumstances. It cannot be recommended for routine use.

DISSOCIATIVE ANALGESIA

The IM or preferably IV administration of a small dose (approximately 0.25 mg/kg) of ketamine produces a state known as dissociative analgesia. This state is characterized by intense analgesia and amnesia, usually without loss of consciousness or protective airway reflexes. Dissociative analgesia is accompanied by a dreaming phenomenon that may be unpleasant. While superficially it is a very attractive technique, several cautions are in order. First, rare patients will lose consciousness when this technique is used, and airway reflexes may be obtunded sufficiently so that aspiration is possible.[47] This is probably more likely when the patient has received narcotic analgesics during labor. Second, some patients, particularly patients with pre-eclampsia, become extremely hypertensive secondary to the cardiovascular stimulation produced by ketamine.[48] Finally, some patients may experience terrifying hallucinations, even at this low dose of ketamine.[49] Therefore, in my opinion this is not a technique acceptable for routine use, but it may be useful in selected circumstances, such as in the extremely uncooperative patient who requires an emergency obstetric procedure and refuses regional anesthesia. It is also a useful adjunct to the induction of general anesthesia in the hypovolemic or asthmatic patient and is frequently used for this purpose.

GENERAL ANESTHESIA

General anesthesia may be used in obstetrics for both vaginal and cesarean delivery. The technique should not be used without endotracheal intubation and is usually reserved exclusively for use in emergency procedures because of the risk of aspiration of gastric contents. The technique is outlined in the appendix to this chapter, in the section on high-risk obstetrics.

REGIONAL ANESTHESIA IN OBSTETRICS

As described previously, the pain of uterine contraction together with that of cervical dilation and effacement is transmitted to the spinal cord by afferent fibers that pass to the spinal cord by way of the posterior roots of the 11th and 12th thoracic nerves, with some contribution from fibers in the 10th thoracic and first lumbar nerves. The pain resulting from distention of the birth canal, vulva, and perineum is conveyed by afferent fibers of the posterior roots of the second, third, and fourth sacral nerves. Both of these pathways must be blocked by one or more regional anesthetic techniques in order to provide satisfactory analgesia during labor and vaginal delivery.

LUMBAR EPIDURAL BLOCK

Anatomy and Landmarks

The spinal cord in the adult usually does not extend below the vertebral body of L-2, and more often it ends at L-1 (Fig 18–3), while the dural sac usually ends at the level of S1–2. Surrounding the dural sac, and delimited by the dura matter on one side and the periosteum of the vertebral bodies and the ligamenta flava on the other, is the epidural space, which extends from the foramen magnum superiorly to the sacral hiatus caudally. Therefore, in theory, epidural anesthesia may be given at any level between C-1 and S-5. The L-2 to L-5 interspaces are usually chosen for obstetric epidural block.

The anatomical landmarks for epidural anesthesia are the same as for spinal anesthesia; the line between the left and right iliac crests crosses either in the spinous process of the L-4 vertebra or the L4–5 vertebral interspace (Figs 18–4 and 18–5; see also Fig 18–3). The selected vertebral interspace for the epidural block can be pinpointed by locating this interspace and then palpating the desired interspace in the cephalad direction.

Patient Position

The position of the patient is identical to that for spinal anesthesia. The patient may be either in the lateral decubitus or the sitting position, but the lateral decubitus position (see Fig 18–4) is preferred in order to displace the gravid uterus from the aorta and the inferior vena cava. I prefer the right lateral decubitus position.

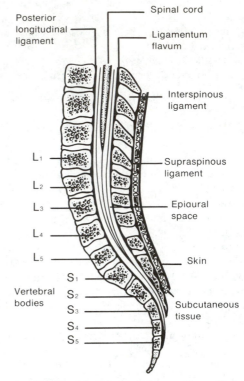

Fig 18–3.—Vertebral column. (From Ostheimer G. (ed.): *Manual of Obstetric Anesthesia.* New York, Churchill Livingstone, 1984. Reproduced by permission.)

Materials

The following materials should be assembled when an epidural block is to be administered:

One pair of sterile gloves.

Antibacterial solution for cleansing the skin.

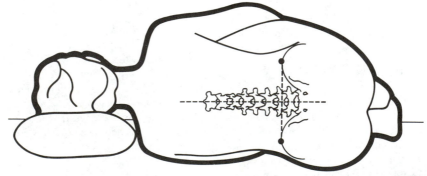

Fig 18–4.—Landmarks in the lateral decubitus position. (From Ostheimer G. (ed.): *Manual of Obstetric Anesthesia.* New York, Churchill Livingstone, 1984. Reproduced by permission.)

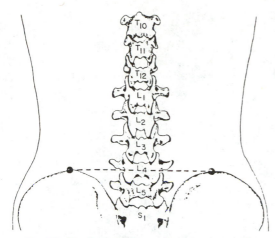

Fig 18–5.—Landmarks in the sitting position. (From Ostheimer G. (ed.): *Manual of Obstetric Anesthesia.* New York, Churchill Livingstone, 1984. Reproduced by permission.)

One sterile cup for the antibacterial solution.
Forceps.
Sterile gauze pads.
Sterile towels for draping the field (if desired).
One 25-gauge, ⅝-inch (1.6-cm) needle for skin infiltration.
One 21- or 22-gauge, 1½-inch (3.8-cm) needle for deep infiltration (if desired).
One 18-gauge needle for use as an introducer (if desired).
One 17- to 19-gauge epidural needle with stylet (I prefer the 17-gauge Weiss modification of the Tuohy needle with the Huber tip).
One 3-ml syringe.
One 5-ml glass syringe.
One 20-ml syringe.
One disposable epidural catheter.
A disposable epidural anesthetic tray usually contains all of the above items.

Technique

Thirty ml of a clear antacid (Bicitra) is administered before an epidural block is initiated. Otherwise, premedication is not given for vaginal delivery. For cesarean delivery, the patient may receive 0.4–0.6 mg of atropine or 0.2–0.4 mg of glycopyrrolate IM and 30 ml of a clear antacid (Bicitra), 30–60 minutes preoperatively. Cimetidine, 300 mg PO before sleep and IM 1 hour preoperatively, may be considered. The technique of epidural anesthesia in

obstetrics is similar to that for the surgical patient, except that special consideration must be given to the condition of the fetus and to the maternal physiologic changes associated with pregnancy and labor.

Arterial blood pressure must be monitored in any patient undergoing regional anesthesia, but the obstetric patient must be particularly carefully observed for changes. The blood pressure is determined in the supine and the lateral decubitus positions before the block is initiated to check for aortocaval compression (supine hypotensive syndrome). An automatic blood pressure monitor is useful but not mandatory. Routine ECG monitoring is mandatory in our institution for the initiation of an epidural block for labor or cesarean delivery.

The obstetric patient selected for epidural anesthesia is acutely hydrated prior to induction of the epidural block by using a large-gauge indwelling plastic catheter to administer 1,000 ml of lactated Ringer's solution or similar crystalloid solution over 10–20 minutes. This hydration helps to prevent the hypotension that may be triggered by the sympathetic block which occurs with epidural anesthesia.[50] The IV infusion is then maintained should the patient require additional hydration or IV medication.

The epidural tray is opened in a sterile manner and the expiration date checked. The gloved anesthetist prepares the skin of the lumbar area with a bactericidal preparation, wiping off the excess solution. The field may be draped with sterile towels. The desired interspace is located. Depending on the special anatomical features of the patient and the requirements of the situation, the second, third, or fourth lumbar interspace may be used. I find that L2–3 is usually the most suitable. The selected entry point into the skin is infiltrated with a small amount of local anesthetic. A 25-gauge needle is used to create the skin wheal. Then a small amount (about 1–2 ml) of local anesthetic is injected into the subcutaneous tissue and the interspinous ligament. Some anesthetists insert an 18-gauge needle through the skin wheal to create a skin opening large enough to allow the epidural needle to pass through without carrying with it a plug of skin on its way to the epidural space. I do not use this technique because I find that subsequent release of the skin will move the hole, and a well-fitted stylet will prevent coring of the skin. If one relies on the position of the skin hole, it may be very difficult to initiate an epidural block.

Various types of epidural needles are available. At my institution, the winged Weiss modification of

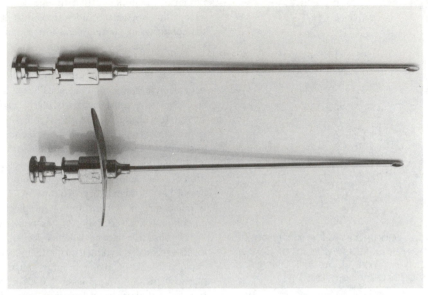

Fig 18–6.—Tuohy needle and its winged modification (Weiss).

the Tuohy needle with a Huber point (Fig 18–6) is preferred; it can be grasped with the index finger and the thumb of both hands at the same time as it is advanced through the tissues. The middle, ring, and little fingers of both hands of the anesthetist rest firmly against the patient's back. This gives a fine control over the movement of the needle unexcelled by any other type of epidural needle. Alternatively, an all-purpose needle such as a 17- to 19-gauge Tuohy needle may be chosen.

The epidural needle is inserted into the intervertebral space and advanced approximately ½ to 1½ inches (1.2–3.7 cm) to a point where the tissue resistance of the interspinous ligament is felt. For this phase of the needle replacement, the shaft of the needle is held between the thumb, index, and middle fingers, with the palmar aspect of the thumb resting on the head of the stylet to prevent its displacement (Fig 18–7). I place the needle in the in-

tervertebral space with the wings "up and down," not parallel. This is to avoid any further movement of the needle after the epidural space is identified. Rotation of the epidural needle in the epidural space may result in "coring the dura," producing a dural perforation. The wings of the needles are grasped, and the anesthetist's hands are steadied by the middle, ring, and little fingers resting on the patient's back, as shown in Figures 18–8 and 18–9.

Any further movement of the needle is halted when the resistance of the interspinous ligament is felt. Advancing the needle only a small distance at

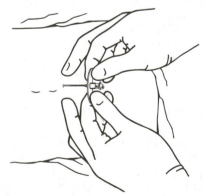

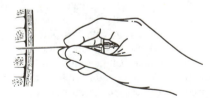

Fig 18–7.—Hand position for needle insertion. (From Ostheimer G. (ed.): *Manual of Obstetric Anesthesia.* New York, Churchill Livingstone, 1984. Reproduced by permission.)

Fig 18–8.—Hand position for hanging-drop technique using the winged epidural needle. (From Ostheimer G. (ed.): *Manual of Obstetric Anesthesia.* New York, Churchill Livingstone, 1984. Reproduced by permission.)

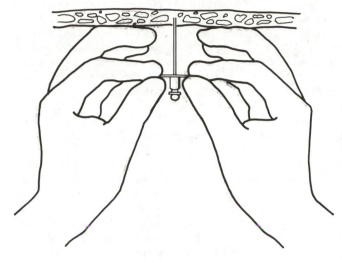

Fig 18–9.—The hanging-drop technique; view from above. (From Ostheimer G. (ed.): *Manual of Obstetric Anesthesia.* New York, Churchill Livingstone, 1984. Reproduced by permission.)

this point will result in its passing through the ligamentum flavum into the epidural space. This area measures only 0.2 inches (5 mm) at its widest extent (in the lumbar area), so that the advancing needle can easily overshoot this distance, pierce the dura, and enter the subarachnoid space. Therefore, it is important that the advancing movement of the epidural needle is delicately controlled. There are two methods of identifying the epidural space: the "hanging drop" method (see Figs 18–8 and 18–9) provides visual identification, while the "loss-of-resistance" method (Fig 18–10) gives tactile evidence of entry.

The "hanging drop" technique depends on the concept that a "negative pressure" exists in the epidural space. This method was discovered by Janzen[51] in 1926 and rediscovered by Heldt and Moloney[52] in 1928. In 1933, Gutierrez[53] used negative pressure to find the epidural space by placing

a drop of saline into the hub of the advancing needle.

While the drop is watched constantly, the needle is slowly and continuously advanced. As soon as the ligamentum flavum is pierced and the bevel enters the epidural space, the drop is suddenly sucked into the needle as if by a negative pressure in the epidural space. This sign occurs about 80% of the time, but the reasons for it are not clear. There are four major theories:

1. A cone of depression may form that would register a negative pressure when a blunt needle impinges on the dura. If this were true, it would occur almost 100% of the time.

2. Expansion of the thoracic cage on inspiration results in negative pressure that may be transmitted through the paravertebral spaces and the intervertebral foraminae to the epidural space. There are no data to support this theory.

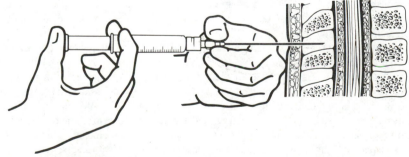

Fig 18–10.—Loss-of-resistance technique with the Tuohy needle. (From Ostheimer G. (ed.): *Manual of Obstetric Anesthesia.* New York, Churchill Livingstone, 1984. Reproduced by permission.)

3. The epidural space may be only a potential space in the erect posture, developing only when the back is flexed and the two layers of dura mater separate. There is some evidence for this theory.

4. The pull of the abdominal viscera on the posterior thoracic and abdominal walls can cause a "negative pressure," but proof of this is lacking. It is probable that the "negative pressure" in the epidural space is due to more than one factor. Slow, continuous movement of the needle is essential instead of a rapid, jerky motion.

Other mechanical devices are available that can aid in the placement of the epidural needle and help reduce the failure rate of the visual technique.

At my institution, the hanging drop technique is used with the Weiss needle and the needle position is confirmed by using the loss-of-resistance technique with air or fluid.

The loss-of-resistance technique, in which the thumb of the anesthetist exerts continuous positive pressure on the end of the piston of the syringe containing air or preservative-free saline, depends on the sudden loss of resistance as the advancing needle point leaves the ligamentum flavum and enters the epidural space. This method was introduced by Sicard and Forestier[54] in 1921 and was used to administer anesthesia for surgical procedures by Pages in the same year. Its success rate is over 90% if the dura is not entered. This technique is usually associated with Dogliotti's name.

The needle is advanced to the level of the interspinous ligament, the stylet is removed from the epidural needle, and a small (5- or 10-ml) syringe filled with air or sterile saline solution is attached. The right-handed anesthetist holds the epidural needle firmly between the index finger and the thumb of the left hand. The back of the left hand rests firmly against the patient's back. This steadies the left hand so that it has fine control over the advancement of the needle (see Fig 18–10). The right hand controls the syringe; with the body of the syringe between the right index and the middle fingers, the thumb applies hard, *steady* pressure to the plunger of the syringe while the left hand slowly advances the epidural needle through the tissues. None of the syringe contents will be expelled as long as the point of the needle is in an interspinous ligament or the ligamentum flavum. As soon as these structures are pierced, however, and the needle enters the epidural space, resistance suddenly disappears and the entire contents of the syringe are suddenly discharged. The movement of the epidural needle is halted immediately.

It is advisable to perform confirmatory tests to identify the needle position in the epidural space. These include an aspiration attempt with a small (5-ml) glass syringe and then injection of 5 ml of air, or an aspiration attempt with a small (5-ml) syringe and slow injection of 3 ml of normal saline or anesthetic solution as a test dose.

If the aspiration test yields a bloody return, the probability is that one of the veins of the epidural plexus has been punctured. To avoid intravascular injection of the relatively large amount of local anesthetic needed for an epidural block, another interspace should be chosen and the procedure repeated. If the aspiration test results in the return of cerebrospinal fluid (CSF), then another interspace is chosen for a repeated attempt to place the needle in the epidural space. Because of this potential problem, I like the L2–3 interspace, so that if there is a dural perforation, one can move caudad and be away from the initial hole by one to two interspaces. It has been reported that a spinal block may rarely result from an epidural block performed after the puncture of the dura at another interspace.[55] In a surgical setting, if it is noted that the dura has been punctured, it may be feasible to continue the procedure as a spinal anesthetic at the same interspace. However, spinal anesthesia is not performed during the first stage of labor.

The first confirmatory test after aspiration consists of attaching a small (5-ml) empty syringe to the epidural needle with the plunger positioned at the 4–5-ml mark. Air is then briskly injected into the epidural space. Pressure on the plunger is released immediately after discharge of the total air volume. Ease of injection of the air and failure of the plunger to move back more than to the 0.5–1.0-ml mark usually indicate that the needle point is in the epidural space. If there is resistance to the air injection or if there is significant return of air into the syringe, then the bevel of the needle may still be located in subcutaneous tissue, the interspinous ligament, or the ligamentum flavum.

Injecting a small amount (3 ml) of local anesthetic solution should not result in any major anesthetic effect if the needle is in the epidural space. However, if the dura mater has been pierced and the local anesthetic is injected into the subarachnoid space, extensive sensory and motor block may be noted. A timed period of 3 minutes is allowed for any anesthetic effect to appear.

If these tests indicate that the needle is in the epidural space, then an aspiration test is performed before each incremental or fractional (3–5-

TABLE 18–1.—LOCAL ANESTHETICS AND DOSAGES FOR SINGLE-DOSE EPIDURAL BLOCK FOR VAGINAL DELIVERY

LOCAL ANESTHETIC*	DOSAGE†		ONSET OF ACTION (min)	DURATION OF ACTION (min)
	(ml)	(mg)		
Bupivacaine (Sensorcaine, Marcaine), 0.25%–0.5%	8–20	20–100	5–10	60–180
2-Chloroprocaine (Nesacaine-CE), 2.0%–3.0%	8–20	160–600	3–5	40–60
Lidocaine (Xylocaine), 1.0%–2.0%	8–20	80–400	5–10	60–75
Mepivacaine (Carbocaine), 1.0%–2.0%	8–20	80–400	5–10	60–75

*All without epinephrine. Marcaine and Carbocaine are registered trademarks of Breon Laboratories, Inc. Nesacaine and Xylocaine are registered trademarks of Astra Pharmaceutical Products, Inc.

†Dose range depending on the patient's height; total milligram dose of the local anesthetic.

ml) dose which is injected every 60–90 seconds until the total dose is administered for a "single shot" epidural block. The indicated dosages have been reduced by about 25% when compared to those that are appropriate for a similar epidural block in a surgical patient (Tables 18–1 and 18–2). After the epidural needle is withdrawn, the patient is allowed to rest in a comfortable position favoring left uterine displacement, i.e., usually a semisitting position with the right hip elevated by a wedge. I prefer to initiate an epidural block with the parturient in the right lateral decubitus position. Thus, with left uterine displacement, the dependent side will receive an adequate amount of drug. Vital signs and the spread of anesthesia are carefully monitored.

Technique for the Placement of an Epidural Catheter

The anatomical landmarks and the initial steps are the same as in the single-dose method of epidural block. An epidural needle must be selected that is large enough to admit the catheter for passage into the epidural space. The needle is positioned in the epidural space using the same techniques as previously described. Either the hanging drop technique or the loss-of-resistance method may be used to identify the epidural space. I administer a test dose of 3 ml of local anesthetic through the needle before inserting the catheter into the epidural space.

The plastic catheter is examined for imperfec-

TABLE 18–2.—LOCAL ANESTHETICS AND DOSAGES FOR SINGLE-DOSE EPIDURAL ANESTHESIA FOR CESAREAN SECTION

LOCAL ANESTHETIC*	DOSAGE†		ONSET OF ACTION (min)	DURATION OF ACTION (min)
	ml	mg		
Bupivacaine (Sensorcaine, Marcaine) 0.75%	12–20	90–150	5–10	120–180
2-Chloroprocaine (Nesacaine-CE) 3%	12–20	360–600	3–5	40–60
Etidocaine (Duranest) 1%	12–20	120–200	5–10	60–90
Lidocaine (Xylocaine) 2%	12–20	240–400	5–10	60–90
Mepivacaine (Carbocaine) 2.0%	12–20	240–400	5–10	60–90

*All without epinephrine.

†Dose range depends on patient's height; total milligram dose of the local anesthetic should not exceed manufacturer's recommendations.

tions. The depth markings are noted and compared with the length of the epidural needle. It is preferable that the tubing be used with a stylet, which facilitates passage of the catheter through the needle. The stylet is withdrawn from the tip of the catheter about 1 inch (2–3 cm). The catheter is uncurled and held by the fingers of the left hand and the tip is inserted through the hub of the epidural needle by the right hand (for a right-handed anesthetist). As the leading point of the tubing contacts the directional bevel of the epidural needle, a sudden resistance is felt. This is usually at the first mark on the epidural catheter. This resistance is gently but aggressively overcome and the tubing is advanced through the needle so that it will project about ¾– 1½ inches (2–4 cm) beyond the bevel of the epidural needle into the epidural space. Then the needle is removed from the tissues in the following manner: the catheter is held firmly approximately an inch (about 2.5 cm) from the hub of the needle while the "wings" or shaft and hub of the needle are held between the index and middle fingers and thumb of the other hand (Fig 18–11). While the catheter is held in place with positive forward pressure, the needle is carefully pulled out so that the thumbs of the two hands meet. Forward pressure should be applied to the catheter at all times. The maneuver is then repeated by grasping the tubing another inch (2.5 cm) distal to the hub of the needle and repeating the same procedure. Finally, the tip of the needle will emerge from the skin. The tubing is prevented from being dislodged by applying firm pressure with the thumb and index finger of the left hand to the tubing at the point where it emerges

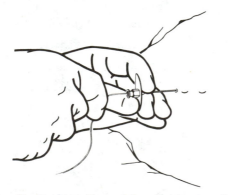

Fig 18–11.—Insertion of the epidural catheter and removal of the epidural needle over the epidural catheter. (From Ostheimer G. (ed.): *Manual of Obstetric Anesthesia.* New York, Churchill Livingstone, 1984. Reproduced by permission.)

from the skin. The needle is then moved back over the catheter. The thumb and index finger may now move some distance up the catheter and hold the catheter firmly to prevent its dislodgment while the needle and stylet are removed from the catheter by the right hand. Always work close to the back to avoid dislocating the catheter.

An adapter is attached to the end of the catheter or a blunt, small-gauge needle is inserted in the tubing. Forward positioning of the needle is impossible once the catheter is advanced beyond the bevel. If forward repositioning is necessary, the needle and the catheter are both completely withdrawn and the block is repeated from the beginning. It is important to remember that once the catheter has advanced beyond the bevel of the epidural needle, any attempt to withdraw the catheter can result in shearing off the catheter. I measure the distance from the hub of the needle to the skin, note the marking on the catheter, and then pull back the catheter to this measured distance after the needle has been removed from the catheter.

Before the catheter is taped in place, a careful, gentle aspiration test is performed to ensure that the catheter is not in the subarachnoid space or in an epidural vein. Another test dose of 3 ml of the local anesthetic solution is then injected and the patient is observed for cardiovascular changes, sensory or motor alterations, or CNS toxic reaction over a period of time not less than 2 minutes. Sterile gauze pads or a Band-Aid are placed above and below the catheter as it emerges out of the skin, and the catheter and pads are secured by pieces of tape. The entire catheter is then taped to the back of the patient and the patient is placed in a semisitting position with a wedge under the right hip to displace the pregnant uterus to the left.

If vital signs remain satisfactory and no significant anesthesia develops after this second test dose, another aspiration test is done and the fractional doses of local anesthetic (3–5 ml) are administered with a minimum interval of at least 60 seconds until the full epidural dose is injected. I do not inject more than 5 ml of local anesthetic at a time, which produces a maximum dose of 25 mg of bupivacaine or 100 mg of lidocaine.

In order to obtain continuous analgesia from T-10 to S-5, the first intermittent epidural dose is the same as in the single-dose method. When the desired level of anesthesia has been achieved with the initial dose, a subsequent "top-up" of about two thirds the initial dose will maintain this sensory level. Top-up doses are added as necessary. An aspiration test must be done prior to each reinforcement because perforation of the dura mater or one of the epidural veins by the catheter has been reported and may have occurred since the last administration of the anesthetic. Fractional doses of local anesthetic (3–5 ml) are administered until the appropriate top-up dose has been given. Dosage schedules are listed in Tables 18–3 and 18–4.

With the patient resting comfortably, the spread of anesthesia is checked frequently by gentle repeated pinpricks or by a cotton swab moistened with alcohol. Since the loss of pain and temperature sensation progresses simultaneously, the use of alcohol to check the spread of anesthesia may be more pleasant for the patient. Repeated pinpricks may not accurately differentiate the area of complete loss of pain sensation from that of spinal analgesia.

Precautions

Aspiration must precede the injection of the local anesthetic solution for two reasons: to avoid accidental subarachnoid injection and to avoid IV injection. The epidural dose is a large multiple of that needed for subarachnoid block. Unintentional injection of such an amount of local anesthetic solution into the subarachnoid space would unavoidably result in high or total spinal block. The epidural venous plexus offers a potential for an intravascular injection of a large volume of local anesthetic which may be followed by central venous system excitation and convulsions. Full cardiopulmonary resuscitative equipment must be immediately available, as is customary for any regional block.

The pharmacologic action of the local anesthetic that is absorbed by the neonate during epidural anesthesia is minimal and the fetal narcotization that may be seen with systemic analgesia is less likely to occur. However, maternal hypotension with a concomitant decrease in uteroplacental perfusion producing fetal hypoxia and acidosis is a possibility and must be treated immediately.

Monitoring of vital signs is mandatory for both mother and fetus. Maternal blood pressure must be checked frequently. If a decrease of 10 mm Hg or more occurs, an immediate response is necessary. Therapy consists of an immediate change in the position of the parturient to a more pronounced left (sometimes right) lateral decubitus position, oxygen by face mask, and an increase in the IV infusion rate initiated by a 200- to 300-ml bolus of an appropriate IV crystalloid solution such as lactated Ringer's. If these measures fail to improve the blood pressure, then 5–10 mg of ephedrine may be injected IV and repeated as necessary.

TABLE 18–3.—LOCAL ANESTHETICS AND DOSAGES FOR CONTINUOUS (INTERMITTENT) EPIDURAL BLOCK FOR VAGINAL DELIVERY

LOCAL ANESTHETIC*	DOSAGE†				ONSET OF ACTION (min)	DURATION OF ACTION (min)	TIME BETWEEN TOP-UP DOSES (min)
	First Dose‡		Top-up Dose§				
	ml	mg	ml	mg			
Bupivacaine‖ (Sensorcaine, Marcaine) 0.25%–0.5%	8–15	20–75	6–10	15–50	5–10	90–180	Approx. 120
2-Chloroprocaine (Nesacaine-CE) 2.0%–3.0%	8–15	160–450	6–10	120–300	3–5	40–60	Approx. 45
Lidocaine (Xylocaine) 1.0%–2.0%	8–15	80–300	6–10	60–200	5–10	60–75	Approx. 60
Mepivacaine (Carbocaine) 1.0%–2.0%	8–15	80–300	6–10	60–200	5–10	60–75	Approx. 60

*All without epinephrine.
†Total milligram dose of the local anesthetic should not exceed manufacturer's recommendations.
‡Dose range depends on patient's height.
§The top-up dose is two thirds of the first dose if the initial dose resulted in a satisfactory level of analgesia and if this level is to be maintained.
‖Some authors have described the use of 0.125% bupivacaine for vaginal delivery. I have not had any personal experience with this concentration.

TABLE 18–4.—LOCAL ANESTHETICS AND DOSAGES FOR CONTINUOUS (INTERMITTENT) EPIDURAL BLOCK FOR CESAREAN SECTION

| LOCAL ANESTHETIC* | DOSAGE† | | | | ONSET OF ACTION (min) | DURATION OF ACTION (min) | TIME BETWEEN TOP-UP DOSES (min) |
| | First Dose‡ | | Top-up Dose§ | | | | |
	ml	mg	ml	mg			
Bupivacaine (Sensorcaine, Marcaine) 0.75%	12–20	90–150	8–12	60–90	5–10	120–180	Approx. 150
2-Chloroprocaine (Nesacaine-CE) 3.0%	12–20	360–600	8–12	240–360	3–5	40–60	Approx. 45
Etidocaine (Duranest) 1.0%	12–20	120–200	8–12	80–120	5–10	75–105	Approx. 75
Lidocaine (Xylocaine) 2.0%	12–20	240–400	8–12	160–240	5–10	60–90	Approx. 60
Mepivacaine (Carbocaine) 2.0%	12–20	240–400	8–12	160–240	5–10	60–90	Approx. 60

*All without epinephrine.
†Total milligram dose of the local anesthetic should not exceed manufacturer's recommendations.
‡Dose range depends on patient's height.
§The top-up dose is two thirds of the first dose if the initial dose resulted in a satisfactory level of analgesia and if this level is to be maintained.

The Test Dose

Moore and Batra[56] have effectively demonstrated that 3 ml of a local anesthetic solution with 1:200,000 epinephrine is an effective test dose prior to epidural block since the epinephrine will increase the heart rate and, possibly, the blood pressure if it is unintentionally injected into an epidural vein, while the local anesthetic will produce sensory analgesia if injected subarachnoid. However, I believe that the most efficient test dose is 1.5% lidocaine hyperbaric solution with 1:200,000 epinephrine. Why? Three milliliters of this solution will give absolute evidence of sensory blockade if placed in the subarachnoid space without the worry of how high the block will go, which has been a matter of concern with hypobaric or isobaric solutions. A test dose including 15 μg of epinephrine is mandatory for all major regional blocks of any type, including cesarean delivery.

How about a test dose for epidural anesthesia for labor and vaginal delivery? Matadial and Cibils[57] demonstrated a significant decrease in uterine activity when epinephrine (1:200,000) was added to the anesthetic solution (1.5% lidocaine), mainly a lessening of intensity. Wallis et al.[58] found a decrease in uterine artery blood flow in pregnant ewes when lumbar anesthesia with chloroprocaine with epinephrine 1:200,000 was administered. Albright et al.[59] have postulated that chloroprocaine with epinephrine 1:200,000 does not alter intervillous blood flow, as demonstrated by the ^{133}Xe technique. However, if the observer omits two patients from that study who had extremely large increases in intervillous blood flow, the increases in intervillous blood flow are of borderline significance due to the range in the reproducibility of the technique and may be due to the effect of epinephrine on the heart of the parturient (heart rate changes before and after epidural block were not reported). Uterine activity measured in Montevideo units usually decreased after the epidural block in 9 of 12 patients, but the mean decrease was apparently not statistically significant. More recently, Hood et al.[60] have demonstrated a significant dose-related reduction in uterine blood flow with 5-, 10-, and 20-μg doses of epinephrine in the chronically instrumented gravid ewe.

For labor and delivery at the Boston Hospital for Women, Division of Brigham and Women's Hospital, the maximum allowable dose of local anesthetic at any one injection is 5 ml, which translates to 5 ml of 0.5% bupivacaine (25 mg) or 5 ml of

1.5%–2.0% lidocaine (75–100 mg), without epinephrine. Since our test doses, delivered by epidural needle or catheter, are 3 ml, and our maintenance injections are a 3-ml test dose and 3–5 ml of local anesthetic, we would be continually administering epinephrine and accumulating large amounts which would most certainly adversely affect labor, especially since we will initiate an epidural block during the latent phase of labor at the request of the parturient and her obstetrician.

Therefore, we do not use epinephrine in our local anesthetic solutions for labor and delivery.

What about the supposed decrease in uterine activity after the initiation of epidural analgesia? Schellenberg[61] has demonstrated that aortocaval compression is an essential factor contributing to or responsible for the temporary depression of uterine activity that has been observed after epidural injection of local anesthetic agents.

With our fractional or incremental injection technique, we have virtually eliminated CNS toxic reactions secondary to the unintentional intravascular injection of local anesthetic during obstetric epidural anesthesia. We have seen the prodrome of a CNS toxic reaction but, with aspiration before each incremental injection, have avoided any sequelae. In effect, all our injections have become test doses. One interesting side effect of an unintentional intravascular injection, besides transient CNS effects, is that the parturient may complain of increased pain with her next contraction. Increased intravascular concentrations of local anesthetic can produce uterine hypertonus[62] and result in the parturient perceiving more discomfort. Figure 18–12 demonstrates an increase in uterine activity after an unintentional intravascular injection of approximately 50 mg of bupivacaine added to whatever circulating concentration of local anesthetic was present. In this instance, an epidural anesthetic utilizing 0.5% bupivacaine has been in place for several hours and has had three reinjections.

At the arrow, after aspiration, 5 ml of 0.5% bupivacaine (25 mg) was administered via an epidural catheter. After 1 minute had passed and another aspiration test performed, another 5 ml of 0.5% bupivacaine (25 mg) was administered, and the parturient had prodromal signs of a CNS toxic reaction but no convulsions. Repeated aspiration of the epidural catheter yielded frank blood. With the next two contractions, the patient complained bitterly of pain and discomfort, which then subsided. Reinsertion of the epidural catheter was successful, and satisfactory analgesia was obtained for the remainder of the labor and delivery.

Complications

Life-threatening complications should be rare. The unintentional accidental subarachnoid injection

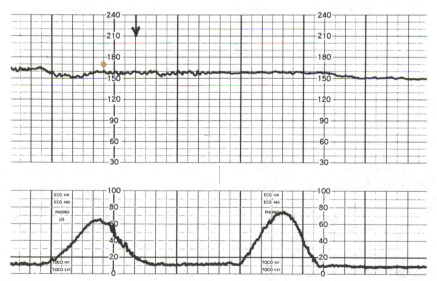

Fig 18–12.—Fetal effects of accidental intravascular injection of 50 mg of bupivacaine. (From Ostheimer G. (ed.): *Manual of Obstetric* *Anesthesia*. New York, Churchill Livingstone, 1984. Reproduced by permission.)

of a large volume of drug resulting in a total spinal block is heralded by nausea and hypotension and may progress to respiratory and cardiac arrest.

Unintentional injection of a large portion of the epidural dose into an epidural vein may result in signs of CNS toxicity, including convulsions.

Other serious complications include extradural hematoma at the puncture site and breakage of the needle while it is positioned in the epidural space.

Indications

Epidural block is a very useful procedure that has many important applications in diagnostic as well as therapeutic medicine. It is of special value for the obstetric patient for vaginal or cesarean delivery. It has obvious advantages for patients with pulmonary, cardiovascular, renal, or hepatic disease, diabetes, toxemia of pregnancy, or other conditions that may require an alternative to general anesthesia.

An epidural block, providing anesthesia that extends from the level of T-10 to S-5 inclusively, gives total relief of pain during the final stages of labor and delivery and therefore is suitable as a single-dose technique if the anesthetist expects that the estimated duration of action of the local anesthetic is sufficient to cover the remaining portion of labor and delivery. The patient should have strong contractions about 3 minutes apart, the cervix should be dilated to 5 cm or more in the multigravida and 6 cm or more in the primigravida, and the presenting fetal part should be engaged in the pelvis.

Continuous epidural anesthesia is a versatile technique because it extends the duration of analgesia obtainable and permits modifying the extent and type of effect by adjusting the top-up dose of local anesthetic according to the current requirements of the patient.

As discussed in the beginning of this chapter, pain of the first stage of labor is due primarily to the dilation of the cervix and to the contractions of the uterus. It is mediated by the T-11 and T-12 innervation, with some fibers from T-10 and L-1. Pain of the second and third stages of labor is perceived via S-2, S-3, and S-4. Epidural anesthesia makes it possible to individualize the block according to the stage of labor: a segmental block may be given in the first stage, limiting the extent of anesthesia to the lower three thoracic and the upper lumbar segments. This leaves Ferguson's reflex intact and avoids the motor block and premature relaxation of the perineum. Since flexion and internal rotation of the presenting part are not interfered with, pain relief can be offered at an earlier stage when the continuous epidural technique is used as a segmental block.

As labor progresses to the second and third stages, anesthesia can be extended to block the sacral innervation. The practice of allowing an epidural to "wear off" during the time is indefensible and in fact *increases* the number of forceps deliveries.[63] In order to provide sacral anesthesia, a full top-up dose is given for this purpose while the patient is in the sitting position for about 5 minutes. A higher concentration of local anesthetic may be selected to achieve motor block and perineal relaxation, especially if a forceps delivery is planned or if abdominal delivery becomes necessary. However, some obstetricians prefer to have their patients pain-free with a block from T-10 to S-5 throughout active labor and delivery.

Because of the versatility of achievable anesthetic effect and the duration of anesthesia obtainable, the continuous epidural technique is well suited for obstetric complications such as cervical dystocia or prolonged labor.

Segmental epidural block can also be used in patients in whom the feasibility of vaginal delivery is uncertain, such as those undergoing a trial of labor after previous cesarean delivery. Epidural analgesia is compatible with the judicious use of IV oxytocin to augment and coordinate labor. If such delivery proves inadvisable, the segmental block can be extended to T-4, which makes cesarean delivery possible under epidural block.

In my experience, even with the epidural catheter tip placed caudad (as in our practice), the "perineal" dose for a segmental epidural block may not always provide appropriate perineal anesthesia. At my institution, a complete block is sought initially from T-10 to S-5 since a top-up dose is not always necessary with bupivacaine.

Good nursing care is essential to the effective management of continuous epidural block for labor and delivery. Careful continuous monitoring of maternal vital signs, fetal heart rate, and uterine contractions is mandatory. A busy obstetric service cannot function at peak effectiveness without the cooperative interaction of the anesthesiologist, obstetrician, and labor nurse, or, in some institutions, nurse midwives. Parturients with epidural analgesia do not have to be delivered by forceps if a competent labor nurse helps the mother coordinate her bearing-down efforts with the contractions of the uterus.

Contraindications

Assuming that the anesthetist is experienced in the technique and in the treatment of the possible complications, the following are relative contraindications to epidural block: the obstetrician's failure to appreciate how the epidural block may affect the management of labor, the need for immediate anesthesia, and the patient's fear of "spinal puncture." Absolute contraindications are injection at the site of the planned puncture, acute CNS disease, and blood coagulopathies.

Comparison With Subarachnoid Block

ADVANTAGES.—Epidural anesthesia offers a greater versatility of effect. For the first stage of labor, analgesia for uterine contractions can be obtained without perineal relaxation. For the second and third stages of labor, perineal relaxation and perineal anesthesia can be given if a continuous technique is used. The onset of hypotension is slower and the degree of hypotension is less than with subarachnoid block. No postdural puncture headache occurs.

DISADVANTAGES.—Technically, epidural anesthesia is slightly more difficult to achieve. Failure rates may be somewhat higher, even for experienced anesthetists. The onset of anesthesia is slower than with subarachnoid block.

Continuous Lumbar Epidural Infusion Anesthesia

A variant of intermittent injections of local anesthetic drugs during epidural analgesia for labor and delivery is the use of a continuous infusion of these drugs throughout labor. This technique has been and is currently being studied[64] and shows considerable promise. It appears to allow the use of a more dilute local anesthetic solution, producing lower blood levels of local anesthetic than intermittent techniques. Motor blockade develops more slowly when bupivacaine is used and the sequelae of migration of the catheter into either an epidural vein or the subarachnoid space are less severe than when a large bolus of local anesthetic is injected. The continuous technique is actually an example of the use of incremental injection of local anesthetic carried to its furthest extreme and is an extremely safe technique. It must be realized, however, that one cannot merely use the continuous infusion technique to allow the insertion of an epidural, the starting of an infusion, and leaving the patient, because significant complications and problems do occur. Patients receiving a continuous infusion of local anesthetic must be monitored frequently for signs of complications of the technique. At a minimum, a labor nurse must be with the patient at all times, with frequent (at least hourly) visits by the anesthesiologist.

Hardware and Supplies

Travenol Weiss epidural tray (with catheter).
Bupivacaine 0.5%, 30-ml vial; 0.25%, 30-ml vial × 2; or 50 ml ampule.
Betadine.
Gloves.
One 60-ml syringe.
Short high-pressure extension tubing.
Volumetric infusion pump.

Block Induction

1. After the routine history and physical examination are completed, the patient is positioned on her side. The lumbar region is prepared with betadine.
2. The epidural catheter is inserted via a No. 17 Weiss needle after proper identification of the epidural space by hanging drop and loss-of-resistance testing.
3. The catheter is tested for unwanted subarachnoid or intravascular placement by injection of 3 ml of 0.5% bupivacaine and the parturient is observed for signs of subarachnoid block or the symptoms of intravascular injection (tinnitus, metallic taste in the mouth, nausea, etc.).
4. An epidural block is then established using incremental 3-ml doses of 0.5% bupivacaine to a total of 6–10 ml for an approximate T-10 level block.
5. Once a stable block with normal maternal and fetal hemodynamics has been established (15–20 minutes), the infusion is started.

Beginning the Infusion

1. Draw up 60 ml of 0.25% bupivacaine in a syringe and attach the syringe to high-pressure infusion tubing. Flush the tubing to create a continuous

column of anesthetic and connect it directly to the epidural catheter. Tape all connections and separately label the tubing. Mount the syringe in the pump.

2. Set the volumetric infusion pump to deliver the desired dose rate and begin the infusion. A selection of dosages of 0.25% bupivacaine is shown below.

> 5 ml/hour = 12.5 mg/hour
> 6 ml/hour = 15 mg/hour
> 7 ml/hour = 17.5 mg/hour
> 8 ml/hour = 20 mg/hour
> 9 ml/hour = 22.5 mg/hour
> 10 ml/hour = 25 mg/hour

For patients over 5'7" tall, begin infusion at a rate of 8–10 ml/hour. For patients less than 5'3" tall, begin infusion at a rate of 5–7 ml/hour. Patients should be positioned supine with left uterine displacement.

Monitoring

The block must be checked at least hourly to ensure uniformity, to rule out subarachnoid or intravascular migration of the catheter, to assess adequacy of analgesia, to monitor any changes in fetal well-being, and to check the level of local anesthetic in the reservoir syringe.

The hourly check must include a *bilateral* evaluation for level of sensory blockade, a review of the fetal heart tracing, and a bladder examination for retention of urine.

Differential Diagnosis of Infusion Problems

ASSYMETRIC SENSORY BLOCKADE.—If a patient lies continuously on one side, the level of sensory blockade may become assymetric. The situation may be corrected by repositioning the patient, disconnecting the pump, repeating a small bolus injection of 0.5% bupivacaine after appropriate testing (3–5 ml), and restarting the infusion. The patient should be encouraged to turn from side to side.

THE CASE OF THE DISAPPEARING LEVEL.— Progressive diminution of sensory blockade and ablation of the block may have a number of causes.
1. The pump on/off switch may be off.
2. The tubing is disconnected.
3. The reservoir syringe is empty and has been for a while.
4. The catheter is no longer in the epidural space, and may be intravascular.

Differential diagnosis consists of rechecking the hardware set-up, then testing to determine where the tip of the catheter is positioned. Disconnect the pump and test the catheter placement. Aspirate, inject a 3-ml test dose, observe, and attempt to reestablish the block with incremental 3-ml doses of 0.5% bupivacaine. If the block cannot be reestablished or if testing indicates intravascular migration of the tip, the catheter must be withdrawn. Depending on the clinical setting, either another catheter may be inserted via a second puncture or alternative analgesia may be initiated. (NOTE: at the above infusion rates, 0.25% bupivacaine will *not* produce symptoms of intravascular injection. The only clue may be a disappearing level.)

DENSE MOTOR BLOCKADE.—Patients on continuous infusions of 0.25% bupivacaine usually exhibit mild to moderate motor blockade of the lower extremities. *If* a progressive dense motor blockade resembling subarachnoid block ensues, the catheter must be disconnected immediately and testing done again. If the catheter appears to be in the subarachnoid space, it should be withdrawn and reinserted at another site, if indicated.

PATCHY BLOCKADE.—Attempt to solidify the block by disconnecting the pump, testing the catheter, and repeating a bolus injection of either 3–5 ml of 0.5% bupivacaine or 1.5%–2.0% lidocaine with 1:200,000 epinephrine. Reconnect the pump.

If a patient requires an acute change in level for cesarean delivery, simply changing the infusion rate will not produce a sufficient block. The patient must be disconnected from the infusion, the catheter tested, and incremental injections of 0.5% bupivacaine or 2% lidocaine with or without epinephrine given to achieve the desired level of sensory blockade.

Often 0.25% bupivacaine does not provide solid perineal analgesia. At the time of delivery the patient may require a supplemental injection of 0.5% bupivacaine or 2% lidocaine to provide sufficient analgesia for forceps delivery or episiotomy. Placing the parturient in the semi-Fowler's position for "pushing" also helps achieve complete perineal analgesia.

Bupivacaine 0.375% may also be used for continuous infusion, which provides a more dense sensory blockade and often eliminates the need for additional perineal blockade at the time of delivery.

SINGLE-DOSE CAUDAL BLOCK

Anatomy and Landmarks

The caudal space is the most distal extension of the epidural space, delimited by the periosteum covering the first four fused sacral vertebrae and the sacrococcygeal ligament crossing the unfused fifth sacral vertebra.

Caudal block is performed by injecting local anesthetic solution through the sacral hiatus into the caudal canal. Developmentally, the sacral hiatus is formed because the spinous process of the fifth sacral vertebra usually fails to fuse. The two unfused parts of the spinous process can be palpated as the two sacral cornua, which constitute an important landmark for caudal block. The sacral hiatus between the sacral cornua is covered by the flat sacrococcygeal ligament (Fig 18–13) which is pierced by the caudal needle. If the cornua cannot be identified, the end of the coccyx is located. It can be assumed that the hiatus lies approximately 2 inches (5 cm) proximal to this point.

In adults, the dural sac extends to about the level of S-2, or about ½ inch (1.5 cm) caudad to a line drawn between the left and right posterior superior iliac spines. Therefore, the caudal needle should not be advanced beyond this level. The caudal canal contains the cauda equina in addition to the epidural venous plexus and the loose areolar tissue generally present in the epidural space.

The hemodynamic changes consistent with term pregnancy produce an engorgement of the venous plexus that reduces the capacity of the epidural space, including that of the caudal canal. This fact must be kept in mind because the extent of caudal anesthesia is largely determined by the volume of the local anesthetic injected. Although, theoretically, the level of anesthesia may be extended to much higher levels, in actual practice it is used for procedures at and below the level of T-10 because of the large volume of local anesthetic required for higher levels of anesthesia.

Patient Position

For the obstetric patient, either the Sims position or the modified Bowie knee-chest position may be found suitable. In the latter, the patient may be positioned prone and flexed, with a pillow folded under the abdomen so as to raise the sacrum and make the parturient more comfortable. This position makes the sacral cornua more prominent and the sacral hiatus easier to identify. In practice, the Sims position is most commonly used.

Materials

When a patient is scheduled for single-dose caudal block, the following materials are needed:

One pair of sterile gloves.
Antibacterial solution for cleansing the skin.
One sterile cup for the antibacterial solution.
Forceps.
Sterile gauze pads.
Sterile towels for draping the field.
One 25-gauge, ⅝-inch (1.6-cm) needle for skin infiltration.
One 21- or 22-gauge, 1½-inch (3.8-cm) needle for deep infiltration.

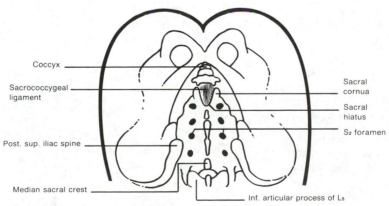

Fig 18–13.—Landmarks for caudal block. (From Ostheimer G. (ed.): *Manual of Obstetric* *Anesthesia.* New York, Churchill Livingstone, 1984. Reproduced by permission.)

One 18-gauge needle for use as an introducer (if desired).

One 19-gauge, 3-inch (7.6-cm) caudal needle with stylet or one 19-gauge, 1½-inch (3.8-cm) short beveled needle.

One 3-ml syringe.

One 5-ml glass syringe.

One 20-ml syringe.

One disposable caudal catheter.

A disposable caudal anesthetic tray usually contains all of the above items.

Technique

Thirty ml of a clear antacid (Bicitra) is administered before the initiation of a caudal block. Otherwise, premedication is not given for vaginal delivery. For cesarean delivery (although caudal anesthesia is rarely used), the patient may receive 0.4–0.6 ml of atropine or 0.2–0.4 mg of glycopyrrolate IM and 30 ml of a clear antacid (Bicitra), 30–60 minutes preoperatively. Cimetidine, 300 mg PO before sleep and IM 1 hour preoperatively, may be considered. The technique of caudal anesthesia in obstetrics is similar to that for the surgical patient, except that special consideration must be given to the condition of the fetus and to the maternal physiologic changes associated with pregnancy and labor.

Arterial blood pressure must be monitored in any patient undergoing regional anesthesia, but the obstetric patient is carefully observed for changes. The blood pressure is determined in the supine and the lateral decubitus positions before the block is initiated to check for aortocaval compression (supine hypotensive syndrome). An automatic blood pressure monitor is useful but not mandatory. Routine ECG monitoring is mandatory in our institution for the initiation of a caudal block for labor or cesarean delivery.

The obstetric patient selected for caudal anesthesia is acutely hydrated prior to the induction of the caudal block by using a large-gauge indwelling plastic catheter to administer 1,000 ml of lactated Ringer's solution or similar crystalloid solution over 10–20 minutes. This hydration helps to prevent the hypotension that may be triggered by the sympathetic block which occurs with caudal anesthesia. The IV infusion is then maintained should the patient require additional hydration or IV medication.

The caudal tray is opened in a sterile manner and the expiration date checked. The gloved anesthetist prepares the skin of the lumbar area with a bactericidal preparation, wiping off the excess solution. The field may be draped with sterile towels.

To create analgesia at the puncture site for the caudal block, the skin overlying the sacral hiatus, i.e., the area between the sacral cornua, is infiltrated with local anesthetic solution using a 25-gauge needle. A 21- or 22-gauge, 1½-inch (3.8-cm) needle may be used to infiltrate the deeper tissues at the entry point for the caudal needle, the subcutaneous tissues over and around the sacral hiatus, and the periosteum of the sacral cornua. A large-bore (18-gauge) needle may be used as an introducer to create an opening in the skin overlying the sacral hiatus. I do not do so because I find that subsequent release of the skin will move the skin hole, resulting in difficult insertion of the caudal needle.

The 3-inch (7.6-cm), 19-gauge caudal needle may be used for this block. The relationship of the notching in the hub to the bevel of the needle is noted. The caudal needle is inserted into the skin with the stylet locked in place and with the bevel turned up. The needle is controlled with the right hand. The shaft is firmly held between the thumb and the middle finger. Pressure is exerted by the index finger on the head of the stylet (Fig 18–14). The initial entry angle for the caudal needle is 70°–80°. The needle is advanced to the level of the sa-

Fig 18–14.—Technique of caudal block. (From Ostheimer G. (ed.): *Manual of Obstetric Anesthesia.* New York, Churchill Livingstone, 1984. Reproduced by permission.)

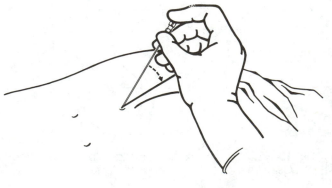

crum. The needle must not be forced against the bone; instead, it is slightly withdrawn, the entry angle reduced by a few degrees, and then the needle is advanced to the level of the sacrococcygeal ligament. Depending on the body type of the patient, the resistance of the sacrococcygeal ligament is met at a depth of approximately ¼–1½ inches (0.5–3.8 cm). At this point, the bevel of the caudal needle is turned ventrally and a shallow entry angle is chosen (Fig 18–15). In the obstetric patient—and in the female patient generally—an angle of 30°–40° is assumed. In the male patient (mentioned here for the sake of completeness) an even shallower angle is used, the needle forming an angle of about 20° because of the lesser angulation of the male sacrum.

The needle is then advanced through the sacrococcygeal ligament and about 1–1½ inches (2.5–3.8 cm) into the caudal canal. The depth of the caudal needle is checked by withdrawing the stylet and holding it over the skin in approximately the same position as the inserted needle. The needle should be below the S-2 level to avoid puncturing the dural sac.

Another method for avoiding puncture of the dural sac involves the use of a 1½-inch (3.8-cm) 19-gauge short bevel needle for the caudal injection. Although the short length of the needle may be a disadvantage in the obsese patient, most patients have little subcutaneous fat overlying the sacrococ-

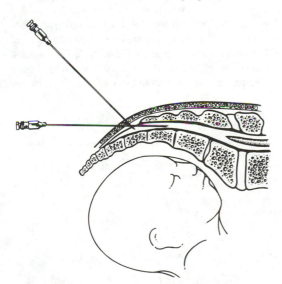

Fig 18–15.—Technique for caudal anesthesia. Note proximity of fetal head. (From Ostheimer G. (ed.): *Manual of Obstetric Anesthesia.* New York, Churchill Livingstone, 1984. Reproduced by permission.)

cygeal ligament. The short length of the needle does not guarantee that puncture of the dural sac or of an epidural blood vessel will be avoided. Aspiration tests in all four quadrants must be performed before the local anesthetic may be injected.

Any needle without a stylet—such as the 19-gauge needle recommended above—may carry a tissue plug into the epidural space. This, however, is not of great importance unless local infection is present. The latter is a contraindication to use of this technique.

After the needle is placed, if the aspiration test yields CSF, an alternate anesthetic technique must be chosen. A bloody return necessitates repositioning of the caudal needle: the needle is withdrawn by about ½ inch (1.5 cm), the stylet is locked in place, and a period of at least 2 minutes is allowed for the traumatized epidural veins to stop bleeding. If repeated aspiration tests after this 2-minute interval continue to produce a bloody return, then the caudal approach must be abandoned in favor of another type of block. A negative aspiration test is an encouraging sign that the needle has been properly placed in the caudal canal. Confirmatory tests, however, must be performed to exclude the possibility of malposition of the needle. The needle may be either lodged under the periosteal layer of the sacrum or along the dorsal surface of the sacrum, and yet give the appearance of proper positioning. Injecting 10 ml of air will identify a malpositioning along the posterior surface of the sacrum since a maneuver will create crepitus in the subcutaneous tissue surrounding the tip of the needle.

A second confirmatory test must be performed to ensure that the caudal needle is positioned correctly. A small syringe is filled with 3 ml of sterile normal saline or local anesthetic solution and attached to the caudal needle. The solution is injected and the plunger of the syringe is quickly released at the very end of the downstroke when the syringe is empty. An easy injection of the fluid without any significant (more than 0.2 ml) return into the syringe and without the appearance of tissue swelling over the sacrum suggests that the needle has been correctly placed. The syringe is detached from the caudal needle, the stylet is locked in place, and the patient's blood pressure and general condition are evaluated. If a test dose of local anesthetic is administered, a period of no less than 2 minutes is allowed for the appearance of any anesthetic effect.

If extensive anesthesia is produced, it may be concluded that the dura has been punctured and that unintentional spinal anesthesia is achieved. In this case, the plans for a caudal block should be abandoned, but it is likely that the sensory block created may be useful for the obstetric procedure at hand. If these tests indicate that the needle is in the caudal canal, then an aspiration test is performed before each incremental or fractional (3–5 ml) dose, which is injected every 60 seconds until the total dose is administered for a "single-shot" caudal block. The caudal needle is then withdrawn and the patient is placed in a comfortable semisitting position. Dosages are listed in Table 18–5.

Technique for Placement of a Caudal Catheter

The technique used to position the caudal needle and to confirm its placement is the same as in the single-dose method.

As in other continuous techniques, it is preferable that the catheter be equipped with a stylet, which makes the passage of the catheter through the needle easier. The plastic catheter is examined for imperfections. The depth markings are noted and compared with the length of the caudal needle. The stylet is withdrawn from the tip of the catheter about 1 inch (2–3 cm). The uncurled catheter is held by the fingers of the left hand and the tip of the catheter is inserted into the hub of the caudal needle by the right hand (for a right-handed anesthetist). The catheter is advanced through the needle, which is held by the left hand so that about 1 inch (2–3 cm) projects past the bevel of the needle into the caudal space. It is important not to force the passage of the catheter since this could result in injury of a nerve

root, trauma to a blood vessel, or puncture of the dura mater.

The needle is removed from the tissues in the following manner: the catheter is held firmly by the right hand approximately an inch (about 2–3 cm) from the hub of the needle while the shaft and hub of the needle are held between the index and middle fingers and thumb of the left hand. While the catheter is held in place with positive forward pressure, the needle is carefully pulled out so that the thumbs of the two hands meet. Forward pressure should be applied to the catheter at all times. The maneuver is then repeated by grasping the tubing another inch (2.5 cm) distal to the hub of the needle and repeating the same procedure. Finally, the tip of the needle will emerge from the skin. The tubing is prevented from being dislodged by applying firm pressure with the thumb and index finger of the left hand to the tubing at the point where it emerges from the skin. The needle is then moved back over the catheter. The thumb and index finger may now move some distance up the catheter and hold the catheter firmly to prevent its dislodgment while the needle and stylet are removed from the catheter by the right hand.

An adapter is attached to the end of the catheter or a blunt small-gauge needle is then inserted into the tubing. Forward repositioning of the needle is impossible once the catheter is advanced beyond the bevel. If forward repositioning is necessary, the needle and the catheter are both completely withdrawn and the block is repeated from the beginning. It is important to remember that once the catheter has advanced beyond the bevel of the epidural needle, any attempt to withdraw it can result in shear-

TABLE 18–5.—LOCAL ANESTHETICS AND DOSAGES FOR SINGLE-DOSE CAUDAL BLOCK FOR VAGINAL DELIVERY

LOCAL ANESTHETIC*	DOSAGE†		ONSET OF ACTION (min)	DURATION OF ANALGESIA (min)
	ml	mg		
Bupivacaine (Sensorcaine, Marcaine) 0.5%	15–25	75–125	5–10	90–180
2-Chloroprocaine (Nesacaine-CE) 2.0%–3.0%	15–25	300–750	3–5	40–60
Lidocaine (Xylocaine) 1.0%–2.0%	15–25	150–500	5–10	60–90
Mepivacaine (Carbocaine) 1.0%–2.0%	15–25	150–500	5–10	60–90

*All without epinephrine.
†Dose range depends on patient's height. Total milligram dose of the local anesthetic should not exceed manufacturer's recommendations.

ing off the catheter. I measure the distance from the hub of the needle to the skin, note the marking on the catheter, and then pull back the catheter to this measured distance after the needle has been removed from the catheter.

Before the catheter is taped in place, a careful aspiration test is performed to ensure that the catheter is not in the subarachnoid space or in an epidural vein. Another test dose of 3 ml of the local anesthetic solution is then injected and the patient is observed for cardiovascular changes, sensory or motor alterations, or CNS toxic reactions over a period of time not less than 2 minutes. Sterile gauze pads are placed above and below the catheter as it emerges out of the skin, and the catheter and pads are secured by pieces of tape. The entire catheter is then taped to the back of the patient and the patient is placed in the left lateral decubitus position with a wedge under the right hip to displace the pregnant uterus to the left.

If vital signs remain satisfactory and no significant anesthesia develops after this second test dose, another aspiration test is done and the fractional doses of local anesthetic (3–5 ml) are administered with a minimum interval of at least 60 seconds until the caudal epidural dose is injected. I do not inject more than 5 ml of local anesthetic at a time. This practice translates to a maximum dose of 25 mg of bupivacaine or 100 mg of lidocaine.

In order to obtain analgesia from T-10 to S-5, the first intermittent caudal dose is the same as in the single-dose method. When the desired level of anesthesia has been achieved with the initial dose, a subsequent top-up dose of about two-thirds the initial dose will maintain this sensory level. Top-up doses are added as necessary. An aspiration test must be done prior to each reinforcement because perforation of the dura mater or of one of the epidural veins by the catheter has been reported and may have occurred since the last administration of the anesthetic. Fractional doses of local anesthetic (3–5 ml) are administered until the appropriate top-up dose has been given. Dosage schedules are listed in Table 18–6.

With the patient resting comfortably, the spread of anesthesia is checked frequently by gentle repeated pinpricks or by a cotton swab moistened with alcohol, in a procedure similar to that with epidural anesthesia, as mentioned previously.

Precautions

Aspiration must precede the injection of the local anesthetic solution for two reasons: to avoid accidental subarachnoid injection and to avoid IV injec-

TABLE 18–6.—LOCAL ANESTHETICS AND DOSAGES FOR CONTINUOUS (INTERMITTENT) CAUDAL BLOCK FOR VAGINAL DELIVERY

| LOCAL ANESTHETIC* | DOSAGE† | | | | ONSET OF ACTION (min) | DURATION OF ACTION (min) | TIME BETWEEN TOP-UP DOSES (min) |
| | FIRST DOSE‡ | | TOP-UP DOSE§ | | | | |
	ml	mg	ml	mg			
Bupivacaine (Sensorcaine, Marcaine) 0.5%	15–25	75–125	8–17	40–85	5–10	90–180	Approx. 120
2-Chloroprocaine (Nesacaine-CE) 2.0%–3.0%	15–25	300–750	8–17	160–510	3–5	40–60	Approx. 45
Lidocaine (Xylocaine) 1.0%–2.0%	15–25	150–500	8–17	80–340	5–10	60–90	Approx. 60
Mepivacaine (Carbocaine) 1.0%–2.0%	15–25	150–500	8–17	80–340	5–10	60–90	Approx. 60

*All without epinephrine.
†Total milligram dose of the local anesthetic should not exceed manufacturer's recommendations.
‡Dose range depends on patient's height.
§The top-up dose is one half to two thirds of the initial dose if this resulted in a satisfactory level of analgesia and if this level is to be maintained.

tion. The caudal dose is a large multiple of that needed for subarachnoid block. Unintentional injection of such an amount of local anesthetic solution into the subarachnoid space would unavoidably result in high or total spinal block. The epidural venous plexus offers a potential for an intravascular injection of a large volume of local anesthetic, which may be followed by CNS excitation and convulsions. Full cardiopulmonary resuscitative equipment must be immediately available, as is customary for any regional block. Maternal hypotension with a concomitant decrease in uteroplacental perfusion producing fetal hypoxia and acidosis is a possibility and must be treated immediately.

Monitoring of vital signs is mandatory for both mother and fetus. Maternal blood pressure must be checked frequently. If a decrease of 10 mm Hg or more occurs, an immediate response is necessary. Therapy consists of an immediate change in the position of the parturient to a more pronounced left (sometimes right) lateral decubitus position, oxygen by face mask, and an increase in the IV infusion rate initiated by a 200–300-ml bolus of an appropriate IV crystalloid solution such as lactated Ringer's. If these measures fail to improve the blood pressure, then 5–10 mg of ephedrine may be injected IV and repeated as necessary.

It is especially important to identify the anatomical landmarks accurately in the obstetric patient. If the tip of the coccyx is mistaken for the sacrococcygeal joint, then the entry point will be distal to the coccyx rather than through the sacral hiatus, and the needle may pierce the rectum and even the presenting part of the fetus. Although rare, accidental injection of the local anesthetic into the fetal head instead of into the caudal canal has been reported. It is obvious that this possibility is increased if caudal block is initiated when the fetal head is low in the pelvis.

Caudal block, along with the subarachnoid, lumbar epidural, and pudendal block techniques, has the potential of eliminating the reflex urge to bear down during the second stage. In the obstetric setting, this may be a liability in that the perineal resistance is needed for a normal internal rotation to occur. To prevent this possible perineal relaxation and the resulting increased incidence of forceps deliveries, the labor nurse will monitor the patient's contractions and the patient is instructed to bear down with each uterine contraction.

Complications

Life-threatening complications should be rare. The unintentional accidental subarachnoid injection of a large volume of drug resulting in a total spinal block is heralded by nausea and hypotension and may progress to respiratory and cardiac arrest.

Unintentional injection of a large portion of the caudal dose into an epidural vein may result in signs of CNS toxicity, including convulsions.

Other serious complications include extradural hematoma at the puncture site and breakage of the needle while positioned in the epidural space.

Hypotension is one possible complication that may arise secondary to the sympathetic block, and it occurs with greater frequency in the obstetric patient. Although the frequency and the degree of hypotension are less with caudal block than with subarachnoid block, the complication does arise in a certain number of patients and the frequency varies with the level to which the caudal block is carried.

Temporary urinary retention may occur as with other blocks and in general anesthesia. The patient may have to be catheterized once or twice, after which she is usually able to void voluntarily.

Indications

The caudal block technique can be modified so as to fill a variety of obstetric anesthesia needs. Properly administered, it gives complete pain relief in 90%–95% of obstetric patients, with the remaining 5%–10% experiencing residual mild discomfort despite analgesia.

A caudal block up to T-10 may be chosen either as a single-dose technique to give anesthesia for the second and third stages of labor or as the catheter technique to manage the whole active phase of labor, including delivery. A caudal block to T-6 may be used for cesarean section in rare instances. However, the mass (volume × concentration) of drug required is approximately twice that needed for lumbar epidural block of the same area.

In addition, the caudal block technique may be used for a wide variety of genitourinary and perineal surgical procedures, therapeutic indications (temporary pain relief as in sciatica, vasodilation as in frostbite of the lower extremities, etc.) and differential diagnostic blocks (e.g., arterial vasospasm of the lower extremities vs. intrinsic vascular pathology).

Contraindications

Absolute contraindications to caudal block include infection at the puncture site involving the skin or deeper tissues (pilonidal cyst), blood dyscrasias or coagulopathies, and active neurologic disease. If sacrococcygeal deformities would make the caudal puncture technically too difficult and therefore potentially traumatic, a lumbar epidural approach may be considered as an alternative.

SPINAL ANESTHESIA (SUBARACHNOID BLOCK)

Anatomy and Landmarks

The subarachnoid space may be safely entered through one of the interspaces between L-2 and L-5 (see Fig 18–7). The dural sac extends to the level of S-2 and the enclosed spinal cord usually extends down to L-1, rarely to L-2. Therefore, a puncture below this level should not encounter the spinal cord. The puncture point for subarachnoid block is established in the following manner. After the most prominent points of the left and right posterior iliac crests have been located, an imaginary line is drawn between these points. It usually crosses the L-4 interspace, i.e., the interspace between the L-4 and L-5 vertebrae (see Fig 18–3). This interspace and the two interspaces above it are usually chosen as points of entry for subarachnoid block. The Taylor approach utilizing the interspace of L5–S1 is rarely used in obstetric anesthesia. In the midline, the entering spinal needle (see Fig 18–2) traverses the skin, the subcutaneous tissue, the supraspinous ligament, the interspinous ligament, and then the ligamentum flavum, which connects the laminae of vertebral arches. The needle then crosses the epidural space filled with loose areolar tissue containing the epidural venous plexus. Finally, the needle pierces the dura and the adherent arachnoid, thus entering the subarachnoid space.

Patient Position

Of the different patient positions for spinal anesthesia, the left or right lateral decubitus position (see Fig 18–3) is generally the most comfortable one for the parturient for vaginal delivery. Because the pregnant patient's hips are frequently wider than her shoulders, care must be taken that the line of the spinous processes of vertebrae is horizontal. To open up the vertebral interspaces, the patient is asked to flex her back by drawing her knees toward her chest. Her head is supported by a small pillow, and her neck should be flexed so that the chin touches the chest.

The obstetric patient usually requires a low block (L10–S5) for an uncomplicated vaginal delivery. At my institution, the lateral decubitus position is the position of choice for the initiation of the block using a hyperbaric solution.

The sitting position may also be used. The obese patient may be easier to block in the sitting position because the line of the spinous processes is not obscured by the subcutaneous fat fold drooping over it. For the sitting position to be most effective for spinal block, the patient sits on the edge of the table with her feet resting on a stool. The neck is flexed so that the chin touches the chest. It is best that the arms are folded across the abdomen, but they may rest loosely supported in the lap. A nurse or an assistant should steady the patient from the front. This support prevents the patient from falling if neurogenic syncope should occur.

It is best to perform the injection of the spinal anesthetic for cesarean delivery with the patient in the right lateral decubitus position. This will prevent concentrating the hyperbaric local anesthetic solution on the left side of the dural sac. Such left-sided pooling of the anesthetic solution occurs when left uterine displacement by right hip elevation is used after initiating the spinal block with the parturient in the left decubitus position. This "puddling" effect may result in an inadequate block on the right side of the patient.

Materials

The following materials should be ready for use when the patient is to be given a subarachnoid block:

One pair of sterile gloves.
Antibacterial solution for cleansing the skin.
One sterile cup for the antibacterial solution.
Forceps.
Sterile gauze pads.
Sterile towels for draping the field.
One 25-gauge, ⅝-inch (1.6-cm) needle for skin infiltration.
One 21- or 22-gauge, 1½-inch (3.8-cm) needle for deep infiltration.

One 18-gauge needle for use as an introducer (if desired).

One 25- or 26-gauge, 3½-inch (8.9-cm) spinal needle with stylet.

One 3-ml syringe.

One 5-ml glass syringe.

One disposable spinal anesthetic tray usually contains all of the above items.

Technique

Thirty ml of a clear antacid (Bicitra) is administered before initiation of the block; otherwise premedication is not given in obstetric anesthesia for vaginal delivery. For cesarean delivery, the patient may require 0.4–0.6 mg of atropine or 0.2–0.4 mg of glycopyrrolate IM and 30 ml of clear antacid (Bicitra) 30–60 minutes preoperatively. Cimetidine, 300 mg PO before sleep and IM 1 hour preoperatively, may be considered. The technique of epidural anesthesia in obstetrics is similar to that for the surgical patient, except that special consideration must be given to the condition of the fetus and to the maternal physiologic changes associated with pregnancy and labor.

Arterial blood pressure must be monitored in any patient undergoing regional anesthesia, but the obstetric patient is carefully observed for changes. The blood pressure is determined in the supine and in the lateral decubitus positions before the block is initiated to check for aortocaval compression (supine hypotensive syndrome). An automatic blood pressure monitor is useful but not mandatory. Routine ECG monitoring is mandatory in our institution for the initiation of an epidural block for labor or cesarean delivery.

The obstetric patient selected for spinal anesthesia is acutely hydrated prior to the induction of the spinal block by using a large-gauge indwelling plastic catheter to administer 1,000 ml of lactated Ringer's solution or similar crystalloid solution over 10–20 minutes before induction of subarachnoid block for vaginal delivery and at least 1,500 ml for cesarean delivery. This hydration helps to prevent the hypotension that may be triggered by the sympathetic block which occurs with spinal anesthesia. The IV infusion is then maintained should the patient require additional hydration or IV medication. In practice, approximately 1,500–2,000 ml of crystalloid solution is usually administered to combat the hypotension before delivery during cesarean delivery. The key to the use of major regional block in obstetrics is to maintain adequate uteroplacental per-

fusion which can be directly monitored via maternal arterial pressure. Decreased perfusion of the intervillous space can place the fetus in jeopardy.

The spinal tray is opened in a sterile manner and the expiration date checked. The gloved anesthetist prepares the skin of the lumbar area with a bactericidal preparation, wiping off the excess solution. The field may be draped with sterile towels. The desired interspace is located and the correct position of the patient is checked. In the decubitus position, the line of the spinous processes must be parallel to the table and the surface of the back must be vertical. This will align the spinous processes in the horizontal plane. Depending on the special anatomical features of the patient, the second, third, or fourth lumbar interspace may be found most suitable. The selected entry point is infiltrated with a small amount of local anesthetic using a 25-gauge needle to create the skin wheal. Then a small amount (about 1–3 ml) of local anesthetic may be injected into the subcutaneous tissue and the interspinous ligament. When satisfactory analgesia of the entry point has been created, an 18-gauge needle is used as an introducer and is inserted through the skin wheal. The index and the middle fingers of the free hand straddle the interspace to fix the tissues of the underlying structures (Fig 18–16). The introducer is used to create a passage for the spinal needle and, theoretically, prevent carrying a plug of skin or fat into the subarachnoid space. However, some anesthetists prefer not to use an introducer.

The introducer is inserted into the interspinous area with this horizontal position maintained. An improperly inserted introducer makes it impossible

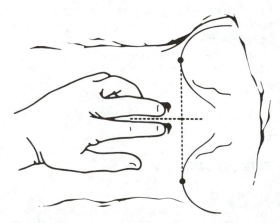

Fig 18–16.—Identification of intervertebral space. (From Ostheimer G. (ed.): *Manual of Obstetric Anesthesia.* New York, Churchill Livingstone, 1984. Reproduced by permission.)

to point the needle in the correct direction. It is preferable to select a thin-gauged (No. 25 or 26) spinal needle for the procedure to reduce the incidence of spinal headache to a minimum. The needle must first be examined for any imperfections or weaknesses. It should be noted that the bevel of the needle is on the same side as the key notch for the stylet in the hub of the needle. Once the physician is satisfied with the needle, he should insert it in such a fashion that the bevel does not cut across the longitudinal fibers of the dura. In practice, this may not be possible. Therefore, the bevel, as indicated by the key notch, should face laterally during its passage through the dura. The spinal needle is held between the thumb, index, and middle fingers and inserted through the introducer (Fig 18–17). The spinal needle is then slowly advanced. Its progress through the tissues is followed by noting the variations in resistance as the various structures are penetrated. First, the firm resistance of the interspinous ligament and the ligamentum flavum is felt, after which a lessening of resistance is observed as the needle crosses the epidural space. This is followed by the characteristic "pop," an abrupt disappearance of a last resistance, as the needle pierces the dura to enter the subarachnoid space. The anesthetist now may check his needle position by withdrawing the stylet to see if CSF appears (Fig 18–18) at the hub of the needle and by aspirating with a syringe, as CSF may not immediately appear because of the small diameter of the spinal needle.

There are several other reasons why CSF may fail to appear:

1. A nerve root or the dura may block the bevel

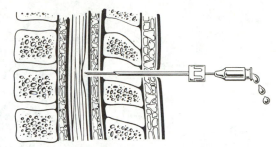

Fig 18–18.—Subarachnoid puncture, followed by appearance of cerebrospinal fluid. (From Ostheimer G. (ed.): *Manual of Obstetric Anesthesia.* New York, Churchill Livingstone, 1984. Reproduced by permission.)

of the needle. After withdrawing the stylet, try rotating the needle 90°–180° to see if the bevel can be freed of this obstruction.

2. The CSF pressure may be too low to push the fluid through the needle. The anesthetist should always confirm the needle position by achieving free flow of CSF when aspirating with a syringe.

3. A tissue plug may be blocking the bevel. This also will be dislodged by an aspiration attempt.

4. The bevel may still be in the epidural space, at least partially. Therefore, the anesthetist should replace the stylet in the needle and then slowly advance the needle a small distance. Then the above maneuvers are repeated.

If contact with bone has been made, stop. The needle must not be forced against this resistance because the lumen of the needle can be easily blocked and the needle point can become "barbed." If you think that the needle lumen is plugged, take the needle out and flush it with normal saline or local anesthetic solution. Contact with bone usually means that the vertebral lamina has been encountered. This necessitates a small change of the direction of the spinal needle. To do this effectively, the needle point is withdrawn completely into the introducer and then a fresh attempt is made for a puncture in a different direction (usually cephalad). Success is indicated by the appearance of CSF in the hub of the spinal needle. When this is achieved, the hub of the spinal needle is held firmly between the index finger and thumb of the left hand of the right-handed anesthetist to prevent any displacement of the needle from its proper location. Aspiration is performed with a syringe to ascertain free flow of CSF. The back of the anesthetist's hand is steadied against the patient's back (Fig 18–19). A syringe filled with the appropriate dose of local anesthetic solution is attached to the spinal needle.

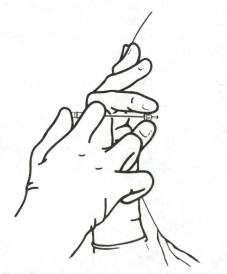

Fig 18–17.—Insertion of spinal needle.

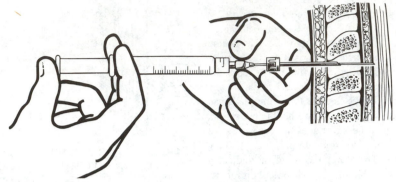

Fig 18–19.—Proper hand position for injection of spinal anesthetic. (From Ostheimer G. (ed.): *Manual of Obstetric Anesthesia.* New York, Churchill Livingstone, 1984. Reproduced by permission.)

Negative pressure is applied to the syringe to draw up a small amount of CSF to ascertain that the proper position of the needle bevel has been maintained. Mixing of the CSF and anesthetic will occur during aspiration. Then the contents of the syringe are injected slowly so as not to create a jet effect in the subarachnoid space. I prefer a small volume (0.2 ml) of aspiration and reinjection after the local anesthetic has been injected to rule out accidental movement of the needle during the insertion of the drug.

The appropriate dose of local anesthetic for the obstetric patient (Tables 18–7 and 18–8) is 30%–50% less than that given to a surgical patient. Incidentally, this dosage reduction is indicated for any patient with increased intra-abdominal pressure, including surgical patients with ascites or large intra-abdominal tumors.

Following the injection of the local anesthetic, the needle and the introducer are withdrawn together and the patient is immediately placed in the supine position. Her uterus is displaced to the left by placing a wedge or a folded blanket under the right hip. Oxygen is administered by face mask and the blood pressure is monitored.

With the patient resting comfortably, the spread of anesthesia is checked frequently by gentle repeated pinpricks or a cotton swab moistened with alcohol. Since the loss of pain and temperature sensation progresses simultaneously, the use of alcohol to check the spread of anesthesia may be more pleasant for the patient. Repeated pinpricks may accurately differentiate the area of complete loss of pain sensation from that of partial analgesia.

When the block reaches the desired segmental level, the patient may be positioned so as to prevent any further spread of the anesthetic. The local anesthetic drug "fixes" to the neuronal elements, so that usually no further spread of anesthetic effect is seen after a "fixation time" of 7–10 minutes.

The spread of the local anesthetic depends on specific gravity relationships, the baricity between

TABLE 18–7.—LOCAL ANESTHETICS AND DOSAGES FOR SUBARACHNOID ANESTHESIA FOR VAGINAL DELIVERY

| LOCAL ANESTHETIC | BARICITY | DOSE BY PATIENT HEIGHT | | | ONSET OF ACTION (min) | DURATION OF ACTION (min) |
		5'	5'6"	6'0"		
Lidocaine 5% (Xylocaine) in 7.5% dextrose in water (premixed)	Hyperbaric	35 mg (0.7 ml)	40 mg (0.8 ml)	45–50 mg (0.9–1.0 ml)	1–3	45–75
Tetracaine 1% (Pontocaine*) and equal volume of 10% dextrose in water	Hyperbaric	5 mg (0.5 ml) + 0.5 ml	6 mg (0.6 ml) + 0.6 ml	7 mg (0.7 ml) + 0.7 ml	3–5	120–180
Total volume		1.0 ml	1.2 ml	1.4 ml		

*Pontocaine is a registered trademark of Breon Laboratories.

TABLE 18–8.—LOCAL ANESTHETICS AND DOSAGES FOR SUBARACHNOID ANESTHESIA
FOR CESAREAN SECTION

LOCAL ANESTHETIC	BARICITY	DOSE BY PATIENT HEIGHT					ONSET OF ACTION (min)	DURATION OF ACTION (min)
		5′	5′3″	5′6″	5′9″	6′0″		
Lidocaine 5% (Xylocaine) in 7.5% dextrose in water (premixed)	Hyperbaric	50 mg (1.0 ml)	55 mg (1.1 ml)	60 mg (1.2 ml)	65 mg (1.3 ml)	70 mg (1.4 ml)	1–3	45–75
Tetracaine 1% (Pontocaine) and equal volume of 10% dextrose in water	Hyperbaric	7 mg (0.7 ml) + 0.7 ml	8 mg (0.8 ml) + 0.8 ml	9 mg (0.9 ml) + 0.9 ml	10 mg (1.0 ml) + 1.0 ml	11 mg (1.1 ml) + 1.1 ml	3–5	120–180
Total volume		1.4 ml	1.6 ml	1.8 ml	2.0 ml	2.2 ml		

the local anesthetic solution used and that of the CSF. Normally, the specific gravity of CSF is 1.003–1.009.

A hyperbaric solution has a higher specific gravity than CSF so that it will move to low-lying parts of the subarachnoid space. If anesthesia of just the perineal area is desired ("saddle block"), this is achieved by placing the patient in the sitting position, as previously described, and allowing her to remain sitting for 30 seconds to 1 minute following injection.

A hypobaric solution has a specific gravity less than that of CSF and it will, therefore, spread to higher lying areas within the subarachnoid space. An isobaric solution, with a specific gravity matching that of CSF, tends to remain at the injection point, even after the fixation time.

Precautions

To ensure safety and success of spinal anesthesia, several precautions should be taken. The entry point for the needle should be below the level of L-2 so as to avoid injury to the spinal cord.

The spinal needle on occasion may puncture one of the epidural vessels, resulting in a blood-tinged return of CSF at the hub of the needle. If this occurs, the anesthetist should wait until the return clears. If the CSF return fails to clear, an attempt is made to repeat the block through the same or another interspace, using a new spinal needle.

The vital signs must be monitored continuously, especially in the initial 10 minutes, i.e., during the fixation of the block, with close attention paid to any fall in blood pressure. In the obstetric patient, uterine displacement and IV hydration will help to prevent hypotension due to aortocaval compression by the gravid uterus and subsequent uteroplacental

hypoperfusion.[50] Oxygen administration by mask to the mother is helpful to combat cerebral hypoxia, which will manifest itself by the appearance of nausea. When a hyperbaric solution is used, a modified head-up position, with a pillow under the head, is advisable in order to prevent an excessive cephalad spread of the block and to make the parturient more comfortable.

Complications

The most common complication of spinal anesthesia in obstetrics is maternal hypotension secondary to the combined effect of the decreased venous return produced by blockade of the sympathetic vascular tone and the aortocaval compression by the gravid uterus.

Should vasopressor therapy be needed, pure receptor stimulating agents should be avoided because these drugs correct the systemic blood pressure by vasoconstriction. Such an effect reduces uteroplacental perfusion and thereby compromises the fetus.[65]

Ephedrine (increments of 10 mg IV) is the best choice at present because it corrects the blood pressure predominantly by myocardial stimulation without compromising the placental circulation. It should be administered immediately when a significant (>10 mm Hg) decline in blood pressure develops, to minimize nausea and preserve fetal well-being.[66]

Life-threatening complications are rare and for the most part are due to an excessive cephalad spread of the local anesthetic causing total spinal anesthesia. This occurrence is heralded by nausea secondary to cerebral hypoxia and hypotension and can progress to respiratory and cardiac arrest. This highlights the importance of meticulous monitoring of the vital signs and of the spread of anesthetic effect after the block is initiated. Standard cardiopulmonary resuscitation must be begun at once should a respiratory or a cardiac arrest occur. If aortocaval compression is thought to be interfering with resuscitative efforts, immediate delivery of the fetus should be performed by cesarean delivery.

Neurologic complications secondary to needle trauma are very rare but have occurred if the dural puncture is performed above the level of L-2, resulting in spinal cord injury. If a paresthesia is elicited, no injection should be made. The needle should be immediately repositioned.

Minor complications include the possibility of postpartum urinary retention and post-dural puncture headache. The tendency to urinary retention is present with most types of anesthesia, including general anesthesia. The condition is temporary, and it is managed by a bladder assessment and catheterization until normal bladder function resumes. Post-dural puncture headache (spinal headache) occurs in a small percentage of patients and it is most troublesome when the patient must resume normal activity as soon as possible. Unfortunately, the parturient is in the group that has the highest incidence of post-dural puncture headache. The diagnosis is made by having the patient sit up or stand up. Headache commences within a few minutes and is relieved by lying down. Its incidence is diminished when the patient is acutely hydrated before the block and when thin-gauged (25- or 26-gauge) needles are used. Persistent severe post-dural puncture headache not responding to hydration, bed rest, and analgesics may be treated with an epidural blood patch.

Meningitis, although rare, may result from contamination of the subarachnoid space during the initiation of spinal anesthesia in the presence of septicemia, local superficial injection of the lumbar area, or contaminated equipment.

Indications

This technique provides excellent anesthesia for vaginal and cesarean delivery.

Contraindications

Absolute contraindications to spinal anesthesia include infection of the meninges of the spinal cord, septicemia, local cutaneous infections at the puncture site, blood dyscrasias or coagulopathies, and acute neurologic disease. Proved allergy to a local anesthetic agent mandates the choice of a local anesthetic drug from a different chemical family.

In other situations, e.g., in the cardiac patient, the advantage of spinal anesthesia must be weighed against problems arising from the potential cardiovascular side effects of the block.

Several deformities of the lumbosacral spine may make spinal anesthesia technically so difficult that the potential for trauma may be unacceptably high.

Continuous (Intermittent) Spinal Anesthesia

Continuous spinal block is not suitable for obstetric anesthesia. The incidence of post-dural puncture headache after this block can be expected to be unacceptably high because the nature of the procedure is liable to make the loss of CSF clinically significant. The spinal needle must be of a large gauge, and therefore it will produce a relatively large dural defect; the presence of the catheter inserted through the dura also potentiates the loss of CSF by a wicking effect.

PUDENDAL NERVE BLOCK

Anatomy and Landmarks

The pudendal nerve originates from S2–4 (Fig 18–20). It leaves the pelvis by way of the lower part of the greater sciatic foramen, curves around the spine of the ischium, crosses the sacrospinous ligament close to its attachment to the ischial spine, and then reenters the pelvis alongside the internal pudendal artery at the lesser sciatic foramen. The pudendal nerve then branches into the inferior hemorrhoidal (rectal) nerve, the perineal nerve, and the dorsal nerve of the clitoris. These nerves are best blocked at the ischial tuberosity. Because it is also easily palpable, the ischial tuberosity is an important anatomical landmark.

The perineal area also derives additional innervation from the pudendal branch of the posterior femoral cutaneous nerve, which supplies mostly the posterior labial portion of the perineum.

Although the major innervation to the anterior aspect of the perineum is carried by the perineal nerve and the dorsal nerve of the clitoris, a secondary nerve supply is also provided by the ilioinguinal (L-1) and the genitofemoral (L1–2) nerves. Therefore,

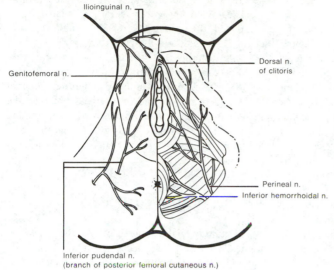

Ilioinguinal n.

Genitofemoral n.

Dorsal n. of clitoris

Perineal n.
Inferior hemorrhoidal n.

Inferior pudendal n.
(branch of posterior femoral cutaneous n.)

Fig 18–20.—Innervation of the female perineum. (From Ostheimer G. (ed.): *Manual of Obstetric Anesthesia.* New York, Churchill Livingstone, 1984. Reproduced by permission.)

these must be blocked by supplemental infiltration if thorough anesthesia of the anterior portions of the labia majora and the mons pubis is needed.

Patient Position

For the pudendal block, the patient is placed in the lithotomy position.

Materials

The following materials are needed:
One pair of sterile gloves.
Antibacterial solution for cleansing the skin.
One sterile cup for the antibacterial solution.
Forceps.
Sterile gauze pads.
Sterile towels.
One 25-gauge, ⅝-inch (1.6-cm) needle for skin infiltration.
One 22-gauge, 3- to 4-inch (7.5–10-cm) short beveled needle for the pudendal block and infiltration of the labia and perineum.
One 10-ml syringe with finger rings. These materials are required for a unilateral pudendal block. In obstetrics, bilateral pudendal blocks are necessary.
If the transvaginal technique is chosen, the special transvaginal needle with the appropriate guide, e.g., the Kobak needle or Iowa trumpet with a 6-inch (15.2-cm), 20-gauge needle, is used.

Technique

The pudendal block can be performed by either the perineal route or the transvaginal route.

The Perineal Technique

The perineal route has the advantage that the branches of both the pudendal nerve and the posterior femoral cutaneous nerve can be blocked from the same injection point as they are both in close proximity to the ischial tuberosity. With the patient in the lithotomy position, the perineal area is cleansed with an aqueous antibacterial solution and the ischial tuberosity is palpated. An intradermal wheal is raised at the site of the ischial tuberosity, injecting a small amount of a local anesthetic through a 25-gauge needle. The 10-ml syringe is filled with the local anesthetic and is attached to the 3- to 4-inch (7.5- to 10-cm) needle. The needle is then inserted through the wheal at a right angle to the skin. The needle is advanced slowly into the tissues, with small amounts of the local anesthetic injected as the needle is advanced. The index finger of the left hand is inserted into the vagina or rectum and the tuberosity of the ischium is palpated.

This index finger now guides the needle toward the ischial tuberosity. This structure is usually encountered at a depth of about 1–1½ inches (2.5 cm) from the skin, depending on the size of the patient. With the needle in place, 5–10 ml of the local anesthetic solution is injected at the anterolateral aspect of the ischial spine as well as under the tuberosity to block the inferior pudendal branch of the posterior femoral cutaneous curve. The syringe now must be detached from the needle, refilled, and reattached. The needle then is advanced to the medial aspect of the ischial spine, where another 5–10 ml of the local anesthetic solution is injected to block the branches of the pudendal nerve. Since the pudendal artery and vein run parallel to the pudendal nerve in this area, the injection of the local anesthetic should be intermittent, with an aspiration performed between the injection of each 2–3 ml of the local anesthetic solution. This will prevent an intravascular injection of a significant amount of local anesthetic drug. If blood is seen on aspiration, the needle should be repositioned until no more blood is observed on aspiration. The syringe is refilled again and about 5–10 ml of the local anesthetic is injected as the needle is advanced about 1 inch (2.5 cm) past the ischial tuberosity into the ischiorectal fossa. This blocks the pudendal nerve in Alcock's canal. The syringe is refilled one last time and the point of the needle is advanced posteriorly to the ischial spine, using the index finger in the vagina or rectum as guide. The finger can palpate the sacrospinous ligament and it guides the needle in this direction until the "popping" sensation indicates that the needle pierced the ligament. The needle is advanced another ¼ inch (0.5 cm) and 5–10 ml of the local anesthetic solution is injected at this point to block the pudendal nerve before it branches. The

needle is now withdrawn. The other side is now blocked. When the contralateral pudendal block is completed, the anesthetist prepares to block the secondary innervation of the perineum.

Using a sterile, 3- to 4-inch (7.5- to 10-cm) needle, one can now proceed to infiltrate the area that is ⅝ inch (1.5 cm) lateral and parallel to the labium majorum, from the middle of the labium to the mons pubis. This blocks the secondary innervation from the iliohypogastric, ilioinguinal, and the genitofemoral nerves. This infiltration, too, is usually performed bilaterally.

The Transvaginal Technique

The transvaginal technique utilizes the same anatomical landmarks. A specialized transvaginal needle and guide assembly is needed, such as the Kobak needle or Iowa trumpet and a 6-inch (15.2-cm), 20-gauge needle.

The patient is in the lithotomy position and the perineum is prepared with an antibacterial solution. The index and middle fingers of one hand are inserted into the vagina until the ischial spine and the sacrospinous ligament can be palpated. With the transvaginal needle withdrawn into the shaft of the guide, the Kobak needle or the Iowa trumpet is inserted into the vagina and its point is positioned on the sacrospinous ligament as it attaches to the ischial spine (Fig 18–21). The needle is then advanced about ⅝ inch (1.6 cm) past the surface of the mu-

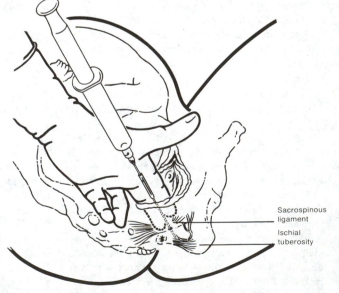

Fig 18–21.—Pudendal block—transvaginal approach. (From Ostheimer G. (ed.): *Manual of Obstetric Anesthesia.* New York, Churchill Livingstone, 1984. Reproduced by permission.)

Sacrospinous ligament

Ischial tuberosity

cosa until it "pops" through the mucous membrane and the sacrospinous ligament. About 5–10 ml of the local anesthetic solution is injected into this location, with aspiration performed after the injection of each 2–3 ml to ensure that the solution is not being injected into the pudendal artery or vein, which lie here in close proximity. If blood return is observed in the syringe, the needle is moved until no such blood return is observed on aspiration. In obstetrics, the block is then repeated on the other side.

A supplementary infiltration of the area lateral to the labia majora to provide analgesia of the anterior perineum may be performed as described previously. See Table 18–9 for dosages.

In practice, the transvaginal technique is most commonly used.

Precautions

Frequent aspirations must be performed when injecting the local anesthetic solution to ensure that the drug is not injected into the pudendal vessels, which lie close to the pudendal nerve.

If the block is done outside the delivery room, cardiopulmonary resuscitation equipment must be immediately available. Delivery rooms must be fully supplied with the same anesthesia and resuscitative equipment as is found in the operating suite (see appendix).

Complications

When the needle is in the vicinity of the ischial spine, care must be taken that the rectal mucosa is not pierced. Although the ischial spine can be pal-

TABLE 18–9.—DOSE PER INJECTION SITE

ROUTE	DOSE (ML)
Perineal	
Anterolateral and inferior aspects of ischial tuberosity	5–10
Medial aspect of ischial tuberosity	5–10
Ischiorectal fossa	5–10
Posterior aspect of sacrospinous ligament	5–10
Transvaginal	
Posterior aspect of sacrospinous ligament	10

pated through the vagina as well as the rectum, the technique of palpating the anatomical landmarks through the rectum is superior since it provides assurance that the rectal mucosa is not pierced.

Indications

There are four indications for pudendal block:

1. Anesthesia of the perineum for the second stage of an uncomplicated obstetric delivery. It should be noted, however, that the uterine contractions are not painless when this method of anesthesia is used, as they would be if a spinal, epidural, or caudal block were performed.

2. Perineal and rectal surgery, with premedication according to the needs of the patient.

3. Differential diagnosis of perineal pain.

4. Relief of pain and perineal pruritis, as in carcinoma of the vulva.

Contraindications

A contraindication to this block is localized injection at the site of needle puncture.

APPENDIX

RESUSCITATION EQUIPMENT

Resuscitative equipment must be immediately available if a regional block is administered outside the delivery room. Of course, the delivery room must have the same type and quality of anesthetic equipment as a surgical operating room.

Adult resuscitative equipment

1. Oxygen apparatus: Including a source of 100% oxygen and a delivery system such as a bag and mask or any one of several commercially available reinflatable bag-and-mask kits.
2. Suctioning apparatus: Essential to help clear the airway of secretions or other material if

regurgitation of gastric contents or active vomiting occurs.

3. Airways, oral, nasal, and endotracheal tubing. If the airway becomes compromised, intubation should be performed with the aid of succinylcholine (1–1½ mg/kg).

4. Laryngoscope: With a variety of blades and sizes.

5. Electrocardiograph/cardiac defibrillator: In combination and portable.

6. Drugs:
   a. General: IV fluids, vasopressors, diphenhydramine, and succinylcholine.
   b. CNS toxic reactions: From accidental intravascular injection or rapid systemic absorption; succinylcholine for endotracheal intubation and diazepam or thiopental for CNS depression.
   c. Cardiopulmonary depression or arrest: Vasopressors (epinephrine for myocardial stimulation/ephedrine for hypotension unresponsive to bolus infusion of IV fluids), sodium bicarbonate, calcium chloride, lidocaine, propranolol, isoproterenol, potassium chloride, digoxin, etc. Cardiopulmonary resuscitation must be initiated if a CNS toxic reaction or myocardial depression leads to severe cardiopulmonary collapse or arrest.

INTRAVASCULAR INJECTION

Treatment of CNS reaction secondary to unintentional intravascular injection:

1. Maintain an adequate airway for effective ventilation (endotracheal intubation may be necessary).

2. Administer 100% oxygen by mask or bag or by intermittent positive pressure ventilation if necessary.

3. Use succinylcholine to facilitate endotracheal intubation if necessary.

4. Administer diazepam IV in incremental doses of 2.5 mg or an ultrashort-acting barbiturate, e.g., thiopental, in incremental doses of 50 mg to stop the convulsions.

5. Monitor maternal vital signs.

6. Monitor fetal heart rate.

7. Place the parturient in the lateral decubitus position and continue to administer oxygen.

8. Treat hypotension with an infusion of crystalloid solution and/or ephedrine in 10-mg increments IV, as needed.

9. Expedite delivery if the fetus is in jeopardy; otherwise delay delivery to permit maternal disposal of local anesthetic.

10. Continue cardiopulmonary resuscitation as needed.

Oxygenation is the key to the successful management of this problem. It is mandatory that resuscitative equipment and appropriate drugs be immediately available when any local anesthetic is administered by any route.

SUBARACHNOID INJECTION

Treatment of massive subarachnoid injection:

1. Utilize the same technique as stated above for treatment of intravascular injection, with the exception that CNS depression with diazepam or thiopental is not necessary. Thiopental may be used to induce sleep, however, which is then maintained by an inhalation technique.

2. Place the patient in the Trendelenberg position as soon as possible after the injection occurs to attempt to limit the spread, as most epidural anesthetic solutions are hypobaric in the subarachnoid space.

3. Attempt to aspirate at least 10 ml of CSF and local anesthetic from the subarachnoid space, if possible, to decrease the amount of local anesthetic in contact with the spinal cord and nerves.

ANESTHESIA FOR THE HIGH-RISK PARTURIENT

I. Introduction
   Parturients are designated as "high risk" because of various problems that might arise in the antenatal or peripartum periods. Anesthetic management, both the choice and the technique, should be based on a thorough understanding of the physiology of pregnancy and the pathophysiology of the problems which made the parturients "high risk."[67–69]

II. Classification
   A. Maternal
      1. Problems related to pregnancy, labor and delivery:

a. Antepartum hemorrhage: placenta previa, abruptio placentae.

b. Hypertensive disorders of pregnancy.

2. Problems unrelated to pregnancy:
   a. Diabetes mellitus.
   b. Cardiac disorders.
   c. Respiratory disorders.
   d. Neurologic disorders.
   e. Renal disorders.
   f. Hematologic disorders.
   g. Endocrinologic disorders.
   h. Miscellaneous disorders: maternal addiction, history of malignant hyperthermia, obesity, maternal age, etc.

B. Fetal
1. Problems related to pregnancy, labor and delivery:
   a. Prematurity.
   b. Postmaturity.
   c. Multiple gestations.
   d. Abnormal presentations.
   e. Intrauterine growth retardation.
   f. Prolapsed cord.
   g. Placental insufficiency:
      (1) Toxemia.
      (2) Diabetes mellitus.
   h. Maternal addiction.

III. Techniques of Anesthesia (Keys to Successful Management):

A. Subarachnoid Block
1. Nonparticulate (clear) antacid: 30 ml within 1 hour before surgery.
2. Adequate acute hydration (approximately 1,000 ml of Ringer's lactate solution for vaginal delivery; 1,500 ml for cesarean delivery) to expand the circulating intravascular volume before initiation of block. A large-bore IV catheter, 0–16 gauge or larger, is preferred.
3. Avoid supine position to prevent aortocaval compression.
4. Small needle (25 or 26 gauge) to reduce the incidence of post-dural puncture headache.
5. Tetracaine, tetracaine-procaine, lidocaine, or bupivacaine (when approved by FDA).
6. Prompt treatment of hypotension with bolus infusion of crystalloid and 10-mg

increments of ephedrine IV as needed.
7. Oxygen by face mask (≥ 6 L/min).
8. Minimize induction: delivery interval.
9. Minimize uterine incision: delivery interval.

B. Epidural Block
1. Nonparticulate (clear) antacid: 30 ml within 1 hour before surgery.
2. Adequate acute hydration (approximately 1,000 ml of Ringer's lactate solution for vaginal delivery, 1,500 ml for cesarean delivery) before initiation of block via large-bore IV catheter— 16-gauge or larger is preferred.
3. Avoid supine position to prevent aortocaval compression.
4. Proper selection of the local anesthetic: bupivacaine, lidocaine, and chloroprocaine.
5. Prompt treatment of hypotension with bolus infusion of crystalloid and 10-mg increments of ephedrine IV, as needed.
6. Oxygen by face mask (≥ 6 L/min).
7. Minimize induction: delivery interval.
8. Minimize uterine incision: delivery interval.

C. General Anesthesia
1. Nonparticulate (clear) antacid: 30 ml within 1 hour before surgery.
2. Avoid the supine position to prevent aortocaval compression.
3. Preinduction oxygenation for 3–5 minutes and then rapid-sequence IV induction utilizing cricoid pressure.
4. Limit thiopental dosage to a bolus of 4 mg/kg of pregnant body weight.
5. Succinylcholine, 1.0–1.5 mg/kg of pregnant body weight.
6. Minimal inspired oxygen concentration of 50%.
7. Avoid hypoventilation or hyperventilation.
8. Minimize induction: delivery interval.
9. Minimize uterine incision: delivery interval.
10. It is not our practice to use a nondepolarizing agent before induction. We *want* to see fasciculations in order to know *when* to perform intubation. Fasciculations do *not* produce much muscle pain in the parturient. Certainly, their intensity is less.

During general anesthesia, a prolonged induction-to-delivery interval and uterine incision-to-delivery interval are associated with a higher incidence of low Apgar scores and acidotic babies. On the other hand, with spinal anesthesia in the absence of hypotension, a longer induction-to-delivery interval does not alter either Apgar scores or the acid-base values of the neonates.[68] However, a uterine incision-to-delivery interval of more than 180 seconds is associated with a high incidence of low Apgar scores and acidotic infants, possibly related to reduced placental circulation.

IV. Specific Problems
  A. *Antepartum hemorrhage* is the major cause of maternal mortality in the obstetric patient. Severe bleeding during the antepartum period is usually due to (1) placenta previa or (2) abruptio placentae.
    1. Anesthetic consideration for placenta previa:[70]
      a. If actively bleeding: Emergency cesarean section utilizing general anesthesia. Blood, plasma, and crystalloids should be transfused as rapidly as possible at a rate determined by blood pressure, central venous pressure, and urine output. Induction of anesthesia should include either a small dose of thiopental (200 mg or 1–2 mg/kg) and/or ketamine (100 mg or 1 mg/kg) if there is significant hypotension.
      b. If not bleeding: Major regional anesthesia (subarachnoid or epidural block) may be used if the patient so desires, provided there is no evidence of hypovolemia.
    2. Anesthetic considerations for abruptio placentae
    Major problems:
      a. If actively bleeding: Emergency cesarean section under general anesthesia. Blood, plasma, and crystalloids should be infused as rapidly as possible at a rate determined by blood pressure, central venous pressure, and urine output. Induction of anesthesia should include either a small dose of thiopental (200 mg or 1–2 mg/kg) and/or ketamine (100

mg or 1 mg/kg) if there is significant hypotension.
      b. May be associated with defects in blood coagulation.[71] Diagnostic tests include hemoglobin/hematocrit, clotting time, platelet count, prothrombin time, and presence of fibrin split products.

The following are contraindications to epidural or spinal anesthesia in our practice:
(1) Prothrombin time twice laboratory control value.
(2) Partial thromboplastin time twice laboratory control value.
(3) Platelet count less than 100,000 cu/mm.
(4) Bleeding time greater than 10 minutes.
(5) Fibrinogen less than 200 mg/dl.
(6) Presence of fibrin split products.

If there is no evidence of maternal hypovolemia or uteroplacental insufficiency, and if the clotting studies are normal, continuous epidural anesthesia may be used for labor and vaginal delivery. If there is severe abruption, emergency delivery should be performed under general anesthesia. Massive and rapid blood transfusion might be necessary. If the infant is alive at delivery, active resuscitation is usually required because of the maternal and fetal hypovolemia resulting in neonatal shock.

B. Toxemia in Pregnancy
  Toxemia is the major hypertensive disorder seen in pregnancy. Pre-eclampsia is the development of hypertension (systolic BP >140 mm Hg, diastolic >90 mm Hg), proteinuria, or edema before the 20th week of gestation. Eclampsia is the pre-eclamptic condition associated with grand mal seizures not related to any neurologic disorder.
    1. Major problems:
      a. Hypertension.
      b. Diminished plasma volume.
      c. Reduced cardiac output.
      d. Generalized vasoconstriction.
      e. Enhanced reactivity to both vasoconstricting and vasodilating drugs.

f. Uteroplacental insufficiency.

g. CNS hyperexcitability.

h. Hepatic involvement.

i. Possible disseminated intravascular coagulation (DIC).

j. Renal involvement and chances of oliguria or azotemia.

k. Drug interaction: Medications like magnesium sulfate, hydralazine, diazepam, phenobarbital, and diuretics may interact with different anesthetic techniques or drugs.

2. Anesthetic considerations:

a. For labor and delivery, properly administered epidural anesthesia is the method of choice. This will help to control blood pressure, increase renal and uterine perfusion, and control pain, which will prevent endogenous catecholamine secretion and consequently further reduction of placental perfusion.

b. For cesarean delivery, especially when severe hypertension is present, we believe general anesthesia is indicated.

(1) Advantage: Avoidance of hypotension, especially with the presence of inadequately corrected hypovolemia.

(2) Disadvantage: General anesthesia will cause exaggeration of hypertension during intubation. This can be minimized by the judicious IV use of small doses of hydralazine (10 mg) before induction. Trimethophan (6.1%), sodium nitroprusside (200 μg/ml), or nitroglycerin (100 μg/ml) by controlled infusion might be necessary.

(3) IV lidocaine might be considered before intubation.

(4) Remember the augmented action of neuromuscular blockers, both depolarizers and nondepolarizers, in the patient who has been receiving magnesium sulfate.

(5) Spinal anesthesia should be avoided, because of the abrupt hypotension which may develop in these patients.

(6) Epidural anesthesia may be used provided hypovolemia is corrected before the induction of the regional block.

In 1979 Joyce et al.[72] demonstrated the efficacy of volume replacement to return the maternal CVP to a "normal" level prior to the induction of epidural anesthesia. This group also demonstrated that the infusion of albumin was safe when compared to plasmanate for volume expansion in such cases. On the other hand, patients with severe toxemia may present with increased afterload with normal CVP and isolated left ventricular dysfunction. Reduction of afterload with arteriolar vasodilators should be the initial treatment in such cases. Hemodynamically, severe pre-eclampsia has such a variable expression that not all patients with the diagnosis of severe pre-eclampsia should be classified under one diagnostic umbrella.

3. Summary

a. Vaginal delivery: Provided there is no coagulation problem, epidural anesthesia should be used for labor and delivery because this will:

(1) Relieve the pain of contractions.

(2) Help to control blood pressure.

(3) Increase placental perfusion by preventing secretion of endogenous catecholamines.

b. Cesarean delivery:

(1) General anesthesia: Since it is mandatory to prevent an increase in baseline blood pressure (especially if the systolic BP is above 200 mm Hg), the reflex increase of baseline blood pressure should be blocked by using a hypotensive drug before induction. Magnesium sulfate potentiates the action of neuromuscular blockers.

(2) Regional anesthesia: Spinal anesthesia should be avoided because of the possibility of a profound drop in blood pres-

sure, with the onset of sympathetic blockade.

C. Diabetes Mellitus
  1. Major problems:
     a. Placental insufficiency.
     b. Superimposed pre-eclampsia.
     c. Diabetic nephropathy.
     d. Increased tendency to ketoacidosis.
  2. Anesthesia management for labor and vaginal delivery:
     a. Small doses of narcotics will provide moderate pain relief.
     b. Lumbar epidural block can provide excellent pain relief both for labor and delivery. Shnider and Levinson[69] suggested that epidural anesthesia will reduce the maternal endogenous catecholamines during labor, which might benefit placental perfusion. Pearson[73] studied epidural anesthesia for high-risk parturients. She noted that the fetus began the second stage in a less acidotic state when mothers received epidural anesthesia than when mothers did not receive any anesthesia.[27] The acidosis was metabolic in origin and was related to high lactate concentrations.
     c. During labor, 1,000 ml of 5% dextrose in lactated Ringer's solution can be used every 6 hours, together with Actrapid insulin, 1–2 units/hour. The insulin infusion can be adjusted to maintain the blood glucose concentration between 80 and 90 mg/dl.
     d. Spinal anesthesia can be used at the time of delivery.
     e. Use a separate IV line for the rapid infusion of non-dextrose-containing solutions if necessary to treat hypotension without producing hyperglycemia.
     f. Bear in mind that the fetus of a diabetic mother might be quite susceptible to hypoxia secondary to maternal hypotension,[74] since one third of normotensive diabetic women have atherosclerotic lesions of the decidual vessels of the placental bed.
  3. Anesthesia for cesarean delivery

     a. The incidence of cardiovascular depression is higher during regional anesthesia for cesarean delivery and is related to higher levels of sympathetic blockade, accentuated by compression of the aorta and inferior vena cava by the gravid uterus. We compared spinal and general anesthesia for abdominal delivery in healthy mothers and diabetic parturients[75] and found that infants of diabetic mothers receiving spinal anesthesia were more acidotic than infants of nondiabetics. In these patients, umbilical venous lactate concentrations were always less than umbilical artery lactate concentrations, which does not support the hypothesis of placental production of lactate during these acute studies at parturition. We noticed marked acidosis in hyperglycemic animals in the presence of hypoxia in a primate study.[76] Further investigation is necessary to determine the full nature of the interrelationships between blood glucose, oxygen content, and acid-base balance in pregnancies complicated by hyperglycemia.
     b. An additional risk of maternal and fetal hyperglycemia accompanying acute volume expansion with dextrose-containing solutions before cesarean delivery in diabetics is the occurrence of neonatal hypoglycemia. Soler and Malins reported an incidence of over 40% in their series when the mean arterial blood glucose at delivery was more than 130 mg/dl.[77] Recent trials of rigorous control of maternal blood glucose during labor with IV insulin resulted in a low incidence of babies of hypoglycemia in diabetic mothers whose disease was well controlled prior to parturition.[78, 79]

Keys for the use of regional anesthesia for cesarean delivery of the diabetic parturient[80] include:
(1) Acute hydration using a non-dextrose-containing solution. Use a

separate IV line and infuse lactated Ringer's solution or normal saline solution.

(2) Dextrose-containing solutions should be administered by constant infusion pump at 7.5 gm/hour.

(3) Good neonatal outcome can be obtained using a well-conducted general or regional anesthesia.

(4) After the procedure, regular insulin can be administered as needed in small doses. A drop in the insulin requirement is observed in these patients during the postpartum period.

Summary

For labor and vaginal delivery, small doses of narcotics will provide moderate pain relief. Lumbar epidural block can provide excellent pain relief both for labor and delivery. Spinal anesthesia can also be used at the time of delivery. One should use a separate IV line for the rapid infusion of solutions not containing dextrose if necessary to treat hypotension without producing hyperglycemia.

The following criteria should be considered in the use of anesthesia for cesarean delivery in diabetic parturients:

1. Acute hydration by non-dextrose-containing solutions before induction of anesthesia. A separate IV line should be used for this purpose.

2. Routine left uterine displacement starting from induction of anesthesia until the delivery of the baby.

3. Prompt treatment of hypotension with IV ephedrine (10-mg increments).

4. Possible use of an ester-type local anesthetic such as 2-chloroprocaine, which is rapidly hydrolyzed both in maternal and fetal plasma by pseudocholinesterase. However, the risk of unintentional dural puncture and possible neurologic deficits with chloroprocaine must be considered by each individual anesthetist.

5. Amide local anesthetics with long fetal/neonatal half-life, e.g., mepivacaine, should be avoided in these cases.

6. Well-conducted general anesthesia can be used if necessary with good neonatal outcome.

D. Cardiac Disease

1. At present, the incidence of cardiac disease in childbearing women is approximately 0.5%–2.0%.[69]

2. The cardiac patient with a left-to-right shunt will generally tolerate labor and delivery without any serious problems unless systemic hypotension or pulmonary hypertension leads to a shunt reversal.[82]

3. Patients with a right-to-left shunt have a high incidence of fetal demise.

4. Major problems:
   a. Fluctuation of the hemodynamic status during labor.
   b. Patients on anticoagulant medications.
   c. Drug interaction: Medications like digoxin, diuretics, and propranolol might interact with different anesthetic techniques or drugs.

5. Anesthesia management:
   a. Acquired heart disease
      (1) Relief of stress and apprehension should be accomplished during labor by the administration of tranquilizers and possibly narcotics.
      (2) For relief of pain, epidural anesthesia should be considered.
      (3) Hypotension should be avoided by judicious administration of local anesthetic doses and preventing and treating aortocaval compression. If there is hypotension, the underlying pathophysiology should be considered when selecting a vasopressor. In some cases, ephedrine in large doses may increase the heart rate and therefore the cardiac workload.
      (4) Regional anesthesia is contraindicated if the patient receives anticoagulants for any reason. Reversal of anticoagulation, monitored by ACT or PTT, may allow regional anesthesia.
      (5) For cesarean delivery: General anesthesia in most instances is the technique of choice.
      (6) A dilute oxytocin solution

should be infused to prevent postpartum uterine relaxation and needless blood loss. Bolus IV injection of oxytocin may cause serious hypotension, while IM ergonovine preparations may produce severe peripheral vasoconstriction followed by hypertension. Both these drugs should be used carefully in this situation.

(7) Parturients receiving propranolol are always at high risk because anesthesiologists may face problems related to reduction in cardiac output and maternal myocardial reserve, as well as decreased responsiveness to β-adrenergic-stimulating drugs in the presence of hypotension.[83] Patients receiving full β-blocking doses of propranolol therapy are not candidates for major regional anesthesia for labor and vaginal or cesarean delivery. Effects of chronic administration of propranolol on the fetus include intrauterine growth retardation, fetal bradycardia, and neonatal hypoglycemia, so babies need careful postpartum attention in such cases.

E. Respiratory Problems
  1. Respiratory problems like chronic bronchitis and asthma might be expected to improve during pregnancy due to the bronchiolar relaxing effect of progesterone.
  2. Medical therapy of respiratory problems is the same as in nonpregnant patients.
  3. For labor and delivery, one should use continuous epidural block, if indicated.
  4. For cesarean delivery, if regional anesthesia is selected, an epidural block is preferable to spinal anesthesia. If one uses general anesthesia, halothane should be considered for its bronchodilating effect.
  5. Aminophylline in continuous infusion might also be necessary. Continuous blood pressure monitoring is essential because of the possibility of inducing hypotension.

F. Neurologic Problems (Uncommon During the Childbearing Age)
  1. *Infectious disease.*—Regional anesthesia is absolutely contraindicated in the presence of an active inflammatory disease in the spinal canal, such as acute meningitis or superficial infection at the site of the lumbar puncture. However, regional anesthesia is not contraindicated in old inflammatory problems, i.e., the parturient with a history of poliomyelitis.
  2. *Paraplegia.*—The unique phenomenon experienced by paraplegics and quadraplegics is called autonomic hyperreflexia, or mass reflex. Interestingly, the syndrome is not found if the lesion is below T-7. It occurs in 85% of cases with lesions above T-7. Stimulation of the skin below the level of the lesion or the presence of distention or contraction of a hollow viscus like the urinary bladder, uterus, or gut may precipitate the mass reflex. This might present in the form of pilomotor erection, sweating, facial flushing, headache, bradycardia, and severe hypertension leading to convulsions, loss of consciousness, and possible subarachnoid or cerebral hemorrhage. It has been reported[95] that 11% of paraplegic patients may develop severe hypertension during pregnancy due to mass reflex. The incidence of premature labor is high among paraplegics. Administration of succinylcholine may be dangerous because of the possibility of hyperkalemia. Patients with paraplegia or quadraplegia require very little or (most often) no anesthesia, depending on the level of the lesion. Regional anesthesia is useful in these patients, but since the risk of hypotension is greater with spinal anesthesia, epidural anesthesia is preferable. Regional anesthesia will also help control the mass reflex during labor and delivery.
  3. *Cerebrovascular accidents.*—Cerebral hemorrhage can be seen in association with severe eclampsia, or can occur during pregnancy due to a leaking

aneurysm or arteriovenous malformation. Cardiovascular stresses during pregnancy, labor, delivery, and the immediate postpartum period can precipitate or exacerbate subarachnoid hemorrhage. Anesthetic management must prevent wide swings in blood pressure. For labor and delivery, continuous epidural block is advisable. The use of forceps is indicated to shorten the second stage, and the Valsalva maneuvers usually associated with the second stage should not be employed. In the immediate postpartum period, one should be prepared to treat hypertension aggressively if it occurs. For cesarean delivery, epidural block is the choice of anesthesia; however, if there is fetal distress or if general anesthesia is indicated for some other reason, one must be careful about the hypertensive response following endotracheal intubation. This response can be blocked by the use of IV lidocaine given before induction, and antihypertensives such as trimethaphan.

4. *Multiple sclerosis.*—Although the choice of anesthesia is controversial,[84] we would use epidural anesthesia for vaginal delivery in such cases, if it is otherwise indicated. We recommend general anesthesia for cesarean delivery in this condition, because of the relatively large amount of local anesthetics required.

5. *Space-occupying lesions (brain tumors).*—Spinal anesthesia may be relatively contraindicated because of reduction in CSF pressure, which, if it occurs rapidly, may produce cerebral herniation and sudden death. Some anesthesiologists may consider epidural or caudal anesthesia in such cases. However, the possibility of dural puncture and the sequelae secondary to the rapid decrease in CSF remain.

6. *Epilepsy.*—There is no evidence that epileptic patients are more susceptible to local anesthetics than the normal population, and in fact anesthetics have been used in the treatment of status epilepticus. Spinal or epidural anesthesia is not contraindicated in such

patients. For general anesthesia, drugs that have potential convulsive action should be avoided (e.g., enflurane, ketamine).

7. *Myasthenia gravis.*[85, 86]
   a. Major problems:
      (1) Change of prolonged second stage because of muscle weakness.
      (2) Postdelivery pulmonary complications because of respiratory muscle weakness.
      (3) Possible complications during anesthesia.
      (4) Possibility of neonatal myasthenia gravis.
   b. Anesthesia management: For labor and delivery, tranquilizers and narcotics may be used. Epidural anesthesia will reduce the requirements of systemic analgesics. Amide local anesthetics are preferable to esters because the patients are usually taking anticholinesterase drugs to control the disease. For cesarean delivery, because of the need of a higher level of sensory anesthesia, there is always a danger of impairment of the respiratory muscles following regional anesthesia. Succinylcholine should be used to facilitate the intubation when general anesthesia is used. However, the possibility of prolonged blockade after the use of depolarizing drugs should be remembered.

G. Renal Disorders[94]
   1. Major physiologic changes:
      a. Effective renal plasma flow (RPF) and glomerular filtration rate (GFR) increase by 50% by 16 weeks of gestation.
      b. The high RPF and GFR result in an increase in the creatinine clearance rate.
      c. During normal pregnancy, the BUN averages 8–9 mg/dl and the creatinine level averages 0.46 mg/dl. Therefore, during pregnancy, a ''normal'' nonpregnant BUN (10–20 mg/dl) and creatinine level (0.5–1.2 mg/dl) may represent renal compromise.

d. One of the commonest disorders in pregnancy that involves kidney function is toxemia of pregnancy.

e. Acute renal failure in pregnancy can occur in conjunction with hemorrhage, sepsis, or toxemia.

2. Anesthetic management:

a. Nephrotoxicity occasionally follows the use of methoxyflurane and enflurane: therefore, these agents should be avoided in the presence of renal compromise.

b. Spinal and epidural anesthesia does not sufficiently alter renal function unless there is significant hypotension.

c. Because ephedrine can maintain renal blood flow without affecting the uterine blood flow, it should be the vasopressor of choice if there is hypotension.

H. Hematologic Disorders

1. Besides the hereditary clotting defects, the defects of major concern in obstetric patients are the acquired problems.

a. Drugs that interfere with platelet function, i.e., aspirin.

b. Massive transfusion of old banked blood.

c. Liver failure.

d. Disseminated intravascular coagulation, which is associated with abruptio placentae, amniotic fluid embolism, intrauterine fetal death, and severe toxemia of pregnancy. The pathophysiology of DIC consists of nearly simultaneous uncontrolled activation of procoagulants and fibrinolytic enzymes in the microvasculature. The process depletes procoagulants. Plasma (fibrinolysin) is elevated, leading to further digestion of fibrin coats, which releases fibrin degradation products and inhibits polymerization.

2. Anesthetic management:

a. General anesthesia should be the choice because of the clotting deficits.

b. Blood volume replacement and circulatory support are necessary.

c. Fresh whole blood or red cells and fresh frozen plasma which contain all known clotting factors should be used.

d. Administration of procoagulants to replace factors that have been consumed is essential.

3. Sickle cell disease

a. Parturients with sickle cell *trait* usually have no problems during pregnancy; however, women with SS or SC disease are poor obstetric risks. Their anemia becomes more severe during pregnancy and the incidence of toxemia is increased.

b. Anesthetic management: High arterial oxygen concentrations and adequate cardiac output must be assured because of the increased chance of sickling. The patient should be kept warm and well hydrated.

c. For labor and delivery, if regional anesthesia is administered, it must be used cautiously. Oxygen should be administered throughout the procedure and aortocaval compression should be avoided.

d. For cesarean delivery, general anesthesia should be used.

I. Endocrine Disorders

1. Hyperthyroidism

a. Major problems:

(1) Patient might be on propranolol therapy.

(2) If the mother is on antithyroid therapy, fetal goiter may occur.

(3) The myocardium remains hypersensitive to catecholamines in such cases.

(4) Possibility of thyroid storm.

b. Anesthetic management: Regional anesthesia should be avoided, especially for cesarean delivery, if the mother is taking propranolol.

2. Pheochromocytoma. During pregnancy, this entity is associated with high maternal and fetal mortality. Although an epidural block can be used for labor and delivery for cesarean delivery, general anesthesia is safer because of the maintenance of sympathetic tone.

J. Problems Because of Miscellaneous Factors

1. Prematurity[87]

a. Major problems:

(1) Respiratory distress syndrome (RDS) is the major cause of mortality in premature infants. Intrapartum hypoxia and severe maternal stress during labor may increase the severity of this disease.

(2) Intracranial hemorrhage—usually related to:

    (i) Uncontrolled delivery.

    (ii) Other causes of birth trauma.

(3) Ischemic cerebral damage from intrapartum asphyxia, hypoxia, and hypotension.

(4) Prolonged effect of depressant medications because metabolic and excretory systems are immature in the preterm infant. Narcotics, sedatives, and tranquilizers have greater effect in such cases.

(5) Hypoglycemia is more common than in term infants. Corticosteroids and anesthetic agents may enhance this condition in prematurity.

b. Premature delivery. Cesarean delivery is performed with increasing frequency in prematurity, especially when complicated by a breech presentation. Decreased neonatal mortality and morbidity rates have been reported as a result of this practice.

c. Anesthesia for premature delivery:

(1) No data exist to suggest a specific advantage to any form of anesthesia in this situation.

(2) Spinal anesthesia may be a preferable regional anesthesia technique, as the local anesthetic concentration will be less than with epidural anesthesia. However, no definitive data exist.

(3) Of interest are the problems that may arise in such patients who have been treated with β-mimetic drugs to retard or arrest premature labor.[88, 89] Such therapy may result in tachycardia and decreased maternal cardiac output and may predispose to maternal hypotension.

Therefore, if the patient has significant tachycardia, regional anesthesia may be contraindicated and general anesthesia should be the method of choice for cesarean delivery.

(4) For labor and delivery, continuous epidural or spinal anesthesia must be considered for a controlled delivery to avoid intracranial hemorrhage.

(5) Pulmonary edema can occur in patients treated with β-mimetics to arrest labor or with corticosteroids to accelerate fetal lung maturation in utero.[89]

2. Breech presentation. Cesarean deliveries for breech presentation are being performed more often in contemporary practice. Unless an emergency exists, e.g., prolapsed cord, for which general anesthesia should be administered, spinal or epidural anesthesia can be utilized. For labor and delivery with a small but near term fetus, a continuous epidural infusion is ideal. However, obstetricians may prefer administering spinal anesthesia just before delivery to avoid dysfunctional labor and the need for oxytocin stimulation.

3. Multiple gestations:

a. *Twins.*—For labor and delivery, continuous epidural infusion offers the better approach. This method obviates the use of depressant drugs like narcotics or tranquilizers and allows a controlled delivery over a relaxed perineum. Occasionally, however, general anesthesia is needed for version or extraction, especially for the second baby. Halothane should be used for proper relaxation of the uterus if necessary. For cesarean delivery, spinal or epidural anesthesia can be used if there is no contraindication. For emergency cases, general anesthesia should be used.

b. *Triplets or quadruplets.*—Cesarean delivery is usually employed in these cases.

(1) Major problems:

    (a) More profound aortocaval compression and higher incidence of hypotension than in singleton gestations.

   (b) Increased tendency toward hypoxemia because of the greater upward displacement of the diaphragm.

   (c) In the presence of a grossly enlarged uterus, gastric emptying may be even further compromised, increasing the risk of aspiration in these patients.

   (d) Fetuses in multiple gestations are often premature and may have growth retardation.

(2) Anesthetic management:

   (a) Spinal anesthesia should be avoided because of the high incidence of hypotension and the possibility of higher spread with involvement of respiratory muscles.

   (b) Epidural anesthesia has been used.[90]

   (c) A well-conducted general anesthesia might also be used. The induction-to-delivery and uterine incision-to-delivery intervals should be minimized because of the chances of partial separation of the placenta.

4. Maternal narcotics addiction[91]
This can bring problems both to mothers and neonates.

   a. Major problems:

   (1) Withdrawal symptoms if parturients do not receive narcotics.

   (2) Increased chance of perinatal mortality from maternal narcotic addiction because of prematurity and low birth weight.

   (3) Maternal withdrawal may trigger fetal withdrawal, leading to fetal hyperactivity, increased oxygen consumption, and fetal hypoxemia.

   (4) Acute drug overdose may cause hypotension and fetal death.

   (5) Hypotension in the mother during anesthesia is frequent because of adrenal insufficiency, associated hypovolemia, or

possibility of maternal overdose from narcotics.

   (6) Difficulty in starting an IV infusion.

   (7) Associated cardiovascular, respiratory, neurologic, and liver problems.

   b. Anesthetic management:

   (1) Labor and delivery: A continuous epidural is preferred because it eliminates the use of addicting drugs.

   (2) Cesarean delivery: The presence of cardiovascular, respiratory, or neurologic problems secondary to addiction may present problems. General anesthesia can be given in such situations but, as a majority of these patients have hepatic problems, halothane should be avoided and N_2O, enflurane, or isoflurane used instead.

   c. Postoperative pain relief: Always a problem in these cases because of chance of readdiction. We administer whatever narcotics are necessary and try to withdraw the women after the initial postpartum period. Use of epidural anesthesia for postoperative pain relief might be beneficial in such cases.

   d. Active resuscitation of the neonates may be necessary.

5. Maternal alcohol addiction[92]

   a. Major problems:

   (1) Medical complications like bleeding problems because of esophageal varices and clotting abnormalities due to abnormal liver function, myocardiopathy, neuropathy, and the possibility of increased gastric acidity will make the administration of anesthesia difficult.

   (2) Possibility of the fetal alcohol syndrome.

   b. Anesthetic management: For both labor-delivery and cesarean delivery, epidural anesthesia is safe as long as there are no clotting abnormalities. Regional anesthesia will help to minimize the chances of the aspiration.

6. Amphetamines[95]
   a. CNS stimulants.
   b. Anesthetic management: Amphetamine causes depletion of CNS catecholamines and might result in a poor response to indirectly acting sympathomimetic agents like ephedrine.
      (1) Increased anesthetic requirement is a possibility if general anesthesia is used.
      (2) Epidural anesthesia might be a better choice in this situation.
      (3) Questions remain about the choice of vasopressors.
7. Malignant hyperthermia
   a. Anesthetic management: Both spinal anesthesia and epidural anesthesia have been used successfully in such patients. The choice of drug is controversial, but it appears that the ester local anesthetics should be considered as the first choice.
8. Obesity
   a. Major problems:
      (1) Associated medical problems like cardiopulmonary or vascular problems, diabetes, etc.
      (2) Larger volume of gastric contents with low pH.
      (3) Technical difficulty with regional anesthesia.
      (4) Obstetric complications are high in this group of patients.
      (5) Laryngoscopy may be difficult in such cases.[93]
   b. Anesthetic management:
      (1) For labor and delivery, an epidural block is preferable and should be used if technically possible.
      (2) For elective cesarean section, if one considers regional anesthesia, spinal anesthesia should be used cautiously if at all, because:
         (a) Control of spinal anesthesia level is unpredictable.
         (b) There is a very high incidence of hypotension.
         (c) Spinal anesthetic can reach higher levels, causing further compromise of the already abnormal pulmonary function. For epidural anesthesia, the volume of the local anesthetic might have to be reduced.
      (3) If general anesthesia is necessary, one should carefully check the airway before the induction of anesthesia. Laryngoscopy may prove difficult in these patients because the chest and large breasts often impede the use of the usual laryngoscope handle. Use of a short-handled instrument (Datta-Briwa) may circumvent this problem.

Summary

There is need for further studies on anesthetic needs for high-risk parturients. Successful anesthesia will depend on the technical skills of the anesthetist and an understanding of maternal and fetal physiology, the pathophysiology of the disease, and the pharmacology of different drugs and their interactions with the anesthetic techniques.

REFERENCES

1. Scott J.R., Rose N.B.: Effect of psychoprophylaxis on labor and delivery in primiparas. *N. Engl. J. Med.* 294:1205–1207, 1976.
2. Hew E.M., Rolbin S.H., Cole A.F.D., et al.: Obstetrical anaesthesia practice. *Can. Anaesth. Soc. J.* 28:158–166, 1981.
3. Adams M.M., Oakley G.P., Marks J.S.: Maternal age and births in the 1980's. *JAMA* 247:493–494, 1982.
4. Cogan R.: Comfort during prepared childbirth as a function of parity. *J. Psychosom. Res.* 19:33–37, 1975.
5. Ueland K., Hansen J.M.: Maternal cardiovascular dynamics: III. Labor and delivery under local and caudal analgesia. *Am. J. Obstet. Gynecol.* 163:8–17, 1969.
6. Shnider S.M., Wright R.G., Levinson G.: Uterine blood flow and plasma norepinephrine changes during maternal stress in the pregnant ewe. *Anesthesiology* 50:30–34, 1979.
7. Zador G., Willeck-Lund G., Nillson B.A.: Acid-base changes associated with labor. *Acta Obstet. Gynecol. Scand. Suppl.* 34:41–49, 1974.
8. Motoyama E.K., Rivard G., Acheson F.: Adverse effect of maternal hyperventilation on the fetus. *Am. J. Obstet. Gynecol.* 122:47–55, 1975.
9. Huch A., Huch R., Lindmark G., et al.: Transcutaneous oxygen delivery measurements in labor. *Br. J. Obstet. Gynaecol.* 81:608–614, 1974.
10. Pearson J.F., Davies P.: The effect of continuous epidural analgesia on maternal acid-base balance and ar-

terial lactate concentration during the second stage of labor. *Br. J. Obstet. Gynaecol.* 80:225–229, 1973.

11. American Society of Anesthesiologists: *Guidelines for Anesthetic Practice*. Chicago, American Society of Anesthesiologists, 1979.

12. American College of Obstetricians and Gynecologists: *National Survey of Maternity Care*. Chicago, American Society of Obstetricians and Gynecologists, 1970.

13. American College of Obstetricians and Gynecologists: *National Survey of Maternity Care*. Chicago, American Society of Obstetricians and Gynecologists, 1980.

14. Rochat R.W.: Maternal mortality in the United States of America. *World Health Stat. Q.* 34:2–13, 1981.

15. Tompkinson J., Turnbull A., Robson G.: *Report on confidential enquiries into maternal deaths in England and Wales, 1973–1975*. London, Her Majesty's Stationery Office, 1979.

16. Bonica J.J.: Anesthetic deaths, in Bonica J.J. (ed.): *Principles and Practice of Obstetric Anesthesia*. Philadelphia, F.A. Davis Co., 1972, p. 752.

17. Dick-Read G.: *Childbirth Without Fear*. New York, Harper & Row, 1959.

18. Jacobsen E.: *How to Relax and Have Your Baby*. New York, McGraw-Hill Book Co., 1959.

19. Lamaze F.: *Painless Childbirth—Psychoprophylactic Method*. London, Burke, 1974.

20. Bradley R.A.: *Husband-coached Childbirth*. New York, Harper & Row, 1974.

21. Beazley J.M., Leaver E.P., Morewood J.H.M.: Relief of pain in labour. *Lancet* 1:1003–1005, 1967.

22. Saling E., Ligidas P.: The effect on the fetus of maternal hyperventilation during labour. *Br. J. Obstet. Gynaecol.* 76:877–881, 1969.

23. Zador G., Nillson B.A.: Low dose intermittent epidural analgesia with lidocaine for vaginal delivery. *Acta Obstet. Gynecol. Scand. Suppl.* 34:17–21, 1974.

24. Moya F., James L.S.: Medical hypnosis for obstetrics. *JAMA* 174:2026–2027, 1960.

25. Flowers C.E., Littlejohn T.W., Wells H.B.: Pharmacologic and hypnoid analgesia. *Obstet. Gynecol.* 16:210–214, 1960.

26. Wahl C.W.: Contraindications and limitations of hypnosis in obstetrics. *Am. J. Obstet. Gynecol.* 84:1869–1874, 1962.

27. Wallis L., Shnider S.M., Palahniuk R.J.: An evaluation of acupuncture analgesia in obstetrics. *Anesthesiology* 41:596–599, 1974.

28. Bundsen P., Peterson L.E., Selstam U.: Pain relief in labor by transcutaneous nerve stimulation. *Acta. Obstet. Gynecol. Scand.* 60:459–468, 1981.

29. Stewart P.: Transcutaneous nerve stimulation as a method of analgesia in labour. *Anaesthesia* 34:361–364, 1979.

30. Dundee J.W.: Alterations in response to somatic pain associated with anesthesia: The effect of thiopentone and pentobarbitone. *Br. J. Anaesth.* 32:407–411, 1960.

31. Powe C.E., Kiem I.M., Fromhagen C.: Propioma-
zine hydrochloride in obstetrical analgesia. *JAMA* 181:290–291, 1962.

32. Cree J.E., Meyer J., Hailey D.M.: Diazepam in labour. *Br. Med. J.* 4:251–256, 1973.

33. Pert C.B., Kuhar M.J., Snyder S.H.: Opiate receptor: Autoradiographic localization in rat brain. *Proc. Natl. Acad. Sci. USA* 73:3729–3733, 1976.

34. Yaksh T.L.: In vivo studies on spinal opiate receptor systems mediating antinociception. *J. Pharmacol. Exp. Ther.* 226:303–316, 1983.

35. Wolozin B.L., Pasternak G.W.: Classification of multiple morphine and enkephalin binding sites in the central nervous system. *Proc. Natl. Acad. Sci. USA* 78:6181–6185, 1981.

36. Snyder S.H.: Drug and neurotransmitter receptors in the brain. *Science* 224:22–30, 1984.

37. Bullingham R.E.S.: Opiate development: New opiates and the future. *Clin. Anesthesiol.* 1:139–142, 1983.

38. Shnider S.M., Moya F.: Effects of meperidine on the newborn infant. *Am. J. Obstet. Gynecol.* 89:1009–1011, 1964.

39. Kay B.: Alfentanil. *Clin. Anesthesiol.* 1:143–146, 1983.

40. Bennet R.L., Batenhoirst R.L, Bivins B.A., et al.: Patient controlled analgesia. *Ann. Surg.* 195:700–704, 1982.

41. Cousins M.J., Mather L.E.: Intrathecal and epidural opioids. *Anesthesiology* 61:276–310, 1984.

42. Hughes S.C.: Intraspinal narcotics in obstetrics. *Clin. Perinatol.* 1:167–75, 1982.

43. Justins D.M., Francis D., Houlton P.G., et al.: A controlled trial of extradural fentanyl in labour. *Br. J. Anaesth.* 54:409–414, 1982.

44. Naulty J.S.: Unpublished data.

45. Quilligan E.J., Keegan K.A., Donahue M.J.: Double-blind comparison of intravenously injected butorphanol and meperidine in parturients. *Int. J. Gynaecol. Obstet.* 18:363–370, 1980.

46. Booker P.D., Wilkes R.G., Bryson T.H.L.: Obstetric pain relief using epidural morphine. *Anaesthesia* 35:377–379, 1980.

47. Lanning C.F., Harmel M.H.: Ketamine anesthesia. *Int. Anesthesiol. Clin.* 16:137–144, 1975.

48. Cryc J.J.: Anesthesia for the high risk obstetrical patient. *Clin. Perinatol.* 9:113–134, 1982.

49. Bovill J.G., Dundee J.W., Coppell D.L., et al.: Current status of ketamine anesthesia. *Lancet* 1:1285, 1971.

50. Eckstein K.L., Marx G.F.: Aortocaval compression: Incidence and prevention. *Anesthesiology* 40:381–384, 1965.

51. Janzen E.: Der negativ Vorschlag bei Lumbalpunktion. *Dtsch. Z. Nervenheilk.* 94:280–288, 1926.

52. Heldt H.J., Moloney J.C.: Negative pressure in the epidural space. *Am. J. Med. Sci.* 175:371–376, 1928.

53. Gutierrez A.: Valor de la aspiracion liquida en el espacio peridural en la anestesia peridural. *Rev. Chir. Buenos Aires* 12:225–230, 1933.

54. Sicard J.A., Forestier J.: Radiographic method for exploration of the extradural space using lipiodol. *Rev. Neurol.* 28:1264–1268, 1921.

55. Gavin R.: Continuous epidural analgesia: An unusual case of dural perforation following catheterization of the epidural space. *N.Z. Med. J.* 64:280–283, 1965.

56. Moore D.C., Batra M.S.: The components of an effective test dose prior to epidural block. *Anesthesiology* 55:693–696, 1981.

57. Matadial L., Cibils L.A.: The effect of epidural anesthesia on uterine activity and blood pressure. *Am. J. Obstet. Gynecol.* 125:846–854, 1976.

58. Wallis K.L., Shnider S.M., Hicks J.S.: Epidural anesthesia in the normotensive pregnant ewe: Effect on uterine blood flow and fetal acid-base status. *Anesthesiology* 44:481–487, 1976.

59. Albright G.A., Joupilla R., Holmen A.I.: Epinephrine does not alter human intervillous blood flow during epidural anesthesia. *Anesthesiology* 54:131–135, 1981.

60. Hood D.D., Dewan D.M., Rose J.C.: Maternal and fetal effects of intravenous epinephrine containing solutions in gravid ewes. *Anesthesiology* 59:A393, 1983.

61. Schellenberg J.S.: Uterine activity during epidural anesthesia with bupivacaine. *Am. J. Obstet. Gynecol.* 127:26–31, 1977.

62. Morishima H.O., Covino B.G., Ych M.: Bradycardia in the fetal baboon following paracervical block anesthesia. *Am. J. Obstet. Gynecol.* 140:775–780, 1971.

63. Phillips K.C., Thomas T.A.: Second stage of labour with or without extradural analgesia. *Anaesthesia* 38:972–976, 1983.

64. Rosenblatt R., Wright R., Denson D., et al.: Continuous epidural infusions for obstetric analgesia. *Reg. Anaesth.* 8:10–15, 1983.

65. Shnider S.M., deLorimer A.A., Asling J.H.: Vasopressors in obstetrics. *Am. J. Obstet. Gynecol.* 106:680–690, 1970.

66. Datta S., Ostheimer G.W., Alper M.H., et al.: Nausea and vomiting after induction of spinal anesthesia for cesarian delivery: Effects of intravenous ephedrine. *Anesthesiology* 56:68–69, 1982.

67. Alper M.H., Roaf E.R.: Anesthetic management of high risk pregnancy. *Clin. Obstet. Gynecol.* 16:347–360, 1973.

68. Datta S., Alper M.H.: Anesthesia for cesarean section. *Anesthesiology* 50:142–160, 1980.

69. Shnider S.M., Levinson G.: *Anesthesia for Obstetrics.* Baltimore, Williams & Wilkins Co., 1979.

70. Hibbard L.T.: Placenta previa. *Am. J. Obstet. Gynecol.* 104:172, 1969.

71. Bonnar J.: Coagulation disorders. *J. Clin. Pathol. Suppl.* 10:35, 1976.

72. Joyce T.H., Debnath K.S., Baker E.A.: Pre-eclampsia: Relationship of CVP and epidural analgesia. *Anesthesiology* 51:5297, 1979.

73. Pearson J.F.: The effect of continuous lumbar epidural block on maternal and foetal acid-base balance during labor and at delivery, in *Proceedings of the Symposium on Epidural Analgesia in Obstetrics.* London, H.K. Lewis & Co., Ltd., 1972, p. 26.

74. Hollmen A.I., Jouippila R., Koivisto M., et al.: Neurologic activity of infants following anesthesia for cesarean section. *Anesthesiology* 48:350, 1978.

75. Datta S., Brown W.U.: Acid-base status in diabetic mothers and their infants following general or spinal anesthesia for cesarean section. *Anesthesiology* 47:272–276, 1977.

76. Kitzmiller J.L., Phillippe M., VonOeyen P., et al.: Hyperglycemia, hypoxia and fetal acidosis in rhesus monkey, abstract. *Proc. Soc. Gynecol. Invest.* 169:98, 1981.

77. Soler N.G., Malins J.M.: Diabetic pregnancy: Management of diabetes on the day of delivery. *Diabetologica* 15:441–446, 1978.

78. Valachokosta F.: Personal communication.

79. West T.E.T., Lowy C.: Control of blood glucose during labor in diabetic women with combined glucose and low dose insulin infusion. *Br. Med. J.* 1:1252, 1977.

80. Datta S., Kitzmiller J.L., Naulty J.S., et al.: Acid-base status of diabetic mothers and their infants following spinal anesthesia for cesarean section. *Anesth. Analg.* 61:662–665, 1982.

81. Lev Ran A.: Sharp temporary drop in insulin requirement after cesarean section in diabetic patients. *Am. J. Obstet. Gynecol.* 120:905, 1974.

82. Ostheimer G.W., Alper M.H.: Intrapartum anesthetic management of the pregnant patient with heart disease. *Clin. Obstet. Gynecol.* 18:81–97, 1975.

83. Datta S., Kitzmiller J.L., Ostheimer G.W., et al.: Propranolol and parturition. *Obstet. Gynecol.* 51:577–581, 1978.

84. Warren T., Datta S., Ostheimer G.W.: Lumbar epidural anesthesia in a patient with multiple sclerosis. *Anesth. Analg.* 61:1022–1023, 1982.

85. Drachman D.B.: Myasthenia gravis (first of two parts). *N. Engl. J. Med.* 298:136, 1978.

86. Drachman D.B.: Myasthenia gravis (second of two parts). *N. Engl. J. Med.* 298:186, 1978.

87. Fedrick J., Anderson A.B.M.: Factors associated with spontaneous preterm birth. *Br. J. Obstet. Gynaecol.* 83:342, 1976.

88. Barden T.P., Peter J.B., Merkatz I.R.: Ritodrine hydrochloride: A betamimetic agent for use in preterm labor. *Obstet. Gynecol.* 56:1–12, 1980.

89. Stubblefield P.G.: Pulmonary edema occurring after therapy with dexamethasone and terbutaline for premature labor: A case report. *Am. J. Obstet. Gynecol.* 132:341–343, 1978.

90. Datta S., Poreda M., Naulty J.S., et al.: Epidural anesthesia for cesarean delivery of quadruplets. *Reg. Anaesth.* 7:69–71, 1982.

19 / Pain Due to Trauma

CRAIG HARTRICK, M.D.
CHARLES E. PITHER, M.B.B.S.

MORE THAN 50 million accidental injuries occur annually in the United States. Of these, more than one third are associated with moderate to severe pain. Approximately 400,000 patients incur partial or permanent disability, and more than 100,000 die, usually from shock.[1]

Bonica, reviewing cases in which pain was the predominant symptom,[2] found that more than one third of all Americans experience persistent or recurrent pain requiring medical therapy. For these patients, it is the pain and not the underlying pathology that is the primary reason for their being nonproductive. The cost to the American society in terms of work days lost, health care expenses, and compensation was estimated at $60 billion in 1980 and was projected to be $80–$90 billion in 1983.[3]

It is important to distinguish between acute and chronic pain since chronic pain is managed differently from acute pain. The inadequate management of acute pain may also be a cause of chronic pain problems.

PATHOPHYSIOLOGY OF ORGAN FUNCTION AND PAIN IN THE INJURED

The interpretation of pain following nociceptive input from the periphery usually serves a protective function. Whereas withdrawal reflexes and muscle guarding act initially to avoid further injury, the perception of pain permits learned avoidance behavior. Diagnostically, pain helps identify sites of somatic or visceral anatomical disruption and the topography of physiologic dysfunction. Pathophysiologically, tissue injury and concomitant pain evoke an endocrine metabolic response. The stress response is characterized by increased catecholamine and cortisol levels that can be essential to the maintenance of homeostasis in the absence of appropriate intervention.

Once the process of injury has been identified and halted and the diagnostic delineation of the injury is complete, further nociceptive information serves no protective role. In fact, continued pain may serve only to increase anxiety and the stress response, which taxes physiologic reserves.

The treatment of posttraumatic pain, therefore, encompasses more than humanitarian considerations for analgesic administration if morbidity secondary to trauma is to be minimized. Reduction of stress, restoration of function, and prevention of subsequent complications are all intimately related to posttraumatic analgesia and must be addressed.

CURRENT MANAGEMENT OF PAIN DUE TO ACUTE INJURY

When the trauma patient arrives in the emergency room, attention is at once directed toward initial resuscitation and stabilization. Priority is given to establishing ventilatory and cardiovascular stability, control of external hemorrhage, and restoration of fluid and blood volume. Depending on the sites of injury, attention may then shift to intra-abdominal or intrathoracic bleeding and the repair of hollow viscus injury, followed by urologic, neurosurgical, and orthopedic intervention. Yet, following the institution of therapeutic intervention, pain relief often continues to have low priority. The first attempt to improve pain relief is often a single dose of an analgesic, usually a narcotic, administered preoperatively. This is despite prolonged periods of pain between admission of the patient to the emergency room and subsequent surgical procedure. Analgesics should not be delayed once the initial assessment is complete; however, the choice of analgesic and the route of administration must be carefully selected with due consideration of the prevailing hemodynamic, respiratory, and neurologic circumstances, as well as the possibility of aspiration of gastric contents.

While most preliminary diagnostic and therapeutic procedures (tracheal intubation, paracentesis, chest tube insertion, etc.) can be performed with local or topical anesthetics, systemic or regional techniques may be required for optimal performance of certain radiologic or CT studies and painful procedures such as fracture splinting or reduction. Aside from facilitating specific diagnostic and therapeutic interventions, there is now ample evidence that pain relief can minimize both patient anxiety and stress response.[4–12]

Stress Response Due to Injury and Pain

The stress response is a complex hormonal and neurologic sequence mediated via adrenergic sympathetic pathways thought to be evoked to promote survival. Elevated sympathetic efferent activity along with elevated epinephrine, norepinephrine, growth hormone, cortisol, renin, aldosterone, and antidiuretic hormone levels lead to tachycardia, hypertension, increased muscle blood flow with decreased renal and splanchnic blood flow, decreased glomerular filtration rate, and sodium and water retention.[13] The predominance of catabolic response leads to hyperglycemia secondary to increased glycogenolysis, lipolysis, and proteolysis in the face of decreased glucose turnover. Vasoconstriction and tachycardia may be important compensatory life-sustaining mechanisms prior to therapeutic intervention. However, once treatment is initiated, further stress or amplification of existing stress is unnecessary[10] and can be dangerous to patients at risk for end-organ ischemia or infarction.[14, 15]

Effect of Regional Anesthesia on Stress Response

Since the endocrine metabolic response to stress is initiated via afferent neurogenic stimuli, local anesthetic neural blockade can abolish the stress re-

sponse by interrupting afferent pathways.[6, 7] As adrenal innervation originates from T-6 through L-2, epidural anesthesia that includes these levels has been particularly effective.[5–8, 16] Epidural blockade to T-5 has been less effective in abolishing stress response during upper abdominal surgery than during lower abdominal surgery. This has been attributed to considerable unblocked afferent pathways transmitted via the vagus.[17] A study reported by Traynor et al. disputes the mechanism.[18] Systemic or epidural narcotics are effective in eliminating pain; however, they are far less effective in eliminating the stress response.[19] Regional anesthesia with local anesthetics seems to be more effective in eliminating or decreasing the stress response by blocking all other pathways.[6]

Moller et al.[7] demonstrated that preoperative institution of epidural blockade to T-4, to include adrenal and hepatic innervation, prevented the normal postoperative increase in cortisol and glucose following hysterectomy, whereas initial increases were observed when epidural anesthesia was initiated after the incision (Fig 19–1). Once afferent blockade was established, no further increases in cortisol or glucose were observed. While resting en-

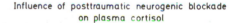

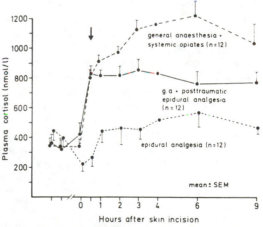

Fig 19–1.—Graph showing the influence of posttraumatic neurogenic blockade on plasma cortisol response to abdominal hysterectomy. *Arrow* indicates the commencement of epidural block 30 minutes after skin incision. Posttraumatic epidural block inhibits a further rise in the plasma cortisol level. (From Moller I.W., Rem J., Brandt M.R., et al.: *Acta Anaesthes. Scand.* 26:56–58, 1982. Reproduced by permission.)

docrine metabolic activity was not reestablished, a major portion of the stress response was indeed inhibited by posttraumatic conduction blockade. Brandt et al.[8] found that postoperative epidural block maintained for just 24 hours was associated with a sustained decrease in the negative nitrogen balance over the 4 days of the study period. Reduced glucose and cortisol levels were presumed to account for the relative improvement in nitrogen balance in patients receiving epidural analgesia.

Effect of Injury and Pain on Respiratory Function

Oxygenation can be impaired in the trauma patient for a variety of reasons. Pulmonary injury as a result of direct penetrating wounds, parenchymal contusions, or aspiration of gastric contents and parenchymal compression as a result of hemothorax or pneumothorax are frequent. Hypoventilation and atelectasis due to reduced respiratory excursion can result from pain following upper abdominal and thoracic incisions or from anatomical disruption of chest wall mechanics secondary to rib or sternal fractures. Johnson[20] studied forced vital capacity (FVC) and forced expiratory volume in 1 second (FEV_1) in patients undergoing elective thoracic and abdominal procedures and reported reductions in preoperative pulmonary function on the first postoperative day of 75% for thoracic, 68% for xyphoid to pubic abdominal, 61% for paramedian upper abdominal, 53% for subcostal, and 38% for midline lower abdominal incisions. Postanesthetic respiratory failure is most prominent when these insults are complicated by preexisting chronic obstructive pulmonary disease. Posttraumatic and postoperative pain relief in these patients is often critical to the restoration of pulmonary function, prevention of further deterioration, and weaning from mechanical ventilatory support.

Effect of Regional Anesthesia on Changes in Pulmonary Function Due to Injury and Pain

Spence[21] demonstrated that while nerve block with intercostal or epidural techniques does not affect the reduction of functional residual capacity (FRC), hypoxemia, or decreased ventilation, regional block does decrease the retention of secretions, preserves ciliary activity, and makes the cough more effective through a reduction in pain. Bromage et al.[22] have demonstrated improved FEV_1 postoperatively with segmental analgesia produced by epidural narcotics. Benhamou et al.[23] demonstrated that intravenous (IV) morphine in high-risk patients with respiratory disease following upper abdominal surgery was unable to alter any objective pulmonary function. However, epidural morphine or epidural lidocaine was able to partially restore VC and FEV_1 to preoperative levels. The other effort-dependent parameters measured, minimal inspiratory and expiratory pressure, remained unaffected, which suggests a contribution from nonanalgesic factors. Rybro et al.[24] compared morphine administered on demand postoperatively following upper abdominal surgery via intramuscular and epidural routes. The epidural morphine group demonstrated significantly reduced radiographic pulmonary changes and significantly higher Pa_{O_2} values with a slower rise in alveolar–arterial oxygen gradient. While Pa_{CO_2} was similar in both groups, the amount of morphine required was far less via the epidural route. Rawal et al.[25] compared postoperative pain relief with intramuscular narcotic, bupivacaine intercostal block, and single-bolus epidural morphine and found that postoperative Pa_{O_2} and Pa_{CO_2} values reflected changes in peak expiratory flow rate. The greatest reductions in peak expiratory flow were seen following intramuscular drug administration and the least were seen following epidural drug administration.

Parbrook et al. studied 50 male patients undergoing elective gastric surgery. They assessed personality, postoperative pain, and subsequent changes in VC.[26, 27] A highly significant correlation was found between high neuroticism scores and increased postoperative pain and pulmonary changes.

Effect of Regional Block on Thromboembolism

The local anesthetic techniques decrease thromboembolic phenomena by providing hyperkinetic blood flow, increased fibrinolysis, decreased coagulation, and inhibition of WBC invasion as well as preservation of endothelial cells in autogenous vein grafts.[28–31] These effects, combined with early mobilization, decrease posttraumatic and postoperative morbidity.[32]

RATIONALE FOR MANAGEMENT

An important goal in posttraumatic pain management is the early restoration of function. Cellular function depends on blood flow for delivery of nutrients to the tissues. Vasoconstriction, whether secondary to pain or direct vascular injury resulting from trauma or surgical manipulation, interferes with nutrient supply. Sympathetic blockade can be employed to decrease vascular resistance and improve skin and vascular graft flow while decreasing pain-mediated vasoconstriction.[33] Regional block for relief of pain can permit improved mobilization of the injured part.[34-36] Early mobilization contributes to preservation of normal myofascial function and normal gastrointestinal function. In one study improved nutrient supply, as measured by gastric emptying time, was significantly better with epidural analgesia than with systemic narcotic administration.[37]

A second goal in posttraumatic pain management is the prevention of delayed sequelae due to injury by early pain relief. The development of late posttraumatic pain syndromes may be partially dependent on initial pain management. Myofascial pain syndromes resulting from injury to musculoskeletal structures and disuse secondary to pain and muscle spasm might well be minimized with early ambulation and mobilization of injured regions. While sympathetic blockade has been of benefit for causalgia and reflex sympathetic dystrophy, whether pretraumatic or early posttraumatic blockade of sympathetic pathways would tend to prevent subsequent occurrence of these syndromes requires further study. There is some evidence that pretraumatic sympathectomy may prevent the development of phantom limb pain following amputation.[38]

MANAGEMENT OF ACUTE PAIN DUE TO TRAUMA

Analgesic therapy of the injured patient is not a major priority until primary resuscitative measures have been applied; however, analgesia is all too often ignored even when the patient has been adequately resuscitated. Whereas this is often rationalized in terms of the basic principles of management of trauma patients, these principles are often wrongly applied. The patient with a severe fracture who is denied analgesia because of a minor head injury, or the patient awaiting surgery, frightened and in pain, without the benefit of any analgesia, is familiar to anyone who evaluates patients in emergency rooms.

The principles and rationale of analgesic management of this group of patients are as follows:

1. The goal is to provide tolerable pain relief.
2. The treatment must be compatible with deranged physiology of vital organ systems.
   a. *Cardiovascular:* The circulation may be severely deranged due to hypovolemia. Drugs given systemically must not interfere with normal physiologic responses or decompensation may occur. The reduced cardiac output and plasma volume may considerably alter the pharmacokinetics of administered drugs. Normal doses of drugs given at conventional rates may produce extremely high plasma levels, causing undesirable side effects. Similarly, muscle blood flow may be seriously impaired, preventing uptake of drugs administered by this route. Organ perfusion may also be altered, and this can affect the clearance and elimination rates of analgesics, causing them to have prolonged effects.
   b. *Respiratory:* Oxygenation may be compromised at several levels in the oxygen cascade. Therapy that interferes with the mechanics of respiration (chest muscle function, airway patency, etc.) or with central control should be avoided. A rise in Pa_{CO_2} caused by hypoventilation will cause cerebral vasodilation; this must be prevented in cases where the intracranial pressure is already raised.
   c. *Neurologic:* The conscious state may be altered and intracranial pathology may be present. Drugs that mask or imitate the signs of raised intracranial pressure such as sedation, vomiting, or pupillary dysfunction are contraindicated.
   d. *Gastrointestinal:* The stomach may be full and gastric emptying delayed. Drugs should not be given by the oral route. Narcotics can cause vomiting and delay gastric emptying even further. This is particularly inappropriate if a general anesthetic is needed.
3. The patient may have pain from more than one site.
4. The patient may be intoxicated or have other drugs in the system.

5. The analgesic management should be based on an individually tailored regimen, in a well-monitored environment.

Treatment of Acute Posttraumatic Pain: Medications

Systemic Analgesics

Narcotic analgesics are the mainstay of the analgesic armamentarium for the trauma victim. Many injuries are associated with severe pain, and powerful agents must be used. The exact choice of agent is probably less important than its mode of administration. The intramuscular route is not suitable for the patient with poor tissue perfusion, IV administration being the route of choice.

IV doses of up to 10 mg of morphine are administered. Small doses are given every 10 minutes until analgesia is adequate.[39] Surprisingly, large doses of up to 30 mg of morphine may be needed,[40] a phenomenon confirmed in battle casualties.[41] The duration of action of the drug is not critical, since additional doses can be given as required.

The IV route gives immediate access to the circulation and therefore allows rapid onset of drug action. Rapid distribution and elimination of IV drugs may, however, produce a shorter effect than for the same dose given intramuscularly. To overcome this problem drugs can be given as an infusion. The infusion rate can be altered to produce the desired plasma level or clinical effect (Fig 19–2). This can be achieved with either a conventional IV set and an infusion pump or a power-driven syringe. Many drugs have been given by this route, including meperidine,[42] papaverine,[43] and morphine,[44] and there is little doubt as to the vastly improved analgesia of this method.[45] A steady state can be rapidly achieved with either a bolus dose or a two-rate infusion. Further refinements of the technique have utilized patient-controlled demand apparatus.[46, 47]

In head injury patients, all narcotics have undesirable side effects. These drugs should be avoided in all but the most trivial of head trauma cases. Less efficacious drugs such as codeine phosphate, 30–60 mg, have been used in an attempt to reduce the side effects of more potent drugs, such as respiratory depression and pupillary constriction. But all too often, such agents produce only minimal analgesia, even in modest doses, and analgesia for this group is provided by alternative methods.

Ketamine produces a profound analgesia and may be used in high dosage as the sole agent for emergency and trauma surgery.[48] At lower dosages it can be used as an analgesic.[49] This agent possesses sympathomimetic action, which may be beneficial in injured patients with a depressed cardiovascular system due to shock.[50] Ketamine, however, increases intracranial pressure and is contraindicated in head injuries.

Fig 19–2.—Computer-simulated plasma meperidine levels following four different routes of administration. *Dotted lines* represent a therapeutic range above which toxic effects are likely to be seen and below which analgesia is unlikely to be adequate. The doses are *(a)* intravenous injections, 50 mg q3h; *(b)* oral, 100 mg q4h; *(c)* intramuscular, 100 mg q4h; and *(d)* infusion, 50 mg in 45 minutes, then 25 mg/hour. (From Mather L.E., Lindop M.J., Tucker G.T., et al.: *Br. J. Anaesth.* 47:1269, 1975. Reproduced by permission.)

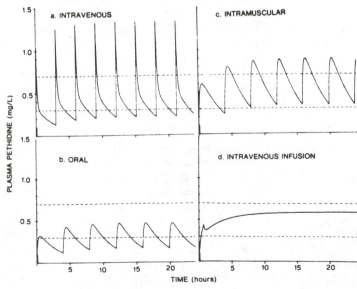

Inhalational Agents

Nitrous oxide is a powerful analgesic and at inspired concentrations of 20%–40% can produce pain relief equivalent to that achieved with 10–15 mg of morphine.[51] N_2O is often available in the emergency department on an anesthetic machine or premixed 50:50 with oxygen as entonox. Administration is simple via a face mask or nasal prongs, and the drug effectively produces analgesia for trauma victims.[52] In many countries entonox is available in ambulances for administration by paramedics, and such early use of the agent has been shown to actually increase survival rates in trauma victims.[53] This may in part be due to the high inspired O_2 concentration. Although some cardiodepressant action has been demonstrated with 60% N_2O,[54] its chief advantage is that any clinical deterioration can be treated by removal of the agent with very rapid reversal of effects. N_2O, however, also causes an increase in intracranial pressure.[55]

Treatment of Acute Posttraumatic Pain: Nerve Blocks

Use of Local Anesthetic Agents for Nerve Block

Many of the general constraints discussed above apply equally well to the use of local anesthetic agents. In the patient with compromised cardiovascular function, care must be exercised when administering drugs that will have further depressant effects on cardiac or cerebral functions. Routes of administration that produce sympathetic blockade are inappropriate in the hypovolemic patient, and this precludes spinal or epidural analgesia until the blood volume is restored to normal. Equally inappropriate are long-acting peripheral nerve blocks when assessment of limb function and pain is important for diagnostic purposes (compartment syndromes, plaster casts). However, the use of regional anesthesia in trauma victims not only avoids the systemic effects of narcotics (sedation, vomiting) but diminishes the stress response. These facts, combined with the completeness of the pain relief afforded by the placement of only a few milliliters of local anesthetic on a nerve, confer immutable advantages of this technique in the injured patient.

What is more, therapeutic measures including surgery can often be carried out with this technique alone. This obviates the need for a general anesthetic in patients with potentially full stomachs.

Local anesthetics can be administered by the following routes: infiltration, IV regional, peripheral nerve block, and conduction blockade.

INFILTRATION.—Local anesthetics can be administered by subcutaneous infiltration for analgesia of minor wounds or by injection into a fractured hematoma for reduction; e.g., for colles fracture, 5–10 ml of 1% lidocaine is injected into the hematoma. The technique does not always produce perfect analgesia but can be used when staff or resources are limited.[56]

IV REGIONAL ANESTHESIA.—Although seldom used for analgesia per se, the IV regional or Bier block is an extremely useful technique for manipulation of limb fractures or simple surgical procedures. The advantages of the technique are that it is simple, has a rapid onset and controllable duration of action, provides good muscle relaxation, and, if certain basic criteria are adhered to, is very safe. The use of a double-cuffed tourniquet allows the duration of block to be extended to 1½ hours.[57] Drugs of low toxicity should be used. Prilocaine 0.5% is probably the drug of first choice,[58, 59] although lidocaine 0.5%, up to 3 mg/kg, also produces adequate analgesia. In the upper limb, the technique is best suited to fractures around the wrist but can be used for supracondylar fractures with care. In the lower limb, the large volumes required (up to 100 ml) impose limitations on its use, but these may be overcome by using a calf tourniquet.[57] Exsanguination with an Esmarch bandage is difficult in the traumatized limb but satisfactory conditions can usually be obtained by elevating the limb for 2–3 minutes or by applying an inflatable limb splint.[60] IV regional anesthesia is ideally suited for the treatment of simple fractures in children.[61]

PERIPHERAL NERVE BLOCKS.—The benefits of peripheral nerve block to trauma patients are often not fully exploited, either because of inexperience of available personnel in performing the blocks or because of surgical time constraints. These techniques deserve better utilization since they usually produce total and long-lasting analgesia with minimal side effects. Furthermore, they often obviate administration of a general anesthetic and shorten the hospital stay of the patient.[34]

Technique for Upper Limb Analgesia.—Brachial plexus block can be performed by the axillary,[62] infraclavicular,[63] interscalene,[64] and supraclavicular routes.[65] The supraclavicular route is less suitable for outpatient or trauma victims because of the inherent risk of pneumothorax.

The exact choice of the technique depends on the site of injury and the patient's ability to move the arm. In general, higher lesions (upper arm injury, dislocated shoulder) require analgesia extending into the C-5 dermatome, and this is best achieved with an interscalene block.[66] This technique is also perhaps the most suitable for colles fracture,[67] as the anatomical snuffbox is often difficult to cover adequately in lower approaches to the brachial plexus. The axillary route has also been used satisfactorily in both adults and children (Fig 19–3).[68–70] The infraclavicular approach rapidly lends itself to continuous infusion when a catheter technique is employed (Fig 19–4).

Patchy analgesia in the hand with any of the above techniques can often be remedied by blockade of the individual nerves at the elbow or wrist, as a tourniquet is seldom required and inadequate analgesia in the upper arm is of little import.

The use of the peripheral nerve stimulator has greatly facilitated the performance of all of these blocks.[71]

Technique for Lower Limb Analgesia.—Although the lower limb is more difficult to block peripherally with a single injection, there are still worthwhile techniques available. In particular, femoral nerve block can be performed simply and easily and can provide excellent analgesia for femoral fractures.[72] The exact extent of the analgesia depends on the fracture site; excellent relief can be obtained for midshaft fractures, good relief for lower third fractures, and partial relief for upper third fractures.[73] The method is also recommended for children[74] and can be extended to give continuous analgesia for several days by the insertion of a catheter.[75] By increasing the volume of injectate and encouraging its cephalad spread, femoral nerve block can be extended to include the lateral femoral cutaneous nerve of thigh and the obturator nerve, thus providing more complete analgesia for the upper thigh.[76]

Except for injuries to the foot, blockade of the sciatic nerve alone is of little value in providing analgesia for trauma, and the traditional (Labat) approach requires the patient to adopt the Sims posi-

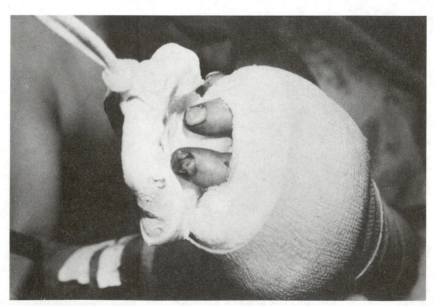

Fig 19–3.—A 38-year-old industrial worker suffered a crush injury to his left hand resulting in traumatic amputation of all fingers except the thumb. Reimplantation of the index, middle, and ring fingers resulted in what appeared to be nonviable digits on the second postoperative day. An axillary catheter was placed and continuous brachial plexus blockade established. The infusion was continued for 1 week. This resulted in improved local blood flow and viability was maintained. Photograph was taken 12 days after trauma.

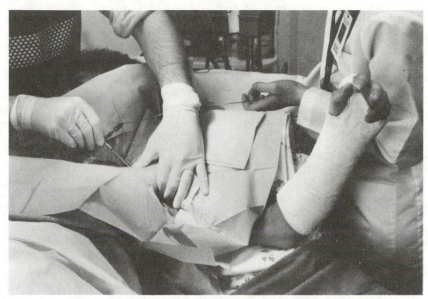

Fig 19—4.—Neuritis. A 54-year-old woman suffered a colles fracture with median nerve contusion requiring open reduction and internal fixation with exploration of the median nerve. She experienced burning pain secondary to median nerve neuritis initially, with the subsequent development of dystrophic changes six weeks following the injury. Figure shows a brachial plexus catheter being placed for continuous infusion with the aid of a nerve stimulator using the infraclavicular approach. The patient responded very well to seven days of continuous analgesia and intensive physical therapy.

tion, which is not always possible with an injured limb. The anterior approach is less reliable but suitable.[77] A lateral approach may be an improvement.[78]

Combined femoral and sciatic blocks can provide excellent analgesia below the knee and can be used for Pott's fractures and dislocations around the ankle.[79] Nerve block of saphenous, common peroneal, and tibial nerves at the knee, a rather neglected technique, can produce excellent analgesia below the upper third of the leg.[80]

Lumbar epidural infusion is an effective means of producing continuous analgesia for the lower extremity without resorting to multiple nerve blocks (see below). As such, this approach is by far the most common regional approach employed in hemodynamically stable patients.

Technique for Trunk Analgesia.—The severity of the pain from fractured ribs often necessitates intubation and ventilation because of inadequate respiration secondary to the injury. Opiate analgesia is inappropriate in these cases because of its respiratory depressant and cough suppressant actions. Epidural blockade can provide complete analgesia while leaving the patient awake and cooperative. This can often prevent the development of secondary changes that would require intermittent positive pressure ventilation. Initially, thoracic epidural was suggested for patients in whom pain was the dominant pathology,[81] but it is now also appreciated that epidural blockade can improve the diminished compliance, increase the vital capacity and functional residual capacity, and decrease the high bronchial resistance seen in these patients.[82, 83] This has led to a more aggressive approach to the treatment of such fractures based on the recognition that the problem is primarily a functional rather than an anatomical derangement.[84] Dittman et al.[85] recommended that all patients with multiple rib fractures have thoracic epidurals, providing the patient is conscious, has a vital capacity greater than 15 ml/kg, and has a Pa_{O_2} above 60 mm Hg on room air. They have shown this regimen to be highly effective in a series of about 250 patients.

A thoracic epidural block should be undertaken with care in a patient who has other injuries and should not be performed until hypovolemia has been corrected. It has been recommended that not more than five or six dermatomes be blocked, and if more than this number are fractured, it should be the lower ribs that are preferentially blocked, as these tend to be more painful and a lower block will interfere less with the cardioaccelerator fibers.[82] Blockade can be maintained with intermittent dosing or continuous infusion, of which the latter has many advantages.

The intermittent bolus technique is often unsatisfactory due to breakthrough pain every few hours, intermittent sympathetic blockade causing hypotension, and the development of tachyphylaxis.[86] Furthermore, the burden of such injections on the medical staff are outside the staffing levels of most hospitals. Continuous infusions offer a much more logical approach from both the pharmacologic and the manpower viewpoints.[87] By adjusting the concentration and the volume of the infusate one can alter the intensity and extent of the blockade. Once the block has been established it is often possible to maintain it with a relatively weak solution, and this diminishes the minimal chances of toxic effects. Abdominal or thoracic wounds often require larger volumes of stronger solutions, at least initially, and the catheter position in the center of the wound is more critical in these patients. In these patients, severe pain can be engendered by regression of the block by as little as one segment, and in the early stages this can occur rapidly with the resultant development of severe pain. In these cases, addition of a narcotic (meperidine, 5–10 mg/hour) to the infusate does not detract from the advantages of the local anesthetic agent but rather improves the analgesia without requiring the use of a dense motor block.[88]

Another approach often used is the intercostal block. Usually the intercostal block must be repeated as required, although when bupivacaine is used, analgesia as long as 16 hours has been obtained.[89] There is also the risk of causing a pneumothorax in patients who may already be respiratorily compromised. It is possible to insert a catheter percutaneously into the intercostal space and, by injecting a large volume, block several segments. This has also been done in patients with fractured ribs.[90, 91]

CHRONIC PAIN FOLLOWING TRAUMA

Pain persisting beyond the normal recovery period, often greatly exceeding that which might be anticipated relative to the residual pathosis, can be considered chronic posttraumatic pain.

General Principles of Management

The treatment of posttraumatic pain that persists due to deranged patterns of healing, the development of altered pain pathways, chronic ischemia, or the misuse or disuse of myofascial structures is far more complex than the treatment of acute pain syndromes. The contribution of psychological factors to the interpretation and outward expression of pain must always be considered in the chronic pain patient; resultant behavioral changes often contribute to the perpetuation of pain. Consequently, a multidisciplinary approach, such as the one proposed by Bonica, should be utilized if consistent success is to be realized.[92] Such an approach requires not only accurate medical diagnosis, but also behavioral and functional considerations utilized in concert with medical and physical therapeutic modalities. No single mode of treatment can be expected to consistently provide satisfactory results.

The complexity of chronic pain mechanisms is such that, in comparison to the acute pain syndromes previously described, one generally is forced to accept lesser degrees of therapeutic success. Reasonable goals should be discussed frankly with the patient at the onset of treatment and frequently reiterated. Chronic pain management should be directed toward pain control rather than cure, with specific goals that include the following:

1. Reduction in pain and elevation in pain threshold.
2. Emphasis on improved function and rehabilitation.
3. Reduction in reliance on medication, with the elimination of potentially addictive drugs.

Chronic Pain Syndromes and Their Mechanisms

Myofascial Pain

Perhaps the most common persistent pain following trauma is that emanating from myofascial (musculoskeletal) structures, i.e., muscle, bone, tendon, ligament, and other soft tissues of mesodermal origin. The myofascial pain may be due to one or more of the following causes: reflex muscle spasms, ischemia of the myofascial structures, decreased nutrition, fatigue of the muscle due to excessive use, and muscle injury. In most instances, the mechanisms of pain involve an interference with oxidative process in the muscle because of decreases in oxygen, enzymes, and other nutrients necessary for muscle metabolism. When fatigue follows overexertion, pain and soreness are experienced hours or days later. This may be due to increased cellular metabolites and water, which stimulate nociceptive nerve endings. Once the painful state is produced, it can be perpetuated by feedback cycles from myofascial trigger points.[93]

Afferent pain signals secondary to muscle spasm enter the spinal cord through the dorsal route where communication via internuncial neurons leads to hyperactivity in the anterior and anterolateral horn cells. This hyperactivity results in efferent traffic, causing more muscle spasm and vasoconstriction. Exercise exaggerates this relative ischemia; thus the pain is intensified.[92]

Trigger points are regions of hyperirritability within myofascial structures that, when stimulated by direct pressure, elicit tenderness and, depending on the severity of the stimulus, referred pain. These regions of focal muscle spasm present a limitation to active and passive motion with apparent shortening and weakening of the involved musculature. Pain from deep somatic structures is typically dull and diffuse in character. The ability to localize precise trigger areas decreases with increasing tissue depth. Diffusion and radiation can be indicators of severity, with muscle spasm and tenderness in zones of reference (to be distinguished from trigger points) often appearing at sites distant from the lesion. The intense nature of these hyperirritable regions makes them relatively resistant to systemic muscle relaxants or analgesics. Injection of a local anesthetic into specific zones of reference will decrease tenderness in that region; however, injection into trigger points not only decreases tenderness, but also reduces muscle spasm and spontaneous pain. Long-standing persistence of this positive feedback cycle can lead to sympathalgic involvement with vasomotor disturbance.

Fibrositis is a term used to characterize the chronic aseptic inflammatory reaction within these soft tissues which can result in fibrosis and contracture. The importance of maintaining function as a means of ultimately reducing pain cannot be overemphasized. Yet mobilization of the affected body parts and physical therapy are often difficult or impossible without first alleviating attendant pain.

Nonmuscular structures such as tendons, ligaments, and fasciae are also common sources of myofascial pain. Thoracic fasciitis following thoracotomy, bursitis and tenosynovitis, and traumatic arthritis as well as ligamentous strains and sprains are but a few of the myriad common examples.

Sympathalgias

This syndrome is characterized by hyperactivity of either or both afferent and efferent C fibers. It is generally classified into two syndromes: causalgia and reflex sympathetic dystrophy. There are three popular theories accounting for the pain associated with causalgia: (1) the gate control theory, (2) a vicious cycle of reflexes, and (3) the artificial synapse theory. The most credible is the artificial synapse theory.[94] It is based on the fact that when a nerve lesion destroys the electrical insulation between different fibers, or alters the anatomy in some way, efferent C fibers stimulate afferent somatic fibers. Constant orthodromic bombardment is interpreted as pain. In addition, antidromic depolarization sensitizes the peripheral nerve endings. This also results in increased transmission of impulses and thereby is interpreted as pain. Thus the nociceptive pain model describing acute pain with afferent pain information being transmitted via C and A delta fibers does not necessarily apply in chronic pain states. In fact, chronic pain information may be transmitted in the fashion described over even the very large A alpha fibers if the afferent traffic is sufficient. These pathways can be delineated by differential nerve blocking techniques and provide a focus for therapeutic intervention.

The syndromes known as the reflex sympathetic dystrophies are sometimes categorized according to which symptoms from within the complex tend to predominate in a given clinical circumstance. However, certain features are considered characteristic. Burning, aching pain initially localized, then spreading proximally, cold sensitivity, hyperesthesia, as well as vasomotor and sudomotor disturbances are typical. When they occur as the result of traumatic insult, the onset of such changes is usually relatively rapid, often beginning within days or weeks of the injury.[95]

Early signs are often thought to include vasodilatation with resultant rubor, color, and edema. Sudomotor changes such as hyperhidrosis also occur but are somewhat less constant. Signs that are generally believed to represent later stages are those of vasoconstriction, i.e., cyanosis and cold skin distally. Trophic changes, such as thin glossy skin, nutritional nail changes, coarse-appearing or actual loss of hair, muscle atrophy, and bone demineralization are noted late in the disease course. As these changes are essentially the result of nutritional deficit imposed by perpetual vasoconstriction, they tend to present distally, where tissues are most vulnerable to ischemic insult, being farthest from the nutritive source. While sympathetic blockade and aggressive physical therapy are well-proven techniques for promoting repair and decreasing pain once reflex sympathetic dystrophy has developed, the notion that early analgesic block in conjunction with early active motion and early sympathetic block might prevent the development of reflex sympathetic dystrophy holds tremendous logical appeal.[96, 97] Controlled studies, however, have yet to be completed.

The term causalgia describes a similar syndrome of burning pain with hyperesthesia and accompanying vasomotor and sudomotor disturbances occurring soon after a partial nerve injury. Penetrating wounds, especially high-velocity missiles, seem to predispose to the development of causalgia, but other forms of nerve injury also produce causalgic states. The pain is usually constant, severe, and spontaneous, but it can be precipitated by emotional stress or by peripheral stimuli and relieved with sympathetic blockade. Often hyperpathia, an extreme degree of hyperesthesia, is seen. Pathologically, ruptured axons seem to heal with endoneural fibrosis rather than discrete neuromas. Why some partial nerve injuries result in neuritis and others in causalgia is not known. Whether the nature of the insult affects either the mode of healing or the subsequent symptoms is also unclear.

Neuralgias and Neuromas

Partial nerve injuries resulting from mechanical trauma sometimes result in an irritative state associated with perineuritis or neuritis. Pain that is burning, lancinating, worse at night, and aggravated by stretching the affected nerve is typical for neuritis. Other irritative phenomena such as fascicular muscle twitching or spasm, hyperesthesia, paresthesia, or dysesthesia may be present. Vasomotor or sudomotor changes are not seen in the absence of significant sympathalgia.

There are numerous examples of postoperative and posttraumatic injuries to peripheral nerves resulting in mononeuritides. Well described are the host of postoperative neuralgias relating to mechanical nerve trauma in the form of pressure due to improper positioning of the patient on the operating room table. Intercostal neuralgia following thoracotomy or chest wall injury is particularly common.

Nerve entrapment or involvement in scar tissue also gives rise to pain. Irritation of sympathetic fibers around the spermatic cord, or injury to the genitofemoral nerve following herniorrhaphy or other inguinal operation, is often unusually resistant to treatment.

Plexalgias do occur posttraumatically in both the upper and lower extremities. Cervical plexalgia can give rise to extensive myofascial neck and shoulder pain. Sudden stretching of the upper extremity at the shoulder can cause brachial plexalgia. Lumbar plexalgia, while usually of viral origin, can occur with trauma because of the considerable mobility present in the lumbar spine. Early sympathetic blockade is probably useful in the prevention of sympathalgias following these injuries.

Following complete disruption of a peripheral nerve, the severed ends of the axons continue to grow in an effort to reunite. Anatomical disruption often precludes proper realignment of each proximal axon with its corresponding distal component. This may result in dysesthesias. Additionally, abnormal afferent impulses emanating from the dorsal root ganglion following nerve injury probably contribute to production of abnormal sensation. Furthermore, in trauma, or in the case of amputation of a body part, the cut ends of the neurons search in vain for the missing nerve trunk and eventually may curl around themselves in whorl-like fashion or become embedded in scar or other soft tissue. These bulbous collections of nonmyelinated neurons are called neuromas. Neuromas do not behave as normal sensory receptors but instead, when appropriately stimulated, often generate an exaggerated response with sharp lancinating pain in the distribution of the affected nerve. Protracted, often clonic muscular contractions over the affected stump can result. Neuromas can be quite labile, giving rise to spontaneous discharge, especially when large and tender, as can be the case when infection complicates the postamputation period.

Central Mechanisms: Deafferentation and Phantom Limb Pain

Dysesthesia following denervation is thought to be due to abnormal neuronal activity at central sites resulting from either the loss of or a relative imbalance of afferent input.[98] This may relate to a relative predominance of small fibers in the absence of input from larger fibers.[99] As in other central pain states, therapies resulting in further peripheral denervation are of no value.

Postamputation phantom sensations occur in most amputees; however, it is said that only 5%–10% report pain in association with these phenomena. A recent study suggests that the incidence may be in fact much higher (72%).[100] The pain can be burning, crushing, shooting, throbbing, or related to the impression that the missing part is fixed in an abnormal and uncomfortable position in space. This is particularly true if pain or abnormal posture was present prior to amputation.[101, 102]

Despite the appearance of vasomotor and sudomotor changes in some patients with phantom limb pain, sympathetic interruption rarely is of lasting value.[103] Furthermore, while these painful sensations can be aggravated by irritation of neuromas within the stump, such peripheral mechanisms cannot fully explain this form of deafferentation pain. Neither the time course of neuroma formation nor the anatomical distribution of the affected nerves is consistent with phantom sensation. Phantom sensations usually correspond to the areas with the greatest representation in the sensory cortex, with gradual shortening of the phantom limb until only the hands or feet remain attached to the stump just prior to resolution. The presence of pain prevents this usual shrinkage. Emotional upset and fatigue can also trigger phantom pain.

Increasing evidence now suggests that reorganization of neural pathways at spinal as well as thalamic and cortical levels takes place following peripheral deafferentation.[104, 105] Melzack proposed a central biasing mechanism.[106] This concept is similar to the central mechanism of deafferentation mentioned previously. Sensory loss creates a relative predominance of small fibers, which results in the release of normal tonic inhibition from central sites. This presumably predisposes to self-perpetuating neuronal activity at spinal and higher centers in the CNS.

Treatment of Chronic Pain

Oral medications, nerve blocks, stimulation-produced analgesia, psychological techniques, physical therapy, and ablative neurosurgery are all used in the treatment of chronic pain following trauma. The treatment of chronic pain utilizing each of these modalities is discussed elsewhere in this text and summarized in Table 19–1.

A few points relevant to posttraumatic pain de-

TABLE 19–1.—TREATMENT MODALITIES

Oral medications
Nonsteroidal anti-inflammatory agents
Tricyclic antidepressants
Tricyclics + phenothiazines
Centrally acting muscle relaxants
Carbamazepine and phenytoin
L-Tryptophan
Nerve blocks
Central
Peripheral
Sympathetic
Stimulation-produced analgesia
TENS
Acupuncture
Periaqueductal gray and thalamus
Dorsal column
Ablative neurosurgery
Cordotomy
DREZ* lesions
Psychological techniques
Cognitive behavior therapy
Biofeedback
Relaxation therapy
Hypnosis
Operant conditioning
Physical Therapy
Mobilization and exercise
Heat and cold

*DREZ = dorsal root entry zone.

serve emphasis. In general, local anesthetic nerve blocks are initially performed as prognostic or diagnostic maneuvers. In certain syndromes such as phantom limb pain, causalgia, and sympathetic dystrophy, such a block, usually of the sympathetic system, will provide relief of longer duration than the action of the local anesthetic agent used. This relief can be extended by repeating the block. In most of the syndromes in which blocks have been shown to be of value, the results are usually better if the block is performed relatively early following the injury. Sometimes blocks with reversible agents provide only transient relief, and one must contemplate the use of a neurolytic agent.[107]

In myofascial dysfunction the use of nerve blocks can relieve the muscle spasm, increase the blood flow by sympathetic block, relieve the pain, and allow aggressive physical therapy. In severe cases such blocks are often needed, at least initially. Milder cases can be managed with trigger point injections.

Various neurosurgical techniques have been devised for the treatment of intractable pain and many of these have been applied to persistent and severe posttraumatic pain. In general the approach that patients often suggest of "cutting the nerves" seldom produces pain relief and can produce a sensory deficit with deafferentation pain that is worse or no better than the original state. Destruction of the dorsal root entry zone has been used in persistent phantom limb pain with some success.[108]

SUMMARY

Posttraumatic pain encompasses acute posttraumatic and subsequent chronic pain states. The pathophysiology of pain varies with chronicity. Consequently, appropriate therapeutic intervention requires consideration of both prevailing perturbations in hemodynamic and respiratory physiology as well as resultant alterations in pain mechanisms. Furthermore, posttraumatic complications and the late development of chronic pain states can be altered by the choice of analgesic technique.

Acute pain management should promote early mobilization and therefore a reduction in posttraumatic and postoperative complications. The complexity of chronic pain, however, requires a multidisciplinary approach to management, with an emphasis on improved function and rehabilitation.

REFERENCES

1. Marks B.M., Sachar E.J.: Undertreatment of medical inpatients with narcotic analgesics. *Ann. Intern. Med.* 78:173–181, 1977.
2. Bonica J.J.: Pain research and therapy: Past and current status and future needs, in Ng L.K.Y., Bonica J.J. (eds.): *Pain, Discomfort and Humanitarian Care.* New York, Elsevier, 1980, pp. 1–64.
3. Chapman C.R., Bonica J.J.: *Acute Pain: Current Concepts.* Scope Monograph. Kalamazoo, Mich., Upjohn Company, 1983.
4. Wikland C.: Regional blockade versus analgesic therapy. *Acta Anaesthesiol. Scand. Suppl.* 74:169–172, 1982.
5. Beran D.R.: Modification of the metabolic response to trauma under extradural analgesia. *Anaesthesia* 26:188–191, 1971.
6. Kehlet H.: The endocrine-metabolic response to postoperative pain. *Acta Anaesthesiol. Scand Suppl.* 74:173–175, 1982.
7. Moller I.W., Rem J., Brandt M.R., et al.: Effect of post-traumatic epidural analgesia on the cortisol and hyperglycemic response to surgery. *Acta Anaesthesiol. Scand.* 26:56–58, 1982.
8. Brandt M.R., Fernades A., Mordhorst R., et al.: Epidural analgesia improves postoperative nitrogen balance. *Br. Med. J.* 1:1106–1108, 1978.
9. Pflug A.E., Halter J.B., Tolas A.G.: Plasma catecholamine levels during anesthesia and surgical stress. *Reg. Anaesthes. Suppl.* 7:S49–56, 1982.
10. Kehlet H.: The modifying effect of general and regional anesthesia on the endocrine-metabolic response to surgery. *Reg. Anaesthes. Suppl.* 7:S38–48, 1982.
11. Brandt M.R., Olgaard K., Kehlet H.: Epidural analgesia inhibits the renin and aldosterone response to surgery. *Acta Anaesthesiol. Scand.* 23:267–272, 1979.
12. Bonnett F., Harari A., Thibonnier M., et al.: Suppression of antidiuretic hormone hypersecretion during surgery by extradural anaesthesia. *Br. J. Anaesth.* 54:29–36, 1982.
13. Gann D.S.: Endocrine and metabolic responses to injury, in Schwartz S.E. (ed.): *Principles of Surgery,* ed. 3. New York, McGraw-Hill, 1979, pp. 1–63.
14. Epstein S.E., Redwood D.R., Goldstein R.E., et al.: Angina pectoris: Pathophysiology, evaluation and treatment. *Ann. Intern. Med.* 75:263, 1971.
15. Braun W.E., Maroko P.R.: Protection of the ischemic myocardium, in Braunwald E. (ed.): *The Myocardium: Failure and Infarction.* New York, H.P. Publishing, 1974, pp. 329–342.
16. Bonica J.J.: Autonomic innervation of viscera in relation to nerve block. *Anesthesiology* 29:739–813, 1968.
17. Bromage P.R., Shibata H.R., Willoughby H.W.: Influence of prolonged epidural blockade on blood sugar and cortisol responses to operations upon the upper part of the abdomen and the thorax. *Surg. Gynecol. Obstet.* 132:1051–1056, 1971.
18. Traynor C., Paterson J.L., Ward I.D., et al.: Effects of extradural analgesia and vagal blockade on the metabolic and endocrine response to upper abdominal surgery. *Br. J. Anaesth.* 54:319–323, 1982.
19. Jorgensen B.C., Andersen H.B., Engquist A.: Influence of epidural morphine on postoperative pain, endocrine-metabolic and renal responses to surgery: A controlled study. *Acta Anaesthesiol. Scand.* 26:63–68, 1982.
20. Johnson W.C.: Postoperative ventilatory performance: Dependence upon surgical incision. *Am. Surg.* 41:615–619, 1975.
21. Spence A.A.: Pulmonary changes after surgery. *Reg. Anaesthes. Suppl.* 7:S119–121, 1982.
22. Bromage P.R., Comporesi E., Chestnut D.: Epidural narcotics for postoperative analgesia. *Anesth. Analg.* 59:473–480, 1980.
23. Benhamou D., Samii K., Noviant Y.: Effect of analgesics on respiratory muscle function after upper abdominal surgery. *Acta Anaesthesiol. Scand.* 27:22–25, 1983.
24. Rybro L., Schurizer B.A., Petersen T.K., et al.: Postoperative analgesia and lung function: A comparison of intramuscular with epidural morphine. *Acta Anaesthesiol. Scand.* 26:514–518, 1982.

25. Rawal N., Sjostrand U.H., Dahlstrom B., et al.: Epidural morphine for postoperative pain relief: A comparative study with intramuscular narcotic and intercostal nerve block. *Anesth. Analg.* 61:93–98, 1982.

26. Parbrook G.D., Steel G.F., Dacrymple F.G.: Factors predisposing to postoperative pain and pulmonary complications. *Br. J. Anaesth.* 45:21–33, 1973.

27. Eysenck S.B., Eysenck H.J.: The measurement of psychoticism: A study of factor stability and reliability. *Br. J. Soc. Clin. Psychol.* 7:286, 1968.

28. Modig J., Malmberg P., Karlstrom G.: Effect of epidural versus general anaesthetic on calf blood flow. *Acta Anaesthesiol. Scand.* 24:305–309, 1980.

29. Stewart G.J., Ritchie W.G., Lynch P.R.: Venous endothelia damage produced by massive sticking and emigration of leukocytes. *Am. J. Pathol.* 74:507–532, 1974.

30. Giddon D.B., Lindhe J.: In vivo quantitation of local anesthetic suppression of leukocyte adherence. *Am. J. Pathol.* 68:327–338, 1972.

31. Cazenave J.P. Benveniste J., Mustard J.F.: Aggregation of rabbit platelets by platelet-activating factor is independent of the release reaction and the arachidonate pathway and inhibited by membrane active drugs. *Lab. Invest.* 41:275, 1979.

32. Modig J., Hjelmstedt A., Sahlstedt B., et al.: Comparative influences of epidural and general anaesthesia on deep venous thrombosis and pulmonary embolism after total hip replacement. *Acta Chir. Scand.* 147:125–130, 1981.

33. Cousins M.J., Wright C.J., Graft, muscle, skin blood flow after epidural block in vascular surgical procedures. *Surg. Gynecol. Obstet.* 133:59–69, 1971.

34. Bridenbaugh P.O.: Anesthesia and influence on hospitalization time. *Reg. Anaesthes. Suppl.* 7:S151–155, 1982.

35. Noller D.W., Gillenwater J.Y., et al.: Intercostal nerve block with flank incision. *J. Urol.* 117:759, 1977.

36. Pflug A.E., Murphy T.M., Butler S.H., et al.: The effects of postoperative peridural analgesic on pulmonary therapy and pulmonary complications. *Anesthesiology* 41:8–17, 1974.

37. Nimmo W.S., Littlewood D.G., Scott D.B., et al.: Gastric emptying following hysterectomy with extradural analgesia. *Br. J. Anaesth.* 50:559–561, 1978.

38. Cousins M.J., Reeve T.S., Glynn C.J., et al.: Neurolytic lumbar sympathetic blockade: Duration of denervation and relief of rest pain. *Anaesth. Intensive Care,* 7:121–135, 1979.

39. Churchill-Davidson H.C.: *A Practice of Anaesthesia,* ed. 4. Philadelphia, W.B. Saunders Co., 1978.

40. Vickers M.D., Woodsmith F.G., Stewart M.C.: *Drugs in Anaesthetic Practice,* ed. 5. London, Butterworths, 1973.

41. Jowitt M.D., Knight R.J.: Anaesthesia during the Falklands campaign. *Anaesthesia* 38:776–783, 1983.

42. Stapleton J.V., Austin K.L., Mather L.E.: A pharmacokinetic approach to postoperative pain: Conscious infusion of peridine. *Anaesth. Intensive Care* 7:25–36, 1979.

43. Fry E.N.: Postoperative analgesia using continuous infusion of popovech. *Ann. R. Coll. Surg. Engl.* 61:371–372, 1979.

44. Orr I.A., Keenan D.J., Dundee J.W.: Improved pain relief after thoracotomy: Use of cryoprobe and morphine infusion. *Br. Med. J.* 283:945–948, 1981.

45. Mather L.E.: Parenteral opiates for postoperative analgesia. *Reg. Anaesth.* 7:144, 1982.

46. Evans J.M., MacCarthy J., Rosen M., et al.: Apparatus for patient controlled administration of intravenous narcotics during labor. *Lancet* 1:17, 1976.

47. Hull C.J., Sibbald A.: Control of postoperative pain by interactive demand analgesia. *Br. J. Anaesth.* 53:385–391, 1981.

48. Bond A.C., Davies C.K.: Ketamine and pancuronium for the shocked patient. *Anaesthesia* 29:59, 1974.

49. Grant I.S., Nimmo W.C., Clements J.H.: Pharmacokinetics and analgesic effects of IM and oral ketamine. *Br. J. Anaesth.* 53:805, 1981.

50. Corssen G., Domino F.F.: Dissociative anesthesia: Further studies and first clinical experience with the phencyclidine derivative CI 581. *Anesth. Analg.* 45:29, 1966.

51. Parbrook G.D.: Techniques of inhalation analgesia in the postop period. *Br. J. Anaesth.* 39:730, 1967.

52. Parbrook G.D.: Therapeutic uses of N_2O. *Br. J. Anaesth.* 40:365, 1968.

53. Smolinski K.T.: N_2O anaesthesia as a means of prevention and early treatment of traumatic shock. *Khirurgica (Mon.)* 37:16, 1961.

54. Eisele J.H., Trenchard D., Stubb J., et al.: The immediate cardiac depression by anaesthetics in conscious dogs. *Br. J. Anaesth.* 41:86, 1969.

55. Moss E., McDowall D.G.: I.C.P. increases with 50% nitrous oxide in oxygen in severe head injuries during controlled ventilation. *Br. J. Anaesth.* 51:757, 1979.

56. Atkinson R.J., Rushman G.B., Lee J.A.: *A Synopsis of Anaesthesia,* ed. 8. Bristol, England, John Wright & Sons, Ltd., 1977, p. 417.

57. Holmes C. McK.: Intravenous regional blockade, in Cousins M.J., Bridenbaugh P.O. (eds.): *Neural Blockade.* Philadelphia, J.B. Lippincott, Co. 1980, p. 343.

58. Kerr J.A.: Intravenous regional anesthesia. *Anaesthesia* 22:562, 1967.

59. Eriksson E.: The effects of intravenous local anaesthetic agents on the central nervous system. *Acta Anaesthesiol. Scand. Suppl.* 36:79, 1967.

60. Winnie A.P., Ramamurthy S.: Pneumatic exsanguination for intravenous regional anesthesia. *Anesthesiology* 33:664, 1970.

61. Carrell E.D., Eyring E.J.: Intravenous regional anesthesia for childhood fractures. *J. Trauma* 11:301, 1971.

62. deJong R.H.: Axillary block of the brachial plexus. *Anesthesiology* 22:215, 1961.

63. Raj P.P., Montgomery S.J., Nettles D., et al.: Infraclavicular brachial plexus block: A new approach. *Anesth. Analg.* 52:897, 1973.

64. Winnie A.P.: Interscalene brachial plexus block. *Anesth. Analg.* 52:897, 1973.

65. Moore D.C.: *Regional Block,* ed. 4. Springfield, Charles C Thomas, 1971.

66. Hefington C.A., Thompson R.C.: The use of interscalene block anesthesia for manipulative reduction of fractures and dislocations of the upper extremity. *J. Bone Joint Surg.* 559:836, 1973.

67. Hughes T.J., Desgrand D.A.: Interscalene block for colles fracture. *Anaesthesia* 38:149–151, 1983.

68. Webling D.D.: Anaesthesia of the upper arm for casualty procedures. *Med. J. Aust.* 2:496, 1960.

69. Clayton M.L., Turner D.A.: Upper arm block anesthesia for children with fractures. *JAMA* 169:99–327, 1959.

70. Eriksson E.: Axillary brachial plexus anaesthesia in children with citanest. *Acta Anaesth. Scand. Suppl.* 16:281, 1965.

71. Raj P.P., Rosenblatt R., Montgomery S.J.: Use of the nerve stimulator for peripheral blocks. *Reg. Anaesth.,* vol. 14, April–June 1980.

72. Berry F.R.: Analgesia in patients with fractured shaft of femur. *Anaesthesia* 32:576, 1977.

73. Tondare A.S.: Femoral nerve block for tracheal shaft of femur. *Can. Anaesth. Soc. J.* 53:1055–1058, 1982.

74. Grossbard G.D., Love B.R.T.: Femoral nerve block: A simple and safe method of instant analgesia for femoral fractures in children. *Aust. NZ J. Surg.* 49:592, 1979.

75. Rosenblatt R.M.: Continuous femoral anesthesia for lower extremity surgery. *Anesth. Analg.* 59:631–633, 1980.

76. Winnie A.P., Ramamurthy S., Durani Z.: The inguinal perivascular technique of lumbar plexus anesthesia: The 3 in 1 block. *Anaesth. Analg.* 52:989, 1973.

77. Beck G.P.: Anterior approach to sciatic nerve block. *Anesthesiology* 26:222, 1963.

78. Ichiyanagi G.: Sciatic nerve block: Lateral approach with the patient supine. *Anesthesiology* 20:601–604, 1959.

79. Berry F.R., Kirchoff J.A.: Neural blockade in the outpatient clinic, emergency room and private office, in Cousins M., Bridenbaugh P.O. (eds.): *Neural Blockade.* Philadelphia, J.B. Lippincott, Co. 1980, p. 501.

80. Rorie D.K., Byer D.E., Nelson D.O., et al.: Assessment of block of the sciatic nerve in the popliteal fossa. *Anaesth. Analg.* 59:371–376, 1980.

81. Gibbons J., James O., Quail A.: The relief of pain in chest injury. *Br. J. Anaesth.* 45:1136, 1975.

82. Lloyd J.W., Rucklidge M.A.: The management of closed chest injuries. *Br. J. Surg.* 56:721, 1967.

83. Dittman M., Keller R., Wolff G.: A rationale for epidural analgesia in the treatment of multiple rib fractures. *Intensive Care Med.* 4:193, 1976.

84. Johnson J.R., McCaughey G.J.: Epidural morphine: A method of management of multiple fractured ribs. *Anaesthesia* 35:155, 1980.

85. Dittman M., Steenblock G., Kranzlin M., et al.: Epidural analgesia or mechanical ventilation for multiple fractures. *Intensive Care Med.* 8:89–92, 1982.

86. Bromage P.R., Pettigrew R.T., Crowell D.E.: Tachyphylaxis in epidural analgesia. Augmentation and decay of local analgesia. *J. Clin. Pharmacol.* 9:30, 1969.

87. Raj P.P., Finnsson R., Denson D.: Epidural analgesia—intermittent or continuous? in Meyer J., Nolte H. (eds.): *Die kontiniuerliche Periduralanasthesie.* Stuttgart, Georg Thieme Verlag, 1983, pp. 26–37.

88. Raj P.P., et al.: Unpublished data.

89. Telivoo L., Perttala Y.: Use of x-ray contrast medium to control intervertebral nerve blocks. *Am. Chin. Cyraecol. Fem.* 55:185, 1966.

90. O'Kelly E., Garry B.: Continuous pain relief for multiple fractured ribs. *Br. J. Anaesth.* 53:987–991, 1981.

91. Murphy D.F.: Intercostal nerve blockade for fractured ribs and postoperative analgesia. *Reg. Anaesth.* 8:151–153, 1983.

92. Bonica J.J.: *The Management of Pain.* Philadelphia, Lea & Febiger, 1953.

93. Raj P.P., McLennan J.E., Phero J.C.: Assessment and management planning of chronic low back pain, in Stanton-Hicks, Boas R. (eds.): *Chronic Low Back Pain.* New York, Raven Press, 1982, pp. 71–99.

94. Miller R.D., Munger W.L., Powell P.E.: Chronic pain and local anesthetic, in Cousins M.J., Bridenbaugh P.O. (eds.): *Neural Blockade.* Philadelphia, J.B. Lippincott Co., 1980, pp. 616–636.

95. DeTakats G.: Nature of painful vasodilation in causalgic states. *Arch Neurol. Psychiatry* 50:318, 1943.

96. Betcher A.M., Bean G., Casten D.R.: Continuous procaine block of paravertebral sympathetic. *JAMA* 151:288, 1953.

97. Tyson M.D., Gaynor J.S.: Interruption of the sympathetic nervous system in relation to trauma. *Surgery* 19:167, 1946.

98. Melzack R., Wall P.D.: Pain mechanisms: A new theory. *Science* 150:971, 1965.

99. Nathan P.W., Noordenbos W., Wall P.D.: Ongoing activity in peripheral nerve: Interactions between electrical stimulation and ongoing activity. *Exp. Neurol.* 38:90, 1973.

100. Jensen T.S., Krebs B., Nielsen J., et al.: Phantom limb, phantom pain and stump pain in amputees dur-

ing the first 6 months following amputation. *Pain* 17:243, 1983.

101. Melzack R.: Phantom limb pain: Implications for treatment of pathologic pain. *Anesthesiology* 35:409, 1971.
102. Riddock G.P. Phantom limbs and body shape. *Brain* 64:197, 1941.
103. Kallio K.E.: Permanency of results obtained by sympathetic surgery in the treatment of phantom pain. *Acta Orthop. Scand.* 19:391, 1950.
104. Devor M., Wall P.D.: Reorganization of spinal cord sensory map after peripheral nerve injury. *Nature* 276:75, 1978.
105. Wall P.D., Eggerr M.D.: Formation of new connections in adult rat brain after partial deafferentation. *Nature* 232:542, 1971.
106. Melzack J.: Central neural mechanisms in phantom limb pain. *Adv. Neurol.* vol. 4, 1974.
107. Wood M.: The use of phenol as a neurolytic agent: A review. *Pain* 5:205–225, 1978.
108. Nashold B.S., Urban B., Zorub D.S.: Phantom pain relief by local destruction of the sub. gerat. of Rolando, in Bonica J., Albe-Fessard D. (eds.): *Advances in Pain Research and Surgery.* New York, Raven Press, 1976, vol. 1.

20 / Cancer

20A / Rational Management of Cancer-Related Pain

THERESA FERRER-BRECHNER, M.D.

OF 700,000 PATIENTS diagnosed to have cancer in the United States yearly, 400,000 die, making cancer the second leading cause of death in the American population. Worldwide, approximately 5 million people die of cancer each year.

How many of these cancer patients suffer from pain? Although the incidence of cancer-related pain has not been systematically studied on a large scale, some isolated studies state that pain occurs in 58%–80% of patients hospitalized with cancer.[1–4] With advancement of disease, the figure increases to as much as 87% before death.

The burden of cancer-related pain is overwhelming, especially because recent advances in cancer therapy have succeeded significantly in increasing survival time after the initial cancer diagnosis. Predisposition to the occurrence of pain in cancer patients with longer survival times behooves us to reevaluate our management of cancer-related pain.

Pain clinics have mushroomed throughout the United States in the past 10 years, but their emphasis has been on the management of chronic noncancer or benign pain. Although chronic benign and cancer pain patients both experience prolonged pain and therefore need similar physical and psychological approaches in a systematized treatment program, there are distinct differences between the two groups. In the cancer patient, the somatic origin of pain is easily identified by the usual diagnostic tools. In contrast, the somatic origin of pain is often difficult to identify in the patient with chronic benign pain. The cancer pain patient usually has recurrent acute exacerbation of pain corresponding to the progression of the disease, while chronic benign pain patients usually describe continuous intractable pain, most often without evidence of disease progression. In addition to chronic pain, the cancer patient's concomitant symptoms such as nausea and vomiting, constipation, and anorexia must be addressed if acceptable pain relief is to be obtained.

In contrast to the behavior modification programs typically undertaken for the chronic benign pain patient, the management of chronic cancer pain includes providing sympathy and caring, addressing the issue of dying, prescribing adequate nonnarcotic and narcotic analgesics, and utilizing various neuroablative procedures.

Because of these differences, the management of the cancer patient with pain must be considered as a distinct program from the management of chronic noncancer or benign pain patients.

It is not difficult to imagine why the patient with cancer tends to develop pain. A survey of several hundreds of patients hospitalized at the Sloan-Kettering Memorial Institute indicates a category of pain syndromes resulting either from direct tumor invasion or from the therapy. In Table 20A–1, the various pain syndromes commonly seen in the cancer patient are classified, with the usual symptoms.

In surveying the causes of pain in patients referred to the UCLA Cancer Pain Clinic, one finds that 61.7% of patients had pain due to direct tumor invasion, mostly due to bone or neural invasion; 30.8% of patients had pain due to the antineoplastic therapy.[5] The remaining patients (7.5%) had pain unrelated to tumor invasion or therapy (e.g., low back pain due to chronic osteoarthritis which commenced prior to the onset of cancer) (Table 20A–2).

TABLE 20A–1.—CAUSES OF CANCER-RELATED PAIN

CAUSE	SYMPTOMS
Secondary to Direct Tumor Involvement	
Bone involvement	Localized to area, progressive increase in intensity
Neural invasion	Burning pain, hyperesthesia, dysesthesia
Brachial plexus	Radicular pain from C-8 to T-1, paresthesias, Horner's syndrome
Lumbar plexus	Radicular pain in L1–3 (groin, thigh)
Sacral plexus	Perianal pain, bowel and bladder dysfunction
Meningeal carcinomatoses	Headache, neck stiffness, low back pain
Epidural/spinal	Pain along invaded vertebral body or neural distribution
Visceral	
Pleural	Interscapular pain to shoulder or anterior chest
Liver	Right upper quadrant abdominal pain radiating to lower ribs
Pancreatic	Midepigastric knife-like pain through to back
Secondary to Cancer-Directed Therapy	
Postsurgical	Occurs 1–2 mo. after surgery
Postsurgical	Burning pain in posterior arm, axilla, chest (intercostobrachial neuritis)
Postthoracotomy	Dysesthesias over area of sensory loss (intercostal neuritis)
Phantom limb	Burning pain over stump
Postchemotherapy	
Postherpetic neuralgia	Pain along a dermatomal distribution, common in patients over 50 years old with depressed immune response
Toxic neuropathy (e.g., vincristine)	Dysesthesia over hands and feet
Postirradiation	Can occur 6 mo. to 20 yr after irradiation
	Progressive motor weakness; radiation injury to adjacent luna, rib, or humerus

Most patients referred to the cancer pain centers with pain secondary to direct tumor invasion are in progressive stages of the disease. Therefore, they usually require prompt and more aggressive attempts in alleviating pain, such as the early use of neuroablative procedures.

Patients with pain following cancer therapy usually have longer histories of pain and their disease is usually nonprogressive when they are referred for pain management. Often these patients require a program geared toward long-term pain management, somewhat similar to that for chronic benign or noncancer pain.

The most common primary sites of cancer among the patients referred to UCLA cancer clinic are shown in Table 20A–3.

TABLE 20A–2.—INCIDENCE OF PAIN SYNDROMES IN AN OUTPATIENT CANCER PAIN CLINIC (N = 120)

PAIN SYNDROME	NO. (%) OF PTS.
Direct tumor invasion	74 (61.7)
Bone metastasis	34 (18.3)
Neural invasion	19 (15.8)
Visceral invasion	21 (10)
Therapy related	37 (30.8)
Postsurgical	20 (16.6)
Postchemotherapy	6 (5)
Postherpetic	7 (5.8)
Postirradiation	5 (4.2)
Unrelated to cancer or therapy	9 (7.5)

TABLE 20A–3.—SITE OF PRIMARY IN AN OUTPATIENT CANCER PAIN CLINIC (N = 120)

SITE	NO. (%) OF PTS.
Breast	26 (21.7)
Colon	18 (15)
Lung	17 (14.2)
Cervix and uterus	12 (10)
Urinary system	12 (10)
Lymph and blood	8 (6.6)
Primary bone	6 (5)
Head and neck	6 (5)
Malignant melanoma	6 (5)
Liver and pancreas	6 (5)
CNS	3 (2.5)

EVALUATION

In evaluating the cancer patient with pain, a physician must determine if the pain is a symptom or a disease entity in itself.

Pain is considered a symptom if it is secondary to an expanding or metastatic lesion that may be appropriately managed by cancer-directed therapy (i.e., chemotherapy or radiation therapy). Therapy that decreases tumor size may effectively reduce pain.

If the pain is due to a malignant lesion that cannot be managed by appropriate cancer-directed therapy or if the pain is a result of cancer-directed therapy (e.g., postherpetic neuralgia, vincristine neuropathy, postmastectomy pain), the pain should be regarded as a disease entity in itself and appropriate pain-directed therapy be applied. Figure 20A–1 summarizes the evaluation of cancer pain as a symptom or a disease, in relation to treatment strategies.

An evaluation checklist for the cancer pain patient is given below.

PRIOR TO FIRST VISIT:

    Self-history questionnaire
    Psychological Distress Index (Brief Symptom Inventory [BSI])

    Pain scales (McGill's)
    Review of available records, x-ray films, laboratory tests

AT FIRST VISIT:

    Pain scales
    Complete history
    Physical examination, including complete neurologic examination
    Interview for degree of psychological distress
    Review of records and x-ray films brought in by patient
    Clarify patient's goals
    Plan therapy immediately

AT SUBSEQUENT VISITS:

    Pain scales (McGill's, BSI)
    Monitor for abrupt changes in neurologic status
    Monitor analgesic intake for efficacy and side effects

A self-history questionnaire sent to the patient prior to the first visit is extremely helpful in decreasing the amount of time spent by these particularly debilitated patients during their first visit. Such forms can contain some brief psychological test material such as the McGill's pain scale[6] and the Brief Symptom Inventory (BSI).[7] Both these tests are ideal for the cancer patient with pain who is unable to complete lengthy psychological tests such as the 560-item Minnesota Multiphasic Personality Inven-

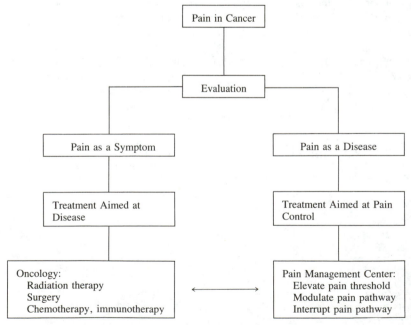

Fig 20A–1.—Evaluation of cancer pain as a symptom or disease, in relation to treatment strategies.

tory, which is used for chronic benign pain patients. The McGill pain scale and the BSI in such patients correlates with scales derived from testing of chronic benign pain patients.[8] No matter what type of psychological tests are used, it is important that they be brief and easily administered with each visit.

During the first visit, baseline pain scales are helpful to ascertain the ability of the patient to effectively express the degree of pain he or she feels and for use as a monitor of therapeutic response. Examples of such scales and the mean response obtained from the cancer pain patients on entry into the pain clinic follow:

1. If the worst pain you have ever experienced is 100%, how much did you feel, on the average, last week? $x = 67\%$ (SE = 5.3%) (n = 36)

2. Rate your average pain level during the past week by placing a mark on the line:

Least possible pain $\underline{\quad 57.0\% \quad}$ Worst possible pain
SE = 5.1% (n = 36)

3. If you have received any treatment for your pain in the past 2 weeks, please rate the level of pain relief that resulted:

Complete relief $\underline{\quad 33\% \quad}$ No relief
SE = 5.6% (n = 36)

These scales can be administered easily with every visit to monitor the patient's response to the various treatment modalities instituted. Such tests can be administered by an office nurse or receptionist and handed to the physician before the physician sees the patient.

A complete neurologic examination is mandatory during the first visit to establish what neural pathways are compressed by tumor tissue or affected by previous radiation and/or chemotherapy. Since cancer is not a static disease, it is essential to do repeated neurologic examinations, especially to rule out any impending spinal cord compression, which is considered an emergency. During the past year, of 85 patients followed up in the Cancer Pain Clinic, 4 patients were diagnosed to have impending spinal cord compression in the pain clinic and therefore were admitted for emergency myelography, radiation, and steroid therapy, thus avoiding irreversible paraplegia or quadriplegia. In all 4 patients the symptoms were a sudden escalation of pain intensity and an abrupt decrease in motor function below the area of impending cord compression. Rapid inter-

vention was instrumental in decreasing the pain and reversing the motor loss.

During the first visit the psychologist must interview all patients to determine what coping skills the patient and the family still possess to deal with the stress of cancer disease. In contrast to chronic benign pain patients, cancer pain patients primarily have shattered coping skills and higher degrees of reactive depression.[9]

After the history and physical examination, psychological interview, and review of records are completed, the physician and psychologist should briefly meet and immediately plan the patient's treatment program.

In planning the treatment modality, the patient's goals must be established. In the initial questionnaire two goals are identified by the patients: a pain relief goal and an activity goal. The pain relief goal is elicited by the following question: If we are unable to take away your pain completely, what would be a level acceptable to you (100% being the worst pain you have ever felt)? The majority of our patients place their pain relief goal at 20%–30%. When such a goal is achieved as seen with our weekly pain scales, the therapy is considered successful. One finds that one could achieve the pain relief goal in 75% of patients after 6 weeks.[10]

The activities goal is elicited by asking the patient the following question: If we were able to diminish your pain, what would you like to be able to do now that you cannot do because of your pain? The activities goal listed by the patient is often unrealistic, perhaps related to a strong denial of the progression of their disease. In our experience, less than 50% of patients who achieve their pain relief goal also achieve their activities goal.[10]

In the initial contact with the patient, the physician must maximize his relationship with the patient by expressing belief in the patient's pain, explaining explicitly to the patient the cause of each pain, shedding the authority figure, and helping the patient establish effective pain communication and realistic goals.

In planning the therapy, the patient and family must be educated to the various options for pain management so that they can understand the risk-benefit ratio for each option. It is also important to list all the alternatives that can be used in the future so that the patient feels secure that other therapies are available if the chosen therapy fails.

On subsequent visits it is helpful to administer the pain scales with every visit and the McGill pain scale and BSI less frequently. The analgesic intake can be monitored effectively by having the pharmacist devise a flow sheet indicating the dose, frequency, and total amount of analgesic obtained by the patient on each visit. One should encourage patients to obtain medications from the clinic pharmacy for two reasons: effective monitoring, and assurance that the prescribed medications are available.

In general, there are two distinct groups of cancer patients who are referred to a pain clinic. In one group are patients whose pain is essentially chronic benign pain, since the pain is chronic and the patient's life expectancy can extend to years. The mainstay of therapy for these patients should be noninvasive, and principles in the management of chronic benign pain should be followed. In the second group are patients with advanced illness and in whom cancer-directed therapy has been exhausted. Rapid invasion of bone, nerves, or viscera induces acute pain, and drug dependence is usual. Therapy focuses on the appropriate dosage and timing of analgesic and invasive somatic therapy, such as neurolysis or cordotomy (Table 20A–4).

THERAPEUTIC INTERVENTION

General Principles

There are four principal modalities used in the management of cancer-related pain:
1. Attacking the pathology causing the pain.
2. Raising the pain threshold.
3. Modulating the pain pathway.
4. Interrupting the pain pathway.
Which one (or more) of these modalities will be

used depends on factors such as progression of the disease, localized or generalized pain location, life expectancy, and the risk-benefit ratio of the modality applied to the individual patient.

The choice of therapy must be individualized for each patient. Alterations of therapy from time to time for each individual patient is necessary because of the expected changes in the primary disease process. A commitment to continue pain management for as long as necessary, often until the patient's death, is expected. When a cancer patient is initially evaluated for pain management, it is necessary to identify immediately whether the cause of pain can still be treated by tumor-directed therapy. For example, a patient with localized bone metastasis from radiation-sensitive breast carcinoma may still be a candidate for radiation therapy. The pain experienced by such a patient will diminish with radiation therapy. However, an adequate analgesic regimen is necessary early in the course of radiation therapy, since it takes several days for effective tumor reduction by radiation therapy to occur.

In such patients radiation therapy may eventually fail, and the patients continue to have pain secondary to progressive bone metastasis. The pain then must be treated as a disease entity itself and treated aggressively with one or more of the pain-directed therapies. Table 20A–5 outlines the modalities used for treating pain as a disease.

Pharmacologic Tailoring

The effective use of narcotic and nonnarcotic analgesic agents is the physician's strongest weapon against cancer pain.

TABLE 20A–4.—CLASSES OF CANCER PATIENTS REFERRED TO PAIN CLINIC

CLASS 1	CLASS 2
Description of Patients	
Ambulatory outpatients	Nonambulatory inpatients
No obvious active progression of cancer	Rapid progression of cancer
Pain usually due to therapy received	Pain usually due to rapid bone, nerve, or visceral invasion
Future therapy against cancer still possible	Exhaustion of therapy against cancer growth
General Principles of Management	
Time-contingent oral nonnarcotic analgesics	Time-contingent oral narcotic analgesics
Noninvasive somatic therapy: minor nerve block and stimulation-produced analgesia	Invasive somatic therapy, chemical neurolysis, or cordotomy
Physical and psychological rehabilitation	Psychological intervention for patient and family to deal with death and dying

TABLE 20A–5.—Cancer Pain as a Disease: Treatment Aimed at Pain Control

Elevating the pain threshold
  Pharmacologic approach:
    Analgesics: nonnarcotic and narcotic
    Adjuvant drugs: antidepressants, anxiolytics, steroids, antiemetics
    Management of drug-related side effects: antacids, laxatives
  Nonpharmacologic approach:
    Psychological support: sympathy and understanding
    Psychological techniques: hypnosis, guided imagery, biofeedback
Modulating the pain pathway
  Increasing endogenous opiates
    Peripheral low frequency stimulation: TENS or acupuncture
    Central PAG stimulation
  Stimulation of spinal gating
    Peripheral high-frequency stimulation (TENS)
Interrupting the nociceptive pathway
  Chemical nerve blocks
  Neurosurgical ablation
    Rhizotomy
    Myelotomy
    Cordotomy
    Thalamotomy
    Hypophysectomy

Certain general principles must be adhered to in utilizing analgesics for cancer pain patients. First, the dosage (amount and timing) of each drug must be tailored to the individual patient. Textbook dosages, often successful for acute pain management, are ineffective for the management of chronic cancer pain. The development of tolerance with prolonged use and/or progression of disease necessitates periodic readjustment of the dosage. The development of tolerance is *not* synonymous with drug addiction. Drug addiction is characterized by an intense craving for drugs primarily because of psychological reasons, and intake ceases to be supervised medically. Most patients with cancer and chronic pain eventually develop tolerance and physical dependence (i.e., physical withdrawal symptoms will occur on drug cessation), and these two conditions should not be confused with drug addiction. Explicit education, not only of patients but also of family members involved with patient care, regarding these differences can result in dramatic improvement in analgesic compliance.

Second, medication must be prescribed on a time-contingent basis instead of on the traditional pain-contingent basis, for several reasons. An adequate analgesic level can be sustained more effectively with the time-contingent approach after an initial trial indicates the frequency and dose necessary to *prevent* pain escalation in the individual patient. The patient's anxiety is also markedly diminished with this approach since there is less anticipation of pain occurring before medication can be obtained, and external control (by nurses, relatives) is less likely. This preventive time-contingent approach is the mainstay of effective analgesic tailoring. Its value should never be underestimated. Changing from pain-contingent to time-contingent medication intake can make the difference between ineffective and effective pain relief and can also result in a diminished total daily analgesic dose.

For pharmacologic tailoring to be successful, the physician must get a detailed history of previous analgesics utilized, whether such drugs were used on a time-contingent basis, whether the drug was totally or partially effective, and, if the drug was effective, how long efficacy lasted. It is often helpful to have the patient attempt to quantify, using the clinical pain estimate or the visual Analog Scale for Pain, the amount of pain relief that was achieved. Individualized pharmacologic tailoring on an outpatient basis is often ineffective for 1–2 weeks. Close monitoring by weekly or biweekly visits is often necessary. Some means of telephone communication for the patient to report inadequate pain relief and/or side effects must be established. The patient should be encouraged to fill out a daily diary indicating his or her response to prescribed medications on an hourly basis. Intake of medications during sleep hours depends on whether or not the patient is awakened by pain during the night. If there is inadequate pain relief at night and on awakening in the morning, the patient should be encouraged to continue time-contingent analgesic intake for 24 hours. A simple alarm clock and bedside location of medication are sufficient to ensure analgesic intake during the sleep hours.

Dose and frequency titration of analgesia until acceptable pain relief should be individualized for each patient. It is often more advantageous to start with a low dose and then increase it gradually to maximize patient compliance. Starting with high doses often results in undesirable side effects and immediately decreases compliance. The initial optimal and equianalgesic dosages are merely guidelines and should not limit the physician in increasing a given drug by small increments to achieve adequate analgesia.

Table 20A–6 is a list of commonly used narcotic and nonnarcotic analgesics and suggested starting dosages. It is presented in a ''ladder'' approach, as

TABLE 20A–6.—STEPLADDER APPROACH
TO ANALGESIC TAILORING

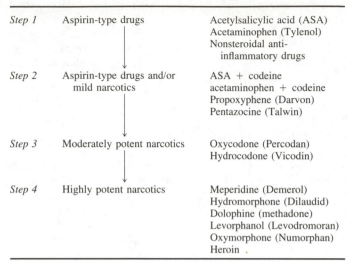

Step 1	Aspirin-type drugs	Acetylsalicylic acid (ASA) Acetaminophen (Tylenol) Nonsteroidal anti-inflammatory drugs
Step 2	Aspirin-type drugs and/or mild narcotics	ASA + codeine acetaminophen + codeine Propoxyphene (Darvon) Pentazocine (Talwin)
Step 3	Moderately potent narcotics	Oxycodone (Percodan) Hydrocodone (Vicodin)
Step 4	Highly potent narcotics	Meperidine (Demerol) Hydromorphone (Dilaudid) Dolophine (methadone) Levorphanol (Levodromoran) Oxymorphone (Numorphan) Heroin

suggested by Twycross.[11] The principle is to start with simple nonnarcotic analgesics first, and then more potent narcotic analgesics. This ladder approach is essential to prevent the rapid development of tolerance to potent narcotics, which would diminish their efficacy during the terminal stages. The maximal utilization of analgesics at each step of the ladder will help expand the time of analgesic efficacy, especially in patients with a long life expectancy. Different combinations of the analgesics in the ladder are sometimes useful in increasing the analgesic efficacy while preventing increase of the primary analgesic's side effects. For example, the co-administration of methadone with a nonsteroidal anti-inflammatory drug can increase analgesia without increasing the CNS side effects often seen with methadone.

In titrating the analgesic in patients with terminal disease, one must remember that large dosages are necessary to obtain relief in at least 75%–80% of patients.[12] Unfortunately, tolerance to analgesic develops more rapidly than tolerance to side effects, and therefore it is important to titrate the dose within the limits of tolerable side effects. There is no single drug dose or route of administration that is appropriate for *all* patients with advanced cancer. To be successful, one must understand the patient's underlying disease and recognize that pain will not be a static problem. Repeated adjustment of drug dosage, frequency, and route of administration may be necessary to parallel the progression or, for more fortunate patients, the stabilization of disease.

Because of the possibility that the analgesics will be needed for a long period of time, extending to months, oral administration should be used as long as possible. Even patients with advanced disease can still take drugs orally and effectively.[13] The early use of intramuscular injection often results in painful, "leathery" muscles at injection sites; more importantly, it is difficult for close relatives involved with patient's care to cope with.

In summary, the principles of effective analgesic tailoring are as follows:

1. Individualize type of drug, dose frequency, and route of administration for each patient.

2. Educate patient and close relatives involved with care regarding myth of addiction and difference from tolerance and physical dependence.

3. Prescribe medications on time-contingent, around-the-clock regimen instead of on an as-needed or pain-contingent basis.

4. Obtain a detailed history of the analgesics previously utilized.

5. Titrate to acceptable analgesia and tolerable side effects.

6. Familiarize yourself with analgesics that are available and utilize such analgesics in a "ladder" approach, from nonnarcotic to potent narcotic analgesics.

7. Utilize the oral route as long as possible.

8. Establish a communication line for patients to report efficacy and side effects.

Adjuvant Drugs

Other medications are often necessary adjuncts to analgesics in the pharmacologic management of the cancer patient with chronic pain. Specifically, antidepressants and anxiolytic agents are frequently utilized.[14] Reactive depression to the prolonged illness is known to accompany cancer disease[15] and therefore must be addressed before effective analgesia can be achieved. The use of antidepressants such as doxepin or amitriptyline in doses of 25–50 mg is often adequate for this group of patients. In contrast to psychiatric patients, higher dosages are not recommended in cancer pain patients because of increased CNS side effects, especially when the patients are taking high dosages of narcotic analgesics. Increased availability of serotonin can also be encouraged by use of L-tryptophan (1–3 gm/day) and D-phenylalanine (300–600 mg/day). The decrease in maximal pain thresholds with nutritional manipulation and L-tryptophan supplement in normal subjects has been demonstrated to be significant.[16]

When anxiety levels become a factor in increased pain reports, anxiolytic agents may be used. Diazepam can be used on a short-term basis, but its prolonged use may aggravate depression. If prolonged anxiolytic use is indicated, alprazolam (Xanax) is probably a more appropriate drug because of its combined anxiolytic-antidepressant effect.

Adjuvant medications to control side effects from analgesics, such as antacids for salicylates and laxatives or stool softeners for the constipating effects of narcotics, must also be administered on a preventive time-contingent approach.

Modulating Pain Pathways

Modulation of the pain pathways by use of modalities that encourage the release of endogenous opiates and/or stimulation of the spinal gating mechanism[17] has been widely used in the chronic benign pain patient. The efficacy of such modalities in patients with intractable pain due to cancer has not been adequately studied. The release of endogenous opiates by stimulation of the periventricular gray area has been found to be effective in relieving midline and bilateral cancer-related pain.[18] However, recent double-blind studies indicate there is no difference between sham and real stimulation of such central sites, even in patients in whom presurgical morphine tests show naloxone reversal or mor-

phine analgesia.[19] Although this study was done in chronic benign patients, the mechanism of previously reported pain relief with this procedure is now open to question. Obviously, additional studies with larger numbers of patients need to be done.

Dorsal column stimulation in an attempt to induce a descending inhibition has been shown to be only 50% effective in cancer patients.[20] It is more effective for phantom pain than for peripheral nerve lesions and acute pain.[21]

Peripheral stimulation-induced analgesia, by percutaneous acupuncture or transcutaneous electrical nerve stimulation (TENS), widely used for chronic noncancer pain, is found to be 96% effective the first 10 days in cancer pain patients, decreasing to 11% after 1 month of use.[22] Such decreased efficacy is probably due to the concomitant use of exogenous opiates, which occupy the opiate receptors, making them unavailable for the released endogenous opiate to occupy. High-frequency stimulation (TENS: 80–120 Hz) might be more appropriate for the cancer patient on narcotic intake since it acts by inhibition of nociceptive pathway by the spinal gating mechanism instead of by increasing endorphins.[23]

Injection of opiates into the epidural, intrathecal, and intraventricular space has shown to induce profound analgesia in patients with cancer pain. Morphine, in dosages much lower than that used for systemic administration, produced analgesia when injected into the intrathecal space of patients with cancer pain.[24] However, recent studies in cancer patients taking high-dose narcotics indicate decreased efficacy[25] with epidurally injected narcotic, even in doses only 25% of systemic doses. In addition, pharmacokinetic studies indicate that morphine, being less lipid soluble than other narcotics, probably exerts its effect by bulk distribution to the ventricular system instead of by the presumed binding in the spinal cord opiate receptors.

The advantage of using morphine rather than local anesthetics or neurolytic agents is that there is no accompanying motor or sensory loss with morphine.

Complications reported consist of pruritis (dermatomal or generalized), nausea and vomiting, urine retention, and, most serious of all, delayed respiratory depression several hours after injection. Respiratory depression is more common after intrathecal than after epidural injection and in narcotic-naive patients than in the usually narcotic-tolerant cancer pain patient. The longest duration of single morphine injection epidurally or intrathecally is reported to a maximum of 27 hours, which necessitates repeated injection or injection through the more recently developed subcutaneously implanted precision pumps.[26]

Preservative-free morphine is used for both epidural and intrathecal injection. The role of centrally deposited morphine should not be overestimated in the cancer pain patient. If a decision is made to employ this technique in the cancer pain patient, consideration must be given to the systemic narcotic intake and the physical condition of the patient. Prior to injection of morphine, a test dose of lidocaine 1% (2–3 cc) must demonstrate the presence of dermatomal block. After the block wears off, morphine can be injected in doses ranging from 2 to 5 mg, in 1 mg/cc concentration. Various other narcotics can be used, such as methadone, fentanyl, or meperidine, but morphine is favored because of its longer duration of action.[27]

After initial injection, the patient should be closely monitored in an intensive care unit or by a trained nurse who is adequately informed of the possibility of delayed respiratory depression. An ampule of naloxone, 0.4 mg, can be drawn in a syringe and taped in front of the patient's chart.

Interrupting Pain Pathways

Interruption of the nociceptive pathway, perhaps used most extensively in the cancer pain patient, can be achieved by injection of temporary or "permanent" chemical substances or by neurosurgical procedures.

Over the past 50 years various chemical substances have been injected into the nociceptive pathway in an attempt to alleviate cancer pain. A classification of such substances and their reported duration of action is given in Table 20A–7.

Before a nerve block is performed in a cancer pain patient, some physiologic considerations must be taken into account, such as the following:

1. A decreased platelet count (<100,000/cu mm) contraindicates the use of nerve block since the needle insertion might provoke an inordinate amount of bleeding and hematoma.

2. The cancer patient, because of decreased oral intake due to nausea and anorexia, may have a decreased circulating volume so that he or she is subject to hypotension following a sympathetic block.

3. Tumor invasion may distort or "sheath" the nociceptive pathway to be blocked. This nerve root incasement may be secondary to radiation or previous nerve block causing arachnoiditis.[28]

4. Compromised pulmonary function after a thoracic epidural block, especially in patients with primary or metastatic lung disease, may further deteriorate, resulting in loss of intercostal muscle function. Arterial blood gases must be measured before and after a diagnostic epidural block.

5. Since most cancer pain patients are already receiving potent narcotics when they become candidates for neural blockade, a successful block with phenol or alcohol should not mean abrupt cessation of the patient's narcotic analgesics. To prevent physical withdrawal, a systematic withdrawal regimen should be planned.

The role of neural blockade in the cancer patient with pain can be diagnostic or therapeutic. Diagnostic nerve blocks are done to define the segmental distribution of pain, to differentiate central versus peripheral pain, and to define the role of somatic, autonomic, or musculoskeletal components in the patient's total pain complaint. In addition, a diagnostic nerve block can be used to predict the success of a planned neurolytic block in decreasing pain to an acceptable level, or if the accompanying loss of sensation and side effects are acceptable to the patient.

A diagnostic nerve block is mandatory prior to a more permanent block with neurolytic agents. Only after a 75% decrease in pain, and after the patient's acceptance of accompanying numbness and possible

TABLE 20A–7.—DURATION OF ACTION OF SUBSTANCES USED
FOR NEURAL BLOCKADE

CLASS	DURATION	EXAMPLES
I Short-acting	Minutes to hours	Local anesthetics
		Opiates (single injection)
II Prolonged	Days to months	Cryoanalgesia
		Hypertonic saline
		Opiates (by continuous infusion with a pump)
III Permanent	Months to years	Phenol
		Alcohol
		Ammonium sulfate

motor loss, should a neurolytic block be performed.

A diagnostic block must be done with precision and meticulous attention to detail. Error in needle placement, especially with paravertebral somatic nerve blocks,[29] can lead to a wrong conclusion and an unsuccessful therapeutic nerve block. Fluoroscopy should be used for precise needle placement when performing celiac plexus, paravertebral somatic, and sacral root blocks. Figure 20A–2 illustrates the location of the needle tip for a somatic nerve block. A lateral or oblique view is mandatory to ensure that the depth of the needle tip is accurate. In the study at UCLA it was found that in 40% of somatic nerve blocks, the needle tip was improperly placed when fluoroscopy was not used. When a celiac plexus block is performed, lateral fluoroscopy must be used to ensure that the tip of the needle is located anterior to the vertebral body. Since 40–50 cc of local anesthetic or alcohol solution is used for this procedure, precise needle location, confirmed by fluoroscopy, is of paramount importance in ruling out the possibility of a catastrophic intraspinal injection.

In contrast to regional block for surgical anesthesia, smaller volumes and lower concentrations of local anesthetic are used for diagnostic nerve blocks since the primary aim is to block small autonomic and nociceptive neural fibers. For example, in autonomic blocks, 0.5% lidocaine or 0.25% bupivacaine is used, and for sensory blocks, 1% lidocaine or 0.5% bupivacaine.

Continuous epidural catheterization for diagnostic segmental block of trunk pain with specific dermatomal distribution (e.g., pain in thoracic chest wall secondary to second or third rib metastasis). Placement of the epidural catheter as close to the segmental distribution of pain as possible and the incremental injection of 3–6 cc of 1% lidocaine can be both diagnostic and therapeutic. Such neural blockade can be beneficial in patients with excruciating pain while undergoing radiation therapy, in patients with acute herpes zoster neuralgia, and in patients with unmanageable pain after radical surgery. In the author's experience, 9 of 32 patients who received epidural local anesthetic injections while undergoing radiation therapy experienced pain remission after 4–5 days of radiation therapy, and the epidural injections were discontinued without return of the pain.

Continuous epidural catheterization can lead to diagnostic information resulting in afferent interruption by chemical or neurosurgical technique (14/32), successful narcotic withdrawal (2/32), and comfort until death (3/32). In the UCLA series, 28 of 32 patients were benefited by the continuous epidural catherization with intermittent injection of local anesthetics.

After the epidural catheter is inserted at the desired level, the catheter must be securely taped to the skin to ensure nondislodgment for a period of days. Dislodgment occurs frequently when the patient is moved from the hospital bed to the transporter or x-ray table. Thereafter, if possible, definitive therapy must be undertaken within 24–48 hours of catheter placement.

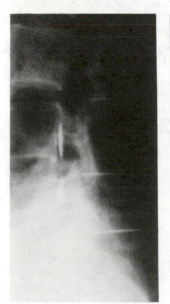
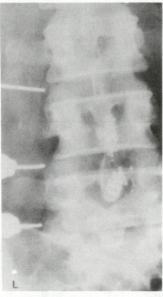

Fig 20A–2.—The location of the needle tip for somatic nerve root block, anteroposterior *(left)* and lateral *(right)* views. A lateral or oblique view is mandatory to ensure that the needle tip is at the level of the intervertebral foramen.

A bacterial filter must be attached to the injection port of the catheter. However, such filters do not block the tracking of bacteria through the outside wall of the catheter. In the author's experience, abscesses developed in two patients. In one patient the abscess was located subcutaneously; in the other patient, it was located in the epidural space and necessitated a laminectomy and drainage of the abscess. In the latter patient, culture of the abscess fluid indicated contamination from sources outside the catheter. Both patients had some intermittent urinary incontinence which probably encouraged the wicking effect of the epidural catheter. Therefore, urinary incontinence is a relative contraindication for continuous epidural catheter placement for days, unless the patient's urinary bladder can be catheterized to diminish leakage into the epidural catheter when the patient is supine.

Intrathecal erosion of the catheter can occur several days after placement. In the author's series, signs of intrathecal block developed in two patients 3 and 4 days after catheter placement during the test dose injection of 3–4 ml of 1% lidocaine. It is therefore important always to administer small test doses of a local anesthetic prior to administration of full dose, even if the epidural catheter has been in place for several days.

The role of nerve blocks in the total management of specific pain syndrome will be described later. However, one must recognize that nerve blocks are only one of the many tools available for the management of cancer pain and should not be used as the sole therapy.

Permanent Blocks

Over the past 20–30 years, chemical neurolysis with various concentrations of phenol or alcohol has been used to manage cancer pain. Since chemical neurolysis is associated with complications in 2%–16% of patients,[30] strict criteria must be adhered to prior to entertaining the possibility of performing a neurolytic block:

1. Exhaustion of tumor-directed palliative therapy for pain control.

2. Inadequate pain control despite high dosages of narcotic, and drug-related side effects.

3. A diagnostic nerve block with local anesthetic provides at least 75% pain relief.

Some chemical neurolytic blocks commonly used for cancer pain are listed in Table 20A–8, along with the site of injection, agents used, dosages, and reported success. Of note is the high success rate (94%) reported with celiac plexus block.[31] This block is particularly helpful in patients with pancreatic carcinoma or retroperitoneal metastasis.

Although injection of phenol or alcohol into various sites has been done, the success rate has not been adequately studied. Intrathecal alcohol injection was initiated by Dogliotti in 1936. Despite 50 years of use, the success rate is only 46%–63%.[32] Intrathecal phenol injection, initiated somewhat later by Maher, in 1960, also has the same range of success, despite 20 years of use.

The differences between phenol and alcohol when used intrathecally are listed in Table 20A–9. Understanding these basic differences between alcohol and phenol will maximize their efficacy. The difference in their baricity will influence the positioning of the patient during injection. With phenol, the patient is positioned so that the somatic nerve roots to be blocked are in the most dependent position, whereas with alcohol, the dorsal roots to be blocked are in the most superior position. Since phenol is dissolved in absolute glycerol, it is extremely viscid and requires at least a 20-gauge spinal needle. With phenol, the prolonged latency after injection allows

TABLE 20A–8.—CHEMICAL NEUROLYSIS WITH NERVE BLOCKS

TYPE OF BLOCK	AGENT(S)	DOSE	% SUCCESS REPORTED
Lumbar sympathetic	50% alcohol	5–10 cc	NA*
	10% phenol in glycerol	5–10 cc	NA
	7% phenol in water	5–20 cc	NA
Celiac plexus	50% alcohol	50 cc	94
Epidural	30% alcohol	3–10 cc	NA
	10% phenol in glycerol	3–10 cc	33
	7% phenol in water	3–10 cc	NA
Subarachnoid	100% alcohol	.5–.75 cc	45–60
	4%–5% phenol in glycerol	.5–.75 cc	48–62
Pituitary ablation	100% alcohol	1–2 cc	70

*NA, not available.

TABLE 20A–9.—INTRATHECAL INJECTION OF PHENOL AND ALCOHOL

PARAMETER	PHENOL	ALCOHOL
Baricity	Hyperbaric	Hypobaric
Concentration	4% phenol in absolute glycerol	100% alcohol
Site of action	Dorsal ganglion at intervertebral foramen	Dorsal sensory root as it takes off from spinal cord
Onset of neurolytic action	15–20 min	Immediate
Pain on injection	+	+ + + +

for repositioning if the feeling of ''warmth'' experienced by the patient after the initial contact of phenol with neural tissue spreads to other dermatomes besides the desired levels. Alcohol acts immediately on contact and therefore does not provide this advantage. In addition, unlike phenol, alcohol produces burning pain on injection. Because of this difference, phenol is the preferred solution for intrathecal neurolysis.

If the upper side of the patient is tilted 45° backward, the anterior motor roots can be preserved. However, in reality, such selective blocking may not occur since phenol is known to destroy all types of fibers it comes in contact with.[33]

Complications of intrathecal neurolysis are primarily those of bladder, bowel, and motor paresis.[34] The patient must be informed of these possible complications before one proceeds.

Intrathecal hypertonic saline has also been used for neurolysis but has been successful in less than 50% of cases and is quite painful on injection.

Epidural neurolysis with phenol has recently been introduced as an alternative to intrathecal neurolysis. In our experience, this block is useful when a wide segmental block is necessary (for example, for extensive chest wall pain) and in treating pain in upper extremities (brachial plexus neuropathy from Pancoast tumor). Favorable results at the cervical and thoracic levels have been reported.[35] The advantage of epidural neurolysis is its simplicity and controllability and the lower risk of extensive spinal cord injury as compared to the intrathecal method.

The differences between spinal and epidural neurolysis in terms of drug utilized, position, and site of action are shown in Figure 20A–3.

Neurosurgical Procedures for Cancer Pain

Various neuroablative procedures have been performed in the patient with cancer-related pain despite lack of well-controlled studies indicating their relative efficacy compared to other nonsurgical methods for controlling pain. Neurosurgical procedures for cancer pain management are classified in Table 20A–10.

Before neurosurgical ablative procedures are proposed, the patient must first have received an adequate trial of analgesic tailoring, pain-modulating techniques, and chemical neural blockade. A diagnostic nerve block should be done to predict the effect of neuroablative procedure in the spinal cord and peripheral level.

Neurostimulation techniques have only been applied to a small number of cancer patients with pain and therefore it is still premature to suggest a wide application. For further details of neurosurgical procedures, see chapter 39C.

The reported efficacy of the various neurosurgical procedures range from 33% to 100% with a mean of 50%–60%, strikingly similar to results seen with intrathecal neurolytic blocks. However, risks are often greater with neurosurgical procedures because of the patients' physical condition, which often renders them poor candidates for neurosurgery and anesthesia. For a further description of each procedure, the reader is referred to standard textbooks of neurosurgery. Two particular procedures warrant special attention, percutaneous cordotomy and pituitary ablation, since these procedures are commonly used for the management of cancer-related pain.

Percutaneous cordotomy is the interruption of the ascending spinothalamic tract, usually at the cervical level. The procedure is usually done by stereotactic technique and a needle is inserted on the lateral aspect of the neck, guided by fluoroscopy to the target site. After confirmation of proper needle placement, a lesion is made by radiofrequency. Efficacy is reported to be 80% immediately postoperatively but decreases to 60% in a few weeks.[36]

The indication for entertaining the possibility of cordotomy is unilateral pain in a patient who still has intact bowel and bladder function and motor

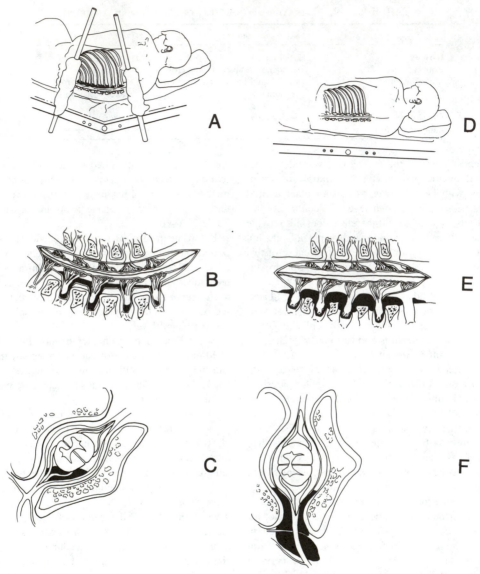

Fig 20A–3.—A, proper positioning for intrathecal neurolysis; the area to be blocked is in the most dependent portion. The table is flexed and rotated 45° backward. **B,** horizontal view of phenol layering in the intrathecal canal. **C,** cross section illustrating layering of phenol in spinal canal; 45° backward tilt allows concentration of solution in dorsal roots.

D, positioning for epidural neurolysis by simple lateral decubitus position with painful side being dependent. **E,** horizontal view of phenol layering in epidural space. **F,** cross section illustrating layering of phenol in epidural space. (From Ferrer-Brechner T.: *Anesthesiol. Rev.* 8:15, 1981. Used with permission.)

function and a life expectancy of 6 months to 1 year. It is relatively contraindicated in patients who have poor pulmonary function (e.g., those with lung carcinoma) on the ipsilateral side of the pain. Since the spinothalamic tract decussates contralaterally while motor fibers do not, cordotomy might result

in impairment of the intercostal muscles on the remaining functional lung.

In patients who are poor candidates for percutaneous cordotomy, neurolytic nerve blocks should be presented as an immediate alternative. One protocol to follow is to insert an epidural catheter along the

TABLE 20A–10.—NEUROSURGICAL PROCEDURES FOR CANCER PAIN MANAGEMENT

NEUROSURGICAL PROCEDURE	REPORTED SUCCESS	INDICATIONS	COMPLICATIONS	REFERENCES
NEUROABLATION				
Spinal dorsal rhizotomy	40/72		"Anesthesia dolorosa"	42
			Complete motor loss	43
				44
Commisural myelotomy	27/80	Vaginal and visceral pain	Recurrence of pain in 2 mo.	45
				46
				47
Cordotomy	60%–80%	Sacral and lower limb pain	Recurrence of pain in 3–4 mo.	36
				40
Medullary tractotomy	45/56	Upper limb path		48
				49
Mesencephalic tractotomy	NA	Pain in face, neck, upper limb	High mortality	50
			Recurrence of pain in weeks	51
				52
Stereotaxic thalamotomy		Head, face, neck, upper limb	Central pain in 70%–80%	53
				54
			Recurrence of pain in weeks	55
Psychosurgery:				
Lobotomy	45/48		Psychic disturbances	56
Angulotomy	37%		Recurrence of pain	57
Hypophysectomy	74% (radiofrequency)		Diabetes insipidus	41
	94% (alcohol)		CSF rhinorrhea	37
	80% (yttrium)			39
NEUROSTIMULATION				
Central gray stimulation	5/6	Widespread and bilateral pain		58
Thalamic and hypothalamic stimulation	NA			59
Dorsal column and peripheral nerve stimulation	NA 50%		CSF fistula, infection, hematoma, spinal cord compression	60

dermatomal distribution of pain, and to inject local anesthetics to differentiate whether pain is central or peripheral. If pain is adequately relieved, the epidural catheter is left in place and a neurosurgical consultation is sought to determine if the patient is a good candidate for cordotomy. If the patient is not a good candidate, epidural phenol neurolysis can be carried out immediately because the catheter was left in place.

Hypophysectomy has been recommended for the management of bone pain secondary to hormone-dependent breast or prostate cancer. Various approaches have been used, including a transphenoidal approach with injection of various destructive substances such as alcohol,[37] water,[38] or yttrium,[39] the application of cryogenic probe,[40] and radiofrequency.[41] Success rates have been quoted as 74%–94%, but long-term follow-up to death has not been carried out successfully. When approached with this alternative and apprised of the procedure, most patients prefer to have less invasive procedures. Complications, which include diabetes insipidus and CSF rhinorrhea, can be severe and are usually not acceptable to the patient. Therefore, in our cancer pain clinic, hypophysectomy plays a minor role in the overall management of the patient with cancer pain.

INTEGRATION OF VARIOUS MODALITIES

For the pain physician to effectively apply the various modalities available for management of cancer-related pain, a decision tree is proposed (Fig 20A–4). This flow chart is ideal primarily for outpatients. In essence, the first step is to apply analgesic tailoring for 2 weeks, and if inadequate pain relief occurs, peripheral stimulation can be added. If pain relief is still inadequate, neurostimulation or neuroablation by chemical or surgical techniques can be sought. In our first series of 120 patients, the

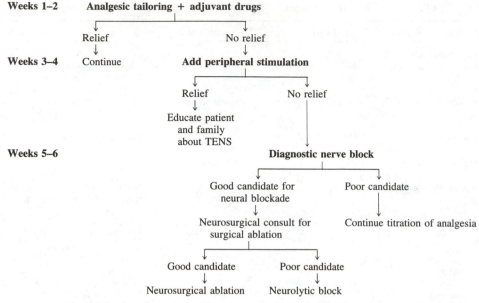

Fig 20A–4.—Suggested management of cancer-related pain.

use of such a ladder approach resulted in acceptable pain relief in 75% of patients after 6 weeks. Such a graduated approach to the somatic management of cancer-related pain can be adjusted for the individual patient according to the timing and duration of each step, depending on the progression of disease. Such an approach can also be adjusted according to the availability of various modalities to the physician managing the pain problem. It cannot be overemphasized that psychological intervention must go hand-in-hand with the somatic modalities at all times.

REFERENCES

1. Foley K.M.: Pain syndromes in patients with cancer, in Bonica J.J., Ventafridda V. (eds.): *Advances in Pain Research and Therapy*. New York, Raven Press, 1979, vol. 2.
2. Pannuti F., Martone A., Rossi A.P., et al.: The role of endocrine therapy for relief of pain due to advanced cancer, in Bonica J.J., Ventafridda V. (eds.): *Advances in Pain Research and Therapy*. New York, Raven Press, 1979, vol. 2.
3. Twycross R.G.: Clinical management with Diamorphine in advanced malignant disease. *Int. J. Clin. Pharmacol.* 93:184–198, 1974.
4. Wilkes E.: Some problems in cancer management. *Proc. R. Soc. Med.* 67:23–27, 1974.
5. Ferrer-Brechner T., Brechner V.L.: Evaluation of graduated multi-modality pain management of outpatient cancer patients, in *Abstracts of the Third World Congress on Pain of the International Association for the Study of Pain*. Edinburgh, International Association for the Study of Pain, 1981.
6. Melzack R.: The McGill pain questionnaire: Major properties and scoring methods. *Pain* 1:277–299, 1975.
7. Derogatis L.R.: *Brief Symptom Index*. Baltimore, Johns Hopkins University, 1978.
8. Cohen R.S., Brechner T.F., Reading A.E.: A survey of the subjective parameters of pain in cancer patients (abstr.). *Am. Pain Soc.* 1982, p. 18.
9. Gitelson J.S., Brechner T.F., McCreary C., et al.: Psychological aspects of cancer pain: Correlation with response to standard medical treatment for relief of pain (abstr.). *Am. Pain Soc.,* 1980, p. 25.
10. Ferrer-Brechner T., Clark W.C., Wagner J.M., et al.: Pain, contentment and psychological distress in oncology outpatients: A sensory decision theory approach (abstr.) *Am. Pain Soc.,* 1982, pp. 29–31.
11. Twycross R.G.: Medical treatment of chronic cancer pain. *Bull. Cancer* 67(2):209–216, 1980.
12. Gerbershagen J.: Non-narcotic analgesics, in Bonica J.J., Ventafridda V. (eds.): *Advances in Pain Research Therapy*. New York, Raven Press, 1979, vol. 2, pp. 255–262.
13. Twycross R.G.: Rehabilitation in terminal cancer patients. *Int. Rehabil. Med.* 3(3):135–144, 1981.
14. Ventafridda V., Sganzeria E.P., Fochi C.: Use of psychotropic substances with antidepression action in pain control. *Minerva Med.* 70(9):667–674, 1979.
15. Gitelson J., Brechner T., McCreary C.: Psychological predictors of response to treatment for cancer pain, in *Abstracts of the Third World Congress on Pain of the*

International Association for the Study of Pain. Edinburgh, International Association for the Study of Pain, 1981.

16. Seltzer S., Stoch R., Marcus R., et al.: Alteration of human pain thresholds by nutritional manipulation and L-tryptophan. *Pain [Suppl.]* 13:385–393, 1982.

17. Melzack R., Wall P.D.: Pain mechanisms: A new theory. *Science* 147:150–171, 1965.

18. Meyerson B.A., Boethius J., Carlsson A.M.: Percutaneous central gray stimulation for cancer pain. *Appl. Neurophysiol.* 41(1–4):57–65, 1978.

19. Walskie P.J., Gracely R.H., Greenberg R.P., et al.: Comparison of effects of morphine and deep brain stimulation on chronic pain (abstr.). *Am. Pain Soc.* 1982, p. 36.

20. Long D.M., Erickson D.E.: Stimulation of the posterior columns of the spinal cord for relief of intractable pain. *Surg. Neurol.* 4(1):134–141, 1975.

21. Krainick J.R., Thoden U.: Experience with dorsal column stimulation (DSC) in the operative treatment of chronic intractable pain. *J. Neurosurg. Sci.* 18(3):187–189, 1974.

22. Ventafridda V., Sganzeria E.P., Fochi C., et al.: Transcutaneous stimulation in cancer pain, in Bonica J.J., Ventafridda V. (eds.): *Advances in Pain Research and Therapy*. New York, Raven Press, 1979, vol. 2, pp. 509–515.

23. Sjolund B.H., Eriksson M.B.F.: Stimulation techniques in the management of pain, in Kosterlitz H.W., Terenius L.Y. (eds.): *Pain and Society*. Basel, Verlag Chemie, 1980, pp. 415–430.

24. Gebert E., Sarubin J., Yosung K.A.: Morphine intrathecally in postoperative and cancer-induced pain (author's transl.). *Anaesthesist* 29(12):653–655, 1980.

25. Max M.: Pharmacokinetic correlates of epidural and intrathecal opiates (abstr.). *Am. Pain Soc.* Miami, 1982, p. 26.

26. Poletti C.E., Cohen A.M., Todd D.P., et al.: Cancer pain relieved by long-term epidural morphine with permanent indwelling systems for self-administration. *J. Neurosurg.* 55(4):581–584, 1981.

27. Bromage P.R., Camporesi E., Chestnot D.: Epidural narcotics for postoperative analgesia. *Anesth. Anal.* 59:473–480, 1980.

28. Maher J.A. R.M. neuron selection in relief of pain: Further experience with intrathecal injections. *Lancet* 1:16, 1957.

29. Brechner T., Brechner V.: Accuracy of needle placement during diagnostic and therapeutic nerve block, in Bonica J.J., Albe-Fessard D. (eds.): *Advances in Pain Research and Therapy*. New York, Raven Press, 1976, vol. 1, pp. 679–683.

30. Wood K.: The use of phenol as a neurolytic agent: A review. *Pain* 5:205, 1978.

31. Thompson G.E., Moore D.C., Bridenbaugh L.D., et al.: Abdominal pain and alcohol celiac plexus nerve block. *Anesth. Analg.* 56(1):1–5, 1977.

32. Swerdlow M.: Subarachnoid and extradural neurolytic block, in Bonica J.J., Ventafridda V. (eds.): *Advances in Pain Research and Therapy*. New York, Raven Press, 1979, vol. 2, pp. 325–337.

33. Hansebout R.R., Cosgrone J.B.R.: Effects of intrathecal phenol in man: A histological study. *Neurology* 16:277, 1966.

34. Swerdlow M.: Current views on intrathecal neurolysis. *Anaesthesia* 33:733, 1978.

35. Colpitts M.R., Levy B.A., Lawrence M.: Treatment of cancer-related pain with phenol epidural block (abstr.). *World Congress on Pain*. Montreal, 1978.

36. Rosamoff H.F., Carrall F., Brown J., et al.: Percutaneous radiofrequency cervical cordotomy technique. *J. Neurosurg.* 23:639, 1965.

37. Katz J., Levin A.B.: Treatment of diffuse metastatic cancer pain by instillation of alcohol into the sella turcica. *Anesthesiology* 46(2):115–121, 1977.

38. Lipton S., Miles J., Williams N., et al.: Pituitary injection of alcohol for widespread cancer pain. *Pain* 5(1):73–82, 1978.

39. Fitzpatrick J.M., Gardiner R.A., Williams J.P., et al.: Pituitary ablation in the relief of pain in advanced prostatic carcinoma. *Br. Med. J. (Clin. Res.)* 284:75–76, 1981.

40. Rand R.W., Dashe A.M., Paglen D.E., et al.: Stereotactic cryohypophysectomy. *JAMA* 189:255–259, 1964.

41. Lloyd J.W., Rawlinson M.A., Evans P.J.: Selective hypophysectomy for metastatic pain: A review of ethyl alcohol ablation of the anterior pituitary in a regional pain relief unit. *Br. J. Anaesth.* 53(11):1129–1133, 1981.

42. Loeser J.D.: Dorsal rhizotomy for the relief of chronic pain. *J. Neurosurg.* 36:745–750, 1972.

43. Coggeshall R.E., Applebaum M.L., Facem M., et al.: Unmyelinated axons in human ventral roots, a possible explanation for the failure of dorsal rhizotomy to relieve pain. *Brain* 98:157–166, 1975.

44. Barrash J.M., Leavens M.E.: Dorsal rhizotomy for the relief of intractable pain of malignant tumor origin. *J. Neurol.* 38:755–757, 1973.

45. Wertheimer P., Lecuire J.: La myelotomie commissurale posterieure: A propos de 107 observations. *Acta Chir. Belg.* 52:568–574, 1953.

46. Lembke W.: Uber die mediolongitudinale Chordotomie in Halsmarkbereich. *Zentrabl. Chir.* 89:439–443, 1964.

47. Papo I., Luongo A.: High cervical commissural myelotomy in the treatment of pain. *J. Neurol. Neurosurg. Psychiatry* 39:705–710, 1976.

48. Birkenfeld R., Fisher R.G.: Successful treatment of causalgia of upper extremity with medullary spinothalamic tractotomy. *J. Neurosurg.* 20:303–311, 1963.

49. White J.C., Sweet W.H.: *Pain and the Neurosurgeon: A 40 Years Experience*. Springfield, Ill., Charles C Thomas, 1969.

50. Mazars G., Merienne L., Cioloca C.: Etat actuel de

la chirurgie de la douleur. *Neurochirurgie* 1(suppl.):1–164, 1976.

51. Nashold B.S., Wilson W.B., Slaughter D.G.: Stereotactic midbrain lesions for central dysaesthesia and phantom pain. *J. Neurosurg.* 30:116–126, 1969.

52. Wycis H.T., Spiegel E.A.: Long-range results in the treatment of intractable pain by stereotaxic midbrain surgery. *J. Neurosurg.* 19:101–107, 1962.

53. Pagni C.A.: Place of stereotactic technique in surgery for pain, in Bonica J.J. (ed.): *Advances in Neurology,* vol. 4, *International Symposium on Pain.* New York, Raven Press, 1974, pp. 699–706.

54. Sano K.: Intralaminar thalamotomy (thalamolaminotomy) and posteromedial hypothalamotomy in the treatment of intractable pain, in Krayenbuhl H, Maspes P.E., Sweet W.H. (eds.): *Pain—Its Neurosurgical Management: II. Central Procedures.* Basel, S. Karger, 1977, pp. 50–103.

55. Steiner L., Foster D., Leksell L., et al.: Gammathalamotomy in intractable pain. *Acta Neurochir.* 52:173–184, 1980.

56. Lindstrom P.A.: Prefrontal sonic treatment—16 years' experience, in Laitinen L., Vaernet K. (eds.): *Psychosurgery Procedures: Second International Congress on Psychosurgery.* Springfield, Charles C Thomas, 1972, pp. 357–376.

57. Foltz E.L., White L.E.: Rostral cingulotomy and pain "relief" in Knighton R.S., Dumke P.R. (eds.): *Pain.* Boston, Little Brown, 1966, pp. 469–491.

58. Richardson D.E., Akil H.: Pain reduction by electrical brain stimulation in man. *J. Neurosurg.* 47:178–183, 1977.

59. Fairman D.: Thalamic and hypothalamic stimulation advances, in Bonica J.J., Ventafridda V. (eds.): *Pain Research and Therapy,* vol. 2. New York, Raven Press, 1979, pp. 493–498.

60. Loeser J.D.: Dorsal column and peripheral nerve stimulation, in Bonica J.J., Ventafridda V. (eds.): *Pain Research and Therapy,* vol. 2. New York, Raven Press, 1979, pp. 499–507.

20 / Cancer

20B / Recent Developments in the Treatment of Cancer Pain

RICHARD M. ROSENBLATT, M.D.

FOR THE PAST 50 years, cancer—its diagnosis and treatment—has persisted as one of the foremost topics in the medical literature. Nevertheless, treatment of cancer pain in the dying patient has not received the attention it merits. Only with the development of thanatology as a scientific discipline and, concurrently, the establishment of hospice facilities to care for the dying patient have changes come about in the way physicians manage terminal cancer pain. We are just now beginning to witness the potential for comprehensive approaches to deal with the cancer pain. As a consequence, it is no longer acceptable simply to placate the cancer patient with ineffective doses of analgesics during the preterminal phase and then render him stuporous prior to death. The patient's physician must now take into consideration the etiology of the pain, its level of intensity, and the functional impairment that it produces. The therapeutic modalities must be selected on the basis of both their analgesic properties and their potential impact on the functional status of the patient. Thus, in selected patients, pain control measures like neurolytic blocks or spinal narcotics may be preferable to more potent systemic narcotics. In other cases analgesics, both narcotic and nonnarcotic, may be the treatment of choice but administered on a prophylactic schedule rather than on demand.

Therefore, physicians who treat cancer patients must now be familiar with the various analgesic modalities available. Unfortunately, this is a subject that is not within the domain of any particular specialty at the present time. Anesthesiologists can play an active role in this area because of their familiarity

with most of the current pain control modalities and extensive experience with narcotic analgesics. Whether anesthesiologists will emerge in the future as specialists in the management of terminal pain remains to be seen; the need is certainly there.

A number of articles have been published on the treatment of cancer pain. Several comprehensive reviews are recommended reading.[1-3] This chapter is limited to a review of selected topics of direct import to anesthesiologists: the epidemiology of cancer pain, the optimal narcotic and nonnarcotic analgesics, advances in neurolytic blocks, and the use of chronic spinal narcotics. The chapter concludes with a brief discussion of the hospice concept and the potential role of anesthesiologists in such a facility.

EPIDEMIOLOGY OF CANCER PAIN

Despite the prevalence of cancer in our society, there are limited statistical data on the pathogenesis and development of pain among patients. Certainly there is nothing comparable to the Framingham Study with its wealth of information. The incidence of cancer pain in large series of patients has been variously reported, as follows: 29% (Shepard),[4] 38% (Foley),[5] 58% (Wilkes),[6] 60% (Foley),[5] 64% (Pannuti et al.),[7] 68% (Haram and Saunders),[8] and 87% (Cartwright et al.)[9] The wide range of incidence can be attributed in part to differing methods for defining pain. There is also a marked variation in the incidence of pain according to the site of the primary and metastatic lesions. For example, leukemia rarely produces pain (5% incidence), whereas osteolytic tumors are typically painful (85% incidence).[5] Overall, it is estimated that nearly one third of cancer patients will have moderate to severe pain during the intermediary phase and nearly two thirds will have such pain during the terminal phase.[10] Even this statistic is somewhat misleading since it does not reveal the entire picture. Approximately one half of those patients with cancer pain are thought to die with severe intractable pain uncontrolled by current therapy.[11] This has prompted Bonica to deem this reservoir of human suffering one of the most pressing health problems in the United States.[10]

THE OPTIMAL NARCOTIC FOR CANCER PAIN

Narcotic analgesics are the principal means to control moderate to severe cancer pain. Despite their long history of use, there is no consensus regarding the optimal narcotic for cancer patients or the best schedule of administration. Brompton's mixture has been widely utilized in this application because of its analgesic properties, ease of administration, and patient acceptance. There exist several different formulations for the Brompton's solution. The mixture typically contains 15 mg of morphine hydrochloride, 10 mg of cocaine hydrochloride, 2 ml of alcohol 90%, 4 ml of syrup, and chloroform water to 15 ml.[12]

Melzack and associates have studied the use of Brompton's mixture to alleviate cancer pain and have verified its effectiveness.[13] In a subsequent study, however, it was noted that there was no significant difference in clinical results when Brompton's mixture was compared with oral morphine.[14] The results suggested that the addition of cocaine, alcohol, and chloroform water to the mixture was superfluous and potentially dangerous since it increased the amount of sedation produced by the narcotic and introduced the potential for local anesthetic toxicity. Several authors have recommended the deletion of these additives.[15, 16]

Morphine is widely regarded as the standard of comparison for potent narcotic analgesics in cancer pain patients. Other narcotics have also been advocated. Heroin was presumed to be a superior drug because of its greater potency, enhanced solubility, and increased narcotic-induced euphoria in comparison to morphine. Twycross, on comparing morphine and heroin in a Brompton's mixture, found no appreciable difference.[17] This finding was subse-

quently confirmed by Mount et al.[18] Thus, currently available data on heroin do not indicate it to be superior to morphine.

Methadone, with its long duration of action and excellent oral absorption, would seem to be another ideal narcotic. Ettinger et al., however, reported three cases in which excessive drug accumulation was produced by the administration of methadone in accordance with the manufacturer's recommendations.[19] The half-life of the drug averages 25 hours (range, 13–47 hours). There appears to be a marked divergence, however, in the plasma levels and analgesic response, the latter usually lasting 4–6 hours. Chronic administration of methadone therefore warrants careful titration of the drug over a 4- to 5-day period until equilibrium is reached. Methadone, it should be noted, is superior to both morphine and the Brompton's mixture in terms of cost: the estimated cost for 100 methadone tablets is nearly half that for morphine.[20] Whether morphine will ultimately be replaced in the future by methadone or some other synthetic narcotic remains to be seen. At present, most centers continue to use morphine as their primary analgesic, either alone or in a Brompton's mixture to treat cancer pain.

Most authors are in agreement on the need to give narcotics on a fixed-interval basis rather than an as-needed schedule. Administration of narcotics on a regular schedule avoids the peaks and valleys in analgesic blood levels and ensures a constant level of analgesia. The primary objective with this approach is the prophylaxis of pain and prevention of analgesic regression. Varying intensities in the level of pain are best managed by altering the dosage of the drug without changing the dosing interval. This approach virtually necessitates the use of oral agents and active participation by the patient in determining the dose of drug to be taken.

The prolonged use of narcotics does entail some risks to the patient: habituation, tolerance, and the potential for drug abuse. The distinction among habituation, tolerance, and drug abuse must be clarified. Habituation certainly occurs in cancer patients whose pain is controlled by narcotics. The important point to consider is that these patients are habituated to the prophylaxis against pain. The drug is a necessary means to achieve this state and should not be denied them merely because of their dependency relationship. The situation is somewhat analogous to what occurs in a patient with an endocrinopathy being treated by hormonal replacement. When viewed in this context, habituation has a decidedly less ominous connotation. Furthermore, there is indirect evidence to support this specific conceptualization. Endorphins are now perceived as hormone-like substances with biologic activity similar in nature to the other more traditional hormonal peptides.[21] Chronic intractable pain appears to be due to a deficiency state of endorphins relative to the level of substance P (sP), a nociceptive neurotransmitter recently shown to correlate with the level of pain and need for narcotics in a group of postsurgical pains.[22] There are further supporting data in that pain fluctuates in a diurnal pattern in keeping with other endocrine disorders such as diabetes or hypothyroidism.[23]

Tolerance to narcotic analgesics does appear in cancer patients and can pose a significant management problem. Despite the contention by Twycross that this phenomenon does not occur,[17] both Houde[24] and Foley et al.[25] have demonstrated its existence. Both Houde and Foley et al. recommended that the problem of tolerance to narcotics be managed by increasing the dosage of drug, switching to alternative drugs, or using a combination of drugs.

Narcotic abuse by cancer patients is a real problem, but one whose magnitude has been overstated. Very few cancer patients have been found to use their analgesics in a sociopathic manner.[24] There are only isolated instances of drug abuse among these patients. As an example, the intravenous abuse of illicitly obtained Brompton's mixture (intended for oral use) was just reported recently.[26]

NONNARCOTIC ANALGESICS

In spite of the need for new narcotics with improved characteristics, the major advances in the field at the present time pertain to the recent introduction of potent nonnarcotic analgesics and the administration of narcotic analgesics either intrathecally or epidurally. The latter method is proving to be efficacious for alleviating severe pain in the terminal patient and is discussed later in this chapter.

Nonsteroidal anti-inflammatory analgesics have become the principal drugs within the nonnarcotic analgesic group. Aspirin and acetaminophen have been the standard nonsteroidal anti-inflammatory analgesic agents up to the present time and are sufficiently potent to alleviate mild to moderate pain. The more potent nonsteroidal anti-inflammatory analgesics compounds like indomethacin or phenylbutazone are rarely used as analgesics because of their greater incidence of side effects and toxicity. A number of new nonsteroidal anti-inflammatory an-

algesics have been introduced recently. These include zomepirac, meclofenamate, naproxen, and diflunisal. These drugs, in general, have analgesic activity superior to that of either aspirin or acetaminophen and are better tolerated by the patient, with a lower overall incidence of side effects and toxicity.

Zomepirac* (Zomax) is representative of this group of drugs and will be discussed in detail. The drug was derived from tolmetin, has neither opioid agonist nor antagonist activity, and is unrelated to salicylates in chemical structure. Its exact mechanism of action is somewhat speculative, although it has been shown to be a potent prostaglandin synthetase inhibitor. By inhibiting the function of this enzyme, the formation of prostaglandin E_2 (PGE_2) is blocked. This particular compound is produced when cell membranes are disrupted and the arachidonic acid is converted by prostaglandin synthetase to PGE_2. This latter compound is a potent activator of peripheral pain receptors. Zomepirac, by reducing the amount of PGE_2 formed, presumably reduces the intensity of nociceptive stimulus transmitted to the CNS and in this manner decreases the perception of pain by the patient.[27] The analgesia produced by zomepirac cannot be reversed with naloxone, and physical dependence with the drug has not been observed.[27]

Zomepirac's analgesic activity has been tested extensively under a variety of clinical conditions. The findings have been relatively consistent. A 100-mg oral dose of zomepirac produced analgesia equal to or greater than that achieved with 60 mg of codeine (either alone or in combination with APC),[28] 50 mg of pentazocine,[29] or 8 mg of parenteral morphine.[30] Parenteral zomepirac is currently under investigation and may be even more efficacious.

The incidence of side effects and toxic effects from zomepirac is relatively low and the effects are generally benign. Gastrointestinal intolerance was far less with zomepirac than with aspirin;[31] the effect on platelet function,[32] bleeding times,[33] and fecal blood loss[34] was similarly reduced. Zomepirac thus possesses an analgesic profile markedly different from its predecessors, yet the incidence of adverse reactions associated with its use is substantially lower by comparison. Moreover, not being an opioid derivative obviates the dual problems of respiratory depression and drug addiction. Conse-

---

*Zomepirac is now withdrawn by the FDA for regular use in the USA, but can be approved by the FDA for use on a specific physician request.

quently, zomepirac is proving to be a useful drug for control of mild to moderate pain. Further investigations are warranted to determine if it is the optimal drug in its class and the degree of analgesic potentiation when it is combined with a narcotic analgesic.

Nonsteroidal anti-inflammatory analgesics appear to be particularly useful in cancer patients with metastatic bone pain. Osteolytic tumors have been shown to secrete prostaglandins, including PGE_2, thereby exacerbating the pain from the growth of the tumor and accelerating bone resorption due to their osteoclastic activity. The administration of a nonsteroidal anti-inflammatory analgesic seems to be particularly effective as a means of controlling metastatic bone pain. Ventafridda et al. reported that 55% of 763 cancer patients (personal series) had significant relief with the administration of a nonsteroidal anti-inflammatory analgesic.[35] The authors concluded that nonsteroidal anti-inflammatory analgesics "have an important role in the treatment of pain of all degrees of severity associated with neoplastic disease. The effect of these drugs on the progress of the tumors needs further clarification. New compounds (aspirin and indomethacin were studied) with fewer adverse effects and greater analgesic efficacy already in development will offer welcome additional treatment options." Nonsteroidal anti-inflammatory analgesics offer the clinician a pharmacologic means to treat mild to moderate pain in an efficacious manner without resorting to the use of narcotic analgesics early in the course of a malignancy. Furthermore, these drugs may prove to be ideal adjuvants for use with narcotic analgesics in the treatment of severe pain, thus combining the mechanism of action of the nonsteroidal anti-inflammatory analgesics with the centrally acting narcotic analgesics.

SPINAL NARCOTICS IN THE TREATMENT OF CANCER PAIN

The most innovative and potentially useful advance in the field of analgesics is the recognition that narcotics can be effective when administrated directly into the epidural or intrathecal space. The resulting analgesia is superior to that produced by systemic administration and, unlike the effect produced by local anesthetics, there is no impairment of motor function. This recent development can be traced to the report by Yaksh and Rudy in which they demonstrated the direct action of narcotics on the spinal cord.[36] The presence of narcotic receptors in the spinal cord has since been confirmed by others.[37, 38]

This has prompted numerous investigators to use epidural narcotics to relieve pain under actual clinical conditions for postoperative, chronic benign, and terminal pain. The results have been uniformly encouraging in terms of the quality of analgesia. The technique's acceptance for routine clinical use has been tempered, however, by the observation that respiratory depression of delayed onset can occur following injection.[39, 40] In addition, urinary retention and pruritis have been noted with spinal narcotics. These problems constitute less of a constraint in the dying patient with severe pain than in the postoperative patient or patient with chronic benign pain.

It is not surprising, therefore, that clinicians have attempted prolonged analgesia by repetitive epidural injections of narcotics. Several methods exist to accomplish this. The simplest method entails the insertion percutaneously of an epidural catheter and subsequent top-up injections of narcotic given by the patient or his family. Wishart maintained two cancer patients pain-free—one for 4 weeks and the other for 6 weeks—by this technique.[41] He covered the insertion site with antibiotic ointment and "Opsite" to maintain sterility. The distal end of the catheter was taped to the patient's shoulder and connected to a microfilter, and the patient or his family administered 5 mg of morphine in a 10-ml volume every 10–12 hours, as needed. This particular technique, although simple to perform, may lead to retrograde infection of the epidural space via the catheter. For this reason, most authors have used a totally implanted system with either intermittent or continuous infusion of drugs.

Poletti and co-workers, after an initial experience with a Broviac catheter placed epidurally, went to an indwelling system consisting of a morphine reservoir connected to a shunt pump and an on-off Hakim valve.[42] This permitted the patient to self-administer the narcotic as required. However, the method necessitates refilling the reservoir every 2–12 months, depending on the usage of drug. It also is somewhat limiting in the amount of drug that can be delivered and its accurate disbursement.

These two deficiencies are overcome by implanting an Ommaya reservoir connected to the proximal end of an epidural catheter. The reservoir, placed subcutaneously in a convenient site, can be filled by the patient, who gives himself an injection of the desired amount of drug. Leavens et al. has used this system on six patients for up to 7 months without any major problems.[43] Pruritis did occur in several patients but was easily controlled with diphenhydramine (Benadryl).

As an alternative to giving narcotics on an intermittent basis, several authors have implanted continuous infusion devices. Onofrio, Yaksh, and Arnold surgically placed an Infusaid (Metal Bellows Corporation, Sharon, Mass.) drug delivery system in a patient with severe intractable pain produced by a sacral chordoma.[44] The intrathecal infusion of morphine, 0.6 mg/24 hours, provided ample analgesia. No problems were encountered with the system, and the 50-ml reservoir could be refilled by percutaneous injection every 2–4 weeks on an outpatient basis. Similar results were obtained by Coombs et al. in two patients followed up for 6 months with an identical system.[45]

Caution must be exercised in interpreting these results since the reports are somewhat preliminary in nature and the technique is new. Nevertheless, the quality of analgesia produced by spinal narcotics cannot be disputed, and this method appears to be the treatment of choice for terminal cancer patients with severe pain that is poorly controlled by oral narcotic analgesics. Further investigations are urgently needed to delineate the long-term efficacy, dosing schedules, and optimal technique. Despite these reservations about the use of prolonged spinal narcotic analgesia, it would be inhumane to deny this intervention to the dying patient. (See chapter 38 for further information).

NEUROLYTIC BLOCKS AND CANCER PAIN

Interest in neurolytic blocks has been subdued in comparison to that generated by spinal narcotics. Several articles have been published recently on this subject and merit consideration. Swerdlow[46] and Gerbershagen[47] each reviewed the technique and results of intrathecal neurolysis.

Significant new developments or improved methods for neurolytic blocks have been decidedly sporadic. Several recent articles have refined the technique for celiac plexus block. The impetus for this resurgence in interest can be traced to a definitive anatomical and radiologic study of the celiac plexus undertaken by Moore, Bush, and Burnett.[48] Their report is mandatory reading for the clinician with an interest in celiac plexus blocks. The efficacy of celiac plexus neurolysis was determined by Hegedus[49]

and Singler,[50] who reported their experience in a series of 36 and 11 patients, respectively. Although there were minor differences in the techniques used and the volume of neurolytic solution injected, the results were relatively comparable: nearly 50% of the patients had marked relief of pain following neurolytic block. These results pertain to patients with terminal cancer; in the case of chronic benign pain from the chronic pancreatitis, the results were somewhat less.

The potentially most useful advance in neurolytic blocks has been made in the ablation of the pituitary using a stereotactic approach. The technique was pioneered by Moricca[51] in 1963; a subsequent report was published in 1981 on his cumulative experience.[52] The same technique has been used by Levin, Katz and their co-workers to ameliorate severe intractable pain in 29 patients with either prostatic cancer or widely metastatic disease.[53] They instilled absolute alcohol into the sella turcica under stereotactic control and succeeded in destroying the function of the pituitary gland, as evidenced by a lack of antidiuretic hormone (ADH). In addition, neurolysis of the pituitary stalk and degeneration of the supraoptic and paraventricular nuclei of the hypothalamus and the median eminence were observed at autopsy in some patients. Of the 17 patients with prostatic carcinoma, 94% obtained good to excellent pain relief by this technique. In the remaining 12 patients with mixed tumors, 11 patients benefited from the procedure and had good to excellent pain relief. The longest survival in each group was 9 and 7 months, respectively, and there were no untoward complications attributable to the neurolytic blocks. The authors concluded that the analgesia resulted from the suppression of ADH production by chemical destruction of the hypothalamic nuclei and that this effect could not be reversed with naloxone.

Based on the analgesic efficacy of celiac plexus block and pituitary neurolysis, it is evident that these two techniques are potentially quite beneficial in select circumstances. For pancreatic carcinoma, neurolytic celiac plexus block appears indicated for the patient with advanced disease and moderate to severe pain. In those instances where patients with prostatic cancer or widely disseminated tumors have intractable pain that is poorly localized, pituitary ablation appears to be the treatment of choice. The major limitation to both procedures is the relative lack of individuals trained to perform these blocks. This impediment should not prevent the primary physician from considering either block for his patient. These two neurolytic blocks nicely complement the analgesic capabilities of spinal narcotics and for the first time afford the physician sufficient therapeutic flexibility to effectively manage cancer patients with highly advanced disease and intractable pain.

THE HOSPICE MOVEMENT AND THE ROLE OF THE ANESTHESIOLOGIST

"Hospice" has become a ubiquitous term in the medical and lay literature and has lost much of its specificity in meaning. The term originally designated lodging facilities for crusaders during the Middle Ages. The modern connotation can be traced to St. Christopher's Hospice. This facility was developed to care for the terminally ill patient. This, together with increased interest about death and dying, has prompted a marked change in the manner in which the dying patient is managed.

The loss of specificity in use of the term relates to the nature and objectives of the hospice. The common usage implies a free-standing facility that resembles more a hotel than a modern hospital. The facility and the care it renders to the patient deliberately eschew the vestiges of modern society and its dependence on high technology.

This is where the confusion has arisen. The hospice movement really entails an objective: to provide the highest quality of life for the dying patient. Whether the care is provided within a separate free-standing facility, a specialized unit within an acute care hospital, or on an outpatient basis does not alter the concept, or is abandonment of modern medicine a central issue. In order to produce the best quality of life for the terminally ill patient, some of the most sophisticated patient management is required. What is abhorred and consequently avoided is the overreliance on diagnostic tests and needless procedures which characterizes the modern hospital, along with its depersonalizing aspects.

The primary attribute of a hospice, irrespective of the physical facility in which it is housed, is its personnel. Management of the dying patient is a very involved and taxing enterprise. It requires a team approach in order to be successful. The team consists of a variety of medical and paramedical professionals, including doctors, nurses, medical social workers, physical therapists, psychologists, pharmacists, occupational therapists, and dietitians, among others. A successful cancer pain center will also have an administrative director to coordinate its overall activities. Individual patients, however, are followed and managed by a patient coordinator who calls on the various services provided by members of the team. Thus, one may find a neurosurgeon handling the surgical therapy, an anesthesiologist the nerve blocks, and a pharmacist the medications. The patient's coordinator may be one of these individuals or someone entirely different. Variations in the quality of care rendered are minimized by collective review of patient management regimens.

The involvement of anesthesiologists in a hospice program can span from performing nerve blocks to overseeing the total care for individual patients or acting as administrative head of the program. The potential role of anesthesiologists in a hospice thus depends on the individual involved. Just as many chronic pain clinics are run by anesthesiologists, it is not inconceivable that many cancer pain centers likewise will have anesthesiologists in the chief administrative position. This reflects in part the prior training of anesthesiologists in pharmacology and physiology and their leadership role in the operating room. What remains to be developed is fellowship programs in anesthesia to train residents who have a career goal in this subspecialty.

The hospice movement therefore represents a challenge to American anesthesiology for participation by its members in an activity outside of the operating room environment. When viewed in this context, the hospice movement offers a chance to diversify and broaden the specialty. If the experience in similar endeavors such as the preceding involvement in intensive care units is any indication, the specialty will not only make a valuable contribution but will be enriched in the process.

REFERENCES

1. Twycross R., Ventafridda V.: The continuing cancer patients, in *Proceedings of an International Seminar on Continuing Care of Terminal Cancer Patients.* New York, Pergamon Press, 1979.
2. Gybels J., Adriaensen H., Cosyns P.: Treatment of pain in patients with advanced cancer. *Eur. J. Cancer* 12:341–351, 1976.
3. Catalano R.: The medical approach to management of pain caused by cancer. *Semin. Oncol.* 2:379–392, 1975.
4. Shepard D.A.: Principles and practice of palliative care. *Med. Assoc. J.* 116:522–526, 1977.
5. Foley K.M.: Pain syndromes in patients with cancer, in Bonica J.J. (ed.): *Advances in Pain Research and Therapy.* New York, Raven Press, 1979, vol. 2, pp. 59–75.
6. Wilkes E.: Some problems in cancer management. *Proc. R. Soc. Med.* 67:23–27, 1974.

7. Pannuti F., Martoni A., Rossi A.P., et al.: The role of endocrine therapy for the relief of pain due to advanced cancer, in Bonica J.J. (ed.): *Advances in Pain Research and Therapy*. New York, Raven Press, 1979, vol. 2, pp. 145–165.

8. Haram J., Saunders C.M.: Facts and figures, in *The Management of Terminal Disease*. London, Edward Arnold, 1978, pp. 12–18.

9. Cartwright A., Hockey L., Anderson A.B.: *Life Before Death*. London, Routledge & Kegan Paul, 1973.

10. Bonica J.J.: Importance of the problem, in Bonica J.J. (ed.): *Advances in Pain Research and Therapy*. New York, Raven Press, 1979, vol. 2, pp. 1–12.

11. Parks C.M.: Home or hospital? Terminal care as seen by surviving spouses. *J. R. Coll. Gen. Pract.* 28:19–30, 1978.

12. Noyes R. Jr.: Treatment of cancer pain. *Psychosom. Med.* 43(1):57–70, 1981.

13. Melzack R., Ofeish J.G., Mount B.M.: The Brompton mixture: Effects on pain in cancer patients. *Can. Med. Assoc. J.* 115:125–129, 1976.

14. Melzack R., Mount B.M., Gordon J.M.: The Brompton mixture versus morphine solution given orally: Effects on pain. *Can. Med. Assoc. J.* 120:435–438, 1979.

15. Howrie D.L.: Brompton's mixture for pain relief. *J. Pediatr.* 99:666–667, 1981.

16. Twycross R.G.: The effect of cocaine in the Brompton cocktail, in *Pain Abstracts,* vol. 1. Montreal, Second World Congress, August 1978, p. 78.

17. Twycross R.G.: Choice of strong analgesic in terminal cancer: Diamorphine or morphine. *Pain* 3:93–104, 1977.

18. Mount B.M., Ajemian I., Scott J.F.: Use of the Brompton mixture in treating the chronic pain of malignant disease. *Can. Med. Assoc. J.* 115:122–124, 1976.

19. Ettinger D.S., Vitale P.J., Trump D.L.: Important clinical pharmacologic considerations in the use of methadone in cancer patients. *Cancer Treat. Rep.* 63(3):457–459, 1979.

20. Moertel C.G.: Treatment of cancer pain with orally administered medications. *JAMA* 244(21):2448–2450, 1980.

21. Roth J., LeRoith D., Shiloach J., et al.: The evolutionary origins of hormones, neurotransmitters, and other extracellular chemical messengers. *N. Engl. J. Med.* 306(9):523–527, 1982.

22. Neumann P.B., Henriken H., Grosman N., et al.: Plasma morphine concentrations during chronic oral administration in patients with cancer pain. *Pain* 13:247–252, 1982.

23. Macek C.: Bihormonal theory of diabetes gets solid backing. *JAMA* 247(12):1685–1686, 1982.

24. Houde R.W.: Systemic analgesics and related drugs, in Bonica J.J. (ed.): *Advances in Pain Research and Therapy*. New York, Raven Press, 1967, vol. 12.

25. Foley K.M., Tyler H.R.: The management of pain of malignant origin, in *Current Neurology*. Boston, Houghton Mifflin, 1979, vol. 2, pp. 279–302.

26. Fischbeck K.H., Mata M., D'Aquisto, R., et al.: Brompton mixture taken intravenously by a heroin addict. *West. J. Med.* 133:80, 1980.

27. Pruss T.P., Gardock J.F., Taylor R.J.: Evaluation of the analgesic properties of zomepirac. *J. Clin. Pharmacol.* 20:216–222, 1980.

28. Baird W.M., Turek D.: Comparison of zomepirac, APC with codeine, codeine and placebo in the treatment of moderate and severe pain. *J. Clin. Pharmacol.* 20:243–249, 1980.

29. DeAndrade J.R., Honig S., Ciccone W.J., et al.: Clinical comparison of zomepirac with pentazocine in the treatment of post-operative pain. *J. Clin. Pharmacol.* 20:292–297, 1980.

30. Wallenstein S.L., Roger A., Kaiko R.F., et al.: Relative analgesic potency of oral zomepirac and intramuscular morphine in cancer patients with postoperative pain. *J. Clin. Pharmacol.* 20:250–258, 1980.

31. Ruoff G.D., Andelman S.Y., Cannella J.J.: Long-term safety of zomepirac: A double-blind comparison with aspirin in patients with osteoarthritis. *J. Clin. Pharmacol.* 20:377–384, 1980.

32. Mielke C.H., Kahn S.B., Muschek L.D.: Effects of zomepirac or hemostasis in healthy adults and on platelet function in vitro. *J. Clin. Pharmacol.* 20:409–417, 1980.

33. Minn F.L., Zimny M.A.: Zomepirac and warfarin: A clinical study to determine if interaction exists. *J. Clin. Pharmacol.* 20:418–421, 1980.

34. Johnson P.C.: A comparison of the effects of zomepirac and aspirin on fecal blood loss. *J. Clin. Pharmacol.* 20:401–405, 1980.

35. Ventafridda V., Fochi C., Conno D., et al.: Use of non-steroidal anti-inflammatory drugs in the treatment of pain in cancer. *Br. J. Clin. Pharmacol.* 10:343S–346S, 1980.

36. Yaksh T.L., Rudy T.A.: Analgesia mediated by a direct spinal action of narcotics. *Science* 192:1357–1358, 1976.

37. Atweh S.F., Kuhar M.J.: Autoradiographic localization of opiate receptors in rat brain: Part I. Spinal cord and lower medulla. *Brain Res.* 124:53–67, 1977.

38. Lamotte C., Pert C.B., Snyder S.H.: Opiate receptor binding in primate spinal cord: Distribution and changes after dorsal roof section. *Brain Res.* 112:407–412, 1976.

39. Davies G.K., Tolhurst-Cleaver C.L., James T.L.: CNS depression from intrathecal morphine. *Anesthesiology* 52:280, 1980.

40. Glynn C.J., Mather L.E., Cousins M.J., et al.: Spinal narcotics and respiratory depression. *Lancet* 2:356–357, 1979.

41. Wishart J.M.: Epidural morphine at home, letter. *Can. Anaesth. Soc. J.* 28(5):492, 1981.

42. Poletti C.E., Cohen A.M., Todd D.P., et al.: Cancer pain relieved by long-term epidural morphine with

permanent indwelling systems for self-administration. *J. Neurosurg.* 55:581–582, 1981.

43. Leavens M.E., Stratton-Hill C. Jr., Cech D.A., et al.: Intrathecal and intraventricular morphine for pain in cancer patients: Initial study. *J. Neurosurg.* 56:241–245, 1982.

44. Onofrio B.M., Yaksh T.L., Arnold P.G.: Continuous low-dose intrathecal morphine administration in the treatment of chronic pain of malignant origin. *Mayo Clin. Proc.* 56:516–520, 1981.

45. Coombs D.W., Saunders R.L., Gaylor M.S., et al.: Continuous epidural analgesia via implanted morphine reservoir, letter. *Lancet* 2(8243):425–426, 1981.

46. Swerdlow M.: Intrathecal neurolysis. *Anaesthesia* 33:733–740, 1978.

47. Gerbershagen H.V.: Neurolysis: Subarachnoid neurolytic blockage. *Acta Anaesthesiol. Belg.* 1:45–57, 1981.

48. Moore D.C., Bush W.H., Burnett L.L.: Celiac plexus block: A roentgenographic, anatomic study of technique and spread of solution in patients and corpses. *Anesth. Analg.* 60:369–379, 1981.

49. Hegedus V.: Relief of pancreatic pain by radiography-guided block. *AJR* 133:1101–1103, 1979.

50. Singler R.C.: An improved technique for alcohol neurolysis of the celiac plexus. *Anesthesiology* 56:137–141, 1982.

51. Moricca G.: Chemical hypophysectomy for cancer pain. *Adv. Neurol.* 4:707–714, 1974.

52. Moricca G., Arcuri E., Moricca P.: Neuroadenolysis of the pituitary. *Acta Anaesthesiol. Belg.* 1:87–99, 1981.

53. Levin A.B., Katz J., Benson R.C.: Treatment of pain of diffuse metastatic cancer by stereotactic chemical hypophysectomy: Long term results and observations on mechanism of action. *Neurosurgery* 6:258–262, 1980.

21 / Phantom Limb Pain

RICHARD M. ROSENBLATT, M.D.

THE SYNDROME of phantom limb pain is one of the more enigmatic problems in medicine. For the patient who has experienced the physical and psychological trauma of an amputation, phantom limb pain must seem demonic. Just as perplexed and frustrated is the physician, because of the recalcitrance of the problem to therapy. It therefore comes as no surprise that there has been a continuing interest in this clinical entity, as evidenced by numerous articles in the medical literature. What is surprising is the limited number of scientific investigations on this subject. Until recently most publications were conjectural or anecdotal in nature. There still exists a paucity of information on phantom limb pain regarding its epidemiology, pathogenesis, mechanism of action and controlled therapeutic trials. These deficiencies can be attributed, for the most part, to the obtusive and nebulous properties of the syndrome. Nevertheless, phantom limb pain is neither a new entity nor one that has gone unobserved until now.

The first written record of the phenomenon of phantom limb is credited to Pare Ambroise, who in 1634 wrote a remarkably accurate description, even by today's standards. He noted, "following the loss of a limb, the victim may continue to be conscious of the lost part with the same or even greater clarity than the real one."[1] This compares rather favorably with a more modern description by Melzack:[2]

[M]ost amputees report feeling a phantom limb almost immediately after amputation of an arm or leg. The limb is usually described as having a tingling feeling, a definite shape, and moves through space much the same way the normal limb would move when the person walks, sits down, or stretches out on a bed. At first, the phantom limb feels perfectly normal in size and shape—so much so that the amputee may reach out for objects with the phantom hand, or try to get out of bed by stepping on the floor with the phantom leg. As time passes, however, the phantom limb begins to change shape. The leg or arm becomes less distinct and may fade away altogether, so that the phantom foot or hand seems to be hanging in mid-air. Sometimes, the limb is slowly "telescoped" into the stump until only the hand or foot remains at the stump tip.

The association of pain with a phantom limb seems not to be an inevitable occurrence following amputation. It was not until 1872 that the entity of phantom limb pain was described by Mitchell, based on his experiences during the Civil War.[3] The attributes of phantom limb pain contrast markedly with the prior benign descriptions. Sunderland has written the following description of phantom limb pain:[1]

After the amputation of a limb almost all patients experience a vivid sense of the presence of the whole or part of the limb which has been lost and this sensory illusion may be retained for many years. . . . [I]n most cases the phantom is not particularly troublesome, the amputee rapidly adapts to the new situation, the image soon fades and disappears, and at no stage does it become a therapeutic problem. In a few, however, the phantom becomes the seat of severe and unrelenting pain which may defy all attempts to terminate or relieve it.

Other authors have used the following adjectives to describe the specific qualities of phantom limb pain: burning, cramping, aching, and stabbing;[4] tingling, shooting, and crushing.[5] The extreme severity of the pain is vividly captured by another quotation from Sunderland: "the patient may feel that his fingernails are digging into the palm or are being torn off."[1]

The phenomenon of phantom limb pain encompasses a wide spectrum of symptoms. On one end of the continuum is the mildest, least noxious discomfort. At the other end is an intense, excruciating pain often having a bizarre, seemingly sadistic quality. Rather than dwell on the descriptive features of phantom limb pain, Sunderland has proposed a system of taxonomy to classify patients with this disorder. Phantom limb pain is subdivided into four classes, according to the severity of the pain and its functional attributes:

   I. Mild intermittent paresthesia that has no appreciable impact on the individual's level of functioning.

  II. Moderate intermittent paresthesia that occasionally interferes with the normal daily routine.

 III. Severe paresthesia that occurs intermittently and is debilitating in nature.

 IV. Severe paresthesia that occurs continuously

or sufficiently frequent to grossly impair the individual's life-style.

The incidence and severity of phantom limb pain among amputees are not known. Most authors regard the phenomenon of phantom limb perception among amputees as nearly universal. In contrast, the number of individuals reported to experience phantom limb pain after amputation ranges from 2% to 64%.[6–13] Certain patients do seem to be predisposed to the development of phantom limb pain. These are usually patients who have experienced a traumatic amputation, have postoperative complications in the stump, are from a lower socioeconomic class, and have an immobile frozen phantom limb.[1] Also implicated are patients who experience war-time amputations, are retired from work, develop stump neuromas, have high scores for neuroticism on the Eysenck Personality Inventory, or have organic and

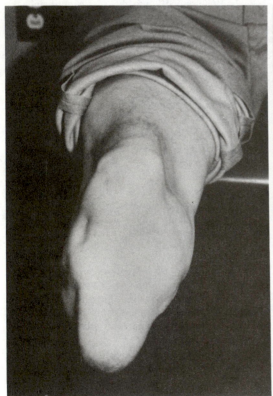
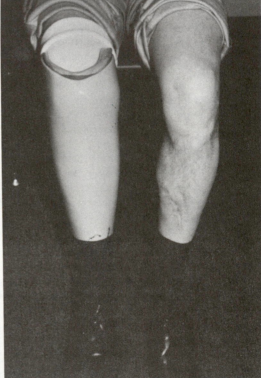

Fig 21–1.—A 78-year-old man had phantom limb sensation and pain following amputation 2 years earlier. Cramping pain radiated to the foot and increased with the use of a prosthesis and with weight-bearing. The patient was treated with a series of lumbar sympathetic blocks, local infiltration of the stump with neurolytic agents, and readjustment of the prosthesis. Six months after treatment he was able to cope with the pain and was functional. *Left*, amputated right leg 2 years earlier. *Right*, the prosthesis in use by the patient.

psychosomatic symptoms as noted on the Cornell Medical Index.[14] The presence of a behavioral or psychiatric disorder might be presumed to be a factor predisposing to the development of phantom limb pain, but this does not appear to be the case. Psychiatric disorders have been shown to occur with the same frequency in amputees whether they have phantom limb pain or not.[1, 13]

Not only is the incidence of phantom limb pain poorly documented, its pathogenesis can often be highly unpredictable and change over time. First, phantom limb pain does not always manifest immediately after an amputation. The majority of patients who develop phantom limb pain do so during the interval extending from the first month after the amputation up to 1 year later (Fig 21–1).[1] There are several reports of the delayed appearance of phantom limb pain some 13, 25, and 30 years after amputation.[6, 15, 16] Second, phantom limb pain may change markedly in its mental image, varying in both the intensity and quality of the pain. Acute exacerbations are not uncommon, with a concomitant increase in the severity and frequency of pain. The phantom limb may also take the form of a grossly malformed, convoluted extremity whose perceived image is fixed in space.

Two perturbations in the mental picture of the phantom limb are commonly described by amputees and are thought to be associated with the healing process. "Telescoping" describes the shortening of the phantom limb localized to the midportion of the extremity. "Fading" denotes the gradual disappearance of the phantom limb altogether. These two processes can be active simultaneously and play an important though poorly understood role in the regression of the phantom limb and the cessation of pain.

Accurate statistics on the longevity of phantom limb pain do not exist; a single study has reported that 70% of amputees who experience phantom limb pain do so for at least 1 year or more.[1]

TREATMENT OF CHRONIC PHANTOM LIMB PAIN

Over the past several decades an exceedingly large number of therapeutic modalities have been tried in an effort to alleviate phantom limb pain. Listed in Table 21–1 are the various conservative and surgical methods that have been tried. It is not necessary to review each modality on an individual basis. Most reports in the literature are anecdotal

and have consisted of an uncontrolled clinical trial involving a small number of patients followed up for a short period of time; in most instances subsequent investigations have failed to substantiate the initial laudatory findings. For the reader who is interested in a recent analysis of the literature, a comprehensive review article has been published on this subject.[17]

More germane is the survey on the treatment of phantom limb pain in the United States conducted recently by Sherman et al.[18] They sent questionnaires to Veterans Administration hospitals, medical schools, pain clinics, and pain specialists to determine which treatments are in current use, their rate of success, and delineation of treatments that had previously proved unsuccessful in controlling phantom limb pain. They sent out 835 questionnaires and received back 328 (41%). Completed questionnaires were returned from 73% of the VA hospitals and 75% of the medical schools in the country. They found that the number of phantom limb patients seen by a composite of the various institutions within a state correlated well with the relative population of the state. As would be expected, VA hospitals saw more patients with phantom limb pain than medical schools. The majority of patients in the survey with phantom limb pain were treated by specialists in physical medicine and rehabilitation (25.9%), anesthesiology (14.3%), orthopedic surgery (10.4%), or psychiatry and psychology (10.1%).

Each respondent in the survey rated the modalities he used to treat phantom limb on a scale of 0 (no success) to 10 (entirely successful). The various treatments were then subdivided into three classes: conservative therapy alone, conservative therapy plus surgery, and surgical therapy alone. When the average ratings were calculated for the three groups, the conservative therapy only group had a statistically better result than either the conservative therapy plus surgery or the surgical therapy only group. The efficacy of specific treatments was then determined. Although acupuncture, nerve blocks, relaxation training, biofeedback, stump conditioning, ultrasound, supportive therapy, and prosthetic revision all produced high success scores, they were also found to have similarly high rates of prior failure. Transcutaneous electrical nerve stimulation (TENS) was used by most respondents but was marginally successful and had a high rate of prior failure. The surgical procedures without exception were associated with uniformly low success scores and dismally high prior failure rates. There was even a negative

TABLE 21–1.—CONSERVATIVE THERAPEUTIC MODALITIES AND SURGICAL PROCEDURES
USED IN THE TREATMENT OF PHANTOM LIMB PAIN

Conservative Modalities

Acupuncture	Massage
Analgesics	Neurolytic block of the stump or peripheral nerves
Anticonvulsants	Percussion therapy
Antidepressants	Phantom limb exercises
Barbiturates	Phenothiazines
Behavior modification	Placebo therapy
Biofeedback	Psychotherapy
Curare	Prosthesis modification
Electroshock therapy	Radiotherapy
Electrosleep	Relaxation therapy
Epidural or spinal block	Steroids
Hypnotherapy	Stump desensitization
Intravenous procaine	Supportive therapy
Intravenous regional with guanethidine	Sympathetic blocks
Local anesthetic block of the stump or peripheral nerves	Transcutaneous electrical nerve stimulation (TENS)
Local heat	Tranquilizers
LSD	Ultrasound
	Vasodilators
	Vitamin therapy

Surgical Procedures

Anterior cingulate lesion	Neurectomy
Cervical tractotomy	Parietal lobotomy
Cordotomy	Peripheral nerve stimulation
Dorsal column stimulation	Posterior central gyrus ablation
Dorsal root ablation	Prefrontal lobotomy
Excision of neuroma	Rhizotomy
Intraspinal stimulation	Stump revision
Lobectomy	Sympathectomy
Lumbar tractotomy	Substantia Gelatinosa ablation
Midbrain lesion	Thalamic lesion
Midbrain stimulation	Thalamic stimulation
Nerve strangulation	

correlation among individual surgeons in regard to the number of patients with phantom limb treated by them and their utilization of surgical therapy.

Based on the results of this study, Sherman et al. concluded that no single method of treatment was particularly efficacious in phantom limb pain. Most interventions produced results comparable to those achieved with placebo therapy. They recommended a multidisciplinary approach to the patient with phantom limb pain, utilizing exclusively a combination of conservative modalities. Emphasis should be directed toward maximizing the functional level of the individual and away from modalities that foster chronic pain behavior. The findings of this single survey are consistent with the bulk of the literature published on phantom limb pain, and the recommendations of the authors are not altogether surprising when viewed in this context. Surgery, except when there is definite stump pathology or a reflex dystrophy, has been shown to be ineffective and po-

tentially hazardous. Resorting to a combination of treatments appears, at the present time, to be a reasonable approach, although it likewise remains to be determined whether a multimodality treatment program is any more efficacious than the respective constituents by themselves.

My approach to the treatment of chronic phantom limb pain is somewhat more involved than that enumerated by Sherman et al.[18] and reflects a personal bias in that I believe that phantom limb pain, like most pain problems, has two active components: the primary organic disorder and a secondary behavioral component. Unilateral treatment of either the organic or behavioral problem is usually predestined to fail. Thus, I pursue concurrently two differing avenues of evaluation and treatment, shown in algorithmic form in Table 21–2. The algorithm is divided into four levels: an initial evaluation phase and three levels of treatment for pain of increasing intensity (based on Sunderland's classification) and

TABLE 21–2.—ALGORITHM FOR EVALUATION AND
TREATMENT OF CHRONIC PHANTOM LIMB PAIN

Initial Patient Evaluation	History and physical examination Appropriate laboratory tests Behavioral assessment Medical-surgical consultations
LEVEL 1 Treatment	Diagnostic sympathetic, sensory nerve blocks Trigger point injections TENS Physical therapy
LEVEL 2 Treatment	Repetitive nerve blocks Nonnarcotic analgesics Anticonvulsants Membrane stabilizing drugs Beta-blockers
LEVEL 3 Treatment	Psychotropic medications L-tryptophan Maintenance narcotics Epidural narcotics Epidural stimulation

resistance to prior therapy. Each level is further subdivided into two parts, reflecting the dualistic—organic and behavioral—nature of pain.

The initial screening of the patient with phantom limb pain should entail a comprehensive and detailed review of both his physical and behavioral status. Consultations by an orthopedist, a neurologist, and a specialist in physical medicine are essential in order to exclude an otherwise treatable systemic disorder or pathologic lesion of the amputee's extremity. The patient's mental condition and level of functioning should be determined in consultation with a psychiatrist, and appropriate psychometric testing should be performed by a psychologist. Psychometric testing is somewhat controversial, since there is no consensus regarding the optimal psychometric test to assess patients with chronic pain. At the very minimum a Minnesota Multiphasic Personality Inventory (MMPI) should be administered. Based on information thus obtained during the preliminary evaluation phase, one can make several judgments: a possible etiology for the pain, an estimation of its severity, and the relative contribution of the behavioral component to the problem as a whole.

The initial treatment of a patient with phantom limb pain should endeavor to correct any underlying or predisposing conditions. Among the entities to be specifically pursued and excluded are the following: a neuroma or painful bone spur in the stump, an

ulcerated or redundant flap, occult osteomyelitis, a peripheral neuropathy, or vascular impairment of the distal extremity. In addition, all amputee patients with phantom limb pain should undergo a diagnostic sympathetic block to exclude a reflex dystrophy. This condition responds quite favorably to repeated local anesthetic blocks, chemical neurolysis, or surgical ablation.

In most instances neither a predisposing condition nor an autonomic dystrophy will be elicited. In these cases a gradual approach is required to control the pain. The initial treatment of phantom limb pain should make use of conservative modalities that do not reinforce chronic pain behavior. Physical therapy using massage, diathermy, vibratory, or percussion treatments is the prime modality that should be tried initially. Patients should also be prescribed a TENS unit for use at home. Although the results with TENS therapy have been highly variable, the simplicity, noninvasiveness, low cost, and lack of complications with TENS make the intervention particularly desirable and worth trying in all patients with phantom limb pain (Fig 21–2).

Pain of moderate intensity or pain unresponsive to prior therapy requires a more aggressive approach. Intermittent or continuous nerve blocks (epidural, brachial, femoral, sciatic) of the affected extremity or specific trigger point injections can often be quite beneficial and reduce the intensity of the pain. An intravenous regional block of the limb with guanethidine or the systemic administration of procaine likewise merits consideration. In contrast, drug therapy with narcotic analgesics (i.e., Darvon, codeine, pentazocine) should be avoided at this stage of treatment. The use of a nonnarcotic analgesic, however, may be indicated. Aspirin and acetaminophen have been the traditional drugs of choice as nonnarcotic analgesics. They are being superceded by more potent prostaglandin-inhibitory analgesics that have analgesic potency superior to codeine and are nonaddictive. Other classes of drugs (anticonvulsants, beta blockers) have been tried for phantom limb pain but seem to be ineffective.

Severe intractable pain presents a particularly troublesome dilemma. The syndrome of phantom limb pain is essentially benign in terms of its effects on life expectancy, but it can be totally debilitating to the patient. One must take into account this dichotomy when selecting a treatment for intense phantom limb pain. Many modalities have potentially serious sequelae and do not warrant the risk they impose when the probability of success is taken into consideration. Consequently, one should ap-

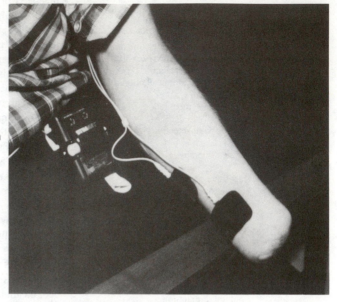

Fig 21–2.—Patient had phantom limb pain following traumatic injury and amputation of the wrist and hand. Pain was relieved with the use of transcutaneous electrical nerve stimulation.

proach this problem in a sanguine manner and attempt to secure the highest level of functioning by the patient, while recognizing that one is only palliating the pain, not ablating it. In selected patients maintenance therapy with a narcotic analgesic may be indicated. My preference is to prescribe oral methadone, 2.5–5 mg q6h, in combination with a tricyclic antidepressant. The psychotrophic drug seems to reduce the patient's narcotic requirement by modifying his perception of the pain. It must be emphasized that this regimen necessitates periodic assessment of the patient and his drug usage. With judicious supervision, however, this palliative approach can often facilitate the patient resuming a normal life-style.

It may be possible to abstain from systemic narcotics and yet achieve profound, sustained relief of the phantom limb pain. In a recent report, two patients were injected with meperidine into the lumbar epidural space.[19] The phantom limb pain was alleviated in both instances for a period of 2 months. Whether epidural narcotics will prove to be a superior method for the treatment of phantom limb pain remains to be seen.

As discussed earlier, the behavioral consequences of phantom limb pain must not be overlooked. They can result in considerable functional impairment that is far in excess of the deficit produced by the organic pathology. Just as one structures the treatment of phantom limb pain according to its severity, the same sequential approach should be utilized to deal with the behavioral component. The initial evaluation of the patient should include a comprehensive review of his behavioral status. Any functional or psychiatric abnormality noted during the screening evaluation should be dealt with in the standard fashion. It has been my observation that most recent amputees benefit from participation in a program of group therapy or supportive counseling. In more severe cases behavioral modification, hypnosis, or biofeedback is indicated. Patients with severe pain and an attendant behavioral problem merit individual psychotherapy and a course of antidepressant medication. This latter drug, as indicated earlier, is prescribed for both its antidepressant activity and as an adjuvant to methadone. It should not be forgotten that phantom limb pain can be highly deleterious to the patient's relationship with his family and his pursuit of an occupation. An evaluation by a medical social worker and occupational counselor can often be quite helpful. One may find that the actual focus of the problem resides in this domain, and with its resolution the pain becomes a more manageable secondary consideration.

TREATMENT OF ACUTE PHANTOM LIMB PAIN

Most authors have confined their remarks on the treatment of phantom limb pain to individuals in whom the syndrome has been present for an extended period of time—several months to years. It may be more efficacious to institute aggressive therapy at the first appearance of the phenomenon rather than in its chronic phase, in an effort to abort its development. This prophylactic approach has been used by Raj and myself on several occasions. In Figure 21–3 one can see an example of this approach. In another example, the most dramatic response was elicited in a teenager who mangled both legs in an accident involving a manure spreader. The patient sustained a severe injury and had bilateral above-knee amputations performed under general anesthesia. He awoke with marked pain that required large doses of narcotics for control. The phantom limb pain was similarly quite severe but unrelieved by narcotics. The patient perceived the severed legs as being grossly malformed and contorted. To manage the acute phantom pain, lumbar epidural analgesia was begun in the postoperative period by a continuous infusion of .25% bupivacaine, 10 ml/hr, using a volumetric infusion pump (Abbott Laboratories).[20] An upper sensory level of T8–9 was produced by this means and afforded total pain relief and allowed for discontinuance of the narcotics. Of prime interest, the perception of the phantom limb gradually changed over the first 2

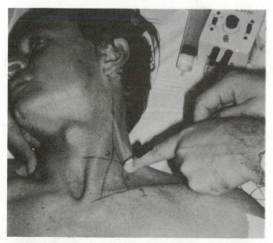

Fig 21–3.—A 32-year-old man had phantom limb pain of the left hand 1 day after surgery following traumatic amputation of the left upper arm. An interscalene block was done with the use of a nerve stimulator to relieve the pain in the early postoperative period. After prolonged bupivacaine infusion for 1 week, the phantom limb pain was relieved, although the phantom limb sensation remained for 3 months thereafter.

days of the epidural analgesia to a more benign image with the legs in a neutral posture at rest, similar to that described by Bromage and Melzack in volunteers administered epidural anesthesia.[21] The regional analgesia in this patient was continued for the ensuing 5 days. After discontinuation of the regional anesthesia, only minor pain reappeared at the surgical site. The favorable image of the phantom limb and the absence of pain have persisted in this individual.

At present there is very limited experience with the acute treatment of phantom limb pain. It has been a long-standing recommendation in the practice of anesthesiology that prospective amputees receive a regional anesthetic to minimize the incidence of phantom limb pain in the postoperative period. The validity of this practice has never been verified. The observation by Raj and myself that a prolonged regional block can alter the mental image of the phantom limb in the acute phase and the degree of pain in the chronic phase lends partial validity to this recommendation and warrants further study.

It is conceivable that this salutary result may give us an insight into the development of phantom limb pain. Several theories to date have been advanced and are differentiated primarily on whether they are central, peripheral, or mixed in site of action. The central site of action for phantom limb pain is currently the predominant theory. It was postulated by Head and Holmes in 1912,[22] who described a central body schema whose perceptual image could be altered by peripheral input. The theory has since been substantiated by Bromage and Melzack, based on their finding of a remarkably constant latent body schema in normal individuals given a regional block.[21] The occurrence of a traumatic amputation with its intense neuronal stimulation during and after the event most likely imparts a new body image. A regional block, by interrupting the peripheral input for sufficient periods of time, ablates this process and restores the preexisting latent body image, one that is devoid of pain and in which the amputated limb exists in a position of orthopedic rest.

Given the recalcitrance of chronic phantom limb pain to treatment, a prompt and vigorous intervention in the acute period appears to be indicated. Whether all prospective amputees should be administered a prolonged block remains to be seen. At the very least, however, those patients who develop phantom limb pain immediately after amputation should be considered.

CONCLUSION

Having reviewed the history, epidemiology, pathogenesis, and treatment of phantom limb pain, one is struck by the perversity of the syndrome and the fact that it persists as one of the more enigmatic problems in clinical medicine. The limited ability to deal with this disorder cannot be ascribed merely to a lack of interest, but rather to a more fundamental deficit in our knowledge regarding the neurophysiologic basis for phantom limb pain. Until the basic science aspects of this disorder are elucidated, it is doubtful that truly substantive progress will be made in its management.

REFERENCES

1. Sunderland S.: *Nerves and Nerve Injuries*. New York, Churchill Livingstone, 1978.
2. Melzack R.: Phantom limb pain. *Anesthesia* 35:409–419, 1971.
3. Mitchell S.W.: *Injuries of Nerves and Their Consequences*. London, Smith, Elder & Co., 1872.
4. Wilson R.R.: Neurologic mechanisms of pain: Modifications by neural blockade, in Cousins M.J., Bridenbaugh P.O. (eds.): *Neural Blockade*. Philadelphia, J.B. Lippincott Co., 1980, p. 576.
5. Miller R.D., Munger W.L., Powell P.E.: Chronic pain and local anesthetic neural blockade, in Cousins M.J., Bridenbaugh P.O. (eds.): *Neural Blockade*. Philadelphia, J.B. Lippincott Co., 1980, p. 627.
6. Browder E.J., Gallagher J.P.: Dorsal cardotomy for painful phantom limb. *Ann. Surg.* 128:456–469, 1948.
7. Cauty T.J., Bleck E.E.: Amputation stump pain. *IS Armed Forces Med. J.* 9:635, 1958.
8. Cronholm B.: Phantom limbs in amputees. *Acta Psychiatr. Scand.* 72(S):1–310, 1951.
9. Cwalt J.R., Randall G.C., Morris H.: The phantom limb. *Psychosom. Med.* 9:118–123, 1947.
10. Henderson W.R., Smyth G.E.: Phantom limbs. *J. Neurol. Neurosurg. Psychiatry* 11:88–112, 1948.
11. Hermann L.G., Gibbs E.W.: Phantom limb pain. *Am. J. Surg.* 67:168–180, 1945.
12. Little J.M., Petritsi-Jones D., Kerr C.: Vascular amputees: A study in disappointment. *Lancet* 27(1):793–795, 1974.
13. University of California: Progress Report to the Advisory Committee on Artificial Limbs. Berkeley, University of California Press, vol. 11, 1952.
14. Morgenstern F.S.: Chronic pain, in Hillow G. (ed.): *Modern Trends in Psychosomatic Medicine*. London, Butterworths, 1970.
15. Bailey A.A., Moersch F.P.: Phantom limb. *Can. Med. J.* 45:37–42, 1941.
16. Leriche R.: *The Surgery of Pain*. London, Balliere, Tindall & Cox, 1939.
17. Sherman R.A.: Published treatments of phantom limb pain. *Am. J. Phys. Med.* 59:232–242, 1979.
18. Sherman R.A., Sherman C.J., Gall N.G.: A survey of current phantom limb treatment in the United States. *Pain* 8:85–99, 1980.
19. Gorski D.W., Chinthagada M., Rao R.L.K., et al.: Epidural meperidine for phantom limb pain. *Reg. Anes.* 7(1):39–41, 1982.
20. Rosenblatt R.M., Raj P.P.: Experience with volumetric infusion pumps for continuous epidural analgesia. *Reg. Anaesth.* 4:3–5, 1979.
21. Bromage P.R., Melzack R.: Phantom limbs and the body schema. *Can. Anaesth. Soc. J.* 21:267–274, 1974.
22. Head H., Holmes G.: Sensory disturbances from cerebral lesions. *Brain* 34:102–254, 1912.

22 / Pain of Herpes Zoster and Postherpetic Neuralgia

GLORIA E. MAYNE, M.D.

MARK BROWN, M.D.

PATRICIA ARNOLD, B.S. Ed.

FRANK MOYA, M.D.

ACUTE HERPES ZOSTER

HERPES ZOSTER, commonly known as shingles, is an acute infectious viral disease which primarily affects the posterior spinal root ganglion of the spinal nerves. A single posterior spinal root ganglion or a small number of adjacent ones may be affected, usually on the same side. The corresponding ganglia of the cranial nerves may also be similarly affected. The causative virus, varicella zoster, belongs to the group of host-specific DNA viruses. This same virus produces chickenpox or varicella in children and young people.[1]

Herpes zoster most frequently occurs in adults who have previously had chickenpox. It is thought that the virus remains dormant in the dorsal root ganglia until, many years later, the virus is reactivated and produces herpes zoster. The fall in immunity which permits reactivation may be due to infection or malignancy, or it may occur in the iatrogenically immunosuppressed patient, but in the majority of cases there is no known reason.[1] Patients with herpes zoster occasionally give a history of recent contact with the virus exogenously, but it is rare that infection so develops. Indeed, the incidence of herpes zoster does not increase during seasonal chickenpox epidemics (Fig 22–1).[2]

It is thought that after the virus multiplies in the dorsal foot ganglion it is transported along the sensory nerves to the nerve endings, where the herpes zoster lesions are formed (Fig 22–2). In the immunocompetent patient, the disease is confined to a local distribution, as there is a rapid mobilization of defense mechanisms.[3] In 55% of cases infections occur in the area supplied by the thoracic spinal nerve, in 20% in the area supplied by the cervical nerves, in 15% in the area supplied by the lumbar and sacral nerves, and in 15% in the area supplied by the ophthalmic division of the trigeminal nerve.[2]

Although the posterior root ganglia of the spinal and cranial nerves are most commonly affected, any part of the entire CNS may be involved. For example, the anterior motor horn may be affected or the patient may develop myelitis or encephalomyelitis. In rare cases only the sympathetic ganglia are involved, resulting in a syndrome resembling reflex sympathetic dystrophy.

The location of the herpes zoster infection may be determined by the site of a primary inflammatory disease, malignancy, or trauma. Patients with neoplasms, especially lymphomas, are more susceptible to herpes zoster. It is estimated that as many as 25% of patients with Hodgkin's disease develop herpes zoster. This high incidence may be the result of recent irradiation of affected nodes, advanced disease, and possibly splenectomy.[2] Other associated diseases include meningitis, spinal cord tumors, anterior poliomyelitis, syringomyelia, tabes dorsalis, intoxications from arsenicals and carbon monoxide poisoning, and other malignant neoplasms such as those of breast, lung, or the gastrointestinal tract.[3] Patients undergoing cardiac, bone marrow, and renal transplants are also susceptible to herpes zoster infection.

345

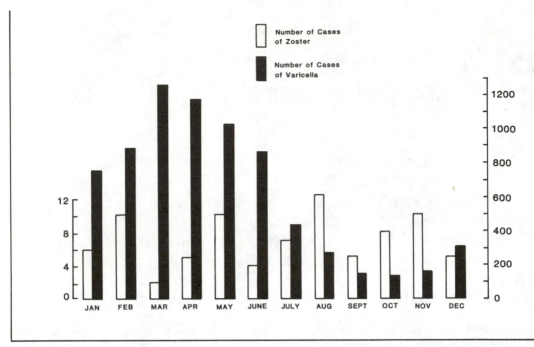

Fig 22–1.—Seasonal comparison of number of diagnosed cases of varicella or herpes zoster. The incidence of varicella is higher in the months of January to June, whereas the incidence of herpes zoster is higher in the months of August to November.

Males are affected more frequently than females. Herpes zoster is more common in debilitated individuals.

POSTHERPETIC NEURALGIA

Postherpetic neuralgia is a continuation of herpes zoster in older patients. Although spontaneous resolution of herpes zoster may be expected in most patients, a significant number experience intractable pain. Postherpetic neuralgia, which persists for months or years after the skin lesions have healed, occurs in about 10% of patients over 40 years of age and in 20%–50% of patients over 60 years of age.[7, 8] Some young patients may experience postherpetic neuralgia for 1 or 2 weeks after the herpes zoster lesions heal, although hypoesthesia or hyperesthesia may persist.

Postherpetic neuralgia is one of the most difficult problems encountered by physicians. Few other conditions create such agonizing pain and suffering for the patient. Many patients consider suicide as a means of relief from the torturous pain.

DIFFERENTIAL DIAGNOSIS

Acute Herpes Zoster

The diagnosis of herpes zoster is usually difficult to make in the pre-eruptive stage. Once the lesions appear, the clinical features are so typical that the diagnosis is easy to make. Prior to eruption, herpes zoster is often mistaken for other pain-causing conditions such as coronary disease, pleurisy, pleurodynia, cholecystitis, neural disease, appendicitis, peritonitis, and collapsed intervertebral disk. Occasionally, a localized herpes simplex infection along the distribution of a segmented nerve is confused with herpes zoster. Differentiation between the two herpes virus conditions can be made with virus isolation procedures in the laboratory.

To confirm the diagnosis of herpes zoster, virus can be isolated from the vesicular fluid, but not usually from pustules or crusting lesions, 7–8 days after eruption. Specific antigens can also be demonstrated in vesicular fluid and in the crusts of lesions by the use of a simple gel precipitin technique.

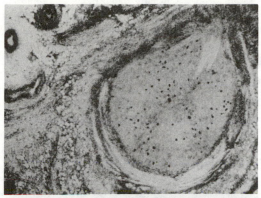

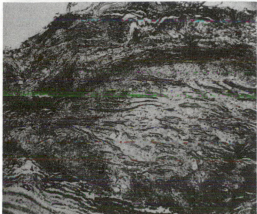

Fig 22–2.—Inflammatory reaction in the ganglion due to herpes zoster. *Top,* ganglion and satellite cells show intranuclear inclusions. *Bottom,* the ganglion is swollen and hemorrhagic.

Epithelial cells with eosinophilic intranuclear inclusions with multinucleated giant cells can be identified in material scraped from the base of a vesicular lesion. The white blood cell count is normal in uncomplicated herpes zoster. Mononuclear pleocytosis is present in the cerebrospinal fluid of patients with herpes zoster, particularly those with cranial nerve involvement.

Visceral pain can be differentiated from herpes zoster pain by a somatic sensory nerve block, which will not relieve visceral pain.

Postherpetic Neuralgia

Postherpetic neuralgia can also be confused with other problems, but the patient usually has a history of a previous unilateral skin eruption, and there may be residual scarring of the skin. Hyperesthesia, dysesthesia, and anesthesia may also be present in the affected area. Skin eruption may be minimal relative to that associated with herpes zoster so that few or even no scars are present with postherpetic neuralgia (zoster sine herpete). In these patients, the CNS was damaged by the original infection, resulting in a neuralgia that did not produce any scars in the skin. A rising zoster antibody titer in the acute stage confirms the zoster virus infection.[1]

SIGNS AND SYMPTOMS

Acute Herpes Zoster

Acute herpes zoster usually presents with pain which is localized to the dermatome distribution of one or more affected posterior root ganglia. The pain may be accompanied by fever and malaise. The pain is usually mild at first but may grow more severe over the succeeding few days. It can be dull, sharp, burning, aching, or shooting. Paresthesia is also commonly present. Skin lesions usually appear 4–5 days later, but they may appear immediately (Fig 22–3, Plate 3).

At first there is local redness and swelling, followed by the appearance of red papules which progress through vesicles, blebs, pustules, and then to the crusting stage over the succeeding 2–3 weeks (Fig 22–4, Plate 4; and Fig 22–14, A, Plate 8). The lesions are characteristically unilateral, running along the dermatome distribution in band form. In mild cases the skin lesions may not affect the whole dermatome, but sensory involvement of the whole dermatome is usually present. In severe cases larger blebs cover the whole dermatome and tend to coalesce. The whole area is likely to be extremely painful and is aggravated by contact or movement.

Occasionally, motor paralysis in the intercostal and abdominal muscles, arms, legs, and muscles innervated by cranial nerves may be associated with herpes zoster infection (Fig 22–5, Plate 5). These motor defects may be reversible over a period of years.

If the trigeminal (gasserian) ganglion is affected, there is usually pain in the nerve distribution, headache, weakness of the eyelid muscles, and occasionally Argyll Robertson pupil. Lesions may appear on the face, cornea, mouth, and tongue. Scarring and anesthesia of the cornea may occur. The first division of the trigeminal nerve is most often affected (Fig 22–6, Plate 5). If there is involvement of the geniculate ganglion, there may be Bell's palsy, vertigo, disorders of hearing, and lesions of the external ear and canal and anterior portion of the tongue (see Fig 22–6, Plate 5).

The crusts generally fall off by about the fifth week, leaving irregular pink scars. These scars are eventually hypopigmented and anesthetic. They form characteristic pocks which are usually surrounded by mottled pigmentation and which may last for years (Fig 22–7, Plate 6). The hyperesthesia and pain usually subside and disappear at about the same time the crusts fall off.

Postherpetic Neuralgia

In 10%–50% of patients with herpes zoster, pain and hyperesthesia persist after the lesions are healed. This condition, called postherpetic neuralgia, may improve slowly, but once it has been present for 6 months, complete spontaneous cure is unlikely.

The discomfort of postherpetic neuralgia is of two types: pain and dysesthesia. The persistent, intractable pain, which is constant and never varying, often has a feeling of heat. It is variously described as burning, shooting, twisting, lancinating, pressing, and gripping. A feeling of tightness may also be present. Relief is usually found in sleep. In chronic postherpetic neuralgia, the patient commonly suffers from hyperpathia, often associated with damage to a peripheral nerve, the spinothalamic tract, or the thalamus. It may be due to a reduction in the number and proportion of conducting nerve fibers.

Dysesthesia is often interpreted as pain. Uncomfortable, unpleasant sensations make the patient unable to bear the lightest contact with the skin. Some patients even cut holes in their clothing to eliminate the problem. A slight breath of wind can incite a paroxysm of pain. Curiously, most patients can tolerate firm pressure on the affected area but not light pressure, and some may wear especially tight clothing or keep their hands pressed over the painful region. Patients may complain of the sensation of worms under the skin or of ants crawling over the skin (formication).

MECHANISM OF PAIN: HISTOPATHOLOGY

Acute Herpes Zoster

Early lesions of herpes zoster are minute, unilocular vesicles involving the epidermis and corium. There is a ballooning degeneration of the involved epithelial cells, and intranuclear inclusion bodies are

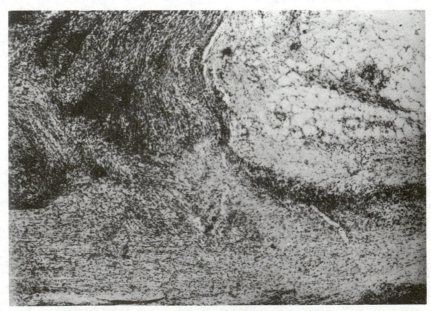

Fig 22–8.—The histopathologic appearance of dorsal root ganglion, showing edema and hemorrhage. There is round cell infiltration with neuronal destruction.

often present. Huge giant cells with multiple inclusions are often found in mature lesions. There may be necrosis and hemorrhages into the uppermost portion of the dermis if there is destruction of the germinal layer. The typical varicella vesicles are formed from serum that collects around the damaged cells. The fluid in the vesicle soon becomes cloudy from polymorphonuclear leukocytes, multinucleated giant cells, degenerated cells, and fibrin. A scab is formed when the fluid is absorbed.[4]

The dorsal root ganglion of the affected nerve is hemorrhagic and swollen. There is round cell infiltration and eventually neuronal destruction. Ganglion and satellite cells may have intranuclear inclusions (Fig 22–8). Maximum degeneration is seen in the posterior nerve root about 2 weeks after the dermal lesions first appear. Similar changes may be seen in the posterior column and sensory nerves (Fig 22–9). Rarely, the anterior horn may be involved, or a localized meningitis may also occur. Eventually the ganglion may be replaced by scar tissue.[7]

Postherpetic Neuralgia

Many theories have been proposed to explain the intractable nature of postherpetic neuralgia. Noxious impulses may become established in centrally located, closed, self-perpetuating loops, and progressive facilitation develops in these synapses. Eventually, pain that is entirely unaffected by surgical section of peripheral pathways occurs spontaneously. The possibility also exists that the infection involves higher pathways in the cord and brain than was formerly believed. If such is the case, the infection is outside the reach of extradural and intrathecal medication, and possibly beyond cordotomy.

The gate control theory might explain some of the features involved in the production and persistence of postherpetic neuraglia. It is postulated that pain is carried by small unmyelinated and small myelinated nerve fibers to the CNS, where the input is modified via pathways in larger myelineated nerve fibers. Nerve impulses are transmitted faster in large myelinated nerve fibers than in small unmyelinated nerve fibers. In acute herpes zoster, there is a tendency for proportionately more of the large fibers to be damaged and destroyed than the small fibers. Large fibers regenerate more slowly than small fibers, and their diameter after regeneration is usually smaller than originally. Hence, there is an increase in the percentage of smaller fibers relative to large fibers.[9]

According to the gate control theory, this is exactly the situation in which minimal small fiber stimulation might produce the sensation of pain because the normal modulation of large nerve fiber stimulation is no longer present. It is important to note that the older patient has fewer large fibers to

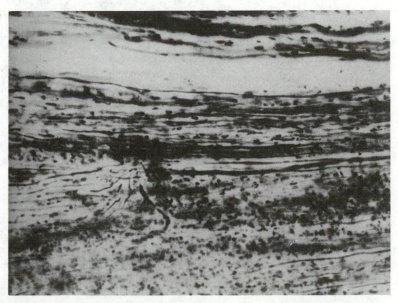

Fig 22–9.—Sensory nerve showing pleomorphism, edema, and hemorrhage due to neuritis caused by herpes zoster.

begin with and loses more through the herpes zoster infection. Therefore, the older patient is more likely to feel a greater degree of pain than the younger patient, and to be more susceptible to the intractable pain of postherpetic neuralgia.

MANAGEMENT

Acute Herpes Zoster

The goals of treatment of herpes zoster are early resolution of the acute problem and prevention of postherpetic neuralgia. The earlier treatment is started, the less likely it is that the disease will progress to postherpetic neuralgia. Because no treatment can reliably relieve the pain and discomfort of postherpetic neuralgia, it is essential for the physician to treat early in the disease course so as to reduce the incidence of this complication. Aggressive management is imperative in the older patient, who is at greater risk of developing postherpetic neuralgia.

Some physicians do not treat acute herpes zoster because they believe it will resolve spontaneously if left alone. They institute treatment only if postherpetic neuralgia develops. This is a great disservice to patients. Treatment during the early stages of acute herpes zoster is the best means of preventing needless pain and suffering.

No treatment mode is effective in all cases. Success is usually limited with any method. Many methods of management have been tried for acute herpes zoster and postherpetic neuralgia.

Drug Therapy

Various drugs that have been used in the treatment of the acute stage of herpes zoster are listed in Table 22–1 and described below.

ANTIVIRAL AGENTS.—The herpes zoster virus, like all viruses, is a parasite that takes over healthy cells and uses their DNA to reproduce itself. It is believed that if viral DNA synthesis can be slowed or inhibited, specific host immune systems might have more time to help control the viral infection. Some substances which grossly inhibit DNA synthesis and which were developed as possible anticancer drugs have been found to have a more significant antiviral activity than anticancer activity. Theoretically, these agents could either kill the virus or alter

TABLE 22–1.—DRUG
THERAPY FOR ACUTE
HERPES ZOSTER

Antiviral agents
  Cytosine arabinoside
  Adenine arabinoside
  Idoxuridine
  Acyclovir
  Thymidine analogues
  Interferon
  Zoster immune globulin
  Adenosine monophosphate
Analgesics
Anti-inflammatory agents
  Prednisone
Antidepressants and tranquilizers
  Amitriptyline and fluphenazine
  Doxepin
Other
  Vitamin B12
  B-complex vitamins
  L-Tryptophan

---

its replication. To be effective, the agents must be given before significant tissue damage occurs.

Such agents include cytosine arabinoside (Ara-C), adenine arabinoside (Ara-A), acyclovir, and idoxuridine. Experimental trials employing systemic administration of Ara-C in various dosage schedules have yielded conflicting results. These results ranged from apparent success in early uncontrolled studies to no benefit or apparent worsening of infection in controlled therapeutic trials.[7] Controlled studies of Ara-A in the treatment of herpes zoster in immunosuppressed patients have reported promising results. Therapy was most successful when administered early and to patients under 38 years of age or to those with reticuloendothelial malignancy. Cutaneous healing was accelerated, pain was acutely relieved, and the incidence of postherpetic neuralgia was low.[10]

Most recently, intravenous (IV) acyclovir has been found to be effective in acute herpes zoster infection by workers at the University of Minnesota. Acyclovir masquerades as one of the building blocks of the DNA needed by the herpes virus to reproduce itself. This stops the chain and the virus ceases to replicate.

Some ophthalmologists have used idoxuridine for treating herpes zoster lesions of the conjunctiva and cornea. Prompt treatment is necessary, and the best results are obtained when idoxuridine is used within 4–5 days of the onset of infection. The effects of idoxuridine are variable, and it will not prevent postherpetic neuralgia.[2] Varying concentrations of idoxuridine in dimethyl sulfoxide (DMSO) have been used in New Zealand in patients with herpes zoster, and it has been shown that pain decreased faster and that fewer vesicles developed after topical application. Early initiation of treatment is necessary.[11] Similar positive results have been reported from Denmark.[12]

Idoxuridine in 35%–40% DMSO has been used in Great Britain on herpes zoster skin lesions. It is reported that there is faster healing of lesions and a shorter duration of postherpetic neuralgia, and that late sequelae are uncommon. Success depends on early institution of treatment. DMSO decreases inflammation and edema and has a bacteriostatic action. DMSO is an extremely strong solvent that has not been approved by the FDA for this use.[2]

Thymidine analogues have been found to have some inhibitory effect on certain strains of varicella zoster virus.[13]

Interferon, which is produced by the body's immune system, appears to have a role in the control of disease. It seems to work most effectively in tandem with other components of the body's immune system. Large doses, however, can cause adverse side effects. It has been reported that interferon production in vesicle fluid of patients with disseminated herpes zoster is delayed in comparison with that of patients with localized disease.[7] When human leukocyte interferon has been administered, it has been shown to increase circulating interferon levels.[7] It may, therefore, be used in cases in which there is a risk of herpes zoster dissemination.

The development of a vaccine against herpes virus is currently underway. Scientists have isolated the gene which makes a major protein in the sheath or coat of the virus. It is hoped that with the introduction of a harmless part of the virus into the system, the body will produce antibodies against it. Testing is still in the preliminary stages.

Zoster immune globulin has been found to be ineffective in altering the clinical course of herpes zoster in immunocompromised adults. It is presently used, however, for the passive protection of susceptible leukemia patients who have been exposed to chickenpox. It is also recommended for use in any immunocompromised children at risk of chickenpox.[8, 14]

Adenosine monophosphate (My-B-Den) given intramuscularly (IM) has also been used in the treatment of acute herpes zoster.[15] The exact mechanism by which it provides certain therapeutic benefits is not understood. It may act by correcting underlying biochemical imbalances or defects at the cellular level. Beneficial effects may also occur as a result of the vasodilating effect of the drug and its ability to decrease tissue edema and inflammation.

We believe that the ultimate answer to the problem of herpes zoster and its sequela, postherpetic neuralgia, lies in antiviral therapy. An antiviral agent is needed that will safely and reliably kill the virus before there is neurologic damage.

Much investigative work must be done to find suitable antiviral agents against the varicella zoster virus. Other agents being studied as antiviral agents are isoprinine, ribavirin, and BUDA.

ANALGESICS.—Analgesics are an important adjunctive therapy to antidepressants. Analgesic drugs may be categorized as nonaddictive, moderately addictive, or strongly addictive.[16] Selecting the optimal agent for a specific patient involves consideration of a variety of factors, the most important of which are the quality, intensity, duration, and distribution of pain.

Nonnarcotic, nonaddictive drugs are useful for the control of mild pain. Acetylsalicylic acid (aspirin) and acetaminophen (Tylenol) are effective drugs with a low incidence of side effects. However, they are not effective in controlling severe pain.

Codeine, propoxyphene (Darvon), pentazocine (Talwin), and oxycodone (Percodan) are examples of moderately addictive drugs. The incidence of addiction is relatively low, except for Percodan, but dependence may occur with any of them. They are good analgesic agents, but they sometimes produce adverse side effects such as constipation.

When used properly, the strongly addictive narcotics are effective in the treatment of severe refractory pain. They provide relief to varying degrees. In acute herpes zoster infection, strong medication may be needed to control severe pain. Since the acute stage is short, strongly addictive drugs may be used for a limited period of time. In such cases, the narcotic is tapered off as treatment decreases the degree of pain. When pain is at a level which can be controlled by nonnarcotic drugs, the narcotics should be discontinued. (The assessment of the degree of pain is based on both objective and subjective findings as a means of preventing addiction.) Examples of strongly addictive drugs are morphine, hydromorphone (Dilaudid), and meperidine (Demerol).

Anti-inflammatory Agents

The effects of corticosteroid therapy on herpes zoster are still unclear, but reports are encouraging.

Gelfand reported dramatic relief of pain in less than 2 days in patients treated with oral cortisone.[17] Appleman obtained equally good pain relief in about the same time period with intradermal or IV corticotropin.[18] Elliot obtained excellent results after treating severely painful zoster with high doses of prednisone. The average duration of pain following early prednisone therapy was 3½ days, while pain lasted an average of 3½ weeks in untreated controls.[19] These studies, however, involved only a small number of patients and few or no controls. Eaglstein et al. found that oral corticosteroids did not shorten the course of the infection or affect pain during the first 2 weeks, but did shorten the duration of postherpetic neuralgia (Fig 22–10). Best results are obtained when treatment is started early in the course of the disease.[20] Inflammation and scarring are reduced with use of the anti-inflammatory agents. Despite uncertainty as to the effects of corticosteroid therapy on herpes zoster, corticosteroids have been extensively used to treat this infection.[2]

Steroids are usually used within the first 10 days and continued for as long as 3 weeks. Prednisone is usually the agent of choice. It may be given orally in doses of 60 mg/day the first week, 30 mg/day the second week, and 15 mg/day the third week.

Subcutaneous infiltration of steroids and a short- or long-acting local anesthetic has been used with encouraging results (see below). Skin lesions dry up and heal faster with this approach.

ANTIDEPRESSANTS AND TRANQUILIZERS.—Antidepressants are believed to have two clinical effects: they relieve pain and depression. Tricyclic drugs are known to block serotonin reuptake. They would, therefore, be expected to enhance the action of this neurotransmitter at synapses, and such enhancement produces analgesia in laboratory animals. One of the mechanisms active in the central pain states is that of some defect in the transmission system, the neuraxis, and specifically a deficit in serotonin.[21]

There is a strong consensus among clinical investigators that centrally active antidepressants deserve a trial in any patient in whom pain is not relieved, whether or not the patient appears depressed. Tricyclics and anxiolytics are commonly given together because, although depression is not common in acute herpes zoster, many patients experience anxiety along with severe pain. The most widely used combination is Elavil and Prolixin.

In addition to their antidepressant and analgesic properties, tricyclics are also sedative (for sleep regulation). Elavil and Sinequan may correct the sleep disturbances, frequent awakening, and early morning awakening that are common in severe chronic pain states.

Adverse side effects of the tricyclic antidepressants include hypotension or hypertension, tachycardia, arrhythmias, drowsiness, confusion, disorientation, dry mouth, blurred vision, increased intraocular pressure, urinary retention, and constipation.

OTHER DRUG THERAPIES.—It is thought that the host immune system is incompetent during the acute outbreak. At the very least, then, vitamins, minerals, and improved general nutrition may help improve the immunologic system or make available a missing element.

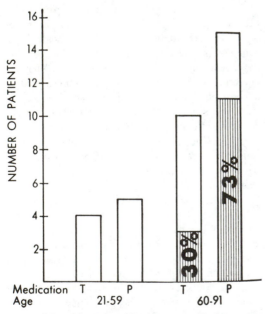

Fig 22–10.—Triamcinolone results in a significant decrease in the incidence of postherpetic neuralgia in elderly patients. (From Eaglstein W.H., Katz R., Brown J.A.: *JAMA* 211(10):1681–1683, 1970. Copyright 1970, American Medical Association; reproduced by permission.)

Nerve Blocks

LOCAL INFILTRATION.—In a large group of patients, Epstein injected 0.2% triamcinolone in normal saline subcutaneously in the areas of eruption and the sites of pain and itching. He obtained excellent results, which approached 100%, and the development of postherpetic neuralgia was reduced to 2%. This study suggests that subcutaneous injection of steroids and local anesthetics is an effective treatment for acute herpes zoster. No significant complications were recorded, the technique is simple and inexpensive, and the response to treatment is fairly predictable.[22, 23] Our own experience with this technique corroborates these results (Figs 22–11, 22–12, Plates 6 and 7).

SOMATIC NERVE BLOCKS.—Since nerve root involvement is suspected in acute herpes zoster, somatic nerve blocks have been used in its treatment. These blocks can include brachial plexus, paravertebral, intercostal, and sciatic blocks. Regrettably, they have been found to be of limited value in the acute phase and of no value in the postherpetic stage.

SYMPATHETIC NERVE BLOCKS.—As understanding of the pathology of herpes zoster developed, attention was directed toward the sympathetic ganglia. Sympathetic blocks have been performed to relieve the vasospasm thought to cause the pain and nerve damage. Evidence suggests that sympathetic blockade performed during the acute phase of herpes zoster can help the immediate pain problem, often dramatically. Of greater value, however, is the possibility that it can prevent the development of postherpetic neuralgia. Although the evidence for this is less clear, it is probably a worthwhile prophylactic measure that should be used as early as possible.[24]

Trigeminal herpes zoster has been treated with a bupivacaine block of the ipsilateral stellate ganglion in a small study. Dramatic and lasting relief of all dysesthesia was obtained in about 77% of patients; some discomfort and paresthesia of the affected area persisted for several weeks in about 22%. Pain recurred after initial relief in about 22%. Vesicular skin lesions dried more quickly than in untreated patients (Fig 22–13, Plate 7). Transient side effects included hoarseness, paresis of the ipsilateral arm, and paresis of the hemidiaphragm. The investigators were unable to draw any conclusions because of the informality of the study, but believe that these preliminary results justify further investigation.[25]

In one large study, more than 90% of patients with herpes zoster were treated successfully with one sympathetic block: the course of the disease showed definite improvement; pain disappeared or diminished within 15 minutes and lasted 20–45 minutes initially, with spontaneous diminution of pain

in 8 hours and complete relief in 24 hours; and blisters dried within 48 hours. Successfully blocked patients did not develop postherpetic neuralgia. Complete failure, in only a few patients, occurred when treatment was begun after the patient had been suffering for 10 days or longer and the disease had extended to a number of segments. A similar study reported complete recovery in 75% of patients after one block, while the rest responded to a second block 2 days later.[26]

Winnie has written that the incidence of success with sympathetic block depends on how soon after the onset of the disease the block is performed. If a sympathetic block is performed within the first 2–3 weeks, virtually 100% success is achieved. The success rate drops after that point. As postherpetic neuralgia supervenes, after 4–6 weeks, the success rate falls to about 20%. Thereafter, the incidence of success associated with sympathetic blocks decreases even more over the years.[27]

It is clear that if favorable results are to be obtained, it is absolutely necessary for patients to be treated in the first 2–3 weeks of the disease. This therapy also apparently prevents the disease from progressing to the postherpetic syndrome, at least in younger patients (Fig 22–14, Plate 8).

EPIDURAL BLOCKS.—Epidural blocks using local anesthetic have been successful in acute herpes zoster. The duration of the infection is shorter, the lesions dry faster, and pain is relieved. In patients with herpes zoster of 7 weeks' duration or less, Perkins and Hanlon, in a small series, achieved 70%–100% immediate relief, 90%–100% relief 24 hours after treatment, and 100% relief in a 1- to 5-month follow-up. There was no subsequent report of postherpetic neuralgia. Their studies suggested that local anesthetic alone was effective and that the inclusion of corticosteroids did not increase benefits.[28]

SPINAL BLOCKS.—Spinal blocks are not usually indicated because they are not as specific as epidural blocks. A patient who has had a laminectomy in the affected area would be an exception.

NEUROLYTIC BLOCKS.—Neurolytic blocks are not indicated in acute herpes zoster.

COMPLICATIONS.—Complications that may result from any nerve block procedure include pain, local hemorrhage, infection, soreness at the needle insertion site, sterile abscess (usually in the immunosuppressed patient), vertigo, and Cushing's syndrome.

Psychosocial Therapy

Since the acute phase of herpes zoster is short, psychosocial therapy is not mandatory. Patients with severe anxiety and fright may benefit from such a support program.

Other Therapies

Transcutaneous electrical nerve stimulation (TENS) is not usually used in the treatment of acute herpes zoster. Ice therapy is a counterirritation technique that is based on the gate control theory. It is sometimes used alone in the acute stage to cool the area. Acupuncture and hypnosis are not usually used in acute herpes zoster, as other, conventional methods are more appropriate. Surgery and neurosurgery are not indicated. The acute stage is self-limiting and does not call for such drastic measures.

Postherpetic Neuralgia

Drug Therapy

Drugs used in the treatment of postherpetic neuralgia are listed in Table 22–2. A threefold purpose governs the role of drug therapy in the patient with postherpetic neuralgia: (1) to provide analgesia for pain, (2) to reduce depression and anxiety, and (3) to decrease insomnia. Since a considerable degree of depression, anxiety, and insomnia accompanies all chronic pain syndromes, hypnotics, tranquilizers, antidepressants, and anticonvulsants have frequently been used as analgesic adjuvants in the management of postherpetic neuralgia. These include the barbiturates, flurazepam hydrochloride (Dalmane), rauwolfia alkaloids, phenothiazine derivatives, benzodiazepines (Valium, Librium), amphetamines, tricyclic antidepressants, diphenylhydantoin (Dilantin), and carbamazepine (Tegretol).

It is important to warn the patient of the potential

TABLE 22–2.—DRUG THERAPY
FOR POSTHERPETIC NEURALGIA

Analgesics
Antidepressants and tranquilizers
Anticonvulsants
    Diphenylhydantoin
    Carbamazepine
    Sodium valproate and amitriptyline

---

side effects of any drug. A patient who knows that certain unpleasant effects are to be expected is less likely to stop taking the prescribed medication. It is equally important for the physician to adopt a positive approach regarding the medication. On the average, 35% of patients benefit significantly from the placebo effect.[29] This can be used to advantage by enthusiastically describing the sought-after effects of each drug which, with time, may be obtained in some individuals. Patients are also less likely to stop taking their medication before it has had time to give the desired effect.

ANTIVIRAL AGENTS.—As a rule, antiviral agents are inappropriate in the treatment of postherpetic neuralgia. Exceptionally, they may be used to prevent the possible recurrence of herpes zoster infection in a susceptible patient. For example, the patient with Hodgkin's disease is predisposed to the development of recurrent herpes zoster. In this case, antiviral agents may be given prior to treatment of the primary disease (e.g., chemotherapy and radiation therapy), when reactivation of the virus is most likely.

ANALGESICS.—Analgesics may be required to control the severe intractable pain of postherpetic neuralgia. Narcotics should be used with extreme caution, if at all, because (1) they are addictive, (2) the problem is chronic, (3) patients are not usually terminally ill, (4) side effects such as nausea, loss of appetite, and constipation usually make these patients miserable, (5) there may be adverse drug interactions with antidepressants and other drugs, and (6) most important, adequate pain relief may be obtained with other drugs. The temporary, initial use of narcotics to relieve extreme pain may be necessary, however, until the patient begins to respond to therapy.

ANTIDEPRESSANTS AND TRANQUILIZERS.— Antidepressants and tranquilizers are frequently used in conjunction with analgesics. Some patients become depressed as a reaction to pain. The signs of depression may be subtle and missed. Lindsay found that as many as 90% of the patients whom he had seen were depressed. About 85% of these patients responded to the antidepressant drugs.

Tricyclic antidepressants are the most commonly used drugs and are the most effective single drugs used in the management of postherpetic neuralgia. Antidepressants may act at a higher level than the neurotransmitters, perhaps on pressure molecules in the hypothalamus or pituitary. This could explain why only some depressed patients fit the catecholamine hypothesis, which holds that a deficit of serotonin or norepinephrine is the cause of the problem. It could also be that both chronic pain and depression represent neurotransmitter deficiencies and that the antidepressants restore these. The drugs should be given in appropriate dose levels and several different drugs should be tried before it is concluded that there is no response.

Tricyclics and anxiolytics are commonly given together because many patients experience anxiety along with depression. This feeling may be caused by anticipation of painful spasms, social obligations which may exacerbate pain by increasing stress, fear of having a painful episode in public, or fear that the pain may never leave.

Many patients who did not obtain relief with tricyclics alone were benefited when a phenothiazine was added.[30] Phenothiazines may therefore have analgesic properties of their own. For lasting pain relief, treatment must be continued throughout life. Elavil, 50–75 mg/day, and Prolixin, 1 mg t.i.d. or q.i.d., are the usually recommended drugs.

As a last resort, Nathan obtained immediate and great relief in about one third of hospitalized patients who had not responded to any other therapy. A short course of high-dose chlorprothixene (Taractan), 50 mg every 6 hours for 5 days, was used. The prominent side effects of this high dose made hospitalization during the course of therapy necessary, and many patients stopped taking the medication because they were unable to tolerate the side effects. This treatment is recommended only if all other methods fail and if pain is severe, as pain often returned in a few weeks or months.[31]

ANTICONVULSANTS.—Anticonvulsants are sometimes useful when other medications have failed. Phenytoin (Dilantin), 100 mg t.i.d. or q.i.d., or carbamazepine (Tegretol), 500–1,000 mg/day in three to four divided doses, can be used to relieve sharp pain.[29, 32]

Raftery reported success with sodium valproate (Depakene), 200 mg b.i.d, and amitriptyline, 10–25 mg b.i.d. He characterized pain in four ways: stabbing or lancinating, burning, a dull ache, and hyperesthesia. If the stabbing component of pain continued, he increased the dosage of sodium valproate to 200 mg t.i.d. If the burning and hyperesthesia remained, he increased the dosage of amitriptyline. He found the dull ache component of pain to be most resistant to therapy. If it persisted, he infiltrated the scar with local anesthetic and steroids or started TENS.[33]

The side effects of anticonvulsants tend to limit their use. These effects include bone marrow depression, ataxia, diplopia, nystagmus, abnormal liver function tests, nausea, lymphadenopathy, confusion, and vertigo.[29]

Nerve Blocks

The pathogenesis of postherpetic pain is unknown. Autopsy studies have shown that the entire sensory pathway, including the brain and sympathetic ganglia, may be involved.[8] There appear to be multiple areas along this pathway which are capable of initiating pain. This provides a rationale for the various methods of treatment and an explanation of treatment failures.

Analgesic blocks can be used as prognostic, therapeutic, and prophylactic tools in managing pain. As prognostic tools, blocks help predict the effects of prolonged interruption of nerve pathways achieved by injection of neurolytic agents or surgery. By interrupting pain pathways, therapeutic blocks influence the autonomic response to noxious stimulation. They break the vicious cycle of the disease. Patients with severe intractable pain who are not suited to other treatment regiments gain relief with blocks with neurolytic agents (Fig 22–15, Plate 9).[34]

LOCAL INFILTRATION.—Epstein used subcutaneous infiltration of steroids and obtained relief in about 64% of his patients. He injected a 0.2% solution of triamcinolone in normal saline daily under all areas of pain, burning, or itching until the desired effect was obtained. Maximum benefit was achieved within the first 12 treatments.[22] In a comparison study, Tio et al. used subcutaneous infiltration of 0.25% bupivacaine and 0.2% triamcinolone alone or in conjunction with medication and sympathetic blockade. Overall results showed moderate to significant improvement in 70% of patients. They noted a difference in response to treatment in relation to the duration of symptoms: patients with symptoms of less than 1 year's duration responded markedly better (85% success) than patients with symptoms of more than 1 year's duration (55% success).[34]

These studies suggest that subcutaneous infiltration of steroids offers an effective treatment of postherpetic neuralgia. No significant complications were recorded; the technique is simple and inexpensive; the response to treatment is fairly predictable. Most important, it offers relief for some patients suffering from postherpetic neuralgia for many months.

SOMATIC NERVE BLOCK.—Because nerve root involvement is an obvious characteristic of postherpetic neuralgia, sensory nerve blocks were used in early attempts to relieve its pain. Results were limited and depended primarily on the duration of the blocks, although there were some reports of success in managing pain in the early stages of the disease. Coincidental spontaneous resolution may have been responsible. Nerve blocks are primarily used in postherpetic neuralgia for diagnosis and prognosis, especially as a prognostic block prior to neurolytic block. Steroids injected around the dorsal nerve have had unpredictable and limited success.

SYMPATHETIC NERVE BLOCK.—Thirty-four patients with postherpetic neuralgia for an average of 2 years, and ranging in age from 52 to 82 years, were treated with regional sympathetic blocks. Each patient received an average of three or four blocks. This treatment, however, seemed to be without any effect.[35]

Bonica reported good but temporary results with a series of paravertebral somatic sympathetic blocks using 0.2% procaine at 4-day intervals. The best results were obtained in patients with postherpetic neuralgia of less than 2 months' duration.[3]

EPIDURAL BLOCK.—Because epidural steroids have been successful in treating a variety of lumbosacral conditions, Forrest experimented with this technique on postherpetic neuralgia. In a well-controlled study, he obtained a progressive decrease in pain. Patients began to have relief after the first steroid injection. One month after the third steroid injection, 57% were pain-free. At 6 months, 86% were pain-free. Nine patients were followed up for 1 year, and of these, eight were completely pain-free. Forrest first identified the affected dorsal roots with segmental epidural injections of 0.5% bupivacaine, 2 ml in the lumbar and thoracic regions and 1 ml in the cervical area. This provided *complete* temporary relief. A series of three epidural steroid injections was then given 1 week apart. Methylprednisone, 80 mg, was used for single root involvement, 60 mg per root for two root involvement, and 40 mg per root for three root involvement, the total dose for any one visit not exceeding 120 mg. The patients were kept in a lateral position for 30 minutes and discharged 6 hours later. Complications included minor weight gain and a slight increase in resting blood pressure.[36] Other investigators using a

significantly different technique have not had much success with epidural injections.

NEUROLYTIC BLOCK.—Neurolytic blocks may be considered when other blocks have not given the patient significant relief. They should only be performed after a prognostic block has demonstrated that an effective block of the appropriate area can be achieved. Neurolytic agents are used in cases of prolonged destruction of nerves. These blocks include 50% ethyl alcohol in aqueous solution, absolute alcohol 95% concentration in aqueous solution, and 6% phenol. Ethyl alcohol causes a higher incidence of neuritis than phenol. This is primarily due to incomplete peripheral nerve block resulting from inaccurate needle placement or to spillage of the agent on somatic nerve fibers. The duration of effects may vary from days to years, but usually ranges from 2 to 6 months.

Ammonium compounds can also be used for peripheral nerve block. Pain relief is due to selective destruction of unmyelinated C fibers by the ammonium ion. A solution of 10% ammonium sulfate in 1% lidocaine or 15% ammonium chloride is used. The duration of effect ranges from 4 to 24 weeks. Neuritis does not occur with either ammonium sulfate or chloride. The most annoying side effect is numbness, which can be as bad as the pain for some patients.[16]

Psychosocial Therapy

It is especially important to treat the patient with postherpetic neuralgia as a whole patient, not just as an area of skin. The emotional stability of the patient is almost always affected by the disease, and the stresses involved for the patient and all members of the household require thoughtful management.

Severe depression is seen in more than 50% of these patients, and suicide is commonly considered by those with long-term intractable pain. Counseling by a psychologist or clinical social worker who is experienced in pain management is a valuable adjunct to drug therapy. Training the patient in stress management and relaxation techniques is important. Anxiety and stress can exacerbate and prolong the pain. By practicing relaxation techniques, the patient may be able to control the pain to some degree.

In some patients, the pain-tension-anxiety cycle can convert acute pain symptoms into a chronic condition. Very often, no matter what is done to treat these patients, the pain is not relieved unless the stress factors are also removed. Basically, two types of persons are susceptible to chronicity: the tense, hard-driving, conscientious perfectionist, and the dependent individual unable to cope with life while burdened with repressed anger and hostility. Pain-reinforcing behavior, such as moaning, grimacing, asking for medication, and remaining in bed, and the favorable consequences, such as attention, expressions of sympathy, and perhaps the occasion to manipulate others, may lead to chronic pain behavior, which eventually becomes independent of the original underlying pathology.

The most important guideline in preventing chronicity is complete honesty with the patient. The patient must be made aware of the relationship between psyche and pain, and must be relieved of the fear of organic disease. Once the patient can fully accept the emotional causes of pain, he or she can then learn to relieve the pain by controlling anxiety and tension.

Family and friends should be included in counseling sessions. They, too, must cope with the pain a loved one is experiencing. The counselor not only can ease their anxiety, but also can teach them how to provide effective emotional support to the patient during an extremely difficult period in his life. Concentrating on the special needs of the families may require extra effort on the part of the staff, but it should result in a greater number of patients who recover, with the physical and emotional well-being of the family intact.

Many patients are elderly and live alone and are unable to turn to family and friends to provide the assistance they need to perform routine daily tasks. The counselor should contact the appropriate social service agencies, which can provide transportation and other necessities such as prepared meals, grocery shopping, housework, and regular contact with the patient to check on his well-being.

Other Therapies

Since many patients continue to have residual pain of varying degrees that can be aggravating, they may require management with other techniques. The following techniques are used when all other modalities have failed (Table 22–3).

TENS.—TENS has been used in an attempt to relieve the intractable pain of postherpetic neuralgia. Winnie reported a success rate of only 20%, but relief was sufficient to permit a return to normal activity without analgesic therapy.[23]

TABLE 22–3.—OTHER THERAPIES
FOR POSTHERPETIC NEURALGIA

Transcutaneous electrical nerve stimulation
Cold therapies
    Ice
    Ethyl chloride
    Cryocautery with dry ice
Acupuncture
Hypnosis
Surgery and neurosurgery

Ice and other cold therapies.—Ice is applied to the skin for 2–3 minutes several times a day, starting with the least sensitive area and approaching the most sensitive area. A vibrator is then used in the same manner. This is used in conjunction with psychotropic drugs. Ethyl chloride or other cold spray is used by itself as treatment. Fluid is sprayed over the whole painful area, beginning at the upper area and working down. Evaporation cools the area. The procedure is repeated twice at 1-minute intervals until the skin is thoroughly cooled. When of value, treatments relieve the pain for varying lengths of time. When pain returns to nearly its former intensity, the treatment can be repeated. If the patient responds satisfactorily, pain is relieved by two or three periods of spraying per day.[1, 32] Good to excellent pain relief was maintained in about 66% of patients with refractory postherpetic pain using cyrocautery with a stick of solid carbon dioxide (dry ice) applied directly to the hyperesthetic skin areas of the cutaneous scars.[37]

Acupuncture.—In a preliminary report, significant pain relief was achieved in 40% of postherpetic neuralgia patients treated with acupuncture. Many of these patients had already had invasive or destructive procedures prior to acupuncture. Further investigation is underway.[38]

Hypnosis.—Hypnosis acts at the level of the cerebral cortex. Impulses are sent down from higher centers to close the neurophysiologic gate controlling pain. Pain relief through hypnosis is sometimes complete, but more often is not. Hypnotism is reported to be of help in patients with chronic unbearable pain which changed to bearable discomfort by breaking up patterns of suffering.

DMSO.—The therapeutic value of DMSO in postherpetic neuralgia is unknown. It may be tried as a benign last resort. Only states, however, have approved DMSO for medical use.

Surgery

Surgery is the treatment of last resort for severe intractable postherpetic pain. It is not always successful. More effective management techniques learned in recent years have further limited this option.

Surgery usually attacks the pain pathway in stages at progressively higher divisions. Because it was suspected that the origin of the pain lay in the scar and peripheral receptors, wide excision and skin grafting was tried. This was found to be ineffective and is rarely tried today.

Rhizotomy of the somatic afferents and sensory root ganglia has also had poor results. Investigators who have had some success recommend that ablation include several segments above and below the affected area. Sympathectomy has not been successful in treating postherpetic neuralgia.

Cordotomy has been used with good results. In most cases, however, the pain returns. Early recurrence has been blamed on failure to ablate all of the nerves in the pathway, which resume function once the swelling has decreased. Stereotactic ablation of the conducting paths in the thalamus and mesencephalon and frontal lobotomy have been used. These should only be tried in patients with a very short life expectancy who have not had success with any other methods. Dorsal root entry zone lesions (DREZ) have also been tried recently. It is too early to say if this procedure is superior to cordotomy.

Because of the finality of surgery and the unpredictable responses, many surgeons in recent years have taken advantage of the technological advances in other areas to replace destructive procedures. These include electronic stimulators used to block transmission of nerve impulses. An implantable electrode placed over the dorsal columns of the spinal cord has been tried with some success. More recently, deep brain stimulators which are patient-activated have been applied to the mesencephalic medial lemniscus.[39] The purpose is to block the pain-conducting systems and to stimulate endorphine secretion, the body's natural pain reliever. Good pain relief is found in 42% of postherpetic pain patients.

A THERAPEUTIC REGIMEN IN PRACTICE

Approximately 13% of the patients seen in the Pain Center servicing the greater Miami region have herpes zoster or postherpetic neuralgia. Since southern Florida is a popular retirement area, these patients are older, on average (72 years), than patients seen in many other practices. Because of our patient population, we have the widest experience in the nation in handling these patients. Depression is found in most of our herpetic patients. A history of drug abuse or surgery related to postherpetic neuralgia is rare.

Sympathetic nerve blocks and/or subcutaneous infiltration of a local anesthetic–steroid mixture are the preferred initial treatments. If the area affected with herpes zoster is very infected or if the acute attack is very severe, and if the duration of the pain is less than 2–3 months, then a series of two to three sympathetic nerve blocks is indicated. Otherwise a series of five to six subcutaneous infiltrations of triamcinolone and bupivacaine is carried out.

Subcutaneous infiltrations have three advantages: (1) less risk of complications, (2) results are as good, and (3) patient acceptability is greater. In the acute stage, treatments are usually given twice a week and then tapered to once a week.

Either sympathetic block or subcutaneous infiltration can be done within the first 2 months, depending on the physician's preference and the accessibility of the area. If the patient does not respond to the first approach, we quickly shift to a series of treatments with the other technique. However, if a good trial series of subcutaneous infiltration with triamcinolone and bupivacaine is done and there is no improvement, sympathetic blocks usually will not help, even within the initial 2-month period. On the other hand, if sympathetic nerve blocks are not beneficial during this period, subcutaneous infiltration of triamcinolone and bupivacaine following these blocks can be helpful in many patients.

Depending on the region of the body affected, stellate ganglion blocks, epidural sympathetic blocks, or paravertebral lumbar sympathetic blocks may be done. Stellate ganglion blocks require 10–15 cc of 0.25%–0.5% bupivacaine. Epidural sympathetic blocks require 4–6 cc of 0.25% bupivacaine, depending on the age, size, and physical status of the patient. If the single-needle lateral approach for paravertebral lumbar sympathetic block is chosen, approximately 20 cc of 0.35% bupivacaine is used.

Antidepressants with tranquilizers are sometimes added to the treatment regimen if the patient does not respond well to therapy. The type of medication chosen is based on the patient's medical history, the type of pain, and the presence of other problems (e.g., sleep disorders). Several different types are tried before it is decided that the therapy is ineffective. The combination most commonly used is Elavil, 25–50 mg orally at bedtime, with Prolixin, 1 mg orally twice a day. Sinequan, 25–50 mg orally at bedtime, can also be used. Triavil, Norpramin, and other antidepressants can also be tried.

L-Tryptophan, 1–3 gm/day, a food supplement, is used in combination with a multivitamin or B-complex. It returns normal function to the CNS by being available for the body to use in making serotonin, a neurotransmitter, as needed. L-Tryptophan supplementation reduces anxiety, depression, and pain sensitivity and improves sleep.

Analgesics are used as necessary. However, sometimes even the most potent narcotics are of little help to some patients. Strongly addictive narcotics are used only for refractory pain, and then tapered off as quickly as possible when other treatment methods begin to take effect. Narcotics usually can be eliminated in a short time. If the patient shows improvement but significant pain remains, efforts are made to replace the strong narcotic with a mild narcotic and mild analgesic combination.

Patients are advised to take the pain medication as soon as they need it—when the pain is distracting and before it becomes severe. The more severe pain becomes, the more medication is required to quell it.

Psychosocial counseling is routinely given to most patients, with family involvement when appropriate. Elderly patients need a lot of support. Appointments with the counselor are scheduled once a week or as needed.

If the above initial therapeutic methods do not work, or if residual pain still troubles the patient, alternative treatments are considered. These include TENS, ice therapy with psychotropic drugs, hypnosis (important for refractory pain), and adenosine monophosphate. Occasionally, acupuncture or vibrator therapy may be tried. Remarkable results have been unofficially reported in burns and other skin problems treated with Willard Water, a catalyst-altered water (immediate decrease in pain, redness, and itching, and prevention of scarring).[40] Its value in treating herpes zoster has not been tested, but it may be tried when all else fails. Rarely, patients have been referred for neurosurgery; the results were unsatisfactory.

Kindness, understanding, and patience are particularly important with these elderly patients. Many are separated from their families and live alone, so the traditional support roles are nonexistent. Senility, confusion, and pure fright are not uncommon.

The disease is carefully explained to each patient. An honest prognosis is given. While false hopes are not transmitted, a positive outlook is encouraged. Patients are asked to estimate their progress by using an assessment chart at each visit. They are encouraged to call any time they have a question or a problem; all calls are returned within a reasonable period.

RESULTS

Estimates of the degree of pain relief obtained are based primarily on the patient's self-evaluation. Family and staff ratings are also considered, based on modification of the patient's attitude, reduction in medication, and improvements in physical function. Occasional patients may claim no reduction in pain but will admit that they require less medication and that they are able to do things which the pain previously prohibited. When the duration of the acute herpes zoster is less than 2–3 weeks, complete or definite relief is obtained in nearly 90% of cases using the therapeutic regimen followed at our pain center. If the duration of the problem is less than 1 year, 80% of patients report complete or definite relief. If the duration is longer than 1 year, only 55% of patients have complete or significant relief. Overall results at the last visit showed 70% definite improvement. In follow-up calls (6 months to 2 years later), 70% of that group continued to report complete or definite improvement.

COMPLICATIONS

Acute Herpes Zoster

The most common complications of acute herpes zoster usually appear following the eruption of the rash. They include neuralgia, facial or oculomotor palsy, paralysis of motor nerves, myelitis, meningoencephalitis, postherpetic neuralgia, systemic lexicity (dissemination), fevers, chills, bacterial sepsis, and varicella pneumonia. Meningoencephalitis, which has its onset either during or 2–4 days after the rash appears, can also be a complication. Postherpetic neuralgia seems to occur more frequently and is more protracted in the immunosuppressed patient, especially in those with Hodgkin's disease or other lymphomas.

There is a marked increase in the incidence of infection in the immunosuppressed or immunoincompetent patient. The clinical course in these patients is exaggerated, acutely disabling in many cases, and it may become life-threatening if visceral involvement occurs with dissemination. In the early stages, the infection is similar to that in the immunocompetent patient. In the immunosuppressed patient, however, the infection often spreads segmentally to involve ipsilateral and, less frequently, contralateral dermatomes. It is usually associated with fever and increasing debilitation. While some of the old lesions are healing, new lesions continue to appear. Many patients develop dissemination and visceral involvement which may ultimately prove fatal.

Generally, patients in whom the disease remains localized for 4–6 days do not experience complications. The greatest morbidity and mortality usually occur with visceral involvement through dissemination, especially in patients over 40 years of age.

Systemic toxicity, fever, chills, and sometimes secondary bacterial sepsis occur. Varicella pneumonia, which is associated with a high mortality, occurs less frequently.

Postherpetic Neuralgia

Whereas primarily physical complications occur with acute herpes zoster, the complications of the postherpetic stage are primarily emotional. Depression is common and may include suicidal tendencies. Destruction of the patient's life-style (inability to work, breakup of the family, restricted mobility which prohibits former social activities) may be the tragic human consequence affecting the long-term pain patient.

Physical function may be further impaired, beyond that seen with the acute stage, because of the longer period of immobility.

PROGNOSIS

There is a close relationship between the duration of the neuralgia and therapeutic efficacy: prompt treatment shortens the progressive course of the disease and also decreases its severity. There appears to be a correlation between the age of the patient and the response to therapy. Patients less than 60 years old generally respond better to therapy and, even untreated, have a lower incidence of postherpetic neuralgia than patients older than 60. In addition, older patients do not respond as well as young patients to therapy and specifically to sympathetic

nerve blocks. For unknown reasons, postherpetic neuralgia lesions in the ophthalmic division of the trigeminal nerve are often the most difficult lesions to treat successfully. The psychological makeup of the individual patient is also important. Lastly, one fifth of patients with neoplasms who have had herpes zoster will experience at least one recurrence.[2]

TECHNIQUE OF HERPETIC NEURALGIA BLOCK BY SUBCUTANEOUS INFILTRATION

Careful questioning of the patient is necessary to determine which dermatomal areas are afflicted with intractable pain. The length and the area of the skin involved vary greatly from patient to patient. The area is marked with a skin-marking pen and is surgically prepared and draped.

A solution of 0.2% triamcinolone in 0.25% bupivacaine is freshly prepared under sterile conditions. Alternatively, a 50-ml solution is prepared containing 0.25% or 0.125% bupivacaine mixed with 16 mg of dexamethasone. With sterile technique observed, the solution is injected subcutaneously throughout the area of most intense pain (the marked area). A 22-gauge, 3.5- to 4-inch spinal needle is used to tunnel immediately below the dermal layer of the skin, and the solution is infiltrated along the previously drawn line. The volume of solution used with each treatment varies from 5 to 50 cc. The number of separate introductions of the needle ranges from 3 to 20. Following administration, local pressure is applied to reduce hemorrhage.

The total number of such treatments ranges from one to ten, the average being four to six injections. In acute herpes zoster, treatments are usually given two or three times weekly and tapered to one a week if the patient is responding well.

REFERENCES

1. Lipton S.: Post-herpetic neuralgia, in *Relief of Pain in Clinical Practice*. Oxford, England, Oxford Scientific Publications, 1979, pp. 231–248.
2. Raj P.P.: Herpes zoster: Preventing post-herpetic pain. *Consultant*, March 1981, pp. 71–76.
3. Bonica J.J.: Thoracic segmental and intercostal neuralgia, in Bonica J.J. (ed.): *The Management of Pain*. Philadelphia, Lea & Febiger, 1953, pp. 861–867.
4. Champlin R.E., Gale R.P.: The early complications of bone marrow transplantation. *Semin. Hematol.* 21(2):101–108, 1984.
5. Rubin R.H., Rolkoff-Rubin N.E.: Viral infection in

the renal transplant patient. *Proc. Eur. Dial. Transplant Assoc.* 19:513–526, 1983.

6. Preiksaitis J.K., Rosno S., Grumek C.: Infections due to herpes viruses in cardiac transplant recipients. Role of the donor heart and immunopressive therapy. *J. Infect. Dis.* 147(6):974–981, 1983.

7. Hines J.D., Nankervis G.A.: Herpes zoster infection. *Hosp. Med.* 8:72–84, 1977.

8. Frengly J.D.: Herpes zoster: A challenge in management. *Primary Care* 8(4):715–731, 1981.

9. Haas L.F.: Postherpetic neuralgia: Treatment and prevention. *Trans. Ophthalmol. Soc. NZ* 29:133–136, 1977.

10. Dolin R., Reichman R.C., Mazur M.H., et al.: Herpes zoster-varicella infections in immunosuppressed patients. *Ann. Intern. Med.* 89:375–388, 1978.

11. Burton W.J., Gould P.W., Hursthouse M.W., et al.: A multicentre trial of Zostrom (5 percent idoxuridine in dimethyl sulphoxide) in herpes zoster. *NZ Med. J.* 94:384–386, 1981.

12. Esmann V., Wildenhoff K.E.: Idoxuridine for herpes zoster, letter. *Lancet* 2:474, 1980.

13. Machida H., Kuninaka A., Yoshino H.: Inhibitory effects of antiherpesviral thymidine analogs against varicellazoster verus. *Antimicrob. Agents Chemother.* 21(2):358–361, 1982.

14. Gunby P.: Leukemia patients to be given varicella vaccine. *JAMA* 247(17):2340–2341, 1982.

15. Sklar H.S., Blue W.T., Alexander E.J.: Herpes zoster: The treatment and prevention of neuralgia with adenosine monophosphate. *JAMA* 253(10):1427–1430, 1985.

16. Tio R., Moya F., Usubiaga L.: Management of intractable pain, in Lichtiger M., Moya F. (eds.): *Introduction to the Practice of Anesthesia.* Hagerstown, Md., Harper & Row, 1978, pp. 485–501.

17. Gelfand M.L.: Treatment of herpes zoster with cortisone. *JAMA* 154:911–912, 1954.

18. Appleman D.H.: Treatment of herpes zoster with ACTH. *N. Engl. J. Med.* 253:693–695, 1955.

19. Elliot F.A.: Treatment of herpes zoster with high doses of prednisone. *Lancet* 2:610–611, 1964.

20. Eaglstein W.H., Katz R., Brown J.A.: The effects of early corticosteroid therapy on the skin eruption and pain of herpes zoster. *JAMA* 211(10):1681–1683, 1970.

21. Murphy T.: Drugs for chronic pain, in *Advances and Update in Pain Therapy.* Presented at the ASA Annual Meeting, Las Vegas, Oct. 25, 1982.

22. Epstein E.: Triamcinolone-procaine in the treatment of zoster and postzoster neuralgia. *Calif. Med.* 115(2): 6–10, 1971.

23. Epstein E.: Treatment of herpes zoster and postzoster neuralgia by subcutaneous injection of triamcinolone. *Int. J. Dermatol.* 20:65–68, 1981.

24. Murphy T.: Herpes zoster, in *Advances and Update in Pain Therapy.* ASA Annual Meeting, Oct. 25, 1982, p. 40.

25. Olson E.R., Ivy H.B.: Stellate block for trigeminal herpes zoster, letter. *Arch. Ophthalmol.* 98:1656, 1980.

26. Rosenak S.S.: Paravertebral block for the treatment of herpes zoster. *NY State J. Med.* 56:2684–2687, 1956.

27. Winnie A.P.: The patient with herpetic neuralgia, in Moya F., Gion H. (eds.): *Postgraduate Seminar in Anesthesiology,* program syllabus. Miami Beach, 1983, pp. 165–170.

28. Perkins H.M., Hanlon P.R.: Epidural injection of local anesthetic and steroids for relief of pain secondary to herpes zoster. *Arch. Surg.* 113:253–254, 1978.

29. Moore M.E.: Use of drugs in the management of chronic pain. *Anesthesiol. Rev.* 43:14–18, 1975.

30. Taub A.: Relief of postherpetic neuralgia with psychotropic drugs. *J. Neurosurg.* 39:235–239, 1973.

31. Nathan P.W.: Chlorprothixene (Taractan) in postherpetic neuralgia and other severe chronic pains. *Pain* 5:367–371, 1978.

32. Crue B.L. Jr., Todd E.M., Maline D.B.: Postherpetic neuralgia: Conservative treatment regimen, in Crue B.L. Jr. (ed.): *Pain Research and Treatment.* New York, Academic Press, 1975, pp. 289–292.

33. Raftery H.: The management of postherpetic pain using sodium valproate and amitriptyline. *J. Irish Med. Assoc.* 72(9):399–401, 1979.

34. Tio R., Moya F., Vorasaran S.: Treatments of postherpetic neuralgia. *Anesth. Sinica* 16(4):151–153, 1978.

35. Colding A.: The effect of regional sympathetic blocks in the treatment of herpes zoster. *Acta Anaesth. Scand.* 13:133–141, 1969.

36. Forrest J.B.: Management of chronic dorsal root pain with epidural steroid. *Can. Anaesth. Soc. J.* 25(3):218–225, 1978.

37. Suzuki H., Ogawa S., Nakagawa H., et al.: Cryocautery of sensitized skin areas for the relief of pain due to postherpetic neuralgia. *Pain* 9:355–362, 1980.

38. Lewith G.T., Field J.: Acupuncture and postherpetic neuralgia, letter. *Br. Med. J.* 281:622, 1980.

39. Mundinger F., Salamao J.F.: Deep brain stimulation in mesoencephalic lemniscus medialis for chronic pain. *Acta Neurochir. Suppl.* 30:245–258, 1980.

40. U.S. Congress, House, Subcommittee on Health and Long-Term Care, Select Committee on Aging: Catalyst altered water. 96th Cong., 2d sess., 1980, Comm. Pub. No. 96-240.

PART IV

Regional Pain

23 / Pain in the Head and Face

MATT J. LIKAVEC, M.D.
JAMES C. PHERO, D.M.D.
JOHN S. McDONALD, D.D.S., M.S.
GARY S. ROBINS, D.M.D.
JOHN STEINER, M.D.
P. PRITHVI RAJ, M.D.

Introduction

CHRONIC HEAD AND facial pain follows physiologic and behavioral changes initiated by its acute counterpart, as progression toward three or more months of continuous pain. These changes generally alter the intensity of pain in regional or distant regions and reinforce the patient's belief that a serious problem exists. Pain behavior develops during this period of reinforcement, which may be further aided by such complicating factors as drug dependence and financial gain. A progression from one pain syndrome to another is common in patients with chronic head and neck pain. A thorough assessment is necessary because therapeutic options vary for each syndrome.

A full history must be obtained and must include the following essential information: the onset of the pain, its initial presentation, pain characteristics, and therapeutic interventions, including the effect of such interventions. A complete physical examination with special emphasis on the head, neck and upper extremity anatomy should include likely tissues of pain origin and should search for physiologic changes due to chronicity. In an attempt to define which structures hurt and why they hurt, the physical examination should begin with the patient's

description of the site, patterns, and varying intensities of pain. The patient's perception of pain may be disproportional to the pathologic condition and may not correlate with the structures actually producing or modifying the pain. Evaluation of the CNS is important and should include somatic, sympathetic, and parasympathetic systems in the involved region. In general, somatic pain pathways for intracranial structures above the tentorium are in the trigeminal (V) nerve with the pain usually referred to the frontotemporal, parietal, or orbital regions of the skull. The pain pathways below the tentorium are contained in the glossopharyngeal (IX) nerve, the vagus (X) nerve, and the upper cervical sensory roots. Pain referred from these structures is usually felt in the occipital region of the skull. Postganglionic sympathetic fibers transverse the stellate or superior cervical ganglion, while postganglionic parasympathetic fibers traverse the oculomotor, facial, glossopharyngeal, and vagus nerves.

The workup incorporates radiographic evaluation of the involved areas, including x-ray films of the cervical spine, basal skull, sinuses, teeth, and temporomandibular joints. Basal skull views are obtained to check for integrity of the foramina. X-ray

365

films of the temporomandibular joints and carotid angiograms might be indicated, particularly if the pain is unilateral. Computerized tomograms and brain scans may be indicated when a focal neurologic disorder is suspected.

A thorough psychological evaluation is useful as many of these patients do suffer from depression and hysteria. The details of psychometric testing and diagnosis of various psychosomatic syndromes are found elsewhere in this book.

23A / Intracranial Pain

MATT J. LIKAVEC, M.D.

THE PAIN-SENSITIVE STRUCTURES in the head consist of (1) the skin, subcutaneous tissue, muscle, arteries, and the periosteum of the skull; (2) the structures around the eye, the ear, and the nasal cavities; (3) the intracranial venous sinuses and tributaries and large veins; (4) parts of the dura at the base of the brain and arteries within the dura mater and the pia-arachnoid; and (5) the trigeminal nerve, the glossopharyngeal nerve, the vagus nerve, and the first three cervical nerves.

The tumor cells, glial scar tissue, or abnormal blood vessels do not by themselves cause pain as they do not contain nociceptive nerve endings. The pain of intracranial disease is referred to specific areas based on the anatomical distribution of the nerves that innervate the head. The trigeminal, glossopharyngeal, vagal, and first three cervical nerves transmit pain from intracranial structures. The supratentorial anterior and middle fossa is innervated by the sensory nerve endings from the fifth cranial nerve. The posterior fossa and the infratentorial structures are innervated partly by cervical nerves C-1, C-2, and C-3, and partly by glossopharyngeal and vagal nerves.

In examination of the patient with intracranial pain, one must determine the innervation and the pain-sensitive structures it supplies. Based on the innervation and the pain-sensitive structures one can diagnose clinical syndromes that determine the anatomical location of the lesion. Figure 23A–1 shows the common distribution of headaches caused by intracranial and extracranial pathologies.

Processes in the supratentorial compartment often localize pain to the orbital or frontal region. A posterior fossa lesion often produces a headache in the occipital-nuchal region. Some posterior fossa tentorial lesions or lesions to the occipital area of the supratentorial fossa refer pain to the ear or to the back of the neck. Usually the location of the pain from a pathologically localized lesion is unilateral.[1–6]

However, this is not always the case.[1] One must realize that there are a number of clinical syndromes with recurrent headache in which no definable neuropathologic process is involved. The cephalic pains not often associated with a neuropathologic process include migraine, cluster headaches, tension headaches, psychiatric headaches, cough and exertion headaches, and occipital neuralgia. Also included in this category are the headaches associated with hypertension, carotidynia, Costen's syndrome, Toloso-Hunt syndrome, retropharyngeal neuralgia, postherpetic neuralgia, acrocyanotic headaches, and temporal arteritides.[4, 6, 7]

After completion of the history and physical examination, the diagnostic workup of a patient with a headache that does not follow classic syndromes begins with a CT scan of the head with and without contrast material. The CT scan should be directed not only toward the intracranial contents, but also through the orbits and the sinuses when indicated. In approximately 90% of patients, the CT scan will be diagnostic except when vascular pathology is suspected.

With vascular lesions (i.e., aneurysm, arteriovenous malformation, or some other vascular malformation), the CT scan will not be diagnostic unless the lesion reaches a certain critical size. In these circumstances a complete cerebrovascular radiographic workup is indicated. In the future, digital subtraction angiography may have a place.[8] If one is still left without an etiology on completion of the CT scan and the vascular workup, one should proceed to a lumbar puncture and appropriate x-ray studies. The new MRI scan is proving very helpful.

After completion of the workup, most of the causes of intracranial pain will have been assessed. Patients without descernible causes of intracranial pain require continued evaluation. With time, one may be able to discern a pathology that was not evident earlier.

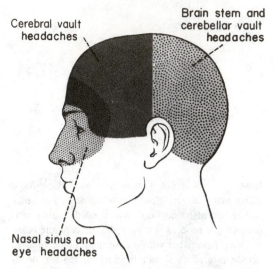

Cerebral vault
headaches

Brain stem and
cerebellar vault
headaches

Nasal sinus and
eye headaches

Fig 23A–1.—Common distribution of headache seen in patients with various pathologies affecting the intracranial structures, eye, and nasal sinuses. (From Guyton A.S. (ed.): *Textbook of Medical Physiology*, ed. 6. Philadelphia, W.B. Saunders Co., 1971. Reproduced by permission.)

HEADACHE AFTER HEAD TRAUMA

Immediately after significant head trauma, it is expected that the patient will have a headache. The reason is quite simple: direct irritation of the nerve endings involving the face, scalp, periosteum, or dura causes pain. This intracranial pain is usually self-evident and is treated with evaluation of the appropriate CNS lesions.

If a patient who is wide awake after an injury begins to complain bitterly of increasing intracranial pain, it can be an indication of a developing blood clot, with intracranial shifts and/or herniation. This complaint is best evaluated by a neurosurgeon.

Some patients after a head injury complain of constant or throbbing headaches, and on workup and evaluation an increased size of the ventricular system is noted. The intracranial pressure will be elevated slightly. Decompression of the increased intracranial pressure by drainage of the cerebrospinal fluid either by lumbar puncture or by shunting relieves the pressure and pain. This type of headache appears to be one that is associated with hydrocephalus and possibly plateau waves.[6, 9, 10]

There are some patients with traumatic headache which is delayed in onset. This has been described by a number of investigators as the postconcussive

syndrome.[11, 12] Fortunately, in the vast majority of cases the headache subsides over the next weeks to months. In a small number of patients the headache continues to persist. One should make sure that there is no significant intracranial pathology, and that the patient does not get addicted to drugs.

HEADACHE DUE TO VASCULAR PATHOLOGY

The true vascular headache can be one of three types. The first type of vascular headache is that of the acute hemorrhage. This could be either from an aneurysm or an arteriovenous malformation. A small jet of blood pours out into the subarachnoid space and stops abruptly. If it does not stop abruptly, the patient dies. When it does stop abruptly, the patient complains of the worst headache of his life.[6] With this history the diagnostic workup is not too difficult. A problem arises with histrionic patients who get a bad tension headache and complain of the worst headache of their lives. Unfortunately, these patients must undergo diagnostic workups, including CT scans and lumbar punctures, to rule out the possibility of subarachnoid hemorrhage. However, it is better to consider this course than to disregard the symptoms and miss the patient with a treatable subarachnoid hemorrhage.

The second type of vascular headache is that associated with a growing vascular lesion, e.g., an aneurysm or arteriovenous malformation. This is usually caused by irritation of the surrounding meninges or stretching of the blood vessels and is usually a throbbing, pounding type headache that is often localizable to one spot. Obviously, an aneurysm stretching or pushing on dura will cause a headache referred to a certain part of the head, depending on the innervation of the area of dura that is irritated.[12]

The third type of headache associated with vascular pathology is that of the vascular headache associated with thrombosis, e.g., intracranial thrombosis of the internal carotid artery. Patients complain bitterly of an aching or throbbing headache located behind the eyes.[13] Unfortunately, this symptom is neither pathognomonic nor diagnostic.

HEADACHE DUE TO TUMOR

The first type of tumor pain is the pain associated with an increased intracranial pressure. This can be either from hydrocephalus secondary to an obstructing lesion or because the mass reaches a critical size. The pain associated with hydrocephalus can be either occipital or bifrontal. It is sometimes described as intermittent, sometimes as constant in nature. The key is the consideration of intracranial pathology, not necessarily a specific description of the headache. The headache associated with the mass reaching the critical size can be due to two reasons: (1) intracranial shifts and the irritation of dura and meninges and the blood vessels that are compromised with the shift of the intracranial contents, and (2) possible dural irritation from the mass reaching such a size that it irritates the nerve endings and the dura in the blood vessels in the area. The last type of headache associated with tumor would be that of the diffuse headache. This really has no specific characteristic and seems to vary from patient to patient with intracranial tumor pathology. The patient may complain of constant headache, or it may be intermittent, throbbing, pounding, sharp, dull, aching, irritating, or lancinating. The key is that the headache is distinctly different from any other the patient has ever had. It is because of the different onset of the headache that one is led to the workup.[3, 4, 6, 12]

In summary, when one is thinking about intracranial pain, one is left with the following approach. First, the history and physical examination may yield clues to a clinical syndrome that is recognizable and at times treatable, or a neurologic deficit, or an anatomically localized area of irritation that would lead one to think of intracranial pathology. On completion of this step, if there is no answer available, neuroradiologic and continued diagnostic workup is indicated. Only if vascular pathology is suspected should angiography be performed because of its associated risks. If the diagnosis is still not evident, one should attempt various nonaddicting therapies, such as tricyclic antidepressants, beta blockers, biofeedback, TENS stimulation, muscle relaxants, and the judicious use of narcotics. With this approach, intracranial pathology can be ruled out and cranial pathology can be diagnosed and treated.

REFERENCES

1. Guttman L.: *Spinal Cord Injuries: Comprehensive Management and Research.* Oxford, England, Blackwell Scientific Publications, 1976.
2. Long D.M.: Pain of spinal origin, in Youmans J.R. (ed.): *Neurological Surgery.* Philadelphia, W.B. Saunders, 1982, vol. 6, pp. 3613–3626.
3. Yonas H., Jannetta P.J.: Neurinoma of the trigeminal root and atypical trigeminal neuralgia: Their commonality. *Neurosurgery* 6:273–277, 1980.
4. Long D.M.: Surgical therapy of chronic pain. *Neurosurgery* 6:317–328, 1980.
5. Ingram W.R.: *A Review of Anatomical Neurology.* Baltimore, University Park Press, 1976.
6. Hosobuchi Y., Adams J.E., Rutkin B.: Chronic thalamic stimulation for the control of facial anesthesia dolorosa. *Arch. Neurol.* 29:158–161, 1973.
7. Turnbull I.M., Shulman R., Woodhurst B.: Thalamic stimulation for neuropathic pain. *J. Neurosurg.* 52:486–493, 1980.
8. Richardson D.E.: Central gray stimulation for control of cancer pain, in Bonica J.J. Ventafuidda V.: *Advances in Pain Research and Therapy.* New York, Raven Press, 1979, vol. 2.
9. Meyerson B.A., Boethius J., Carlsson A.M.: Percutaneous central gray stimulation for cancer pain. *Appl. Neurophysiol.* 41:57–65, 1978.
10. Meyerson B.A., Boethius J., Carlsson A.M.: Alleviation of malignant pain by electrical stimulation in the periventricular-periaqueductal region: Pain relief as related to stimulation sites, in Liebakind J.C., Albe-Fessard D.G. (eds.): *World Congress on Pain,* ed. 2. New York, Raven Press, 1979, pp. 523–533.
11. Swanson S.E., Farhaat S.M.: Neurovascular decompression with selective partial rhizotomy of the trigeminal nerve for tic douloureux. *Surg. Neurol.* 18:3–6, 1982.
12. Freeman L.W., Heimburger R.F.: Surgical relief of pain in paraplegic patients. *Arch. Surg.* 55:433–440, 1947.
13. Tinsley M.: Compound injuries of the spinal cord. *J. Neurosurg.* 3:306–309, 1946.

23B / Common Headaches

JAMES C. PHERO, D.M.D.
JOHN S. McDONALD, D.D.S., M.S.
GARY S. ROBINS, D.M.D.

HEADACHE IS ONE of man's most common pain syndromes. It is estimated that every year at least 80% of the U.S. population experiences headaches.[1] More than 41 million Americans have headaches severe enough to make them seek medical care.

Headaches may be divided into three main groups based on the mechanism by which the pain is produced: vascular headaches, muscle contraction (tension) headaches, and traction/inflammatory headaches. Vascular headaches include headaches caused by the vasoactivity of the cerebral arteries, and particularly by vasodilation. Muscle contraction headaches are produced by persistent contraction of the muscles of the head, neck, and face. Traction and inflammatory headaches include all headaches secondary to organic disease of the skull and its components.

VASCULAR HEADACHE

Migraine

Migraine is a French word that means one-sided headache. Unfortunately, the term is often used generically by many clinicians to include a variety of headache types: chronic recurring headache, tension headache, and headaches for which no adequate etiology can be found. Such an approach to headache confuses all classifications to the extent that they become meaningless.

A classification of migraine that is descriptive as well as based on mechanisms comes from the Ad Hoc Committee on Classification of Headache of the National Institute of Neurological Diseases and Blindness.[2] According to this group, vascular headaches of the migrane type consist of recurrent attacks of headache varying in intensity, frequency, and duration. The attacks are commonly unilateral in onset and are usually associated with anorexia, nausea, and vomiting. In some patients attacks are preceded by sensory, motor, and mood disturbances. There may also be a familial history of migraine. These factors may vary by attack and in each patient.

Neither the headache nor the aura preceding it signals the true beginning of a migraine attack. The symptoms are the end point in a series of psychological changes brought about by the patient's reaction to a variety of stressful situations.

There are varied figures for the prevalence of migraine.[3] About 15% of the population under 40 years of age experiences migraine or one of its variants. Migraine usually begins at puberty. However, the first attack may occur between the ages of 5 and 30. Boys and girls are affected about equally,[4] but the disorder affects more women than men, reaching a 3:2 predominance in women by age 40. Approximately 70% of migraine patients have a family history of the disease. The personality of the migraine patient has been described as compulsive, overconscientious, and ambitious, with an outstanding performance with the emphasis on perfectionism.[5] Migraine can be subdivided into classic migraine, common migraine, and ophthalmoplegic or hemiplegic migraine.

Predisposing Causes for Migraine Attacks

Stress is the major initiating factor in migraine, although the migraine attack does not begin until the stress is over. Another important triggering factor is a rapid change in hormone levels. For example, in some women migraine attacks occur during ovulation or before menstruation,[6] and in hypoglycemic patients the attacks follow a rapid change in blood glucose levels, especially after oversleeping or fasting. Certain foods with a high content of tyramine or other vasoactive substances can trigger an attack (e.g., alcoholic drinks, chocolate, nuts, citrus juice, and aged cheese).[7-9] Physical stimuli such as bright sunlight or stuffy rooms can also precipitate migraine. The presence of illness may increase the frequency and severity of migraine attacks (e.g., depression, moderate or severe hypertension, collagen disorders, and febrile illness).

Drugs that can cause migraine include reserpine (a serotonin releaser), nitroglycerin, and antihypertensive drugs that can cause vasodilation.[10] Excessive amounts of ergotamine intake can cause rebound headaches. Estrogen commonly given to menopausal women or when used in oral contraceptives can worsen the migraine headaches in 50% of women.

Signs and Symptoms

Migraine attacks may be moderate, severe, or incapacitating and may occur once every 2 years or as frequently as three times a week.

Classic Migraine

An attack of classic migraine has three stages: the aura, the headache, and the postheadache period. The aura is an episode of focal neurologic symptoms that lasts 15–30 minutes and is usually premonitory, although in some patients these symptoms occur during the headache. The most common focal neurologic symptoms are visual disturbances, numbness or weakness on one side of the body, transient aphasia, thickness of speech, and vertigo. In addition to experiencing an aura, some patients have symptoms the day before an attack, such as abnormally increased hunger, nervousness, or other alterations of mood. At the onset of the attack, the migraine headache may be limited to half the head, but later it may spread to include the other side. The headache is frequently accompanied by nausea, photophobia, vomiting, diarrhea, vertigo, tremors, excessive perspiration, and chills (Fig 23B–1). During the postheadache phase the skull on the side of the attack remains tender and the patient may feel exhausted.

The neurologic symptoms of classic migraine may persist beyond the headache phase. When this occurs the headache is described as "complicated" migraine.[13] It is thought that migrainous manifesta-

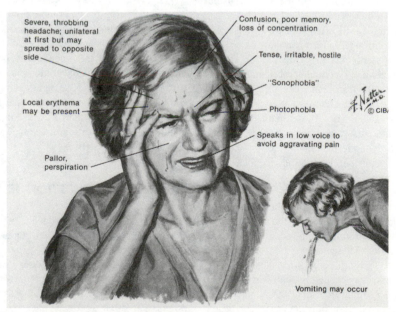

Severe, throbbing headache; unilateral at first but may spread to opposite side

Local erythema may be present

Pallor, perspiration

Confusion, poor memory, loss of concentration

Tense, irritable, hostile

"Sonophobia"

Photophobia

Speaks in low voice to avoid aggravating pain

Vomiting may occur

Fig 23B–1.—Common clinical manifestations of migraine attack. (© Copyright 1981, CIBA Pharmaceutical Company, Division of CIBA-GEIGY Corporation. Reprinted with permission from *Clinical Symposia,* illustrated by Frank H. Netter, M.D. All rights reserved.)

tions may imitate cerebrovascular disease.[14] However, the majority of patients in whom complicated migraine occurs are young and have a well-established history of migraine.

Common Migraine

In common migraine, the vasoconstrictive phase is not severe enough to produce an aura of focal neurologic deficits. In between typical attacks, patients with either form of migraine may also have "migraine equivalents"—episodes of focal neurologic disturbances, vomiting, or abdominal pain that occur without any headache.

Ophthalmoplegic and Hemiplegic Migraines

Ophthalmoplegic and hemiplegic migraines tend to be complicated forms of migraine.[11] The usual disturbances of ophthalmoplegic migraine (e.g., paralysis of the oculomotor nerve) may last for weeks. This causes extraocular paralysis, ptosis, ocular muscle weakness, and pupillary changes. Because these symptoms occur on the same side as the headache, this type of migraine may resemble the symptoms of carotid aneurysm. Angiography is a useful diagnostic aid in these cases.

Hemiplegic migraine often causes aphasia and confusion in addition to sudden hemiparesis or hemiplegia. These symptoms may precede or accompany an ipsilateral or contralateral headache and usually last less than an hour. The fact that hemiplegic migraine is often familial may help in establishing the diagnosis. These patients should have a computerized tomography (CT) scan with contrast and a dynamic radionuclide brain scan. In patients with persistent neurologic sequelae from complicated migraines, CT scan may show small infarcts.

In basilar artery migraine, the preheadache phase reflects circulatory disturbances of the basilar artery in the brain stem and in thalamic, occipital, and cerebellar regions.[12] These areas are supplied by branches of the vertebrobasilar arterial system. The prodromal period may include visual loss and brain stem symptoms ranging from paresthesias to vertigo and ataxia. Severe throbbing occipital pain and vomiting follow, with some patients losing consciousness for a brief period.

Cluster Headache

Attacks due to cluster headache generally occur at night. They are generally brief (4 hours or less), but occur every 24 hours during the cluster period. The clusters usually occur for several weeks or months during the spring and fall and then disappear for 6–12 months. In some patients attacks last continuously for years. Most cluster headaches occur in persons aged 20–30 years, and most (90%) occur in males. In more than 65% of patients with cluster headaches, the facial thermogram reveals multiple spotted areas of dense coolness in the ipsilateral supraorbital region. These areas are not found in other forms of vascular headaches.[15]

Predisposing Causes

Cluster headaches are most often brought on by consumption of alcoholic beverages. An injection of histamine or the administration of nitroglycerin can also trigger a cluster headache.

Signs and Symptoms

The cluster headache is characterized by an excruciating boring pain located behind or around one eye and spreading over the affected side. Some patients have described this type of headache as a knife cutting into their head. The pain is of such intensity that patients have attempted suicide during periods of attacks. Associated symptoms include conjunctival injection, tearing, nasal congestion, rhinorrhea, partial Horner's syndrome, and sweating or flushing on the portion of the face where the pain is prominent (Fig 23B–2).

MUSCLE CONTRACTION HEADACHES

Muscle contraction headache is a generalized, steady, nonpulsatile headache often accompanied by a sensation of tightness in the suboccipital regions bilaterally. Well-defined tender muscle trigger points may be noted on palpation of the diffusely aching muscle. Pressure on these tender trigger points will often aggravate the headache pain and may cause spread or referral of pain to other areas of the head (Fig 23B–3).

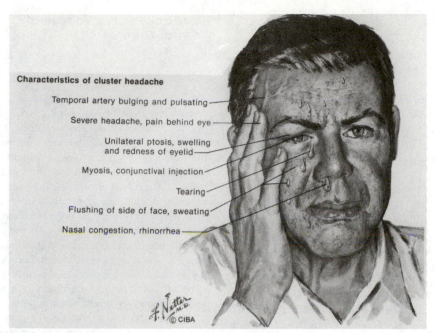

Fig 23B–2.—Common clinical manifestations of cluster headache. (© Copyright 1981, CIBA Pharmaceutical Company, Division of CIBA-GEIGY Corporation. Reprinted with permission from *Clinical Symposia,* illustrated by Frank H. Netter, M.D. All rights reserved.)

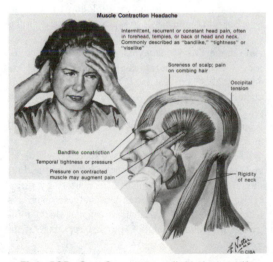

Fig 23B–3.—Common clinical manifestations of muscle contraction headache. (© Copyright 1981, CIBA Pharmaceutical Company, Division of CIBA-GEIGY Corporation. Reprinted with permission from *Clinical Symposia,* illustrated by Frank H. Netter, M.D. All rights reserved.)

Predisposing Causes

Emotional factors may play a primary role in the development of muscle contraction headaches. No single contributory factor has been implicated. Multiple factors, including anxiety, stress, fatigue, depression, repressed hostility, emotional conflicts, unresolved dependency, and psychosexual conflicts, may cause muscle contraction headaches.

Markovich[16] reported that 90% of all headaches are muscle contraction in origin and are precipitated by anxiety, depression, or cervico-occipital neuralgia. He proposes that when the head in homo sapiens changed its position from the quadruped to the erect posture, the relationship between the cervical spine and the head also changed. This produced undue strain on neural structures exiting from the cervical spine at that level.

Mechanism of Pain

Muscle contraction headaches are perpetuated by the "vicious cycle" generated by the abnormal and painful contraction of the cervico-nuchal muscles, mainly the trapezius. The localized muscle ischemia produces chronic muscle spasm. This may trap the greater and lesser occipital nerves as they travel through the bulk of the muscle, ascending into the back of the head. They innervate the posterior scalp region, the temporal areas, and the lobes of the ears, sending terminal branches into the angle of the jaw, the back of the eye, and the vertex of the head.

Occipital Headache

Occipital neuralgia is a chronic recurrent headache pain that is usually bilateral. It is characterized by a long-lasting, recurrent type of pain, the intensity of which may vary from minimal to severe in nature. It is regionalized in the occipital region but may extend to the neck and over the head to the frontotemporal region. Sometimes it may involve the eyes. There is an associated decreased range of motion, stiffness of the muscles of the neck, and tender trigger points over the affected musculoskeletal areas.

A much less common form of occipital headache is due to inflammation, injury, or pressure on the occipital nerves, upper cervical spinal roots, dorsal horn, or dorsal root ganglia. It is described as a long-lasting, sustained, nonthrobbing ache of moderate intensity. It is always associated with muscle contraction and tenderness, which make it difficult to separate from muscle contraction headache. Its characteristic feature is paresthesia or algesia of the tissues of the scalp and the skin of the neck.

TRACTION AND INFLAMMATORY HEADACHE

This type of headache is intracranial in origin and is most often produced by inflammation or traction leading to displacement or distention of multiple pain-sensitive structures of the head. Most often displacement is the result of traction. This may be caused by cerebrovascular disease, brain tumor, changes in intracranial pressure, infections, or inflammation. Conditions related to cerebrovascular disease include stroke, hypertension, aneurysm hemorrhage, and arteriovenous malformation. Headaches related to inflammatory processes may be due to meningitis, intracranial arteritis, and phlebitis. This is described in chapter 23A.

Headaches of Extracranial Arterial Origin

Temporal Arteritis

Headache caused by temporal arteritis (giant cell arteritis, cranial arteritis) is described as intense, deep, aching, throbbing, burning, and persistent.[17] The headache is worse when the patient lies down and is diminished when the patient is in an upright position. There is hyperalgesia of the scalp, and the distended arteries are extremely tender. Some patients may experience pain on mastication. There is often pain in the teeth, ear, jaw, zygoma, and nuchal and occipital regions. The presenting complaint may be ocular symptoms. Of importance to the practitioner is that temporal arteritis may progress to partial or complete loss of vision in more than a third of patients. If loss of vision is threatened, there is an urgent need for immediate treatment. Temporal arteritis affects women twice as frequently as men, occurs around age 55, and is associated with polymyalgia rheumatica in about 25% of cases.[18]

Cellulitis occurs over the swollen nodular artery, accompanied by photophobia, diplopia, transient or permanent blindness, low-grade fever, chills, weight loss, anorexia, profuse sweating, malaise, and fatigue. Mild leukocytosis is present. The erythrocyte sedimentation rate is elevated. Histologic examination of an involved artery reveals arteritis characterized by intimal hyperplasia and destruction plus fragmentation of the internal elastic membrane. A granulomatous inflammatory reaction involves all arterial coats.

Therapeutic management is directed toward decreasing the inflammation by steroid therapy and removing the affected segment of the artery by surgical endarterectomy. Appropriate analgesics are also recommended along with nerve blocks (local infiltration or stellate ganglion blocks) for acute management of pain.

Carotidynia Syndrome

Carotidynia refers to pain that arises from either or both extracranial carotid arteries and which may radiate to the ipsilateral side of the face and ear. At times, head and facial discomfort may be the primary manifestation of carotidynia. Although the pharynx may exhibit slight hyperemia, the exudative changes of bacterial infection are absent. Regional lymph nodes are not enlarged. Most patients complain of sore throat, which may be erroneously treated with antibiotics.

Dilation, distention, or displacement of a segment of the artery stimulates pain-sensitive receptors in the adventitia. Head movement, swallowing, chewing, coughing, yawning, and sneezing may elicit the pain. The diagnosis is established by applying digital pressure on the involved carotid segment with slight posterior displacement. This pressure elicits the pain pattern of a spontaneous attack. The specific etiology is obscure, but a viral origin appears likely.

Initial treatment is conservative and consists of reassuring the patient and prescribing a soft diet and mild analgesics. Intractable cases have been treated surgically by interruption of the cervical sympathetic fibers and excision of the carotid sheath.

MANAGEMENT AND PREVENTION OF HEADACHES

As with other syndromes of chronic pain, the treatment is multifaceted. Proper adjustment of medication and dosing intervals helps to break the patient's pain cycle. This can be done with a combination of a nonsteroidal anti-inflammatory agent such as ibuprofen and a muscle relaxant such as methocarbamol. The tricyclic antidepressants, such as amitriptyline or doxepin, may be useful to decrease the patient's pain and to alleviate inadequate sleep. Beta blockers such as propranolol have proved useful in some cases.

Appropriate myoneural blocks are of both diagnostic and therapeutic value (Fig 23B–4). They break the sustained muscle contraction, relieving the muscle tension. This allows increased blood flow to the neuromuscular structures, helping them to maintain the muscle relaxation.

Physical therapy is essential and includes range of motion exercises, muscle balance, strengthening exercises, spray-and-stretch procedures, manual traction, and ultrasound with electrical stimulation. Although physical therapy and transcutaneous electrical nerve stimulation (TENS) play an adjunctive role in the initial phase of treatment, they help decrease the need for medications and/or myoneural blocks.

Relaxation therapy, hypnosis, and biofeedback

may help decrease the stress factor. Surgical ablation of the occipital nerves should be avoided, as it is rarely curative and may produce a denervation dysesthesia.

Drugs in the Management of Vascular Headaches

Vascular headaches of the migraine type are related to changes in the caliber of vessels supplying the meninges and brain. The prodromal period is accompanied by vasoconstriction, which changes to vasodilation with the onset of headache. With the release of histamine from the wall of the vessel, the vessel wall develops edema, which results in prolonged vasodilation. Therapy for patients with vascular migraine headaches is directed toward producing vasoconstriction in the affected vessels.

Ergot Derivatives

Ergot is produced by certain parasitic fungi that grow on rye and other grains. Stole in 1918 succeeded in isolating the active alkaloid constituent of ergot, ergotamine, which was found to have predictable effects in the management of migraine.

The ergot derivatives may be used in the management of acute migraine attacks. The typical adult dose is 1 mg of ergot immediately at the onset of the headache and 1 mg every 30 minutes thereafter, to a maximum of 6 mg of ergot per attack. Ergot is often found compounded with other "headache relievers." The most common combination is ergot and caffeine. Caffeine is a cerebral vasoconstrictor that reduces cerebral blood flow. It has a synergistic effect when combined with ergot. Belladonna alkaloids are also compounded with ergot to provide relief in those individuals suffering from migraine-induced nausea and vomiting. When severe nausea and vomiting prevent the oral ingestion of medication, ergot preparations are available as rectal suppositories and nasal sprays.

Drugs for Prevention of Migraine

Preventative treatment of migraine may be considered in patients with a high frequency of attacks, contraindications to common abortive drugs, poor response to ergotamines, predictable attack occur-

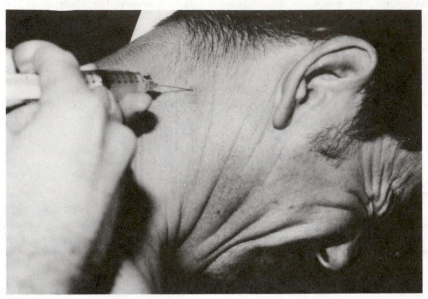

Fig 23B—4.—A 35-year-old man involved in a motor vehicle accident had neck and back injuries and chronic muscle contraction tension headaches that began shortly after the accident and still persisted 15 years later. Headaches were often accompanied by severe nausea and vomiting, for which the patient was sometimes hospitalized. Myoneural junction blocks and physical therapy effectively relieved the headache pain for long periods. However, the best relief was subsequently afforded by a series of IV 2-chloroprocaine infusions.

rence, and repeated morning migraine.[19,20] Several agents are available. Patients can benefit from a sequential implementation of prophylactic drugs.[21]

β Blocking Agents for Prophylaxis of Migraine

The exact mechanism of the migraine attack is unknown. The attack is mediated by vasodilation in the extracerebral circulation. Dilation of these peripheral arteries can occur in response to adrenal mechanisms and is mediated by β_2 receptors in the vessel wall. On a theoretical basis, β-adrenergic blocking agents could prevent dilation of these vessels.

β-adrenergic receptors are located in the regions supplied by the external and internal carotid arteries. β blockers may serve to abolish vasodilation in these regions during the headache phase of migraine.

β blockers also inhibit reuptake of serotonin by the platelets. Levels of serotonin increase before an attack of migraine and fall to low levels during the headache phase. The use of β blockers may serve to diminish the preheadache rise in serotonin, leading to a reduction in the frequency and severity of headaches.

PROPRANOLOL.—Propranolol should be prescribed judiciously and with caution. Clinically, the patient should be informed to watch for dizziness, lethargy, depression, nausea, diarrhea, muscle aching, and asthmatic wheezing. The serious and significant toxic effects of propranolol are congestive heart failure, hypotension, bradycardia, bronchiolar constriction, and intensified hypoglycemic response in diabetic patients.

The initial starting dose is 80 mg/day orally in divided doses. The usual effective dose range is 160–240 mg/day. The dosage should be increased gradually to achieve optimum migraine prophylaxis. Propranolol therapy should be discontinued in 6 weeks if satisfactory results have not been obtained. It is suggested that when decreasing or stopping this drug, the decrease should be done gradually over a period of 2 weeks.

NADOLOL.—Nadolol is the only other β blocker that currently appears useful in the treatment of migraine. The side effects of this drug are similar to those of propranolol. In addition, chronic pain patients receiving nadolol should be observed for increasing depression, which can be a side effect of this drug.

Initial adult oral dose of nadolol is 40 mg/day for migraine prevention and management. This dose may be gradually increased. It is usually not necessary to exceed 160 mg/day. If after 6 weeks the response is not satisfactory, the drug should be gradually stopped.

Methysergide

Methysergide inhibits the effects of serotonin, a substance which appears to mediate vascular headaches. Methysergide is used for preventing or reducing the intensity and frequency of vascular headaches. The usual adult dose is 4–8 mg/day. If after a 3-week trial period efficacy has not been demonstrated, the drug should be discontinued. Continuous administration should not exceed 6 months. There must be a drug-free interval of 3–4 weeks after each 6-month course of treatment, as retroperitoneal fibrosis, pleuropulmonary fibrosis, and fibrotic thickening of cardiac valves may occur with long-term therapy. The dosage should be gradually reduced during the last 2–3 weeks of each treatment course to avoid headache rebound.

Calcium Channel Blockers

Focal brain hypoxia has been proposed as having a key role in the origin of classic migraine.[22] The antihypoxic properties of selective calcium entry blockers have been postulated to be of value in the prophylaxis of migraine. According to Amery's hypoxia hypothesis, a short episode of focal cerebral hypoxia may be the instigator in the development of migraine. The exact mechanism is unknown but is thought to include excess sympathetic drive. An imbalance is produced between the oxygen supply and the metabolic requirements of the brain. The resulting cerebral hypoxia leads to cortical depression causing the aura. Further depression initiates biochemical, vascular, and hematologic changes that result in migraine.

Calcium entry blockers for prophylactic treatment of migraine decrease the calcium thought to enter and intoxicate cells exposed to hypoxic conditions. A secondary property of these agents is prevention of vasoconstriction without modifying the myogenic activity inherent in vascular smooth muscle cells.

Calcium channel blockers, including verapamil, diltiazem, nifedipine, and flunarizine, are currently under study for the prophylaxis of migraine. While this category of drug shows promise, these agents have not yet been approved for migraine management in the United States.

Lithium

Lithium has been utilized not only for the management of manic episodes of manic-depressive illness but also to prevent attacks of cluster headache.[37] Lithium treatment is an alternative in therapy-resistant chronic cases of cluster headache. The initial adult dosage of lithium is 300 mg twice a day. Serum blood levels of lithium must be regularly measured; the optimal serum concentration is 0.4–1.2 mEq/L, depending on clinical response. Unfortunately, lithium toxicity is closely related to serum lithium levels and can occur at doses close to therapeutic levels. Adverse reactions are seldom encountered at serum levels below 1.5 mEq/L. Patients should be warned to discontinue lithium if such clinical signs of lithium toxicity as diarrhea, vomiting, tremor, mold ataxia, drowsiness, or muscular weakness occur. Treatment duration is typically 16–24 weeks.

Tricyclic Antidepressants

The headache-prone patient tends to be depressed and/or anxious. The efficacy of treating depression in the patients with headaches with tricyclic antidepressants has been fairly well documented for this group of patients. These agents are described in detail in section V.

REFERENCES

1. Plum F.: Headache, in Beeson P.B., McDermott W.: *Cecil-Loeb Textbook of Medicine*, ed. 13. Philadelphia, W.B. Saunders, Co. 1971, pp. 154–160.
2. Ad Hoc Committee on Classification of Headache: Classification of headache. *Arch. Neurol.* 6:173–176, 1962.
3. Waters W.E.: Prevalence of migraine. *J. Neurol. Neurosurg. Psychiatry* 38:613–616, 1975.
4. Bille B.S.: Migraine in school children. *Acta Paediatr.* 51(suppl. 136):1, 1962.
5. Wolff H.G.: Personality factors and reactions of subjects with migraine. *Arch. Neurol. Psychiatry* 37:895–903, 1937.

6. Ziegler D.K., Hassanein R.S., Couch J.R.: Characteristics of life headache histories in a nonclinic population. *Neurology* 27:265, 1977.

7. Sandler M., Youdin M.B., Hannington E.A.: A phenylethylamine oxidizing defect in migraine. *Nature* 250:335–337, 1974.

8. Henderson W.R., Raskin N.H.: Hot dog headache. *Lancet* 2:1162–1163, 1972.

9. Schaumberg H.H., Byck R., Gerstl R., et al.: Monosodium 1-glutamate: Its pharmacology and role in Chinese restaurant syndrome. *Science* 163:826–828, 1969.

10. Kinball R.W., Friedman A.P.: Further studies of neurohumoral agents in patients with vascular headaches. *Neurology* 11:116–119, 1961.

11. Friedman A.P., Harter D.H., Merritt H.H.: Ophthalmoplegic migraine. *Arch. Neurol.* 7:82–87, 1962.

12. Bickerstaff E.R.: Basilar artery migraine. *Lancet* 1:15–17, 1961.

13. Bruyn G.W.: Complicated migraine, in Vinken P.J., Bruyn G.W. (eds.): *Handbook of Clinical Neurology.* Amsterdam, North Holland Publishing Co., 1968, vol. 5, pp. 59–95.

14. Dorfman L.J., Marshall W.H., Enzmann D.R.: Cerebral infarction and migraine: Clinical and radiological correlations. *Neurology* 29:317, 1979.

15. Friedman A.O., Wood E.H.: Thermography in vascular headache, in *Medical Thermography Theory and Applications.* Los Angeles, Brentwood Publishing, 1975, pp. 80–85.

16. Markovich S.E.: Pain in the head: A neurological appraisal, in Gelb H.: *Clinical Management of Head, Neck and TMJ Pain and Dysfunction.* Philadelphia, W.B. Saunders Co., 1977, pp. 126–139.

17. Wilkinson I.M.S., Russell R.W.F.: Arteries of the head and neck in giant cell arteritis. *Arch. Neurol.* 27:378–391, 1972.

18. Hauser W.A., Ferguson R.H., Holley K.E., et al.: Temporal arteritis in Rochester, Minnesota, 1951–1967. *Mayo Clin. Proc.* 46:597–601, 1971.

19. Saper J.R.: Migraine: II. Treatment. *JAMA* 239:2480–2484, 1978.

20. Kronby M.H.: Prophylaxis of migraine. *Can. Fam. Physician* 26:961–965, 1980.

21. Raskin N.H., Schwartz R.K.: Interval therapy of migraine: Long-term results. *Headache* 20:336–340, 1980.

22. Amery W.K.: Brain hypoxia: The turning point of the migraine attack? A hypothesis. *Cephalgia* 2:83–109, 1982.

23C / Trigeminal Neuralgia

JOHN STEINER, M.D.

TRIGEMINAL NEURALGIA (tic douloureux) is a common clinical syndrome, not a disease.[1] This painful facial condition can be reliably diagnosed by history alone, and the closer the patient adheres to the criteria for classic trigeminal neuralgia, the better the prognosis. The goals of therapy include accurate diagnosis, exclusion of secondary or symptomatic causes of the disorder, and initiation of proper therapy. An appreciation of the natural course of the syndrome allows the physician to advise the patient in effective management.

During acute episodes, the patient may be so desperate for relief he may accept surgical procedures that might not be necessary and will be regretted later. Effective medical and surgical treatments with high rates of success are available, and the condition has a much better prognosis than other types of facial pain.

ETIOLOGY

Tic douloureux occurs more often in women than in men (60:40 female-male ratio) and begins most often in the fifth decade. The right side seems to be more frequently involved (60% of cases). Bilateral involvement is rare and its occurrence suggests that the underlying problem is multiple sclerosis. The pain is confined to the distribution of the trigeminal (V) nerve, and most often involves the maxillary (V_2) and mandibular (V_3) divisions, either singly or in combination. About 10% of patients have pain in all divisions of the nerve, while 2%–4% have pain exclusively in the ophthalmic (VI) division. Although some patients may experience the tic bilaterally, during a single attack only one side is involved.

SIGNS AND SYMPTOMS

Tic douloureux is an episodic syndrome, prone to exacerbations and remission. It is characterized by the sudden onset of severe paroxysmal pain, usually without warning, although some patients describe a premonitory awareness seconds before the pain strikes. The pain builds up in a crescendo manner, wanes, and recurs. Patients can clearly describe the pain, using terms such as "shock-like," "electrical," and "lancinating." They wince and often cry out when it strikes.

Pain paroxysms often are triggered by a light touch on the face, particularly around the nares and corner of the mouth. The patient will cover that area with the hand or with a handkerchief to maintain a constant pressure stimulation and prevent the more devastating paroxysm brought on by such a light stimulus as a breeze. Sometimes patients find that they can precipitate attacks by touching the trigger zone and endure the pain, as they find that the paroxysm more quickly builds to a climax, and they then have a refractory period of relative freedom from pain for a time. The patient then can shave or apply makeup. The attack has an abrupt onset and abrupt termination, although attacks may occur hundreds of times daily. On occasion, attacks can be precipitated by head position. Sometimes they awaken the patient from sleep, or are so thoroughly agonizing that the patient has difficulty sleeping and exhibits symptoms of sleep deprivation. When trigger zones are circumoral, patients become reluctant to eat.

Patients often become incapacitated from the prolonged period of pain, which affects their eating and sleeping habits, makes impossible prolonged mental concentration, and decreases creative effort. They may also become depressed and desperate, and sometimes they feel suicidal after recurrent episodes. They are fully conscious and retain voluntary

379

control of motor activity at all times. The older patient may exhibit mental confusion as a result of the sleep deprivation, lack of nourishment, dehydration, and the side effects of medication.

The closer the patient's clinical characteristics adhere to the classic syndrome, the less frequently are structural lesions found. Van Loveren et al., in their experience with 1,000 patients, have never found an unsuspected tumor, arteriovenous malformation, or aneurysm in a patient with typical trigeminal neuralgia.[2]

PHYSICAL EXAMINATION

On physical examination, the classic tic patient is often normal. Patients resist being examined during an attack and often protect their face from the examiner's testing. The corneal reflex is always preserved. Janetta has reported that as many as one third of his patients have sensory abnormalities primarily about the nares and lips, the only area where the trigeminal nerve has exclusive territory. He finds abnormalities in light touch, and must often use a single cotton wisp moving from the abnormal to normal area. Others have reported considerably lower frequency.[3] Other cranial nerves are normal, and there is no specific localized tenderness on the scalp or along the jaw. Hearing in particular, as well as balance, are normal.

DIFFERENTIAL DIAGNOSIS

Classic tic douloureux can be diagnosed by history and by the almost immediate response, albeit sometimes brief, to carbamazepine (Tegretol). Entities to be considered in the differential diagnosis are listed in Table 23C–1. One should consider co-existing multiple sclerosis, especially in the younger person, when the patient has episodes of tic bilaterally.

The history and physical examination findings can usually help the physician sort out secondary causes of tic douloureux. Most workers believe there is a peripheral etiology for trigeminal neuralgia. Terrence et al. described a patient with a brain stem stroke[4] who had the clinical attributes of tic and responded to carbamazepine. Patients with lateral medullary syndrome describe sharp, jabbing, or burning pain in the ipsilateral eye or face at the onset of the stroke, probably related to involvement of sensory neurons in the nucleus of the descending

TABLE 23C–1.—DIFFERENTIAL DIAGNOSIS
OF TIC DOULOUREUX

Tic douloureux (trigeminal neuralgia)
  Primary
    Aberrant vascular contact with demyelination
    Herpes simplex?
  Secondary
    Brain stem stroke
    Brain stem ischemia
    Basilar impression—Paget's disease
    Cerebellar-pontine angle tumor
      Cholesteotoma
      Trigeminal neuroma
    Carotid-basilar artery anastomosis
    Multiple sclerosis
    Empty sella syndrome
    Pseudotumor cerebri
    Hydrocephalus
Other facial pain
  Postherpetic neuralgia
  "Tic convulsif"
  Cluster migraine
  Chronic paroxysmal hemicrania
  Chronic migrainous neuralgia
  Glossopharyngeal neuralgia
  Temporomandibular joint dysfunction and related
    disorders
  Greater occipital neuralgia
  Thoracic outlet syndrome
  Atypical facial pain

tract of cranial nerve V, a rostral extension of the substantia gelatinosa of the spinal cord.[5] Caplan and Gorelick reported three patients who described a peculiar and shocking sensation in the face "as if salt and pepper had been thrown into my eyes and face."[6] While the symptoms were predominantly one-sided, there was bilateral involvement, and associated left-sided weakness.

When an altered corneal reflex, evidence of facial, auditory, or vestibular dysfunction, or unilateral cerebellar signs are noted, a cerebellopontine angle tumor must be considered. A history of mastoid infection and the finding of a scarred tympanic membrane should suggest the presence of a cholesteotoma with extension. An audiometric examination is often useful in determining whether a sensorineural hearing loss exists.

Infrequently the patient gives a history of facial muscle movement at the time of paroxysmal pain. Cushing described "painful tic convulsif,"[7] and Kempe and Smith reported a case in which a persistent carotid-basilar anastomosis was compressing trigeminal, facial, nervus intermedius, and glossopharyngeal nerves and giving rise to expected pain in those distributions.[8] Sometimes involuntary facial movement during the painful experience is very slight, and the diagnosis can often be made if the physician is present when the patient's paroxysms begin and is able to witness these movements, usually about the inferior orbicularis oculi and rizorius muscles.

Often patients are seen by their dentist for trigeminal pain because they identify the course of the pain along the mandibular or maxillary divisions of the nerve and believe it originates from a tooth. Extractions are often done, but offer no relief. Dental conditions do not produce, but might act as a trigger for, the paroxysmal pain.

Downward traction on the trigeminal nerve has been suggested as the mechanism for tic in patients with hydrocephalus,[9] the empty sella syndrome,[10] and pseudotumor cerebri,[11] and should be suspected in an overweight woman who also complains of headache and has episoldes of obscured vision.

Postherpetic neuralgia should be considered when the patient describes unilateral, usually ophthalmic division aching, burning jabs of pain, and there is either a history of a herpetic zoster eruption or evidence of scarring on the skin and/or cornea. The pain, while often variable in intensity, is never paroxysmal, nor is the person free of pain. This pain can be increased by contact over the site and by eyelid movement.

Cluster migraine, characterized by the onset of unilateral, high-intensity pain, often localized behind or around the eye, shifting from side to side, lasting 30–45 minutes, associated with autonomic phenomena such as unilateral lacrimation and pupillary asymmetry, and often awakening the patient from sleep, presents little problem in the differential diagnosis of tic douloureux. However, another type of headache, recently described and considered to occur only infrequently, is chronic paroxysmal hemicrania. It was first described by Saagsted and Dale in 1974 and is characterized by the sudden onset of high-intensity pain, usually beginning in the occipital area, but radiating forward behind the eye. It lasts about 10 minutes and recurs 20 to 30 times per day. It is unresponsive to major analgesics but is brought under quick control with indomethacin.

Tic is sometimes confused with the temporomandibular joint (TMJ) syndrome, although the entities are quite different. Although patients with tic often do not eat while having periods of pain, they have no tenderness in the pain-free intervals, nor do they complain of soreness. The pain of TMJ syndrome is constant, often of only moderate severity, and sometimes spreads into the neck and scalp. There is tenderness over the TMJ or along the coronoid process. The patient often reports that his jaw locks or that he has had trauma to the jaw. Teeth malocclusion, asymmetric jaw opening and closing, and a noisy TMJ are frequently seen. Joint noise, associated with reported pain, can often be identified clearly by listening over the joint as the person chews or palpated by placing the tips of one's little fingers in the patient's external auditory meatus and having the patient move his jaw. Sometimes a cluster-like unilateral vascular headache coexists with the TMJ syndrome and must be treated before it is realized that the TMJ syndrome is the inciting process.

Constant progressive pain with alteration of corneal reflex and involvement of adjacent cranial nerves often indicates direct involvement of the nerve as a result of nasopharyngeal malignancy.

Greater occipital neuralgia, which arises from compression of the posterior branch of the second cervical root, and lesser occipital neuralgia, which arises from compression of its anterior root, give rise to a pain syndrome beginning around the insertion of the trapezius and scalenius muscles and radiating along the course of the nerves. Patients often describe a high-intensity pain followed by a dull ache, and often find a tender spot on their scalp over the exit of the nerve. Persistent scalp paresthesias are often described. The pain referral pattern of greater occipital neuralgia can sometimes be confused with pain syndromes arising from the higher cranial nerves. Kerr has defined an anatomical pathway in which ephaptic transmission at the point of the root entry zone of the second cervical root connects with the descending spinal root of the trigeminal nerve, which is laminated so that the first division of the trigeminal nerve is located more laterally.[12] The patient will sometimes discover that self-induced pressure over the sore nuchal-occipital area will also increase retro-ocular pain, and expresses considerable amazement when that pain disappears as the physician infiltrates the areas with local anesthetic.

Palpation of a small mass at the exit of the greater occipital nerve is an indication for skull radiography as a diagnostic test before local anesthetic is injected. Infrequently a primary bone tumor, such as a plasmacytoma, can be detected in this manner. As the greater occipital nerve lies adjacent to an artery and lymph node, enlargement of the artery, such as sometimes occurs during the development of collateral posterior fossa circulation in vascular disease, or the development of local lymphadenopathy will occasionally produce this painful scalp syndrome.

Glossopharyngeal neuralgia has many of the characteristics of tic douloureux, but the pains occur in the posterior half of the tongue, tonsil, and pharyngeal area and are often precipitated by swallowing. These pains are described as a stabbing, jolting pain, of high intensity, with periods of exacerbation and remission. The patient may also experience syncopal attack, related to bradycardia as a result of vagal stimulation.[13] Regional swabbing of the pharynx with a cocaine solution often helps differentiate this problem from that of trigeminal neuralgia.[14] Essential glossopharyngeal neuralgia responds to carbamazepine. Secondary causes of this type of pain must be found.

A seldom considered cause of unilateral hemicrania, with pain radiating into the face, jaw, and scalp, is the thoracic outlet syndrome. Patients describe a unilateral "vascular" headache resistant to antimigraine drugs. In addition to the hemicrania, patients describe pain and paresthesias in the affected limb that are aggravated or precipitated by maneuvers that require shoulder abduction, lifting, or holding, and they report they are awakened from sleep by the "dead arm" several times weekly.[15] Headache is seldom relieved unless the patient undergoes resection of the first rib.[16]

Atypical facial pain is sometimes misidentified as tic douloureux. Pain, usually in women, is generally constant, described as aching and boring, and does not conform to the anatomical distribution of the trigeminal nerve. It is often maximal in the second division of that nerve. It is usually unilateral but can spread and involve both sides. This pain is generally associated with an unrecognized or unaccepted depression and sometimes responds to antidepressant medication.

PATHOPHYSIOLOGY

The pathophysiology of pain generation in trigeminal neuralgia is unclear, but different pathologic entities have as a common factor compression or stretching of the nerve along its course. This results in segmental demyelination of large diameter A alpha and beta fibers in this region and results in artificial synapses with ephaptic transmission between these fibers. These abnormalities occur most often at the root entry zone of the portio major of the trigeminal nerve. Gardner and Miklos believe that the most common cause of trigeminal neuralgia is compression of the nerve root by an aberrant branch

of the superior cerebellar artery or by angulation over the petrous apex.[17] This association was first noted by Dandy.[18]

The understanding of the pathophysiologic process has followed the development of methods for more detailed visualization of the nerve, both at the time of operative intervention as well as in the postmortem specimen, and the availability of increasingly sophisticated neurophysiologic techniques applied to experimental animals to record transmissions both from the nerve and from higher neural centers.

Evidence exists for both a central and a peripheral site of pain generation and transmission in trigeminal neuralgia, and Fromm et al. put it best when they said that there was "both a peripheral etiology and a central pathogenesis. . . . Trigeminal neuralgia occurs in individuals with a central nervous system susceptibility when disease or irritation of a peripheral causes increase nerve firing to the point of triggering paroxysmal discharges in the trigeminal nuclei."[19] They also demonstrated that several drugs (carbamazepine, baclofen, phenytoin) effective in the treatment of trigeminal neuralgia not only depressed excitatory synaptic transmission in the spinal trigeminal nucleus, but also markedly facilitated segmental inhibition in this nucleus. Phenobarbital, an anticonvulsant drug not effective in trigeminal neuralgia, did not have this effect.[19–21]

Gardner indicated that "hemifacial spasm was the seventh nerve counterpart of trigeminal neuralgia. Each may be considered the equivalent of a focal seizure at the nerve root level."[1] He also suggested that the paroxysms of pain represented "backtalk" conduction in that nerve. Iwakuma et al. believe that transaxonal short-circuiting of the action current of efferent to efferent fiber was a more reasonable theory for the development of facial twitching than the theory of anatomical misdirection of fibers.[22]

In trigeminal neuralgia, Calvin et al. suggested that the peripheral nerve impulse might be reflected back along the course of the nerve.[23] Burchiel demonstrated abnormal impulse generation in focally demyelinated trigeminal roots of experimental animals. This activity was independent of brain stem connections of nerve, and areas of experimentally demyelinated roots have been shown to produce repetitive action potential firing, lasting in some cases for minutes.[24]

Haines, Jannetta, and Zorub reported that there is continuity between an artery or vein and the trigeminal root, which is the proximate cause for the neuralgia, and reported neurovascular contacts in

35% of normal cadavers. In 31 of 40 trigeminal nerves exposed surgically, vascular compression by adjacent arteries was noted.[25] Earlier (1967) Haines and Jannetta found no neurovascular contacts in 56 fresh cadaver brains, and resolved the issue by reporting that neurovascular contacts are increasingly recognized by more subtle criteria.[26] Hardy and Rhoton demonstrated vascular contact at the trigeminal root entry zone in more than 50% of unselected autopsies.[27] Tew's group[2] attempted to differentiate between incidental and significant vascular contact at the time of posterior fossa exploration and noted that while vascular contact was identified in 82% of their patients, it was considered significant in less than half (46%). This observation was important in their view, because it then led to partial section of the sensory root appropriate to the division, according to the work of Emmons and Rhoton.[28]

It is unclear what conditions predispose the nerve to set up the repetitive aberrant firing rate when it is compressed or stretched. Jannetta reports that when the adherent pia arachnoid that binds the artery and nerve together is divided, the artery assumes a different relationship. It is unclear what causes the pia arachnoid to bind these structures together. The coexistence of herpes simplex eruptions at the time of trigeminal nerve section has been noted since the time of Cushing.

Behrman and Knight have noted the frequent finding of herpetic lesions in patients who develop trigeminal neuralgia.[29] Ellison et al. noted recurrent herpes simplex infections following section of the trigeminal nerve.[30] Whereas Beaver found no evidence of viral particles on electron microscopic examination of the root or ganglia, Baringer and Swoveland cultured herpes simplex from the ganglia but not from the root of the trigeminal nerve in persons known not to have facial pain and in one person with trigeminal neuralgia.[31]

DIAGNOSTIC STUDIES

Radiologic Studies

Sobel et al.[32] and Van Loveren et al.[2] have found plain skull films to be of no value. CT studies to exclude masses in the posterior fossa are indicated if the patient's clinical picture deviates from the classic picture and if any physical signs that would cause one to suspect a posterior fossa mass, such as

a clear-cut sensory loss, altered corneal reflex, unilateral hearing deficit, or unilateral cerebellar ataxia, are present. Angiograms seldom demonstrate the aberrant course of small posterior fossa vessels and should be reserved for the patient in whom a larger aneurysm or arteriovenous malformation is suspected.

Electrophysiologic Studies

Electrophysiologic studies typically include electromyography (EMG), somatosensory evoked responses, and related audiometric examination. While potentially useful in helping to define the pathophysiology of tic douloureux, electrophysiologic tests to measure trigeminal sensory conduction are not routinely used in evaluating patients with facial pain, and there are no studies now that correlate electrophysiologic findings with operative findings or clinical course.

Masseter and temporalis muscle EMG was reported by Saunders et al., who found signs of denervation in 7 of 18 patients, attributed to compression of the motor root. They postulated that sensory fibers were also involved in the motor root in addition to the adjacent sensory fibers in the portio major sensory part.[33]

Somatosensory evoked potential determinations may have an important role in determining whether a conduction block exists, but correlative studies have yet to be reported. Stohr et al. reported abnormalities in latency and amplitude in 7 of 17 patients with trigeminal neuralgia who did not undergo operation.[34] They applied stimulation to the corner of the mouth—in essence stimulated both V_2 and V_3 divisions—and recorded the cortical evoked potential over the contralateral hemisphere, but did not report correlative operative findings or results.

Standard audiometric examination and occasionally brain stem auditory evoked responses are useful in determining whether there is involvement of the statoacoustic nerve in posterior fossa tumors arising from that nerve and in continuity with the trigeminal nerve.

TREATMENT

The form of therapy offered to persons with trigeminal neuralgia is dependent on the experience of the treating physician. It is generally agreed that patients with trigeminal neuralgia should be started on carbamazepine.[35–37] Almost all patients report immediate and significant improvement when given carbamazepine and, depending on dosage, respond within 5 days. It is not a cure. The natural course of the disease is variable. After the patient is symptom free, the dosage is gradually reduced or stopped, and the patient may remain asymptomatic for a time, until the next exacerbation, when he seeks another solution. Often after relief is achieved, breakthrough pain develops while the patient is on the same dosage, and when the dosage is increased, more side effects are experienced.

Most neurologists report that younger patients with seizures have few side effects when treated with carbamazepine, but the response of patients with tic is different. Patients are older and less tolerant of side effects. It must be started slowly, at perhaps 100 mg twice daily, and increased to 600–800 mg/day. Pain relief often occurs at low dosages and at drug levels lower than those established for therapeutic efficacy in epilepsy.

The older tic patient often has coexisting multiple sensory deficits: cataracts, hearing loss, cervical spondylosis, peripheral neuropathy. They are often more unsteady because of marginally functioning preprioceptive input systems. Young patients sometimes report diplopia and unsteadiness at peak dosage times, which are transient. When these effects are added to the multiple subliminal deficits of the older patient, the drug can be intolerable.

Some physicians are unfamiliar with the use of carbamazepine and secure their knowledge of it through information listed in the *Physician's Desk Reference,* which urges extreme caution in its use. It is not infrequent to see an elderly patient perhaps months after he has heard a negative comment from another physician about the drug; the patient stops taking the drug, even though he had no side effects and it stopped the pain. While there have been 17 fatal cases of aplastic anemia associated with carbamazepine, few patients were taking only that drug, and the incidence of such a catastrophe has been estimated to be 1 in 250,000.[38] Recent investigators have suggested that elaborate by-protocol drug monitoring does not guarantee safety of drug usage, as the toxicity is of sudden onset. Hart and Easton noted the uncommon hematologic toxicity and questioned the need for vigorous laboratory testing as recommended by the manufacturer.[38]

Baclofen, an antispasticity drug well tolerated by most patients, has been found to be effective in some patients with tic douloureux.[39] It is given as a 10-mg tablet twice daily and increased slowly to about 60 mg. Rapid withdrawal has been associated with visual hallucinations. Phenytoin has also been reported to be beneficial in the tic patient. Clonazepam, an anticonvulsant, has been reported to be useful in other patients with tic douloureux, but is a frequently sedating drug.[40, 41]

Nerve Blocks

Nerve blocks using local anesthetics and/or steroids may be effective. However, neurolytic blocks or rhizotomy may be necessary in cases of severe tic doulourex, especially if the patient has become extremely depressed and suicidal.

Although many chemicals (e.g., alcohol, phenol) have been injected into the trigeminal ganglion, the results were often short-lived and were frequently associated with unpleasant facial dysesthesias, corneal anesthesia, corneal ulceration, and sometimes nasal ala ulceration.

Glycerol Injections

During the development of the stereotactic technique for γ-irradiation of the trigeminal ganglion and root in the treatment of trigeminal neuralgia, glycerol was used as a vehicle to introduce tantalum dust into the trigeminal cistern for permanent identification of the cistern. Quite unexpectedly, the observation was made that the glycerol injection often provided significant pain relief without producing any major sensory loss.

Hakanson found the injection of 0.2–0.4 ml of sterile glycerol into the trigeminal cistern using the anterior percutaneous route via the foramen ovale gave 86% of 75 patients complete pain relief. He visualized the cistern with the aid of metrizamide as the x-ray contrast medium. It is thought that gycerol acts mainly on partly demyelinated nerve fibers, which are assumed to be involved in the trigger mechanism of the pain.

Trigeminal Thermocoagulation

Controlled thermocoagulation of the trigeminal ganglion and rootlets for differential destruction of pain fibers can be used in treating severe chronic trigeminal neuralgia. This technique is fairly sophisticated in that it provides for selective control in the destruction of the affected nerves. Sweet and coworkers have reported their results in 350 patients without mortality or morbidity. In 6% of the patients, the initial treatment gave inadequate sensory loss and repetition was required. Twenty-two percent of the patients with trigeminal neuralgia had a late recurrence, but again, Sweet et al. thought the procedure could be repeated for pain relief. Using this technique, the small myelinated and unmyelinated fibers, carrying the pain impulses, can be destroyed with carefully regulated increments of heat, leaving larger nerve fibers intact to preserve some sense of touch and resulting in a low incidence of analgesia, hypoalgesia, and dolorosa.

Radiofrequency Percutaneous Rhizotomy

In 1974, Sweet and Wepsic refined Kirschner's percutaneous coagulation technique to accomplish controlled thermocoagulation of the trigeminal ganglion under short-acting anesthetic agents, which permitted the patient to awaken rapidly for sensory testing during the operation.[42] Under x-ray control the needle was placed into the foramen ovale and advanced according to the localization desired. This method introduced a reliable radiofrequency current for production of reproducible lesions, had electrical stimulation for more precise localization, and had temperature monitoring for better control of lesion size. Complications in the procedure included carotid artery puncture, anesthesia dolorosa, and corneal anesthesia. Methods for more accurate needle placement have been emphasized by Tew and coworkers.[43]

Surgical Management

Middle European surgeons had suggested section of various sites of the trigeminal nerve beginning in the mid-1700s,[43] and Cushing reported on a large series of patients to whom gasserian ganglion section was performed.[7] Permanent facial numbness and lack of corneal sensitivity were often unacceptable to the patient postoperatively.

While intracranial section of the trigeminal nerve was proposed at the turn of the century, Dandy was the first to describe a large series of patients with partial section of the sensory root at the pons.[44] He attributed his success to the development of electrocautery instrumentation, which enabled him to operate on 215 patients with trigeminal neuralgia using the suboccipital craniectomy approach and with

most of the patients under local anesthesia. He found either a tumor, enlongated basilar artery, or cavernous angioma adherent to and compressing the trigeminal nerve in 10.7%; in 66 (30.7%) patients the superior cerebellar artery was attached in the same way, while the petrosal vein crossed or passed through the trigeminal nerve. In 87 patients (40%) he found no lesion to explain the pain.

Jannetta and Rand, using microsurgical techniques through a posterior subtemporal transtentorial approach, visualized an aberrant tortuous artery compressing the trigeminal nerve to less than half its normal diameter.[45] When the pia arachnoid adhesions binding the artery were released, the artery assumed a new position away from the nerve. Gardner in 1959 was the first to insert a piece of Gelfoam between an artery and the trigeminal root. Gardner and his colleagues reported the successful treatment of facial hemispasm as a result of neurovascular compression in 1962. Jannetta and Rand, using microsurgical techniques at the time of suboccipital exploration, reported finding arterial compression of the trigeminal nerve at the pons in patients with trigeminal neuralgia.[46] Pathologic confirmation via electron microscopy of the marked deterioration of the myelin sheaths of the posterior roots were described by Kerr in 1967,[47] and other authors have reported areas of demyelination and hypermyelination in the symptomatic area.

Efficacy of Posterior Fossa Exploration

Posterior fossa exploration has the advantage of direct visualization of anatomical variants, exclusion of other causes of pain, and the ability to visualize other causes. Its obvious disadvantage is the operative procedure itself, which requires inpatient hospitalization. In experienced hands the mortality is very small, and the brain itself is not disrupted.

There are a number of comparisons between the radiofrequency rhizotomy (RF) and microvascular decompression (MVD); some have multiple authors and a small number of cases; others have a dominant author and a significantly greater number of cases treated one way.

Jannetta used the posterior fossa approach primarily and reviewed his surgical experience on 411 patients in 1980. He reported visualizing arterial anomalies in 241 patients, venous anomalies in 57 patients, mixed arteriovenous anomalies in 96 patients, 15 tumors, and one aneurysm. Of the 411 patients, 328 did well after one microvascular decompression; 14 required a second procedure, and one a third procedure. Jannetta performed radiofrequency rhizotomy on 17 after microvascular decompression, and 38 needed medication. Two patients had slight pain without medication, 5 patients had severe pain, 5 died (3 postoperatively), and one each died of suicide and an accident.

Van Loveren et al. reported that 90% of their patients responded initially to carbamazepine, but a surgical procedure was offered when the patient had objectionable side effects, recurrence of the tic, or became refractory to the drug.[2] They favored radiofrequency rhizotomy because of its efficacy and because it requires minimal anesthesia, can be done on an outpatient basis, and can be repeated easily. Posterior fossa exploration is offered to those in whom radiofrequency rhizotomy fails and in whom a posterior fossa lesion is suspected.

Van Loveren et al. reported on 700 patients treated with percutaneous stereotactic rhizotomy and 50 patients treated with posterior fossa decompression coupled with partial sensory rhizotomy when vascular contacts were not clearly identified. There was a 20% recurrence rate in patients who underwent percutaneous stereotaxis rhizotomy and were followed for 6 years after the procedure, while 61% had excellent results, 13% had good results, 5% had fair results, and 1% had poor results. Three years after posterior fossa decompression 12% had recurrence of neuralgia, 84% were pain free, and excellent results were achieved in 68%, good results in 12%, fair results in 4%, and poor results in 1%.[2]

Nugent emphasized the choice of placement of the radiofrequency electrode more central to the ganglion. In his experience with more than 800 patients, he reported a recurrence rate of 21% in 8 years.[48] In most series there is a 2% mortality from posterior fossa decompression. Burchiel and coworkers reported on their 75 patients: 55 underwent radiofrequency rhizotomy and 20 underwent microvascular decompression; 4 underwent both. In the radiofrequency rhizotomy group, 42% had recurrent pain and six required further surgery. Neurologic deficit was confined to the trigeminal nerve, with one patient developing anesthesia dolorosa and four having corneal anesthesia. Of the 20 patients that underwent microvascular decompression, three failed to achieve complete relief and two required further surgery.[37]

Patients with multiple sclerosis who have bilateral tic often respond adversely to carbamazepine and do better with percutaneous radiofrequency rhizotomy.[49] Transient sensory alterations added to the already compromised nervous system often cannot be tolerated by the patient with multiple sclerosis.

GENERAL MANAGEMENT

The treatment of patient with tic douloureux depends on accurate diagnosis, identification, and treatment of secondary causes of the syndrome, and on the experience of the neurosurgeon. The closer the patient's disease adheres to the classic picture, the better is the prognosis.

The patient with classic tic douloureux initially should be given carbamazepine in small doses, with the dosage increased to tolerance and the medication continued only if there is significant response, although not necessarily complete control, after 8–10 days. Patients must be educated about the use of Tegretol and must be aware of differing opinions within the treating community about its use. If there is incomplete control the physician can shift to Dilantin or baclofen (Lioresal). After several weeks of complete control, medication should be reduced or stopped. Recurrence of tic should be expected, and the patient should be educated not to become angry that the treatment did not cure him. Some patients focus on the intensity of the pain and seek surgical relief because they fear its recurrence in a quiescent period.

The surgical approach to trigeminal pain depends on the surgeon's skill, experience, and preference. The primary pain physician should be aware of the surgeon's experience and preference. Stereotactic radiofrequency procedures potentially offer the least mortality, least hospitalization, avoidance of the problems of general anesthesia, and can be repeated more easily. Painful anesthesia, corneal insensitivity, and carotid puncture are known complications of that disease, but the incidence of complications is less as techniques for more accurate probe placement and thermal control are developed.

Microvascular decompression has an overall mortality of about 2%, and requires general anesthesia, inpatient hospitalization, and the operation itself. It has the advantage of allowing the surgeon to visualize abnormalities within the posterior fossa that might cause or contribute to the genesis of facial pain. Continued follow-up of the patient is essential after any treatment.

REFERENCES

1. Gardner W.J.: Concerning the mechanism of trigeminal neuralgia and hemifacial spasm. *J. Neurosurg.* 19:947–958, 1962.

2. Van Loveren H., Tew J.M. Jr., Keller J.T., et al.: A 10 year experience in the treatment of trigeminal neuralgia: A comparison of percutaneous stereotactic rhizotomy and posterior fossa exploration. *J. Neurosurg.* 57:575–764, 1982.

3. Hussein M., Wilson L.A., Illingsworth R.: Patterns of sensory loss following fractional posterior fossa trigeminal nerve section for trigeminal neuralgia. *J. Neurol. Neurosurg. Psychiatry* 45:786–790, 1982.

4. Terrence C., Costa R., Fromm G.: An unusual case of paroxysmal facial pain. *J. Neurol.* 221:73–76, 1979.

5. Fisher C.M.: Headache in cerebrovascular disease, in Vinken P.J., Bruyn G.W. (eds.): *Handbook of Clinical Neurology.* Volume 5: *Headache and Cranial Neuralgias.* Amsterdam, North Holland, 1968, pp. 124–156.

6. Caplan L., Gorelick P.: Salt and pepper on the face: Pain in acute brainstem ischemia. *Ann. Neurol.* 13:344, 1983.

7. Cushing H.: The major trigeminal neuralgias and their surgical treatment based on experiences with 332 gasserian operations. *Am. J. Med. Sci.* 160:157–184, 1920.

8. Kempe L.G., Smith D.R.: Trigeminal neuralgia, facial spasm, intermedius and glossopharyngeal neuralgia with persistent carotid-basilar anastomosis. *J. Neurosurg.* 31:445–451, 1969.

9. Findler G., Feinsod M.: Reversible facial pain due to hydrocephalus with trigeminal somatosensory evoked response changes: Case report. *J. Neurosurg.* 57:267–269, 1982.

10. Neelson F., Goree J.A., Lebovitz H.E.: The primary empty sella: Clinical and radiographic characteristics and endocrine function. *Medicine* 52:73–92, 1973.

11. Hart R.G., Carter J.E.: Pseudotumor cerebri and facial pain. *Arch. Neurol.* 39:440–442, 1982.

12. Kerr F.W.L.: The divisional organization of afferent fibers of the trigeminal nerve. *Brain* 86:721–732, 1963.

13. Morales F., Albert P., Alberca R., et al.: Glossopharyngeal and vagal neuralgia secondary to vascular compression of the nerves. *Surg. Neurol.* 8:431–433, 1977.

14. Selby G.: Diseases of the fifth cranial nerve, in Dyck P.J., Thomas P.K., Lambert E.H. (eds.): *Peripheral Neuropathy.* Philadelphia, W.B. Saunders Co., 1975, pp. 533–569.

15. Raskin N.H., Howard M.W., Ehrentfeld W.K.: Headaches as the presenting symptom of the thoracic outlet syndrome. *J. Neurol.* 33(suppl. 2):191, 1983.

16. Roos D.B.: Experience with first rib resection for thoracic outlet syndrome. *Ann. Surg.* 173:429–442, 1921.

17. Gardner W.J., Miklos M.V.: Response of trigeminal neuralgia to decompression of sensory root: Discussion of cause of trigeminal neuralgia. *JAMA* 170:1773–1776, 1959.

18. Dandy W.E.: Concerning the cause of trigeminal neuralgia. *Am. J. Surg.* 24:447–455, 1934.

19. Fromm G.H., Chattha A.S., Terrence C.F., et al.: Role of inhibitory mechanisms in trigeminal neuralgia. *Neurology* 31:683–687, 1981.

20. Fromm G.H., Killiam J.M.: Effect of some anticonvulsant drugs on the spinal trigeminal nucleus. *Neurology* 17:275–280, 1967.

21. Fromm G.H., et al.: Baclofen in trigeminal neuralgia. *Arch. Neurol.* 37:768–771, 1980.

22. Iwakuma T., Matsumoto A., Nakamura N.: Hemifacial spasm: Comparison of three different operative procedures in 110 patients. *J. Neurosurg.* 57:753–756, 1982.

23. Calvin H.S., Loeser J.D., Howe J.F.: A neurophysiological theory for the pain mechanism of tic douloueux. *Pain* 3:147–154, 1977.

24. Burchiel K.J.: Abnormal impulse generation in focally demyelinated trigeminal roots. *J. Neurosurg.* 56:674–683, 1980.

25. Haines S.J., Jannetta P.J., Zorub D.S.: Microvascular relations of the trigeminal nerve: An anatomic study with clinical correlation. *J. Neurosurg.* 52:381–386, 1980.

26. Haines S., Jannetta P.: Microvascular relationships of the trigeminal nerve. *J. Neurosurg.* 53:416, 1980.

27. Hardy D.G., Rhoton A.L. Jr.: Microsurgical relationships of the superior cerebellary artery and the trigeminal nerve. *J. Neurosurg.* 49:669–678, 1978.

28. Emmons W.F., Rhoton A.K. Jr.: Subdivision of the trigeminal sensory root: Experimental study in the monkey. *J. Neurosurg.* 35:585–591, 1971.

29. Behrman S. Knight G.: Herpes simplex associated with trigeminal neuralgia. *Neurology* 4:525–530, 1954.

30. Ellison S.A., Carton C.A., Rose H.M.: Studies of recurrent herpes simplex infections following section of the trigeminal nerve. *J. Infect. Dis.* 105:161–167, 1959.

31. Baringer J.R., Swoveland P.: Recovery of herpes simplex virus from human trigeminal ganglions. *N. Engl. J. Med.* 288:664–665, 1973.

32. Sobel D., Norman D., Yorke C.H., et al.: Radiography of trigeminal neuralgia and hemifacial spasm. *Am. J. Neuroradiol.* 135:93–95, 1980.

33. Saunders R.L., Krout R., Sachs E.: Masticator electromyography of trigeminal neuralgia. *Neurology* 21:1221–1225, 1971.

34. Stohr M., Petruch F., Scheglmann K.: Somatosensory evoked potentials following trigeminal nerve stimulation in trigeminal neuralgia. *Ann. Neurol.* 9:63–66, 1981.

35. Blom S.: Trigeminal neuralgia: Its treatment with a new anticonvulsant drug (G32883). *Lancet* 1:839–840, 1962.

36. Crill E.: Carbamazepine. *Ann. Intern. Med.* 79:79–80, 1973.

37. Burchiel K.J., Steege T.D., Howe J.F., et al.: Com-

parison of percutaneous radiofrequency gangliolysis and microvascular decompression for the surgical management of tic douloureux. *Neurosurgery* 9:111–119, 1981.

38. Hart R.G., Easton J.D.: Carbamazepine and hematological monitoring. *Ann. Neurol.* 11:309–312, 1982.

39. Fromm G.H., Terrence C.S., Chattha A.S., et al.: Baclofen in trigeminal neuralgia: Effect on the spinal trigeminal nucleus: A pilot study. *Arch. Neurol.* 37:768–771, 1980.

40. Court J.E., Kase C.S.: Treatment of tic douloureux with a new anticonvulsant (Clonazepam). *J. Neurol. Neurosurg. Psychiatry* 39:297–298, 1976.

41. Smirne S., Scarlato G.: Clonazepam in cranial neuralgias. *Med. J. Aust.* 1:93–94, 1977.

42. Sweet W.H., Wespic J.G.: Controlled thermocoagulation of trigeminal ganglion and roots for differential destruction of pain fibers: I. Trigeminal neuralgia. *J. Neurosurg.* 39:143–157, 1974.

43. Tew T.M. Jr., Keller J.T., Williams D.S.: Application of stereotactic principles to the treatment of tri-geminal neuralgia. *Appl. Neurophysiol.* 41:146–156, 1978.

44. Dandy W.E.: An operation for the cure of tic douloureux: Partial section of the sensory root at the pons. *Arch. Surg.* 18:687–734, 1929.

45. Jannetta P.J., Rand R.W.: Transtentorial retrogasserian rhizotomy in trigeminal neuralgia by microneurosurgical technique. *Bull. LA Neurol. Soc.* 31:93–99, 1966.

46. Jannetta P.J., Rand R.W.: Arterial compression of the trigeminal nerve at the pons in patients with trigeminal neuralgia. *J. Neurosurg.* 26(suppl.):159–162, 1976.

47. Kerr F.W.L.: Evidence for a peripheral etiology of trigeminal neuralgia. *J. Neurosurg.* 26:168–174, 1967.

48. Nugent G.R.: Comment on article by Burchiel et al. *Neurosurgery* 9:118–119, 1981.

49. Brett D.C., Ferguson C.G., Ebers G.C., et al.: Percutaneous trigeminal rhizotomy: Treatment of trigeminal neuralgia secondary to multiple sclerosis. *Arch. Neurosurg.* 39:219–221, 1982.

23D / Orofacial Pain

GARY S. ROBINS, D.M.D.
JAMES C. PHERO, D.M.D.
JOHN S. MCDONALD, D.D.S., M.S.

PAIN OF DENTAL ORIGIN

TOOTHACHE IS THE MOST common cause of pain in the jaw. Pain due to exposure of the dentin is provoked by cold or sweet food. The pain of pulpal irritation is provoked by hot food or drink. The pain of dental abscess is often caused by pressure in the inflamed tissues surrounding the affected tooth. Odontalgia usually results from pulp irritation related to dental caries. Other causes of odontalgia include abrasion and erosion of the teeth, apical periodontitis, occlusal trauma, and unerupted teeth that cause pressure on branches of the trigeminal nerve by the periodontal membranes. Localized jaw pain can be due to infected cysts or carcinoma in the mandible or maxilla.

Pains of dental disease can be related to infected teeth or periodontal disease. Teeth can be tested by placing hot or cold materials on them or by using an electrical pulp tester, palpation, percussion, or periodontal probing of the supporting structures. If dental disease is suspected, the patient should be referred to a dentist for evaluation. X-ray series of the teeth should show any obvious infections. Symptoms related to the teeth usually become localized with time.

TEMPOROMANDIBULAR JOINT DISORDERS

A differential diagnosis is the first step in the workup of a patient with pain that may be of craniomandibular origin and is related to the dental apparatus. Besides looking for obvious odontologic or periodontal disease, the practitioner evaluates the condition to see if a relationship exists among the functioning movements of the jaw, temporomandibular joint (TMJ), muscles, ligaments, and the occlusion. If the pain appears related to the TMJ, the examiner must ascertain whether the problem is extracapsular or intracapsular. Extracapsular problems of the masticatory apparatus are mainly muscular in origin. Also, the dentition plays a role in causing referred pain to facial structures. (An example would be a third molar referring pain to the ear.) Intracapsular problems could be arthritic conditions, ankylosis, or displacement or dislocation of the temporomandibular disk, any of which could result in inflammation or dysfunction of the jaw and pain. Other diagnostic possibilities in the evaluation of facial pain include trauma-related fractures, infections, gout, bony cavities, ankylosis, neoplasia, cervical problems, sinus problems, ear disease, eye disease, oropharyngeal problems, neurologic problems, psychogenic pain from anxiety and depressive states, intracranial problems, conversion hysteria, vascular problems (temporal arteritis, internal carotid occlusion), migraines and other vascular problems, arterial hypertension, developmental abnormalities (hypoplasia, hyperplasia, chondroma, Eagle's syndrome), diseases of the TMJ (degenerative arthritis, osteochrondritis, rheumatoid arthritis, psoriatic arthritis, infections, gout), and a host of others.

Most of the disorders of the masticatory system manifest either as pain or as dysfunction of jaw movements. Many patients treated for TMJ disorders have multifactorial problems, such as malocclusion, psychological stress, joint disease, pain, dysfunction, vertebral entrapments, poor body mechanics, and myofascial pain from cervical trapezius.

389

Anatomy and Physiology

In investigating TMJ problems, one should have a basic knowledge of the anatomy and physiology of the TMJ including the biomechanics of joint movement (Figure 23D–1). The TMJ is a synarthrodial joint, composed of fibrocartilage rather than the hyaline cartilage that is found in most other joints. This fibrocartilage has regenerative capabilities which include remodeling at the articular surfaces. The lower compartment of the TMJ has a rotary movement. This occurs up to approximately 27 mm of mouth opening when measured from the incisor edges of the anterior teeth. The remainder of the opening occurs within the range of 27 to 45 mm and is accomplished by the upper compartment, which is involved with translatory movement. A disk is connected to the mandibular condyle by collateral ligaments attaching to its medial and lateral aspect. The articular surfaces are not innervated by nerves or blood vessels. Posteriorly, a bilaminar zone[1] is found, that is highly innervated and vascularized. The bilaminar zone contains a superior stratum of elastin and an inferior stratum of collagen fibers. The upper stratum is stretched when the condyle and disk are translated forward in wide opening or lat-

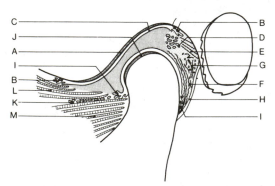

Fig 23D–1.—Sagittal view of the temporomandibular joint. *A,* articular surface of the temporal bone; *B,* synovial membrane of the superior cavity; *C,* superior cavity; *D,* vascular knee; *E,* superior stratum of bilaminar zone; *F,* inferior stratum of bilaminar zone; *G,* loose areolar connective tissue; *H,* posterior capsule; *I,* inferior cavity synovial membrane; *J,* articular surface of condyle; *K,* blood vessels; *L,* superior belly of lateral pterygoid; *M,* inferior belly of lateral pterygoid muscle. (Originally from Travell,[6] reproduced in Gelb.[15] Reproduced here by permission of W.B. Saunders Co.)

eral movements of the jaw. For a proper knowledge of joint mechanics, it is important that lateral pterygoid function be well understood. Anteriorly, the lateral pterygoid muscle is attached to the disk and condyle. Recent evidence suggests that the superior belly of the lateral pterygoid is involved in stabilizing the disk on the condyle as the mouth is closed. Moreover, the inferior belly of the lateral pterygoid contracts on mouth opening and is connected to the condyle. This muscle is relaxed during mouth closure;[2] therefore, the lateral pterygoid muscle has two separate functions.[3]

Other masticatory muscles may also be involved in TMJ pain. The main muscles of jaw closure are the masseter, internal pterygoid, and temporalis muscles, along with the superior belly of the lateral pterygoid muscle. The inferior belly of the lateral pterygoid, along with the digastric, myelohyoid, and genohyoid, is involved with opening of the mandible. Lateral movements of the jaw are controlled by the contralateral external pterygoid muscle, the inferior portion of the contralateral lateral pterygoid muscle, and the posterior portion of the ipsilateral temporalis muscle. Protraction of the mandible is controlled mainly by the internal pterygoid, masseter, and suprahyoid muscles.[4] Retraction of the mandible occurs from contraction of the temporalis muscle bilaterally (middle and posterior fibers) and both bellies of the digastric and the deep fibers of the masseter.[5]

Causes of TMJ Dysfunction

Extracapsular Problems

Extracapsular problems may be related to occlusion of the teeth, psychological stress, trauma to the joint, and habit patterns, such as sleeping on the face with pressure to the jaw. All of these may result in muscle dysfunction, leading to spasms, hypomobility, loss of or decrease in function, pain, and limitation of mandibular motion.

TRIGGER AREAS IN MASTICATORY MUSCLES.—Travell[6] has observed in muscles, areas called trigger zones, which are responsible for referred pain patterns. She suggests that these trigger areas, "which are a small zone of hypersensitivity located within the muscle in spasm or in fascia, deep pressure on the trigger area, or touching it with a needle, reproduces a spontaneous pain at a distance, and infiltrating it locally with procaine eliminates the related reference of pain.'' She has shown that different parts of a skeletal muscle will have a specific referred pain pattern, a pattern that is consistent from one person to another. Travell has mapped these referred pain patterns of the head, illustrated in Figures 23D–2 through 23D–6, by experimentally injecting hypertonic saline intramuscularly in these areas and observing referred pain patterns from the injection sites. She has classified these areas located within the masticatory muscles as follows:

1. *Masseter muscle:* Superficial layer refers pain to the jaws, molar teeth, and gums. From the anterior border of the masseter muscle and upper part of this division of the muscle, pain is referred to the upper teeth; from the lower part, pain is referred to the lower molars. From trigger areas at the angle of the mandible, pain travels upward in and over the temporalis and around the outer portion of the eyebrow. Trigger areas in the deep layer of the masseter refer to the TMJ and deep in the ear.

2. *Temporalis muscle:* This muscle refers to the side of the head and to the maxillary teeth, depending on which area of the temporalis is injected. The anterior temporalis refers to the supraorbital ridge and maxillary incisors. The medial temporalis refers to the bicuspid area. The posterior temporalis refers to the upper molars and occiput.

3. *External pterygoid muscle:* Refers pain deep into the TMJ and maxillary region.

4. *Internal pterygoid muscle:* Refers mainly to structures within the mouth, tongue, and hard palate, and the TMJ neck muscles.

5. *Trapezius:* Suprascapular portion refers to the angle of the mandible, posterolateral neck, and mastoid process, temporal area, and back of orbit.

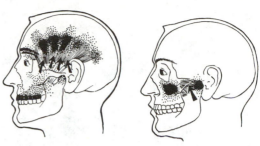

Fig 23D–2.—Left, composite pain reference pattern of the temporalis muscle. Trigger areas are indicated by *arrows;* their reference zones are indicated by the *stippled* and *black regions.* **Right,** composite pain reference pattern of the external pterygoid muscle. (Originally from Travell,[6] reproduced in Gelb.[15] Reproduced here by permission of W.B. Saunders Co.)

Spasms of the trapezius muscle causes ''stiff neck,'' with limitation of motion on the contralateral side.

6. *Sternocleidomastoid:* Refers to the forehead, supraorbital ridge, inner angle of the eye, middle ear, posterior auricular region, the point of the chin, and the pharynx, with diffuse pain in the cheek.

MYOFASCIAL PAIN DYSFUNCTION.—Laskin et al. have suggested a psychophysiologic theory of myofascial pain dysfunction, according to which stress and dental irritation may cause muscle hyperactivity, leading to muscle fatigue and myospasm (Fig 23D–7). They list four clinical signs of the TMJ dysfunction syndrome: pain, muscle dysfunction, clicking of the TMJ, and deviation or limited motion on opening.[7] Along with absence of radiographic changes in the TMJ are lack of tenderness

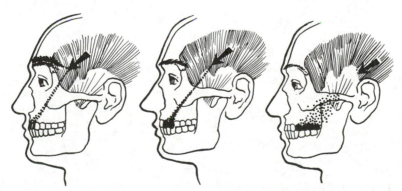

Fig 23D–3.—Specific trigger areas at three sites in the temporalis muscle, as observed in a case of facial neuralgia. Trigger areas were located at *arrows,* and pain was referred to the *black* and *stippled zones.* (Originally from Travell,[6] reproduced in Gelb.[15] Reproduced here by permission of W.B. Saunders Co.)

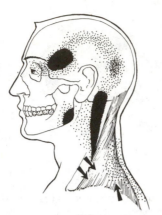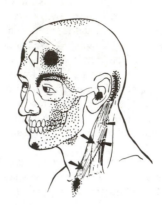

Fig 23D–4.—Left, composite pain reference pattern of the trapezius muscle, suprascapular region. Trigger areas are indicated
by *arrows;* pain reference zones are indicated
by *stippled* and *black* regions. **Right,** composite pain reference patterns of the clavicular and sternal divisions of the sternomastoid.
The sternal division refers pain mainly to
the cheek, eyebrow, pharynx, tongue, chin,
throat, and sternum. The clavicular division refers pain mainly to the forehead bilaterally, to
the posterior auricular region and deep in the
ear, and infrequently to the teeth. Trigger
areas are indicated by *arrows;* pain reference
zones are indicated by the *stippled* and *black*
regions. (Originally from Travell,[6] reproduced
in Gelb.[15] Reproduced here by permission of
W.B. Saunders Co.)

and pain in the TMJ on palpation through the external auditory meatus. Patients with psychological
stress may have increased clenching of the teeth or
bruxism, which may increase the intracapsular pressure in the TMJ, leading to a disturbance of proper
joint movement. This can result in internal derangements in the TMJ.

Teeth should interdigitate during swallowing and
mastication. When the teeth are in occlusion, the
TMJ and masticatory muscles must be relaxed. If
interference in the bite occurs as the mouth is
closed, the lower jaw will be proprioceptively
moved by the sensory input of the periodontal ligaments of the teeth, the TMJ, and the CNS. Efferents
to the masticatory muscles through the trigeminal
mechanism will position the jaw where the bite feels
good to the patient (habitual bite). However, the jaw
position, if due to malocclusion, drifted teeth, or
high dental fillings, may not be where the muscles
are relaxed. This complex behavior of the masticatory apparatus can set up referred pain patterns and
trigger points in the muscles, leading to chronic fatigued muscles, joint dysfunction, and pain. A removable, intraoral orthopedic repositioning appliance can be placed over the maxillary or mandibular
teeth, preventing interdigitation of the teeth and allowing the muscles of mastication to relax, thereby
resulting in improved muscle function. As a diagnostic tool, this apparatus will determine if the occlusion is a causative factor in the pain pattern.

Habit patterns have been shown to cause TMJ
disorders. Examples of this behavior include fingernail biting, pencil/pen chewing, or any habit that
keeps the jaw in a forward position. This can create
pain in the masticatory muscles, as a referred pain
pattern may be set up from the abnormal jaw posture over long periods of time. Another example
may be a secretary holding the telephone on the
shoulder for hours at a time or typing with the head

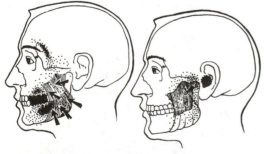

Fig 23D–5.—Pain reference patterns of the
masseter muscle. **Left,** superficial layer;
right, deep layer. Trigger areas are indicated by *arrows;* their pain reference zones
are indicated by *black* and *stippled* regions.
(Originally from Travell,[6] reproduced in Gelb.[15]
Reproduced here by permission of W.B. Saunders Co.)

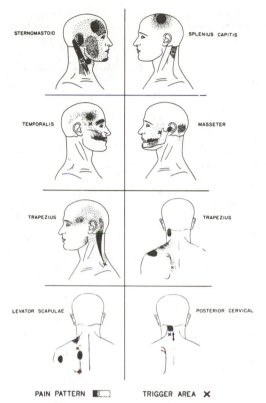

PAIN PATTERN ▨   TRIGGER AREA ✗

Fig 23D–6.—Zones of reference in the head and neck. *Solid black areas* indicate so-called essential zones, while *stippled areas* indicate spillover zones. The heavier the stippling, the more frequently this area is a zone of reference. (Originally from Travell J., Rinzler S.H.: *Postgrad. Med.* 11:425–427, 1952; reproduced in Gelb.[15] Reproduced here by permission of W.B. Saunders Co.)

in a flexed position. This can result in cervical problems with referred head pain.

Gelb and Tarte have evaluated symptoms of 200 TMJ dysfunction patients (Table 23D–1). The muscles most frequently found to be involved by spasm were the external pterygoids, the internal pterygoids, the masseter, and the temporalis. Gelb and Tarte also showed that preauricular pain was the major ear symptom, along with clicking as the next frequent TMJ symptom. Moreover, they showed that the temporalis muscle was the muscle most often associated with head pain in these patients.

Intracapsular Problems

Derangements of the TMJ can be caused by the articular disk being displaced anteriorly or anteromedially to the mandibular condyle, resulting in joint noises (clicking and popping), pain, dysfunction of jaw movements (limitation, deviation in movement, or catching), with the possibility of eventual osteoarthritic changes. This can be observed by arthrography of the TMJ.

A progressive degenerative process develops when the articular disk is displaced anteriorly.[8] Farrar and McCarty suggest that in the beginning of an internal derangement of the TMJ, posterior capsulitis is the initial finding. Later, an intermittent clicking can occur, which may be classified as early, intermediate, or late, depending on jaw opening position. This can eventually lead to a breakdown of the joint structures over a period of time. Moreover, if the articular disk is dislocated anteriorly without reduction, a chronic closed lock can occur. Eventually the condyle becomes seated more supe-

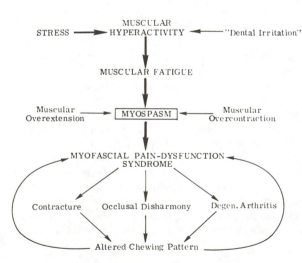

Fig 23D–7.—Etiology of the myofascial pain-dysfunction syndrome. Although three means of entry into the syndrome are shown, the *broad arrows* indicate the most common path. The mechanism whereby stress leads to myospasm is termed the psychophysiologic theory of the myofascial pain-dysfunction syndrome. (Modified from Laskin D.M.: Etiology of the pain-dysfunction syndrome, in Sarnat, Laskin: *The Temporomandibular Joint.* Springfield, Illinois, 1979. Used by permission.)

TABLE 23D–1.—SYMPTOMS OF 200 PATIENTS WITH TEMPOROMANDIBULAR JOINT DYSFUNCTION*

	AGE GROUP (YR)								
	1–10	11–20	21–30	31–40	41–50	51–60	61–70	71–80	TOTAL
Men	1	6	10	19	11	9	1	0	57
Women	0	14	31	32	32	24	8	2	143
Muscles in muscle spasm									
Internal pterygoids	1	20	38	44	38	30	7	0	178
External pterygoids	1	20	41	50	41	32	8	2	195
Masseter	0	13	30	39	36	30	9	1	158
Temporalis	1	16	29	35	35	27	6	2	151
Sternomastoid	1	12	34	28	33	25	3	2	138
Posterior cervical	1	9	31	41	37	27	5	2	153
Mylohyoid	0	4	16	23	32	27	3	1	106
Trapezius	1	6	18	33	26	16	9	2	111
Others	0	12	31	31	23	17	2	0	116
Ear symptoms									
Tinnitus	0	0	6	26	27	25	7	1	92
Hearing loss	0	0	1	0	4	5	8	2	20
Preauricular pain	1	10	35	22	25	28	3	2	103
Auricular pain	0	3	10	2	6	7	4	0	32
TMJ symptoms									
Clicking	1	15	24	21	38	8	16	1	124
Crepitation	0	0	0	4	7	5	8	2	26
Pain	0	11	10	14	12	9	5	2	63
Bruxism	0	8	17	13	4	6	3	0	51
Head pain									
Facial	0	0	5	4	2	1	2	0	14
Occipital	0	0	3	6	3	4	2	0	16
Cervical	1	14	20	30	11	8	4	2	90
Temporal	1	8	27	47	32	14	4	1	134
Vertigo	0	4	2	6	3	3	4	1	23

*From Gelb H., Tarte J.: A two-year clinical evaluation of 200 cases of chronic headache: The craniocervical-mandibular syndrome. *JADA* 91:1230, 1975. Reproduced by permission.

riorly in the fossa, leading to possible herniation of posterior ligaments with degenerative changes of the condyle. This change can be observed radiographically. At this point, the patient usually has pain and limited opening with deviation of opening toward the affected side. The disk will not retract back to its normal position, and over a period of time degenerative arthritis may occur.

Arthritis

Osteoarthritis (degenerative arthritis) of the TMJ can occur from prolonged displacement or distraction of the articular disk, as was just mentioned. Kreutziger and Mahan[9] suggest that osteoarthritis with pain and tenderness can occur over the head and the posterior aspect of the condyle. Pain may also be present with function and is most severe with wide opening. This discomfort usually increases during the day and is found to be exacerbated by fatigue or emotional stress. In later stages, pain may be present continually.

Radiographically, one may find changes in the joint space, anatomical changes in the mandibular condyle or eminence, and changes in the subchondreal bone. It has been suggested that the etiological factors for osteoarthritis of the TMJ are usually multiple, "with a degeneration of the joint probably due to repetitive impulse loading.[9] Degenerative changes with aging and cumulative trauma, abusive oral habits, occlusal imbalances, traumatic injuries, psychogenic factors, and endocrine imbalances are the most common causative agents."

Rheumatoid arthritis can cause similar pains as osteoarthritis. The differentiation between the two will show the following characteristics, as described by Kreutziger and Mahan.[10] Rheumatoid arthritis tends to be a more symmetric disease, whereas osteoarthritis is usually unilateral. In rheumatoid arthritis the disease progresses in the synovial tissues initially, and these tissues are converted to pannus cells, which release enzymes that destroy the articular surface of the mandibular condyle. Thus, erosion of the condyle and rheumatoid arthritis begin at the periphery and extends toward the center. In osteoarthritis, the process of degeneration begins at the center of the condyle, with subsequent flattening of the articular surface and occasionally the formation of osteophytes at the anterior margins. Fibrosing ankylosis of the TMJ, which is rarely observed in osteoarthritis, is found in rheumatoid arthritis. Moreover, in rheumatoid arthritis one may find shortening of the mandibular condyle, which will result in an anterior open bite. Therefore, an adult with a normal occlusion but who is developing an anterior open bite or a unilateral open bite should be suspected of having an arthritic condition unless proved otherwise.

Bony Cavities

Ratner et al.[11] have found a relationship between postextraction sites, idiopathic trigeminal neuralgia, and atypical facial pains. His research has shown that bony cavities may be found in the alveolar bone in patients who have had teeth extracted and later experience atypical facial pain. In these patients, histopathologic examination has shown that the extraction sites were composed of a highly vascular bone with an abnormal healing response, along with mixed aerobic and anaerobic flora. Recommended treatment consists of vigorous curettage of the bony cavities and the administration of antibiotics to aid in repair of these sites.

Radiographic Examination of the TMJ

In the radiographic investigation of patients with TMJ disease, the following modalities have been used: transcranial x-rays, tomographic x-rays, segmental vertex, lateral pharyngeal view, and computerized tomography (CT). The transcranial view shows the condyle at a 25° angle to the sagittal plane and usually shows more of the lateral aspect of the condyle, where degenerative changes most often occur. There is controversy as to the validity of the transcranial radiograph in evaluating condylar position relative to the temporal fossa. However, when one correlates clinical findings with this radiographic investigation, useful diagnostic information

can be gained. Posterior positioning of the condyle viewed on a transcranial x-ray film along with posterior capsulitis and pain on dysfunction with clicking may suggest an anterior disk displacement. Segmental vertex views will show if there is impingement of the coronoid process. Also, panoramic x-ray films will show if hyperplasia or hypoplasia of the condyle is present along with an elongated coronoid process. At present, tomography is the best technique for evaluating arthritic changes in the TMJ in reference to arthritic changes. CT is being used as the most recent x-ray procedure for evaluating TMJ displacements. It is possible with this modality to observe an anterior thickening that may correlate with arthrographic and tomographic changes.[12] However, the CT scan will not show a perforation of the posterior ligament or the dynamics of disk movement, as can be seen with fluoroscopy during arthrography.

Arthrography

At present, arthrography is the main diagnostic procedure for evaluating disk displacement. Recently Wilkes[13] and McCarty,[14] using arthrography, showed that it is possible to diagnose disk displacement or dislocation by this method. The arthrographic technique yields much diagnostic information. Either the lower joint space or both joint spaces are injected with a small amount of water-soluble iodine dye, which will outline the articular disk. With a normal disk position, a small amount of dye will protrude in the anterior compartment. As the jaw is opened, a sigmoidal configuration in the posterior portion with complete absence of dye in the anterior portion is observed. However, as progressive changes occur in the TMJ, there will be prolonged stagnation of dye in the anterior compartment on mouth opening until a click occurs, indicating a reduction of an anteriorly displaced TMJ disk, at which point the sigmoidal configuration in the posterior compartment will be present. However, in the locked position, the anterior compartment will have a considerable amount of dye present, and without reduction, this dye will not return to the posterior compartment. It should be noted that there is a possibility of false positive results on arthrography. Therefore, not only should one be able to compare arthrographic findings with clinical findings, but surgery on the TM joint should not be contemplated based on x-ray films and arthrograms alone. The technique for arthrography of the TMJ is sometimes difficult. Even the skilled examiner may experience problems with patient management or technique. Therefore, if an arthrogram is obtained that does not clearly show classic findings, surgery on the TMJ should not be attempted until a repeated arthrogram shows typical appearances. A CT scan may also be useful in this situation for providing additional information when surgery is in question. Our criteria for TMJ surgery is not a displacement of the disk, but the severity of the patient's pain and amount of dysfunction in jaw movements (chewing, talking, etc.).

Examination

When examining the facial pain patient, one should assess the muscles of mastication and their relationship to occlusion and TMJ dysfunction. Dysfunction of the masticatory apparatus is usually due to some discrepancy in the manner in which the muscles, teeth, and TMJ interact. When one or all of the closing muscles of the mandible are in spasm, there is limited jaw opening. This opening is measured at the incisal edges of the anterior teeth, normally within the range of 35–45 mm. However, one must determine whether the restrictive motion is due to muscle dysfunction, disk derangements, etc. If the patient can move his mandible laterally approximately 8–10 mm from the normal closing position and has limited opening, then it is likely the problem is in the muscle. As in other areas of the body, diagnostic injections of a local anesthetic into the muscle in question and subsequent relief of pain or dysfunction may be used to differentiate this pain pattern in the deeper muscles of the face. The patient can be asked to clench his teeth for a short period of time, and if the pain increases with this maneuver, then the problem may involve the closing masticatory muscles, periodontal structures, and/or teeth abscesses. When a tongue blade is held between the posterior teeth on the painful side, resulting in a decrease in the pain, dental disease or closing muscles involved in the patient's pain pattern may be excluded, since biting on the tongue blade would only increase this pain sensation.

Disk displacement and joint disease should be evaluated as follows. If opening of the mouth results in deviation of the mandible to one side, one should first determine whether the patient's dysfunction is on the ipsilateral side of jaw deviation. Popping or clicking of the TMJ can be indicative of internal disk derangements. One should note the timing of the click, which may occur on opening and/or closing. A late opening click may be indicative of chronic ligament problems, which may not be treatable on a conservative basis. Normal joints have no noise or restrictive motion. If the noise is present without pain, there should be an investigation on a conservative basis since further problems may result later in life. Grating noises of crepitus in the TMJ may be indicative of changes in the condylar head or disk as a result of arthritic changes.

In the differential diagnosis of TMJ disorders, a removable dental orthopedic appliance that allows the muscles of mastication to relax and change the position of the jaw joint in the fossa should be utilized to evaluate the patient's pain. If the pain decreases with this apparatus, it is possible that the problem is caused by a discrepancy in the occlusion, TMJ, or muscles that were not in proper harmony. No change in the patient's symptoms should make one hesitant to manage this problem aggressively. Irreversible procedures have at times been performed, including capping of the teeth, surgical procedures, reshaping of the teeth (equilibration), and orthodontics.

One of the most difficult areas to evaluate is the split tooth syndrome. Here, the pain occurs with chewing, and clinically one cannot see the situation on x-ray films or through diagnostic testing of the teeth, since many times the fractures are internal. One can become suspicious if, when the subject bites on a hard object, the pain is reproduced. A split tooth can refer pain to the head and neck and be a continual source of pain. If the previously mentioned procedures in the diagnostic workup of facial pain does not stop or change the patient's symptoms, one should consider causative factors not related to the dental apparatus.

Treatment of Orofacial Pain Related to TMJ Disorders

In the treatment of TMJ disease, one should initially utilize reversible palliative therapeutic procedures. In the palliative approach, the patient is asked to follow a soft diet, restrict jaw movement, and use hot and cold packs on the area. The physician may inject trigger points and use coolant spray-and-stretch techniques. Oral medications such as anti-inflammatory agents, muscle relaxants, and pain medications are considered palliative treatment, as are muscle therapy modalities such as high-voltage galvanic stimulation and ultrasound of the TMJ area, along with jaw exercises to harmonize muscle dysfunction. If the pain or dysfunction is decreased following muscle therapy modalities, muscle dysfunction was probably the cause of the problem. If such modalities do not correct the problem, the primary etiology of the pain may be intracapsular or a stress-related psychological problem. Vitamin therapy may be instituted if the patient has a dietary deficiency. Biofeedback and acupuncture are used along with myofunctional therapy to change tongue posture, which may play a role in head and neck pain. Also, TENS units may be used to alter the pain pattern experienced, as is done for other types of pain throughout the body.

For definitive dental treatment of pain, the following irreversible procedures are available: equilibration of the teeth (reshaping the teeth to follow the harmony of the TMJ muscles), restoring the teeth to proper vertical dimension for control of myofascial tension, orthodontics, dental restorative procedures, permanent splints, orthognathic surgery, or a combination of these procedures. If the patient has an intracapsular problem, such as bony or fibrous ankylosis or a dislocated disk, oral surgery may be the treatment of choice. Cortisone can be injected along with a local anesthetic into the TMJ for control of acute inflammatory reaction and pain exacerbation. Not more than one or two injections should be given because of possible osteonecrosis. Chronic subluxation (in which the mandibular condyle is held beyond the articular eminence and is locked in an open position) may require surgical intervention. In patients with arthritis, especially juvenile rheumatoid arthritis, there is destruction of the condylar head, resulting in exacerbation and an open bite with continual changes in the occlusion due to muscle spasm. Definitive treatment should not be done to this particular patient. A dental orthopedic appliance can be helpful in providing masticatory muscle relaxation. This appliance can be periodically adjusted as the patient's bite changes due to their rheumatoid problem.

Tumors of the TMJ are rare but do occur. Also, psychological factors alone could cause the patient to clench the teeth and could result in myofascial pain and dysfunction. Although the symptoms occur in the dental apparatus, the cause is psychological. This must be treated by the appropriate medical specialist (psychologist or psychiatrist). The patient will not get better with dental treatment in this case.

The oral surgical procedure for an anterior disk dislocation usually involves plication of the posterior diskal ligament.[14] When the disk is repositioned over the condyle, the mandible may be repositioned down approximately 1–2 mm from the space now occupied by the disk in the fossa. This results in an occlusal opening on the operative side in an unbalanced bite. This should be temporarily corrected by a dental orthopedic appliance for stabilization of the jaw-joint complex. Once surgery has been performed on the TMJ, physical therapy should be undertaken as soon as possible to prevent fibrosing ankylosis from occurring and to break up any adhesions that may have formed from the surgical procedure. Patients should be instructed in daily exercises to open at least 40 mm, or more if possible. Eventually some type of dental treatment will be necessary to restore the occlusion to proper function.

REFERENCES

1. Rees L.A.: The structure and function of the mandibular joint. *Br. Dent. J.* 96:125–133, 1954.
2. Munro R.L.: Electromyography of muscles of mastication, in Griffin C.J., Harris R. (eds.): *The Temporomandibular Joint Syndrome.* Basel, Karger, 1975, pp. 87–116.
3. McNamara J.A.: The independent functions of the two heads of the lateral pterygoid muscle. *Am. J. Anat.* 138:197–206, 1973.
4. Vitti M., Basmajian J.V.: Integrated actions of masticatory muscles: Simultaneous EMG from eight intramuscular electrodes. *Ant. Rec.* 187:173–189, 1977.
5. Basmajian J.V.: *Muscles Alive,* ed. 4. Baltimore, Williams & Wilkins G., 1978, p. 385.
6. Travell J.J.: Temporomandibular joint pain referred from the head and neck. *Prosthet. Dent.* 10:745–763, 1960.
7. Laskin D.M., Sarnat B.G., Laskin D.M.: *The Temporomandibular Joint,* ed. 3. Springfield, Ill., Charles C Thomas, publisher, 1975, p. 234.
8. Farrar W.B., McCarty W.L.J.: *A Clinical Outline of Temporomandibular Joint Diagnosis and Treatment,* ed. 7. Montgomery, Alabama, Normandie Publications, 1982, p. 87.
9. Kreutziger K.L., Mahan P.E.: Temporomandibular degenerative joint disease. *Oral Surg.* 40:165–182, 1975.
10. Kreutziger K.L., Mahan P.E.: Temporomandibular degenerative joint disease. *Oral Surg.* 40:297–319, 1975.
11. Ratner E.J., Person P., Kleinman D.J.: Jaw bone cavities and trigeminal and atypical facial neuralgias. *Oral Surg.* 48:3–20, 1979.
12. Helms C.A.: Computerized tomography of the meniscus of the temporomandibular joint: Preliminary observations. *Radiology* 145:719–722, 1982.
13. Wilkes C.H.: Structural and functional alterations of

the temporomandibular joint. *Northwest Dent.* 57:287–294, 1978.

14. McCarty W.L.: Diagnosis and treatment of internal derangements of the articular disc and mandibular condyles, in Solberg W.K., Clark G.T. (eds.): *Temporomandibular Joint Problems*. Chicago, Quintessence Publishing Co., 1980, pp. 145–178.

15. Gelb H.: *Clinical Management of Head, Neck and TMJ Dysfunction: A Multidisciplinary Approach to Diagnosis and Treatment*. Philadelphia, W.B. Saunders Co., 1977.

23E / Facial Pain of Sympathetic Origin

JAMES C. PHERO, D.M.D.
JOHN S. McDONALD, D.D.S., M.S
GARY S. ROBINS, D.M.D.

COMMON CAUSES OF pain of sympathetic origin in the region of the face are causalgia, reflex sympathetic dystrophy, herpes zoster, and postherpetic neuralgia and psychogenic states. Management of psychogenic pain is described elsewhere in this book.

CAUSALGIA

The pain of causalgia is continuous, with variable intensity. On the superficial burning sensation in the region are superimposed deep shooting, stabbing or crushing pains. The pain is aggravated by any stimulus to the region that increases sympathetic outflow. Trophic changes similar to those seen in reflex sympathetic dystrophy are a striking feature of the condition. The skin is often warm, dry, and erythematous, but periods of vasoconstriction and hyperhidrosis occur frequently.

Causalgia is thought to involve a combination of peripheral and central mechanisms. In peripheral tissues, an abnormal interaction between sensory and sympathetic nerve endings or the release of pain-producing substances may play a role. Injured nerve segments may produce spontaneous neural activity which may spread to sensory fibers across demyelinated axons. Selective damage to large afferent fibers could lead to self-sustaining or spontaneous activity within pain systems of the CNS.

REFLEX SYMPATHETIC DYSTROPHY

Following trauma or surgery, or spontaneously in some disease states, patients may develop pain, autonomic dysfunction, delayed functional recovery, and dystrophic changes. Reflex autonomic changes have been proposed as the pathologic basis of the syndrome, but other factors such as alterations in central pain transmission and altered production, release, or reuptake of neurotransmitters may be involved.

Management of Causalgia and Reflex Sympathetic Dystrophy

Patients generally experience pain disproportional to the extent of injury, and the pain is usually burning in quality. Hyperesthesia is the most consistent finding. Hyperhidrosis, cool skin, edema, and cyanosis are common findings but are not always present. Early in the course of the disease the affected region may be warm and dry. Smooth shiny skin, altered hair growth patterns, and bone dermineralization occur late in the process. Differences in skin temperature between involved and uninvolved extremities help to confirm the diagnosis.

Treatment consists of stellate ganglion blocks for unilateral facial and upper extremity involvement. Pain relief after sympthetic blocks confirms the diagnosis, particulary if there is little or no response to placebo injection. Initial management involves a series of six blocks 3–7 days apart. If there is a positive response, the blocks are continued until symptoms are minimal to absent or until no further improvement is obtained. Three to six blocks will usually produce dramatic and lasting improvement if treatment is started early. Long-standing cases tend to be resistant to blocks but may respond to transcutaneous electrical nerve stimulation (TENS), psychotropic medication, and psychotherapy.

Rationale for Sympathetic Nerve Blockade

Signs of hyperpathia (hyperesthesia and/or hyperalgesia), neurovascular instability (vasoconstriction with cyanosis and edema or vasodilation), sudomotor disturbances (hyperhidrosis, hypohidrosis, or anhidrosis), and pilomotor changes are indications for diagnostic or therapeutic sympathetic nerve blocks. The quality of pain is burning, throbbing, dull, or in some cases even sharp and stabbing.[1] Characteristically, the pattern of distribution of this constant pain and of the hyperpathic area does not correspond to the pattern of segmental or peripheral nerve innervation. Therefore, physicians who are not familiar with these pain syndromes do not accept the patient's symptom report and search for neurotic or hysterical traits. Nonrecognition and nontreatment of these conditions regularly result in trophic tissue changes which eventually become irreversible. It is therefore essential to initiate treatment with sympathetic blocks promptly after the onset of pain and related symptoms.

When a local anesthetic block is effective, the patient notes a long effective period of relief. The local anesthetic blocks pain receptors (nociceptors) and thus prevents transformation and coding of nociceptive impulses in these specialized nerve endings; it blocks nociceptive impulse transmission in those efferent fibers associated with sympathetic fibers and thus prevents such impulses from reaching

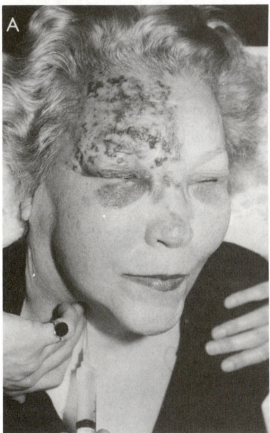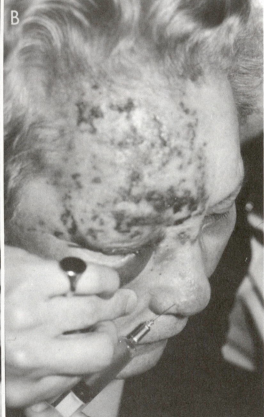

Fig 23E–1.—A 72-year-old woman reported a 1-week sensation of "dullness" over the nose and earache, followed in 5 days by vesicle formation over the right forehead, eye, and nose. She was treated with intralesional injections of bupivacaine and dexamethasone *(left)*, as well as a series of seven stellate ganglion blocks using a bupivacaine/lidocaine mixture *(right)*. Medications included ibuprofen q.i.d. and amitriptyline h.s. Healing was uneventful, with no loss of motor function and no evidence of postherpetic neuralgia. (Courtesy of John McDonald, D.D.S.)

the CNS; it blocks sympathetic pathways and thus interrupts sympathetic reflex mechanisms, which act as positive feedback mechanisms and are usually active in painful conditions.[3] It also reduces or eliminates the increased skeletal muscle activity, which contributes to maintaining the vicious cycle of pain. Regional anesthetic blocks possibly influence higher cortical functions.[3] The pain-relieving effects of regional anesthetic blocks often outlast the pharmacologic impulse-blocking effect of the local anesthetic.[4, 5] This prolonged analgesic effect is presumably due to interruption of the vicious cycle. In the treatment of pain, the goal of regional analgesia is interruption of C and A delta fibers and of efferent sympathetic fibers.[6] This requires only low concentrations of local anesthetics such as 0.5% lidocaine or mepivacaine or 0.125%–0.25% bupivacaine. Because of the long duration of action of bupivacaine, an almost continuous small fiber blockade can be achieved with blocks performed once daily.[4, 7] The technique of stellate ganglion blocks is described in chapter 34.

ACUTE HERPES ZOSTER AND POSTHERPETIC NEURALGIA

Clinically, the virus causes an acute vesicular eruption along the trigeminal nerve, most commonly along its first division. Before or with the eruption of vesicles, there is often severe pain in the distribution of the affected nerve that is exacerbated by touching or stimulating the skin. After a period of several weeks, postherpetic neuralgia may develop in the scarred region from healed herpetic lesions where the skin is hyperpathic. The pain is described as burning and is often quite severe. The duration of pain without treatment is variable, but is usually self-limiting within several years.

Herpes zoster may also affect the facial nerve. The Ramsay Hunt syndrome occurs when inflammation of the geniculate ganglion causes vesicular eruption confined to the pinna, external auditory meatus, and ear drum. This results in severe otalgia with associated facial paralysis and vertigo (see Fig 22–6, Plate 5).

There is increasing evidence that sympathetic blocks performed during the acute stage of herpes zoster shorten the eruptive phase of the disease and decrease the incidence of postherpetic neuralgia. Early treatment is especially important in elderly patients, in whom the incidence of long-lasting postherpetic pain is extremely high. Stellate ganglion blocks should be performed repeatedly. Subcutaneous infiltration with a local anesthetic–steroid mixture provides relief and promotes healing. The subcutaneous infiltration is performed on a regular basis and may be combined with TENS, analgesics, and psychotropic drugs (Fig 23E–1) (Chap. 22).

REFERENCES

1. Schenk C: *Objektivierung Sympathischer Blockaden,* thesis. Mainz, West Germany, Johannes Gutenberg-Universitat, 1978.
2. Zimmerman M.: Neurophysiology of Nociception. Pain and pain therapy, in Bonica J.J., Ventafridda V. (eds.): *Advances in Pain Research and Therapy.* New York, Raven Press, 1979.
3. Turk H., Frey R., Gerbershagen H.U.: Regional anesthesia as a psychotherapeutic method: A new approach to the psychic system (an experimental study). Read before the First World Congress on Pain, Florence, Italy, Sept. 5–8, 1975.
4. Gerbershagen H.U., Panhans C., Schwarz R. (eds.): *Regionalanasthesia in Schmerzdiagnostik und Therapie.* Berlin, Acron, 1978.
5. Gross D: *Therapeutische Lokalanasthesia.* Stuttgart, Hippokrates Verlag, 1972.
6. de Jong R: Theoretical aspects of pain: Bizarre pain phenomena during low spinal anesthesia. *Anesthesiology* 24:628, 1963.
7. Nolte H., Meyer J., Kopf B., et al.: Klinische und Elektrophysiologische Parameter zur Differenzierung der Wirkung von Lokalanesthetika. *Anaesthesist* 23:165, 1974.

23F / Less Common Syndromes Causing Pain in the Head and Neck

JAMES C. PHERO, D.M.D.
JOHN S. McDONALD, D.D.S., M.S.
GARY S. ROBINS, D.M.D.

SYNDROMES may be classified as eponymic, i.e., bearing the name of one or more individuals who contributed to the description of the subject, etiologic-descriptive. Currently the tendency is to use the etiologic description of the syndrome. Syndromes may be caused by tumors, trauma, or congenital or hereditary conditions, or may be the result of genetic abnormalities.

AURICULOTEMPORAL NERVE SYNDROME

In auriculotemporal nerve syndrome, also known as the Frey, Frey-Baillarger, and Dupuy syndrome,[1, 3] the patient experiences flushing and sweating on the involved side of the face, chiefly in the temporal area, during eating. The severity of the sweating may be increased by eating tart foods. Sometimes pain and sensory disturbances occur in the tragus and mandible.

The syndrome is caused by trauma to the auriculotemporal nerve, such as that incurred in suppurative parotitis, a gunshot wound to the parotid gland, septicemia, mandibular resection, or conservative parotidectomy (reported in 80% of cases). Following the trauma to the auriculotemporal nerve, the sweat glands and vessels of the skin over its distribution are denervated producing sensory disturbances. In the process of regeneration, parasympathetic nerves become misdirected and grow along sympathetic pathways. Because the sympathetic endings on the sweat glands are cholinergic, the parasympathetic nerves activate the glands. Therefore, a gustatory stimulus produces sweating and flushing. The fully developed syndrome appears 2 months to 2 years following the trauma and usually remains for life. Treatment by intracranial division of the auriculotemporal nerve has been reported to be successful.

CHARLIN'S SYNDROME

Charlin's syndrome, also known as ciliary neuralgia, nasal nerve syndrome, nasociliary neuralgia, and supraorbital neuralgia,[4, 6] is a form of migraine caused by vasomotor spasm of the middle meningeal artery that result in a violent pain affecting the orbit, temple, forehead, nose, and maxillary regions. The attacks may last 15–60 minutes, tend to spread to the lower half of the head, and may be accompanied by emesis. Suicide because of pain has been reported.

Essential features of Charlin's syndrome are paroxysmal pain in one eye and on the ipsilateral side of the face; profuse watery rhinorrhea, keratitis, and iritis; congestion of the nasal mucosa; and immediate relief of ocular pain and rapid disappearance of keratitis and iritis after cocainization of the anterior half of the lateral wall of the affected nostril.

Treatment for relief of symptoms is cocainization of the anterior ethmoidal nerve in the anterior part of the nasal fossa.

COSTEN'S SYNDROME

Costen, an otolaryngologist, attempted to relate cases of impaired hearing, tinnitus, facial and temporal neuritis, otalgia, and glossodynia to temporomandibular joint dysfunction caused by overclosure of the mandible. The current consensus is that the concept of Costen's syndrome should be abandoned, because the anatomical and physiologic foundation for the various symptoms cannot be substantiated.[7, 9] Temporomandibular joint dysfunction was discussed in detail in chapter 23D.

CRANIOFACIAL PAIN SYNDROME

Craniofacial pain syndrome, alternatively primary atypical facial neuralgia,[10, 11] is a controversial term denoting craniofacial pain somewhere at the transition between classic migraine and trigeminal neuralgia. Many investigators regard it as a variant of vascular headache. Engle classifies it as a hysterical conversion syndrome.

Classic features of this syndrome are a constant aching, throbbing, burning pain of mild to severe nature in the face, scalp, and neck which may spread to the arms; exacerbation during the night; predominance in middle-aged women under stress; absence of trigger zone; and no familial tendency.

Treatment by aggressive procedures is futile. A rational approach to treatment consists of a careful, conservative, multidisciplinary pain management program. Underlying local disease (ear, nose, throat, dental, or neurologic) must be excluded. In this condition, the entire state of the patient and the emotional components of the illness require detailed evaluation and management. Pharmacologic therapy that includes antidepressants and psychosedatives may be indicated.

STYLOID-STYLOHYOID SYNDROME

The pain of styloid-stylohyoid syndrome, also known as Eagle's syndrome, is classically experienced as constant throughout convalescence following tonsillectomy. A sore throat persists during ensuing years. The patient has a foreign body sensation in the throat and difficulty swallowing. Pain is often referred to the ear.[12-14]

An elongated styloid process or processes is the cause of this syndrome. The pharyngeal pains result from stretching or fibrosis that occurs during the posttonsillectomy healing in the sensory nerve endings of cranial nerves V, VII, IX, and X. The diagnosis of an elongated styloid process is made by palpation of the tonsillar areas and by x-ray. Treatment is surgical excision of the elongated styloid process.

If this syndrome is accompanied by headache, the styloid process is impinging on the internal or external carotid artery. This diminishes the caliber of these vessels and irritates sympathetic nerve fibers in the arterial wall.

Impairment of the internal carotid artery results in parietal pain and symptoms along the distribution of the ophthalmic artery. Impairment of the external carotid artery produces pain suborbitally along the path supplied by the artery.

GLOSSOPHARYNGEAL NEURALGIA

Paroxysmal stabbing pain of about 30 seconds' duration followed by a burning sensation lasting 2–5 minutes is characteristic of glossopharyngeal neuralgia. The pain is felt in the posterior tongue, pharynx, and soft palate and extends to the ear.[15-17] A trigger zone is usually located on the lateral wall of the pharynx, at the base of the tongue, or in the area of the external ear posterior to the mandibular ramus. Movement of the tongue, yawning, or coughing may trigger the pain. The resulting pain is intense and severe. It is usually followed by homolateral tearing and salivation. Cocainization of the lateral pharyngeal wall is useful in ascertaining the presence of a true glossopharyngeal neuralgia syndrome.

An idiopathic type of this syndrome exists in which the majority of symptoms subside after the fifth decade. In younger patients, organic causes may be anomalous arteries at the cerebellopontine angle, arachnoiditis, perineural fibrosis, elongation of the styloid process, or viral infection. In persistent cases, surgical correction may be indicated.

HORNER'S SYNDROME

Horner's syndrome is characterized by miosis due to paresis of the dilator fibers of the pupil, ptosis due to paresis of the smooth muscle elevator of the upper lid, anhidrosis and vasodilation over the face due to interruption of sudomotor and vasomotor control, and facial pain.[18-20]

Horner's syndrome is an indication of a primary disease process. Lesions in the brain stem or the cervical or high thoracic cord can produce this syndrome. Involvement of the carotid sympathetic plexus by lesions of the gasserian ganglion or internal carotid artery aneurysm may also produce a Horner's response. Treatment entails surgical elimination of the cause.

HUNT'S SYNDROME

Hunt's syndrome, also known as geniculate ganglion syndrome, herpes zoster oticus, herpes zoster auricularis, Ramsey-Hunt syndrome, involves herpes zoster infection of the geniculate ganglion. Zoster lesions of the external ear and the oral mucosa are observed. A deep pain occurs in the cleft behind the ear between the pinna and the mastoid process. Pain may then radiate to involve the face, ear, neck and occipital areas. The pain may be unilateral, paroxysmal, or constant. The pain usually precedes the appearance of the zoster vesicles. Intraorally the zoster vesicles may involve the peritonsillar region, oropharynx, and posterolateral third of the tongue, with associated pain.[21]

As the disease progresses, swelling of the ganglion in the bony facial canal may produce facial palsy of the Bell type.

The geniculate ganglion of the nervus intermedius supplies cutaneous and mucosal regions as well as the ganglia of cranial nerves IX and X. The peripheral sensory distribution of the nervus intermedius lies in areas also supplied by sensory fibers of cranial nerves V and X. This results in a possible overlap of symptoms.

PAIN OF THE EAR

Otalgia can be either primary or secondary in origin. Primary otalgia is caused by pathologic conditions involving the ear, while secondary otalgia is pain referred to the ear from another site. At least 50% of all pain experienced in the ear originates from another site. Although otalgia may signify serious disease, in many cases the amount of pain experienced is out of proportion to the seriousness of the disease causing it. Also, earaches may have multiple causes, necessitating a thorough ear examination before a definitive diagnosis is reached.

Any structure innervated by the nerves supplying the ear (cranial nerves V, IX, and X, cervical nerves I, II, and III, as well as sympathetic and parasympathetic nerves) can refer pain to the ear. Pain may be referred to the ear from the larynx, pharynx, oral cavity (deep masseter, sternocleidomastoid, facial muscles), temporomandibular joints, sinuses, esophagus, bronchus, lung cervical plexus, and thoracic vasculation.[22]

Disorders of the temporomandibular joint are a frequent cause of otalgia, with the patient often perceiving pain deep within the ear and not in the joint itself. Traumatic occlusion of the teeth, tooth sensitivity, dental infection, and even impacted or unerupted teeth may present as otalgia. Elongation of the styloid process or ossification of the stylohyoid ligament may have ear pain as one of the presenting symptoms.

The essential step in therapy lies in correct diagnosis. Treatment is dictated by the etiology of the pain.

PLUMMER-VINSON SYNDROME

Plummer-Vinson syndrome, also known as iron deficiency syndrome, is a manifestation of iron deficiency that occurs chiefly in women in the fourth and fifth decades of life. Symptoms include a smooth painful tongue, fissures at the corner of the mouth, dysphagia resulting from esophageal stricture, a lemon-tinted pallor of the skin, achlorhydria, and atrophy of the buccal, glossopharyngeal, and esophageal mucous membranes. The cause of the syndrome is achlorhydria in the stomach resulting in the faulty absorption of iron. Treatment of the anemia consists of iron therapy and high protein diets.[23-25]

RAEDER'S SYNDROME

Raeder's syndrome, also known as paratrigeminal neuralgia, paratrigeminal paralysis, and paratrigeminal syndrome, is rare and is characterized by pain in or around the eye accompanied by an incomplete Horner's syndrome (miosis and ptosis without enophthalmos and sweating of the face) and paralysis of the trigeminal nerve. This syndrome also bears a close relationship to cluster headache, except that Raeder's syndrome is due to lesions near the base of the middle cranial fossa with damage to cranial nerve V.

Two symptom groups occur. Patients with the migrainous and reflex type have a past history of headache with recurrence of symptoms. The cause of this type is focal irritation, usually from infection (antrum, dental abscess, otitis).

The second type is a symptomatic type with no history of headache and a sudden onset of symptoms. The cause is an internal carotid aneurysm, congenital abnormality of the carotid, trauma to the base of the skull, metastatic tumors, or primary tumors.

SLUDER'S SYNDROME

Sluder's syndrome, also known as lower-half headache, lower facial neuralgia syndrome, Sluder's neuralgia, and sphenopalatine ganglion neuralgia, is an uncommon facial neuralgia characterized by severe pain in the lower half of the face, below the eyebrows. The pain is unilateral, constant, and boring. It may be referred to the eye, nose, maxillary teeth, ear, zygoma, palate, pharynx, shoulder, and arm. Rhinorrhea, lacrimation, sneezing, photophobia, and salivation may occur. No trigger zone is present. The distribution and duration of pain vary and may simulate Horton's histaminic syndrome. There is some controversy at this time as to whether Sluder's syndrome is a distinct clinical entity.[28]

The cause of Sluder's syndrome is thought to be involvement of the sphenopalatine ganglion from an irritation such as sinusitis. The resulting pain is thought to be neurovascular in distribution and therefore visceral in origin and type. Involved areas correspond to areas supplied by blood vessels receiving autonomic motor and visceral sensory fibers by route of the sphenopalatine ganglion.

VAIL'S SYNDROME

Vail's syndrome, or vidian neuralgia, is characterized by severe paroxysmal attacks of pain involving the nose, face, eye, ear, head, neck, and shoulder. Women are most commonly affected, and the pain is usually nocturnal. It is thought that this condition arises from an infection of the sphenoidal sinus, with inflammation of the vidian nerve, which spreads to the sphenopalatine or geniculate ganglion. Another theory suggests vasodilation of the internal maxillary artery as the causative factor.[29]

REFERENCES

1. Frey L.: Le syndrome du nerf auricolotemporal. *Rev. Neurol. (Paris)* 2:97–104, 1923.
2. Daly R.F.: New observations regarding the auriculotemporal syndrome. *Neurology* 17:1159–1168, 1967.
3. Ven Dishoeck H.A.E.: The auriculo-temporal or Frey syndrome and tympanic neuroectomy. *Laryngoscope* 78:122–131, 1968.
4. Charlin C.: Sindrome del neavionasal. *Dia Médico-Buenos Aires* 2:839, 1970.
5. Chernikova T.V.: Charlin syndrome: Case. *Vêstnic Oftalmologii* 7:398–401, 1935.
6. Ferrannini G.: Charlin's syndrome. *Ann. Ophthalmol.* 95:807–811, 1969.
7. Costen J.B.: A syndrome of ear and sinus symptoms dependent upon disturbed function of the temporomandibular joint. *Ann. Otol. Rhinol. Laryngol.* 43:1–15, 1934.
8. Costen J.B.: Classification and treatment of temporomandibular joint problems. *J. Michigan Med. Soc.* 55:673–677, 1956.
9. Freese A.S.: Costen's syndrome: A reinterpretation. *Arch. Otolaryngol.* 70:309–314, 1959.
10. Harris W.: *Neuritis and Neuralgia.* London, Oxford, 1926.
11. Harris W.: An analysis of 1,433 cases of paroxysmal trigeminal neuralgia (trigeminal-tic) and end-results of gasserian alcohol injection. *Brain* 63:209–224, 1940.
12. Gossman J.R., Yansitano J.J.: Styloid-stylohyoid syndrome. *J. Oral Surg.* 35(7):555–560, 1977.
13. Eagle W.W.: Elongated styloid processes. *Arch. Otolaryngol.* 25:548–587, 1937.
14. Christiansen T.A., Meyerhoff W.L., Quick C.A.: Styloid process neuralgia. *Arch. Otolaryngol.* 101:120–122, 1975.
15. Peet M.M.: Glossopharyngeal neuralgia. *Ann. Surg.* 101:256–268, 1935.
16. Shaheen O.H.: A surgical technique for the relief of glossopharyngeal neuralgia. *Ann. Otol.* 72:873–884, 1963.
17. Barton S., Williams J.D.: Glossopharyngeal nerve block. *Arch. Otol.* 93:186–188, 1971.
18. Horner F.: Über eine Form von Ptosis. *Klin. Monatsbl. Augenheilkd.* 7:193–198, 1869.
19. Langham M.E., Weinstein G.W.: Horner's syndrome: Ocular supersensitivity to adrenergic amines. *Arch. Ophthalmol.* 78:462–469, 1967.
20. Fuoukawa T., Toyokura Y.: Alternating Horner's syndrome. *Arch. Neurol.* 30:311–313, 1974.
21. Hunt J.R.: On herpetic inflammations of geniculate ganglion: A new syndrome and its aural complications. *Arch. Otol.* 36:371–381, 1907.
22. Paparella W.M.: Otalgia, in Paparella M.M., Shumrick D.A. (eds.): *Otolaryngology.* Philadelphia, T.B. Saunders Co., 1980.
23. Plummer H.S.: Diffuse dilation of the esophagus without anatomic stenosis (cardiospasm): a report of ninety-one cases. *JAMA* 58:2013–2015, 1912.
24. Vinson P.P.: HA case of cardiospasm with dilation and angulation of the esophagus. *Med. Clin. North Am.* 3:623–627, 1919.
25. Wintrobe M.M.: Idiopathic hypochronic anemia. *Medicine* 12:187–243, 1933.
26. Raeder J.G.: Paratrigeminal paralysis of oculopupillary sympathetic. *Brain* 47:149–158, 1924.
27. Law W.R., Nelson E.R.: Internal carotid aneurysm as a cause of Raeder's paratrigeminal syndrome. *Neurology* 18:43–46, 1968.
28. Sluder G.: The role of sphenopalatine (Meckel's) ganglion in nasal headaches. *NY State Med. J.* 87:989–990, 1908.
29. Vail H.H.: Vidian neuralgia, with special reference to eye and orbital pain in suppuration of petrous apex. *Ann. Otol. Rhinol. Laryngol.* 41:837–856, 1932.

23G / Pain Due to Cancer of the Head and Neck

JAMES C. PHERO, D.M.D.
JOHN S. McDONALD, D.D.S., M.S.
GARY S. ROBINS, D.M.D.

CANCER IS NOT USUALLY painful at its onset or during the early phases of the disease. A significant percentage of patients are cured by surgery, radiation, or chemotherapy. However, many patients with recurrent or metastatic cancer eventually experience pain, which becomes progressively worse.[1]

About 35% of malignant tumors of the head and neck, with the exception of cancer of the lips and larynx, can be successfully treated. The rest will recur or metastasize. Of these, 50%–60% will be associated with pain. Pain localized to the head and neck depends more on the structures involved than on the histology of the tumor. Epidermoid carcinoma tends to ulcerate and deeply infiltrate surrounding structures. Glandular tumors and lympho-

mas generally grow by enlargement, so that pain is less frequently encountered in these tumors. On the whole, the histologic types of malignant tumors, in decreasing order of importance in causing pain, are epidermoid squamous cell carcinoma, undifferentiated carcinoma, adenoid cystic carcinoma, bone sarcoma, fibrosarcoma, chondrosarcoma, lymphoma, and melanoma. Specific pain syndromes associated with cancer of the head and neck are listed in Table 23G–1.

There is no situation more frustrating than the management of the patient with chronic head and neck pain due to cancer. Treatment varies with the diagnosis, past history of treatments, characteristics of the individual patient, and the experience and ex-

TABLE 23G–1.—SPECIFIC PAIN SYNDROMES*

SITE AND TYPE OF LESION	MECHANISM OF PAIN
Carcinoma of the floor of the mouth, with bone involvement, with or without radionecrosis	Lingual or inferior alveolar neuralgia, complicated by pain caused by the superimposed infection
Carcinoma of the glossopalatine arch, with involvement of the tongue and the tonsil, with or without trismus	Glossopharyngeal neuralgia, with mandibular nerve involvement
Carcinoma of the maxillary antrum	Maxillary neuralgia
Carcinoma of the nasopharynx, with invasion of the base of the skull	Dull painful syndrome in the nape of the neck and occipital region
Carcinoma of the nasopharynx, with invasion of the ethmoidal structure	Trigeminal pain
Advanced neck node metastases or recurrences	Cervical pain and/or Arnold's nerve neuralgia

*Adapted from Bonica J.J., Ventifridda V. (eds.): *Pain of Advanced Cancer*. New York, Raven Press, 1979, by permission.

pertise of the personnel responsible for prescribing and carrying out the treatment. A multidisciplinary approach will avoid patient dependence on individual professionals.

PAIN MECHANISMS AND SYNDROMES

The mechanisms by which head and neck cancer can cause pain include stimulation of mucosal and submucosal nerve endings, ulceration and superimposed infection, compression and involvement of sensitive nerve branches, bone invasion, postirradiation damage, functional problems, psychogenic causes, and pain unrelated to cancer.

Stimulation of Mucosal and Submucosal Nerve Endings

This mechanism is mainly responsible for local burning sensations, superficial pain, and reflex neuralgic pain, such as otalgia in exophytic or erosive lesions (Fig 23G–1).

Ulceration and Infection

Most of the cancers that arise from mucosal membranes, such as squamous cell carcinoma of the mouth and pharynx, tend to ulcerate because of central necrosis and microtraumatisms. Ulceration due to carcinoma in the absence of local irritant agents is usually not painful unless secondary infection is present. Necrotic tissue and alimentary deposits are excellent culture grounds for bacteria, which can grow and cause subsequent inflammation and edema in these ulcerated areas. Exacerbation by function is minimal in static regions such as the cheek, floor of mouth, hard palate, nasal/paranasal cavities, and naospharynx but is severe in the dynamic structures such as the tongue, soft palate, and faucial arch (Fig 23G–2).

Tumor Infiltration of Peripheral Nerve

The deeply infiltrating malignancies of the head and neck frequently involve nerve branches and trunks, with painful symptoms generally corre-

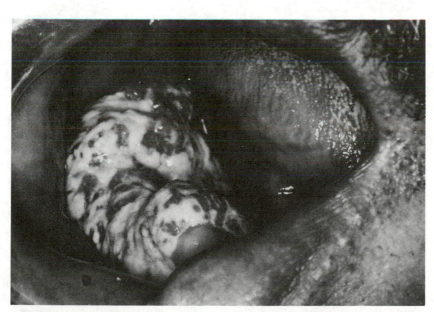

Fig 23G–1.—Squamous cell carcinoma of the right mandibular alveolar ridge in a 47-year-old black man with a 12-month history of sore mouth, a 40 pack-year history of smoking, and heavy ETOH consumption. In June 1982 a $T_2N_0M_0$ carcinoma was diagnosed that involved the right alveolar ridge, gingival buccal sulcus, and ventral tongue. The patient refused treatment; 2 months later the lesion status was $T_4N_0M_0$. A right jaw neck dissection that included the mandible was performed.

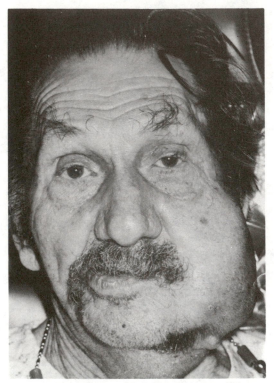

Fig 23G–2.—Squamous cell carcinoma of the left mandible with tumor necrosis and chronic draining fistula in an 84-year-old white man with a 6-month history of "bad breath" and a "6-week" history of swelling of the left jaw. Endoscopy revealed a $T_4N_0M_0$ carcinoma of the left mandibular alveolar ridge, extending to the buccal mucosa, maxillary alveolar ridge, and left lateral nasopharyngeal wall.

ṡponding to the anatomical site of the tumor. The most frequently involved nerves are the lingual nerve (by carcinoma of the anterior two thirds of the tongue and floor of the mouth), the inferior alveolar nerve (by carcinoma of the alveolar ridge, retromolar trigone, and glossopalatine arch), and the glossopharyngeal nerve (by carcinoma of the tonsil and the lateral portion of the base of the tongue).

Important sensitive nerve branches are not present in the laryngeal and hypopharyngeal regions, so problems of pain are unusual in these regions. Malignant tumors of nasal and paranasal origin can involve branches of the maxillary nerve, including the infraorbital and superior alveolar nerves. Advanced nasopharyngeal carcinomas result in a motor nerve palsy and trigeminal neuralgias.

Constant, burning pain with hypoesthesia and dysesthesia in the area of sensory loss is the usual clinical presentation. Tumor compression of a peripheral nerve proximally occurs most commonly in association with paravertebral or retroperitoneal tumor. The pain is radicular and unilateral, and a careful sensory examination can often delineate the site of nerve compression. Metastatic tumor in rib often produces intercostal nerve involvement. In this entity, pain is the earliest symptom, with progressive sensory loss distal to the site of nerve compression (Fig 23G–3).

Meningeal Carcinomatosis

This is a clinical entity in which there is tumor infiltration of the cerebrospinal leptomeninges with or without concomitant invasion of the parenchyma of the nervous system. Pain occurs in 40% of patients and is generally of two types: headache with or without neck stiffness, characterized by a constant pain, and back pain, most commonly localized to the low back and buttock regions. Pain results from traction on tumor-infiltrated nerves and meninges.

The differential diagnosis varies with the site of neurologic involvement. However, in patients with known cancer, signs and symptoms of neurologic dysfunction at several levels of the neuraxis should suggest this possible diagnosis. Alternate considerations may include fungal meningitis, cauda equina epidural tumor, and arachnoiditis.

Lumbar puncture is the procedure of choice to detect malignant cells in the cerebrospinal fluid (CSF) of such patients. An elevated CSF protein concentration and low glucose concentration are often associated findings. In patients with low back and buttock pain, myelography can help delineate tumor nodules along the nerves in the cauda equina.

Tumor Infiltration of Bone

Direct involvement of the bone is usually not painful. Pain arises when tumor progression involves nerve branches, as with cancer of the alveolus, or when the path of neoplastic infiltration is followed from the surface by bacterial infection with consequent osteomyelitis, as seen in alveolar ridge and in carcinoma of the maxillary antrum, where a superimposed obstructive sinusitis may result in bony infection (Fig 23G–4).

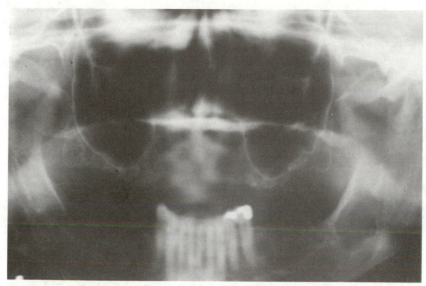

Fig 23G–3.—Recurrent mucoepidermoid carcinoma of the left angle of the mandible. A 41-year-old black woman was seen 3 years following excision of a mucoepidermoid carcinoma involving the left retromolar trigone. Surgery entailed a continuous left radical neck dissection. She reported a 6-month history of paresthesia and anesthesia of the left tongue and mandible, with occasional pain radiating over the entire left face and into the left ear; radiograph was made at this presentation.

Metastases to the Base of the Skull

The syndromes reported here all share two common features. Pain is the earliest complaint, often preceding neurologic signs and symptoms by several weeks to months, and documentation with routine radiographs is often difficult.

Jugular

JUGULAR-FORAMEN SYNDROME.—Occipital pain, often referred to the vertex of the head and ipsilateral shoulder and arm, is an early presenting symptom. The pain is often exacerbated by head movement and associated with local tenderness over the occipital condyle. The patient's signs and symptoms vary with the cranial nerve involved but can include hoarseness, dysarthria, dysphagia, neck and shoulder weakness, and ptosis. The neurologic examination can help to localize the lesion by determining the function of cranial nerves IX, X, XI, and XII, since involvement of all four of these nerves suggests jugular foramen and hypoglossal canal involvement with secondary nerve dysfunction. The presence of Horner's syndrome suggests sympathetic involvement extracranially but in close proximity to the jugular foramen.

CLIVUS METASTASES.—Pain characterized by a vertex headache exacerbated by neck flexion is a common presentation of this entity. Lower cranial nerve dysfunction (nerves VI–XII) usually begins unilaterally but often progresses to bilateral lower cranial nerve dysfunction.

SPHENOID SINUS METASTASES.—Severe bifrontal headache radiating to both temples, with intermittent retro-orbital pain, suggests this entity. The patient often complains of nasal stuffiness or a sense of fullness in the head, with a concomitant diplopia. The neurologic signs of unilateral or bilateral seventh nerve palsy further suggests the diagnosis.

Cervical Vertebrae Metastases (Subluxation of the Atlas)

Metastatic disease involving the odontoid process of the axis (C-1 vertebral body) can result in a pathologic fracture with secondary subluxation, resulting in spinal cord or brain stem compression.

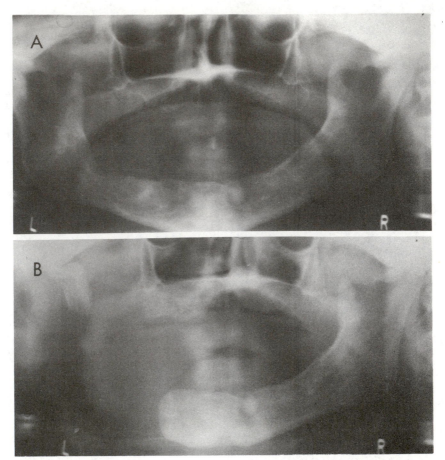

Fig 23G—4.—Carcinoma of the left retromolar trigone. A 52-year-old black man presented with a 2-month history of "pain in the mouth" and a 37-pack-year history of smoking, in addition to the daily consumption of 2–3 pints of ETOH. Panendoscopy revealed involvement of the left retromolar trigone, buccal sulcus, and mandibular alveolar ridge. **A,** radiograph showing invasion of bone by tumor. **B,** appearance following left jaw neck dissection and postoperative irradiation.

Early symptoms include severe neck pain radiating over the posterior aspect of the skull to the vertex and exacerbated by movement, particularly flexion of the neck. Neurologic signs include progressive sensory and motor signs beginning in the upper extremities with associated autonomic dysfunction. Neck manipulation in these patients is dangerous, and tomography is generally necessary to confirm the diagnosis.

FOIX'S SYNDROME (CAVERNOUS SINUS-LATERAL WALL SYNDROME).—The cause of this syndrome is tumor involving the lateral wall of the cavernous sinus or sphenoid bone, intracranial aneurysms, or thrombosis of cavernous and lateral sinuses. A paralysis of cranial nerves III, IV, and VI occurs, resulting in proptosis and edema of the eyelids and conjuctivae. Involvement of cranial nerve V results in a trigeminal neuralgia. Treatment if possible is eradication of the pressure-producing tumor.

GODT FREDSEN'S SYNDROME (CAVERNOUS SINUS-NASOPHARYNGEAL TUMOR SYNDROME).—This syndrome is characterized by anesthesia or neuralgia in cranial nerve V, and paralysis of the tongue on the affected side resulting from a compression of the hypoglossal nerve by enlargement of involved retropharyngeal lymph nodes. Unilateral involvement is pathognomic for invasion of the cavernous sinus. Treatment entails elimination of the tumor mass.

PTERYGOPALATINE FOSSA SYNDROME.—This syndrome resembles Trotter's syndrome. However, pain with the pterygopalatine fossa syndrome occurs in the maxilla rather than the mandible. Anesthesia of the infraorbital and palatal areas occurs and may be followed by blindness and motor nerve paralysis of the pterygoid muscles.

The cause of this syndrome is tumor of the pterygopalatine fossa. In its expansion, the tumor involves the maxillary division of cranial nerve V and adjacent structures. Primary treatment is directed toward the tumor.

TROTTER'S SYNDROME (SINUS OF MORGAGNI SYNDROME, PERITUBAL SYNDROME).—Pain is experienced in the mandible and tongue, with headache on the affected side. Unilateral deafness, deviation of the palate, defective mobility of the palatal and internal pterygoid muscles, and cervical adenopathy occur.

The cause of this syndrome is a neoplasm that originates deep in the lateral wall of the nasopharynx and involves the sinus of Morgagni. It is seen most often in men during the third and fourth decades of life. Treatment is directed toward the tumor and its symptoms.

Postirradiation Damage

Sequelae of radiation therapy range from simple mucositis to radionecrosis. Postirradiation damage, when associated with persistent or recurrent tumor, may give rise to further patient distress. Radiation-induced tumor necrosis provides a rich medium for superimposed infection, which secondarily involves healthy tissues that contain sensitive nerve fibers not previously affected by the cancer. Additionally, radiation induces reactive fibrosis, which can cause painful muscular contractions, for example, trismus. The combination of neoplastic recurrence with radionecrosis accounts for about 70% of the major problems of pain in cancer of the head and neck (Fig 23G–5).

Functional Problems

Functions such as phonation, breathing, and deglutition are frequently affected in patients with cancer of the larynx and hypopharynx. Problems of pain are rarely present in these regions. In cancer of the nasal and paranasal cavities, pain is mainly due to involvement of bony structures and branches of the fifth nerve. Cancer of the nasopharynx is very frequently associated with palsy of one or more cra-

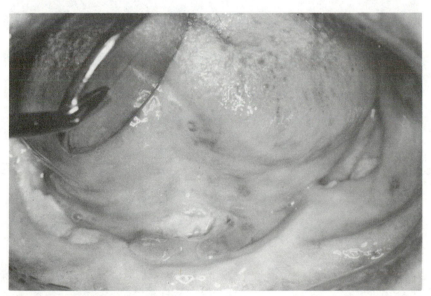

Fig 23G–5.—Radionecrosis. A 62-year-old black woman presented with radionecrosis of the tissues of the floor of the mouth, as well as extensive radionecrosis of the body of the mandible bilaterally.

nial motor nerves. Functional disorders make persistent pain less tolerable in this situation. One of the worst combinations of pain and functional disorders is seen in cancer of the oral cavity and oropharynx, where hyperalgesia and neuralgia during chewing and swallowing may severely compromise the eating process (Fig 23G–6).

Psychological Problems

All the previously mentioned mechanisms may be intensified by particular psychological reactions, both basic and progressively acquired. In addition, the great majority of the patients with cancer of the

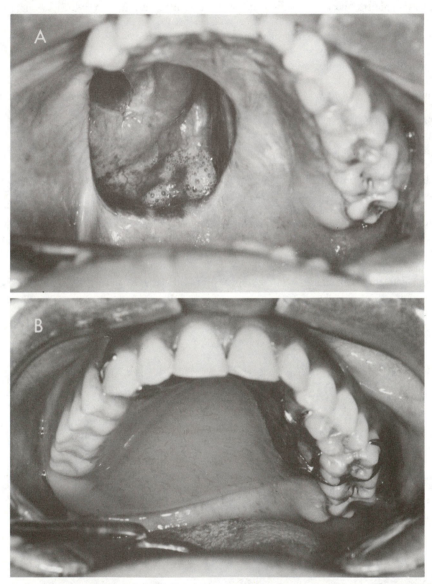

Fig 23G–6.—A, surgical defect following partial maxillectomy for adenocarcinoma of the right posterior hard palate in a 32-year-old black woman. The defect severely compromised the patient's deglutition and speech. **B,** an obturator was fabricated that restored good swallowing function and the ability to speak clearly. (Courtesy of G.P. Huntress, D.D.S., Cincinnati.)

mouth and pharynx are heavy drinkers and smokers, with their attendant psychological problems. The combination of pain and functional disorders often worsens the psychological conditions, creating a vicious cycle. A particularly negative aspect of cancer in the head and neck is that these tumors are visible, so the patient observes, day by day, the disfigurement and progression of the disease.

Pain Associated With Cancer Therapy

This category includes clinical pain syndromes that occur in the course of or subsequent to cancer therapy.

Post-radical Neck Dissection Pain

Pain following radical neck dissection occurs from surgical injury or interruption of the cervical nerves. The pain is characterized by a constant burning sensation in the area of sensory loss. Dysesthesias and intermittent shock-like pain may also be present.

Diagnostic workup should include a careful history of the onset of pain and appropriate x-ray films of the painful area to rule out recurrent disease. Recurrent tumor involving the cervical spine or base of the skull is the major differential diagnosis.

Postchemotherapy Pain

This group includes a series of pain problems which occur in cancer patients receiving chemotherapy. The major features of each of these entities are described below.

STEROID PSEUDORHEUMATISM.—A pseudorheumatism may follow either rapid or slow withdrawal of steroid medications in patients taking these drugs for short or long periods of time.[2] The syndrome consists of prominent diffuse myalgias and arthralgias, with muscle and joint tenderness on palpation, but without objective inflammatory signs. A sense of generalized malaise and fatigue is a common feature of this entity. These signs and symptoms revert with reinstitution of the steroid medication.

POSTHERPETIC NEURALGIA.—In patients with cancer, herpes zoster infection commonly occurs due to several precipitating factors which include malnutrition, decreased immune response and general deliberation. The true incidence of postherpetic neuralgia in patients with cancer is unknown, but it appears to be more common in patients who develop the infection after age 50. There are generally three types of pain: a continuous and/or burning pain in the area of sensory loss, painful dysesthesias, and intermittent, shock-like pain.[3]

RADIATION MYELOPATHY.—Pain is an early symptom of 15% of patients with radiation myelopathy.[4] The pain may be localized to the area of spinal cord damage or may be referred pain, with dysesthesias below the level of injury. Clinically, the neurologic symptoms and signs are that of a Brown-Sequard syndrome (ipsilateral motor paresis with contralateral sensory loss at a cervical or thoracic level) which progresses to a complete transverse myelopathy. The diagnostic workup should include x-ray films of the spine and myelography, both of which are usually unremarkable. Occasionally, widening of the cord at the injured area may be noted. The differential diagnosis includes intramedullary tumor, epidural spinal cord compression, arteriovenous malformation, and transverse myelitis.

Pain Unrelated to Cancer or Cancer Therapy

Approximately 3% of the pain syndromes that occur in cancer patients have no relationship to the underlying cancer or cancer therapy. Degenerative disk disease, thoracic and abdominal aneurysms, and diffuse osteoporosis are the most common non-cancer-related pain syndromes observed in patients with cancer. This category emphasizes that pain in a cancer patient does not necessarily imply recurrent or persistent disease, and it supports the thesis that a careful diagnostic evaluation in the cancer patient is necessary to define the specific pain syndrome before one embarks on a therapeutic course.

RATIONALE FOR MANAGEMENT

The importance of a multidisciplinary team approach to the management of patients with cancer, especially in the terminal phase, is well established. For many years, cancer centers and cancer units of general hospitals have had oncology groups consisting of oncologic surgeons, radiation therapists, medical oncologists, and pathologists to deal with the pathologic process. More recently, the importance of treating the whole patient rather than just the lesion has become appreciated. Consequently, oncology teams have added nutritionists, nurses, physical therapists, psychologists, dolorologists, social workers and various other health professionals, and chaplains with special interest and expertise in cancer management. Consideration of the numerous mechanisms of chronic pain in general and of cancer pain in particular, as well as of the various modalities currently available for therapy, helps one appreciate that no one individual has the knowledge, expertise, and skill to provide optimal relief to each and every patient.

Patient Evaluation

A careful history of the patient's pain complaint can often provide insight into the etiology of the pain. One must attempt to elicit a clear description of the onset of pain, its characteristics, the referral pattern, and exacerbating and relieving factors.

There is no substitute for a complete physical and neurologic examination to provide objective data and to substantiate the clinical history. The neurologic examination is particularly useful in differentiating local pain from referred pain, and peripheral nerve involvement from plexus or cord involvement.

Since the diagnosis of metastatic disease may be elusive, the limitations of the available diagnostic procedures should be recognized by the physician ordering such studies. Basic x-ray films are a useful screening procedure. However, the bone scan is a more sensitive method and may demonstrate abnormalities 3–4 months before changes appear on routine radiographs. Routine radiographs also are inadequate to assess certain areas of the body where bone shadows overlap, such as the base of the skull, the C7–T1 area, and the sacrum. Tomography is necessary to discern bony changes in such areas. Computerized tomography (CT) allows even more detailed visualization of soft tissues and bone and is rapidly becoming the procedure of choice for evaluating the paravertebral and skull-base areas. Cisternal and lumbar myelography and CSF cytologic evaluation are other diagnostic procedures which can further help to delineate the pain diagnosis.

A thorough evaluation of the extent of metastatic disease may help to confirm the diagnosis of a specific pain syndrome. It is important to remember that the incidence of a second primary tumor is increased in patients with a previous history of cancer. Patients in whom the presentation is atypical or the response to therapy different from predicted will have an increased incidence of persistent recurrent or metastatic disease. A needle biopsy or surgical exploration should be performed to establish a tissue diagnosis in these cases.

Establishing an accurate diagnosis is the key to providing appropriate therapy, and a cooperative patient is necessary to facilitate this workup. Generally, analgesics are the mainstay of initial therapy, and adequate pain control will allow the patient to undergo the necessary diagnostic procedures.

Management of Cancer Pain

Chemotherapy

The rationale of anticancer chemotherapy in patients with severe pain is the assumption that a correlation does exist between regression of the tumor and reduction of the pain. In head and neck cancer, this correlation has been clearly demonstrated and is probably due to the fact that the tumor mass is generally smaller than it is in other regions of the body.

Many drugs have been tested, including methotrexate, bleomycin, cisplatin, Adriamycin, and hydroxyurea. Unfortunately, results have been inconsistent and quite poor. The best results obtained in tumor and pain management with chemotherapy have been achieved by combining different drugs (polychemotherapy) or by increasing the dose of single drugs. When treatment is successful, remission of pain is generally prompt even when the objective regression of the tumor is partial or absent.

Radiation Therapy

Radiation therapy is often the initial treatment used in advanced cases of head and neck cancer. Radiation therapy alone can resolve problems of pain secondary to radiosensitive tumors. These include undifferentiated carcinoma of the nasopharynx and tonsil, ulcerating carcinoma of the tongue and floor of the mouth, and undifferentiated tumors of the nasal and paranasal cavities. In the great majority of cases, however, persistent pain is the consequence of recurrent cancer previously treated with surgery or radiation therapy. Repetition of radiation therapy must be carefully thought over and performed only if very poor results can be expected from alternative treatments or as a palliative treatment for pain management. Radiation therapy as a pain management technique appears most beneficial in controlling pain due to infiltration of bone or metastatic bone involvement in the head and neck patient.

Symptomatic and Palliative Surgery

Management of head and neck cancer pain can frequently be achieved by surgery. Recurrence with bone invasion, especially in the setting of osteoradionecrosis, is a frequent cause of pain. Postoperative complications due to previous radiation therapy must be considered in order to avoid life-threatening situations or protracted postoperative periods. The evaluation of these risks depends on the personal experience of the surgeon, who must sometimes reject radical treatment in favor of a shorter and uneventful course with an acceptable expectancy of life with minimal problem of pain.

Surgery after radiation therapy is useful in many clinical situations, but mainly in the case of recurrent cancer of the oral cavity; osteoradionecrosis of the jaws, with or without neoplastic recurrence; recurrence of oropharyngeal cancer (tonsil, base of the tongue, retromolar trigone, or anterior tonsillar pillar); recurrence of tumors of the nasal and paranasal cavities; and recurrence of neck node metastases, after both radiation therapy and surgery.

Surgical therapy useful in the management of head and neck pain due to cancer may include ablative surgery, single or multiple rhizotomies, tractotomy, thalamotomy, and psychosurgery. Details of the procedures are discussed in chapter 39.

Nerve Blocks

In patients with moderate to severe pain due to cancer of the head and neck, nerve blocks can be used to control the pain for a prolonged period of time. Diagnostic blocks are used to determine the mechanism and pathways of the pain, whereas prognostic blocks are used to predict the effects of neurolytic block or neurosurgical section. The physician should not hesitate to inject the gasserian ganglion, because relief of pain must be obtained for the patient even at the price of producing keratitis from block of the ophthalmic branches of the trigeminal

nerve. The problem here is quite different from that in patients who have tic douloureux or other benign, chronic pain, in whom the life expectancy is long and a corneal ulcer is a serious complication. Gasserian ganglion block is particularly useful if the lesion involves structures that are supplied by more than one of the major divisions of the fifth cranial nerve. In such cases, it is preferable to carry out a gasserian ganglion block at the onset of pain to produce a wide field of analgesia into which the cancer can spread without producing much pain subsequently.

The severe pain that accompanies cancer of the oropharynx is often effectively relieved by neurosurgical section of the sensory roots of the glossopharyngeal nerve and a portion of the vagus nerve. Blocks of these nerves with local anesthetics may be used as diagnostic and prognostic tools, but since such blocks also involve motor nerves, neurolytic blocks are contraindicated because they produce prolonged paralysis of pharyngeal and laryngeal muscles, resulting in the loss of the patient's ability to swallow and phonate. This is an especially serious complication if the block is done bilaterally. Unilateral neurolytic block of the glossopharyngeal nerve of the most painful side may be considered in patients with excruciating pain not adequately relieved by narcotics and whose physical condition is too poor to permit neurosurgical section. Pain in the back of the head and upper neck may require a block of C-2 and C-3, first with a local anesthetic to ascertain the pain pathways and subsequently with a neurolytic agent. In many instances, cancer of the mouth, tongue, or lower jaw spreads laterally and posteriorly to produce moderate to severe pain and sometimes trismus, which can be effectively relieved by block of the mandibular nerve combined with paravertebral block of the upper two cervical nerves.

Occasionally, tumors of the face and head cause a burning discomfort in addition to the severe neuralgia and deep, aching pain. The burning pain is usually located over one side of the head, the eye, teeth, lower and upper jaw, the temporal region, and the nape of the neck. This is not relieved by block of the somatic nerves. In such cases, cervical sympathetic block should be carried out, first with a local anesthetic, and if it relieves the burning pain, the procedure is repeated with phenol or alcohol as a supplement to a somatic block.

Advanced cancer of the orbit usually spreads to the entire area supplied by the ophthalmic and maxillary divisions of the trigeminal nerve. When the division affected cannot be blocked, it is necessary to perform a block at the gasserian ganglion level. Advanced cancers originating in the upper half of the maxillary antrum can expand laterally to involve the malar bone and medially to invade the ethmoidal and orbital structures. Moreover, they can pass the midline, affecting practically the entire face and requiring a bilateral gasserian ganglion block.

BLOCKS WITH LOCAL ANESTHETICS IN THE TREATMENT OF CANCER PAIN.—Regional block procedures for the relief of cancer pain are usually performed with neurolytic substances such as alcohol or phenol. There are, however, pain states associated with neoplastic disease which do not require destructive nerve blocks with their inherent side effects and complications. Local anesthetic blocks useful for cancer pain include sympathetic block, somatic nerve block, and extradural block.

SYMPATHETIC NERVE BLOCKADE.—Cancer pain amenable to local anesthetic blocks is characterized by symptoms of so-called carcinomatous (or sarcomatous) neuritis, identical to the signs and symptoms of reflex sympathetic dystrophy. These include pain, hyperpathia (hyperesthesia and/or hyperalgesia), neurovascular instability (vasoconstriction with cyanosis and edema or vasodilatation), su-

domotor disturbances (hyperhidrosts, hypohidrosis, or anhidrosis), and pilomotor changes (Fig 23G–7).

The quality of pain is burning, throbbing, dull, and in some cases even sharp and stabbing. Characteristically the pattern of distribution of this constant pain and of the hyperpathic area does not correspond to the pattern of segmental or peripheral nerve innervation. Therefore, physicians who are not familiar with these pain syndromes do not accept the patient's symptom report and search for neurotic or hysterical traits. Nonrecognition and nontreatment of these conditions almost regularly result in trophic tissue changes which eventually become irreversible. It is therefore essential to initiate treatment with sympathetic blocks promptly after the onset of pain and related symptomatology.

In the initial state of tumor-induced reflex sympathetic dystrophy, which usually occurs 6–10 months after radical and effective tumor surgery, objective signs of tumor recurrence are lacking.[5] In many instances, carefully performed sweat tests[6] are helpful because tumor infiltration of the cervicothoracic and lumbar sympathetic chains results quite early in hypohidroses or anhidroses in the upper and lower limbs, respectively.[7] These changes, which precede any x-ray evidence of tumor recurrence by months and sometimes years, are particularly likely

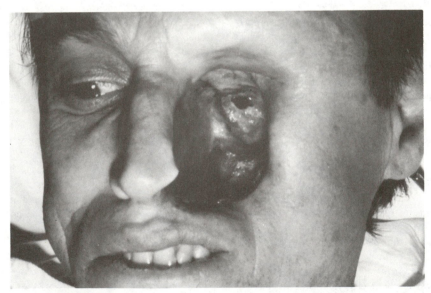

Fig 23G–7.—Appearance of a 44-year-old white man following radical maxillectomy for antral carcinoma in July 1981, with orbital exenteration in January 1982. The patient complained of progressive "burning, stinging" pain, paresthesia, and anesthesia over all three divisions of the trigeminal nerve, secondary to involvement of base of skull by tumor. His pain was tolerable with left stellate ganglion blocks.

to occur with lymphogenous spread of Pancoast tumors.[8, 9]

Another clinical entity frequently observed with cancer pain is the quadrant syndrome or vascular zone disturbance.[10] These conditions present with burning, dull pain; nonsegmental sensory disturbances; vasomotor, sudomotor, and pilomotor changes; and a special quality of pain that can be detected on careful physical examination. Patients indicate either a latency between a nociceptive stimulus with pinprick and the perception of pain or immediately feel a sharp pain on stimulation followed by a dull, severe burning pain.

The distribution of the pain follows the typical sympathetic vascular innervation pattern. Thus, the pain distribution can correspond to one or more quadrants of the body in accordance with the sympathetic nervous system distribution of subclavian arteries, or to the vascular zone of one arterial branch such as the external carotid arteries.

Diagnostic sympathetic block with a local anesthetic prior to planned neurolytic injections relieves the burning cancer pain and the associated muscle tension pain for days and even weeks. This unexpectedly long effective duration of a local anesthetic block is explained by the following actions of local anesthetics on pain mechanisms. The local anesthetic blocks pain receptors (nociceptors) and thus prevents transformation and coding of nociceptive impulses in these specialized nerve endings, and it blocks nociceptive impulse transmission in those efferent fibers associated with sympathetic fibers and thus prevents such impulses from reaching the CNS. Additionally, it blocks sympathetic pathways and thus interrupts sympathetic reflex mechanisms, which act as positive feedback mechanisms and are usually active in painful conditions. Increased skeletal muscle activity, which contributes to the sustenance of the vicious cycle of pain, is also reduced or eliminated.

The pain-relieving effects of regional anesthetic blocks often outlast the pharmacologic impulse-blocking effect of the local anesthetic. This prolonged analgesic effect, which is obtained even in neoplastic disease, is presumably due to interruption of the vicious cycle. In the treatment of pain, the goal of regional analgesia is interruption of C and A

delta fibers and of efferent sympathetic fibers.[11] Sympathetic blocks performed for management of burning cancer pain of the face, head, and neck are the stellate ganglion and cervicothoracic blocks. These require only low concentrations of local anesthetics such as 0.5% lidocaine or mepivacaine, or 0.125%–0.25% bupivacaine. Because of the long duration of action of bupivacaine, an almost continuous small fiber blockade can be achieved with blocks performed once daily.[12] The results achieved with local anesthetics in tumor-induced reflex sympathetic dystrophy are often comparable to those attained with neurolytic blocks, i.e., 1–6 months of pain relief.

REFERENCES

1. Bonica J.J.: Cancer pain: A major national health problem. *Cancer Nurs. J.* 4:313–316, 1978.
2. Rotstein J., Good R.A.: Steroid pseudorheumatism. *Arch Intern. Med.* 99:545–555, 1957.
3. Nordenbos W.: *Pain: Problems Pertaining to the Transmission of Nerve Impulses Which Give Rise to Pain.* New York, Elsevier, 1959, p. 182.
4. Jellinger K., Strum K.W.: Delayed radiation myelopathy in man. *J. Neurol. Sci.* 14:389–408, 1971.
5. Bues E.: Gezielte Grenzstrangresektion: Hohendiagnostik des Sympathikusgrenzstranges und ihre chirurgische Bedeutungen. *Chirug* 25:443, 1954.
6. Moberg E.: Objective methods for determining the functional value of sensibility in the hand. *J. Bone Joint Surg.* 3:454, 1958.
7. Schliack H., Schiffer R.: Anhidrose der Fuss-sohle: Symptom retroperitonealer Tumor invasion. *Dtsch. Med. Wochenschr.* 96:977, 1971.
8. Chiappa S., et al.: Lymphangiography in the diagnosis of retroperitoneal node metastasis in rectal cancer. *Br. J. Radiol.* 40:584, 1967.
9. Dargent M.: Role of the sympathetic nerve in cancerous pain: Inquiry into 300 cases. *Br. Med. J.* 1:440, 1948.
10. Pette H.: Das Problem der wechselseitigen Beziehungen zwischen Sympathicis und Sensibilität. *Dtsch. Z. Nervenkh.* 100:143, 1927.
11. de Jong R.: Theoretical aspects of pain: Bizarre pain phenomena during low spinal anesthesia. *Anesthesiology* 24:628, 1963.
12. Nolte H., et al.: Klinische und elektrophysiologische Parameter zur Differenzierung der Wirkung von Lokalanasthetika. *Anaesthesist* 23:165, 1974.

24 / Cervical Pain

SOMAYAJI RAMAMURTHY, M.D.

THE PATIENT COMPLAINING of neck and shoulder and arm pain should be examined for anatomical location of the pain, derangement of mechanical structures, and an underlying pathologic condition. A careful history and examination are important to reach a diagnosis. X-rays and laboratory tests are necessary but have limited value in arriving at the diagnosis.

The cervical spine and the thoracic outlet are composed of numerous sensitive structures: nerves, vessels, muscles, ligaments, joints, and their capsules. All these structures are compacted into small areas and are subject to numerous movements, stresses, and strains. Pain in this region results from the encroachment of space and impairment of movement.

The sites at which tissues are compressed are the intervertebral foraminae and within the spinal canal. Movement of the neck requires that the disks be strong to withstand distortion and recovery, the ligaments have laxity to allow motion, and the posterior joints be sufficiently separated and have smooth articular surfaces to permit neck movement in all directions. Impairment of movement of any part of the cervical spine can produce pain, discomfort, and disability. Injury, stress, and faulty mechanics of the neck cause irritation of soft tissues, leading to encroachment of space, limitation of movement, and pain.

PAIN-PRODUCING SITES IN THE NECK

The neck contains many pain-sensitive tissues in a compact area. Pain can result from irritation, injury, inflammation, or infection of any of these tissues.[1] The normal cervical disk is not a pain-sensitive structure since increasing intradiskal pressure does not produce pain. On the other hand, a degenerated or damaged disk causes pain that can be abolished by locally anesthetising the posterior longitudinal ligament. The posterior longitudinal ligament, which is innervated by the recurrent meningeal nerve, is the cause of the pain.[1]

The nerve root within the spinal canal and at the intervertebral foramina is a pain-sensitive structure. Stretching the nerve causes impaired vascularity and ischemic pain in the distribution of the nerve.[2] The ligamentum flavum and the interspinous ligaments are nonsensitive to pain. The synovial lining of the posterior zygapophyseal joints, when irritated or compressed, can produce moderately severe pain. However, these joints are not the common source of pain in the cervical region.

Muscle can cause pain in many ways. The nerve root pressure can cause reflex muscle spasm and pain. Muscle pain can also be produced by ischemia secondary to chronic muscle spasm and by stretching and contracting a disused muscle. Ischemic muscle pain results not only from hypoxia but also from an accumulation of acid metabolites.[3–5]

Arthritic pain in the neck is far less significant than the diagnosis of cervical arthritis would imply. Stretching the thickened and contractured periarticular tissues with neck movements causes the pain to be felt in the neck. There is no correlation between the degree of pain felt and the degree of arthritic changes found on radiography.[2]

Torticollis is another cause of neck pain. It can be caused by many conditions. In children torticollis may result from trauma or may be secondary to infection of the laryngopharynx or cervical adenitis. Torticollis in the adult may result from a viral infection, muscle strain, subluxation of a unilateral apophyseal joint, or central neurogenic and psychogenic mechanisms.

418

Cancer in the head and neck region can cause cervical pain. The cause of the pain may vary, depending on whether it produces tissue necrosis, inflammation of pain-sensitive tissues, or pressure on bone, the nerve, or a vessel.

RATIONALE FOR MANAGEMENT OF PAINFUL NECK DISORDERS

A careful history and physical examination are essential for effective physiologic treatment of pain. The examination should ascertain the extent of the pathology and the mechanism of pain. In the acute injury, radiographs should be carefully reviewed for fracture, subluxation, or dislocation. Once fracture or dislocation has been ruled out, the patient should be treated conservatively. Medication is of definite but limited value at this stage. Muscle relaxants and tranquilizers in adequate doses are indicated, but narcotics must be kept to a minimum.

Cervical immobilization with a collar or traction may be helpful in the acute stages, but restoration of the function of the cervical spine and its musculature should be the aim of the treatment. Physical therapy, including exercises, should be encouraged from the very beginning, and the pain should be relieved by any alternative means if analgesics are not sufficient.

If the condition enters the chronic stage, suffering becomes a major component. Adequate psychological support, in addition to pain-relieving procedures and exercises, is necessary for such patients. Surgery should be considered very carefully for such patients and mainly as a last resort. The following guidelines are helpful in this decision: (1) conservation treatment has failed, (2) there is progressive neurologic deficit, and (3) long tract signs attributable to cervical pathology exist. The surgical approach varies from laminotomy and diskectomy to laminectomy and fusion.

PAIN DUE TO DISKOGENIC DISEASE

The cervical disk plays a vital role in many conditions of the neck that cause local neck pain or referred pain in the upper extremities. In its function as a "joint" the cervical disk permits movement and simultaneously helps keep the foramina apart. Nerve root compression from disk herniation is infrequent in the cervical region.[2] The nerve is also completely protected from the bulging disk by the posterior longitudinal ligament. This differs from the lumbar region, where the ligament is incomplete and thin. The nucleus of the disk in the cervical region is located in the anterior wide portion of the disk. This prevents movement of the nucleus pulposus posteriorly, where it is narrow. The annulus fibrosus is also much thicker in the posterolateral portion of the disk. The nerve contact and pressure by the protruded disk are minimized because the nerve roots emerge from the cord opposite to the vertebral bodies and are barely in contact with the inferior margin of the above disk.

When a disk protrusion produces nerve root pain, localization by clinical examination alone is difficult. Myelography, electromyography (EMG), or surgical exploration have been more accurate. Most of the lesions involve C-5, C-6, C-7, and C-8 nerve roots (Table 24–1). Pain in the neck, shoulder, scapula, or interscapular area is nonlocalizing. Similarly, pain in the upper arm is non-specific. Pain in the posterior aspect of the arm is due to C-7 root

TABLE 24–1.—SIGNS AND SYMPTOMS OF NERVE ROOT COMPRESSION OF THE CERVICAL REGION

LOCATION OF LESION	REFERRED PAIN	MOTOR DYSFUNCTION	SENSORY DYSFUNCTION	REFLEX CHANGES
C-5	Shoulder and upper arm	Shoulder muscles (deltoid-supraspinatus-infraspinatus) ↓ abduction and external rotation	↓ Upper and lateral aspect of the shoulder	↓ Biceps reflex
C-6	Radial aspect of forearm	Biceps and brachialis muscles ↓ flexion of the elbow and supination ↓ wrist extensors	Radial aspect of forearm	↓ Thumb reflex and brachioradalis reflex
C-7	Dorsal aspect of forearm	Triceps muscle ↓ extension of the elbow	↓ Index and middle digits	↓ Triceps reflex
C-8	Ulnar aspect of forearm	Intrinsics of the hand ↓ adduction and abduction	↓ Ring and little digits	No change

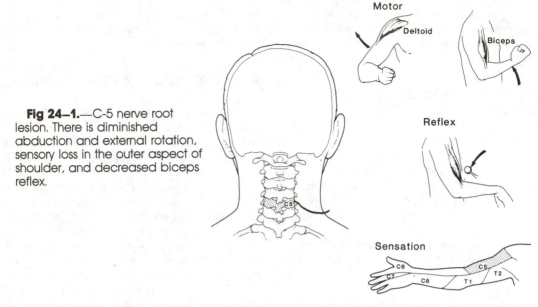

Fig 24–1.—C-5 nerve root lesion. There is diminished abduction and external rotation, sensory loss in the outer aspect of shoulder, and decreased biceps reflex.

lesion, whereas medial anterior or lateral arm pain can be due to C-6 or C-7 nerve roots. Forearm pain usually is due to C-6 or C-7 nerve root lesion. Paresthesia in the hand is more accurately assigned to a particular nerve root. Radiating pain in the thumb usually is due to C-6 nerve root compression. Index and middle finger radiation is due to C-7 nerve root, and paresthesia in ring and little fingers is due to C-8 nerve root (Figs 24–1 through 24–4).

Objective weakness[6] is much more specific for localizing root level. C-5 nerve root lesion is best located by weakness in the deltoid, supraspinatus, and infraspinatus muscles. This can be tested by abduction and external arm rotation. C-6 nerve root lesion is located by weakness of the brachialis and biceps muscle. C-7 nerve root lesion is localized by eliciting weakness in the triceps mainly but also in the flexor carpi ulnaris and radialis, pronator teres, and extensor pollicis longus.

Objective hypoesthesia and hypalgesia in the appropriate dermatomal patterns are useful in localizing nerve root lesions. Testing deep tendon reflexes is of value only if the reflexes are properly tested. A diminished triceps jerk indicates a C-7 root le-

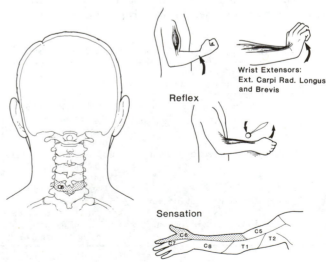

Fig 24–2.—C-6 nerve root lesion. There is diminished flexion of the elbow and wrist extensors, sensory loss in lateral aspect of the forearm, and decreased brachioradialis and thumb reflexes.

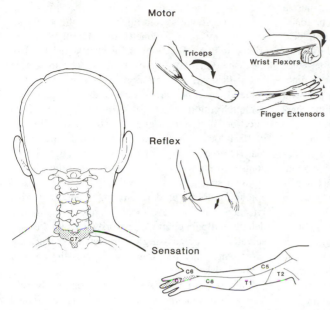

Fig 24–3.—C-7 nerve root lesion. There is weakness of extension of the elbow, wrist flexors, sensory loss in middle finger, and diminished triceps reflex.

sion, or possibly a C-8 nerve root. The brachioradialis reflex may be diminished in C-7 root lesions, but its absence indicates a C-6 root lesion.

Differential Diagnosis

Radicular pain is a shooting, radiating type of pain that is accompanied by objective neurologic signs such as loss of sensation and changes in the reflex and muscle strength. Radiculopathy itself can be caused by other etiological factors such as primary or secondary malignancy of the bone, involvement of the nerve root by carcinoma of the lung, and also by the degenerative changes of the cervical spine itself. Compression of the spinal cord from a herniated disk can produce symptoms very similar to those of nerve root compression. Compression of the spinal cord in the neck produces radicular symptoms in the upper extremities and long tract signs in

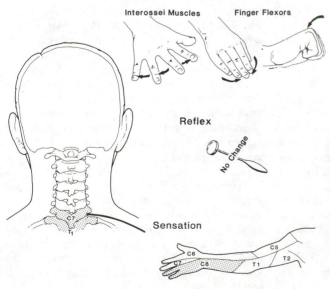

Fig 24–4.—C-8 nerve root lesion. There is weakness in adduction and abduction of fingers, sensory loss in medial aspect of lower half of forearm, and medial 1½ fingers and reflex changes.

the lower extremities. Sensory impairment, muscle weakness, and loss of tendon reflexes may be found in the upper extremities. In the lower extremities, spastic weakness, hyperreflexia clonus and extensor plantar reflexes, and vibratory and position sense may be impaired. Bowel and bladder and their function are not usually impaired. Myofascial pain can also produce pain in the neck and arm, but the character of the pain is different.

Investigations are helpful in differentiating the causes of the neck and arm pain, but through neurologic examination is one of the most important ways of making a diagnosis. X-ray films of the cervical spine, especially lateral and oblique views, are helpful in eliminating the spinal abnormalities. Degenerative changes are commonly seen in asymptomatic individuals, whereas x-ray films of the cervical spine may be normal in patients with a herniated disk. EMG is not useful in the acute stage since it takes at least 3 weeks for the denervation to be detected in the involved muscles. After that period, EMG may be helpful in localizing the level of the lesions and also in differentiating shoulder pain from radiculopathy and muscle disease. Computerized tomographic (CT) scanning is now being employed routinely and has been helpful in differentiating the various causes of nerve root compression. Myelography, especially with the water-soluble contrast medium, is helpful in differentiating the causes of the radiculopathy, and also in differentiating or detecting myelopathy. Not every patient with neck pain requires myelography, and most physicians request myelography only when the surgery is contemplated or a tumor is suspected.

Management

Acute disk herniation is managed conservatively, most commonly with rest, using a cervical soft collar to minimize the movements of the cervical spine. Keeping the muscles relaxed during the acute stage may be beneficial, and drugs such as cyclobenzaprine and diazepam may be useful during the acute stage. Nonsteroidal anti-inflammatory drugs, in addition to decreasing the inflammation, are likely to reduce the pain and swelling. Muscle spasm associated with acute disk herniation can be reduced by ice massage or spray of a vapocoolant such as an ethyl chloride or fluorimethane. Cervical traction could be applied in the hospital or home. Heat followed by gentle limbering movements of the neck and arm may also reduce the pain and muscle spasm.

If symptoms persist despite conservative treatment, an epidural steroid injection should be considered. Methyl prednisolone (Depo-Medrol) 80 mg or triamcinolone 25–50 mg is injected at the level of the disk herniation. Improvement is likely to be seen in 24–48 hours. If there is improvement, no further epidural injections are given. If there is partial or negligible improvement after 10–14 days, a second injection of steroid is given. Two to five milliliters of 1% lidocaine or 0.25% bupivacaine is injected by many workers before or during steroid injection to confirm the correct placement of the drugs in the epidural space. If two injections of steroids placed epidurally do not produce any improvement, further injections are unlikely to be useful. If neurologic deficits and pain continue or worsen despite the conservative treatment, surgical treatment is indicated. Most commonly performed surgery is the anterior cervical diskectomy.

Even if the patient's symptoms completely subside with any of the modalities, the patient should be given appropriate exercises to stretch and strengthen the muscles, watch the precipitating factors, and prevent any recurrence by early evaluation and treatment.

Physical Therapy Program for Cervical Diskogenic Disease

The physical therapy depends on past medical intervention, the extent of the lesion, and the stage of recovery. During the *acute stage,* the patient may be treated with bed rest and immobilization. Cryotherapy and transcutaneous electrical nerve stimulation (TENS) may be used at this stage. Manual therapy of the cervical spine may also be utilized. When the condition reaches the subacute stage, the patient is begun on an exercise program suited to the level and direction of the protrusion. Traction and mobilization techniques may be used in "reducible" lesions where migration of the nuclear fluid from herniated disk is expected. Cyriax and McKenzie believe that disk lesions can be reduced by mobilization/manipulation (Fig 24–5),[7, 8] but others do not agree.

Aggressive physical therapy can begin in the chronic stage, and if the patient is still using a cervical collar for pain relief, wearing time is gradually reduced. Immobilization at this stage will increase muscle weakness, poor postural habits, and tightening of soft tissue structures. The techniques utilized include flexion-extension strengthening and mobilization.

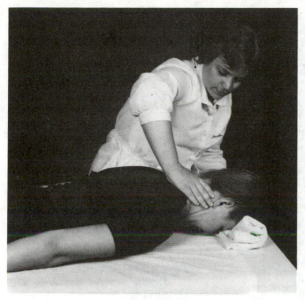

Fig 24–5.—Cervical spine mobilization for cervical diskogenic disease.

PAIN SECONDARY TO DEGENERATIVE DISK DISEASE

Pain secondary to disk degeneration is more common than pain from acute disk herniation. Disk degeneration may be due to many causes; for instance, it may be an end result of disk herniation, annular protrusion, or dehydration of the disk material.[2] Nutrition to the disk is affected by aging, stress, injuries, and strained movements of the spine.

Disk degeneration usually begins with slight tears in annular fibers. This is followed by softening of the nucleus pulposus, which eventually undergoes fragmentation. The encapsulated nuclear material gradually forces its way through the annulus to bulge and press against the posterior longitudinal ligaments. As the disk degenerates the intradiskal pressure decreases, causing the vertebral bodies to approximate secondary to the effects of gravity and muscle contraction. Degenerative changes in the cervical spine deform the intervertebral foramina and the shape of the spinal canal (Fig 24–6).

Degenerative changes can be asymptomatic as well as sympatomatic. The radiologic evidence does not correlate with pain or with nerve root compression due to osteophytes invading the intervertebral foramina. Brain observed that in asymptomatic patients, radiologic degenerative changes are seen in 25% of patients at age 50 and in 75% of patients at age 70.[9] The pain may be local and associated with limitation of neck movements. This would localize the pathologic changes to tissues of the posterior portion of the functional unit. Pain referred to the upper back, shoulders, and upper extremities indicates that the pathology lies in the intervertebral foramina and their adjacent tissues. Patients with spinal cord involvement would have referred pain distally. Management of pain secondary to disk disease is symptomatic and is described elsewhere in this book.

MYOFASCIAL PAIN SYNDROME

Probably the most common cause of neck pain in patients seen in a pain clinic is the myofascial pain syndrome. It is much more common than radiculopathy or the other causes of neck pain. Before attributing the patient's symptoms to myofascial pain syndrome, it is extremely important to rule out other primary problems such as radiculopathy, disk disease, and malignancies of the vertebrae, and referred pain due to visceral disease. Myofascial pain syndromes are characterized by the absence of neurologic signs and the presence of trigger points. Typically, patients complain of neck pain, often pain radiating to the arm. It can be associated with pain referred to different parts of the head. The trigger points are commonly found in the sternocleidomastoid muscle, which can produce pain in the face, behind the eye, and in the neck; in the splenius capitis muscle, which produces pain in the top of the head, suboccipital region, and the upper part of the

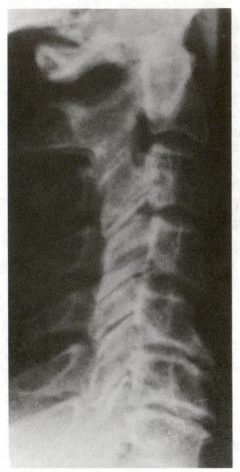

Fig 24–6.—Degenerative arthritis of the cervical spine.

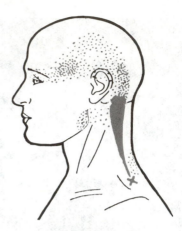

TRAPEZIUS

Fig 24–7.—Distribution of pain due to myofascial pain affecting the trapezius muscle. *X* indicates trigger point; *shaded* and *stippled areas* indicate radiation of pain.

then stretched. In order to stretch the muscle, the neck should be placed in a position opposite to the action of the muscle. For example, the sternocleidomastoid muscle turns the head to the opposite side and tilts it to the same side. In order to stretch the sternocleidomastoid, the chin is turned to the same side as the muscle and the head is tilted away from the painful side. If the relief is temporary with the spray-and-stretch technique, then the trigger points

neck; and in the posterior cervical trigger point region, over the trapezius muscle (Figs 24–7 through 24–9). It is important to know the location of the trigger points in the individual muscles. Their location is fairly constant. With experience, it is easy to locate these points and to feel subtle changes such as nodules, knots, or bands in the involved muscle. If an injection of local anesthetic relieves the pain, the diagnosis of myofascial pain is confirmed.

Management

Treatment of myofascial pain in the acute stage is very effective with vapocoolant spraying (Fig 24–10) and stretching of the involved muscle. This is indicated in the first 2–3 weeks. Ethyl chloride or fluorimethane is sprayed over the muscle, which is

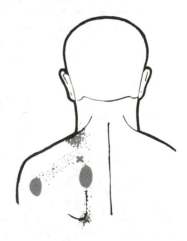

LEVATOR SCAPULE

Fig 24–8.—Distribution of pain due to myofascial pain affecting the levator scapulae. *X* indicates trigger point; *dark* and *stippled areas* indicate radiation of pain.

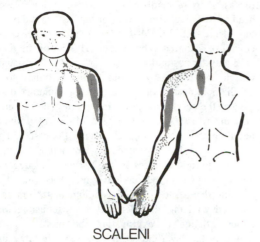

SCALENI

Fig 24–9.—Distribution of pain due to myofascial pain affecting the scalene muscles. *X* indicates trigger point; *dark* and *stippled* *areas* indicate radiation of pain.

are injected with a local anesthetic and steroid. The choice of local anesthetic is not very crucial. The needle injection of saline or injection of any local anesthetic produces equally good results. It is important to reproduce the patient's pain by injecting right into the band or the nodule. Injection of a short-acting local anesthetic such as 1% lidocaine or mepivacaine is less painful than injection of 0.25% bupivacaine. Some prefer to use mixtures containing either 0.25% bupivacaine and 0.5% lidocaine or 0.375% bupivacaine and 0.5% etidocaine. After the injection, the patient is advised to keep the muscle in a relaxed state for 4 days. If this is not done,

muscle spasms are likely to recur. The patient is advised not to drive, since driving puts an excessive strain on the neck and back muscles. Application of heat over the injected area and limbering exercises are beneficial. Physical therapy, with the use of a sine wave current for 15 minutes over the muscles followed by the vapocoolant spray and the limbering exercises for 4 days increases the chances of recovery. After 4 days, stretching and strengthening exercises for the neck muscles should be instituted to prevent recurrence. However, this alone is not sufficient, since many patients who tend to develop myofascial pain are tense individuals. By habit, they tense up their muscles anytime they experience stress. Self-hypnosis relaxation therapy and biofeedback are excellent adjuncts to other modalities on such patients.

FACET JOINT SYNDROME

Pain arising from the facet joint can mimic the neck symptoms of radiculopathy. Usually if the objective evidence of nerve root involvement is absent, tenderness over the affected facet can be identified and the patient's symptoms reproduced. During the acute stage, pain may be associated with significant muscle spasm and also restricted movement of the cervical spine. Conservative measures are the same as the ones outlined above, even though some clinicians prefer manipulation of the cervical spine in order to reduce the facet displacement.

Affected patients respond very well to an injection of local anesthetic–steroid mixture such as

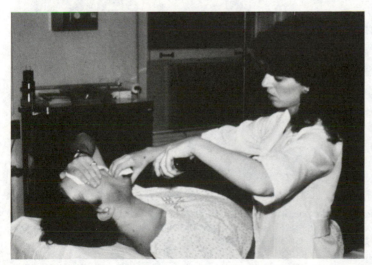

Fig 24–10.—Vapocoolant spray applied to the neck for the treatment of myofascial pain.

0.5% bupivacaine with 2 mg/cc of triamcinolone, 2–4 ml injected over the facet joint. This relieves acute symptoms and is useful even in chronic facet pain. Sometimes more than one injection may be necessary.

Good results have been reported after injection of a local anesthetic–steroid mixture into the facet joint itself. This procedure requires an image intensifier and the help of a neuroradiologist. Since the facet joint space is a potential space, it is difficult to identify needle placement in the joint. Facet joint pain can also be relieved by denervating the joint or blocking the nerve that supplies the joint. The nerve that innervates the joint comes from the corresponding nerve root and one other branch from one level above. In order to block the C5–6 facet joint, facet nerves at the C5–6 level and the C4–5 level must be blocked. This is accomplished by placing a needle at the junction of the superior facet and the transverse process. At this point the nerve curves around the superior facet to innervate the joint. Here it can be stimulated to reproduce the pain. If a local anesthetic injection relieves the symptoms, the nerve can be blocked by a local anesthetic, radiofrequency lesion, cryoprobe, or 0.5 cc of 6% phenol.

TORTICOLLIS

Torticollis is a severe state of contraction of the sternocleidomastoid muscle. It is usually unilateral (occasionally bilateral) and produces a tilting of the head to that side with flexion of the neck and deviation of the face (Fig 24–11).[10] It may be either congenital or acquired. The congenital form of the disease may be postural or muscular, in which striated muscle is replaced by fibrous tissue. Acquired torticollis may result from trauma or inflammatory disease of the cervical spine or may be a neuromuscular disorder (spasmodic torticollis) of either neurologic or psychological origin. Long-standing torticollis produces permanent contracture of the muscle, fibrotic changes in the tissues, and degenerative changes in the cervical spine. There may be variable degrees of pain. Psychological factors associated with this disorder may be responsible for either intiating or aggravating the problem. No treatment has been uniformly successful in alleviating this condition.

Management

Although the pathophysiology of spasmodic torticollis is unknown, most neurologists now feel that it is an extrapyramidal disorder.[11] The lack of understanding of the cause of torticollis is exemplified by the diverse variety of therapeutic approaches which have been proposed. Surgical approaches have been advocated most often and include cervical rhizotomy, thalamotomy, dorsal column stimulation, and excision of the sternocleidomastoid mus-

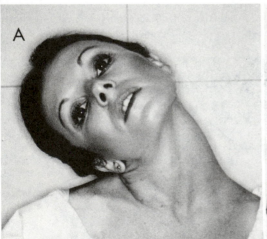
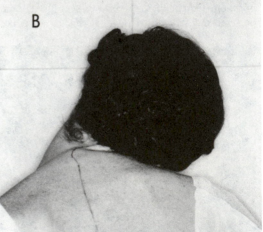

Fig 24–11.—Severe spasmodic torticollis in a 30-year-old woman. The torticollis developed acutely at 6 months of pregnancy after the administration of a phenothiazine. The figure shows the condition one month after developing torticollis. **A,** anterior view; **B,** posterior view.

cle, all of which produce varying degrees of disability and a generally poor therapeutic result. Psychological approaches such as psychotherapy, hypnosis, behavior modification, and biofeedback have been advocated. Drug therapy with amantidine, haloperidol,[12, 13] and more recently apomorphine[14] have generally given poor and unreliable results. Thus, despite much investigation, spasmodic torticollis remains an essentially intractable and disabling condition of unknown cause, with opinion divided as to whether it is an organic psychogenic disease or whether two forms exist.[15] There is some agreement that three stages of the disease may exist:[15, 16] progression for 5 years but with the possibility of remission, a static stage for the next 5 years, and a final stage during which slight improvement might occur.

Block of accessory nerve by relaxing the trapezius and sternocleidomastoid muscles is helpful in evaluating the contribution of these muscles. Frequently other neck muscles are also involved, and a cervical plexus block may be necessary to relieve all the muscle spasm. Once the muscles are relaxed, the degree of fibrotic and bony changes can be evaluated. If the accessory block results in significant improvement, repeated blocks followed by physical therapy to strengthen the opposing muscles are likely to be helpful. Neurolytic block of the accessory nerve may be necessary to provide long-term relief. Psychological factors should be considered and treated concomitantly.

Physical Therapy for Torticollis and Other Muscle Pains

The physical therapeutic approach to cervical musculoskeletal pain differs with the acute or chronic stage of the disease. The treatment plan being highly individualized according to the level and severity of involvement. The following describes the general course of physical therapy for cervical musculoskeletal pain. Note the difference between acute and chronic approaches.

ACUTE STAGE.—At times the patient will need to be immobilized in a soft or hard cervical collar. This helps support the neck musculature and is beneficial in decreasing pain. Care must be taken to maintain or increase the strength of the neck musculature while it is in the collar through exercises performed intermittently without the collar. Use of the collar is gradually eliminated as the pain decreases and the neck musculature and supporting structures become strong.

Exercises consist of gentle passive and active range of motion, i.e., flexion, extension, rotation, and lateral flexion. When the patient can perform these exercises well and relatively painlessly, isometric exercises are begun, followed by active resistive exercises as pain and muscle guarding permits. The patient may also need to perform active range of motion exercises for both upper extremities, especially the shoulders, to prevent adhesive capsulitis. Active exercise will also help increase circulation and prevent contractures and muscle atrophy. The patient is educated in proper posture and neck alignment during sleep and activities of daily living. The patient is encouraged to sleep with a small pillow to prevent hyperextension and increased flexion to prevent stress to cervical structures.

Modalities often beneficial in treating acute cervical pain are traction, cryotherapy, heat therapy, electrical stimulation, and massage. Traction may be positional, manual or mechanical, and static or intermittent. Proper amounts of cervical flexion may be beneficial to decrease pain symptoms by opening the intervertebral joint spaces and facet joints. Patients usually tolerate intermittent traction better, the weight being increased as the patient's tolerance increases. The recent literature suggests variable amounts of weight and different head positions to achieve maximal therapeutic separation of the articulating joint surfaces and musculature. Several types of home traction units are now available. They are usually of the static variety and are used in the supine or sitting positions. Heat or cold treatments and massage are used to promote relaxation, increase circulation, and decrease muscle guarding. Ultrasound is a useful heat modality and may be used by itself for its thermal properties or may be combined with electrical stimulation to enhance the physiologic benefits. Massage of soft tissue and/or trigger points, when present, may be beneficial. Trigger points can also be treated by ultrasound, ultrasound with electrical stimulation, or iontophoresis with an analgesic.

CHRONIC STAGE.—During the chronic stage of musculoskeletal cervical pain, modalities can be an important adjunct to treatment. Mobilization of specific structures in the spine and extremities may be indicated after a thorough evaluation is completed of the articulating surfaces and surrounding soft tissue. However, emphasis is shifted to exercise so that the patient can undertake a more active role in controlling the pain. Involved musculature must be restored to a more "normal" physiologic state, which can be achieved through a specific exercise program carried out in the patient's home, work, and recreational environment. It should be noted that by the time the patient's pain has reached the chronic stage, he has usually received extensive and multimodality treatment that may only have provided temporary relief, if any. The goal of the exercise program is to increase the patient's functional level by increasing his activity level. Another goal is restoration of the functional range of motion and the strength of involved structures and musculature while decreasing muscle guarding.

The patient must be educated in proper body mechanics, posture, and work and sleeping habits. An exercise regimen in conjunction with supportive modalities and treatment techniques is essential for the patient to achieve maximum benefit and return to a higher functioning level.

The physical therapeutic approach to a patient with the diagnosis of torticollis consists of evaluation and determination of a program format. Numerous postural activities in various positions along with maintenance of cervical function are the primary goals. Modalities incorporated in the treatment are ultrasound alone or in combination with electrical stimulation, vigorous soft tissue massage, manual stretching, passive to resistive range of motion exercises, relaxation technique including biofeedback, and cervical mobilization. Patients should also be given a home program to ensure continuation of treatment progress and optimal achievement of goals.

PAIN DUE TO WHIPLASH INJURY

A motor vehicle accident initiates a sequence of events affecting the cervical spine and its joints, ligaments, and musculature. This could be due to abrupt hyperextension or hyperflexion of the neck. The impact abruptly propels the body in a linear horizontal direction. Initially the head remains stationary, then it abruptly moves in the opposite direction. This abrupt movement occurs before the neck muscles can relax to permit the motion. In a rear-end impact the head moves abruptly backward, causing acute hyperextension of the cervical spine and provoking acute stretch reflex of the neck flexors. A head-on collision causes the opposite injury.

A detailed history of the accident as to direction of impact, the awareness of impending collision,

and the direction in which the patient was facing in the moment of the accident must be elicited to localize the tissues injured.

Local pain is caused by deceleration injury, and swelling and edema may irritate nerve roots, causing radiation pain. The subluxation of the cervical vertebrae is limited between C-3 and C-7. Fracture dislocation between atlas and axis can occur. The most confusing of all symptoms are due to irritation of the cervical sympathetics. They are most frequently aural (tinnitus, deafness, postural dizziness) or ocular (blurred vision, pain behind the eyeballs, dilated pupil on the involved side).[2]

The syndrome of acute spinal cord injury may occur after a deceleration hyperextension or hyperflexion injury. Whether the injury is cord contusion or relative vascular insufficiency is not always clear. With cord contusions there is usually a marked sensory and motor loss. The lesion is in the dorsal columns and lateral spinothalamic tracts. With vascular insufficiency the sensory long tracts usually are not involved. The syndrome is frequent in the elderly patient with degenerative osteoarthritis.

A patient with deceleration injury to the spinal cord typically reports a sudden snapping back of the head and numbness of the entire trunk and extremities. The patient is unable to move, or there is tingling of the arms or legs, or an inability to void. Return of power and sensation depends on the lesion (edema or hemorrhage). When the damage is due to edema, function gradually returns in sequence.

Management is symptomatic in the acute stage and is limited by injury to spinal cord, nerve roots, and fracture dislocation of the cervical spine. In the chronic stage the treatment is similar to that described in the section on the "Chronic Stage" of musculoskeletal disorders in this chapter.

ANTERIOR SCALENE SYNDROME

This syndrome can cause numbness and tingling of the arm, hand, and fingers with hypoesthesia and motor weakness of thenar and hypothenar muscles. Pain is usually described as a deep dull ache in the arm and the hand. The symptoms usually occur in the early morning and wake the patient, or after an extended period of activities involving the hand (sewing and knitting).

Physical signs are usually negative and the findings are subjective and reproduced by specific motions and positions. The Adson test is positive. The patient turns the head to the side of the symptoms, extends the cervical spine, abducts the arm, and takes a deep breath. If the radial pulse in the ipsilateral arm disappears and the symptoms reappear, the test is positive (Fig 24–12). The test contracts the scalene muscles and narrows the angle and elevates the rib. The neurovascular bundles at this site are put under traction and compressed.

Spasm of the scalene muscles may result from fatigue or unusual or prolonged physical activity. Occupational stress may produce spasm of the scalene muscles. The presence of a cervical rib or a large transverse process of C-7 has caused an anterior scalene syndrome, but is not generally responsible.

Treatment is similar to the treatment of cervical diskogenic disease. The anterior scalene muscle can be injected with 2–3 ml of a local anesthetic–steroid mixture in the tender portion of the muscle, usually at C-5 or C-6, when the radiating pain is present. If the pain is relieved without further numbness of the arm, the test is positive for relaxing the anterior scalene muscle. A series of neuromuscular block of anterior scalene muscle can be done to maintain mus-

cle relaxation at weekly intervals. Cervical lordosis is decreased with improvements in posture and flexibililty by exercises, postural training, and muscle relaxants. Surgery is not indicated for this syndrome.

CLAVICULOCOSTAL SYNDROME

In this syndrome the neurovascular structures between the first rib and the clavicle are compressed (Fig 24–13). The symptoms consist of paresthesia, numbness, and pain in the arm and the hand, mainly at night or early morning. The diagnosis is made by reduplicating the symptoms by bringing the shoulders down and posteriorly. Treatment entails postural improvement, exercises to increase muscle tone in the shoulder girdle, and psychotherapy for motivation to maintain correct posture.

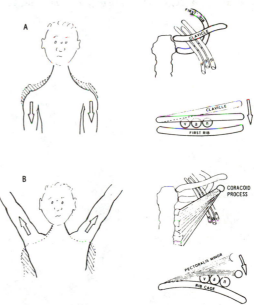

Fig 24–13.—Claviculocostal **(A)** and pectoralis minor **(B)** syndromes. In the claviculocostal syndrome, the neurovascular bundle is compressed between the clavicle and the first rib by retraction and depression of the shoulder girdles. In the pectoralis minor syndrome, the neurovascular bundle may be compressed between the pectoralis minor muscle and the rib cage if the patient elevates the arms in a position of abduction and moves the arms behind the head. (From Cailliet R.: *Shoulder Pain.* Philadelphia, F.A. Davis Co., 1981. Reproduced by permission.)

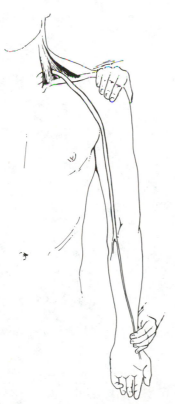

Fig 24–12.—Adson test for neurovascular compression due to the anterior scalene syndrome.

REFERENCES

1. Inman V.T., Saunders J.B. de C.M.: Referred pain from skeletal structures. *J. Nerv. Ment. Dis.* 99:660–667, 1944.
2. Cailliet R.: Functional anatomy, in *Neck and Arm Pain,* ed. 2. Philadelphia, F.A. Davis Co., 1981, p. 26.
3. Barcroft H., Dornhurst A.C.: The blood flow through the human calf during rhythmic exercise. *J. Physiol.* 109:402–411, 1949.
4. Perlow S., Markle P., Katz L.N.: Factors involved in the production of skeletal muscle pain. *Arch. Intern. Med.* 53:814–824, 1934.
5. Baetjer A.M.: The diffusion of potassium from resting skeletal muscles following reduction in blood supply. *Am. J. Physiol.* 112:139–146, 1935.
6. Jackson R.: *The Cervical Syndrome,* ed. 2. Springfield, Ill., Charles C Thomas, Publisher, 1958.
7. Cyriax J.: *Textbook of Orthopaedic Medicine.* Vol. 1: *Diagnosis of Soft Tissue Lesions.* London, Bailliere Tindall, 1978.
8. McKenzie R.A.: *The Lumbar Spine: Mechanical Diagnosis and Therapy.* Waikane, New Zealand, Spinal Publications Limited, 1981.
9. Brain W.R., Knight G.C., Bull J.W.D.: Discussion of the intervertebral disk in the cervical region. *Proc. R. Soc. Med.* 41:509–516, 1948.
10. Hansen D.A.: Torticollis. *South Afr. Med. J.* 40:480–482, 1972.
11. Horton P.C., Miller I.: The etiology of spasmodic torticollis. *Dis. Nerv. System* 33:273–275, 1972.
12. Gilbert G.J.: Spasmodic torticollis treated effectively by medical means. *N. Engl. J. Med.* 285:896–898, 1971.
13. Gilbert G.J.: The medical treatment of spasmodic torticollis. *Arch. Neurol.* 27:503–506, 1972.
14. Tolosa E.S.: Modification of tardive dyskinesia and spasmodic torticollis by apomorphine. *Arch. Neurol.* 35:459–462, 1978.
15. Matthews W.B., Beasley P., Parry-Jones W., et al.: Spasmodic torticollis: A combined clinical study. *J. Neurol. Neurosurg. Psychiatry* 41:485–492, 1978.
16. Meares R.: Natural history of spasmodic torticollis and effect of surgery. *Lancet* 17:149–150, 1971.

25 / Pain in the Extremities

P. PRITHVI RAJ, M.D.
STEPHEN E. ABRAM, M.D.

25A / Pain of Neurogenic Origin

P. PRITHVI RAJ, M.D.

NEUROGENIC PAIN in the extremities consists of cord compression, radiculopathy due to disk prolapse, herpes zoster neuralgia, inflammatory neuritis, and neuropathies. Herpes zoster and postherpetic neuralgia are described in chapter 22.

PAIN DUE TO CERVICAL CORD COMPRESSION

Compression at the cervical level characteristically produces spinal and radicular signs in the upper limbs, with addition of long tract signs in the lower extremities. There is loss of power and bulk in muscles of the shoulder girdle and arms. The biceps, brachioradialis, or triceps jerks mainly depend on the integrity of the C-5, C-6, or C-7 reflex arcs, respectively, and may be diminished or absent. In addition, there can be "inversion" of the brachioradialis reflex: tapping the tendon of this muscle elicits a brisk reflex contraction of the hand and finger flexor muscles and not the usual flexion and supination of the forearm. This unusual response is due to efferent interruption of the segmental reflex arc; the spread of the response and hyperreflexia at lower spinal levels results from pyramidal tract involvement (Figs 25A–1 through 25A–5).

When sensory symptoms extend along the radial border of the forearm and thumb ("numb thumb"), they suggest involvement of the C-6 cord segment or nerve root. Symptoms in the index and middle fingers point to C-7 involvement, and sensory impairment in the ring and little fingers suggests C-8 involvement. Lesions at the cervicothoracic junction can cause unilateral Horner's syndrome which can be associated with wasting of the small muscles of the hand and a sensory deficit on the ulnar border of the hand and forearm (C-8, T-1) (see chap. 24).

The most common causes of compression at this level are cervical spondylosis and protrusion of an intervertebral disk, but intramedullary and extramedullary tumors may also be the cause.

Investigation

To localize and establish the nature of lesions causing intraspinal compression, several diagnostic tests may be used. Roentgenographic investigations are the most important, but electrophysiologic techniques, radioisotope scanning, and cerebrospinal fluid (CSF) examination are also helpful.

Roentgenographic investigation should begin with plain films of the suspected site of spinal cord or

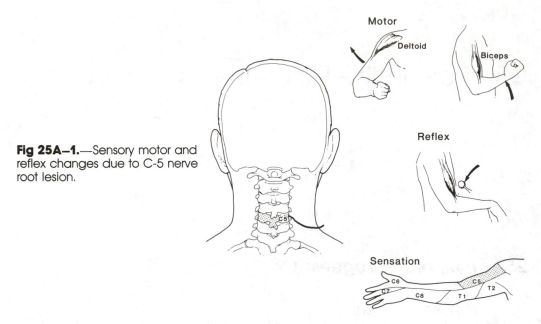

Fig 25A–1.—Sensory motor and reflex changes due to C-5 nerve root lesion.

root compression. Frontal, lateral, and oblique views are required for examination of the cervical spine; frontal and lateral views are generally satisfactory for examination of the thoracic and lumbosacral spine. Lateral films of the cervical spine in flexion and extension are needed if recurrent subluxation is suspected. In certain situations, tomography may be necessary to define a bone lesion more precisely.

Plain films of the spine should be systematically examined, with the examiner noting the number,

shape, density, and alignment of the vertebrae and the contour of the pedicles, the size of the intervertebral foramen, the size and shape of the spinal canal, the width of the disk spaces, and whether abnormal soft tissue shadows or calcifications are present. The anteroposterior depth of the spinal canal is a particularly important measurement. Sagittal diameters of less than 10 mm at any level of the cervical spine usually indicate spinal cord compression; bony compression of the cord is also possible if canals measure 10–13 mm but is improb-

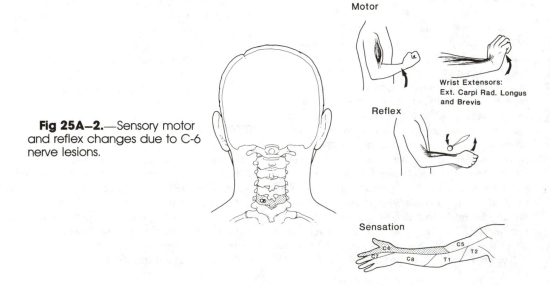

Fig 25A–2.—Sensory motor and reflex changes due to C-6 nerve lesions.

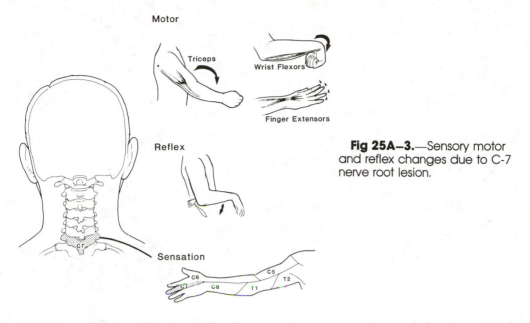

Fig 25A–3.—Sensory motor and reflex changes due to C-7 nerve root lesion.

able if canals are greater than 13 mm. Increases in the transverse diameter of the spinal canal may be associated with thinning of the pedicles and are seen with syringomyelia or intramedullary tumors. Narrowing of the spinal canal with compression of the spinal cord or roots may occur in spondylosis, achondroplasia, and Paget's disease.

Plain x-ray films of the vertebral column may suggest specific conditions. Dumbbell-shaped neu-

rofibromas that enlarge the intervertebral foramen are readily apparent in x-ray films. Congenital anomalies of the vertebral bodies are at times associated with intraspinal teratomas or lipomas. Bone caries suggests an infectious process such as tuberculosis, typhoidal infection, or brucellosis. Vertebral bone destruction by infection often involves the intervertebral disk; conversely, tumor metastases to the vertebral column spare the disks.

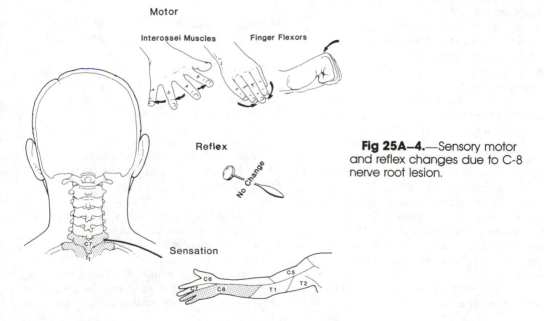

Fig 25A–4.—Sensory motor and reflex changes due to C-8 nerve root lesion.

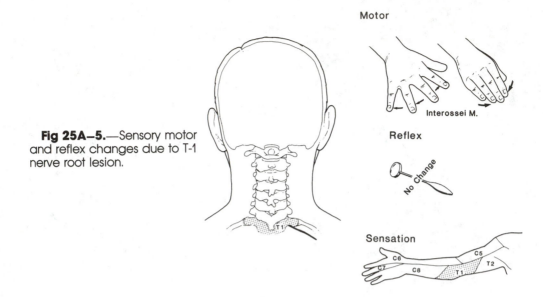

Fig 25A–5.—Sensory motor and reflex changes due to T-1 nerve root lesion.

When surgical treatment is contemplated, myelography by lumbar or cisternal injection is required for precise localization. In expert hands, air myelography is also a useful tool for the assessment of spinal cord size and for diagnosing small tumors. Spinal angiography is a specialized technique necessary for the detailed investigation of tumors and vascular malformations.

Computerized tomography (CT scan) for investigation of lesions in the spinal canal is common practice today and is indicated where myelography is contemplated.

Bone scanning after radioisotope injection may be helpful if metastases are suspected as the cause of bone destruction. However, fractures, infection, and ankylosing spondylitis may also cause increased radioisotope uptake.

Electromyography (EMG) is useful for the localization of intraspinal lesions affecting the motor unit at the anterior horn cell or the nerve root levels.

CSF examination rarely provides specific diagnostic information about compressive spinal cord or root lesions. In general, CSF examination may suggest certain diagnostic possibilities. Xanthochromic fluid is seen with intraspinal hemorrhage or block of CSF circulation. Intraspinal bleeding may originate from vascular malformations, ependymomas, or melanomas. Inflammatory cells indicate an infectious process or chemicomeningitis caused by a ruptured teratoma or dermocyst. Tumor cells may be identified in the CSF of patients with carcinomatous infiltration of the meninges.

In the absence of a block in the circulation of CSF, CSF protein levels above 60 mg/dl suggest intraspinal lesions other than an intervertebral disk protrusion or spondylosis. Spinal fluid blocks are best established by myelography; because irreparable damage to the spinal cord may result from displacement of an intraspinal mass after pressure changes resulting from jugular compression (Queckenstedt test), this procedure should not be done if spinal cord compression is suspected.

Management of Suspected Nerve Root or Spinal Cord Compression

The specific management of intraspinal compression of nerve roots or the cord depends on the suspected diagnosis, the severity of the symptoms, and the extent of the neurologic signs.

Conservative Management Aimed at Reducing Pain and Preventing Future Recurrences

Patients in this category have acute localized pain in the spinal or paraspinal region with or without peripheral radicular radiation; they do not have neurologic deficits indicative of spinal cord or severe root compression. The most likely diagnosis is an acute intervertebral disk protrusion, and with time complete recovery can usually be anticipated. This approach is particularly justified when there is no history of similar previous episodes and when the pain follows minor trauma, effort, or strain.

Patients may stay at home and should rest on a firm bed and make no physical effort. Analgesics and muscle relaxants are given for symptomatic relief. When pain subsides, exercises aimed at strengthening the muscular support of the spinal column may help prevent recurrences.

Plain x-ray films of the involved segment of the spine help ascertain changes in the vertebral bodies or disks. Initially, however, these investigations can be deferred if the patient is in considerable pain.

Conservative Management Aimed at Deciding If the Course of Intraspinal Root Compression is Progressive

Acute pain may be accompanied by signs of moderate sensory or motor deficit in a root distribution. Such signs are represented by some loss of strength, paresthesia, and mild sensory impairment or loss of muscle stretch reflexes. If these signs worsen or do not subside after a trial of conservative treatment, the patient should be admitted to the hospital to ensure immobilization and rest and for further investigation. Epidural steroids or chemonucleolysis have been used at this stage to halt the progress of the nerve root compression.

Management Aimed at Possible Surgical Decompression

This approach is indicated for patients showing signs of spinal cord compression. It is also advisable for patients with nerve root compression if there is intractable or severe recurrent pain or if there are signs of severe neurologic deficit, particularly marked weakness and muscle atrophy. These patients should be admitted to hospital for investigation. If there are no contraindications to surgery, myelography should be performed to establish a diagnosis and determine the site and extent of compression. If indicated, operative treatment should soon follow.

Prompt Investigation and Surgical Decompression

This approach is required for patients in whom spinal cord or cauda equina compression rapidly develops. Impaired bladder or rectal control constitutes an emergency. Patients should be immediately admitted to hospital to undergo only those investigations which enable a localization of the lesion. Such investigations usually include plain films of the spine and an emergency myelogram. In the course of these investigations, patients should be kept fasting to allow the immediate institution of anesthesia if surgical intervention is decided on.

BRACHIAL PLEXALGIA

The brachial plexus can be injured by traction, penetrating wounds, or compression. Acute nontraumatic brachial plexus neuropathy is a disorder of unknown cause. Antecedent needle injections into shoulder muscles, intercurrent infections, and an allergic basis have been suggested as possible etiologic factors. Typically this disorder begins with aching pain in the lateral aspect of the shoulder or, less often, in the region of the elbow or arm. Muscle weakness develops within a few hours or days, and atrophy follows; sensory loss is usually minimal and is restricted to a small patch in the cutaneous distribution of the axillar nerve. The upper brachial plexus is affected more commonly than the lower, and therefore the weakness and atrophy are more often located in the region of the shoulder. In mild cases, improvement begins in a few weeks, and clinical recovery is complete within months. More characteristically, improvement does not begin for several months and may not be complete for years. Nevertheless, eventually complete or almost complete recovery is likely. Rarely, as one side improves, the other brachial plexus becomes affected. Careful EMG examination may reveal more extensive involvement of nerves than was expected from the clinical examination. The CSF is usually normal. There is no known treatment.

COMPRESSION AND ENTRAPMENT OF PERIPHERAL NERVES

The peripheral nerve trunks of the limbs are particularly prone to compression and entrapment, although any nerve passing over a rigid promontory or through a bony canal or tight fascial plane is vulnerable. The degree of compressive damage to nerves depends on the magnitude and duration of the force, whether the force is repeated, whether the nerve is anatomically situated next to soft or hard structures, the physical habitus of the person, and disease susceptibility. Malnutrition, diabetes mellitus, renal disease, and inflammatory neuropathy all are thought to predispose to compression damage. The tendency to compression damage is inherited in some families. For many years, investigators have differed as to whether ischemia or mechanical compression was the factor that produced nerve damage from compression. At an earlier time, the evidence favored ischemia; now it favors mechanical compression. Contusion and hemorrhage and later scarring may complicate some of the comprehensive lesions in man.

The term entrapment denotes the process by which nerves are damaged by repeated compression as they pass over a rigid structure or through a tight bony or fascial canal. Such injury occurs more readily when swelling, inflammation, or degeneration develops in adjacent joints and tendons, as may happen in pregnancy, rheumatoid arthritis, myxedema, and acromegaly. Suggestive evidence that multiple minor episodes of bruising of the nerve may contribute to the development of signs of entrapment comes from the common experience that excessive use of the wrist in knitting or in gardening by the patient with the carpal tunnel syndrome, or prolonged walking by patients with Morton's neuroma, will worsen symptoms. Sites of compression for the median nerve include the pronator teres muscle and the carpal tunnel ligament; for the ulnar nerve, the elbow, wrist, pisohamate tunnel, palm, and metacarpal heads; for the radial nerve, the axilla, posterior aspect of the humerus, the supinator

muscle, and the radial aspect of the distal forearm; for the lateral femoral cutaneous nerve, the pelvic brim; for the femoral nerve, the groin; for the saphenous nerve, the medial side of the knee; for the obturator nerve, the obturator canal; for the common peroneal nerve, the lateral aspect of the knee; for the superficial and deep peroneal nerves, muscle and fascial sheaths near their origin; for the posterior tibial nerve, the tarsal tunnel; and for plantar nerves, the sole of the feet.

The three most common entrapment neuropathies are carpal tunnel syndrome, tardy ulnar palsy, and tardy peroneal nerve palsy.

Carpal Tunnel Syndrome

In the carpal tunnel syndrome the median nerve is compressed as it passes through the canal made by the carpal bones and ligament. Some cases are idiopathic, and in these cases surgeons report a flattening of the median nerve just distal to the crease of the wrist and either thickening of the ligament or, more commonly, noninflammatory thickening of the synovia of the flexor tendons. The median nerve may be compressed within the carpal tunnel by a ganglion or by degenerative joint and synovial changes from rheumatoid arthritis, myxedema, and acromegaly (Figs 25A–6 and 25A–7).

Carpal tunnel syndrome principally affects women. Pricking numbness and pain in the fingers and hands, coming on especially during the night

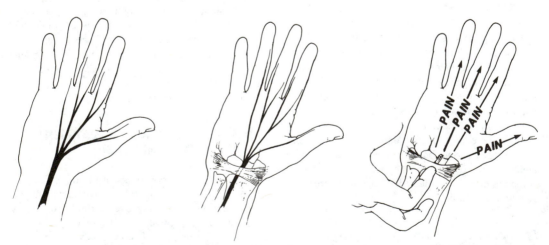

Fig 25A–6.—*Left,* anatomy of the median nerve. *Middle,* the relationship of the carpal ligament to the median nerve at the wrist. *Right,* the distribution of pain when the median nerve is compressed in the carpal tunnel.

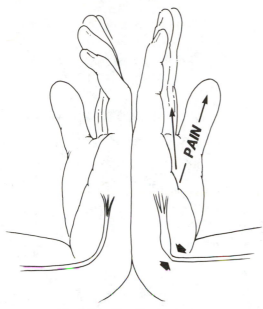

Fig 25A–7.—Phalen's sign.

and relieved by changing the position of the hands (shaking them), are characteristic. It is uncommon for patients to localize the numbness to the exact cutaneous distribution of the median nerve. Furthermore, the aching discomfort that may accompany the numbness may extend up the arm. Atrophy of the muscles innervated by the median nerve (for example, the thenar muscles) is not an early sign. In many cases it is possible to reproduce the painful numbness by holding the wrist in extreme flexion (Phalen's sign). Also, a burst of tingling may occur when the skin over the nerve at the wrist is percussed (Tinel's sign). There may be sensory loss in the distribution of the median nerve, although more frequently none is detected.

Measurement of nerve conduction is an important confirmatory test and consists in determining the time from stimulation of the median nerve at a point above the carpal ligament to the appearance of the thenar muscle action potential. Similarly, one can determine the time from stimulation of digital fibers to the recording of an action potential in electrodes overlying the median nerve above the carpal ligament. In carpal tunnel syndrome, the latency of both responses is usually prolonged.

Since carpal tunnel syndrome may be brought on by an excess of gardening, ironing, sewing, crocheting, or similar activity, relief may follow the discontinuation of these activities. Immobilization

of the wrist during the hours of sleep with a posterior splint of the forearm and hand may give relief. Injections of corticosteroid preparations beneath the carpal ligament sometimes help. Treatment for an associated disease (myxedema, rheumatoid arthritis, acromegaly) may effect an improvement. However, in most instances the treatment of choice is surgical section of the carpal ligament, which usually provides almost immediate relief.

Tardy Ulnar Nerve Palsy

The ulnar nerve may be injured at the elbow, especially in persons with a shallow ulnar groove, those who rest their weight on their elbows excessively, and those who are cachectic and lie in bed (Figs 25A–8; and 25A–9, Plate 10).

Contrary to the findings in the carpal tunnel syndrome, muscle weakness and atrophy characteristically predominate over sensory symptoms and signs, possibly because the ulnar nerve at the elbow has relatively fewer sensory fibers than the median nerve at the wrist. The patient notices atrophy of the first dorsal interosseous muscle or difficulty in performing fine manipulations. There may be numbness of the small finger, the contiguous half of the proximal and middle phalanges of the ring finger, and the ulnar border of the hand. Treatment consists of prevention of further injury. A doughnut-shaped cushion for the elbow may be helpful. Mobilizing and transplanting the nerve to a position in front of the medial epicondyle may prevent further progression of the disorder.

OTHER ENTRAPMENTS OR NEUROPATHIES

Acute and Tardy Peroneal Nerve Palsy

The common peroneal nerve is vulnerable where it crosses the head of the fibula, and can be injured when a person falls asleep in the sitting position with the knees crossed. A more chronic form occurs in cachectic patients who lie for prolonged periods with the legs externally rotated. In this disorder, dorsiflexion of the foot at the angle and extension of the toes are weak, but usually little or no sensory loss is found over the lateral surface of the leg and on the dorsum of the foot.

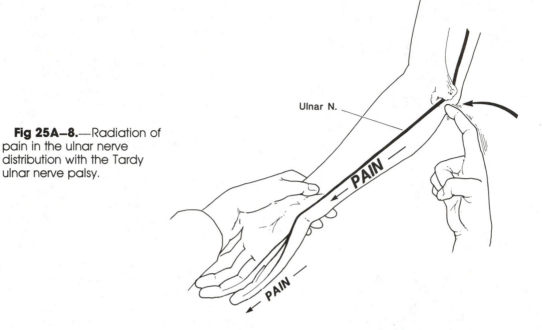

Fig 25A–8.—Radiation of pain in the ulnar nerve distribution with the Tardy ulnar nerve palsy.

Acute Radial Nerve Palsy

The radial nerve may be compressed against a hard edge or surface in persons insensitized by an excess of alcohol or sedatives ("Saturday night palsy") or may be compressed for excessive periods by the weight of a bed-partner's head ("bridegroom's palsy"). Time usually provides complete recovery.

Thoracic Outlet Syndrome

In this syndrome, the brachial plexus is entrapped at the thoracic outlet. This will produce paresthesias of the fingers which is attributed to compression of the brachial plexus by a cervical rib or a tight scalene anterior muscle. Most such patients, however, prove to have either nerve root compression from a cervical disk or carpal tunnel syndrome.

Tarsal Tunnel Syndrome

Fractures of the ankle may compress the posterior tibial nerve, resulting in pain and numbness of the sole of the foot.

Meralgia Paresthetica

Fat persons who wear tight corsets, persons who wear gun belts, and persons with pendulous abdomens may develop superficial paresthesia and burning discomfort in the distribution of the lateral cutaneous nerve of the thigh. Presumably the trouble results from compression of this nerve as it passes beneath the inguinal ligament, but the condition sometimes arises without evident cause.

INFLAMMATORY RADICULAR POLYNEUROPATHY

Acute

Involvement predominantly of the posterior root and spinal ganglion results in a sensory polyradiculoneuropathy which is probably the counterpart of ventral spinal root involvement. As in the motor variety, a preceding infection may antedate the neurologic syndrome by several weeks. Typically the onset is marked by combinations of sensory dysfunction and pain. The sensory dysfunction is most commonly described as unsteadiness in gait or clumsiness in the use of the hands. Even more incapacitating are the painful dysesthesias which develop in some patients. Varying combinations of lancinating pain, prickling hyperesthesia, constricting band-like sensations, and burning or coldness of skin may be described. In most patients the hyperesthetic skin is insensitive, but when the threshold for sensation is exceeded the discomfort is excessive. Any region of the body may be affected, and the disorder involves proximal as well as distal dermatomes. On clinical examination the lower extremities tend to be affected more than the upper, and the various modalities of sensation may be affected to different degrees. Patients often exhibit sensory ataxia, and, because of the severe impairment of joint position, the limbs may be held in distorted positions. Tendon reflexes are often diminished or absent.

Minor degrees of involvement of motor and autonomic neurons are not uncommon. In addition, patients have difficulty in sustaining muscle contraction in the presence of severe involvement of the afferent peripheral nervous system. The CSF changes are similar to those seen in the motor variety. The motor nerve conduction velocity, the amplitude of the muscle action potential, and the distal latency may be within normal limits. By contrast, nerve action potentials cannot be elicited from stimulation of afferent nerve fibers either because the afferent fibers have degenerated or because the action potential is so dispersed.

The prognosis for recovery in sensory polyneuropathy is less good than in the motor variety, and symptoms of cutaneous hyperpathia often persist or recur for many years. The sensory ataxia usually improves but likewise often does not recover completely. This persistence of the neurologic deficit probably is explained by irreversible damage of spinal ganglion neurons. Affected craftsmen and professionals whose work depends on manual dexterity often require retraining in less skilled work.

Chronic

In chronic inflammatory polyradiculoneuropathy the neurologic deficit tends to develop slowly over months or years and persists for years. Some patients have a monophasic course over many years. Others have a stepwise progression to their maximal deficit and then slowly improve. Still others have a recurrent course with ultimate worsening or ultimate improvement. In a few patients the condition progresses slowly to death over several years. As in the acute inflammatory polyradiculoneuropathies, the process tends to involve symmetric proximal body structures and to affect motor, autonomic, and sensory peripheral neurons in varying proportions. The CSF protein level is usually elevated. The pathologic alterations initially resemble those of the acute variety, but with time hypertrophic neuropathy develops. Sural nerve biopsy may show features of the disease without cellular infiltrates. Results of nerve conduction testing and EMG examination are not unlike those of the acute variety, except that normal nerve conduction is preserved in fewer patients. Over a period of years most patients eventually improve beyond their maximal deficit but continue to have a significant neurologic problem.

The use of prednisone often yields dramatic improvement. Regrettably, such effects soon wear off in most instances, and long-term steroid therapy should be avoided because of its complications.

NEUROPATHY ASSOCIATED WITH DIABETES MELLITUS

Frequency and Epidemiology

The reported frequency of neuropathy among diabetic patients ranges widely, from 5% to 60%. The difference is mainly due to differences in the definition of what constitutes neuropathy, and differences in the criteria and techniques to diagnose it. If a mild reduction of nerve conduction velocity is used as a criterion, neuropathy occurs in approximately 60% of diabetics. The frequency of neuropathy increases with age and with the duration of diabetes.

Etiology

It seems unlikely that a single mechanism underlies the various types of diabetic neuropathy. Nerve damage from ischemia to distal lower limbs represents one variety, and compression may be another. The mechanism of nerve fiber damage in the more diffuse types of neuropathy is less well understood. A diffuse microangiopathy of endoneurial capillaries with alteration of the blood-nerve barrier seems a reasonable possibility. Alternative explanations include immunologic or biochemical derangements, insulin deficiency, or phospholipid deficiency. No explanation has been fully supported.

Clinical Symptoms and Classification

The various types of diabetic neuropathy overlap each other, but the following classification illustrates the diverse types.

ASYMPTOMATIC NEUROPATHY.—Although incompletely studied, asymptomatic low nerve conduction velocity is associated with morphological abnormality of nerve fibers.

NEUROPATHY WITH PERIPHERAL VASCULAR DISEASE.—Diabetic patients with severe peripheral vascular disease affecting the distal lower limb may develop a distal stocking-like ischemic neuropathy. Sensory and autonomic symptoms predominate. Only nerves in the territory of the ischemia are affected.

ATAXIC NEUROPATHY (PSEUDOTABES DIABETICA).—A diffuse symmetric distal neuropathy especially affecting the lower limbs is common in diabetics, particularly in those with long-standing disease, but also in patients with mild diabetes mellitus. In most cases the neuropathy involves both large and small afferent fibers, as well as autonomic fibers and motor fibers. Mild cases produce nonpainful numbness of the toes and the front part of the foot. Varying degrees of sensory ataxia are found with more severe cases. The Achilles and, less frequently, the quadriceps reflex disappear. Touch pressure, joint position, and vibration sensations are variably abnormal in the distal lower limb, less so in the upper. Pain and thermal discriminations tend to be spared.

HYPERALGESIC NEUROPATHY.—Patients with hyperalgesic neuropathy have burning painfulness of the skin of the toes, feet, and legs. In addition, lancinating pain, tightness, hypersensitivity of the feet, and deep aching in the limbs may be present. Night pain in the legs, with the features of restless legs, can be improved only by movement such as getting out of bed and moving about. Autonomic involvement resulting in postural hypotension, anhidrosis, and impotence is more common in hyperalgesic than in ataxic neuropathy.

AUTONOMIC NEUROPATHY.—Autonomic symptoms of mild degree are common in diabetes, especially with neuropathy. In the variety called autonomic neuropathy, postural hypotension, impotence in the male, and bladder and bowel incontinence in both sexes are particularly troublesome. These patients tend to have hyperalgesic symptoms as well.

DIABETIC LUMBOSACRAL PLEXUS NEUROPATHY (DIABETIC AMYOTROPHY AND FEMORAL NEUROPATHY).—The terms used to describe this type of diabetic neuropathy draw attention to different clinical presentations. So-called femoral neuropathy often begins suddenly with pain in the anterior aspect of the thigh, followed within a few days by marked weakness, and later atrophy, of the quadriceps muscle. The pattern of EMG denervation reveals that the disorder extends beyond the femoral nerve and involves either the lumbosacral plexus or the roots, or both. A rapid improvement in some cases speaks against the disorder's being due to vascular occlusion. If muscle weakness and atrophy predominate and the disorder affects both legs, the term diabetic amyotrophy has been applied.

Treatment

Only weak evidence indicates that close diabetic control prevents or ameliorates diabetic neuropathy. The pain in hyperalgesic diabetic neuropathy must be approached in several ways. One must allay anxiety and depression, encourage a normal sleep pattern, and find ways of dealing with the pain without addicting the patient. Cool soaks of the feet for 15 minutes twice a day may help. Some patients find relief with phenytoin or carbamazepine. Aspirin with codeine may help others. Sedation should be reserved for night sleep. In the well-adjusted male with impotence, an inflatable prosthesis may allow sexual function.

INVESTIGATIONS OF NEUROPATHY

Electromyography

Nerve conduction velocity testing and EMG have assumed an increasingly important role in establishing the presence and type of neuropathic involvement. As described below, involvement of large alpha motor neurons may be of at least three types: (1) rapid degeneration of the entire neuron (neuronal degeneration), (2) axonal degeneration of the distal axon (dying-back) with or without atrophy and with or without secondary segmental demyelination, and (3) primary segmental demyelination. In neuronal degeneration, nerve conduction velocity tends to remain within normal limits until marked muscle weakness occurs. Needle EMS shows denervation and an increased size of motor unit potentials. In axonal degeneration, low conduction velocity occurs only when the majority of fibers show the features of axonal atrophy and secondary segmental demyelination and remyelination. The EMG features resemble those of anterior horn cell disorders. In primary segmental demyelination, Schwann cell function is altered because of an inborn error of metabolism, by toxin, or by immunologic mechanism. Nerve conduction velocity is reduced and muscle action potentials are reduced in size and dispersed. Special techniques can determine low conduction velocities in both proximal and distal segments of nerve. Denervation, which often accompanies segmental demyelination, implies concomitant axonal degeneration.

The evaluation of an abnormality of the A alpha primary afferent neurons by clinical neurophysiologic techniques is less complete than for alpha motor neurons. A decrease in amplitude and increase in latency of ulnar, median, and sural nerve action potentials provide evidence of such an abnormality. Adequate clinical neurophysiologic evaluation of gamma motor neuron fibers, of A delta and somatic C fibers, and of sympathetic C fibers is not possible at this time. This lack is often not a serious limitation, as most neuropathic conditions also involve A alpha fibers.

Nerve Biopsy

Nerve biopsy can usually provide specific answers to the following questions: Is neuropathy present? What populations of fibers are affected? What type of fiber degeneration is occurring? How severe and how fast is it? Is regeneration or fiber repair occurring? Can specific diagnostic features be recognized? Cutaneous nerve biopsy (usually of the sural nerve) may provide diagnostic information in amyloidosis, in necrotizing angiopathic neuropathy, in leprosy, in sarcoidosis, and in various lipidoses such as metachromatic leukodystrophy and Fabry's disease. A presumptive diagnosis based on nerve biopsy findings may be possible in inflammatory neuropathies, in lymphoproliferative disorders, and in myxedema. Despite its usefulness in diagnosis, however, nerve biopsy should be used sparingly because it may leave a long-lasting, disagreeable, and sometimes painful numbness. Nerve biopsies should probably be performed only in specialized centers.

Peripheral Pathology

To help characterize the pathologic involvement, it is helpful to ask the following questions: Which populations of neurons are affected? What is the level of damage within neurons? What is the type of fiber degeneration? How extensive? What kind of repair or regeneration has occurred?

Several types of nerve fiber degeneration are recognized. In both wallerian and axonal degeneration, involvement of the axon is primary. In wallerian degeneration from crush or section of nerve, the distal axon inevitably degenerates by a series of rapid stereotyped histologic changes. In man, wallerian degeneration occurs from compression, crush, or traction and from transection of fibers, as, for example, in necrotizing angiopathic neuropathy. In axonal degeneration the course may be less rapid than in wallerian degeneration, axonal atrophy may precede degeneration, and electron microscopic abnormalities of axis cylinders may be present prior to dissolution of the myelinated fiber.

At least two types of segmental demyelination are recognized. In primary segmental demyelination, the Schwann cells are affected first and predominantly. For example, in inflammatory polyradiculoneuropathy, involvement of interstitial mononuclear cells results in myelin damage, whereas in lead neuropathy a metabolic poisoning of Schwann cells probably is involved. A secondary segmental demyelination (secondary to axonal atrophy or disease) seems to characterize those neuropathies with axonal atrophy, e.g., in Friedreich's ataxia and in uremia.

The neurologic deficits from demyelinating lesions tend to be less severe and shorter-lived than those from axonal degeneration. Nerve repair following a crush lesion is rapid and more complete than when the nerve trunk is transected. Nerve regeneration tends to be better in the young than in the old.

BIBLIOGRAPHY

1. Aguilar J.A., Elvidge A.R.: Intervertebral disk disease caused by the Crucella organism. *J. Neurosurg.* 18:27, 1961.
2. Ambrose G.B., Alpert M., Neer C.S.: Vertebral osteomyelitis: A diagnostic problem. *JAMA* 97:101, 1966.
3. Charkes N.D., Sklaroff D.M., Young I.: A critical analysis of strontium bone scanning for detection of metastatic cancer. *Am. J. Roentgenol. Radium Ther. Nucl. Med.* 96:647, 1966.
4. DiChiro G., Doppman J.L.: Differential angiographic

features of hemangioblastomas and arteriovenous malformations of the spinal cord. *Radiology* 93:25, 1969.

5. Elsberg C.A., Dyke C.G.: Diagnosis and localization
   of tumors of the spinal cord by means of measurements
   made on x-ray films of vertebrae and the correlation of

clinical and x-ray findings. *Bull. Neurol. Inst.* 3:359,
1934.

6. Hammerschlag S., Wolpert S., Carter B.: Computed
   tomography of the spinal canal. *Radiology* 121:361,
   1976.

25B / Pain of Musculoskeletal Origin

P. PRITHVI RAJ, M.D.

IN GENERAL, pain of soft tissues in the extremities is due to bursitis tenosynovitis and fibrositis. In different regions the same pathologic condition may produce different syndromes, depending on the adjacent tissues involved. Common syndromes are described in this chapter.

BURSITIS

Bursae are closed synovial sacs located at sites of friction between skin, ligaments, tendons, muscles, and bones (Fig 25B–1). Trauma is the most common cause of bursitis, but almost any illness characterized by joint synovitis may be associated with involvement of the lining of bursae. The subdeltoid, trochanteric, olecranon, and prepatellar bursae are commonly involved. Septic or gouty bursitis can be diagnosed by appropriate studies of aspirated fluid. Protection of an inflamed bursa from friction and trauma is the most important aspect of treatment, but moderate doses of salicylates, phenylbutazone, or indomethacin may be helpful. Local injection with an adrenocorticosteroid preparation is indicated if symptoms are severe or refractory to other treatments.

TENOSYNOVITIS[1]

Tendon sheaths, like bursae, have synovial linings and can be involved by any process capable of inducing joint synovitis (Fig 25B–2). Tenosynovitis in the hand or foot is a frequent manifestation of gonococcemia. Calcific tendinitis, a common source of shoulder pain, may be associated with marked inflammatory signs resembling acute gout. Focal thickening of the tendon sheath and adjacent tendon can result in "locking" or "triggering" phenomena. This problem, termed *stenosing tenovaginitis*, is common in the flexor tendons of the fingers. Involvement of the abductor pollicis longus and extensor pollicis brevis tendons of the thumb (de Quervain's syndrome) results in pain and tenderness at the radial aspect of the wrist.[1] There are no general recommendations for management, since tenosynovitis may be a manifestation of various disease states, including rheumatoid arthritis and other connective tissue syndromes, infection, gout, and hypercholesterolemia. The common form of tenosynovitis, unassociated with systemic disease, will often subside with rest. If symptoms are severe or recurrent, local injections of adrenocorticosteroid preparations are usually effective. Surgical excision of the affected tendon sheath is indicated for patients with persistent disability.

FIBROSITIS

This term has been applied to a poorly defined symptom complex characterized by pain and stiffness in varying areas, most often in the neck, shoulder girdle, and posterior aspect of the trunk. Physical signs, except for questionable nodules or thickening of the deep fasciae, are lacking, and laboratory and roentgenographic studies are negative. The term fibrositis is based on vague hypothesis and common usage rather than on anatomical abnormalities. Localized areas of tenderness, commonly in the paravertebral areas medial to the scapula, have been termed "trigger points." The syndrome usually begins in the middle years of life. Because the majority of patients appear tense and anxious and have no recognizable objective basis for symptoms, the syndrome is often considered psychogenic. Since pain and stiffness can be manifestations of a variety of musculoskeletal, neurologic, and systemic disorders, the diagnosis of fibrositis requires the exclusion of more defined illnesses. The patient and his physician tend to share an unhappy experience

443

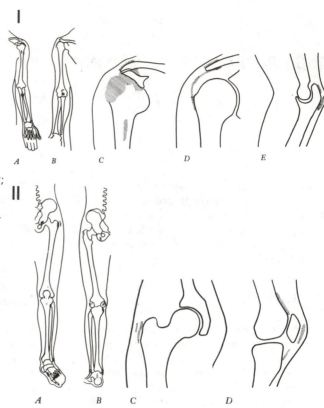

Fig 25B–1.—Sites of the major bursae of the upper extremities. **I** or upper extremity: **A,** in the anterior aspect of the arm; **B,** in the posterior aspect of the arm; **C,** around the shoulder anteriorly; **D,** around the shoulder posteriorly; **E,** at the elbow. **II** or lower extremity: **A,** in the anterior aspect of the leg; **B,** in the posterior aspect of the leg; **C,** around the hip; **D,** in front of the knee. (From Zohn and Mennel.[6] © 1976, Little, Brown & Co.; reproduced by permission.)

in efforts to control symptoms. Even strong reassurance that there is no serious disease has mixed results, as does treatment with salicylates, sedatives, tranquilizers, and muscle relaxants. Temporary relief is occasionally achieved by injection of a local anesthetic into tender points or by chilling the overlying skin with ethyl chloride.

THE PAINFUL SHOULDER

Shoulder pain is frequent and may be caused by diverse mechanisms. Of prime importance in examining patients with pain in the shoulder is that the pain may be referred from cervical, intrathoracic, and diaphragmatic regions. Shoulder motion is limited by the secondary action of muscles through a "joint complex" of independent articulations of the glenohumeral, acromioclavicular, and sternoclavicular joints. For painless shoulder movements, gliding surfaces of periarticular structures—the musculotendinous cuff, the subdeltoid bursa, and the long head of the biceps—should function normally. Any of these structures may be responsible for shoulder

pain. The painful disorders of the periarticular soft tissues of the shoulder are calcific tendinitis, bursitis, bicipital tendinitis, and rotator cuff tears. Arthritis, infections, and traumatic injury of the bone are the usual causes of bony pain of the shoulder (Fig 25B–3).

Calcific Tendinitis and Bursitis

Calcific tendinitis and bursitis are the most common causes of shoulder pain and result from degeneration of the supraspinatus and infraspinatus tendons. Approximately 3% of middle-aged persons have calcific deposits in the rotator tendons. Although most have few or no symptoms, some experience pain because of inflammation of the parietal surface of the overlying subdeltoid bursa. An inflammatory exudate containing calcaneous matter may rupture into this bursa. The symptoms may be acute, subacute, or chronic. The acute syndrome is characterized by the sudden onset of pain in the shoulder area, often with radiation into the neck and proximal arm. Any motion of the shoulder girdle

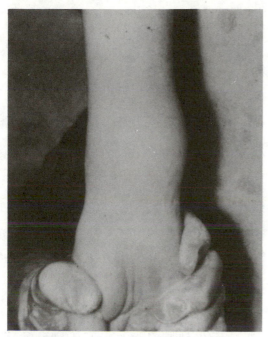

Fig 25B–2.—Painful, swollen wrist due to tenosynovitis. (From Zohn and Mennel.[6] © 1976 Little, Brown & Co.; reproduced by permission.)

elicits pain. There is frequently exquisite local tenderness over the anterior and anterolateral aspect of the shoulder joint. Night pain is a prominent feature. Roentgenographic studies usually demonstrate linear calcific deposits in the involved tendon or a more diffuse calcific pattern in the subdeltoid bursa. In most instances acute symptoms abate after a few days, but in a minority subacute discomfort persists for weeks or months.

Treatment is influenced by the severity and duration of symptoms. Anti-inflammatory agents, such as phenylbutazone or indomethacin, and analgesics are usually sufficient to control acute symptoms. In most patients there is a spontaneous remission of pain and a disappearance of calcific deposits. When the symptoms are very acute, aspiration of calcified material and injection of a local anesthetic–steroid mixture may give prompt relief. The prospects of more chronic discomfort can be minimized by the institution of an active exercise program as soon as the level of discomfort permits. If the patient is not making progress toward regaining normal shoulder motion with a home exercise program, supervised physical therapy is important. A small percentage of patients with refractory pain and persistent roentgenographic findings may require surgical exploration for removal of calcific deposits.

Bicipital Tendinitis

The long head of the biceps originates from the superior surface of the glenoid. It emerges from the glenohumeral bursa to lie in the bicipital groove of the humerus, where it is covered by a synovial sheath. The shoulder pain of bicipital tendinitis frequently radiates along the biceps of the forearm and is aggravated by abduction and internal rotation. Tenderness over the bicipital groove and accentuation of pain with resisted supination of the forearm, with the elbow flexed at 90°, aid in the recognition of bicipital tendinitis. The management is similar to that described for calcific tendinitis: local injection of local anesthetics and steroids, systemic anti-inflammatory agents, and an exercise program. In refractory cases, surgical exploration with tendon transfer usually yields good results.

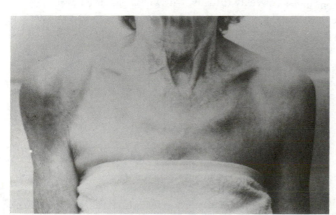

Fig 25B–3.—Patient with right shoulder pain from degenerative arthritis. Note loss of muscle contour. (From Zohn and Mennel.[6] © 1976 Little, Brown & Co.; reproduced by permission.)

Rotator Cuff Tears

The same degenerative changes that underlie the development of shoulder tendinitis can weaken the musculotendinous rotator cuff and predispose it to rupture. Most patients with this problem describe the acute onset of shoulder pain after trauma or strenuous work. If the tear is complete, the patient is unable to abduct the arm, but it can be held in abduction, once elevated to 90°, by the action of the deltoid muscle. With incomplete tears, the patient has only mild pain and moderate weakness. The diagnosis of rotator cuff tears is best established by contrast arthrography. Surgical repair is usually warranted for complete rupture of the supraspinatus tendon. Partial immobilization followed by an exercise program is appropriate for partial tears.

Frozen Shoulder

A minority of patients with any of the shoulder conditions discussed above develop chronic restriction of motion of the glenohumeral joint. When there is no apparent relationship of frozen shoulder to other shoulder disease, such as tendinitis or rotator cuff injury, the condition is sometimes termed adhesive capsulitis. This condition may be clinically indistinct from the shoulder-hand syndrome. Pain is generally less severe and less well localized relative to other conditions causing shoulder pain. The most important aspect of the management of frozen shoulder is prevention. Early attention to the underlying cause of shoulder pain and the institution of an effective exercise program are nearly always successful in combating the progression of shoulder immobility. Management of the chronic frozen shoulder is much more difficult. Manipulation under general anesthesia followed by intensive physical therapy may be indicated when patients are not helped by conservative management. A series of intra-articular injections of local anesthetics and steroids may be helpful in initiating pain relief and physical therapy.

TENNIS ELBOW

Tennis elbow is characterized by pain and tenderness over the lateral epicondyle at the origin of the common extensor tendon (Fig 25B–4). Pain may radiate along the extensors in the forearm. Tennis el-

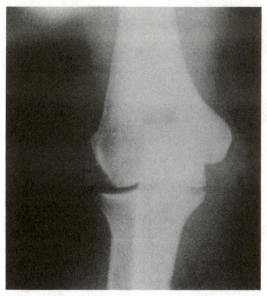

Fig 25B–4.—Lateral epicondylitis in a patient with tennis elbow. (From Zohn and Mennel.[6] © 1976 Little, Brown & Co.; reproduced by permission.)

bow can be caused by subperiosteal hematoma, strain of the extensor origin or the lateral ligament of the elbow, or entrapment of a branch of the radial nerve.[2] Incorrect style in playing tennis, badminton, or golf may initiate and perpetuate tennis elbow.

When pain is present in the medial aspect of the elbow, it affects the common flexor origin; the condition has been termed golfer's elbow. Epicondylitis can also be caused by throwing the baseball.

Treatment of strain at the elbow joint consists of deep heat and rest in the acute stage and a series of local injections of a local anesthetic and steroids weekly (usually 3–6) with a graduated exercise program. In disabling cases, tenotomy of the extensor origin, division of the annular ligament, and radial nerve decompression may be considered. It usually is a self-curing malady, but patients may take several months to recover.[1]

Areas involved by myofascial pain on the upper extremity are shown in Figure 25B–5.

GROIN STRAIN

The commonly affected tendon is the adductor longus at its origin from the pelvis; however, the origins of the rectus femoris, sartorius, and the il-

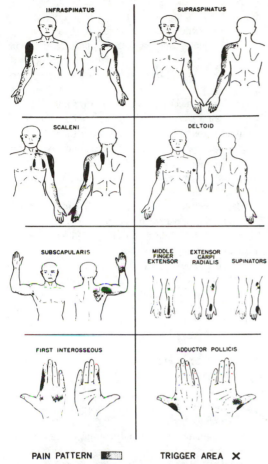

PAIN PATTERN ▨ TRIGGER AREA ✕

Fig 25B–5.—Myofascial pain in the upper extremity. (From Zohn and Mennel.[6] © 1976 Little, Brown & Co.; reproduced by permission.)

lopsoas tendons may be involved. The initial injury is unguarded movement of the hip in a fatigued player which tears the muscle at its insertion to the bone or tendon.

Pain and loss of function are marked. Local tenderness and muscle spasm are found. Stretching the involved muscle aggravates the pain. Initial treatment in the acute stage is directed toward rest, especially of the involved muscles. During the first week deep heat and anti-inflammatory agents are helpful. Local anesthetics with steroids can be injected to obtain pain relief. Ultrasound and resistive exercises can then be planned at 3–6 weeks. In chronic and refractory groin strains, local anesthetics with steroids (a series of six injections weekly), active exercises, and occasionally surgical tenotomy may be necessary.

PAIN IN THE LEG

Areas involved by myofascial pain in the lower extremity are shown in Figure 25B–6.

Pulled Hamstrings

This injury occurs in sports during sprinting or hurdling. Tendoperiosteal tears occur at the ischial origins and musculotendinous tears occur in the

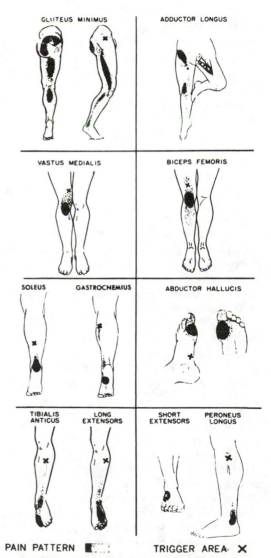

PAIN PATTERN ▰ TRIGGER AREA ✕

Fig 25B–6.—Myofascial pain in the lower extremity. (From Zohn and Mennel.[6] © 1976 Little, Brown & Co.; reproduced by permission.)

lower thigh. Spasms of the hamstrings may accompany low back problems such as spondylolysis or a chronic disk or may accompany meniscal injury, when the hamstring attempts to stabilize the malfunctioning knee.

Pain and tenderness are elicited in the hamstrings. Pain may radiate along the sciatic nerve distribution. Stretching of the affected muscle causes discomfort. The treatment is similar to that for groin strain, i.e., early rest and deep heat followed by trigger point injections and an active exercise program.

Torn Meniscus

Pain in the knee secondary to meniscal injury is common in sports. The minisci act as shock absorbers and allow the femur to glide and rotate over the tibia effortlessly; the menisci also stabilize the knee during this movement.

Injury to the meniscus can occur with minor repetitive trauma, or with twisting strain with the knee flexed and body weight on the knee, or secondary to ligamentous laxity.

In the early stages the torn meniscus may cause no symptoms. Commonly, pain is localized in the joint line on the affected side. There may be loss of movement of a few degrees at the extremes of flexion or extension with swelling and wasting of the vastus medialis. Locking of knee is noticed with a large tear. A locked knee can flex but cannot extend. Muscle spasms may be present. Between attacks the tenderness and pain may disappear.

History is most important to arrive at the diagnosis of torn meniscus. Loose bodies should be excluded by plain radiographs. Arthroscopy is extremely useful in confirming the diagnosis and confirms 95% of medial meniscus tears and 85% of lateral meniscus tears.[3]

A painful swollen knee, with repeated episodes of locking and tenderness over the femoral condyles, warrants meniscectomy. Surgery is rarely required for the first acute episode. After meniscectomy, 30% of patients may have diabling aching stiffness or swelling of the joint.[4] Often the patient may complain of discomfort in and around the knee compartment after meniscectomy. The discomfort is most acute while the patient is running or jumping. There may be a dull ache along the hamstrings. This discomfort is due to capsular or ligament strain relative to ligament laxity secondary to meniscectomy.

Treatment is directed toward prevention of pain by avoiding walking on hard surfaces. A compression bandage is applied to the knee to prevent effusion and provide stability. Acute strains of the capsule, ligaments, and hamstrings are treated with rest, trigger point injection of local anesthetics, ultrasound, and nonsteroidal anti-inflammatory agents.

The key to successful recovery after knee injuries is to develop strong lower limb muscles, especially the quadriceps. This will compensate for weak knee ligaments. The following exercises are instituted: (1) straight leg raising (without and with weights), (2) flexion exercises of the knee, and (3) extension exercises of the knee.

Knee rehabilitation is achieved with patience. Each exercise must be mastered completely before the next one is undertaken. Pain and effusion require a reduction in activity and weights. Sometimes it is advantageous to reapply a plaster cast for a few days to concentrate on straight leg exercises while the effusion and discomfort subside. After a major knee injury 3–6 months may be required for rehabilitation.

Anterior and Posterior Compartment Syndromes

The muscles in both the anterior and posterior compartments of the leg are covered by the fascial sheaths. Skeletal or soft tissue injuries can be accompanied by marked swelling within these compartments. Ischemia followed by infarction in the muscle groups may occur. Commonly the swelling and pain in these compartments begin insidiously as a result of prolonged exercises, such as in long distance running or repeated striking of the foot on a hard surface as in basketball (Fig 25B–7). The tibialis anterior is commonly involved. In young female gymnasts, there is tenderness and traction on the medial border of the tibia and soleal hypertrophy (''junior leg''). Pain in the legs due to athletic overexertion is called ''shin splints.''

Medial Tibial Syndrome

The medial tibial syndrome is due to muscle edema or hypertrophy with pain secondary to ischemia in long distance running. The pains appear during running and disappear at rest. Localized tender trigger points are found at the medial border of the tibia.

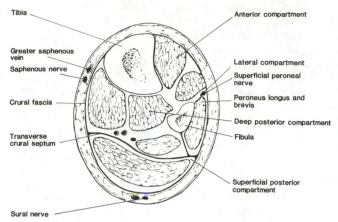

Tibia

Greater saphenous vein

Saphenous nerve

Crural fascia

Transverse crural septum

Sural nerve

Anterior compartment

Lateral compartment

Superficial peroneal nerve

Peroneus longus and brevis

Deep posterior compartment

Fibula

Superficial posterior compartment

Fig 25B–7.—Cross section of the leg showing the various compartments and their contents. (From Zohn and Mannel.[6] © 1976 Little, Brown & Co.; reproduced by permission.)

Anterior Tibial Syndrome

The anterior tibial syndrome causes discomfort and tenderness in the soft tissue on the anterolateral aspect of the leg.[1] There is a painful, tight sensation with weakness on dorsiflexion. Occasionally paresthesias may be elicited to the dorsum of the foot. Findings on physical examination with the patient at rest are often normal. With exercise, muscle tenderness in peroneal group of muscles and weakness in dorsiflexion can be elicited.

The differential diagnosis includes claudication from peripheral vascular disease, tendinitis, and fatigue fractures. Pain which can be eliminated or made tolerable by exercise is not due to a compartment syndrome.

Rest, elevation, massage, and deep heat are helpful in the early stages. In acute stages, decompression may be required, which entails splitting the involved thickened fascia.

Local injection of tender trigger points with a local anesthetic and steroids in the acute and chronic stages help relax the tight muscles and relieve pain. This is done as an adjuvant to physical therapy. In chronic stages, a series of lumbar sympathetic blocks or a continuous infusion of bupivacaine in the lumbar sympathetic chain have been helpful in reducing the activity of afferent C fibers and increasing vascularity to the ischemia areas.

ANKLE AND FOOT PAIN

Repeated trauma from overuse or direct injury will cause areas of focal degeneration in the Achilles tendon and produce pain on exertion; the tendon may rupture. Chronic pain in the tendon may persist, with focal degeneration and secondary thickening of the paratenon.

In the early stages of Achilles tendon pain, deep heat, mobilization, and padding of the heel are indicated. Local injection of steroids is not indicated because they further weaken the collagen of the tendon, leading to eventual rupture.[5] Refractory cases may require surgery to remove the thickened paratenon.

Another common cause of pain at the insertion of the Achilles tendon into the heel is bursitis. A small spur of bone is sometimes found in this region. Injection of a local anesthetic with a steroid at the painful site and the application of deep heat are the first line of treatment. If a spur is present, it could be surgically excised along with the bursa in the later stages. Avoiding high-heeled soles and wearing soft, well-padded soles will help prevent recurrences.

Braised heel, plantar fasciitis, sprain of the spring ligament, and chronic foot strain from wearing unsuitable shoes are other causes of ankle and foot pain. Treatment for these conditions entails intrinsic foot exercises, contrast foot bathing, and correct footwear to minimize pain. If the pain is intolerable, a series of local anesthetics and steroids can be injected in tender spots as an adjuvant technique. In refractory cases lumbar sympathetic blocks and behavior modification may be helpful.

Ankle Sprains

Acute capsular sprains of the ankle are probably the commonest sports injury. Due to invasion and internal rotation, there is a sprain of the lateral ligament. There is local pain and swelling with no radiologic evidence of malleolar fracture. Acute treatment consists of strapping or plaster cast, depending on the severity of pain on weight-bearing. After 2–3 weeks the lesion usually resolves.

Chronic sprained ankle can be treated with deep heat, manipulation, a series of local injections of local anesthetics and steroids, progressive weight-bearing exercises, and soft padded soles. Increased hyperactivity of sympathetic afferent and efferent activity from the region can be decreased by lumbar sympathetic blocks, continuous infusion of bupivacaine in the lumbar sympathetic chain, or epidural blocks.

Foot Pain

Flattening of the longitudinal arch cause plantar fasciitis, strain on the intertransverse ligaments, and bursitis between the metatarsal heads. Neuroma formation can also occur (Morton's neuroma) secondary to flattening of the arch.

Treatment consists of intrinsic foot exercises, surgery or nerve blocks for Morton's neuroma, and surgery for hallux vagus and hallux rigidus.

REFERENCES

1. Duthie R.B., Bentley G. (eds.): *Mercer's Orthopedic Surgery*, ed. 8. Baltimore, University Park Press, 1983.
2. Roles N.C., Maudsley R.H. Radial tunnel syndrome: Resistant tennis elbow as a nerve entrapment. *J. Bone Joint Surg*. 54(B):499, 1972.
3. Jackson R.W., Abe I.: The role of arthroscopy in the management of disorders of the knee. *J. Bone Joint Surg*. [*Br.*] 54:310–322, 1972.
4. Dandy D.J., Jackson R.W.: The diagnosis of problems after menisectomy. *J. Bone Joint Surg*. [*Br.*] 57:349–352, 1975.
5. Gillies H., Chalmers J.: The management of fresh rupture of the tendo Achilles. *J. Bone Joint Surg*. [*Am.*] 52:337–343, 1970.
6. Zohn D.A., Mennel J.: *Musculoskeletal Pain*. Boston, Little, Brown & Co., 1976.

25C / Pain of Sympathetic Origin

STEPHEN E. ABRAM, M.D.

SEVERE BURNING PAIN in an extremity following nerve injuries was described in 1864 in soldiers by Mitchell, Morehouse, and Keen.[1] Mitchell subsequently introduced the term "causalgia" (from the Greek, meaning "burning pain") to describe the syndrome.[2] In the 1920s Leriche demonstrated that the pain of causalgia was often relieved by sympathetic blockade, and that sympathectomy could effect permanent relief.[3] It later became apparent that similar types of pain occurred after trauma or surgery in nonmilitary patients, many of whom had no obvious nerve injury. Vasomotor and sudomotor disturbances and dystrophic changes were reported in patients with and without nerve lesions.

The literature on causalgic pain is confusing not only because the pathophysiology is poorly understood, but also because the terminology is far from uniform. "Causalgia" has been used by some authors to describe all cases of burning posttraumatic pain, while others have employed new terms, including minor causalgia, mimocausalgia, reflex sympathetic dystrophy, Sudeck's atrophy, posttraumatic edema, and shoulder-hand syndrome, to denote posttraumatic pain disorders without major nerve injury. Fortunately, Bonica[4] and many other authorities now use the term "causalgia" to denote the syndrome of pain, autonomic dysfunction, and dystrophic changes following major nerve trauma, and the term "reflex sympathetic dystrophy" to indicate a similar complex of symptoms that arises without obvious nerve injury.

ETIOLOGY

While it is apparent that the sympathetic nervous system plays an important role in the pathogenesis of posttraumatic pain syndromes, our understanding of its contribution to these conditions is incomplete. In fact, it is often unclear whether sympathetic block produces analgesia by interruption of sympathetic efferents or through blockade of afferent fibers traveling in the sympathetic chain.

The Role of Sympathetic Afferents

There is anatomical and physiologic evidence from animal studies that some afferent fibers from the limb travel through the sympathetic chain prior to entering the dorsal horn of the spinal cord.[5-8] Several clinical observations suggest that some types of pain may be mediated by afferent fibers in the sympathetic chain. Echlin described a patient with phantom limb pain who underwent lumbar sympathectomy under local infiltration anesthesia. Following removal of a segment of the chain, mechanical or electrical stimulation of the proximal stump produced severe hip and phantom foot pain.[9] Further clinical evidence of sympathetic afferent contribution to pain is provided by a patient in whom sympathectomy relieved postamputation arm pain after extensive rhizotomy had failed to produce analgesia.[10] Stimulation of arteries in patients under regional anesthesia or with somatic nerve damage has been shown to cause burning pain, which suggests that sympathetic afferents may innervate vessel walls.[3, 11]

The Role of Sympathetic Efferents

The simplest model proposed to explain the role of sympathetic efferents in the pathogenesis of extremity pain is the "vicious circle" hypothesis[12]: noxious stimulation gives rise to segmental and suprasegmental sympathetic discharge, producing vasoconstriction, ischemia, and further nociceptor activation. Impaired perfusion eventually leads to dystrophic changes, such as bone demineralization, skin and nail changes, and muscle atrophy.

451

Another possible model proposes the modulation of nociceptor sensitivity by sympathetic fibers. This might involve the release of pain-producing or pain-modulating substances such as bradykinin, prostaglandins, or 5-hydroxytryptamine.[13] Sympathetic stimulation has been shown to increase the sensitivity of mechanoreceptors[14, 15] and cold receptors,[16] but there is only scant evidence that sympathetic discharge alters nociceptor sensitivity. Matthews[17] showed that sympathetic chain stimulation or close arterial injection of norepinephrine increased the firing frequency of tooth pulp afferents in cats, but evidence of such phenomena in the extremities has not been reported.

Likewise, there is little evidence that sympathetic activity alters conduction in normal peripheral nerves or nerve roots. However, there are several studies which show that sympathetic stimulation facilitates activity in abnormal nerves. Electrical stimulation of the sympathetic chain and direct norepinephrine application have been shown to increase the frequency of spontaneous firing of afferents originating in a neuroma.[18, 19]

Doupe et al.[20] proposed that, following nerve injury, myelin degeneration allows "artificial synapses" to occur, permitting sympathetic (or motor) nerve impulses to activate somatic afferent fibers (Fig 25C–1). Although segmental myelin degeneration has been demonstrated in injured nerves,[21] several lines of evidence indicate that ephaptic transmission is an unlikely explanation in most cases of sympathetic associated pain (Fig 25C–2): (1) causalgic pain from peripheral nerve injury begins immediately, but myelin degeneration does not

occur for several days; (2) resection of the injured nerve segment or extensive dorsal rhizotomy usually fails to relieve the pain of causalgia;[22] (3) depletion of catecholamine stores by intravenous (IV) regional guanethedine injection relieves causalgic pain.[23]

Central Nervous System Mechanisms

Although peripheral mechanisms are important in the pathogenesis of causalgic states, they do not constitute the entire explanation. Numerous case reports of causalgia unrelieved by interruption of both the somatic and sympathetic supply of the limb may be found. One must therefore examine central pain-generating or pain-modulating mechanisms.

Modern concepts of pain perception, including the gate control theory,[24] assume that pain occurs when the number of nerve impulses reaching areas of the brain involved with pain perception exceeds a critical level. Such a level may be reached with injury or noxious stimulation in the periphery. It has been demonstrated in animals and man that loss of peripheral neuronal input produces abnormal bursts of firing in dorsal horn cells which are involved in transmission of nociceptive information.[25, 26] These bursts of activity are similar to those recorded in the dorsal horn and brain stem during noxious stimulation in the periphery. Melzack and Loeser,[27] therefore, proposed that following loss of peripheral input, pain generation takes place in neuronal pools in the dorsal horn and possibly at higher CNS levels. Spontaneous activity in those cells would give rise to pain sensation perceived to arise from the periph-

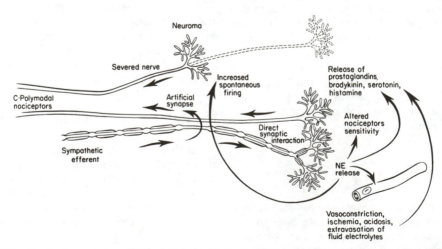

Fig 25C–1.—Some proposed mechanisms of interaction between sympathetic efferent and nociceptive afferent fibers in causalgia.[4]

eral sensory distribution of those cells. That activity can be modulated by descending neuronal input and by visceral, somatic, and autonomic inputs. Thus, treatment that alters peripheral nerve activity or sympathetic discharge may produce analgesia, even though painful impulses arise from within the CNS.

SIGNS AND SYMPTOMS

Causalgia

The term causalgia is generally used to define the condition described by Mitchell: a syndrome of burning pain, vasomotor instability, and trophic alterations following major peripheral nerve injury. Most cases result from lesions of the medial cord of the brachial plexus, the median nerve, or the tibial division of the sciatic nerve, probably because those nerves carry most of the sympathetics and the majority of sensory fibers to the hand and foot.[28] In one study, of 315 nerve lesions complicated by causalgia,[29] 278, or 88%, were caused by injury above the knee or elbow. Most cases are associated with partial nerve injury, although causalgia following total nerve transection is occasionally seen.[30, 31]

It is not surprising that most cases of causalgia are reported during wartime, since the great majority of cases follow high-velocity missile injuries which subject the nerve to rapid violent deformation. There are only a few reports of true causalgia associated with other types of lesions, such as brachial plexus injury after humerus fracture,[32] pelvic fracture,[1] and laceration.[29]

Pain often begins soon after the injury, and many patients report the onset of pain coincident with the trauma. It reaches its peak intensity within a few days to weeks. Superficial burning pain and hyperpathia are universally present. Superimposed on these sensations there is usually deep pain, often of a bizarre quality, described as crushing, tearing, stabbing, or throbbing. A patient with a gunshot wound to the brachial plexus described to me sensations of tight bands around each finger and needles sticking into the fingertips (Fig 25C–3).

Pain is continuous, although there are spontaneous variations in intensity. It is aggravated by any stimulation or movement of the limb and by stimuli that evoke sympathetic responses, e.g., intense auditory or visual stimuli or emotional upset. The extremity is often held away from the body, and contact with clothing or bedsheets is avoided. Cool moist applications may provide some relief. With time, pain may spread to previously unaffected areas. Sunderland states that without treatment the pain gradually subsides and vanishes within 6 months, rarely persisting for more than a year.[28] However, John Mitchell (Weir Mitchell's son, who followed up many of his father's patients) and others have reported pain persisting for years after injury (Fig 25C–4).[33–35]

Vasomotor changes usually accompany causalgia. In a study of 54 patients, the affected extremity was warmer than the normal limb in 25 patients and cooler in 10.[31] Edema is common, and some pa-

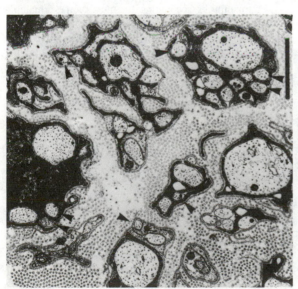

Fig 25C–2.—Electron microgram of cross section of an abnormal human cutaneous nerve. The unmyelinated fibers exhibit abundant miniature axon sprouts *(arrowheads)* next to normal axons. Calibration bar = 2 μ. (From Ochoa J.: Peripheral unmyelinated units in man: Structure, function, disorder and role in sensation, in Kruger L., Liebeskind C. (eds.): *Advances in Pain Research and Therapy.* New York, Raven Press, 1984, vol. 16. Reproduced by permission.)

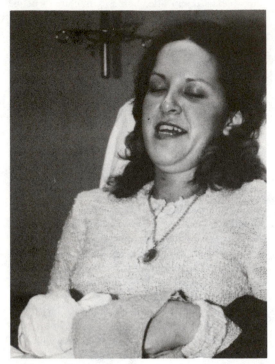

Fig 25C–3.—A 28-year-old woman with a gunshot wound to the right axilla developed severe burning pain following the injury. Not only did she have dysthesia of the right hand, but even touching the left hand provoked a severe burning pain in the right hand. The condition was diagnosed as causalgia.

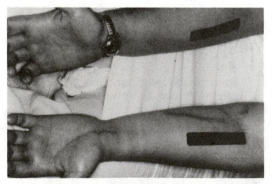

Fig 25C–4.—Patient with ulnar nerve injury of the elbow complained of burning pain in the hand. Condition was diagnosed as causalgia. After ulnar nerve transposition and carpal tunnel release, the constant burning pain persisted.

tients exhibit a mottled cyanotic color, while others demonstrate erythema. Sudomotor disturbances, with either hyperhidrosis or anhidrosis, may be evident.[28]

Dystrophic changes are encountered more frequently and are more severe than those that accompany nerve lesions without causalgia.[28] In 1864, both Mitchell et al.[1] and Paget[36] reported the association of glossy skin with severe pain after nerve injury. Loss or coarsening of hair, bone demineralization, muscle atrophy and fibrosis, and joint stiffness may occur. The incidence of these changes, which may progress to an irreversible state, appears to be related to the length of time between injury and therapy.[4]

Reflex Sympathetic Dystrophy

Following trauma, surgery, or one of several disease states, patients may develop pain, vasomotor and sudomotor abnormalities, delayed functional recovery, and dystrophic changes. The clinical picture resembles that of causalgia except for the absence of major neurologic injury. This group of disorders is clinically important, for it is much more common than causalgia, most patients respond dramatically to appropriate treatment if it is begun early in the course of the process, and pain and disability may be prolonged if treatment is delayed.

Trauma induces the majority of cases of reflex sympathetic dystrophy. Crush injury is a common antecedent, with lacerations, fractures, sprains, and burn injuries accounting for most of the remaining cases.[37] Occasional examples follow injury to minor peripheral nerves. Many of the postoperative cases occur after carpal tunnel decompression and palmar fasciectomy.[37] Reflex sympathetic dystrophy has been reported after several medical diseases, including myocardial infarction[38] and cerebrovascular accident.[39] I have treated a 10-year-old child in whom bilateral reflex sympathetic dystrophy of the upper extremities developed in association with cerebral anoxia.

The pain of reflex sympathetic dystrophy is usually burning in nature, but other qualities, particularly aching or throbbing, are reported. It usually involves the hand or foot but may radiate proximally, often spreading to involve an entire arm or leg. It frequently appears to follow arterial distribution zones rather than dermatomal patterns.[40]

Hyperpathia is frequently noted and may be an important symptom diagnostically. Loh and Nathan

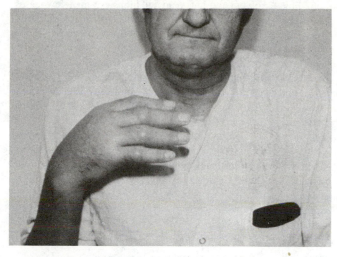

Fig 25C–5.—Patient with reflex sympathetic dystrophy of the right hand. Note edema and stiffness in the wrist and hand.

reported that in a group of patients with a variety of chronic painful disorders, the presence of hyperpathia was useful in predicting which patients would respond to sympathetic blocks.[41] Hyperhidrosis and muscle weakness may also be seen.

Vasomotor instability is often a striking feature of reflex sympathetic dystrophy. Many authors describe warmth and erythema early in the course of the process, while coolness and pallor are seen later,[4, 37] suggesting early sympathetic hypoactivity followed by a hyperadrenergic state. I have noted, however, that many patients with signs of vasodilation admit that the extremity is often cold and cyanotic, particularly with activity. In one such patient, who had reflex sympathetic dystrophy following a Colles fracture, the skin temperature of the affected hand was 8° C warmer than the normal hand, but skin conductivity in the painful limb was much higher, and the sympathogalvanic reflex was

exaggerated, indicating ongoing sympathetic hyperactivity. Hyperemia may be related to periods of relative ischemia following sympathetic discharge with accumulation of CO_2 and lactic acid, which causes arteriolar dilation. Edema, which may be present in the erythematous or vasoconstricted phases, is probably secondary to changes in vascular permeability (Figs 25C–5; and 25C–6, Plate 10).[42]

Dystrophic changes develop during later stages of the disorder. Sudeck's atrophy, the bone demineralization associated with reflex sympathetic dystrophy, has a patchy appearance radiographically and resembles the osteoporosis of disuse.[43] However, the demineralization of reflex sympathetic dystrophy is more severe, develops more rapidly, may occur with only minor changes in motor function, and is not reversed by active or passive exercise (Fig 25C–7).[44]

Joint stiffness and pain on joint movement often

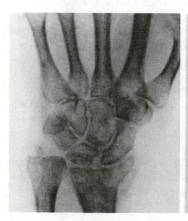
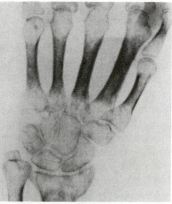

Fig 25C–7.—Patient with Sudeck's atrophy following reflex sympathetic dystrophy. *Left,* early; *right,* late.

develop with time. Articular erosions resembling those of osteoarthritis appear on radiographs of the involved extremity. Histologic examination reveals synovial edema, hyperplasia and fibrosis, capillary proliferation, and mild perivascular inflammation.[43]

The skin becomes smooth and shiny. Hair may become sparse in some cases, coarse in others. Loss of subcutaneous fat pads produces changes in architecture of the digits, which appear thin and tapered. Muscle atrophy, particularly of the interossei, may occur.[4]

Comparison of vasomotor and sudomotor activity of the normal and affected extremity may be helpful diagnostically. Measurement of skin temperature of the volar surface of the thumb or plantar surface of the big toe provides representative measurements. Thermography provides useful documentation of differences in blood flow between extremities and helps assess the efficacy of sympathetic blocks and of clinical progress.

Measurement of sympathogalvanic reflex provides an estimate of sudomotor response to sympathetic stimulation and may demonstrate differences between the extremities. The use of two channels simultaneously, calibrated to record absolute skin conductivity, will frequently show elevated baseline conductivity on the affected side. The sympathogalvanic reflex, or galvanic skin response, which is a transient elevation of skin conductivity following a stimulus that evokes a sympathetic response (skin pinch, electric shock, loud noise, flash of light) is often exaggerated unilaterally.

The Shoulder-Hand Syndrome (Reflex Neurovascular Dystrophy)

This is a poorly understood disorder characterized by pain and stiffness in the shoulder, together with pain, swelling, and vasomotor phenomena in the hand. Involvement of the distal upper extremity is frequently followed by a dystrophic change that resembles Sudeck's atrophy. The syndrome is presumed to result from reflex sympathetic stimulation analogous to that proposed by causalgia. It principally affects patients above the age of 50 and is often associated with acute illness such as myocardial infarction. The significance of associated degenerative change in the cervical spine is uncertain because of its high frequency in the population at risk. When the disease is bilateral the differentiation from acute rheumatoid arthritis may be difficult. Joint symptoms appear to result from periarticular in-

volvement, but synovial biopsies, in a few cases, have disclosed mild histologic abnormalities: edema, proliferation, and disarray of synovial lining cells. There is marked variability in the intensity and duration of acute symptoms and in the extent of dystrophic change. In a small percentage of patients the end result is ''frozen shoulder'' and dystrophic changes in the hands that resemble reflex sympathetic dystrophy.

There is probably no condition for which aggressive physical therapy is more important than for the shoulder-hand syndrome. An active exercise program, facilitated by analgesic medication, should be instituted as soon as possible. When refractory pain impedes progress of the program, nerve blocks should be tried.

DIFFERENTIAL DIAGNOSIS

Several postoperative or posttraumatic conditions have symptoms in common with causalgia and reflex sympathetic dystrophy. Peripheral nerve injuries may produce burning dysesthetic pain without a sympathetic nervous system component. Hyperpathia is frequently encountered within the distribution of transected or entrapped nerves. Pain is limited to the distribution of the involved nerve, and a positive Tinel's sign is often elicited over the site of nerve injury.

Inflammatory lesions such as tenosynovitis or bursitis may produce posttraumatic pain, which may be burning in quality and may persist for months. Myofascial pain often develops after injury or surgery. It is nondermatomal in distribution, may be burning in nature, and is characterized by sensitive trigger points in affected muscles. Although the truncal musculature is most often affected, such problems may also involve the extremities.[45]

Raynaud's disease produces vasospasm of the extremities associated with cold skin, pallor, and often cyanosis (Fig 25C–8, Plate 11). The condition is bilateral, involving the hands and sometimes all four extremities. The vasospasm may be relieved by sympathetic blocks, but most patients are not helped by such treatment. Patients who experience transient vasodilation with sympathetic blocks may benefit from sympathectomy or systemic α-adrenergic blocking agents.

Raynaud's phenomenon, a similar vasospastic disorder, is associated with an underlying pathologic process, frequently one of the connective tissue diseases such as scleroderma, and is often unilateral.

As with Raynaud's disease, sympathetic blocks are helpful in a minority of patients.

Establishing an absolute diagnosis for a chronic pain problem is usually difficult, as multiple pain mechanisms often exist. It is often possible, however, to assess the importance of sympathetic mechanisms by comparing the degree and duration of pain relief achieved by sympathetic blocks with that produced by somatic blocks and placebo injections.

The response to a placebo injection (e.g., intramuscular saline) is often helpful diagnostically. A true placebo response, which is elicited in about one third of chronic pain patients, is usually brief (10–30 minutes). Pain relief persisting for days or weeks probably signifies a psychogenic pain mechanism. A very transitory response to the placebo and a prolonged analgesic effect from a sympathetic block (hours or days) provides some assurance that sympathetics are involved in the pathogenesis of the pain. If no analgesia occurs after sympathetic block and pain is relieved by blocking the appropriate somatic nerves, then a somatic pain mechanism, such as neuralgia, myofascial syndrome, or radiculopathy, is likely. Failure of both sympathetic and somatic block to produce analgesia points to a central type of pain mechanism, which may be psychogenic or may result from neuronal activity within the CNS which is independent of peripheral input.

For lower extremity pain, a differential spinal block may be used to distinguish among sympathetic, somatic, and central pain mechanisms.[46] Following introduction of a needle into the subarachnoid space, and with the patient positioned laterally, 10 ml of normal saline is injected. Relief of pain is interpreted as a placebo response. If no analgesia occurs, 10 ml of 0.25% procaine is injected, which should block preganglionic sympathetic (B) fibers while sparing somatic (A and C) fibers. If signs of sympathetic blockade develop and pain relief ensues, a sympathetic pain mechanism is likely. If no analgesia occurs, 10 ml 0.5% procaine is injected, and pain is reassessed after the onset of somatic blockage. Analgesia is interpreted as evidence of a somatic mechanism. Lack of pain relief points to a central or psychogenic mechanism.

Winnie has suggested a simpler differential block procedure.[47] The placebo saline injection is first carried out. Subsequently, 2 ml of 5% procaine is injected, producing motor, sensory, and sympathetic blockade. If the block produces analgesia and the pain recurs as the somatic block wears off (while sympathetic blockade persists), a somatic mechanism is likely. If it recurs only after sympathetic blockade regresses, a sympathetic mechanism is assumed to be responsible for the pain.

MANAGEMENT

Causalgia

Prior to World War II, treatment was limited mainly to the use of large doses of morphine.[1] Intraneural alcohol injections,[48] dorsal rhizotomy,[49] and periarterial sympathectomy[50] were found to be relatively ineffective. In the 1930s, a few cases of successful treatment by stellate ganglionectomy were reported,[51, 52] and during World War II the importance of sympathectomy became generally recognized. Doupe et al. stressed the importance of local anesthetic blocks in establishing the diagnosis.[20] As sympathectomy became the established mode of therapy, the prognostic value of sympathetic blocks became generally recognized.

Several authors[53, 54] have suggested that sympathetic blocks performed soon after injury may produce lasting improvement in burning pain. Bonica[4] reported complete, permanent relief in 10 of 17 causalgia patients treated with repeated local anesthetic sympathetic blocks. Since the morbidity associated with sympathetic blocks is extremely low, such treatment should be tried as soon as possible after injury. Blocks should be performed daily. A gradual increase in the duration of postblock analgesia and a decrease in the severity of pain when it does recur are encouraging signs. The blocks should be continued until only minimal discomfort persists. Unfortunately, most patients experience pain recurrence as the local anesthetic effect subsides, and no lasting benefit ensues.

Continuous local anesthetic blocks may be used as an alternative to a series of sympathetic blocks. Continuous epidural anesthesia with dilute (0.125%) bupivacaine provides sympathetic blockade of the lower extremities without affecting motor function. Continuous bupivacaine infusion into the interscalene or axillary fascial sheaths can provide continuous sympathetic blockade for the upper extremity (Fig 25C–9).

Hannington-Kiff[23] reported that the IV regional injection of guanethidine in the causalgic limb might produce lasting pain relief. However, he offered little data on the long-term efficacy of the technique in causalgia patients.

Occasional success in the treatment of causalgia

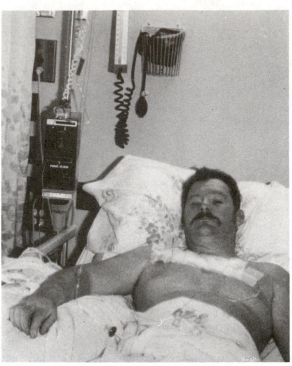

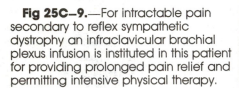

Fig 25C–9.—For intractable pain secondary to reflex sympathetic dystrophy an infraclavicular brachial plexus infusion is instituted in this patient for providing prolonged pain relief and permitting intensive physical therapy.

with oral sympatholytic agents has been encountered. Abram and Lightfoot[35] reported symptomatic improvement of long-standing causalgic pain with oral prazosin. Propranolol has been reported to provide analgesia in causalgia,[55] presumably through blockade of a prejunctional β_2 receptor which, when stimulated, causes norepinephrine release.[56]

Little data are available on the efficacy of transcutaneous electrical nerve stimulation (TENS). I have used TENS in two patients with causalgia following gunshot wounds (brachial plexus and sciatic nerve). Both experienced aggravation of their symptoms.

For those patients who do not experience persistent improvement from sympathetic blocks or other conservative forms of therapy (the majority of cases in most reported series), sympathectomy is the treatment of choice. Bonica[4] has reviewed reports from the literature of 500 patients treated with surgical sympathectomy for causalgia. Eighty-four percent experienced excellent pain relief, 12% fair relief, and 4% no improvement. It is likely that many of the patients who had persistent burning pain after surgery did not have complete sympathectomy. Mayfield[57] reported that 9 of 105 patients did not experience complete analgesia after sympathectomy. All 9 showed evidence of persistent sympathetic activity, all were relieved by sympathetic blocks, and

8 of the 9 had permanent relief from a more extensive sympathectomy.

Clinical sympathectomy with phenol or alcohol is a possible alternative to surgical sympathectomy and may be preferable for extremely debilitated patients. Bonica[4] described three causalgia patients who experienced persistent analgesia from such procedures. He stated that neurolytic blocks produced sympathetic interruption for several weeks to several months, but Boas et al.[58] reported essentially permanent sympathetic denervation in 81% of patients following block with 7% phenol in Conray.

Reflex Sympathetic Dystrophy

Unlike patients with causalgia, most patients with reflex sympathetic dystrophy respond dramatically and permanently to sympathetic blocks if treatment is instituted before irreversible trophic changes occur. Carron and Weller[59] reported that in a series of 123 patients with sympathetic dystrophy, only 6 failed to respond to a series of blocks. Bonica,[4] in reviewing personal data plus reports by six other authors, estimated the success rate with sympathetic blocks to be over 80%. A lower success rate is anticipated if pain has been present for a long time.[60]

While occasional patients experience lasting relief from a single injection, most require a series of three to five and sometimes more injections. Blocks should be performed daily or on alternate days. Pain relief usually outlasts the duration of the local anesthetic, and when the pain does recur, it is usually somewhat diminished. As long as the duration of analgesia increases and the severity of the recurrent pain decreases, blocks should be continued. However, if the pain consistently returns to its previous level as the block regresses, continued injections will probably be ineffective, and alternative forms of therapy should be considered. Recently Raj has used continuous infusion of bupivacaine (6–10 ml in 0.25% concentration) over the sympathetic chain to provide prolonged analgesia (Fig 25C–10).

Physical therapy is an important adjunct to sympathetic blocks and may be effective alone for the treatment of mild cases.[61] For long-standing cases, extensive physical rehabilitation may be necessary. Active and active-assisted range of motion exercises, muscle strengthening and conditioning, massage and heat (whirlpool, paraffin, radiant heat) are particularly useful. Vigorous passive range of motion exercises and the use of heavy weights may retrigger symptoms. Exercises are best performed dur-

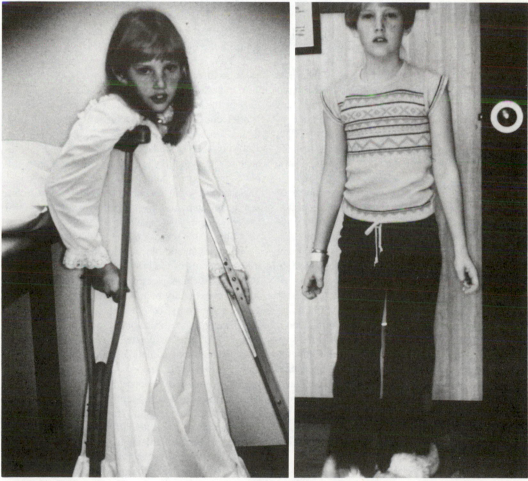

Fig 25C–10.—A, 9-year-old girl had a minor injury to the left foot, which was treated with a cast for 3 months. Following removal of the cast, she was not able to bear weight for one year. At the pain control center she was treated with a continuous infusion with a pump of the lumbar sympathetic chain with a catheter using 0.25% bupivacaine for 7 days. **B** shows full recovery of the patient with this treatment and intensive physical therapy at 1 month. Note that physical therapy with sympathetic block is essential for such success.

ing analgesic periods following sympathetic blocks.

Since Hannington-Kiff [62] introduced the technique of pharmacologic sympathetic blockade using IV regional guanethidine, several other authors[41, 63, 64] have documented its efficacy in the treatment of sympathetic dystrophy. Erickson[64] reported a mean duration of skin temperature elevation of 3 days following the first procedure, and 6 days following the second. Unfortunately, only limited follow-up data are available.

Injectable guanethidine is not available in the United States, but the IV regional use of reserpine has been reported.[65] In my experience, only 3 of 14 patients obtained pain relief with the technique, and two patients experienced syncopal episodes one to several hours after the procedure.[66] Intra-arterial reserpine injection has been reported to provide effective sympathetic blockade in vasospastic disorders[67] and may be more effective than the IV regional route. TENS has been effective as the sole treatment[68] and as an adjunctive therapy for sympathetic dystrophy. Increased skin temperature has been documented during TENS therapy.[69] Pain control may be achieved with the regular use of TENS in some patients with long-standing sympathetic dystrophy who have not responded to sympathetic blocks.

Kozin et al.[70] advocate a several-day course of high-dose systemic corticosteroids. They reported an 82% success rate in patients with "definite" reflex sympathetic dystrophy. Their criteria, however, were not very rigid, and three of the most important ones, burning pain, hyperpathia, and response to sympathetic block, were not among them. Many of the patients who responded to steroids had very chronic pain (mean duration of pain for the group was 25 weeks), and a trial of steroids might be a reasonable form of treatment for patients with long-standing pain who have failed to respond to blocks.

The systemic use of adrenergic blocking agents has met with only limited success. A few patients I have treated, all of whom had pain for more than 6 months, experienced moderate improvement in pain, swelling, and vasoconstriction with oral prazosin. The most gratifying response was in a patient with recurrent foot pain after sympathectomy. IV phentolamine appears to be useful in predicting favorable responses to prazosin, as only those patients who experienced pain relief and increased skin temperature in the affected limb responded to the oral medication. Orthostatic dizziness was seen occasionally with prazosin and precluded its continued use in a few patients. As with causalgia, propranolol

has been reported to be effective in the management of reflex sympathetic dystrophy.[55, 71]

Surgical sympathectomy has been advocated for patients who do not experience permanent relief from blocks or other conservative measures. Kleinert et al.[37] reported on a series of 183 patients with upper extremity sympathetic dystrophy who were initially treated with sympathetic blocks. No demonstrable improvement was seen in 39 patients. Permanent improvement was achieved in 121 patients. In the remaining 23 patients, who experienced only transient relief from blocks, surgical sympathectomy was performed, producing permanent relief in all but four patients.

Prior to electing sympathectomy, several criteria should be met:

1. The patient should experience pain relief from sympathetic blocks on several occasions.

2. Pain relief should last at least as long as the vascular effects of the block.

3. Placebo injection should produce no pain relief, or the relief should be less pronounced and of shorter duration than that achieved with local anesthetic sympathetic blocks.

4. Possible secondary gain motives and significant psychopathology should be ruled out as possible causes of pain complaints.

Neurolytic lumbar sympathetic block may be chosen as an alternative to surgical sympathectomy for lower extremity sympathetic dystrophy. Boas et al.[58] cite 100% success in five patients treated with phenol sympathetic blocks. Because of the proximity of the roots of the brachial plexus to the cervical sympathetic chain, neurolytic sympathetic blockade for upper extremity pain is too hazardous.

Sympathectomy is not without potential problems. Patients are occasionally bothered by dermatologic problems associated with skin dryness. A painful condition, sometimes termed sympathalgia, may begin in the second or third postoperative week.[44] Patients experience muscle fatigue, heaviness, deep pain, and tenderness in the limb, which may continue for weeks. When sympathectomy includes ablation of the stellate ganglion, the resultant ptosis, conjunctival injection, and nasal congestion may be distressing but can usually be controlled by the use of 10% phenylephrine eye drops.

A combination of a tricyclic antidepressant and a phenothiazine may provide analgesia for some patients with long-standing pain of sympathetic dystrophy unresponsive to other types of therapy. Such combinations have been reported to produce analgesia in postherpetic neuralgia[72] and other chronic pain states.[73] The analgesic action of the tricyclics may be related to inhibition of serotinin reuptake at nerve terminals of neurons which act to suppress pain transmission, with resultant prolongation of serotonin activity at the receptor.[74] If that indeed is the mechanism, then amitriptyline, which has the most potent effect on the amine pump, should be the most effective of the tricyclics. The mechanism by which phenothiazines potentiate the analgesic effect of tricyclics is not known. Relatively small amounts of each drug (e.g., amitriptyline, 50–75 mg, and perphenazine, 4–12 mg/day) are often effective.

REFERENCES

1. Mitchell S.W., Morehouse G.R., Keen W.W.: *Gunshot Wounds and Other Injuries of Nerves*. Philadelphia, J.B. Lippincott Co., 1864, p. 164.
2. Mitchell S.W.: On diseases of nerves, resulting from injuries, in Flint A. (ed.): *Contributions relating to the causation and prevention of disease, and to camp diseases*. United States Sanitary Commission Memoirs. New York, 1867, pp. 412–468.
3. Leriche R.: *The Surgery of Pain*, Young A. (trans.-ed.). Baltimore, Williams & Wilkins Co., 1939.
4. Bonica J.J.: Causalgia and other reflex sympathetic dystrophies, in Bonica J.J., Liebeskind J.C., Albe-Fessard D. (eds.): *Advances in Pain Research and Therapy*. New York, Raven Press, 1979, vol. 3.
5. Kuntz A., Farnsworth D.: Distribution of afferent fibers via the sympathetic trunks and gray communicating rami to the brachial and lumbosacral plexuses. *Comp. Neurol.* 53:389–399, 1973.
6. Kuntz A.: Afferent innervation of peripheral blood vessels through sympathetic trunks. *J. South. Med. Assoc.* 44:673–678, 1951.
7. Kuntz A., Saccomanno A.: Afferent conduction from extremities through dorsal root fibers via sympathetic trunks. *Arch. Surg.* 45:606–612, 1942.
8. Threadgill F.D., Solnitzky O.: Anatomical studies of afferency within the lumbosacral sympathetic ganglia. *Anat. Rec.* 103:96, 1949.
9. Echlin F.: Pain responses on stimulation of the lumbar sympathetic chain under local anesthesia. *J. Neurosurg.* 6:530–533, 1949.
10. White J.D., Smithwick R.H.: *The Autonomic Nervous System*. New York, Macmillan Book Co., 1941.
11. Foerster O.: *Die Leitungsbahnen des Schmerzgefuhls und die chirurgische Behandlung der Schmerzzustande*. Berlin, Urban & Schwarzenberg, 1927.
12. Procacci P., et al.: Role of sympathetic system in reflex dystrophies, in Bonica J.J., Able-Fessard D. (eds.): *Advances in Pain Research and Therapy*. New York, Raven Press, 1976, vol. 1.
13. Zimmerman M.: Peripheral and central nervous mechanisms of nociception, pain and pain therapy: Facts and hypotheses, in Bonica J.J., et al. (eds.): *Advances in Pain Research and Therapy*. New York, Raven Press, 1979, pp. 3–32, vol. 3.
14. Calof A.L. et al.: Sympathetic modulation of mechanoreceptor sensitivity in frog skin. *J. Physiol. (London)* 310:481–499, 1981.
15. Loewenstein W.R., Altamirano-Orrega R.: Enhancement of activity in a pacinian corpuscle by sympathomimetic agents. *Nature* 178:1292–1293, 1956.
16. Spray D.C.: Characteristics, specificity and efferent control of frog cutaneous cold receptors. *J. Physiol. (London)* 237:15–38, 1974.
17. Matthews B.: Effects of stimulation on the response of intradental nerves to chemical stimulation of dentin, in Bonica J.J., Albe-Fessard D. (eds.): *Advances in Pain Research and Therapy*. New York, Raven Press, 1976, vol. 1.
18. Wall P.D., Gutnick M.: Ongoing activity in peripheral nerves: The physiology and pharmacology of impulses originating from a neuroma. *Exp. Neurol.* 43:580–593, 1981.
19. Devor M., Janig W.: Activation of myelinated afferents ending in a neuroma by stimulation of the sympathetic supply in the rat. *Neurosci. Lett.* 24:43–47, 1981.
20. Doupe J., Cullen C.R., Chance G.Q.: Post-traumatic pain and the causalgic syndromes. *J. Neurol. Neurosurg. Psychiatry* 7:33–48, 1944.
21. Ochoa J., Noordenbos W.: Pathology and disordered sensation in local nerve lesions: An attempt at correlation, in Bonica J.J., et al. (eds.): *Advances in Pain Research and Therapy*. New York, Raven Press, 1979, vol. 3, pp. 67–90.
22. Sunderland S.: Pain mechanisms in causalgia. *J. Neurol. Neurosurg. Psychiatry* 39:471–480, 1976.
23. Hannington-Kiff J.G.: Hyperadrenergic-effected limb causalgia: Relief by IV pharmacologic norepinephrine blockade. *Am. Heart J.* 103:152–153, 1982.
24. Melzack R., Wall P.D.: Pain mechanisms: A new theory. *Science* 150:971–979, 1965.
25. Loeser J.D., Ward A.A.: Some effects of deafferentation on neurons of the cat spinal cord. *Arch. Neurol.* 17:629–636, 1976.
26. Loeser J.D., Ward A.A., White L.E.: Chronic deafferentation of human spinal cord neurons. *J. Neurosurg.* 29:48–50, 1968.
27. Melzack R., Loeser J.D.: Phantom body pain in paraplegics: Evidence for a central "pattern generating mechanism" for pain. *Pain* 4:195–210, 1973.
28. Sunderland S.: Pain mechanisms in causalgia. *J. Neurol. Neurosurg. Psychiatry* 39:471–480, 1976.
29. Richards R.L.: Causalgia: A centennial review. *Arch. Neurol.* 16:339–350, 1967.
30. Nathan P.W.: On the pathogenesis of causalgia in peripheral nerve injuries. *Brain* 70:145–170, 1947.
31. Shumacker H.B., Spiegel L.L., Upjohn R.H.: Causalgia. *Surg. Gynecol. Obstet.* 86:76–86, 1948.

32. Sunderland S., Kelly M.: The painful sequelae to peripheral nerves. *Aust. NZ J. Surg.* 18:75–118, 1948.

33. Mitchell J.K.: *Remote Consequences of Injuries of Nerves and Their Treatment.* Philadelphia, Lea Brothers, 1895.

34. Barnes R.: The role of sympathectomy in the treatment of causalgia. *J. Bone Joint Surg.* [*Br.*] 35:172–180, 1953.

35. Abram S.E., Lightfoot R.: Treatment of long-standing causalgia with progosin. *Reg. Anaesth.* 6:79–81, 1981.

36. Paget S.: Clinical lecture on some cases of local paralysis. *Med. Times* 1:331–332, 1864.

37. Kleinert H.E., Cole N.M., Wayne L., et al.: Post-traumatic sympathetic dystrophy. *Orthop. Clin. North Am.* 4:917–927, 1973.

38. Steinbrocker, Argyros T.G.: The shoulder-hand syndrome: Present status as a diagnostic and therapeutic entity. *Med. Clin. North Am.* 42:15, 1958.

39. Hathaway B.N., Hill G.E., Ohmura A.: Centrally induced sympathetic dystrophy of the upper extremity. *Anesth. Analg.* 57:373–374, 1978.

40. Gross D.: Pain and autonomic nervous system. *Adv. Neurol.* 4:93–104, 1974.

41. Loh L., Nathan P.W.: Painful peripheral states and sympathetic blocks. *J. Neurol. Neurosurg. Psychiatry* 41:664–671, 1978.

42. Zimmerman M.: Peripheral and central nervous mechanisms of nociception, pain and pain therapy: Facts and hypotheses, in Bonica J.J., et al. (eds.): *Advances in Pain Research and Therapy.* New York, Raven Press, 1979, vol. 3, pp. 3–32.

43. Genant N.K., Kozin F., Bekerman C., et al.: The reflex sympathetic dystrophy syndrome. *Radiology* 117:21–32, 1975.

44. Hermann L.G., Reineke H.G., Caldwell J.A.: Post-traumatic painful osteoporosis: A clinical and roentgenological entity. *AJR,* 47:353–361, 1942.

45. Travell J., Rinzler S.H.: The myofascial genesis of pain. *Postgrad. Med.* 11:425–434, 1952.

46. Winnie A.P., Collins J.J.: The pain clinic: I. Differential neural blockade in pain syndromes of questionable etiology. *Med. Clin. North Am.* 52:123–129, 1968.

47. Winnie A.P.: Differential diagnosis of pain mechanisms. *Refresher Courses in Anesthesiology* 6:171–186, 1978.

48. Lewis D., Gatewood W.: Treatment of causalgia: Results of intraneural injections of 60% alcohol. *JAMA* 74:1–4, 1920.

49. Platt H., Bristow W.R.: Remote results of operations for injuries of peripheral nerves. *Br. J. Surg.* 11:535–567, 1924.

50. Leriche R.: De la causalgie envisagee comme une nevrite du sympathique et son traitement par la denudation et l'excision des plexus nerveux peri-arteriels. *Presse Med.* 24:178–180, 1916.

51. Spurling R.G.: Causalgia of the upper extremity: Treatment by dorsal sympathetic ganglionectomy. *Arch. Neurol. Psychiatry* 23:784–788, 1930.

52. Kwan S.T.: The treatment of causalgia by thoracic sympathetic ganglionectomy. *Ann. Surg.* 101:222–227, 1935.

53. Freeman N.E.: Treatment of causalgia arising from gunshot wounds of peripheral nerves. *Surgery* 22:68–82, 1974.

54. Rasmussen T.B., Freedman H.: Treatment of causalgia. *J. Neurosurg.* 3:165–173, 1946.

55. Simson G.: Propranolol for causalgia and Sudek's atrophy. *JAMA* 227:327, 1974.

56. Stjarne L., Brundin J.: Beta-2 adrenoceptors facilitating noradrenaline section from human vasoconstrictor nerves. *Acta Physiol. Scand.* 97:88–93, 1976.

57. Mayfield F.H.: *Causalgia.* Springfield, Charles C Thomas, Publisher, 1951.

58. Boas R.A., Hatangdi V.S., Richards E.G.: Lumbar sympathectomy—a percutaneous technique, in Bonica J.J., Albe-Fessard D. (eds.): *Advances in Pain Research and Therapy.* New York, Raven Press, 1976, vol. 1, pp. 485–490.

59. Carron H., Weller R.M.: Treatment of post-traumatic sympathetic dystrophy. *Adv. Neurol.* 4:485–490, 1974.

60. Abram S.E., Anderson R.A., Maitra-D'Cruze A.M.: Factors predicting short-term outcome of nerve blocks in the management of chronic pain. *Pain* 10:323–330, 1981.

61. Pak T.J., Martin G.M., Magness J.L., Kavanaugh G.J.: Reflex sympathetic dystrophy: Review of 140 cases. *Minn. Med.* 53:507–512, 1970.

62. Hannington-Kiff J.G.: Intravenous regional sympathetic block with guanethidine. *Lancet* 1:1019–1020, 1974.

63. Holland A.J.C., Davies K.J., Wallace D.H.: Sympathetic blockade of isolated limbs by intravenous guanethidine. *Can. Anaesth. Soc. J.* 24:597–602, 1977.

64. Erickson S.: Duration of sympathetic blockade. *Anaesthesia* 36:768–771, 1981.

65. Bengon H.T., Chomka C.M., Brenner E.A.: Treatment of reflex sympathetic dystrophy with regional intravenous reserpine. *Anesth. Analg.* 59:500–502, 1980.

66. Abram S.E.: Intra-arterial reserpine. *Anesth. Analg.* 59:889–890, 1980.

67. Romeo S.G., Whalen R.E., Tindall J.P.: Intraarterial administration of reserpine: Its use in patients with Raynaud's disease or Raynaud's phenomenon. *Arch. Intern. Med.* 125:825, 1970.

68. Stilz R.J., Carren H., Sanders D.B.: Reflex sympathetic dystrophy in a 6-year-old: Successful treatment by transcutaneous nerve stimulation. *Anesth. Analg.* 56:438–443, 1977.

69. Abram S.E., Asiddao C.B., Reynolds A.C.: Increased skin temperature during transcutaneous electrical stimulation. *Anesth. Analg.* 59:22–25, 1980.

70. Kozin F., Ryan L.M., Carerra G.F., et al.: The reflex

sympathetic dystrophy syndrome (RSDS): III. Scintigraphic studies, further evidence for the therapeutic efficacy of systemic corticosteroids, and proposed diagnostic criteria. *Am. J. Med.* 70:23–30, 1981.

71. Visitunthorn U., Prete P.: Reflex sympathetic dystrophy of the lower extremity: A complication of herpes zoster with dramatic response to propranolol. *West. J. Med.* 135:62–66, 1981.

72. Laub A.: Relief of postherpetic neuralgia with psychotropic drugs. *J. Neurosurg.* 39:235–239, 1973.

73. Kocher R.: Use of psychotropic drugs for the treatment of chronic severe pain, in Bonica J.J., Albe-Fessard D. (eds.): *Advances in Pain Research and Therapy*. New York, Raven Press, 1976, vol. 1, pp. 579–582.

74. Hollister L.: Tricyclic antidepressants. *N. Engl. J. Med.* 99:1106–1109, 1978.

26 / Thoracic and Low Back Pain

SOMAYAJI RAMAMURTHY, M.D.

26A / Pain in the Thoracic Region

SOMAYAJI RAMAMURTHY, M.D.

PAIN IN THE THORACIC REGION can originate in the somatic structures, e.g., the spine, muscles, ligaments, or fasciae, or in the thoracic viscera.

SOMATIC PAIN

Pain of the Spinal Column

Disk herniation is a relatively rare cause of thoracic pain.[1] It gives rise to radicular pain in the distribution of the involved root, with lower limb spasticity. It usually responds well to conservative therapy and epidural steroids when there is no evidence of cord compression.

Facet joints can produce pain that is associated with referred pain in the root distribution and tenderness over the involved facet. Facet joint injection, facet denervation, or injection of local anesthetics and steroids around the involved joint are usually successful in relieving the pain.

Osteoporosis with collapse of the vertebra is a frequent cause of pain and may arise years after the fracture due to the degenerative changes induced in the facet joint (Figs 26A–1 and 26A–2).[2] Patients may be helped with calcium, vitamin D, and fluoride. Local anesthetic nerve root blocks relieve the pain temporarily. Neurolytic nerve root blocks are

indicated for prolonged relief, but the success rate is quite low.

Multiple myeloma of the spine or secondary malignancy from a primary in the lung, breast, or prostate can produce pain (Fig 26A–3). Epidural steroids, by reducing the inflammation of the roots, frequently provide pain relief. Nerve root blocks or the subarachnoid injection of alcohol or phenol may be necessary for prolonged relief of the pain.

Myofascial Pain

Pain arising from paravertebral muscles such as in longissimus and ileocostal muscles is a frequent cause of thoracic pain. Pain can be reproduced by pressure on the trigger area and is relieved by the injection of a local anesthetic–steroid mixture.

Tender trigger points located in the pectoral and serratus anterior muscles accompanied by spasm in those muscles are a frequent cause of chest pain (Figs 26A–4 through 26A–6).[3] This kind of pain may accompany visceral disease but is most frequently associated with coronary artery disease. Pain is reproduced by pressure on the trigger point and relieved by local anesthetic injection. Pain is not relieved by intercostal block, since the pectoral muscles are innervated by the branches of the brachial plexus. Transcutaneous electrical nerve stimulation (TENS) and stretching exercises are helpful in preventing recurrence.

Postthoracotomy Pain

Chronic pain following thoracotomy can be due to various etiological factors, as described below.

ENTRAPMENT OF NERVE FIBERS IN THE SCAR TISSUE.—A light touch on the scar produces intense radiating pain, sometimes accompanied by burning pain due to associated reflex sympathetic dystrophy. Injection of the scar with a local anesthetic is diagnostic. Repeated injections of a local anesthetic mixed with a steroid is likely to provide long-term relief.

NEUROMA.—A palpable neuroma in the scar, loss of pinprick sensation over the skin, and elicitation of pain on palpation are diagnostic. Repeated injection of a local anesthetic–steroid mixture may relieve the pain. Persistent pain from a well-localized neuroma may respond well to neurolytic injection of phenol or to cryolysis.

SYMPATHETIC DYSTROPHY.—Burning pain associated with hyperpathia, decreased skin temperature over the area, and increased sweating characterize this syndrome. Pain is relieved by blocking the sympathetic fibers with a paravertebral sympathetic block, nerve root block, or epidural block. Myofascial trigger points also can be the cause of

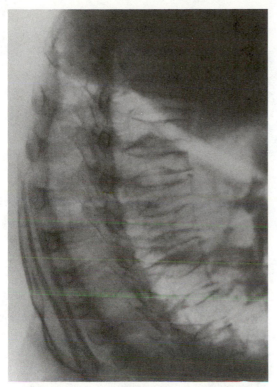

Fig 26A–1.—Lateral view of the thoracic spine in a 61-year-old woman with senile osteoporosis. Note the flat, fish-shaped vertebrae. (From Matzen P.F., Fleissner H.K.: *Orthopedic Roentgen Atlas.* Orlando, Florida, Grune & Stratton, 1970. Reproduced by permission.)

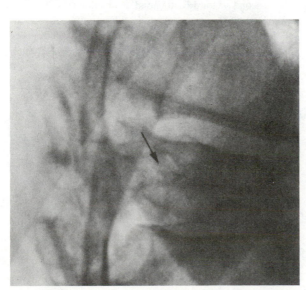

Fig 26A–2.—Lateral view of the 12th thoracic vertebra in a 68-year-old man. *Arrow* indicates complete collapse of the body. (From Matzen P.F., Fleissner H.K.: *Orthopedic Roentgen Atlas.* Orlando, Florida, Grune & Stratton, 1970. Reproduced by permission.)

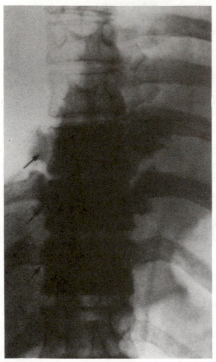

Fig 26A–3.—Osteosclerotic metastases in the 9th, 10th, and 11th thoracic vertebrae (marble vertebrae). (From Matzen P.F., Fleissner H.K.: *Orthopedic Roentgen Atlas.* Orlando, Florida, Grune & Stratton, 1970. Reproduced by permission.)

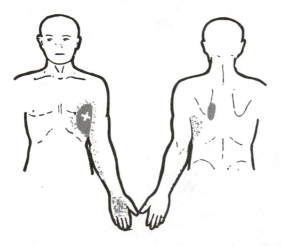

SERRATUS ANTERIOR

Fig 26A–4.—Sites of pain related to the serratus anterior muscle. *X* indicates trigger point; *solid* and *stippled areas* indicate regions of radiating pain.

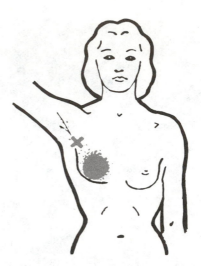

PECTORALIS MAJOR

Fig 26A–5.—Sites of pain related to the pectoralis muscle. *X* indicates trigger point; *solid* and *stippled areas* indicate regions of radiating pain.

postthoracotomy pain. It can be recognized on careful palpation of the paravertebral tissues.

Tietze's Syndrome[4]

Pain and swelling at a costochondral junction characterizes this syndrome. It usually involves the second or third costochondral junction (Fig 26A–7). Swelling is not associated with any evidence of inflammation. The differential diagnosis includes secondary malignancy and sepsis. Spontaneous remission may occur over a long period. Injection of a local anesthetic–steroid mixture and the use of oral nonsteroidal anti-inflammatory drugs are helpful.

THORACIC VISCERAL PAIN

Cardiac Pain

Almost all pain that originates in the heart results from ischemia secondary to coronary sclerosis.[5] This pain is referred mainly to the base of the neck, over the shoulders, over the pectoral muscles, and down the arms. Most frequently the referred pain is on the left side rather than on the right, probably

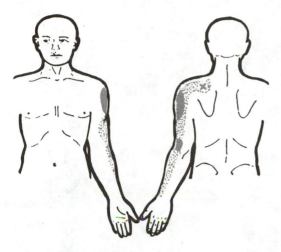

SUPRASPINATUS

Fig 26A–6.—Sites of pain related to the supraspinatus muscle. *X* indicates trigger point; *solid* and *stippled areas* indicate regions of radiating pain.

because the left side of the heart is much more frequently involved by coronary disease than is the right side, but occasionally there is referred pain on the right side of the body as well as on the left.

The pain impulses are conducted through sympathetic nerves passing to the middle cervical ganglia, to the stellate ganglia, and to the first four or five thoracic ganglia of the sympathetic chains. Then the impulses pass into the spinal cord through the second, third, fourth, and fifth thoracic spinal nerves (Fig 26A–8).

Direct Parietal Pain From the Heart

When coronary ischemia is extremely severe, such as immediately after a coronary thrombosis, intense cardiac pain frequently occurs directly beneath the sternum simultaneously with pain referred to other areas. Pain directly beneath the sternum is difficult to explain on the basis of the visceral nerve connections. Therefore, it is highly probable that sensory nerve endings passing from the heart through the pericardial reflections around the great vessels conduct this direct pain.[6]

In addition to pain from the heart, other sensa-

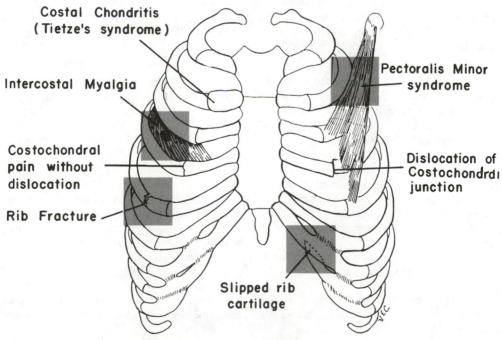

Fig 26A–7.—Tietze's syndrome (after Bonica).

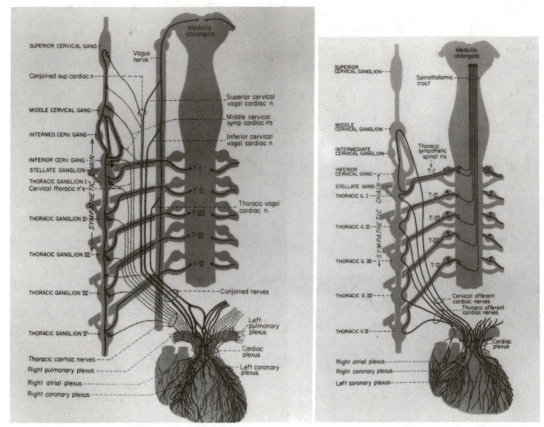

Fig 26A–8.—The autonomic nerve supply to the heart. *Left,* efferent; *right,* afferent nerve supply. (From Bonica J.J. (ed.): *Sympathetic* *Nerve Blocks for Pain Diagnosis and Therapy.* New York, Winthrop Breon, vol. 1. Reproduced by permission.)

tions may accompany coronary thrombosis. One of these is a tight, oppressive sensation beneath the sternum. The exact cause is unknown, but a possible cause is reflex spasm of blood vessels, bronchioles, or muscles in the chest region.[7]

The pain of acute myocardial ischemia is treated conservatively by reducing the myocardial workload, decreasing the oxygen consumption, and increasing the coronary blood flow with drugs such as propranolol, calcium channel blockers, and nitrites. Myocardial revascularization procedures are also indicated.

Chronic intractable pain can be treated by stellate ganglion block by chemical or surgical sympathectomy.

Some workers have utilized continuous epidural infusion to relieve the pain of acute myocardial ischemia and infarction. The myofascial pain in the left chest wall can be treated with trigger point injection with local anesthetics accompanied by TENS and shoulder girdle exercises.

Relief of Referred Cardiac Pain by Sympathectomy[8]

To interrupt pain impulses from the heart one can either cut the sympathetic nerves that pass from the heart to the sympathetic chains or, as is usually performed, cut nerve fibers as they pass through the sympathetic chains into the spinal cord. Cardiac pain can frequently be relieved simply by removing the sympathetic chain from T–2 through T–5 on the left side only, but sometimes it is necessary to remove fibers on both sides in order to obtain satisfactory results.

Lungs

The lungs and the visceral pleura are not sensitive structures and do not give rise to pain with injury. Parietal pleural pain is transmitted along the somatic fibers and interrupted by the intercostal block or thoracic root blocks at the appropriate level. Pain originating from the bronchus and trachea is carried by the vagus and is felt in the suprasternal area. Carcinoma of the lung causes pain when it involves the parietal pleura or metastasizes into the rib or spine.[9] This pain can be relieved by blocking the intercostal nerves or spinal roots. Pain originating from cancer of the bronchus can be relieved by vagotomy.

Esophagus[1]

Sensation from the lower two thirds of the esophagus is transmitted along with the sympathetic fibers and through the T5–10 posterior roots. Sensation from the upper third is transmitted by the vagus. Pain from the esophagus is usually referred to the pharynx, lower neck, arms, or midline chest regions, beginning at the upper portion of the sternum and ending approximately at the lower level of the heart. Irritation of the gastric end of the esophagus may cause pain directly over the heart, although the pain has nothing whatever to do with the heart. Such pain may be caused by spasm of the cardia, the area where the esophagus empties into the stomach, which causes excessive dilation of the lower esophagus, or it may result from chemical, bacterial, or other types of inflammatory irritation.

Pain originating from involvement of the esophagus can be treated with sympathetic blocks or through T5–10 nerve root block or posterior rhizotomy. Pain originating in the upper third of the esophagus is relieved by vagotomy.

REFERENCES

1. O'Brien J.P.: Mechanisms of spinal pain, in Wall P., Melzack O. (eds.): *Textbook of Pain*. Edinburgh, Churchill Livingstone, 1984, pp. 240–251.
2. Gunn D.R.: Degenerative diseases of the thoracic pain, in Ruge D., Wiltse L.L. (eds.): *Spinal Disorders; Diagnosis and Treatment*. Philadelphia, Lea & Febiger, 1977, pp. 323–327.
3. Travel J.: Myofascial trigger points: Clinical review, in Bonica J.J., Albe-Fessard D. (eds.): *Advances in Pain Research and Therapy*. New York, Raven Press, 1976.
4. Bonica J.J.: *The Management of Pain*. Philadelphia, Lea & Febiger, 1953.
5. Zanchetti A., Malliani A.: Neural and psychological factors in coronary disease. *Acta Cardiol. Suppl.* 20:69–89, 1974.
6. Malliani A., Lombardi F.: Considerations of fundamental mechanisms eliciting cardiac pain. *Am. Heart J.* 103:575–578, 1982.
7. Aviado D.M., Schmidt C.F.: Reflexes from stretch receptors in blood vessels, heart and lungs. *Physiol. Rev.* 35:247–300, 1975.
8. Cox W.V., Robertson H.I.: The effect of stellate ganglionectomy on the cardiac function of intact dogs and its effect on the extent of myocardial infarction and on cardiac function following coronary artery occlusion. *Am. Heart J.* 12:285–300, 1936.
9. Procacci P., Zoppi M.: Pathophysiology and clinical aspects of visceral and referred pain, in Bonica J.J., Lindblom V., Iggo A. (eds.): *Advances in Pain Research and Therapy*. New York, Raven Press, 1983.

26B / Low Back Pain

SOMAYAJI RAMAMURTHY, M.D.

PATIENTS with low back pain form the largest group of patients seeking relief in a pain center. About 20% of the U.S. population experiences back pain each year. Fortunately, 80%–90% get better. Presently in the United States, there are 2 million people totally disabled, and another 5 million are partially disabled by back pain. (For a discussion on the epidemiology of low back pain, see Chap. 2.) Many of these patients seek help in pain centers after medical care elsewhere, perhaps from numerous physicians, has failed to alleviate the pain. Most patients have already been exhaustively investigated to rule out primary or secondary pathologic conditions such as tumors, fractures, or infections. The usual etiological factors in patients with low back pain are nerve root irritation, myofascial syndromes, sympathetic dystrophy, and facet joint syndromes. These lesions may be present singly or in combination and often have psychological components. Abdominal and pelvic visceral pathologic conditions should always be considered in the differential diagnosis of low back pain, although they are infrequently causes of it.

RADICULOPATHY DUE TO NERVE ROOT IRRITATION

Radiculopathy due to nerve root irritation is characterized by shooting pain to the ankle, foot, or toes. The roots commonly involved are L-5 and S-1. On examination, straight leg raising reproduces the radiating pain, which is further aggravated by dorsiflexion of the ankle. Appropriate sensory loss, muscle weakness, and absent or decreased ankle jerk reflex may be present. Electromyography (EMG), myelography, or computerized tomography (CT) are likely to indicate the level of the lesion. Radicular pain can be due to herniated disk, spinal stenosis, tumor infiltration of nerves, metastasis,

herpes zoster, and arachanoiditis. Of these, the commonest cause is herniated lumbar disk.

Pain Due to Herniated Lumbar Disk

A history of intermittent chronic backache followed by a twisting maneuver and a popping sensation in the low back with subsequent pain referral to the leg is characteristic of acute lumbar disk displacement.[1] In 95% of patients with lumbar radiculopathy due to disk herniation, pain is the presenting symptom. Paresis in the absence of pain should alert the physician to a possible tumor.[2]

The radicular pain of disk herniation is described as a "toothache-like" pain, aggravated by activity and relieved by rest. However, sleep disturbance is a fairly common symptom of radicular pain. Patients may have some difficulty falling asleep and may be awakened by leg pain, which is relieved by walking. In cases of disk displacement, the sleep disturbance tends to improve with a few days of bed rest. Progressive sleep disturbance despite adequate bed rest should lead one to suspect a space-occupying lesion.[3]

Differential Diagnosis

Mechanical Pain

Segmental insufficiency resulting in mechanical low back pain secondary to degenerative disk disease is a diagnosis of exclusion.[4] Patients report predominantly back pain rather than leg pain. Pain can be referred to the groin, buttocks, and lateral thighs; it is aggravated by activity and relieved by rest. Standing, sitting, or leaning forward for any period of time aggravates the pain. Patients have difficulty pushing or pulling objects, straightening up from a bent position, and twisting. Lifting is impaired by pain, as is sitting in a stressful position—for example, on the floor. Recurrent acute attacks of low back pain, brought on by any activity and relieved by rest, and low back fatigue toward the end of the day are also symptoms of mechanical insufficiency.

Plain x-ray films may show degenerative spondylolisthesis or a pars interarticularis defect with or without spondylolisthesis. The diagnosis may also be confirmed by standing stress films, which show displacement of one vertebra over another or angulation greater than 15°.[5]

Spinal Stenosis

Neurogenic or vascular claudication usually implies a condition other than disk herniation. Unilateral or bilateral leg pain brought on by activity and relieved by rest is most commonly caused by central and/or foraminal spinal stenosis.[6]

It is helpful to differentiate radiculopathy secondary to disk displacement from neurogenic claudication secondary to spinal stenosis on a pathophysiologic basis. The disk displacement results from a mechanical distortion of the nerve root by a relatively rapid high compression force. The result is intraneural injury, edema, inflammation, and the production of ectopic stimulus of pain. Spinal ste-

nosis, on the other hand, produces a slowly and circumferentially applied load (Fig 26B–1). The nerve root is irritated by motion in a tight canal, which causes edema, ischemia, and neurogenic claudication. The pain is aggravated by activity and relieved by rest. Neurogenic claudication may be unilateral (foraminal stenosis) or bilateral (spinal canal stenosis). It can occur at any age and is associated with structural abnormalities (scoliosis or spondylolisthesis) in young patients and with degenerative spondylolisthesis and/or ankylosing hyperostosis (Fournier's disease) in older patients.

Conditions that must be considered in the differential diagnosis of low back pain and/or sciatica from disk displacement include the following:

Degenerative disk disease
Spondylolysis
Spondylolisthesis
Spinal stenosis
Facet joint syndrome
Metabolic bone disease
   Paget's disease
   Osteoporosis
Metastatic tumors
Multiple myeloma
Ependymoma
Neurofibroma
Vertebral osteomyelitis
Herpes zoster (shingles)
Traumatic low back sprain

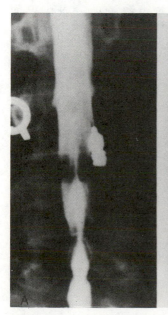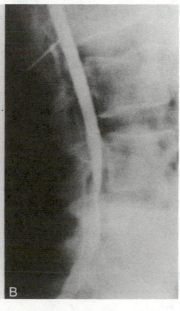

Fig 26B–1.—AP **(A)** and lateral **(B)** myelographic views indicating the presence of stenosis at the L4–5 and L5–S1 levels. (From Kirkaldy-Willis W.H.: *Managing Lower Back Pain.* New York, Churchill Livingstone, Inc., 1983, p. 114. Reproduced by permission.)

Psychogenic back pain
Aneurysm
Myofascial low back pain

Vascular Claudication

Leg pain that results from vascular insufficiency and resulting ischemia can be differentiated from neurogenic claudication by history. Patients with vascular claudication are able to walk a short distance before extremity pain and loss of function force them to stop. They then prefer to stand in place to increase arterial perfusion pressure, rather than to sit. Vascular claudication is usually associated with diminished or absent peripheral pulses.[7] Patients with spinal stenosis and neurogenic claudication would rather sit or flex the lumbar spine for relief when leg pain occurs from walking.

Abdominal pain, tenderness, bruits, and pulsatile masses, particularly in men over age 50, are clues to the diagnosis of a symptomatic abdominal aortic aneurysm. Occasionally an impending rupture of an aneurysm may be preceded by low back pain.

Efficacy of Physical Examination and Other Investigative Methods in Disk Herniation

Hudgins showed that impaired crossed straight leg raising was associated with surgical diagnosis of disk displacement in 97% of patients.[8] Disk displacement at surgery was noted in 90% of patients with weakness of the big toe extensor muscle, indicative of fifth lumbar root involvement. Ninety percent of patients with asymmetric reflexes had a herniated disk at surgery. Sensory deficit in a radicular distribution was least predictive of the physical findings, with only 70% of patients having a disk herniation at surgery (Table 26B–1).

TABLE 26B–1.—USUAL PHYSICAL FINDINGS IN PATIENTS WITH PROVED DISK DISPLACEMENT*

PHYSICAL FINDING	NO. (%) OF PTS.
Painful crossed straight leg raising	97
Weakness	90
Asymmetric reflex	90
Sensory deficit	70

*From Hudgins.[8] Reproduced by permission.

Limitation of forward flexion to less than 20°, straight leg raising impaired at less than 50°, and pain below the knee that is increased by dorsiflexion of the foot are highly predictive of lumbar radiculopathy from herniated disk. Follow-up studies have shown that patients who have one or more of these objective findings will respond better to invasive treatment, e.g., epidural steroid injection, chemonucleolysis, or laminectomy.[9, 11]

The diagnosis of a herniated disk must be confirmed by a good-quality metrizamide myelogram and/or a CT scan.[12] The myelogram enables the surgeon to see the entire subarachnoid space. Good visualization of the normal spinal cord, conus medullaris, lumbar roots, and nerve root sleeves can be obtained with metrizamide myelography (Fig 26B–2). Coincidental nerve root anomalies, lateral recess, and central spinal canal stenosis coincidental with disk displacement can be found most easily by myelography. Multiple disk displacement is also easily recognized on the myelogram (Fig 26B–3). In patients who have already had surgery, the myelogram is imperative to rule out iatrogenic cyst and to help differentiate epidural scar tissue from herniated disks (Figs 26B–4 and 26B–5).

A conus tumor or ependymoma may be detected on myelography and missed on other tests, including CT. Spinal fluid analysis should be correlated with myelographic findings.

The CT scan performed with partially diluted and absorbed contrast dye in the subarachnoid space imparts another dimension to diagnosis when one is trying to determine the exact source of pain. When disk displacement coincides with spinal stenosis and other spinal lesions, the CT scan with contrast has been useful in determining whether invasive procedures like chemonucleolysis will help relieve pain.

In rare instances, radiculopathy confirmed by history and physical examination cannot be demonstrated by a good-quality metrizamide myelogram and CT scan. In such instances, confirmation by epidural venography[13] and/or diskography[14] may be in order (Figs 26B–6 and 26B–7).

Adequate spinal fluid analysis, including cell count and differential as well as spinal fluid protein levels, should be obtained in all but the most straightforward cases of suspected herniated disks. In 186 disk herniations, Hudgins found that the mean spinal fluid protein level was 35 mg/dl (range, 16–80 mg/dl). Patients with tumors had a mean spinal fluid protein level of 173 mg/dl (range, 50–570 mg/dl).[8]

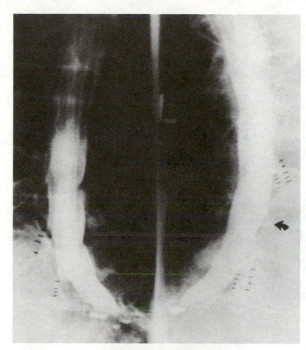

Fig 26B–2.—Metrizamide myelogram showing the subtle nerve root sleeves cut-off of right L–5, indicating compression from a lateral disk herniation. (From Stanton-Hicks M., Boas R.A.: *Chronic Low Back Pain.* New York, Raven Press, 1982. Reproduced by permission.)

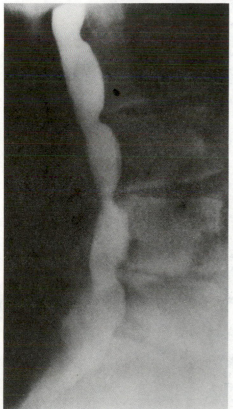

Fig 26B–3.—Myelogram, lateral view, showing multilevel indentations due to degenerative disk disease. (From Kirkaldy-Willis W.H.: *Managing Lower Back Pain.* New York, Churchill Livingstone, Inc., 1983, p. 115. Reproduced by permission.)

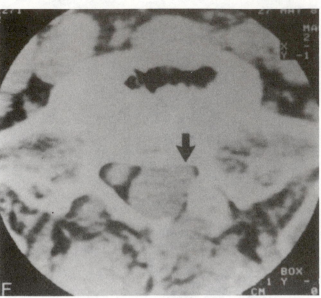

Fig 26B–4.—CT scan at L5–S1 level: *arrow* points to a poorly defined soft tissue shadow. The mean density is too low for herniation but correct for scar tissue. (From Kirkaldy-Willis W.H.: *Managing Lower Back Pain.* New York, Churchill Livingstone, Inc., 1983, p. 119. Reproduced by permission.)

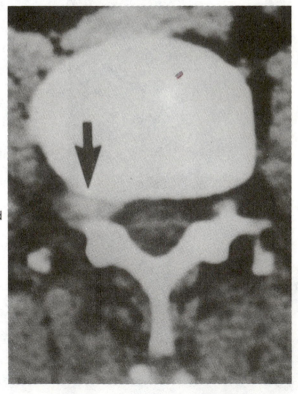

Fig 26B–5.—CT scan of L4–5 showing lateral disk herniation *(arrow).* (From Kirkaldy-Willis W.H.: *Managing Lower Back Pain.* New York, Churchill Livingstone, Inc. 1983, p. 119. Reproduced by permission.)

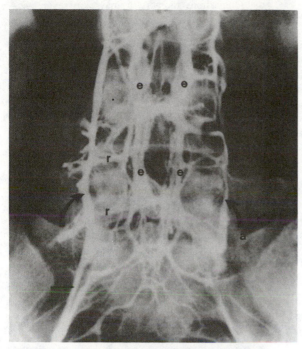

Fig 26B–6.—Normal epidural venogram: *a,* ascending lumbar veins; *r,* radicular venous branches; *e,* symmetric filling. (From Stanton-Hicks M., Boas R.A.: *Chronic Low Back Pain.* New York, Raven Press, 1982. Reproduced by permission.)

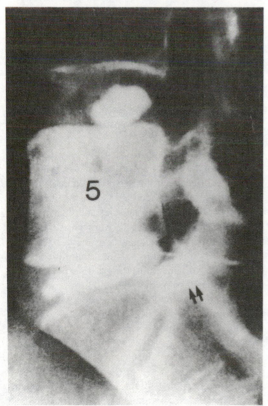

Fig 26B–7.—Diskogram of two levels showing normal biconcave L4–5 disk and elongated extravasation of the dye from the degenerated L5–S1 disk *(arrows).* (From Stanton-Hicks M., Boas R.A.: *Chronic Low Back Pain.* New York, Raven Press, 1982. Reproduced by permission.)

Treatment of Disk Herniation

By the time the patient is referred to a pain clinic, rest, traction, and nonsteroidal anti-inflammatory therapy have already been unsuccessful. Epidural injections of steroids are likely to relieve the pain in 70%–80% of patients, especially if they are treated early (see Chap. 35). In selected cases laminectomy with disk excision has been successful when conservative methods have failed.

MYOFASCIAL SYNDROME

The torso muscles that may cause myofascial low back pain include five thoracolumbar paraspinal muscles, the serratus posterior inferior, the lower rectus abdominis, the quadratus lumborum, and the iliopsoas muscles.

Thoracolumbar Paraspinal Muscles

Myofascial pain due to trigger points in the paraspinous muscles of the lower torso is an important cause of low back pain. The quadratus lumborum is the muscle most commonly involved, but trigger points located there are often overlooked because of inadequate physical examination.

The major thoracolumbar paraspinal muscles fall into two groups. One group includes two superficial muscles with nearly longitudinal fibers; the fibers of the other, deeper group generally run diagonally.[15] Both of the superficial muscle bundles function primarily to extend the spine and are therefore stretched by flexion. The deeper group of muscle fibers, located in the semispinal, multifidi, and rotator muscles, are shorter and become more diagonal. During the stretch-and-spray procedure, the deeper fibers require spinal rotation combined with flexion to stretch them fully.

Referred Pain Pattern

Trigger points in the thoracolumbar paraspinal muscles tend to refer pain caudally.[16–22] Those in the iliocostal muscle of the thorax refer pain anterolaterally to the lower chest and abdomen in a roughly segmental distribution and may refer pain upward through several spinal segments to the scapular region. Referred pain travels downward from trigger points in both the iliocostalis lumborum and the longissimus thoracis; it may skip several segments, sometimes appearing low in the buttock.[16, 23, 24]

The deep paraspinal muscles refer pain and tenderness to the midline from either side.[15, 16, 25]

Diagnosis

Trigger points develop in the iliocostal and deep paraspinal muscles when these muscles are strained during combined flexion and twisting of the torso. The longissimus thoracis is more likely to suffer overload when the patient lifts a heavy object while facing forward. Figure 26B–8 illustrates the three stages of low back pain of myofascial origin.

The patient moves with the spine stiffened protectively. When the superficial paraspinal muscles are involved, tense bands can be palpated against underlying structures. These bands exhibit exquisitely tender trigger points and strong local twitch responses. The trigger points in the multifidi and rotator muscles are characterized by circumscribed deep tenderness adjacent to a spinous process that is sensitive to tapping or to firm pressure (Figs 26B–9 and 26B–10).

Treatment

Treatment consists of spraying and stretching the muscle, a series of myoneural blocks with local anesthetics and steroids, and exercises. To passively stretch the superficial iliocostal and longissimus paraspinal muscles during the spray-and-stretch procedure, the patient sits with the feet on the floor, leans far forward, drops the head, and lets the arms hang loosely between the legs. The operator applies a jet stream of vapocoolant spray in downward sweeps over the affected muscles and their pain reference zones while adding forward pressure on the torso to further flex the spine. For the deep paraspinal muscles—the semispinal, the multifidi, and especially the rotator muscles—a rotary stretch is added to the flexion: the operator firmly grasps the patient's shoulder and rotates the opposite side forward while spraying over the passively stretched muscles with downward sweeps.

Myoneural block with local anesthetic and steroid is described in detail in chapter 33. A home program of active exercises, as described by Cailliet,[26] and an understanding by the patient of the mechanics of the back[27] are often essential to permanent recovery.

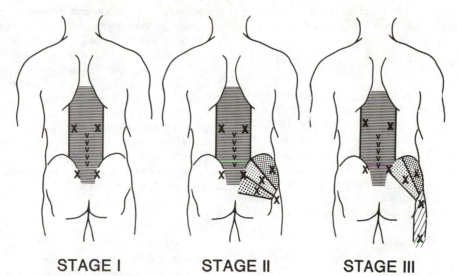

STAGE I   STAGE II   STAGE III

Fig 26B–8.—The myofascial origin of low back pain. Stage I: early muscle spasms of the paravertebral muscles. Stage II: stiffness, tenderness, and spasm in the paravertebral and gluteal muscles, particularly the piriformis, gluteus medius, and gluteus minimus muscles. Stage III: additional involvement of the tensor fasciae latae.

Serratus Posterior Inferior Muscle

The myofascial pain syndrome of the serratus posterior inferior muscle is seen infrequently but is distressing when present. It responds well to trigger point therapy.

This muscle connects *above and laterally* to the last four ribs and *below and medially* to the spinous processes of the last two thoracic and first two lumbar vertebrae. It depresses the ribs during forced expiration and helps to rotate the spine at the thoracolumbar junction, turning the face toward the same side.

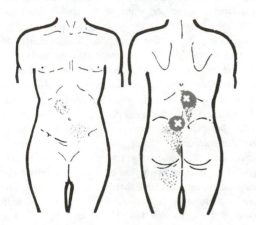

MULTIFIDUS

Fig 26B–9.—Sites of pain related to the multifidus muscle. *X* indicates trigger point; *solid* and *stippled areas* indicate regions of radiating pain.

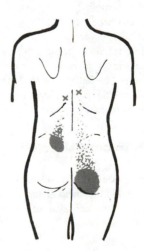

LONGISSIMUS

Fig 26B–10.—Sites of pain related to the longissimus muscle. *X* indicates trigger point; *solid* and *stippled areas* indicate regions of radiating pain.

Aching pain is referred in the region of the trigger point and over the lower ribs posteriorly.[15]

Diagnosis

Referred pain from a trigger point in this muscle is often constant over the lower ribs and is independent of spinal movement. On examination, flexion of the thoracolumbar spine is slightly restricted. Patients with this myofascial pain syndrome often have disharmony between the respiratory muscles of the chest and abdomen, but a deep breath is not painful as a rule. Associated trigger points are often found in adjacent paraspinal and oblique abdominal muscles.

Treatment

To lengthen this muscle by the stretch-and-spray procedure, the patient sits and leans forward to establish maximum flexion of the thoracolumbar spine, with the shoulder on the side of the affected muscle rotated forward. As sweeps of vapocoolant are applied, the patient relaxes, takes a deep breath, exhales, and continues to relax. During additional sweeps, the operator exerts pressure to achieve passive flexion-rotation movement of the spine.

During this passive stretching, parallel sweeps of the jet stream are applied upward and outward over the muscle, covering it and its pain reference zone.[15] A hot pack is then applied.

For complete relief, ischemic compression or injection of the trigger point in this muscle may be required as well. The latter must be done with great care to avoid needle penetration of an intercostal space to prevent pneumothorax.

Rectus Abdominis Muscle

Back pain is occasionally referred from trigger points in the abdominal musculature, chiefly in the terminal fibers of the cephalad and caudal ends of the rectus abdominis muscle.[15]

Functional Anatomy

This muscle attaches *above* to the fifth, sixth, and seventh ribs anteriorly and *below* to the pubis. It strongly flexes the spine and tenses the anterior abdominal wall, helping to retrude the abdomen, as in

expiration, and to increase intra-abdominal pressure.

In the uppermost fibers, trigger points may lie in the angle between the midline and the rib cage at the level of or slightly below the tip of the xyphoid process. On either side, these trigger points project pain horizontally across both sides of the back at the lower thoracic level. Similarly, trigger points in the lowest fibers of the rectus abdominis lie close to the symphysis pubis and from either side refer pain horizontally across the sacrum, iliac crests, and upper gluteal regions. Intermediate trigger points are more likely to refer pain to the corresponding quadrant of the abdomen than to the back.[15]

Diagnosis

The distinctively horizontal pattern of low or mid-back pain, with characteristic trigger point tenderness in the terminal fibers of the rectus abdominis on one or both sides, identifies myofascial pain of the rectus abdominis muscle. The weakness associated with trigger points in this muscle causes abdominal wall laxity; the patient fails to "pull in" the protruded abdomen.

Treatment

For the stretch-and-spray procedure, the patient lies supine with the feet resting on a support below the level of the treatment table; this position extends the lumbar spine and separates the pubis from the rib cage, lengthening the abdominal muscles. The vapocoolant jet stream is applied longitudinally in one direction over the affected muscle, starting at the trigger point. Finally, the patient takes and holds a deep breath with the diaphragm so as to fully protrude the abdomen and further stretch the rectus abdominis muscles. With the patient tilted to the other side, the spray is also swept over the pain reference zone in the back.

A home exercise program ensures more lasting recovery. It starts with pelvic tilts to strengthen the abdominal muscles and then proceeds to slow letbacks (situps in reverse), with the knees held straight to bring the hip flexors into play.[15] The lengthening contraction of the abdominal wall muscles during the letbacks helps greatly to restore the muscles to normal function. When a series of ten slow letbacks can be done comfortably, the patient may progress to partial situps (shortening contraction) with the knees bent, and then to full situps.

The number of these should progress slowly from one to 10 or 15 in a series, with a pause and deep breathing between cycles.

Trigger points in the rectus abdominis are effectively inactivated when injected with local anesthetic solution. Care must be taken to avoid penetrating the peritoneum or the pleura at the superior end of the muscle.

Quadratus Lumborum Muscle

The quadratus lumborum is the most often overlooked source of myofascial low back pain.[28, 29] Many of the fibers in this muscle run nearly vertically deep under the paraspinal muscles. They connect above to the 12th rib and below to the posterior third of the iliac crest and to the iliolumbar ligament. In addition, fibers attach medially to the transverse processes of the upper four lumbar vertebrae; some of these fibers are oriented diagonally upward to the 12th rib and others are oriented diagonally downward to the iliac crest, forming a series of crisscrossing bundles.

Acting unilaterally, the longitudinal fibers flex the spine laterally toward the same side or, if the spine is held straight, elevate the homolateral pelvis; the diagonal fibers flex the spine laterally toward the opposite side. The paired quadratus lumborum muscles depress the 12th ribs during forced expiration and coughing. Acting bilaterally in concert, all quadratus lumborum fibers extend the spine.

Referred Pain Pattern

When located in the lateral, more superficial longitudinal fibers of this muscle, trigger points refer pain downward, mainly over the iliac crest and the greater trochanter and sometimes anteriorly to the lower abdomen and groin. Trigger points in the medial, deeper fibers also refer pain downward, but more posteriorly to the sacroiliac joint and deep in the midbuttock. The complaint of pain referred from these trigger points and the finding of deep tenderness on palpation that they refer to the same area[29] easily lead to an erroneous diagnosis of trochanteric bursitis or sacroiliac joint involvement.[30] Bilateral involvement of the quadratus lumborum may lead to pain on both sides of the back.

The pain caused by this muscle may extend into the lower extremity when it activates satellite trigger points in the gluteus minimus muscle.

Diagnosis

Acute strain of the quadratus lumborum muscle may result from a quick stooping movement when the torso is twisted somewhere to one side or from a fall or other accident. Active trigger points in this muscle may also develop after sustained or repetitive overload, as in gardening or scrubbing the floor. Patients then complain of pain on walking, when formed without heavy loading or sustained effort.

Most patients clearly remember the strain that started their back pain but are unaware of or disregard the mechanical stresses that perpetuate trigger point activity. Low back pain is often relieved by correcting a discrepancy in leg length.[31] Continuing strain of the quadratus lumborum is often caused when standing if one leg is shorter than the other[32, 33] or when sitting if the hemipelvis is small. Either of these asymmetries tilts the pelvis downward on the smaller side and causes a compensatory scoliosis, which in turn tilts the axis of the shoulder girdle.

A discrepancy in leg length of 13 mm may cause no problem if no initiating event has occurred to activate quadratus lumborum trigger points. However, a discrepancy of only 3 mm can be a potent perpetuator of active trigger points in this muscle. The difference in leg length is readily corrected by adding a lift to the heel of the shoe on the short side and/or by cutting down the heel on the long side.

The small hemipelvis is corrected by sitting on a pad placed under the ischial tuberosity on the short side. A normal pelvis can be tilted, or a tilted pelvis corrected, by placing a wallet in a long back pocket of the pants.[34]

Another group of patients have short upper arms in relation to torso height. Frequently throughout the day, they must lean forward or sideways for elbow support, chronically straining the quadratus lumborum and perpetuating its trigger points. Pads added to the armrests of the chair prevent this. Kitchen sponges will serve.

Iliopsoas Muscle

When the iliopsoas muscle is involved in a myofascial pain syndrome, the quadratus lumborum is usually involved as well, and for lasting relief, trigger points in the latter muscle must also be inactivated. Bilateral involvement of the psoas muscle is common, but one side is usually more severely affected.

The psoas muscle attaches cephalad to the sides of the lumbar vertebral bodies, and the iliac muscle attaches to the inner surface of the iliac bone, thereby lining the lateral wall of the pelvis major. Distally, most of the iliac fibers join the psoas tendon, which attaches to the lesser trochanter on the medial aspect of the femur. Acting bilaterally, the psoas muscles flex the lower lumbar spine. Unilaterally, the psoas and iliac muscles flex the thigh and assist external rotation at the hip joint.

Referred Pain Pattern

Pain referred from trigger points in the iliopsoas muscle forms a distinctive *vertical* pattern homolaterally along the lumbosacral spine, extending downward to the sacroiliac region. The pain may also be referred over the front of the thigh on the same side.

Diagnosis

Patients with a taut iliopsoas muscle shortened by trigger point activity walk with the thigh in external rotation and in slight flexion at the hip, which flattens the normal lordotic lumbar curve. They have a stooped posture[34] because of the limited extension and internal rotation of the thigh and restricted extension of the lumbar spine. This posture is distinguished from that due to skeletal kyphosis by x-ray examination of the spine.

On physical examination, exquisite tenderness is found in three sites: (1) immediately above the femoral attachment of the iliopsoas tendon when pressure is applied deeply along the medial wall of the femora triangle toward the lesser trochanter, (2) in the iliac muscle when pressure is applied against the iliac fossa, just inside the brim of the pelvis behind the anterior superior iliac spine, and (3) in the psoas muscle when a medial thrust is added to deep abdominal pressure exerted lateral to the rectus abdominis muscle, just below the level of the umbilicus.

OTHER TRIGGER POINTS OF THE LOW BACK

Pressure just medial to the posterior superior iliac spine produces pain in the majority of low back pain patients. This point overlies many structures which could give rise to pain in the low back, such as the sacrospinal trigger point, L5–S1 facet, liliolumbar fascia, sacroiliac joint, and occasionally a fibrofatty tissue which can act as a trigger point.

GLUTEUS MEDIUS.—The trigger point here is located in the muscle band in the middle of the gluteal area and is present in a majority of patients who have buttock pain (Fig 26B–11).

GLUTEUS MINIMUS AND TENSOR FASCIA LATA.—Trigger points here cause the pain to be referred along the lateral aspect of the thigh. They are palpable in the gluteal area between the greater trochanter and the iliac crest.

PIRIFORMIS TRIGGER POINT.—This can mimic sciatica due to disk disease, with pain along the posterior aspect of the thigh and leg and subjective numbness because of irritation of the sciatic nerve. The trigger point is palpated in the sciatic notch with the patient in the lateral position (Fig 26B–12).

BICEPS TRIGGER POINT.—This trigger point produces pain behind the knee. It is palpatated 6 cm above the knee on the lateral aspect of the posterior thigh.

GASTROCNEMIUS TRIGGER POINT.—The gastrocnemius trigger point produces pain and cramping in the calf muscles. A well-defined band is palpable at the midcalf on the medial side of the gastrocnemius.

FIBROSITIS.—Diffuse subcutaneous tenderness present over the painful area usually responds to infrared therapy followed by massage or sympathetic blocks. Associated tension and endocrine abnormalities should also be treated.

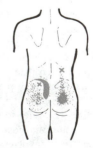

GLUTEUS
MEDIUS   ILIOCOSTALIS

Fig 26B–11.—Sites of pain related to the gluteus medius and iliocostalis muscles. *X* indicates trigger point; *solid* and *stippled areas* indicate regions of radiating pain.

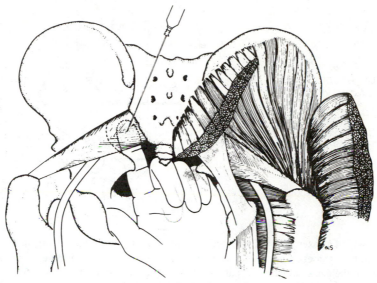

Fig 26B–12.—Technique of piriformis injection. (After Wyant G.M.: Chronic pain syndromes and their treatment: 3. The piriformis syndrome. *Can. Anaesth. Soc. J.* 20:305, 1979. Reproduced by permission.)

SYMPATHETIC DYSTROPHY

Sympathetic dystrophy may be due to mild nerve root irritation secondary to many causes. Signs and symptoms are detailed under reflex sympathetic dystrophy in chapter 25C.

Spinal or epidural diagnostic differential blocks can be performed to diagnose the C pain fiber pathway. The technique is described in chapter 15D.

FACET SYNDROME

Pain originating from the facet joints can mimic nerve root irritation pain. This pain is referred to the leg and is aggravated by a change in position.

Facet pain can be relieved by injection into the joint or around the capsule, or by blocking the nerve supply to the joint (Figs 26B–13 and 26B–14). Injection of a local anesthetic into the joint cavity with the aid of an image intensifier provides good long-term relief. Local anesthetic, 0.5–2 ml, with 10 mg of triamcinolone is injected, usually at 2-week intervals, two to three times for prolonged relief.

Facet Denervation

Each facet joint is supplied by a branch of the nerve root at the same level and one level above.

Good results have been reported after facet nerve block with a local anesthetic followed by neurolysis with phenol, radiofrequency treatment, or treatment with a cryoprobe.

The block is accomplished by placing the needle at the junction of the transverse process and the superior facet. Identification is facilitated if the nerve is stimulated, reproducing the pain. One-half to one milliliter of the solution blocks the nerve.

In patients with acute back pain from facet joint involvement, local anesthetic and steroid injection, 2–3 cm lateral to the level of the top of the corresponding spinous process, and a level above, results in good pain relief.

PAIN AFTER BACK SURGERY

Patients that have undergone multiple surgical procedures on the back commonly complain of low back pain with stiffness and weakness (Fig 26B–15). By the time these patients seek relief in a pain clinic, they have had serious changes in their personal and social life, have had financial problems secondary to inability to work, and may have psychological problems related to depression and chronic pain behavior. These patients must be differentiated from patients with nerve root irritation, myofascial pain syndromes, reflex sympathetic dystrophy, arachnoiditis, and psychological problems.

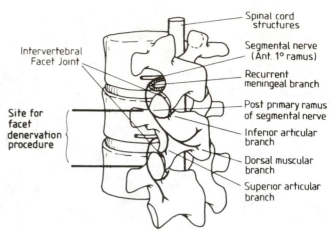

Fig 26B–13.—Segmental innervation of vertebral facet joints. Superior and inferior articular branches supply each facet. (From Stanton-Hicks M., Boas R.A.: *Chronic Low Back Pain.* New York, Raven Press, 1982. Reproduced by permission.)

Treatment consists of an exercise program, beginning with very gentle exercises and gradually adding stretching and strengthening exercises. All narcotics and depressant drugs are withdrawn gradually either by an inpatient or an outpatient method. Often it is necessary to provide continuous pain relief with an epidural catheter, to provide physical therapy, and to allow an alternative method of pain relief as drugs are withdrawn. Most of these patients will benefit by central modalities, e.g., learning self-hypnosis, relaxation techniques, or biofeedback.

Principles of behavior modification should be employed throughout the treatment program. Drugs are given on schedule, not on as-needed basis. Patients are encouraged not to discuss their pain. Pain-independent behavior is encouraged and rewarded. Exercises are prescribed to quota and not to tolerance.

ABDOMINAL VISCERAL PAIN

Visceral fibers from the upper abdominal viscera, liver, stomach, duodenum, spleen, and pancreas travel through the celiac ganglia and sympathetic

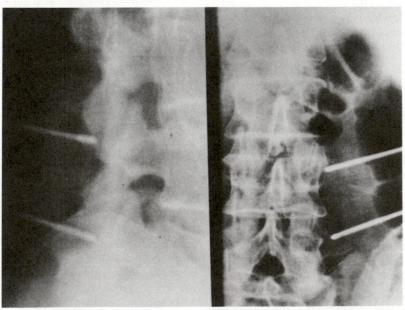

Fig 26B–14.—AP and lateral radiographs showing needle positions for facet denervation. (From Stanton-Hicks M., Boas R.: *Chronic Low Back Pain.* New York, Raven Press, 1982, Reproduced by permission.)

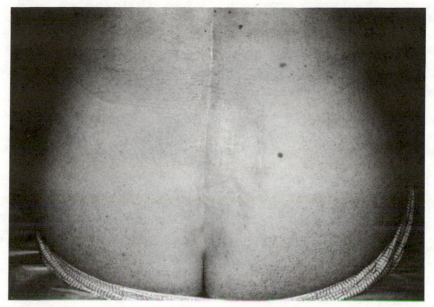

Fig 26B–15.—Patient who has had multiple laminectomies for back pain with fusion. Note the multiple scars, stiffness, and lack of muscle contour.

chain and enter the cord through the roots T5–10.

Even though pain originating from these viscera can be treated by blocking the sympathetic chain or T5–10 nerve roots, celiac plexus block is the commonest procedure performed. Celiac plexus block on the right side with 25 ml of local anesthetic or neurolytic solution relieves the pain originating from the liver biliary tract, head of the pancreas, right kidney, and duodenum. The left-sided block relieves pain from the stomach, spleen, parts of duodenum, and body and tail of the pancreas and left kidney. Bilateral celiac plexus block is commonly used when treating pain arising from malignancy of the upper abdominal viscera.

Gastric Pain

Pain arising in the fundus of the stomach, usually caused by gastritis, is referred to the anterior surface of the chest or upper abdomen, from slightly below the heart to an inch or so below the xiphoid process. This pain is frequently characterized as burning pain; it, or pain from the lower esophagus, causes the condition known as "heartburn."

Most peptic ulcers occur within 1–2 inches on either side of the pylorus in the stomach or in the duodenum, and pain from such ulcers is usually referred to a surface point approximately midway be-

tween the umbilicus and the xiphoid process. The cause of ulcer pain is almost undoubtedly chemical, because when the acid juices of the stomach are not allowed to reach the pain fibers in the ulcer crater, the pain does not exist. This pain is characteristically intensely burning.

Biliary and Gallbladder Pain

Pain from the bile ducts and gallbladder is localized in the midepigastrium almost coincident with pains caused by peptic ulcers. Biliary and gallbladder pain is often burning, like that from ulcers, although cramps often occur too.

Biliary disease, in addition to causing pain on the abdominal surface, frequently refers pain to a small area at the tip of the right scapula. This pain is transmitted through sympathetic afferent fibers that enter the ninth thoracic segment of the spinal cord.

Pancreatic Pain

Lesions of the pancreas, such as acute or chronic pancreatitis, in which the pancreatic enzymes eat away the pancreas and surrounding structures, promote intense pain in areas both in front of and behind the pancreas. The pancreas is located beneath the parietal peritoneum and receives many parietal sensory fibers from the posterior abdominal wall. Therefore, the pain is usually localized directly behind the pancreas in the back and is severe and burning in character.

Chronic pancreatic pain has been relieved in many instances by celiac plexus block with a local anesthetic–steroid mixture. TENS also has been used successfully in some patients.

When a malignancy of the viscera extends into the parietal peritoneum or the diaphragm, the pain is carried by the somatic fibers in the intercostal nerves or phrenic nerve, with referred pain to the shoulder. Interruption of these pathways may be necessary to provide pain relief.

Renal Pain

The kidney, pelvis, and ureters are all retroperitoneal structures and receive most of their pain fibers directly from skeletal nerves. Therefore, pain is usually felt directly behind the ailing structure. However, pain occasionally is referred via visceral afferents to the anterior abdominal wall below and about 2 inches to the side of the umbilicus.

Pain from the bladder is felt directly over the bladder, presumably because the bladder is well innervated by parietal pain fibers. However, pain also is sometimes referred to the groin and testicles because some nerve fibers from the bladder apparently synapse in the cord in association with fibers from the genital areas.

Uterine Pain

Both parietal and visceral afferent pain may be transmitted from the uterus. The low abdominal cramping pains of dysmenorrhea are mediated through the sympathetic afferents, and an operation to cut the hypogastric nerves between the hypogastric plexus and the uterus will in many instances relieve this pain. On the other hand, lesions of the uterus that spread into the adnexa around the uterus, or lesions of the fallopian tubes and broad ligaments, usually cause pain in the lower back or side. This pain is conducted over parietal nerve fibers and is usually sharper in nature rather than the diffuse cramping pain of true dysmenorrhea.

REFERENCES

1. Murphy F.: Sources and patterns of pain in disc disease. *Clin. Neurosurg.* 15:343, 1968.
2. Brown M.D.: Low back strain and rupture of the intervertebral disc: Section 2, Diagnosis of back pain syndromes; Section 4, Treatment of painful back syndromes, in *Practice of Orthopaedic Surgery,* ed. 2, Hagerstown, Md., Harper & Row, 1977.
3. Brown M.D.: The diagnosis of back pain syndromes. *Orthop. Clin. North Am.* 6:233, 1975.
4. Brown M.D.: Lumbar spine fusion, in Finneson B.E. (ed.): *Low Back Pain,* ed. 2. Philadelphia, J.B. Lippincott Co., 1979.
5. Knutsson F.: The instability associated with disc degeneration in the lumbar spine. *Acta Radiol.* 25:593, 1944.
6. Grabias S.: The treatment of spinal stenosis. *J. Bone Joint Surg.* [*Am.*] 42:308, 1980.
7. Hawkes C.H., Roberts G.M.: Neurogenic and vascular claudication. *J. Neurol. Sci.* 38:337, 1978.
8. Hudgins P.W.: The predictive value of myelography in the diagnosis of ruptured lumbar discs. *J. Neurosurg.* 32:152, 1970.
9. Wiltse L.: Chemoneucleolysis in ideal candidates for laminectomy. *Spectator,* June 30, 1978.
10. Winnie A.P., Hartman J.T., Meyers H.L., Ramamurthy S., et al.: Pain clinic: II. Intradural and extradural corticosteroids for sciatica. *Anesth. Analg.* 51:990–1003, 1972.
11. Spengler D.M., Freeman C.W.: Patient selection for lumbar discectomy. *Spine* 4:129, 1979.
12. Haughton V.M., Eldevik O.P., Magnaes B., et al.: A prospective comparison of computed tomography and myelography in the diagnosis of herniated lumbar discs. *Radiology* 142:103, 1982.
13. MacNab I., St. Louis E.L., Grabias S.L., et al.: Selective ascending lumbosacral venography in the assessment of lumbar disc herniation. *J. Bone Joint Surg.* [*Am.*] 58:1093, 1976.
14. Abdulla A.F., Ditto E.W., Byrd E.W., et al.: Extreme lateral lumbar disc herniations. *J. Neurosurg.* 41:229, 1974.
15. Travell J., Simons D.G.: *Myofascial Pain and Dysfunction: The Trigger Point Manual.* Baltimore, Williams & Wilkins Co., 1983, pp. 639–659.
16. Travell J., Rinzler S.H.: The myofascial genesis of pain. *Postgrad. Med.* 11(5):425–434, 1952.
17. Travell J., Travell W.: Therapy of low back pain by manipulation and of referred pain in the lower extremity by procaine infiltration. *Arch. Phys. Med. Rehabil.* 27:537–547, 1946.
18. Travell J.: Basis for the multiple uses of local block of somatic trigger areas (procaine infiltration and ethyl chloride spray). *Miss. Valley Med. J.* 72:13–22, 1949.
19. Kelly M.: The relief of facial pain by procaine (Novocaine) injections. *J. Am. Geriatr. Soc.* 11:586–596, 1963.
20. Bates T., Grunwaldt E.: Myofascial pain in childhood. *J. Pediatr.* 53:198–209, 1958.
21. Kellgren J.H.: Observations on referred pain arising from muscle. *Clin. Sci.* 3:175–190, 1938.

22. Travell J.: Pain mechanisms in connective tissues, in Raga C. (ed.): *Connective Tissues: Transactions of the Second Conference, 1951.* New York, Josiah Macy, Jr. Foundation, 1952, pp. 86–125.

23. Mennell J.M.: *Back Pain.* Boston, Little, Brown & Co., 1960, pp. 109–128.

24. Weber A., Herz R.: The relation between caffeine contracture of intact muscle and the effect of caffeine on reticulum. *J. Gen. Physiol.* 52:750–759, 1969.

25. Livingston W.K.: *Pain Mechanisms.* New York, Plenum Press, 1976, pp. 128–139.

26. Cailliet R.: *Low Back Pain Syndrome,* ed. 3. Philadelphia, F.A. Davis Co., 1981, pp. 115–116, 193–194.

27. Tichauer E.R.: Ergonomics: The state of the art. *Am. Ind. Hyg. Assoc. J.* 28(3–4):105–116, 1967.

28. Sola A.E., Kuitert J.H.: Quadratus lumborum myofascitis. *Northwest Med.* 53:1003–1005, 1954.

29. Travell J.G.: The quadratus lumborum muscle: An overlooked cause of low back pain. *Arch. Phys. Med. Rehabil.* 57:566, 1976.

30. Reynolds M.D.: Myofascial trigger point syndromes in the practice of rheumatology. *Arch. Phys. Med. Rehabil.* 62:111–114, 1981.

31. Sicuranza B.J., Richards J., Tisdall L.H.: The short leg syndrome in obstetrics and gynecology. *Am. J. Obstet. Gynecol.* 107:217–219, 1970.

32. Nichols P.J.: Short-leg syndrome. *Br. Med. J.* 6:1863–1865, 1960.

33. Gould N.: Back-pocket sciatica, letter. *N. Engl. J. Med.* 290:633, 1974.

34. Michele A.A.: The iliopsoas muscle: Its importance in disorders of the hip and spine. *Clin. Symp.* 12(3):67–101, 1960.

PART **V**

Pharmacology of Drugs Used in Pain Management

27 / Pharmacokinetic Considerations for Drug Dosing

LAURENCE E. MATHER, PH.D.
DONALD D. DENSON, PH.D.

EVEN THE MOST clinically oriented medical practitioner is aware of the enormous impact pharmacokinetic research has had in the past decade on our understanding of the time course of drug and drug metabolite concentrations in the body. The literature abounds with illustrations of the pharmacokinetic properties of drugs and how these properties are modified by various diseases. However, fewer reports detail the connection between the reported pharmacokinetic properties and the dosing strategy required for patients. The main reason for this frequent omission is that pharmacodynamic data are lacking for the majority of drugs. Thus, while the relationships between dose and blood (plasma, etc.) drug concentrations and time (pharmacokinetic data) have been derived, the relationship between blood (plasma, etc.) drug concentrations and effects, both therapeutic and toxic (pharmacodynamic data), may not have been derived, or a clear relationship has not been found. Nevertheless, some more recent textbooks of therapeutics do attempt to address available pharmacokinetic and pharmacodynamic data (for example, the textbooks by Gilman, Goodman, and Gilman,[1] and by Avery[2]). This chapter attempts to integrate the pharmacokinetic information available for the systemic analgesic agents without introducing mathematical complexities, but instead focusing on the interpretation and application of this information to pain therapy.

ESSENTIAL DEFINITIONS AND TERMINOLOGY

Basic Information: Clearance and Volume of Distribution

There are two basic terms to be acquired from the pharmacokinetic data for any drug. These are *clearance,* or the efficiency of the body in eliminating drug, and *volume of distribution,* or the degree of dilution of the drug within the body. From these pharmacokinetic properties other more familiar secondary terms, such as half-life, may be derived. These pharmacokinetic terms form the basic vocabulary by which drugs, and recipients of drugs, may be categorized and compared. The remainder of the discussion is based on this terminology.

In physiologic terms, *clearance* by any organ (or tissue) is equal to the product of blood flow to that organ and the extraction ratio by that organ (and therefore it has the dimensions of flow). *Total body clearance* is the desired pharmacokinetic property measured experimentally (and is usually referred to as just "clearance"). It is the sum of all organ clearances. For example, renal clearance is equal to the total body clearance times the fraction of the dose eliminated via the kidneys, and so on for other organs. Clearance is related to time, so it can be thought of as an average of the functional drug "output." If drug "input" is made *over a period of time* (multiple doses, continuous infusion), the ratio of input to output gives the mean steady-state concentrations, and this is an important index of *drug exposure* for pharmacodynamic effects.

Volume of distribution is a little more complicated because there are several varieties. Any volume is a proportionality constant between an amount and a concentration. So too with pharmacokinetic volumes, except that pharmacokinetic volumes are "apparent" volumes. Whereas they express the proportionality between the amount of drug in the body and the concentration of drug in the fluid sampled (blood, plasma, etc.), the actual numerical value increases with time after drug administration. Pharmacokinetic volumes are "apparent" volumes because they are not (generally) homogeneous anatomical and physiologic spaces but rather reflect the aggregate of heterogeneous partitioning of drug into different organs and tissues. Pharmacokinetic volumes are (generally) time dependent because equilibration is governed by the differing rates of delivery to and uptake by different organs and tissues. Therefore, there are two principal volumes of distribution to understand: an *initial dilution volume,* sometimes called a central compartment volume, which reflects dilution and distribution within tissues which rapidly equilibrate with the blood, and a *total volume of distribution,* which measures overall equilibration with all tissues. The latter volume has been the subject of some contention among pharmacokineticists. There are two principal contenders, each with legitimate claims for recognition.

The *volume of distribution at steady-state equilibrium* defines the extent of dilution at the time of peak distribution, irrespective of the rate of elimination. The *volume of distribution during pseudoequilibrium* defines the extent of dilution during the "elimination phase" when blood and tissues are giving up drug in the same proportion (pseudoequilibrium), and its value is referenced to this rate. It is sometimes called volume of distribution (area) or volume of distribution (beta) since it relates the dose, area under the blood (or plasma, etc.) concentration time curve, and the rate of decay of concentrations (often called beta).

Rate of Changes: Half-Life

The familiar term "half-life" (or "half-time") is really only a measure of *how fast* concentrations change and is related both to clearance (inversely) and to the volume of distribution (directly). Again, there may be some ambiguities in the literature, since half-lives (like volumes) depend on the time after drug administration except for those rare cases in which distribution occurs so fast it cannot be detected. Drugs may appear to have many (increasing) half-lives, depending on time after administration, and these are the result of the tissue uptake gradually becoming completed. According to traditional models, when tissue uptake is complete, the concentrations in blood and tissues decay in parallel (pseudoequilibrium), and the half-life is described by a single terminal half-life. This is the commonly referenced value of "half-life" of the drug and provides useful information on *when* the drug dose may need repeating, not on *how much* drug may need to be given.

It will be obvious to the reader trained in acute care that the redistribution phase is not without importance. In fact, in acute care, pseudoequilibrium or steady-state conditions may not occur. Many drugs are used routinely in doses at which their duration of action is terminated by their redistribution into nonresponsive tissue mass, therefore the time (half-lives) of the redistribution phase is important information for acute care. It is well known that patients awaken from thiopental bolus injection because of redistribution from responsive brain tissue into muscle mass. It is equally important that patients stop convulsing after an accidental intravenous (IV) local anesthetic bolus for the same reason. How, then, should these fast ("redistribution" phase) half-lives be interpreted? Foremost, with caution! Because the rate of redistribution decreases with time after drug administration, the redistribution half-lives are sensitive to the time when the samples are taken—one may even miss them altogether. The body responds to the arterial concentration initially, but the duration of response depends on the tissue concentration or the venous concentration draining the responsive tissue. Pharmacokinetic studies, for convenience, rely heavily on samples drawn from a vein in the arm. However, these concentrations also reflect the rate of equilibration of the arm tissue and this may bear no relation whatsoever to responsive tissue. Therefore, in the absence of the other information, arterial concentrations should be the guide, and it is their rate of change that provides valuable information on redistribution rates. Venous concentrations are damped. However, in the general case, it is *not* the arterial *whole blood (or plasma) concentration* that drives the pharmacodynamic response.

Blood Cell and Plasma Protein Binding

For drugs that act by a specific receptor interaction (there appear to be few drugs that do not), the reaction is driven by the *free drug concentration in the blood*, and this is measured by the concentration of drug in plasma water. The remaining part is regulated by the *plasma (protein) binding:* a fraction describing the nondialyzable or nonultrafilterable fraction from plasma (or, preferably, whole blood), and the *blood cell uptake*. The bound fraction is presumed inert pharmacologically but may either aid or prevent elimination, and is considered an important characteristic of the drug. For all drug-protein interactions, the *fraction bound* decreases with increasing drug concentrations due to the reversible nature of the interaction. However, over the range of concentrations of interest clinically, the binding may not change appreciably. If this is the case, then blood cell uptake tends to be constant also, so that whole blood, plasma or serum, or plasma water are all equally valid measures of the driving force for pharmacologic response. However, in some cases (e.g., accidental IV bolus injection of local anesthetic), it is likely that plasma and blood cell binding is temporarily overwhelmed so that the "free drug concentration" is disproportionately high and the response therefore is exaggerated.

PHARMACOKINETIC DIFFERENTIATION OF ACUTE, SUBACUTE, AND CHRONIC THERAPY

Relating Numerical Values

It was indicated above that acute care is often characterized by the lack of steady-state conditions so that doses of many drugs are determined according to a redistribution-governed duration of action. When agents are given IV or by inhalation, blood concentrations may be altered rapidly and the duration of therapy has fewer limitations. However, the real differentiation of acute, subacute, and chronic therapy must be made in relation to the sojourn of the drug in the body. Here, drug half-life(s) provide a useful guide.

By definition, the half-life defines the time required for the blood (etc.) concentration to change by a factor of 2 from an original steady-state condition. This may be an increase if the drug is given by infusion, but most commonly it is a decrease after drug administration. Because most body processes concerning drug absorption, distribution, and elimination occur by first-order rate processes (i.e., their rates are proportional to how much drug there is at that time), there are finite limits on the blood

concentrations attained. This means that a drug given at a constant rate (inhaled, infused, etc.) will not accumulate continuously but will approach a steady-state (plateau) concentration equal to the quotient of rate of administration and clearance. Conversely, after administration, concentration will approach zero at the same rate theoretically in proportion to the existing concentration. Therefore, in one half-life concentrations will change by 50% from the original steady state and in two half-lives concentrations will change again by 50% from the newly reached steady state (i.e., to 75% of the original) and so on, according to Table 27–1.

The redistribution phases make for rapid changes according to the same mathematical rules, and their effects are additive to those of the terminal phase. Therefore, the redistribution effect accounts for tissue filling in the early times after change from the original steady state has been initiated. The magnitude of the influence is directly proportional to the capacity of tissues to absorb drug and fill, and this is quantified by the relative areas under the concentration-time curve for the different phases.

Some specific examples can be used to relate time effects via drug half-lives. During inhalation, the arterial concentration of nitrous oxide rises very rapidly at first and then more slowly. The redistribution (fast) phase and terminal half-lifes are, respectively, approximately 3 and 30 minutes.[3] The fast half-life is responsible for the rapid rise and the slow half-life governs the slower and later approach to steady state. A true steady state of arterial concentrations is achieved only after five to six times 30 minutes, but an approximate steady state is achieved a little after 30 minutes due to the enormous contribution of the fast phase in quickly filling the low capacity of the tissues. Steady state, therefore, can be

TABLE 27–1.—CHANGE IN CONCENTRATION AS A FUNCTION OF (TERMINAL) HALF-LIFE

CUMULATIVE HALF-LIFE (Multiples)	APPROACH TO FINAL STEADY STATE* (% Completed)
0	0
1	50
2	75
3	87.7
4	93.8
5†	96.9
6†	98.4

*Accumulation to or removal from and original steady state.

†Considered to be completed steady state for clinical purposes.

achieved in a patient within the normal time frame of exposure during surgery. The same patient may also receive curare, which has fast and slow half-lives of around 10 and 120 minutes, respectively, and this drug also undergoes marked redistribution.[4] However, it is obvious that a true steady state will not be achieved unless surgery is extensively prolonged. Therefore, the degree of relaxation must be regulated by top-up doses under non-steady-state conditions because blood concentrations are continually dominated by the redistribution phase. Under these circumstances, an alternative is to give a loading dose to fill the tissues plus an infusion to maintain concentrations so that a steady state can be achieved within the given time frame. This, in fact, has been done for curare (and other drugs) with considerable success.[4]

However, if the patient were to be anesthetized with diazepam, could a steady state of sleep-producing blood concentrations be maintained? Diazepam has a redistribution half-life of 1 hour and a terminal half-life of 30 hours.[5] If surgery is short, there is a pseudo-steady state because of the relatively slow rate of change of blood concentrations even during the redistribution phase. Although as surgery progresses, it may be necessary to use top-up doses of diazepam (usually given around 30 minutes apart),[6] but it is not useful to infuse this agent. After redistribution, clinical effects decline slowly, in accord with the prolonged terminal half-life and production of active metabolites, so that complete recovery occurs slowly.

These principles apply to treatment with analgesic agents also. Short-term control of acute pain can be obtained with agents of rapid removal from the blood either more by redistribution (e.g., fentanyl) or by clearance (e.g., alfentanil). The difference becomes apparent when more prolonged control of pain is required. Repeated doses of an agent having a redistribution-limited duration of action leads to cumulation after the redistribution phase has dominated. For agents such as fentanyl, prolonged respiratory depression may occur.[7] In contrast, repeated doses of an agent having a predominantly clearance-limited duration of action does not lead to cumulation at anything like the same rate. Alfentanil may be an example but there are insufficient data as yet. It is difficult to find relevant examples of drugs having purely clearance-limited duration of action, however. Certain examples can be found where a high clearance is responsible for brief action over different periods of time (e.g., succinylcholine—muscle relaxation; propanidid—anesthesia; procaine—antidysrhythmic action; penicillin—antimi-crobial action). However, it is uncertain whether the same relationship would pertain over prolonged periods, i.e., whether the rate of biotransformation or excretion would remain constant at the same rate or whether saturation effects would occur. For the majority of analgesic agents, both redistribution and clearance are important determinants of duration of action and therefore of dosing frequency.

For acute pain therapy, say postoperative pain, there are two fundamental choices in the selection of analgesic agents: many repeated doses of an agent with a higher clearance, or few repeated doses of an agent with a lower clearance. In practical terms, there may be vast differences from the patient's viewpoints. The repeated use of a high clearance agent may mean periods of fluctuating analgesia—from possible overdose to periods of pain between doses—and, of course, the possibility of receiving the inevitable needle pricks whenever analgesia is requested. The use of the low clearance (long-acting) agents avoids the fluctuating analgesia and the frequent needle pricks. However, if complications do occur with the low clearance agents, then the complications, too, are long-acting.

Fortunately, many repeated doses with higher clearance agents can be translated into continuous IV infusions which abolish the fluctuating analgesic response. The important point of infusing high clearance agents is that, should adverse effects occur, cessation of infusion means that no more drug will be admitted to the circulation so that blood concentrations will start to decay immediately. This is in contrast to analgesics given by an absorption route, where absorption will continue relentlessly.

For routine chronic therapy, little use can be made of the IV route except as part of a diagnostic workup of the patient. During chronic therapy, absorption routes require knowledge of absorption rates and bioavailability of the drugs used, in addition to the fundmental properties of clearance and volume of distribution. (Drug absorption and bioavailability are discussed in more detail below.) At this point, two new concepts will be introduced: the minimum effective analgesic (blood) concentration (MEAC) and the use of a "pharmacokinetic profile" of the patient based on an IV administered opiate.

The Minimum Effective Analgesic (Blood) Concentration

The MEAC had been defined as the "lowest (blood) concentration of opiate consistent with the patient's report of complete analgesia.''[8] This is a very useful concept because it provides another way of comparing drugs, of recipients of drugs, and the relationship, in time, of responses to drugs for individual patients. This, then is the primary pharmacodynamic characteristic of the drug. The secondary pharmacodynamic characteristics may be side effects—for example, adverse effects on the respiratory system, which should be quantified with respect to concentration also.

How valid is the concept of the MEAC? There is a widespread impression that analgesic response is not related to blood concentrations. This impression is based on two criticisms: (1) the relationship is not founded at all, and (2) a relationship based on whole blood concentrations is inappropriate.

Probably the first report demonstrating a relationship between time, degree of analgesia, and plasma concentration of an opioid analgesic was that of Berkowitz and co-workers.[9] In their study, analgesic effects and pentazocine plasma concentrations were studied after IV and intramuscular (IM) administration of pentazocine in postoperative patients. Mean data only were reported, and these indicated that 45 mg/70 kg administered IM achieved more sustained plasma concentrations and more sustained analgesia than one half of this dose administered as an IV bolus. On the other hand, reports of studies with morphine (e.g., Laitinen et al.[10]) have indicated that there is no correlation between plasma concentrations and analgesia, and these statements have been repeated as generalities in major textbooks (e.g., Clarke[11]).

Why does this discrepancy exist? There are two probable reasons. First, until very recently there have been great difficulties in assaying morphine reliably in biologic samples. Even now, many of the techniques based on radioimmunoassay, at least partially, comeasure morphine metabolites. Newer techniques based on electrochemical detection for high-performance liquid chromatography may yield entirely different results. Second, although the assay may be put right, morphine may be a poor choice to investigate this relationship. Although morphine has the pharmacologic properties of the prototype opiate agonist, its chemistry is that of a highly water-soluble, poorly lipid-soluble agent—unlike pentazocine, meperidine, and the majority of other opiates. Facile equilibration between blood and receptor sites is enhanced by lipid solubility. Methadone is nearly 100 times more lipid soluble than morphine at physiologic pH (partition coefficient, Table 27–2); therefore, a relationship between plasma concentration and effect is more likely to be demonstrated for methadone (or other lipid-soluble substance) than for morphine.[12]

After administration of an appreciably lipid-soluble opiate which will be transported to its specific receptor sites by the blood, it may be presumed that there is, in fact, a relationship between the opiate concentration in the blood and the concentration at the receptors which produces the pharmacologic effects. If this relationship is considered in terms of receptor occupancy, there must be a minimum occupancy at the time the patient first perceives pain after being analgesic or becomes analgesic in the presence of a painful stimulus. This transition point was defined as the MEAC, although it must be apparent that this represents one point on a continuous relationship between blood concentration and opiate effect, much like the relationship with respiratory depression.[12]

Plainly, it can be argued that the concentration of unbound drug in plasma water, not the whole blood concentration, is the correlate of response. This argument is legitimate, and it must be conceded that anything else is second best. However, in practical terms, the total concentration in blood, plasma, or serum will suffice if (1) the relationship between whole blood and plasma concentrations is essen-

TABLE 27–2.—Some Relevant Physicochemical Properties of Selected Opiates*

DRUG	PARTITION COEFFICIENT† (n octanol: pH 7.4)	pK_a	%IONIZED AT pH 7.4†
Morphine sulfate	1.42	7.93	76
Codeine phosphate	2.28	8.10	83
Meperidine hydrochloride	38.8	8.50	94
Pentazocine hydrochloride	111	9.16	98
Methadone hydrochloride	116	9.26	99
Alfentanil hydrochloride	129	6.50	11
Fentanyl citrate	813	8.43	91
Sufentanil citrate	1778	8.01	80

*See references in Kaufman J.F., et al.: *Lancet* March 6:559–560, 1982, and Mather.[12]
†At 37° C.

tially constant in the clinically important range, and (2) the degree of binding to protein and cells also is essentially constant in this range. For the drug most studied, meperidine, this would appear to be the case.[13, 14] Other drugs have yet to be investigated as thoroughly as meperidine, but data are emerging, especially in postoperative patients and at concentrations at which patients request analgesic medication or access patient-controlled analgesic therapy devices have been measured. It should be noted that the values of MEAC will depend on the fluid sampled, and this is a necessary part of the specified value.

Where it has been assessed, MEAC is noted to vary among patients, but remains reasonably consistent for any given patient over the first 1–2 days after surgery. It is probable that some of the intersubject variability arises because of differences in blood cell and protein binding, and that these differences would be minimized by the use of plasma ultrafiltrate as the reference sample. If patients receiving continuous opioid therapy for postoperative pain suddenly appear to have increased opiate requirements, this can indicate the need for urgent intervention. A case of an apparent "resetting" of the MEAC during meperidine infusion was reported by Stapleton et al.;[15] a patient who had previously been pain free and stable with a meperidine blood concentration of 0.65 mg/L suddenly developed pain associated with a wound hematoma. Increasing the blood concentration to 1.1 mg/L suppressed the pain without side effects and allowed palliation while awaiting intervention by the gynecologist. Three important points emerged from this report: (1) the infusion did not mask additional pain from a different source, (2) the additional pain was controlled by increasing the concentration, and (3) no side effects were apparent while the additional pain was controlled. In patients with intractable pain, the MEAC may remain constant over many months, irrespective of changes in pharmacokinetics for any reason. This may mean that patients can require dose revisions in order to "titrate" to analgesic concentrations.[8] It is important, therefore, that pharmacokinetics and pharmacodynamics be considered together. If this is not done, patients can appear "refractory" or "oversensitive" to opiates without the clinician having any insight into the cause. The "pharmacokinetic cause" of a high clearance preventing adequate blood concentrations from being attained is entirely different from the "pharmacodynamic cause" of an abnormally high MEAC preventing adequate blood concentrations from being

attained from the particular dosage regimen, although both can make a patient seem refractory to the effects of the drug.[8] The importance of drug clearance will be developed further when we consider oral medication for patients with chronic pain, and in the subsequent discussion of comparative clinical pharmacokinetic data useful in selecting agents.

FACTORS INFLUENCING PHARMACOKINETIC RESPONSES

Drug therapy for pain management of the subacute or chronic nature allows the achievement of steady-state or pseudo-steady-state concentrations of a drug. The choice of dosing method and interval depends on how wide a variation is allowable for a given drug. This in part is governed by the magnitude of the difference in the MEAC and the toxic threshold. The achievement of steady-state simplifies the pharmacokinetics of the drug, since the rate of appearance in the plasma becomes equivalent to the rate of disappearance from the plasma. Once a steady-state has been achieved, distribution is still occurring but is masked by absorption and elimination. This phenomenon is independent of route of administration (enteral or parenteral). This section describes the factors influencing interindividual variation for a given drug. In pain therapy, these factors are extremely important, since many of the pain medications are converted to active metabolites. The behavior of the active metabolites is also influenced by the same factors.

As stated above, at steady state, the rate of absorption and the rate of elimination are equal. The amount of drug to be administered is related to the steady-state concentration by the following simple equation:

$$D = Cl \times C_{ss} \times \tau$$

where D is the dose of the drug, Cl is clearance of the drug, C_{ss} is the steady-state concentration, and τ is the dosing interval. It should be remembered that Cl is the product of the apparent volume of distribution (in this case, during the elimination phase) and the elimination rate. Changes causing interpatient variation will be discussed in a general way. For information on the effects of specific disease states on pharmacokinetics, the reader is referred to the text by Benet, Massoud, and Gambertoglio.[16]

What physiologic factors affect each of the variables of interest?

Factors Influencing Clearance

The majority of drugs used in pain therapy are eliminated by metabolic degradation. With the exception of the ester-type local anesthetics, which are also hydrolyzed in the plasma by pseudocholinesterase, these drugs are metabolized in the liver. Hepatic clearance thus becomes an important determinant in blood concentrations of these drugs. Hepatic clearance can be divided into two categories: flow-limited and function- or capacity-limited, representing two extremes, based on whether the clearance is principally dependent on the rate of drug delivery (i.e., blood flow) or activity of drug metabolizing enzymes (i.e., extraction ratio). In fact, most drugs fall between these extremes. Table 27–3 provides examples of the application of these classifications to common pain medications.

For drugs belonging to the flow-limited class, the most important physiologic variable is liver blood flow. Co-administration of drugs known to decrease liver blood flow can cause a dramatic decrease in elimination rate and thus in clearance. For example, co-administration of cimetidine[17][18] or propranolol[19] with lidocaine causes a significant decrease in lidocaine clearance. The decrease associated with the co-administration of propranolol is now thought to be due to both a decrease in liver blood flow and an inhibition of liver metabolism.[20] For drugs of the flow-limited class, small changes in the extent of protein binding do not alter the elimination rate, since the hepatic extraction ratio exceeds the fraction free in blood.

Conversely, drugs of the function- or capacity-limited class can be markedly affected by alterations in the extent of protein binding, since the liver is only capable of removing the free drug. This class is unaffected by modest changes in liver blood flow. Changes in enzymatic activity or the quantity of

liver enzyme have profound effects on the rate of elimination for function-limited drugs. The Michaelis-Menten enzyme kinetic terms, k_m and V_{max}, are the most important terms in the hepatic clearance for these drugs: k_m defines the affinity and capacity and is affected by the quality of the enzyme; V_{max} controls the rate of drug metabolism and is affected by changes in the quantity of the enzyme. For example, co-administration of enzyme-inducing drugs, such as phenobarbital, can accelerate the rate of bupivacaine elimination in patients receiving continuous perineural infusions of bupivacaine for pain relief.

Genetic factors can markedly alter the clearance rate for drugs that must undergo biotransformation for termination of activity. For example, genetically abnormal pseudocholinesterase can lead to prolonged action of succinylcholine in ester-type local anesthetics.[21] Abnormal acetylator traits can cause significant decreases in the clearance for such drugs as isoniazid and procainamide.

Drug metabolism is decreased in the aged. This can account for the pronounced decreases in hepatic clearance in elderly patients. This may be due to either decreases in the amount of available enzyme or, more likely, to subcellular hepatic changes occurring as a function of either age or disease.

Factors Influencing Volume of Distribution

As stated earlier, volumes of distribution are apparent volumes describing the dilution of a given drug within the body. It is important to remember that the volume of distribution of a drug relates the drug concentration in the plasma to the *total amount* of drug in the body. Distribution is a physicochemical interaction between a drug and the body. It is governed on one hand by the physicochemical properties of the drug, such as pK_a or degree of ionization, lipid solubility or polarity, and molecular weight, and on the other hand by physiologic properties of the body, such as pH, tissue composition, permeability of membranes, and blood flow. A combination of the drug properties and characteristics of the body determine the binding to plasma and tissue proteins. For most of the pain medications, plasma protein binding occurs to both albumin and α_1-acid glycoprotein. Albumin may be thought of as a high-capacity/low-affinity protein, and α_1-acid glycoprotein may be thought of as a low-capacity/high-affinity protein. For comparison of different patient populations, volumes of distribution may be

TABLE 27–3.—CLASSIFICATION OF SOME COMMON PAIN MEDICATIONS ACCORDING TO HEPATIC CLEARANCE

LOW	INTERMEDIATE	HIGH
Chlordiazepoxide	Acetaminophen	Etidocaine
Ibuprofen	Alfentanil	Imipramine
Indomethacin	Bupivacaine	Lidocaine
Methadone	Codeine	Morphine
Phenobarbital	Meperidine	Pentazocine
Phenylbutazone	Sufentanil (?)	Phenacetin
Phenytoin		Propoxyphene
Salicylic acid		Salicylamide

expressed in liters per kilogram of either body weight or lean body mass to facilitate a comparison, although direct relationships between volumes and masses have rarely been demonstrated. The lean/fat body ratio aids in estimation of volumes of distribution, particularly in the aged population and in obese patients.

Within a given class of drugs, for example the local anesthetics, the steady-state volumes of distribution tend to increase with the increased apparent partition coefficients. That is, the more lipid soluble the agent, the more it tends to distribute in the fatty tissues. The magnitude of the effect of the apparent partition coefficient is governed to some extent by the extent of protein binding and the pK_a of the parent drug. It must be remembered that only the non-ionized portion of the drug can diffuse across membranes. In addition, in the absence of active or facilitated transport, only the unbound fraction of drug can leave the bloodstream and reach different tissues, and therefore the volume of distribution describes the action of only the free portion of the drug. The extent of binding is dependent on the affinity and the capacity of the binding proteins. In blood, most drugs are rather nonspecifically bound to albumin. For the basic drugs, which include the local anesthetics and opiates, α_1-acid glycoprotein is the most important binding protein. Alterations in protein binding can cause marked increases or decreases in apparent volumes of distribution. An example of this may be seen in cancer patients being treated with continuous epidural infusions of bupivacaine for relief of terminal cancer pain. In metastatic disease, marked increases of α_1-acid glycoprotein are common. For a given infusion rate of bupivacaine, these patients have an extremely high total bupivacaine concentration. However, examination of the free fraction of bupivacaine discloses that it is within a normal range. The net result is a decrease in the total plasma clearance.[22]

Once the drug leaves the systemic circulation, the binding to tissues becomes extremely important since this governs not only the rate at which the drug is available for return to the systemic circulation, but also the extent to which it can be absorbed by tissue. Physiologic changes within the tissue, for example in pH, also contribute to the rate and extent of drug transfer. Table 27–4 demonstrates the relationship between protein binding, volume of distribution, and the body distribution of drugs.

Blood flow and cardiac output are major components of the apparent volume of distribution since drugs are distributed via the bloodstream through

TABLE 27–4.—DISTRIBUTION CHARACTERISTICS OF MORPHINE, MEPERIDINE, AND BUPIVACAINE*

SAMPLE	FRACTION OF DRUG IN BODY		
	MORPHINE†	MEPERIDINE‡	BUPIVACAINE§
Unbound	0.122	0.051	0.024
In extracellular fluids	0.055	0.034	0.101
Outside extracellular fluids	0.946	0.967	0.899
Bound to plasma proteins	0.005	0.034	0.039
Bound to extracellular proteins	0.011	0.015	0.092
Bound to tissues	0.867	0.934	0.884

*Calculated according to the method of Tozer. (Tozer T.N.: Concepts basic to pharmacokinetics. *Pharmacol. Ther.* 12:109–131, 1981.
†V = 224; fu = 0.650.
‡V = 294; fu = 0.360.
§V = 72; fu = 0.041.

the body. Thompson et al.[23] studied the pharmacokinetics of intravenously-administered lidocaine in 11 patients with evidence of advanced heart failure. The volume of distribution at steady state exhibited a significant decrease from 1.3 L/kg in normal patients to 0.9 L/kg in patients with heart failure. Hence measured plasma concentrations were significantly higher than in normals. From this finding, it was concluded that lidocaine plasma concentrations in the toxic range are achieved earlier in patients with heart failure, so that plasma concentration monitoring appears to be useful. Similarly, decreased volumes of distribution are well documented with digoxin. In cases of co-administration of a highly protein bound drug, displacement of another drug with a lesser protein affinity may occur. This will result in an elevated free fraction of drug, and an elevated apparent volume of distribution. Situations which cause an increased volume of distribution without counteractive changes in clearance will result in an increased half-life of the drug.

Importance of Changes in Half-Life

It is important to remember that half-life is a derived-parameter that reflects changes in clearance and/or volume of distribution.[24] The simple relationship shown below serves to illustrate this dependence:

$$t\frac{1}{2} = \frac{0.693 \text{ V}}{Cl}$$

Early studies of drug pharmacokinetics in altered physiologic states were compromised by their reliance on half-life as the sole measure of alterations in drug disposition. Diseases can affect either or both of the physiologically related parameters, volume and clearance. Thus changes in half-life will not necessarily reflect changes in drug disposition. Half-life is important in multiple dosing regimens because it is a determinant of the time required to achieve steady state, the time required to remove the drug from the body, and a means to estimate the appropriate dosing interval.

Steady-State Concentration

As previously described, at steady state, the rate of appearance of drug in plasma and the rate of disappearance of drug from plasma are equivalent. Thus, the following simple relationship holds:

$$\frac{D}{Cl} = C_{ss}$$

It can be seen that for a fixed dose, alterations in clearance will result in changes in the steady-state concentration.

While reported effective steady-state concentrations are valuable guidelines, there is considerable interpatient variation in the steady-state concentration necessary to achieve a desired effect. For each patient, there is a range of plasma levels over which the response passes from threshold (MEAC) to a maximum, and a level which is associated with optimum response. Consideration of dosing adjustments should include the subjective nature of the pain and the MEAC. Additionally, one must consider alterations in the number of receptors and receptor sensitivity associated with the nature, magnitude, and duration of the pain to be treated. The therapeutic range must be taken into account, i.e., the difference between the toxic concentration and the MEAC. For the most part, steady-state concentrations are more useful information for drugs having a central effect, such as the opiates (discussed earlier). Deciding on acceptable steady-state concentrations are far more difficult for drugs used for regional nerve block. In this case, there is little relationship between their plasma concentrations and their actual effect of the drug on the nerve. For long-term continuous epidural infusions of bupivacaine, there is a good correlation between the plasma concentration and the type of nerve fibers blocked in normal patients. This re-emphasizes the need for more interactive pharmacokinetic and pharmacodynamic data. In cases of prolonged perineural block, either by multiple injection or by continuous infusion, knowledge of plasma concentrations can serve to prevent untoward effects. In multiple dos-

ing circumstances such as these, an understanding of the principles of absorption and bioavailability is imperative.

DRUG ABSORPTION AND BIOAVAILABILITY

If a drug is given any other way except IV, two additional and independent pharmacokinetic parameters must be considered: *rate* and *extent* of absorption into the general circulation. Both of these regulate the *magnitude* and the *time course* of blood drug concentrations, and are, therefore, important determinants of the pharmacodynamic response.

Drugs for the relief of pain may be administered extravascularly by a variety of routes, e.g., intramuscularly, subcutaneously, internally, intraspinally, or by inhalation. Because of the diverse anatomical sites involved, it is important to find a unified method of understanding and even predicting the outcome, irrespective of the site used. Such unity is to be found by referring to the perfusion (i.e., flow/volume) of the site used and the physicochemical properties of the drugs in question.

It will be plain that the absorption rate is enhanced by a high perfusion at the site of administration and a high lipid solubility of the drug administered. Superimposed on these basic features, a number of physical factors modify the actual rate of absorption from a particular site, over and above their influences on the physicochemical properties of the drug. For example, absorption appears to be faster from smaller volume, more concentrated solutions than from larger volume, more dilute solutions, but these effects may be opposed by the increased tonicity and viscosity of more concentrated solutions. The liberation of histamine by morphine, for example, causes vasodilation and local edema, both of which affect the absorption rate but in opposite directions. The net outcome depends precisely on the relation of the particular drug in the particular patient. Although the factors have been delineated in principle (see article by Schou[25] and the references therein), little information exists on the microenvironment of drugs likely to be injected by the pain therapist.

Information on the macroenvironment as it relates to perfusion and lipid solubilities of drugs is much easier to obtain and predict. For example, because drugs are readily absorbed in the nonionized (lipid-soluble) form, alteration of local pH to increase the fraction of drug in the nonionized form will enhance the rate of absorption, perhaps by dilution of injectate with body fluids or by addition of exogenous chemical substances to the injectate. Alternatively, movement of the drug from areas of unfavorable pH to areas of favorable pH (e.g., from stomach to small intestine) will enhance absorption rate of drugs more ionized in the stomach than in the small intestine (i.e., basic drugs). At the same time, the greater perfusion of the small intestine favors absorption of all drugs (even acids, which may be more nonionized in the stomach).

The other physicochemical property of note is water solubility and thus also may be pH dependent. Drugs in their nonionized (or neutral) forms are, in general, poorly water soluble. Hence, if a drug exceeds its limiting solubility at a particular pH and precipitates, its rate of absorption may be limited by the rate of redissolving in its biologic environment. Of course, drugs administered, for example, by mouth as solid dose forms also must dissolve to be anything more than a little bulk in the diet. Hence, strict criteria for the rate of dissolution are imposed by drug regulatory authorities.

Having the drug in an "absorbable form" at an "absorption site" is the first stage in achieving pharmacologic effects. The second stage is the combined influences of rates of membrane penetration and the subsequent removal by the blood, unless the drug is to exert its primary action locally (e.g., local anesthetic agents, anti-inflammatory steroids, destructive agents). The secondary action of these agents may be promoted via vascular absorption, so that the rate of systemic absorption should be known for such agents also. While the first two stages have to do with the *rate* of absorption, the third stage has to do with the *extent* of absorption, i.e., the systemic bioavailability of the drug.

Whereas drug dosage from disintegration and the drug dissolution rate can be assessed in vitro, bioavailability can be assessed only in vivo. It is common to see references to three kinds of bioavailability in the literature. The first is *absolute bioavailability:* this is the "generic" bioavailability and is defined by the fraction of dose reaching the general circulation, compared with the same dose administered IV. The second is *relative bioavailability,* which denotes a similar comparison of two different dosage forms, e.g., different formulations (tablets vs. solution), different sites (oral vs. IM), etc. Both of these measurements are based on timed samples drawn from the circulation at identical sampling points. The fractions of dose available to the general circulation are quantified by their areas under the blood (plasma, etc.) concentration-time curve (i.e., the time integral), either measured or mathematically extrapolated to infinite time, so as to account for differences in *rate* rather than *extent* of absorption. Methods based on comparison of peak concentrations only may give spurious estimates because of differences in absorption rate.

The third kind of bioavailability is *physiologic availability,* which is an expression of comparisons based on the effects observed. This measure takes into account cases in which absorption, although complete, may be so slow as to produce little or no drug effects. The first two measures also cannot differentiate the various aspects of the sequence of drug dosage, from disintegration and/or dissolution locally, actual drug absorption across local to capillary membranes, and drug destruction by chemical or enzymatic means both locally and en route to the general circulation. Bioavailability is the continued product of the fractions of dose passing successively through each of these phases (i.e., fraction of dose presenting for absorption times fraction of dose passing across the capillary membrane times fraction of dose escaping local or en route destruction). There are few relevant quantitative data as to the magnitude of the first two of these phases, but considerably more evidence for understanding the third.

In broad terms, the only major barrier to admission of drug to the general circulation comes from enteral administration, where absorption locally results in collection by the portal venous system and presentation to the liver en route to the general circulation. For drugs which are removed from the body by enzymatic biotransformation in the liver, this phase can become the great equalizer and may render perfectly useful drugs (by parenteral administration) totally useless if they are given by mouth. However, this effect can be predicted from the knowledge of the drug. Remember that the total body clearance is made of the sums of clearances by individual organs and tissues. Then, knowledge of the magnitude of the hepatic (i.e., total-nonhepatic) clearance can give an excellent index of predictability of the major determinant of oral bioavailability. Remember too that clearance is given by the product of organ flow and extraction ratio. Therefore the transmission fraction (1 − extraction ratio) can be used to quantify the amount of drug escaping extraction. Turning this around, the transmission ratio equals (1 − hepatic (blood) clearance/hepatic blood flow). Notice that the value for clearance has to be based on drug concentrations in whole blood. Plasma or serum concentrations will not do, because of uncertain drug uptake into blood cells, which also are presented for clearance. Although individual values of organ blood flow may show time-related and patient-related variability, the use of an average value of organ flow (e.g., liver blood flow, 1.5 L/minute) gives a reasonable estimate for purposes of estimating probable drug bioavailability after oral administration. It should be noted that this refers to the portion of clearance related to organs interposing absorption and elimination, most notably the liver for drugs administered enterally, but other organs or tissue as well.

Extraction *between* the site of absorption and the general circulation is commonly called *first-pass extraction,* and the clearance is often called the *first-pass effect.* This concept is vital to determining dose equivalents of drugs given orally. Many older textbooks would refer to drugs being "poorly absorbed" if given orally as the reason for poor effects after usual-sized doses, compared with effects after IM administration. In fact, first-pass extraction, not absorption, generally is the limitation, and this could be overcome by appropriate dose scaling except, in some cases, for one additional problem.

Drugs are extracted by tissues such as the liver in a series of events resulting in their biotransformation to metabolites. As a general rule, metabolites are more polar (i.e., less lipophilic) than their parent drugs and, as a consequence, have less propensity for penetrating the CNS and greater propensity for excretion by the kidney. Compared to the parent drug, metabolites may be inactive, somewhat active, or even be *the* active species for which the drug is given and have the same or totally different pharmacokinetic properties. For a drug dosage schedule to be scaled up to account for drug lost in the first-pass effect, the drug must not be biotransformed to metabolites, which, if accumulated in the blood, lead to adverse effects.

USE OF PHARMACOKINETIC DATA FOR DOSAGE RATIONALIZATION

Because the apparent volumes of distribution can relate dose to blood concentration, they can be used in designing dosage regimens. Remember that there are two kinds of distribution volumes: an initial dilution volume, which relates dose to concentration immediately after (IV) injection, and a total volume of distribution, which relates dose (more correctly, amount of drug in the body) to blood concentration after the redistribution processes. The two are linked

by the rate of change of volume of distribution,[26] which is, as the term suggests, an index of *rate* of redistribution. If drug appears in the general circulation at the rate that it *redistributes* out of the general circulation, then the concentrations in the general circulation change only in response to elimination, and this is usually much slower than redistribution. Therefore, a measure of total volume of distribution is useful to relate blood concentration to dose after an absorption route administration where absorption and redistribution occur simultaneously but in opposing directions. For example, if an analgesic blood concentration of meperidine in a particular patient was 0.5 mg/L, how can the pharmacokinetic properties of the drug be used in designing dosage regimens suitable for routine clinical use?

Pharmacokinetic data reported for meperidine may be as follows:

Initial dilution volume (V) = 80 L
Steady-state distribution volume (V_{ss}) = 250 L
Fast half-life ($t\frac{1}{2}_f$) = 15 minutes
Slow half-life ($t\frac{1}{2}_s$) = 4 hours
Total body clearance (Cl) = 0.6 L/minute

Giving an IV bolus of 50 mg would result in initial concentrations of 50 mg/80 L = 0.63 mg/L, and this is in excess of the required value of 0.5 mg/L. At 15 minutes ($t\frac{1}{2}_f$), the concentration would have decreased to 0.31 mg/L, i.e., considerably less than the target concentration. The patient may or may not report pain since blood concentrations which are *changing rapidly* due to redistribution are poor predictors of analgesic response.[8]

However, the important point is that the duration of response will be short and will require additional doses to replace dose lost by redistribution. If an additional 50-mg dose were given at, say, 30 minutes, when the blood concentration would be approximately 0.16 mg/L, the accumulation would increase the concentration to 0.78 mg/L, and so on. Conversely, the slow half-life only describes the rate of concentration change after many such doses. The total body clearance gives a measure of the rate of drug loss from the circulation, also only after redistribution, and is suitable for calculating the maintenance rate over this period, i.e., average steady-state concentrations = infusion rate/Cl. Hence, 0.5 (mg/L) = infusion rate/0.6 (L/min), so that the infusion rate required to maintain the target concentration is 0.5 mg/L × 0.6 L/min = 0.3 mg/min. This rate will *maintain* the target as an average concentration *only if given continuously.* If intermittent bolus doses are given, then concentrations will be initially more and later less than the target.

If the rates of absorption and redistribution are approximately equal, the steady-state distribution volume is useful to relate dose to concentration, also. An IM dose of 100 mg of meperidine will, therefore, equilibrate in about 250 L, giving a peak blood concentration of 0.4 mg/L (and probably fail to be analgesic).[27] Subsequent doses will result in accumulation so that peak concentrations reach the analgesic range. Because of similar rates of absorption and redistribution, an *obvious* redistribution phase is not always seen with IM or other absorption routes. However, the slow half-life dominates and the concentration will decay to about 0.2 mg/L after about 4 hours. Obviously, doses must be given when the blood concentration fails to match the analgesic concentrations, which, after redistribution, are consistent predictors of pain response (for the lipid-soluble agents). Again, clearance will give a value to relate mean steady-state concentration to dose rate, but it will be obvious that this is not a useful value for analgesic therapy. If the dose is subject to first-pass effect, then the dose must be scaled to the *bioavailable dose* rate.

Drugs given by almost any other route except enteral-portal, i.e., including enteral-sublingual, enteral-buccal, intraspinal, intramuscular, and subcutaneous, are appreciably free from first-pass effects. Although at least some part of the dose may be subjected to a slow absorption process, due, say, to repartitioning out of fat pools, this is not a first-pass effect. The outcome may result in such small blood concentrations from this portion of the dose that no pharmacologic effect can be detected. There is some controversy over the degree of avoidance of first-pass effect from drugs given rectally.[28] This route is especially sensitive to formulation of the drug where hydro/alcoholic formulations result in rapid absorption but suppositories result in slow absorption. Mather and Glynn[8] made use of slow absorption of meperidine from suppositories to provide sustained nighttime analgesia in patients with chronic pain. A bioavailability of meperidine in excess of 80% was estimated, and this compares favorably with 50% from administration by mouth. Detailed information on the design of dosage by infusion using the various recipes for attaining and maintaining target concentrations has been set out elsewhere.[12]

The sections that follow describe the pharmacokinetic properties of drugs. In some cases, however, no data for MEAC are available, or pharmacokinetic data obtained in otherwise healthy volunteers may be the only reliable source available and differ from MEAC data in certain ways. From the data provided, it is possible to rationalize dosage schemes in a similar manner to that presented above. In particular, the reader should note bioavailability factors for oral dosage.

THERAPEUTIC MONITORING

The success of the dosing regimen described in the previous section is limited by the potentially large interpatient variability in terms of volume of distribution, clearance, and therefore elimination half-life, and by variability in absorption and bioavailability. Therapeutic monitoring seems an ideal solution to these problems. However, knowing when and what drug levels to monitor is of utmost importance. Blood concentration determinations cannot substitute for clinical judgment and must always be interpreted in the context of available clinical data. However, by reducing the number of unknown variables, the clinician may apply his or her skills to the maximum by focusing more directly on the disease process and on the physiologic status of the patient. Measurements of plasma drug concentrations may clarify a situation in which usual doses of drug fail to produce a therapeutic benefit or result in unanticipated toxicity. They are particularly useful in patients with renal, hepatic, cardiovascular, or gastrointestinal disease, in whom the relation between dose and plasma concentration may be unpredictable. They may also be of benefit in patients receiving several drugs simultaneously. Richens and Warrington[29] suggested seven major reasons for monitoring plasma drug concentrations: (1) when there is a wide interindividual variation in the metabolism, (2) when saturation kinetics occur, (3) when the therapeutic ratio of a drug is low, (4) when signs of toxicity are difficult to recognize clinically, (5) when gastrointestinal, hepatic, or renal disease is present, (6) when drug interactions are suspected, and (7) when patient noncompliance is suspected.

Before routine monitoring of plasma concentration can be useful, the optimum therapeutic range of levels must be defined. For this purpose, prospective studies in which the dosage increments are made during careful monitoring, both of plasma concentrations and of clinical response, are necessary. However, such studies often are conducted using ''normal patients,'' and the results may not be applicable to all patients for whom the drug is prescribed. In addition, one must be able to adequately interpret the results of therapeutic monitoring, that is, either total drug concentration or free drug concentration.

Consider the pain patient treated with a continuous IV infusion of meperidine. For severe pain, a steady-state concentration of 0.6 mg/L may be required.[13, 14, 30] This concentration of meperidine may be accompanied by evidence of respiratory depression. If this patient were being treated with a continuous epidural infusion of meperidine, adequate analgesia might well be obtained at a plasma steady-state concentration of 0.1–0.2 mg/L, far below the concentration associated with respiratory depression. This example clearly demonstrates the importance of using clinical judgment in association with blood concentration data to determine treatment efficacy. This can be further illustrated by examination of a patient being treated for terminal cancer pain. Clinical experience dictates that a rate of 25 mg/hour of bupivacaine would be required to provide adequate analgesia.[31] Blood concentrations monitored daily revealed that the bupivacaine concentration continued to accumulate reaching 6.5 mg/L at steady state in this patient. However, this patient had an α_1-acid glycoprotein level of 260 mg/dl and a free fraction concentration of bupivacaine of 0.12 mg/L. The increase in α_1-acid glycoprotein resulted in an increase in the binding, which resulted in a decrease in bupivacaine clearance. The free fraction concentration of 0.12 mg/L is well below that required to cause CNS toxicity. The practitioner who obtains bupivacaine blood concentrations of greater than 2–2.5 mg/L of bupivacaine might greatly reduce the infusion rate if not all aspects of the blood concentration data were understood. However, the result of such a reduction in infusion rate would be unsatisfactory analgesia.

The importance of individual monitoring to determine the efficacy of a multiple-dose regimen is illustrated by a recently reported study, in which 23% of the patients were found to be receiving doses below or above the therapeutic range.[32] Accurate and prudent monitoring of selected patients will also allow the practitioner to separate the psychological contributions to pain from the nonefficacy of the selected dosing regimen.

REFERENCES

1. Gilman A.G., Goodman L.S., Gilman A.: *The Pharmacological Basis of Therapeutics*. New York, Macmillan Publishing Co., Inc., 1980.
2. Avery G.S.: *Drug Treatment: Principles and Practice of Clinical Pharmacology and Therapeutics*. Sydney, Australia, Adis Press, 1980.
3. Epstein R.M.: Nitrous oxide, in Papper E.M., Kitz R.J.: *Uptake and Distribution of Anesthetic Agents*. New York, McGraw-Hill Book Co., 1963, pp. 231–250.
4. Ramzan M.I., Somogyi A.A., Walker J.S., et al.: Clinical pharmacokinetics of the non-depolarizing muscle relaxants. *Clin. Pharmacokinet.* 6:25–60, 1981.
5. Klotz U., Avant G.R., Hoyumpa A., et al.: The effects of age and liver disease on the disposition of diazepam in adult man. *J. Clin. Invest.* 55:347–359, 1975.
6. Seow L.T., Mather L.E., Cousins M.J.: A comparison of intravenous diazepam and chlormethaziole as supplementation for regional anaesthesia. *Br. J. Anaesth.* 57:747–752, 1985.
7. Hug C.C. Jr., Murphy M.R.: Fentanyl disposition in cerebrospinal fluid and plasma and its relationship to ventilatory depression in the dog. *Anesthesiology* 50:342–349, 1979.
8. Mather L.E., Glynn C.J.: The minimum effective analgetic blood concentration of pethidine in patients with intractable pain. *Br. J. Clin. Pharmacol.* 14:385–390, 1982.
9. Berkowitz B.A., Asling J.H., Shnider S.M., et al.: Relationship of pentazocine plasma levels to pharmacological activity in man. *Clin. Pharmacol. Ther.* 10:32–38, 1969.
10. Laitinen L., Kanto J.L., Vapaavuoir M., et al.: Morphine concentrations in plasma after intramuscular administration. *Br. J. Anaesth.* 47:1265–1268, 1975.
11. Clarke R.S.J.: Opiate analgesics, in Gray T.C., Nunn J.F., Utting J.E. (eds.): *General Anaesthesia*, ed. 4. London, Butterworths, 1980, pp. 257–271.
12. Mather L.E.: Pharmacokinetic and pharmacodynamic factors influencing the choice, dose and route of administration of opiates for acute pain, in Bullingham R. (ed.): *Clinics in Anaesthesiology: 1. Opiate Analgesia*. London, W.B. Saunders Co., 1983, pp. 17–40.
13. Mather L.E., Meffin P.J.: Clinical pharmacokinetics of pethidine. *Clin. Pharmacokinet.* 3:252–268, 1978.
14. Edwards D.J., Svensson C.K., Visco J.P., et al.: Clinical pharmacokinetics of pethidine: 1982. *Clin. Pharmacokinet.* 7:421–433, 1982.
15. Stapleton J.V., Austin K.L., Mather L.E.: Pharmacokinetic approach to postoperative pain: Continuous infusion of pethidine. *Anaesth. Intensive Care* 7:25–32, 1979.
16. Benet L.Z., Massoud N., Gambertoglio, (eds.): *Pharmacokinetic Basis for Drug Treatment*. New York, Raven Press, 1984.
17. Feely J., Wilkinson G.R., McAllister C.B., et al.: Increased toxicity and reduced clearance of lidocaine by cimetidine. *Ann. Intern. Med.* 96:592–594, 1982.
18. DiFazio C.A., Moscicki J.C., DiFazio C.J.: Cimetidine inhibits lidocaine plasma clearance. *Anesthesiology* 57:A188, 1982.
19. Feely J., Wilkinson G.R., Wodd A.J.J.: Reduction of

liver blood flow and propranolol metabolism by cimetidine. *N. Engl. J. Med.* 304:692–695, 1981.

20. Vu V.T., Chen C.: Effects of dl-propranolol on lidocaine disposition in the perfused rat liver. *Drug Metab. Dispos.* 10:350–355, 1982.

21. Raj P.P., Ohlweiler D., Hitt B.A., et al.: Kinetics of local anesthetic esters and the effects of adjuvant drugs on 2-chloroprocaine hydrolysis. *Anesthesiology* 53:307–314, 1980.

22. Denson D.D., Raj P.P., Finnsson R.: Continuous epidural infusions of bupivacaine for management of terminal cancer pain: Pharmacokinetic considerations. *Anesthesiology* 57:A215, 1982.

23. Thompson P.D., Melmon K.L., Richardson J.A., et al.: Lidocaine pharmacokinetics in advanced heart failure, liver disease and renal failure in humans. *Ann. Intern. Med.* 78:499–508, 1973.

24. Gibaldi M., Koup J.R.: Pharmacokinetic concepts: Drug binding apparent volume of distribution and clearance. *Eur. J. Pharmacol.* 20:299–304, 1981.

25. Schou J.: Subcutaneous and intramuscular of drugs, in Brodie B.B., Gillette J.R. (eds.): *Handbook of Experimental Pharmacology.* Berlin, Springer-Verlag, 1971, pp. 47–66.

26. Niazi S.: Volume of distribution and tissue level errors in instantaneous intravenous input assumptions. *J. Pharm. Sci.* 65:750–752, 1976.

27. Austin K.L., Stapleton J.V., Mather L.E.: Multiple intramuscular injections: A major source of variability in analgesic response to meperidine. *Pain* 847:62, 1980.

28. DeBoer A.G., Moolenaar F., DeLeede L.G.H., et al.: Enteral drug administration: Clinical pharmacokinetic considerations. *Clin. Pharmacokinet.* 7:285–311, 1982.

29. Richens A., Warrington S.: When should plasma drug levels be monitored? *Drugs* 17:488–500, 1979.

30. Austin K.L., Stapleton J.V., Mather L.E.: Relationship between blood meperidine concentrations and analgesic response. *Anesthesiology* 53:460–466, 1980.

31. Raj P.P., Denson D., Finnsson R.: Prolonged epidural analgesia: Intermittent or continuous, in Meyer J., Nolte H. (eds.): *Die Kontinuierliche Periduralanasthesie.* Volume 7 in *Internationales Symposion Über Die Regionalanasthesie.* Stuttgart, George Thieme Verlag, 1983, pp. 26–38.

32. Frewin D.B.: Therapeutic drug monitoring: A survey of sub- and supratherapeutic serum drug levels in a large teaching hospital. *NZ Med. J.* 95:774–776, 1982.

28 / Clinical Pharmacokinetics of Analgesic Drugs

LAURENCE E. MATHER, Ph.D.
DONALD D. DENSON, Ph.D.

FROM THE OUTSET, it should be recognized that while opiate analgesic drugs are first-line medications for the relief of acute pain,[1] they are not recommended for the relief of chronic pain of a nonmalignant origin.[2] However, if other treatment avenues have been excluded or exhausted, it seems unethical to withhold from these patients the pain relief provided by opiates. The main reason for withholding these drugs is the doctor's fear that the patient will become dependent on the drug. However, the important question is to decide, in consultation with the patient, whether the possibility of drug dependence is more of a problem than the pain. Then the patient should decide whether to embark on long-term opiate analgesia for the pain.[3] Therefore, even more than for patients with acute pain, the prescriber of these drugs should be aware of their pharmacokinetic properties and what factors might come into play, mandating dosage revision or other than textbook doses.

MORPHINE

After intravenous (IV) administration of typical premedicant and postoperative doses of morphine sulfate (bolus of 10 mg/70 kg for an adult), venous plasma concentrations between 200 and 700 ng/ml occur initially but decline rapidly according to the redistribution half-lives (Fig 28–1). Within 20–40 minutes, the slower (elimination) phase is apparent, and concentrations now decrease with typical half-lives of 2–4 hours. After a single dose of this size, concentrations remain in the analgesic range for 1–3 hours. There is considerable interpatient variability both in the minimum effective analgesic (blood) concentration (MEAC) and in the plasma concentrations.

From Table 28–1 it will be seen that initial dilution volumes are generally small but that the total distribution is extensive (note the wide range). The size of the ratio between the two relates to the (extensive and rapid) redistribution (see Table 27–1). Since morphine is poorly lipid soluble, it is likely that body distribution is primarily to muscle rather than fat,[4] as is true for the majority of opiates, but redistribution of the more lipid-soluble ones continues into fat.[5] It would be predicted, therefore, that patients having diminished blood flow to muscle might show exaggerated responses to morphine given IV. Conversely, these patients would show delayed or inefficient absorption of morphine given intramuscularly (IM). The data in Table 28–1 also show that pharmacokinetic characteristics do not differ appreciably between various patient groups, with the exception of cancer patients. In this group, it is possible that drug-eliminating mechanisms may be impaired by cytotoxic agents, and this, combined with the large variability in dose requirements, is another reason for careful monitoring.

Otherwise, morphine is absorbed rapidly after IM and oral administration and maximum plasma concentrations occur within 15–60 minutes.[6, 7] After IM injection, 100% bioavailability generally results,[6] but less than 40% (range, 18%–64%) bioavailability after oral administration has been observed in a group of cancer patients.[7] In otherwise healthy patients, oral bioavailability probably is even lower than 30% since the total systemic clearance is close to 1.2 L/minute.

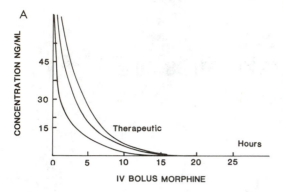

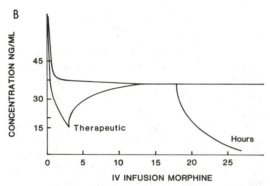

Fig 28–1.—Simulated blood concentration–dose relationships for morphine sulfate given IV: **A,** bolus doses of 10, 15, and 20 mg; **B,** bolus dose of 10 mg followed by infusion of 2.5 mg/hour commencing immediately *(upper trace)* or after 2 hours *(lower trace)*. Simulations show continuation of infusion or cessation at 18 hours. Typical postoperative MEAC values for morphine range from 6 to 33 (average, 16) ng/ml in patients that have undergone major abdominal surgery. (Data from Dahlstrom et al.[8])

Although bioavailability is high and absorption is rapid when morphine is given by IM injection, elimination and redistribution occur while the drug is being absorbed. As a consequence, single IM doses of 10 mg of morphine sulfate produce *maximum* plasma concentrations of 30–60 ng/ml, but the same dose given orally results in only approximately one-half that level. If these values are related to the MEAC, which was shown to vary from 6 to 33 ng/ml, it is easy to see why some patients fail to become analgesic for some or all of the time after normal doses, especially patients with postoperative pain.[8]

For patients with chronic pain, oral morphine has

been advocated.[9] In an attempt to increase the interval between doses of oral morphine, a sustained-release tablet preparation was developed (MST-1). Studies in healthy volunteers have shown that variable and unpredictable plasma concentrations are obtained[10] but that 20-mg tablets may produce concentrations in the effective range at least for several hours. Other studies in postoperative patients indicate that the analgesic response to this preparation was not better than that achieved with morphine sulfate in solution, and that both produced poor results.[11] Plasma concentrations were measured with a method that also partially measured metabolite, and the results indicated wide variability in morphine plasma concentrations but were otherwise unhelpful to the study. Other workers have investigated rectal suppository dose forms of morphine, but these do not show much increase in bioavailability over oral preparations. This finding appears to confirm the information from animal studies that morphine is biotransformed in gastrointestinal mucosa as well as liver.[12] It is notable that cirrhotic patients, who generally have impaired clearance of opiates, do not have impaired clearance of morphine.[13]

Morphine is less bound to plasma protein than are most other opiates. The average bound fraction in normal subjects is 35%, but this figure decreases to 20%–30% in patients with severe renal and hepatic dysfunction.[14, 15] It is theoretically possible that the lower bound fraction contributes to the increased central depression seen in patients with these conditions after administration of the usual clinical single doses of the drug. With chronic dosing, the large distribution volume would probably minimize this influence, since the majority of drug in the body is not present in the plasma. The other difference in plasma binding is that morphine is predominantly bound to albumin. Hence, pathology influencing albumin kinetics may predispose patients to exaggerated effects from morphine.

Renal excretion of unmetabolized morphine accounts for only 10% of the drug. The remainder of the products excreted in urine are morphine conjugates (70%–80%), mostly morphine-3-glucuronide, normorphine, and its conjugates (5%–10%).[16, 17]

MEPERIDINE

Injected IV in adult patients with postoperative pain, a single 50-mg dose of meperidine achieves effective analgesic concentrations for 1–2 hours in most patients, but as short as 30 minutes in some.

TABLE 28–1.—Pharmacokinetic Properties of Morphine in Healthy Volunteers and Clinical Patients*

PARAMETER	HEALTHY VOLUNTEERS‡	INTRAOPERATIVE		POSTOPERATIVE LOW DOSE§	CANCER PAIN‖	CIRRHOTICS (VOLUNTEERS)¶	HEALTHY (CONTROLS)¶
		Lose Dose§	High Dose‡				
$T\frac{1}{2}_{fast}$ (min)	2 (1–4)	1 (1–2)	1 (1–2)	1 (1–2)	NR	5 [3]	10 [8]
$T\frac{1}{2}_{inter}$ (min)	NM	16 (10–30)	20 (10–30)	13 (10–30)	NM	NM	NM
$T\frac{1}{2}_{slow}$ (hr)	3 (2–5)	4 (1.5–9)	2.5 (4–5.5)	2 (1.5–45)	3 (1–8)	2.2 [1.3]	2.5 [1.5]
V (L)	26 (5–50)	16 (5–25)	7 (5–10)†	15 (5–40)	23 (3–30)	44 [35]	72 [65]
V_{ss} (L)	NR	NR	NR	NR	100 (40–270)	180 [100]	220 [100]
V_{area} (L)	230 (190–290)	380 (190–750)	320 (300–400)	220 (140–350)	130 (60–310)	210 [110]	280 [180]
Cl (L/min)	1.1 (0.8–1.3)	1.3 (0.8–1.9)	0.9 (0.7–1.2)	1.2 (0.6–1.8)	0.4 (0.3–0.8)	1.2 [0.4]	1.2 [0.3]

IM DOSE
F	100+
$T\frac{1}{2}_{abs}$ (min)	(5–15)
T_{max} (min)	(10–20)

ORAL DOSE
F	38 (15–64)
T_{max} (min)	(30–90)

*Data are in means (range) [SD] and are derived from venous plasma or serum. NR, not recorded; NM, not relevant to model analyzed.
†Arterial samples.
‡Data from Stanski et al. (1978).[6]
§Data from Dahlstrom et al. (1982).[8]
‖Data from Sawe et al. (1982).[7]
¶Data from Patwardhan et al. (1981).[13]

As with morphine, the duration of analgesia from a single IV dose is short because of extensive redistribution within the body to muscle mass and well-perfused tissues. As is not true of morphine, continued redistribution results in appreciable uptake by fat. This wider uptake evidently is reflected in meperidine having a larger initial dilution volume (rapidly equilibrating tissues) than morphine, and as a consequence of a higher lipid solubility than morphine.

Single IM 100-mg doses of meperidine frequently fail to produce effective analgesia in postoperative patients. Peak concentrations achieved typically are in the range of 0.3–0.4 mg/L after gluteal injection, but may be as much as 50% more or less than this average. Similarly, there is no consistency in the time at which the peak concentration occurs—it may be as short as 10 minutes or as long as 90 minutes after injection. Pharmacokinetic studies performed in healthy volunteers do not show the same degree of variability as in surgical patients, perhaps because of hemodynamic stability (Table 28–2). The duration of effective analgesia from single IM doses, if achieved at all, may be quite short—often only 1 hour or less. The duration of analgesia will, of course, depend on the opiate concentration in relation to the individual patient's MEAC, and this too may vary severalfold among patients. The duration of other central effects such as euphoria and drowsiness will outlast the analgesic effects but also may be short—often only 2 hours. Systemic accumulation from strategically timed subsequent doses may be necessary to achieve effective analgesia of adequate duration.[18–20]

An important point made by Austin et al.[21] is that meperidine plasma concentration response curves are steep. Therefore, fluctuating plasma concentrations will mean fluctuating analgesia. It is logical to devise ways of flattening out the plasma concentration-time curves inherent in intermittent doses (Fig 28–2) as a means of providing prolonged analgesia. Figure 28–2,A simulates an idealized case in which doses are given regularly and are always absorbed at the same rate. Orders written for 4-hourly dosing are more likely to generate irregularity in timing of doses so that the time in excess of effective analgesic concentrations is irregular and incomplete.

Even at steady state IM dosing there are peak-to-trough concentration differences as large as the value of MEAC. For drugs administered intermittently, flattening of the blood concentration time curve can be provided either by prolonging the absorption phase (i.e., "sustained release") so that this is slower than elimination, or by using an agent

TABLE 28–2.—Pharmacokinetic Properties of Meperidine in Healthy Volunteers and Clinical Patients*

PARAMETER	HEALTHY VOLUNTEERS[†]	INTRAOPERATIVE[‡]	POSTOPERATIVE BOLUS[§]	POSTOPERATIVE 32-HR INFUSION[‖]	CHRONIC PAIN[¶]	CIRRHOSIS (VOLUNTEERS)[**]	HEALTHY (CONTROLS)[**]
IV DOSE	(Blood)	(Plasma)	(Plasma)	(Blood)	(Blood)	(Blood)	(Plasma)
$t\tfrac{1}{2}_{fast}$ (min)	NR	3 (3)	8 (7)	30 (28)	4 (5)	16 (7)	
$t\tfrac{1}{2}_{slow}$ (hr)	7 (1)	3 (1)	3 (1)	6 (3)	3 (1)	7 (1)	3 (1)
V_1 (L)	62 (14)	40 (26)	82 (19)	138 (63)	84 (60)	174 (61)	121 (44)
V_{ss} (L)	270 (20)	185 (87)	NR	238 (104)	181 (87)	406 (177)	330 (100)
V_{area} (L)	NR	203 (99)	187 (41)	NR	NR	NR	NR
Cl (L/min)	0.57 (0.09)	0.83 (0.41)	0.73 (0.20)	0.60 (0.14)	0.74 (0.32)	0.66 (0.30)	1.32 (0.38)
IM DOSE							
F		99 (7)					
$T\tfrac{1}{2}_{abs}$ (min)		(7–13)					
T_{max} (min)		(10–20)					
ORAL DOSE							
F		59 (60)					
$T\tfrac{1}{2}_{abs}$ (min)		(11–22)					
T_{max} (min)		(45–90)					

*Data are in mean (SD) and are derived from either venous plasma or venous whole blood samples. Values derived from plasma are up to 30% greater than for whole blood because of drug partitioning into blood cells. NR, not recorded.
†Data from Verbeeck et al. (1981).[20]
‡Data from Mather et al. (1975).[18]
§Data from Tamsen et al. (1982).[95]
‖Data from Austin et al. (1981).[19, 21]
¶Data from Mather and Glynn (1982).[1]
**Data from Klotz et al. (1975).[96]

with slower elimination than meperidine, such as methadone. However, the most logical approach is to give the drug continuously, i.e., by IV infusion. Repeated IV injections (see Fig 28–2,C) produce even greater fluctuations than IM injections.

IV infusion schedules may be constructed empirically or designed from knowledge of pharmacokinetic characteristics. Either way, therapeutically attractive infusion regimens have two components—loading and maintenance—to achieve and then maintain effective steady-state analgesic blood concentrations. Of course, this presupposes knowledge of efficacious blood concentrations. These have been determined for meperidine. An example of a convenient empirical scheme is shown in Figure 28–2,D. A loading infusion dose of 100 mg of meperidine is given over 30 minutes, followed by a maintenance infusion dosage of 25 mg/hour. This regimen is well accepted by clinical staff, because it is simple to remember, and by patients. Although there is a period when the analgesia tends to fade a little, if the schedule is begun when the patient first requests postoperative analgesia, this period does not cause distress. The loading infusion is gentle to the patient and does not cause disorientation and nausea, as bolus doses tend to do. Clinical reports uniformly indicate high efficacy from infusions.[22, 23]

A number of methods for designing infusion regimens have been proposed, and these have been reviewed recently by Rigg and Wong[24] and by Tsuei et al.[25] The majority of regimens use a loading infusion to produce excess plasma concentrations, usually by a factor of 2 or 3, before allowing drug redistribution to reduce the concentrations to those desired at steady state. Steady state, of course, occurs when the drug input rate is exactly balanced by clearance rate. For the opiates, for which there may be only a small separation between minimum analgesic concentration and respiratory depression, the methods based on significantly overloading probably are best avoided.[26] Instead, the method of "separate exponentials" is preferred because it does not produce overloading.[27] Simulated meperidine infusions based on this method are also shown in Fig 28–2,D in comparison to the empirical method. By using a bolus and a loading infusion, the method of separate exponentials allows one to devise a regimen that completely fills the gaps so that the patient should experience effective analgesia continuously.

Orally administered doses of 100 mg of meperi-

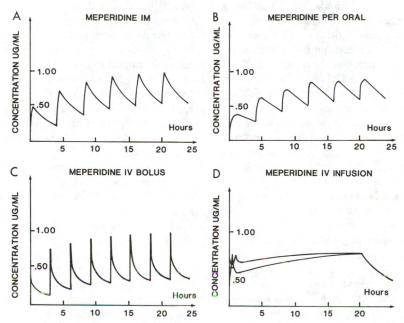

Fig 28–2.—Simulated blood concentration–dose relationships for meperidine hydrochloride given by different regimens: **A,** intramuscular (gluteal) injections, 100 mg every 4 hours; **B,** oral doses, 200 mg every 4 hours; **C,** IV bolus doses, 50 mg every 3 hours; **D,** IV infusions: 100 mg over 30 minutes followed by 25 mg/hour *(lower trace)*, 50 mg bolus plus 100 mg over 30 minutes followed by 25 mg/hour *(upper trace)*. Typical MEAC values in patients that have undergone major abdominal surgery range from 0.25 to 0.75 (average, 0.5) μg/ml. (Data from Mather et al.,[18, 28] Tamsen et al.,[95] and Austin et al.[97])

dine will not achieve effective analgesic concentrations (only 0.1–0.2 mg/L) because of extensive first-pass hepatic extraction and slower absorption than when the drug is given IM. A bioavailability of 40%–60% will occur in most patients with normal liver function.[20, 28–30] Therefore, doses must be scaled to account for the lower bioavailability and slower absorption occurring after oral administration of meperidine. Patients with intractable pain can be treated successfully with oral meperidine under these circumstances,[3] but there are logistical complications. First, most commercially manufactured tablets are only of 50-mg strength. Therefore, a loading dose of 6 tablets and maintenance doses of 4 tablets may be required. Second, doses must be repeated approximately every 4 hours, and a patient may wake at night requiring further doses. Patient acceptance of the dosing schedules is not good. A sustained-release capsule containing a larger dose would be welcome. Investigations have indicated that the nighttime analgesia problem can be circumvented by rectal suppositories containing 300 mg of meperidine. This form of administration gives better

bioavailability than oral administration and it gives slow release which can extend through the night.[3]

The elderly and the young are known to be more sensitive to the narcotic effects of meperidine, just as they seem to be more sensitive to other opiates. With respect to meperidine, the increased sensitivity was thought to be related to diminished plasma protein levels and diminished red cell binding but recent studies have failed to confirm this view. Recent studies with improved methodology suggest that binding is around 30%–50%.[31–33] As is true of many other basic drugs, meperidine binding is strongly directed by the concentration of α_1-acid glycoprotein in the plasma so that physiologic and pathophysiologic modifiers of the concentration of this protein will influence meperidine binding. Likewise, increased production of this protein after trauma or surgery may underlie equal or even increased meperidine requirements at times when postoperative pain would be expected to be diminishing.

Meperidine is primarily metabolized in the liver; hence it would be expected that hepatic dysfunction would cause a lower clearance, longer half-life, and greater oral bioavailability. Indeed, in patients with biopsy-proved alcoholic cirrhosis, clearance is one-half normal, the slow half-life is doubled, and oral bioavailability is increased to around 85%,[29, 30] but distribution volumes and plasma binding are unaltered. In such patients, therefore, initial doses should not be altered but subsequent doses should be spaced farther apart. Oral doses should be reduced as well. Conversely, in patients concurrently receiving enzyme-inducing drugs such as phenytoin, a small (average, 30%) reduction in clearance and half-life occurs that could necessitate slightly shorter dosage intervals. Distribution volumes or oral bioavailability, however, are unaltered, so the dose amount need not be altered.

Renal elimination of meperidine is minor under normal conditions—less than 10% of the dose is excreted in urine. With forced acidification of urine by oral ammonium chloride, this value may be increased to about 20%–25%.[20] However, adjunct treatment of meperidine overdose by this method is not useful clinically, since neither the half-life nor the clearance is affected significantly. By the same token, one would not expect patients with renal disease to require dosage revisions of meperidine. The evidence on this point is conflicting because of the biotransformation of meperidine to normeperidine. The renal clearance of normeperidine exceeds the glomerular filtration rate and this metabolite has a long half-life, causing it to accumulate in patients with renal disease. The propensity for normeperidine to produce a CNS irritability syndrome has been debated,[34] but the potential for this adverse effect from meperidine should be recognized.

FENTANYL

Most doses of fentanyl are given IV, most often intraoperatively. Because of a short duration of action of single doses, fentanyl was thought to have a short half-life in the body. This notion persisted for many years, but recent detailed pharmacokinetic studies have provided data to the contrary. Fentanyl does, however, have an extremely high clearance, but clearance does not regulate the duration of effects after single or infrequent doses. Fentanyl is now recognized as a drug having "redistribution-limited" duration of action, much like thiopental, and for the same reasons. The lipid solubility of fentanyl is extremely high (see Table 27–1). Hence, fentanyl has a rapid onset due to facile CNS pene-

tration, but a short duration, as the drug continues to move down the concentration gradient to muscle and then to fat, where it has high solubility. Drug is readily removed from blood (i.e., high clearance), but slow removal from the fat pools cause the half-life to be longer than the half-life of morphine, despite similar (or even higher) clearances (Table 28–3). Determination of the true value of the half life of fentanyl is difficult because of lack of sensitivity of the assays to the low blood concentrations occurring after normal doses.[9]

There are some discrepancies in the actual values of pharmacokinetic properties of fentanyl,[5] so the data in Table 28–3 are not representative of the range reported.

Because the (slow) half-life is long, accumulation occurs with repeated doses, i.e., the fentanyl blood concentrations fall below the pharmacologically active range during the redistribution phase(s). Subsequent doses are added to a slowly declining background until even the background concentrations remain in the range associated with pharmacologic effects— not just analgesia, but also respiratory depression.[35, 36]

The combination of a high clearance and the capacity for extensive fat uptake makes fentanyl a suitable drug to give by IV infusion.[37] However, it is likely that a fentanyl congener, alfentanil, may become the drug of choice for IV infusions. Alfentanil is not as lipid soluble as fentanyl but is considerably more lipid soluble than meperidine. It has the dual characteristics of rapid onset and short duration

TABLE 28–3.—PHARMACOKINETIC PROPERTIES OF FENTANYL AND TWO OF ITS NEW DERIVATIVES, ALFENTANIL AND SUFENTANIL, IN HEALTHY VOLUNTEERS AND SURGICAL PATIENTS*

PARAMETER	HEALTHY VOLUNTEERS		SURGICAL PATIENTS	
	Fentanyl†	Alfentanil‡	Alfentanil†	Sufentanil†
$t\frac{1}{2}_{fast}$(min)	NR	NR	1.4 (1.3)	1.2 (0.6)
$t\frac{1}{2}_{inter}$ (min)	NM	NM	10 (6)	17 (10)
$t\frac{1}{2}_{slow}$ (hr)	3 (1)	1.5 (0.5)	1.5 (0.3)	2.6 (1.3)
V_1 (L)§	60 (18)	11 (2)	9 (7)	8 (4)
V_{ss} (L)§	335 (143)	27 (7)	57 (53)	98 (34)
V_{area} (L)§	359 (87)	32 (9)	74 (59)	158 (78)
Cl (L/min)§	1.53 (0.25)	0.24 (0.09)	0.56 (0.43)	0.73 (0.20)

*Data are in means (SD), and are derived from venous plasma after an IV dose.
†Data from Bower S., Hull C.J.: *Br. J. Anaesth.* 54:871–877, 1982. Drugs were mixed and injected simultaneously. Hence, data are strictly comparable.
‡Data from Bovill J.G., et al.: *Janssen Report* No. N-23814, 1981. Studies were covered in different patients but under identical protocols.
§Because of different degrees of uptake into blood cells, values for these parameters based on plasma measurements do not give a complete comparative picture. Reported mean values of whole blood:plasma concentration ratios are: fentanyl, 0.97; alfentanil, 0.63; sufentanil, 0.74 (Meuldermans et al.: *Arch. Int. Pharmacodyn. Ther.* 257:4–19, 1982). Therefore, comparable "physiologic" equivalent values can be obtained by dividing these parameters by the whole blood:plasma concentration ratio.

of action. Although its clearance is not as high as that of fentanyl, its distribution volumes are much smaller and its half-life is very short. The latter property allows the clinician excellent control of concentrations during and after infusions.

Sufentanil, an even more lipid-soluble congener than fentanyl, paradoxically has pharmacokinetic properties intermediate between fentanyl and alfentanil. Its claim to clinical significance is related to an apparently higher specificity for control by opiate receptors and fewer peripheral effects than any of the other opioid agents. Its most important use appears to be in opiate/O_2 anesthesia for patients with limited compensatory reserve, such as those undergoing cardiac surgery.

METHADONE

Early clinical studies indicated that methadone was equivalent to morphine in both potency and duration of action. Consequently, it appeared to offer little advantage over morphine. In general terms, methadone is noted for two properties: long half-life and high oral bioavailability. The majority of doses of methadone consumed worldwide are administered as part of opioid abstinence programs or in the treatment of intractable pain by providing a "generic" potent analgesic for pain relief assessments.[38] However, recent developments in analytic methodology have permitted detailed studies of its pharmacokinetics in man, and some investigators have demonstrated the usefulness of methadone in providing postoperative analgesia.

On first principles, it would seem that the often inadequate and generally fluctuating analgesic response obtained with the relatively short half-life opiates such as morphine and meperidine could be improved if a longer half-life agent were used to smooth out the fluctuations. Methadone is the longest half-life opiate commonly available and, if given IV to avoid the vagaries of absorption, it can provide long-lasting and seemingly reliable postoperative analgesia.[39] Gourlay et al.[39] administered 20 mg of methadone over 1 minute shortly after induction of anesthesia so that extensive redistribution would occur quickly into the initial dilution volume while the patient is anesthetized. Therefore, the initially high blood concentrations, which may be undesirable in the awake patient can be dispersed while the patient is anesthetized and ventilated. The median duration of postoperative analgesia was found to be 26 hours, and the median MEAC was 30 µg/L. If

these doses were to be given to awake patients after surgery, the duration of administration would need to be prolonged—perhaps over 20–30 minutes—to avoid any complications of high "peak" concentrations.

Details of pharmacokinetic analysis after IV administration are given in Table 28–4. The terminal half-life is very long, 30–40 hours, and the clearance is much lower than that of other opiates. Distribution volumes appear to be variable, and the source of this variability is uncertain. Although methadone is not as lipid soluble as fentanyl, it too would be expected to penetrate first to muscle and then to fat. The low clearance of methadone, compared to fentanyl, reflects an intrinsically lower ability of the liver to biotransform methadone. If urine is made acidic with ammonium chloride, renal clearance can account for nearly one third of the total clearance of methadone. Total body clearance, however, is 30%–40% higher, and the half-life is nearly one-half the value in volunteers treated with methadone and having urine made acid on one occasion and alkaline on another occasion.[40]

Simulated blood concentration to dose relationships for methadone given IV are shown in Figure 28–3.

Nothing is known of the influence of pathophysiology on the pharmacokinetics of methadone. Being a low clearance drug, its clearance and therefore half-life should be affected by pathology or drugs that influence metabolic functions, e.g., cytotoxic agents that impair drug metabolism, or anticonvulsants that induce cytochrome P-450.

Methadone seems to be the drug of choice for patients with intractable pain and in whom opiate

TABLE 28–4.—PHARMACOKINETIC PROPERTIES OF METHADONE IN VOLUNTEERS AND SURGICAL PATIENTS*

PARAMETER	SURGICAL PATIENTS† (Blood)	OPIATE ABUSER VOLUNTEERS‡ (Plasma)
t½$_{fast}$ (hr)	NR	3 (1)
t½$_{slow}$ (hr)	35 (20)	28 (11)
V₁ (L)§	NR	149 (32)
V$_{ss}$ (L)	416 (151)	NR
V$_{area}$ (L)§	NR	272 (86)
Cl (ml/min)	172 (88)	137 (92)

*Data are in means (SD) and are derived from venous sampling. In the first study, whole blood was used, but in the second study plasma was used.

†Data from Gourlay et al. (1982).[39]

‡Data from Meresaar et al.: *Eur. J. Clin. Pharmacol.* 20:473–478, 1981.

§The whole blood:plasma concentration ratio for methadone reported by Gourlay et al.[39] was 0.73 (0.05). Therefore, multiplying values derived from blood by this number will give the equivalent of plasma-derived values. When this is done, it can be seen that there are no apparent differences for methadone kinetics in the two groups.

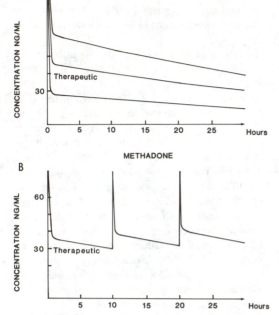

Fig 28–3.—Simulated blood concentration–dose relationships for methadone hydrochloride given IV: **A,** IV bolus doses of 20, 20, and 30 mg; **B,** initial bolus loading dose of 20 mg followed by maintenance bolus doses of 5 mg. Typical MEAC values are 20–50 ng/ml in patients that have undergone lower abdominal surgery and 30–70 ng/ml in patients that have undergone upper abdominal surgery. (Data from Gourlay et al.[98, 99])

therapy is indicated. Although the duration of action of the first dose is often only 4–6 hours, establishment of a dose regimen based on this duration will lead to intoxication due to accumulation. The duration is short because the effect persists only through the redistribution period (half-life of 2–3 hours), but accumulation occurs because of the long terminal half-life.[4] Hansen et al.[41] have suggested that patients be allowed to take 10-mg doses ad libitum for the first 3–5 days in order to titrate themselves into the effective range. Therefore, maintenance therapy can be chosen on the basis of the individual patient's responses, but probably once- or twice-daily dosing will suffice.[4] Twycross[9] has made the point forcefully that dosing should be on a timed schedule, not "as required." The same author has also suggested that oral morphine is likely to be as efficacious as any opiate if given correctly. Like morphine, methadone is metabolized to inactive prod-

ucts. However, the prolonged dosing interval for methadone, coupled with its high bioavailability (median, 80%), would seem to favor methadone if used alone. Combination with psychotropic drugs to treat side effects or act as co-analgesics can further enhance its usefulness.[41]

PROPOXYPHENE

The need for a strong but new narcotic analgesic appeared to be met by dextropropoxyphene. As a consequence it was prescribed widely throughout the 1960s and into the early 1970s, both by hospital and by community practitioners. Even as recently as 1978, 31 million prescriptions were written for propoxyphene in the United States alone.[42] However, concern about the safety of this agent increased in the 1970s. It is now generally recognized that propoxyphene cannot be classified as a nonopiate analgesic. The classic triad of psychological dependence, physical dependence, and tolerance accompanies the use of propoxyphene, especially in circumstances of prolonged and heavy use that are often associated with the intractable pain population. Furthermore, its analgesic efficacy has been deemed to be less than that of aspirin and only barely more than that of placebo.[43] However, with respect to side effects, propoxyphene, like lidocaine, causes functional depression of cardiac-conducting mechanisms, and these probably contribute to its toxicity in cases of overdose.[44] In fact, in animal tests, it is a potent local anesthetic agent with a potency intermediate between dibucaine and lidocaine.[45]

Despite this information, propoxyphene remains a widely used analgesic agent, both singly and (currently more commonly) combined with other agents, typically acetaminophen, sometimes aspirin, but possibly other agents, including antipyrine. It is relevant, therefore, to report information on the pharmacokinetics of propoxyphene as well as on the pharmacokinetic factors known to require modification of its dosage regimens in clinical patients.

There have been many studies of propoxyphene pharmacokinetics. Unfortunately, the majority of pharmacokinetic studies, until very recently, were deficient in the duration of sampling, so that their results may be questionable. The recent studies using more sensitive analysis have been able to follow blood concentrations long enough for precision, but have not set out their pharmacokinetic analysis in a manner directly comparable to those for other drugs tabulated in this chapter. An additional complication occurs since one of the primary pathways of metabolism of propoxyphene is N-dealkylation. One methyl group is lost from the tertiary amine group, producing norpropoxyphene. The clearance of norpropoxyphene is lower and its terminal half-life is longer than that of propoxyphene; hence it is always present in the blood of patients taking propoxyphene, and it contributes to the actions, both therapeutic and adverse, of propoxyphene. The following discussion attempts to integrate important findngs regarding the pharmacokinetics of propoxyphene and norpropoxyphene.

Propoxyphene shares some of the properties of morphine and morphinomimetics, but not all. For example, it has an analgesic effect in morphine-tolerant mice in the hot plate test for analgesia, but naloxone is more effective in antagonizing morphine than propoxyphene in this test.[46] In other animal tests for opiate analgesics, naloxone blocks the effects of both propoxyphene and norpropoxyphene (rat tail flick) or propoxyphene only (writhing test).[44] These animal data provide experimental evidence that narcotic antagonist naloxone will ameliorate but probably not completely abolish adverse effects of too much propoxyphene.

It has been reported that in healthy human subjects receiving IV doses[47] propoxyphene undergoes extensive redistribution and tissue binding since its apparent distribution volume (V_{area}) is much greater than the other opiates—a mean of 960 L (range, 590–1,230 L). Its renal clearance is negligible but its total body clearance is high (mean, 0.96 L/minute; range, 0.59–1.2 L/minute). As a consequence of the extensive tissue distribution, the slow phase half-life is quite long, averaging 15 hours (range, 8–24 hours). Redistribution phase half-lives have not been quantitated, but it is probable that these are not different from redistribution phase half-lives of other opiates such as meperidine or methadone. The slow phase half-life of norpropoxyphene averages around 25 hours, and this is consistent with its having a distribution volume 20%–30% greater than that of propoxyphene.

The vast majority of doses of propoxyphene are ingested orally. Hence its bioavailability is of prime importance. In the same healthy volunteers, Gram and co-workers in 1979 assessed oral bioavailability.[47] When propoxyphene was given by mouth, an average bioavailability of 43% (range, 29%–70%) was found. While norpropoxyphene is produced during first-pass hepatic clearance after oral administration, additional other metabolites that remain undetected in blood must be produced also, since the amount of norpropoxyphene produced did not correlate with the extent of first-pass clearance.[47] It is possible that metabolism of propoxyphene occurs in other parts of the gastrointestinal tract, since experimentally produced portacaval shunts in the dog increased the oral bioavailability from 25% to only 54%.[48] This is possible also for morphine.[12]

Patients with hepatic dysfunction and, more definitively, portacaval shunt are at risk of toxicity from propoxyphene, as their propoxyphene concentrations double those of patients with sound livers who receive the same oral doses. Conversely, their norpropoxyphene concentrations are one third to one fourth of normal. These observations are consistent with reduced first-pass clearance.[49]

In patients with renal failure, propoxyphene and norpropoxyphene accumulate so that their concentrations are many times normal. This is mostly due to diminished first-pass clearance of propoxyphene and decreased renal clearance of norpropoxyphene.[50] Neither propoxyphene nor norpropoxyphene is removed significantly by hemodialysis because of their extensive body distribution and relatively high plasma protein binding (20% for propoxyphene). Therefore this technique would be of no use in treatment of propoxyphene overdose.

It has been indicated already that propoxyphene bioavailability is variable within a patient population.[47, 51] Ingestion of food is known to cause variable bioavailability of many therapeutic substances, but this does not occur for propoxyphene. Hence patients may ingest propoxyphene preparations, including those containing aspirin, with meals, without loss of either agent.[51]

Caution should be observed in patients also taking carbamazepine. It appears that propoxyphene inhibits the metabolism of carbamazepine to the extent that toxicity is possible. This does not appear to be the case for phenytoin or phenobarbital, but phenobarbital appears to hasten the metabolism of propoxyphene.[41]

Taking the pharmacokinetic data for propoxyphene as a whole, the dominant characteristics are a high clearance but also a large distribution volume, giving a long half-life, as well as metabolism to an active compound (norpropoxyphene), which also has long half-life. Therefore, even with normal doses, there is the potential for toxicity to develop days after therapy is initiated, as accumulation takes place commensurate with the long half-life. It is a drug that seems to have little place in analgesic therapy if used alone and not a significantly more important place even if used with a simple antipyretic analgesic. Its pharmacologic role has been said to equate somewhat with that of codeine, but without the gastrointestinal effects of codeine. Its role in the spectrum of contemporary analgesic agents is in doubt, and it certainly cannot compete with codeine preparations on the basis of cost.[52]

AGONIST ANTAGONISTS

Pentazocine

Pentazocine was popularized in the 1960s in the quest for a potent but nonaddicting analgesic agent. The addiction potential of pentazocine is considerably lower that that of the traditional opiate agonists described previously, but it is accompanied by a definite abuse potential. In low doses (40 mg) it produces morphine-like effects, but in high doses (60–80 mg) morphine-like stimulation-debilitation is more prominent. A definite withdrawal syndrome occurs after chronic use. When given in equipotent doses to morphine, pentazocine depresses respiration to the same extent.

The pharmacokinetics of pentazocine have been studied in healthy subjects and patients, but detailed studies correlating with pentazocine analgesia (acute and chronic) may be useful because of the agonist/antagonist nature of the drug. Basically, pentazocine is a high clearance drug, with little drug excreted unmetabolized in the urine. Therefore, one would predict low bioavailability after oral administration, and in fact a bioavailability of 18% has been ob-

served (Table 28–5).[53, 29] Like methadone, pentazocine has a high lipid solubility, and a similar fraction is ionized in plasma. It is not surprising, therefore, that it has a similar large distribution volume, but, because of the high clearance rate, it has a much shorter half-life than methadone, about 3–4 hours, and is more like fentanyl or morphine in this regard.

In patients with hepatic dysfunction, the dosing interval should be prolonged for parenteral administration. Doses given orally should be reduced also, since a threefold increase in bioavailability also occurs.[29] Because renal clearance accounts for only a small percentage of the dose and because metabolites are not known to be pharmacologically active, renal dysfunction should not necessitate dose revision.

Buprenorphine and Butorphanol

There are many similarities between buprenorphine and butorphanol so that they may be considered together although buprenorphine is properly classified as a partial agonist rather than agonist-antagonist. However, most original sources of clinical and research reports on these agents published in the literature reflect their British and American origins, respectively. The pharmacology of each drug has been reviewed at a time when the pharmacokinetic data were at early stages of investigation.[54] There are several important points concerning the pharmacology of these agents to be noted. There appears to be a well-defined dosage rate for *appropriate opiate agonist effects*—for example, 2 mg of butor-

TABLE 28–5.—PHARMACOKINETIC PROPERTIES OF PENTAZOCINE IN HEALTHY VOLUNTEERS
AND CLINICAL PATIENTS*

| SAMPLE PARAMETER | HEALTHY VOLUNTEERS | | | SURGICAL PATIENTS | CIRRHOTIC PATIENTS | |
	Plasma†	Blood‡‖	Blood§	Blood	Blood	Blood§
$t1/2_{fast}$ (min)	8 (7)	NR	NR	5		NR
$t1/2_{slow}$ (hr)	2.4 (1.1)	3.8 (05)	5.1 (1.4)	3.8	6.6 (2)	12 (3)
V_1 (L)	102 (63)	NR	NR	46	NR	NR
V_{ss} (L)	258 (110)	342 (188)	NR	NR	306 (77)	NR
V_{area} (L)	292 (133)	415 (107)	390 (75)	230	356 (94)	390 (86)
Cl (L/min)	1.7 (1.4)	1.2 (0.2)	0.76 (0.13)	1.2	0.68 (0.30)	0.40 (0.12)
F (%)	18 (5)	21 (7)		68 (21)	70 (190)	
B/P		1.13			1.0	

*Data are in means (SD) and are derived from venous plasma or blood. NR = not recorded, F = fraction, B = blood concentration, P = plasma concentration.
†Data from Ritschel W.A., et al.: *Arzneimittelforsch* 32:64–68, 1982.
‡Data from Neal E.A., et al. (1979).[29]
§Data from Pond S.M., et al. (1980).[30]
‖Data from Ehrnebo M., et al. (1977).[53]

phanol produces equivalent analgesia to 80 mg of meperidine when given IV to surgical patients with postoperative pain, while 8 μg/kg of buprenorphine produces similar analgesia to 2 mg/kg of meperidine given under similar conditions. Furthermore, both buprenorphine and butorphanol *depress respiration* to the same extent as the pure agonist when given in equianalgesic doses. The same applies to the incidence of *nausea and sedation*. However, unlike what is seen with the pure agonists, the dose-response curve for respiratory depression is plateau-like, i.e., a ceiling effect is obtained at doses of about twice the analgesic dose (the antagonist effect). Interestingly, there is a well-defined ceiling effect for analgesia as well in patients with pain[54] and in animals, when a reduction in enflurane MAC is used as an objective criterion.[55, 56]

Another important point of the pharmacology of buprenorphine and butorphanol concerns the *antagonism with naloxone:* when co-administered, higher than traditional doses are required. Because naloxone has an extremely high clearance and because these agents dissociate from the opiate receptor very slowly, supplementary doses of naloxone may also be required to reverse the established effects of these agents.

Probably the most important point concerns the *dependence liability*. In a variety of animal models, both buprenorphine and butorphanol demonstrated lower dependence liability than traditional agonists. In man, definitive results are not available, but both agents seem to be more like codeine and propoxyphene than like morphine in regard to dependence liability. Therefore, these agents may be useful in patients requiring long-term use, but may present difficulties in dosage adjustments because of the ceiling effect. Long-term therapy almost always mandates oral administration, hence additional pharmacokinetic issues of bioavailability become important.

Foremost, both buprenorphine and butorphanol are high clearance drugs and have half-lives similar to that of morphine—about 3 hours (Table 28–6). Buprenorphine data reported in Table 28–6 were obtained from arterial sampling and therefore more readily demonstrate three-compartment kinetics than butorphanol, which is adequately described by a two-compartment system. The arterial sampling is the main reason that the initial dilution volume appears so small. Butorphanol, on the other hand, has extremely large initial and total distribution volumes which are comparable to those of propoxyphene. These are consistent with it having a high fat solu-

TABLE 28–6.—PHARMACOKINETIC PROPERTIES OF BUPRENORPHINE AND BUTORPHANOL IN SUBJECTS AS INDICATED*

PARAMETER	BUPRENORPHINE†		BUTORPHANOL‡ Healthy Volunteers
	Intraoperative	Postoperative	
$t1/2_{fast}$ (min)	2 (0.7)	2 (1)	11
$t1/2_{inter}$ (min)	11 (3)	19 (10)	NM
$t1/2_{slow}$ (hr)	2.3 (12)	3.1 (2.0)	3.3
V_1 (L)	9 (4)	14 (7)	250
V_{ss} (L)	97 (38)	188 (112)	600
V_{area} (L)	NR	NR	1,200
Cl (L/min)	0.90 (0.20)	1.3 (0.3)	30

*Data are in means (SD) for buprenorphine and are derived from arterial plasma. Data for butorphanol are derived from analysis of venous plasma data, presented in original report. NM, not modeled; NR, not recorded.
†Data from Bullingham et al. (1980).[57]
‡Data from Gaver et al. (1980).[58]

bility. Its clearance (calculated to be 3 L/minute, from data provided in the only publication concerning its disposition) is extremely high and, coupled with insignificant excretion of unmetabolized drug into urine, may mean appreciable metabolism by tissues other than liver. Similarly, buprenorphine is not excreted significantly into urine and is removed from the body by metabolism (presumably hepatic). Both drugs are absorbed effectively after IM injections, after which maximum plasma concentrations occur within ½–1 hour.[57, 58] Both drugs would be expected to undergo extensive first-pass hepatic elimination after oral administration, and this would limit their usefulness in chronic administration.

In an attempt to avoid the first-pass hepatic extraction, buprenorphine has been used sublingually with considerable efficacy.[57, 59] Postoperative analgesia lasting up to 9 hours has been reported. Patient acceptance is facilitated by the lack of bad taste because the dose of drug is so small. Pharmacokinetic analysis of plasma concentration data after IV and sublingual administration points to variable bioavailability which can be in excess of 90%, but may be very much lower if the sublingual tablets are swallowed. An average of 50%–60% may be expected, but since the absorption rate is slow (average absorption half-life = 76 minutes), a priming parenteral dose would be necessary to achieve onset of analgesia within an acceptable period.

Whether these opiates will have an important role in providing analgesia for intractable pain remains to be determined from continued research and development.[60] Their usefulness by sublingual administration and the importance of any reduced potential for dependence also have yet to be determined in the long run. Acute treatment with these agents is appealing because of their ceiling effects on respiratory depression and the relatively long duration of action of buprenorphine. However, antagonism by the pure antagonist naloxone is not predictable, and this would seem to speak against their use.

SELECTED NONNARCOTIC ANALGESICS

Salicylates

In addition to an analgesic effect, salicylates (sodium salicylate, aspirin, salicylamide) exhibit antiinflammatory, antipyretic, antirheumatic, and uricosuric actions. The analgesic, antipyretic, and antiinflammatory actions may be due to inhibition of prostaglandin synthesis. The analgesic effect is also thought to be due to an inhibitory effect on the pain-producing actions of bradykinin and the antipyretic effect may be due to peripheral vasodilation. In large doses, the uricosuric action has been attributed to preventing tubular reabsorption of uric acid. On the other hand, low-concentration salicylates are not only nonuricosuric, but can counteract the effects of probenecid on uric acid excretion.[61]

Salicylates are gastric irritants and have been implicated in gastric ulceration. It is likely that salicylate-induced gastric bleeding is exacerbated by the inhibitory effects on platelet aggregation. The mode of action of aspirin on platelet aggregation appears to be an inhibitory effect on the release of adenine diphosphate, induced by collagen. In addition, aspirin inhibits the function of cyclic endoperoxides necessary for thromboxane synthesis.[61] Minor effects on respiration and intermediary metabolism have been noted at high doses. Sodium salicylate and aspirin are rapidly and efficiently absorbed from both the stomach and the small intestine, with peak plasma concentrations occurring in about 1 hour following oral administration. Conversion of aspirin to salicylates is extremely rapid following absorption. Rapid conversion of aspirin to salicylates is due to a high first-pass effect which occurs in both the wall of the small intestine and the liver. Salicylic acid is excreted unchanged and as the glycine conjugate. Several other oxidative and conjugated pathways do occur.

The desired steady-state concentration range for salicylates is extremely narrow.[62] This is further complicated by the fact that salicylates exhibit Michaelis-Menten (nonlinear) or dose-dependent kinet-

ics so that the elimination half-life, which ranges from 2½ to 4 hours at low dose, and increases to 16–19 hours at high dose. Salicylates exhibit normal first-order kinetics only when the total amount of salicylate in the body is less than 200 mg. This level, of course, is markedly subtherapeutic.

The dose dependency of salicylates is manifest in both the volume of distribution and the extent of protein binding. Salicylates are characterized by an extremely low volume of distribution (0.07–0.1 L/kg). As discussed in chapter 27, this corresponds to a dilution volume just slightly larger than the blood volume, suggesting that tissue and fat distribution is minimal. The range of salicylate binding is extremely broad (50%–90%) and occurs primarily with albumin. Because the relative half-life increases with increasing dose, the time required to obtain a steady state increases with increasing dose. For example, it has been demonstrated that it takes about 2 days to reach steady-state concentrations when 1.5 gm/day of aspirin is given to adults, while more than 1 week may be required to reach steady-state concentrations when the dose is doubled.[62] Based on available clinical evidence, it has been found that there can be a great deal of flexibility regarding the size and dosing interval, as long as the total daily dose is chosen properly. One recommended conservative dosing regimen is to use 60 mg/kg of aspirin per day in one to six divided doses.[63] However, because of the large interpatient variability and dose-dependent kinetics associated with aspirin and salicylates, doses must be readjusted empirically, based on feedback information and data obtained from plasma concentration monitoring. Salicylates displace naproxen, phenylbutazone, and phenytoin from their plasma protein binding.[64] This results in a higher free fraction of these three drugs when they are administered concomitantly with salicylates. Salicylates have also been demonstrated to decrease the rate and extent of absorption for fenoprofen and indomethacin. When salicylates are administered in conjunction with corticosteroids, salicylate blood concentrations fall, probably because of alterations in glomerular filtration rate. Co-administration of oral anticoagulants and aspirin has been demonstrated to cause enhanced bleeding. This could be due to the salicylate-induced gastrointestinal irritation or impaired hemostasis secondary to platelet aggregation. Enhanced fecal blood loss has also been demonstrated with concomitant ingestion of alcohol and aspirin. Indomethacin-induced uricosuria can be diminished with co-administration of aspirin. The clinical pharmacokinetic profiles for salicylates, aspirin, and acetaminophen are compared in Table 28–7.

Acetaminophen

Acetaminophen is a para-aminophenol derivative with analgesic and antipyretic properties similar to those of aspirin. The antipyretic effect appears to result from a direct action on the hypothalmic heat-regulating centers. Acetaminophen has been shown to be an inhibitor of the action of endogenous pyrogen on the heat-regulating center.[65] At 500–600 mg, aspirin and acetaminophen appear to be equally effective in terms of antipyretic properties.[66] Acetaminophen appears to be equipotent to aspirin in inhibiting central prostaglandin synthesis. However, the peripheral prostaglandin synthetase inhibition noted with aspirin is not found with acetaminophen. This partially explains why acetaminophen is an effective antipyretic and analgesic when used for pain of noninflammatory origin. This is an important consideration in the management of patients with rheumatic or other inflammatory conditions.

The dose-response relationship for acetaminophen analgesia has not been unequivocally established. For example, 500- to 650-mg doses are markedly more effective than 300-mg doses. However, increasing the dose to 1,000 mg may not provide additional analgesia. A ceiling dose for maximum analgesia has not yet been determined.

Unlike aspirin, acetaminophen produces relatively few side effects in a normal dosage range. For example, acetaminophen does not produce gastric irritation and does not interfere with platelet function.[67] Additionally, acetaminophen does not potentiate the action of oral anticoagulants and is nonuricosuric. Hypersensitivity to acetaminophen is rare, and there is no cross-sensitivity between aspirin and acetaminophen.

Acetaminophen is effectively metabolized by liver enzymes. Only about 3% of the parent drug is excreted unchanged in the urine. Conjugation reactions with glucuronic acid and sulfuric acid account for approximately 80% of the metabolism of acet-aminophen. Minor metabolites formed by hydroxylation and deacetylation are responsible for the hepatotoxicity seen with acetaminophen overdose.[68] These metabolites are potent arylating agents and, under normal circumstances, are conjugated by hepatic glutathione and excreted in the urine as cystine and mercapturic acid conjugates.[68, 69] The amount of hydroxylated metabolites formed is determined not only by the amount of glutathione and acetaminophen present, but also by the amount of cytochrome P-450 present in the liver. The rate and extent of toxic metabolite formation are increased by phenobarbital, which is a known inducer of the mixed function oxidase system, cytochrome P-450.[68] Co-administration of acetaminophen with known inducers of hepatic enzymes should be done only with caution. Alcohol, for example, has been demonstrated to dramatically increase the toxicity of acetaminophen in mice.[70]

Acetaminophen is rapidly absorbed from the small intestine following oral administration. Peak concentrations are reached in approximately 1 hour. Unlike aspirin, acetaminophen is not efficiently absorbed through the gastric mucosa, and the rate of acetaminophen absorption is dependent on gastric emptying time. Co-administration of drugs known to prolong gastric emptying time, for example meperidine or pentazocine, causes a significant decrease in the rate of acetaminophen absorption.[71] Conversely, drugs such as metoclopramide, which stimulate gastric emptying, increase the rate of acetaminophen absorption without influencing the bioavailability.[64] Therapeutic concentrations for acetaminophen range from 10 to 30 mg/L. Peak concentrations following oral ingestion of 1 gm reach 30–40 mg/L in about 1 hour.[72] Bioavailability of acetaminophen has been found to be dose dependent, ranging from 0.63 at a dose of 500 mg to 0.87 at a 1,000–2,000 mg.[73] Unlike aspirin, elimination kinetics for acetaminophen are not dose dependent. The elimination half-life is 2.8 hours. Total plasma clearance does exhibit a dose dependency secondary to changes in bioavailability following oral administration. Acetaminophen is not highly protein bound (about 25%) and is characterized by a reason-

TABLE 28–7.—PHARMACOKINETIC PROPERTIES OF ASPIRIN, SALICYLATES, AND ACETAMINOPHEN

DRUG	TIME TO PEAK (hr)	ELIMINATION HALF-LIFE (hr)	VOLUME OF DISTRIBUTION (L/kg)	TOTAL CLEARANCE (L/kg/hr)	BIOAVAILABILITY	EXTENT OF PROTEIN BINDING (%)	FRACTION METABOLIZED	THERAPEUTIC RANGE (mg/L)	ACTIVE METABOLITES	DOSE-DEPENDENT KINETICS
Aspirin	0.25	0.25	0.2	0.55	0.9	50–90	0.99	20–100	Yes	Yes
Salicylates	0.5–1.0	2–3/19–20	0.1	0.03	0.9	50–90	0.90	150–300	Yes	Yes
Acetaminophen	1.0	2.8	1.0	0.25	0.8	~10	0.95	10–20	No	No

ably high steady-state volume of distribution (1.0 L/kg).

The plasma concentration-time profile for acetaminophen following IV administration is characterized by a rapid distribution phase, followed by a slower elimination phase. The half-life of distribution for acetaminophen is 0.3 hour.[75] In patients with cirrhosis of the liver, the elimination half-life is increased by 44%. A corresponding decrease in the total plasma clearance has also been demonstrated.[74] Chronic dosing in cirrhotic patients did not result in accumulation. However, plasma concentrations are two to three times higher than in patients with normal liver function.[76] These higher blood levels in cirrhotic patients did not result in any signs of acetaminophen hepatotoxicity. These data also suggest that a reduction in dosage for patients with cirrhosis of the liver would be appropriate. Decreases in albumin and other plasma proteins associated with liver disease have a minimal effect on acetaminophen pharmacokinetics because of the low extent of protein binding.

A starting chronic dosing regimen based on a minimum steady-state concentration of 10 mg/L and an average bioavailability of 0.8 for a 70-kg person with normal hepatic and renal function is 1,000 mg every 4 hours. A steady-state concentration will be achieved in 1 day, given a fixed dose and dosing interval. This dosing regimen can be simplified to approximately 15 mg/kg every 4 hours. This regimen should result in an average steady-state concentration of 11.5 mg/L, with fluctuation from a minimum steady-state concentration of 6.75 mg/L to a maximum steady-state concentration of 14.2 mg/L.

Pyrrole Acetic Acid Derivatives

Pyrrole acetic acid derivatives appear to have anti-inflammatory and analgesic properties similar to those of aspirin or indomethacin. Two potent derivatives, zomepirac and tolmetin, have been introduced. Both drugs appear to be effective in the treatment of arthritic pain. Zomepirac has been advocated as a "comprehensive, nonaddicting analgesic."[75] Zomepirac and tolmetin are potent prostaglandin synthetase inhibitors. Zomepirac inhibits platelet aggregation to a greater extent than tolmetin, presumably because of its greater lipid solubility.[75–77] Zomepirac and tolmetin do not cause withdrawal symptoms following chronic administration. Fecal blood loss studies revealed that moderate dosages (300 mg/day) of tolmetin caused less loss than aspirin (3,900 mg/day), and patient acceptability was greater than with zomepirac. Large doses of zomepirac (600 mg/day) tended to cause a greater fecal blood loss than high-dose aspirin (4,800 mg/day).[78] Similar studies with tolmetin demonstrated less fecal blood loss with a dose of 1,200 mg/day than with a 3,900 mg/day dose of aspirin.[79] The side effects associated with both tolmetin and zomepirac are similar to those reported for aspirin and salicylates, but on a less frequent basis.[75, 80] Tolmetin has also been reported to exhibit antipyretic properties.[81]

There are many clinical pain studies reported for zomepirac. Zomepirac in 50- and 100-mg doses was found to be superior to 650 mg of aspirin for the relief of oral surgical pain.[82] Zomepirac, 100 mg, was judged equieffective to APC with codeine, 60 mg, for postoperative pain, and clearly superior to codeine, 60 mg.[83] Zomepirac, 100 mg, provided more satisfactory postoperative analgesia than IM morphine, 4–8 mg.[84] In a clinical evaluation of 159 cancer patients being treated for postoperative pain, 100 mg of zomepirac was rated superior to 4–8 mg of IM morphine and roughly equivalent to 16 mg of IM morphine.[85] Zomepirac was judged effective for the management of chronic cancer pain,[86] chronic orthopedic pain,[87] and pain emanating from muscle contraction headache.[88] Somewhat surprising is the relatively poor patient response to zomepirac in osteoarthritic studies.[89, 90] Tolmetin, on the other hand, has been primarily evaluated as an effective drug for the management of rheumatoid arthritis.[80] Therapeutic trials with tolmetin have been conducted using aspirin, indomethacin, phenylbutazone, and members of the profen family as comparative drugs. Tolmetin has been demonstrated to be superior to placebo in all studies. Tolmetin and aspirin appear to be equipotent, but side effects have been less frequent with tolmetin. There has been no significant difference between tolmetin, 800–1,400 mg/day, indomethacin, 100–150 mg/day, or phenylbutazone, 400 mg/day.[80]

Tolmetin and zomepirac are rapidly absorbed following oral administration. Tolmetin reaches a peak plasma concentration at 0.5–1 hour,[91] while zomepirac reaches a peak concentration in 1–1.5 hours.[92] Zomepirac exhibits a rapid distribution phase, followed by elimination, while tolmetin exhibits only a monoexponential decay following its peak, thereby masking the distribution phase. Both zomepirac and tolmetin are extensively protein bound to serum albumin.[75, 93] This leads to a relatively low volume of distribution. The volume of distribution

TABLE 28–8.—PHARMACOKINETIC PROPERTIES OF TOLMETIN AND ZOMEPIRAC

DRUG	TIME TO PEAK (hr)	ELIMINATION HALF-LIFE (hr)	VOLUME OF DISTRIBUTION (L/kg)	TOTAL CLEARANCE (L/kg/hr)	BIOAVAILABILITY	EXTENT OF PROTEIN BINDING (%)	FRACTON METABOLIZED	THERAPEUTIC RANGE (gm/ml)	ACTIVE METABOLITES	DOSE-DEPENDENT KINETICS
Tolmetin	0.5–1.0	0.92	0.09	0.07	1.0	99.0	0.83	20–30	No	Yes
Zomepirac	1.0	4.3	1.0	0.16	0.95	98.5	0.78	0.1–10	No	No

at steady state for tolmetin is an order of magnitude lower (0.09 L/kg) than for zomepirac (0.9 L/kg), which reflects the lower lipid solubility of tolmetin. Tolmetin and zomepirac are metabolized by liver enzymes. The extent of metabolism is extremely variable. The major metabolite of tolmetin is the *d*-carboxylic acid derivative, accounting for 50%–70%. Conjugated tolmetin and other metabolites account for approximately 13%, and only 17% of tolmetin is excreted unchanged.[94] Zomepirac, on the other hand, is highly conjugated by glucuronic acid. The glucuronide accounts for 40%–60% of the dose, with other metabolites accounting for only 4%–6%. Approximately 20% of the dose is excreted unchanged.[75] Elimination of tolmetin is much faster than elimination of zomepirac. However, the volume of distribution at steady state for zomepirac is greatly increased, which results in approximately equivalent total plasma clearances for both drugs. Clinical pharmacokinetic parameters for tolmetin and zomepirac are summarized in Table 28–8. Volumes of distribution have not been corrected for bioavailability, since no absolute bioavailability data are available, because neither drug has been approved for IV administration. The recommended dosing for tolmetin is 600–1,200 mg/day in divided doses.[80] For multiple dosing, tolmetin presents an interesting problem. It has been suggested that dosing should be every 6–8 hours. However, tolmetin has such a short half-life that these intervals lead to tremendous fluctuations in plasma concentrations. For example, a 400-mg dose taken every 8 hours results in a plasma C_{max}/C_{min} ratio of approximately 500, and 300 mg taken every 6 hours results in a plasma C_{max}/C_{min} ratio of 100. A dose of 150 mg taken every 3 hours can be used to minimize the fluctuation. Such dosing results in a C_{max}/C_{min} ratio of approximately 8.

The most common multiple dosing regimen for zomepirac is 50–100 mg/6 hours. This dosing regimen should result in a steady-state concentration between 0.8 and 1.6 mg/L (calculated for a 70-kg individual). Unlike tolmetin, a dosing interval of 6 hours leads to a C_{max}/C_{min} ratio of only 2.6. Tolmetin and zomepirac, being extremely highly pro-

tein bound to serum albumin, may interact with other albumin-bound drugs such as warfarin, sulfonoureas, phenytoin, and aspirin. Drug interaction data for zomepirac and tolmetin are incomplete. Concomitant administration of magnesium aluminum hydroxide liquid antacids with tolmetin did not result in alterations in plasma tolmetin concentrations, time to peak concentration, or area under the plasma concentration-time curve. The renal clearance of tolmetin was also unaltered.[80]

At the time of this writing, zomepirac has been implicated in a series of anaphylactic reactions resulting in death. Thus, the practitioner should prescribe zomepirac only after careful evaluation of patients for a hypersensitivity response.

REFERENCES

1. Mather L.E., Glynn C.J.: The minimum effective analgetic blood concentration of pethidine in patients with intractable pain. *Br. J. Clin. Pharmacol.* 14:385–390, 1982.
2. Bressler D.E., Katz R.L.: Chronic pain and alternatives to neural blockade, in Cousins M.J., Bridenbaugh P.O. (eds.): *Neural Blockade.* Philadelphia, J.B. Lippincott Co., 1980, pp. 651–678.
3. Glynn C.J., Mather L.E.: Pharmacokinetics applied to patients with intractable pain: Studies with pethidine. *Pain* 13:237–246, 1982.
4. Paalzow L.K.: Pharmacokinetic aspects of optimal pain treatment. *Acta Anaesthesiol. Scand. Suppl.* 74(2):37–43, 1982.
5. Mather L.E.: Clinical pharmacokinetics of fentanyl and its newer derivatives. *Clin. Pharmacokinet.* 8:422–446, 1983.
6. Stanski D.R., Greenblatt D.J., Lowenstein E.: Kinetics of intravenous and intramuscular morphine. *Clin. Pharmacol. Ther.* 24:52–59, 1978.
7. Sawe J., Dahlstrom B., Paalzow L., et al.: Morphine kinetics in cancer patients. *Clin. Pharmacol. Ther.* 30:629–635, 1981.
8. Dahlstrom B., Tamsen A., Paalzow L., et al.: Patient controlled analgesic therapy: IV. Pharmacokinetics and analgesic plasma concentrations of morphine. *Clin. Pharmacokinet.* 7:285–311, 1982.
9. Twycross R.G.: Morphine and diamorphine in the terminally ill patient. *Acta Anaesthesiol. Scand. Suppl.* 74(26):128–134, 1982.

10. Leslie S.T., Rhodes A., Black F.M.: Controlled release morphine sulphate tablets: A study in normal volunteers. *Br. J. Clin. Pharmacol.* 9:531–533, 1980.

11. Hanks G.W., Rose N.M., Aherne G.W., et al.: Controlled-release morphine tablets. *Br. J. Anaesth.* 53:1259–1264, 1980.

12. Iwamoto K., Klaasen C.D.: First pass effect of morphine in rats. *J. Pharmacol. Exp. Ther.* 200:236–244, 1977.

13. Patwardhan R.V., Johnson R.F., Hoyumpa A., et al.: Normal metabolism of morphine in cirrhosis. *Gastroenterology* 81:1006–1011, 1981.

14. Olsen G.D.: Morphine binding to human plasma proteins. *Clin. Pharmacol. Ther.* 16:1125–1130, 1975.

15. Olsen G.D., Bennett W.M., Porter G.A.: Morphine and phenytoin binding to plasma proteins in renal and hepatic failure. *Clin. Pharmacol.* 17(6):677–684, 1975.

16. Yeh S.Y.: Urinary excretion of morphine and its metabolites in morphine dependent subjects. *J. Pharmacol. Exp. Ther.* 192:201–210, 1975.

17. Brunk S.F., Delle M.: Morphine metabolism in man. *Clin. Pharmacol. Ther.* 16:51–57, 1974.

18. Mather L.E., Lindop M.J., Tucker G.T., et al.: Pethidine revisited: Plasma concentrations and effect after intramuscular injection. *Br. J. Anaesth.* 47:1269–1275, 1975.

19. Austin K.L., Stapleton J.V., Mather L.E.: Rate of formation of norpethidine from pethidine. *Br. J. Anaesth.* 53:255–258, 1981.

20. Verbeeck R.K., Branch R.A., Wilkinson G.R.: Meperidine disposition in man: Influence of urinary pH and route of administration. *Clin. Pharmacol. Ther.* 30:619–628, 1981.

21. Austin K.L., Stapleton J.V., Mather L.E.: Pethidine clearance during continuous intravenous infusions in postoperative patients. *Br. J. Clin. Pharmacol.* 11:25–30, 1981.

22. Sprigge J.E., East D.S.R., Fox G.S., et al.: Meperidine infusion for postoperative analgesia in grossly obese patients. *Can. Anaesth. Soc. J.* 29:142–150, 1982.

23. Church J.J.: Continuous narcotic infusions for relief of postoperative pain. *Br. Med. Jr.* 1:977–979, 1979.

24. Rigg J.R.A., Wong T.Y.: A method for achieving rapidly steady state blood concentrations of I.V. drugs. *Br. J. Anaesth.* 53:1147, 1981.

25. Tsuei T.E., Nation R.L., Thomas J.: Design of predetermined regimens to achieve and maintain a predetermined concentration range. *Clin. Pharmacol. Ther.* 23:289–295, 1980.

26. Rigg J.R.A., Ilsley A.H., Vedig A.E.: Relationship of ventilatory depression to steady-state blood pethidine concentrations. *Br. J. Anaesth.* 53:613–620, 1981.

27. Shand D.G., Desjardins R.E., Bjornson T.D., et al.: The method of separate exponentials: A simple aid to devising intravenous drug-loading regimens. *Clin. Pharmacol. Ther.* 29:542–547, 1981.

28. Mather L.E., Tucker G.T.: Systemic availability of orally administered meperidine. *Clin. Pharmacol. Ther.* 20:535–540, 1976.

29. Neal E.A., Meffin P.J., Gregory P.B., et al.: Enhanced bioavailability and decreased clearance of analgesics in patients with cirrhosis. *Gastroenterology* 77:96–102, 1979.

30. Pond S.M., Tong T., Benowitz N.L., et al.: Enhanced bioavailability of pethidine and pentazocine in patients with cirrhosis of the liver. *Aust. NZ J. Med.* 10:515–519, 1980.

31. Edwards D.J., Svensson C.K., Visco J.P., et al.: Clinical pharmacokinetics of pethidine (meperidine): 1982. *Clin. Pharmacokinet.* 7:421–433, 1982.

32. Mather L.E.: Pharmacokinetic studies of meperidine, in Foley K., Inturrisi C. (eds.): *Advances in Pain Research.* New York, Raven Press, in press.

33. Nation R.: Meperidine binding in maternal and fetal plasma. *Clin. Pharmacol. Ther.* 29:472–479, 1981.

34. Austin K.L., Stapleton J.V., Mather L.E.: Multiple intramuscular injections: A major source of variability in analgesic response to meperidine. *Pain* 8:47–62, 1980.

35. Hug C.C. Jr., Murphy M.R.: Fentanyl disposition in cerebrospinal fluid and plasma and its relationship to ventilatory depression in the dog. *Anesthesiology* 50:342–349, 1979.

36. Gill K.J., Cartwright D.P., Scoggins A., et al.: Ventilatory depression related to plasma fentanyl concentrations during and after anesthesia. *Br. J. Anaesth.* 52:632P, 1980.

37. Hull C.J., Sibbald A.: Control of postoperative pain by interactive demand analgesia. *Br. J. Anaesth.* 53:385–391, 1981.

38. Murphy T.M.: Treatment of chronic pain, in Miller R.D. (ed.): *Anesthesia,* New York, Churchill Livingstone, 1981, vol. 2, pp. 1459–1490.

39. Gourlay G.K., Wilson P.R., Glynn C.J.: Methadone produces prolonged postoperative analgesia. *Br. Med. J.* 284:630–631, 1982.

40. Nilsson M., Anggard E., Homstrand J., et al.: Pharmacokinetics of methadone during maintenance treatment: Adaptive changes during the induction phase. *Eur. J. Clin. Pharmacol.* 22:343–350, 1982.

41. Hansen B.S., Dam M., Brandt J., et al.: Influence of dextropropoxyphene on steady state serum levels and protein binding of three antiepileptic drugs in man. *Acta Neurol. Scand.* 61:357–367, 1980.

42. Brevik H., Rennemo F.: Clinical evaluation of combined treatment with methadone and psychotropic drugs in cancer patients. *Acta Anaesthesiol. Scand. Suppl.* 74(26):135–140, 1982.

43. Smith R.J.: Federal government faces painful decision on darvon. *Science* 203:857–858, 1971.

44. Holland D.R., Steinberg M.I.: Electrophysiological properties of propoxyphene and norpropoxyphene in canine cardiac conducting tissues in vitro and in vivo. *Toxicol. Appl. Pharmacol.* 47:123–133, 1979.

45. Nickander R., Smits S.E., Steinberg M.I.: Propoxy-

phene and norpropoxyphene: Pharmacology and toxic effects in animals. *J. Pharmacol. Exp. Ther.* 200:245–253, 1977.

46. Neil A., Terenius L.: Propoxyphene acts differently from morphine in opioid receptor-effector mechanisms. *Eur. J. Pharmacol.* 69:33–39, 1981.

47. Gram L.F., Shou J., Way W.L., et al.: *d*-Propoxyphene kinetics after single oral and intravenous doses in man. *Clin. Pharmacol. Ther.* 26:473–482, 1979.

48. Giacomini K.M., Nakeeb S.M., Levy G.: Pharmacokinetics of propoxyphene: I. Effect of portacaval shunt on systemic availability in dogs. *J. Pharm. Sci.* 69:786–789, 1980.

49. Giacomini K.M., Giacomini J.C., Gibson T.D., et al.: Propoxyphene and norpropoxyphene plasma concentrations after oral propoxyphene in cirrhotic patients with and without surgically constructed portacaval shunt. *Clin. Pharmacol. Ther.* 28:417–424, 1980.

50. Roberts S.M., Levy G.: Pharmacokinetic studies of propoxyphene: IV. Effect of renal failure on systemic clearance in rats. *J. Pharm. Sci.* 69:363–364, 1980.

51. Melander A., Berlin-Wahlen A., Bodin N.-O., et al.: Bioavailability of *d*-propoxyphene, acetylsalicylic acid, and phenazone in a combination tablet (Doleron): Interindividual variation and influence of food. *Acta Med. Scand.* 202:119-124, 1977.

52. Jaffe J.H.: Narcotic analgesics, in Goodman L.S., Gilman A. (eds.): *The Pharmacological Basis of Therapeutics,* ed. 2. Toronto, Macmillan, 1970, pp. 237–275.

53. Ehrnebo M., Boreus L.O., Lonroth U.: Bioavailability and first pass metabolism of oral pentazocine in man. *Clin. Pharmacol. Ther.* 22:888–892, 1977.

54. Heel R.C., Brogden D., Speight T.M., et al.: Butorphanol: A review of its pharmacological properties and therapeutic effects. *Drugs* 16:473–505, 1978.

55. Murphy M.R., Hug C.C. Jr.: The enflurane sparing effect of morphine, butorphanol, and nalbuphine. *Anesthesiology* 57:489–492, 1982.

56. Murphy M.R., Hug C.C. Jr.: Anesthetic potency of fentanyl in terms of its reduction of enflurane MAC. *Anesthesiology* 57:485–488, 1982.

57. Bullingham R.E.S., McQuay H.J., Dwyer D., et al.: Sublingual buprenorphine used postoperatively: Clinical observations and preliminary pharmacokinetic analysis. *Br. J. Pharmacol.* 12:117–122, 1981.

58. Gaver R.C., Vasilev M., Wong H., et al.: Disposition of parenteral butorphanol in man. *Drug Metab. Dispos.* 8:230–235, 1980.

59. Bullingham R.E.S., McQuay H.J., Porter E.J.B., et al.: Sublingual buprenorphine used postoperatively: Ten hour plasma drug concentration analysis. *Br. J. Clin. Pharmacol.* 13:665–673, 1982.

60. Kjaer M., Henriksen H., Knudsen J.: A comparative study of intramuscular buprenorphine and morphine in the treatment of chronic pain of malignant origin. *Br. J. Clin. Pharmacol.* 13:487–492, 1982.

61. Levy G.: Pharmacokinetics of salicylate in man. *Drug Metab. Rev.* 9:3–91, 1979.

62. Levy G., Tsuchiya T.: Salicylate accumulation kinetics in man. *N. Engl. J. Med.* 287:430–432, 1972.

63. Levy G., Giacomini K.M.: Rational aspirin dosage regimens. *Clin. Pharmacol. Ther.* 23:247–252, 1978.

64. Hayes A.H.: Therapeutic implications of drug interactions with acetaminophen and aspirin. *Arch. Intern. Med.* 141:301–304, 1981.

65. Clark W.G., Moyer S.G.: The effects of acetaminophen and sodium salicylate on the release and activity of leukocyte pyrogen in the cat. *J. Pharmacol. Exp. Ther.* 181:183–191, 1972.

66. Beaver W.T.: Mild analgesics: A review of their clinical pharmacology. *Am. J. Med. Sci.* 250:577–604, 1966.

67. Mielke C.H., Britten A.F.H.: Use of aspirin or acetaminophen in hemophilia. *N. Engl. J. Med.* 282:1270, 1970.

68. Mitchell J.R., Thorgeirsson S.S., Potter W.Z., et al.: Acetaminophen induced hepatic injury: Protective role of glutathione in man and rationale for therapy. *Clin. Pharmacol. Ther.* 16:676–684, 1974.

69. Mitchell J.R., Jollow D.J., Gillette J.R., et al.: Drug metabolism as a cause of drug toxicity. *Drug Metab. Dispos.* 1:418–423, 1973.

70. Peterson F.J., Holloway D.E., Erickson R.R., et al.: Ethanol induction of acetaminophen toxicity and metabolism. *Life Sci.* 27:1705–1711, 27.

71. Clements J.A., Heading R.C., Nimmo W.S., et al.: Kinetics of acetaminophen absorption and gastric emptying in man. *Clin. Pharmacol. Ther.* 24:420–431, 1978.

72. Wojeicki J., Gawronska-Szklarz B., Kazimierezyk J., et al.: Comparative pharmacokinetics of paracetamol in men and women considering the follicular and luteal phases. *Arzneimittelforsch.* 29:350–352, 1979.

73. Rawlins M.D., Henderson D.B., Hijab A.R.: Pharmacokinetics of paracetamol (acetaminophen) after intravenous and oral administration. *Eur. J. Clin. Pharmacol.* 11:283–286, 1977.

74. Andreasen P.B., Hutters L.: Paracetamol (acetaminophen) clearance in patients with cirrhosis of the liver. *Clin. Pharmacol. Ther.* 23:247–252, 1978.

75. McLeod D.C.: Zomepirac. *Drug Intell. Clin. Pharm.* 15:522–530, 1981.

76. Pruss T.P., Gardocki J.F., Taylor R.J., et al.: Evaluation of the analgesic properties of zomepirac. *J. Clin. Pharmacol.* 20:216–222, 1980.

77. Mielke C.H., Kahn S.B., Muschek L.D., et al.: Effects of zomepirac on hemostasis in healthy adults and on platelet function in vitro. *J. Clin. Pharmacol.* 20:409–417, 1980.

78. Johnson P.C.: A comparison of zomepirac and aspirin on fecal blood loss. *J. Clin. Pharmacol.* 20:401–405, 1980.

79. Johnson P.C., Binachine J.R., Bierne J., et al.: Gastrointestinal blood loss produced by tolmetin aspirin

and indomethacine as measured by (51)Cr technique. *Clin. Res.* 22:642–646, 1974.

80. Brogden R.N., Heel R.C., Speight T.M., et al.: Tolmetin: A review of its pharmacological properties and therapeutic efficacy in rheumatic diseases. *Drugs* 15:429–450, 1978.

81. Wax J., Winder C.V., Tessman D.K., et al.: Comparative activities, tolerance and safety of non-steroidal anti-inflammatory agents in rats. *J. Pharmacol. Exp. Ther.* 192:172–179, 1975.

82. Cooper S.A.: Efficacy of zomepirac in oral surgical pain. *J. Clin. Pharmacol.* 20:230–242, 1980.

83. Baird A.M., Turek D.: Comparison of zomepirac, APC with codeine, codeine, and placebo in the treatment of moderate and severe postoperative pain. *J. Clin. Pharmacol.* 20:243–249, 1980.

84. Forrest W.H.: Oral zomepirac and intramuscular morphine in postoperative pain. *J. Clin. Pharmacol.* 20:259–260, 1980.

85. Wallenstein S.L., Rogers A., Kaiko R.F., et al.: Relative analgesic potency of oral zomepirac and intramuscular morphine in cancer patients with postoperative pain. *J. Clin. Pharmacol.* 20:2502–58, 1980.

86. Stambaugh J.E., Tejada F., Trudnowski R.J.: Double-blind comparisons of zomepirac and oxycodone with APC in cancer pain. *J. Clin. Pharmacol.* 20:261–270, 1980.

87. Mayer T.G., Ruoff G.E.: Clinical evaluation of zomepirac in the treatment of acute orthopedic pain. *J. Clin. Pharmacol.* 20:285–291, 1980.

88. Diamond S.: Zomepirac in the symptomatic treatment of muscle contraction headache. *J. Clin. Pharmacol.* 20:298–302, 1980.

89. Andelman S., Levin J., Simson J., et al.: A double-blind crossover comparison of zomepirac and placebo in pain secondary to osteoarthritis of the knee. *J. Clin. Pharmacol.* 20:364–370, 1980.

90. Ruoff G.E., Andelman S.Y., Cannella J.J.: Long-term safety of zomepirac: A double-blind comparison with aspirin in patients with osteoarthritis. *J. Clin. Pharmacol.* 20:377–384, 1980.

91. Selley M.L., Glass J., Triggs E.J., et al.: Pharmacokinetic studies of tolmetin in man. *Clin. Pharmacol. Ther.* 17:599–605, 1975.

92. Nayak R.K., Ng K.T., Gottlieb S.: Zomepirac kinetics in healthy males. *Clin. Pharmacol. Ther.* 27:395–401, 1980.

93. Selley M.L., Madsen B.W., Thomas J.: Protein binding of tolmetin. *Clin. Pharmacol. Ther.* 24:694–705, 1978.

94. Selley M.L., Thomas J., Triggs E.J.: A gas-liquid chromatographic method for the quantitative determination of tolmetin in plasma and tolmentin and its major metabolite in urine. *J. Chromatogr.* 94:143–148, 1974.

95. Tamsen A., Hartvig P., Fagerland C., et al.: Patient controlled analgesic therapy: Individual analgesic demand and analgesic plasma concentrations of pethidine in post operative pain. *Clin. Pharmacokinet.* 7:164–175, 1982.

96. Klotz U., Avant G.R., Hoyumpa A., et al.: The effects of age and liver disease on the disposition of diazepan in adult man. *J. Clin. Invest.* 55:347–359, 1975.

97. Austin K.H., Stapleton J.V., Mather L.E.: Relationship between blood meperdine concentrations and analgesic response. *Anesthesiology* 53:460–466, 1980.

98. Gourlay G.K., Willis R.J., Wilson P.R.: Postoperative pain control with methadone: Influence of supplementary methadone doses and blood concentration-response relationship. *Anesthesiology* 61:19–26, 1984.

29 / Nonsteroidal Anti-inflammatory Agents

DONALD D. DENSON, Ph.D.
LAURENCE E. MATHER, Ph.D.

NONSTEROIDAL anti-inflammatory agents have received considerable attention during the past decade. Nonsteroidal anti-inflammatory agents as a class have a diversity of chemical structures. However, most agents do possess an organic acid moiety in common. Nonsteroidal anti-inflammatory agents are indicated in the management of rheumatoid and osteoarthritis as well as ankylosing spondylitis.

All of the nonsteroidal anti-inflammatory agents apparently produce their anti-inflammatory effect by the inhibition of prostaglandin synthesis. In addition to the therapeutic actions of the nonsteroidal anti-inflammatory agents, each is capable of producing potentially serious side effects. The major side effects include gastric irritability, gastrointestinal bleeding, and blood dyscrasias. The efforts of researchers to design drugs with maximal therapeutic efficacy and minimal side effects has resulted in the appearance of a large number of new agents in recent years.

A multitude of clinical trials have compared the different nonsteroidal anti-inflammatory drugs, and the results of these studies indicate that the drugs are of comparable efficacy. The relative potencies of the drugs in inhibiting prostaglandin synthesis in vitro do not appear to be related to their comparative efficacy in reducing inflammation. It should be noted that all of the agents reviewed in Table 29–1 are equianalgesic with low-dose aspirin (1–2 gm/day) and have an anti-inflammatory efficacy equivalent to high-dose aspirin (> 5 gm/day). Reported differences in the efficacy of these agents appears to be related more to the comparative dosage utilized in the various studies than to the properties of a specific drug. Few studies have been able to document the relationship between dose, serum concentration, and anti-inflammatory response in patients with rheumatoid arthritis.[1] This is due in part to the lack of accurate methods for assessing the inflammatory process. In clinical practice, therefore, there are no clear guidelines to assist the clinician in the selection of the most appropriate drug for a specific patient. With the exception of drugs that offer twice-daily dosing schedules, such as naproxen, sulindac, and fenbufen, and which are therefore convenient for patients on long-term therapy, the clinician may base the selection of the most appropriate nonsteroidal anti-inflammatory agent on clinical experience, potential for side effects, and relative cost.

The nonsteroidal anti-inflammatory agents possess very similar pharmacokinetic characteristics. The clinical pharmacokinetics of the nonsteroidal anti-inflammatory agents have been recently reviewed.[2] Generally, these agents are rapidly and extensively absorbed following either oral or rectal administration. Distribution is extremely small, owing primarily to the high extent of protein binding. Hence, volumes of distribution for the majority of the nonsteroidal anti-inflammatory agents are on the order of 10 L for a 70-kg individual. The nonsteroidal anti-inflammatory agents are extensively metabolized in the liver, with renal excretion playing a minor role. They have, in general, very low total clearance values and therefore are extremely sensitive to changes in plasma protein binding.

The following sections review the available pharmacokinetic data for the major nonsteroidal anti-inflammatory agents. An effort has been made to include newer agents for which data are available. Table 29–1 summarizes the pharmacokinetic and

521

TABLE 29–1.—PHARMACOKINETIC PROPERTIES OF SELECTED NONSTEROIDAL
ANTI-INFLAMMATORY DRUGS

DRUG	*USUAL DAILY DOSE (mg)	*USUAL DOSING INTERVAL (hr)	*TIME TO PEAK (hr)	**†ELIMINATION HALF-LIFE (hr)	*†VOLUME OF DISTRIBUTION (L/kg)	‡TOTAL CLEARANCE (L/kg/hr)	†EXTENT OF PROTEIN BINDING (%)	*FRACTION METABOLIZED
Alclofenac	300	8	1–4	1.5–5.5	0.10	0.01–0.05	90–99	0.5–0.9
Apazone	1200	6	3–6	10–15	0.16	0.007–0.01	95	0.38
Diclofenac	100	8	1–3	1–2	0.12	0.04–0.08	99	0.99
Fenbufen	600–1,000	12	1–2	10	2–4	0.14–0.25	. . .	0.96
Fenclofenac	900–1,200	12	3–4	20–38	0.2–0.25	.004–.007	96	
Fenoprofen	2,400	6–8	1–2	2–3	0.10	0.02–0.04	99	0.95
Flurbiprofen	150–300	8	1–2	3–4	0.10	0.03–0.04	99	0.85
Ibuprofen	1,600	6–8	0.5–1.5	2–2.5	0.14	0.04–0.05	99	0.99
Indomethacin	75–100	6–12	1–2	6	0.12	0.014	92–99	0.895
Ketoprofen	200	6–8	0.5–2	1.5	0.11	0.07	94	0.99
Naproxen	500–750	12	1–2	12–15	0.10	.005–.006	98–99	0.99
Phenylbutazone	300–400	6–8	2	50–100	0.17	.001–.002	98	0.99
Sulindac	400	12	1	7	. . .	. . .	93	0.93

Data compiled from:

*Data from Verbeeck et al.[2]

†Data from Heel R.C., Avery G.S.: Appendix A: Drug data information, in Avery G.S. (ed.): *Drug Treatment*. New York, Adis Press, 1980, p. 1213.

‡Estimated from volume of distribution and half-life according to: $Cl = \dfrac{0.693 \times VD}{t1/2}$

drug dosing data for the nonsteroidal anti-inflammatory agents to be reviewed in the following section.

INDOMETHACIN AND SULINDAC

Indomethacin is a highly effective antipyretic, anti-inflammatory analgesic. The pharmacologic action of indomethacin stems from its inhibition of prostaglandin synthesis. In addition, indomethacin inhibits the motility of polymorphonuclear leukocytes and uncouples oxidative phosphorylation in cartilaginous and hepatic mitochondria.

Indomethacin is extensively and rapidly absorbed following both rectal and oral administration, with peak blood concentrations occurring 1 hour following rectal administration and 1½–2 hours following oral administration.[3–5] Concentrations of indomethacin for chronic administration can be accurately predicted by the measurement of single-dose values.[3] There are, however, marked interindividual and intraindividual differences in maximum plasma concentrations of indomethacin following oral administration.[6] Maximum blood concentrations following rectal administration are somewhat lower than those achieved following oral administration. Indomethacin enters synovial fluid slowly. The rate of entry is governed by plasma protein binding,

which is extremely high (> 90%) but variable.[5] The high protein binding accounts for the relatively low apparent volume of distribution for indomethacin, generally 0.15–0.2 L/kg. Indomethacin is extensively metabolized, with only 5%–10% of an oral dose recovered as unchanged drug in the urine. Biotransformation involves both oxidative and conjugative pathways in the liver.[4] Considerable interindividual and intraindividual variations occur in the elimination half-life of indomethacin. This may be due in part to the fact that indomethacin undergoes extensive enterohepatic recirculation.[7]

Indomethacin does not exhibit age-related changes in pharmacokinetics. No differences in plasma concentration half-lives or clearance rates were detected when normal volunteers were compared with patients with rheumatoid arthritis.[3] The disposition characteristics of indomethacin do not seem to be significantly altered in renal failure. However, accumulation of the conjugated form of indomethacin in the plasma of patients with severely impaired kidney function has been reported. A good correlation between endogenous creatinine clearance rate and extent of indomethacin excretion in the urine has been reported.[8] While the effect of hepatocellular disease on the disposition of indomethacin has not been investigated, Kunze et al.[9] found a significantly reduced elimination rate in patients with occluded bile ducts. Since indomethacin undergoes extensive biliary recycling, this result is to be expected. Concomitant administration of antacids such as magnesium or aluminum hydroxide will result in the delayed absorption of indomethacin. Sodium bicarbonate, on the other hand, tends to increase the absorption rate, resulting in somewhat higher and earlier peak plasma concentrations, probably because the increased pH of the gastric lumen facilitates the dissolution of indomethacin, which is an organic acid.

Studies on the interaction between indomethacin and aspirin have yielded conflicting results. On the one hand, Jeremy and Towson[10] reported that aspirin reduced indomethacin plasma concentrations in patients with rheumatoid arthritis. Kwan et al.[11] suggested that the decrease in indomethacin concentration with aspirin is attributable to changes in gastrointestinal absorption and resorption and enhanced biliary excretion of the drug. Helleberg et al.[5] reported that aspirin does not alter and may even increase plasma indomethacin concentrations. Co-administration of indomethacin and warfarin does not result in a clinically relevant drug interaction. Co-administration of indomethacin and probenecid results in increased plasma concentrations of indomethacin and this may improve the clinical efficacy of indomethacin. However, an increased plasma concentration also increases the risk of side effects.

Indomethacin has been demonstrated to be efficacious in the management of inflammatory diseases for many years, but its use has been limited by toxicity. Sulindac is a chemically related drug which was synthesized as a result of a search for a compound as effective as indomethacin but less toxic. The reduction in gastrointestinal irritation accompanying sulindac administration may be due to the fact that sulindac is an inactive pro-drug converted by liver microsomal enzymes to sulindac disulfide which appears to be an important anti-inflammatory metabolite. Sulindac reaches peak plasma concentrations in 1–2 hours after oral administration. The active sulfide metabolite reaches maximum levels in the plasma approximately 2 hours after oral ingestion of the parent drug. Oral bioavailability appears to be greater than 88%. Plasma protein binding of sulindac and the sulfide metabolite is extremely high, greater than 90%. Only limited information regarding the distribution characteristics of sulindac are available. The relatively long elimination half-life of both sulindac and its active metabolite make this drug an excellent choice for long-term anti-inflammatory treatment since dosing can be accomplished twice daily. Sulindac undergoes extensive

biotransformation in the liver. In addition to the reversible reduction to sulindac sulfide, an irreversible oxidation to a sulfone derivative is also prevalent. The sulfone derivative and its glucuronide conjugate are the major products excreted in the urine (about 28%). Sulindac and its glucuronide account for about 20% of the dose, while about 25% is excreted in urine as unidentified metabolic products.[12] The complex disposition of sulindac owing to reversible metabolism precludes conventional analysis of its pharmacokinetics.[13]

PHENYLBUTAZONE AND AZAPROPAZONE

Phenylbutazone is a pyrazolone derivative and a highly effective anti-inflammatory analgesic. Phenylbutazone inhibits the synthesis of prostaglandins, a property common to all nonsteroidal anti-inflammatory agents. In addition, phenylbutazone uncouples oxidative phosphorylation and inhibits ATP-dependent biosynthesis of mucopolysaccharide sulfates in cartilage tissue. Phenylbutazone produces a mild uricosuric effect by diminishing tubular reabsorption of uric acid. However, phenylbutazone administration may be accompanied by aplastic anemia and agranulocytosis and these have limited its use in long-term therapy.

Phenylbutazone is rapidly and completely absorbed following either rectal or oral administration. Peak plasma concentrations are generally reached within 2 hours. Phenylbutazone is extensively bound to plasma proteins (approximately 99%), accounting for its low volume of distribution (0.17 L/kg).[14] Concentrations of phenylbutazone in synovial fluid reach 55%–80% of those obtained in plasma. Significant concentrations may persist in the joints for up to 3 weeks following discontinuation of treatment. Phenylbutazone is extensively metabolized in humans. The fraction excreted in urine unchanged is less than 1%. Like indomethacin, phenylbutazone undergoes extensive oxidation and conjugation in the liver. In contrast to indomethacin, however, biliary excretion of phenylbutazone and its metabolites has been found to be extremely low. Although there are large interindividual and intraindividual variations, the elimination half-life for phenylbutazone is approximately 75 hours. Phenylbutazone exhibits dose- and time-dependent pharmacokinetics in man.[15]

Research aimed at developing a newer pyrazole derivative with a spectrum of activity similar to phenylbutazone but without toxicity resulted in the discovery of apazone (azapropazone). Whereas the efficacy of this drug parallels that of phenylbutazone, no evidence of agranulocytosis has been reported with apazone. Apazone is rapidly and completely absorbed from the gastrointestinal tract following oral administration. The peak plasma concentrations, however, are reached somewhat later than for phenylbutazone—approximately 4 hours after administration. Since plasma protein binding of apazone is extremely high (99%), the volume of distribution is relatively low (0.1–0.15 L/kg). The extent of accumulation of apazone in synovial fluids has not been reported. In contrast to many of the nonsteroidal anti-inflammatory agents, 62% of apazone is excreted unchanged in the urine. Total body clearance approaches 1 L/hour, which is relatively high for the nonsteroidal anti-inflammatory agents. The elimination half-life for apazone is about 12 hours, considerably less than that reported for phenylbutazone.

Ritch et al.[16] reported on the pharmacokinetic data for azapropazone in the elderly. The elimination half-life was prolonged secondary to a decrease in total plasma clearance but no change in the volume of distribution between young and old subjects was noted. These changes contrast with those reported for phenylbutazone, where no significant differences in pharmacokinetics for phenylbutazone were found in young and elderly subjects.

Changes in the pharmacokinetics of both apazone and phenylbutazone have been reported in renal failure.[17] Plasma protein binding of phenylbutazone, for example, has been reported to be decreased in patients with acute renal failure. This is a likely explanation of the noted increase in volume of distribution and prolonged half-life of phenylbutazone in uremic patients. Held and Enderle[18] have suggested a reduction in phenylbutazone dosage for patients with renal insufficiency. As noted above, apazone undergoes significant renal clearance (62%).[19] Administration of apazone in patients with renal failure would be expected to result in a decreased total plasma clearance, which would result in an increased half-life. In patients with renal failure, therefore, the dose of apazone should be reduced according to the degree of impairment of kidney function and plasma protein binding of the drug.

In patients with liver disease, both phenylbutazone and apazone would be expected to undergo pharmacokinetic changes, as a result of reduced plasma protein binding. For phenylbutazone, an increase in the free or unbound fraction would increase both the total body clearance and the volume of distribution and result in an apparently normal elimination half-life. In patients with compromised liver function, total plasma clearance for apazone has been reported to be similar to that for healthy subjects, while there was a 2½–fold increase in the free fraction in plasma and a 50% reduction in the free drug clearance. In patients with severe cirrhosis, total plasma clearance was reduced to only 20% of normal. Appropriate dosing reductions should be made in an effort to prevent dose-related side effects, since the pronounced increase in free fraction in plasma and the decrease in plasma clearance can lead to a marked reduction in free drug clearance, resulting in accumulation of free drug in the body. Unlike indomethacin, co-administration of antacids did not alter the rate or extent of apazone absorption.

No studies are available regarding the effects of aspirin and concomitantly administered phenylbutazone or apazone. Unlike indomethacin, phenylbutazone does potentiate the anticoagulative effect of warfarin. This effect may be secondary to both a plasma protein binding displacement interaction and a metabolic inhibition. Apazone behaves similarly, with the interaction between warfarin and apazone being attributed to plasma protein binding displacement interactions. Co-administration of phenylbutazone with sulfonyl ureas used for hypoglycemic therapy can potentially result in hypoglycemic coma. Similar interactions of apazone with oral hypoglycemics have not been reported. Apazone, on the other hand, does result in a significant increase in phenytoin plasma concentrations, presumably through a protein binding displacement interaction.

Equivalent plasma steady-state concentrations for apazone and phenylbutazone would be obtained using a dosing of 1,200 mg/6 hours for apazone and either 300 mg/6 hours or 400 mg/8 hours for phenylbutazone.

NAPROXEN

Naproxen is a propionic acid derivative. As a class, propionic acid derivatives tend to be relatively less toxic but also exert relatively less anti-inflammatory action than full doses of aspirin or indomenthacin. Thus, naproxen appears to be as effective as aspirin as an anti-inflammatory agent but is better tolerated. The mechanism of anti-inflammatory action with the propionic acid derivatives appears to be similar to that described for the other nonsteroidal anti-inflammatory agents.

Naproxen is rapidly and extensively absorbed after both oral and rectal administration. Peak plasma concentrations routinely occur within 2 hours after oral administration.[20] As described for the other nonsteroidal anti-inflammatory agents, naproxen distributes into synovial fluids. Mean synovial fluid concentrations at 3–4 hours after an oral dose are approximately 50% of those in plasma. Naproxen binds to plasma proteins extensively (99.6%) but the binding is concentration dependent. The apparent volume of distribution is low, about 0.1 L/kg, in agreement with the extensive protein binding.

Naproxen depends extensively on hepatic metabolism for termination of activity. Less than 10% of an oral dose is excreted unchanged in the urine. Unlike indomethacin and phenylbutazone for which oxidation is an important pathway, glucuronic acid conjugation is the major elimination pathway for naproxen. The elminiation half-life of naproxen ranges from 12 to 15 hours and is independent of dose.

No data are available with regard to pharmacokinetic changes in the elderly with naproxen. In addition, no reports of changes of naproxen pharmacokinetics in patients with rheumatoid arthritis are available. The effect of renal failure on the pharmacokinetics of naproxen is similar to that noted for phenylbutazone. That is, the total body clearance and apparent volume of distribution of naproxen are significantly increased, resulting in an unchanged elimination half-life. These changes are probably secondary to decreased plasma protein binding.

Segre et al.[21] reported that the simultaneous oral administration of aspirin and naproxen results in lower plasma concentrations of naproxen. This observation may be due to a drug displacement interaction. The naproxen plasma concentration differences are relatively low, however, and may be of limited clinical importance. Unlike phenylbutazone, naproxen has no apparent effect on the steady-state free or total concentrations of warfarin. Naproxen, however, does have a direct inhibitory effect on platelet function, thus it would be prudent to monitor patients concurrently taking naproxen and warfarin. Co-administration of probenecid and naproxen results in a decreased metabolic clearance for naproxen, presumably through metabolic inhibition. Because of this interaction, co-administration of probenecid and naproxen will result in higher steady-state naproxen plasma concentrations. Naproxen pharmacokinetics allow appropriate steady-state concentrations to be achieved with a twice-daily dosing regimen, and therefore naproxen is a convenient drug for patients on long-term therapy.

For example, the average steady-state concentration for 500 mg of naproxen taken twice daily would be approximately 100 μgm/ml.

IBUPROFEN AND RELATED DRUGS

Ibuprofen, like naproxen, also is a propionic acid derivative. Minor structural changes to the ibuprofen nucleus result in fenoprofen, ketoprofen, fenbufen, and flurbiprofen. These derivatives are milder than naproxen but often are better tolerated by patients who cannot tolerate the more active nonsteroidal anti-inflammatory agents. Some patients with rheumatoid arthritis do extremely well on ibuprofen, but, in general, it is more useful for milder cases of inflammatory and degenerative arthritis. Flurbiprofen appears to be more active as an anti-inflammatory agent than ibuprofen but is usually well tolerated. Ketoprofen and fenoprofen occupy much the same place in therapeutics as naproxen. Fenbufen lends itself to twice-daily dosing. In general, these compounds are extremely rapidly and efficiently absorbed following oral administration, with bioavailabilities greater than 85%. Peak plasma concentrations occur between 0.5 and 3 hours, depending on the drug selected (see Table 29–1). All of the drugs in this class are distributed into synovial fluid. Ibuprofen passes slowly into synovial fluid and remains in high concentration after plasma concentrations have decayed. Flurbiprofen distributes relatively rapidly into synovial fluid and concentrations are comparable to plasma concentrations 6 hours following a single oral dose. Fenbufen synovial fluid concentrations are about one third of the corresponding plasma concentrations at 4 and 8 hours following oral administration. Information on the extent of synovial fluid distribution for fenoprofen and ketoprofen is not available. All of the drugs in this class are extensively bound to plasma proteins (95%–99%).

Renal excretion of unchanged drug varies from less than 1% for ibuprofen to 60%–65% for ketoprofen. All members of this group of nonsteroidal anti-inflammatory agents undergo hepatic drug metabolism. With the exception of fenbufen, for which only conflicting data are available, this group of compounds is characterized by a relatively low volume of distribution (0.1–0.12 L/kg).[2] Elimination half-lives are in the range of 0.5 hours for ketoprofen to 10 hours for fenbufen.

No data are available on the pharmacokinetic changes associated with aging for this group of compounds. In addition, no pharmacokinetic changes associated with rheumatoid arthritis have been reported.

Fenbufen is the only drug of this group that has been studied in renal failure. Rogers et al.[22] concluded that renal failure alters the metabolic pattern of fenbufen. Although the elimination half-life was not altered in patients with renal insufficiency, there were decreased amounts of fenbufen and its active metabolite in plasma, probably due to diminished plasma protein binding. The authors concluded that the potential for moderate accumulation in plasma of the more polar urinary metabolites, which are inactive and relatively nontoxic would present little hazard to the patient with renal insufficiency. Studies relating the influence of liver disease on the pharmacokinetics of this group of compounds have not been reported.

Co-administration of aspirin increases the free drug clearance for all members of this class of compounds. The mechanism of this interaction is not known and the clinical relevance is doubtful. Concomitant administration of warfarin and fenbufen for 7 days resulted in slight changes in prothrombin time. These changes were considered to be of no clinical significance. Similar studies with flurbiprofen and ibuprofen demonstrated no effect of co-administration of these compounds. Probenecid has been shown to inhibit the conjugation of ketoprofen and renal excretion of ketoprofen conjugates. Co-administration of phenobarbital and fenoprofen results in significantly lower fenoprofen concentrations in plasma, suggesting accelerated metabolism secondary to phenobarbital. Co-administration of flurbiprofen and antipyrene results in a significant prolongation of the elimination half-life for antipyrine. This raises the possibility that flurbiprofen could alter the metabolism of other drugs that are extensively metabolized by the liver. Normal dosing regimens with the ''profen'' family are usually on a three to four times daily basis, with the exception of fenbufen, which lends itself to twice-daily dosing regimens.

PHENYLACETIC ACID DERIVATIVES

A relatively new class of nonsteroidal anti-inflammatory agents are derivatives of phenylacetic acid. Three members of this family studied to date are diclofenac, fenclofenac, and alclofenac. These compounds are effective anti-inflammatory analgesics in less severe rheumatic conditions. They appear to be comparable to the propionic acid derivatives, possessing similar overall efficacy and side effects. Pharmacokinetic characterization of drug absorption and elimination for this class is relatively sparse. Available data suggest that diclofenac is absorbed rapidly following oral administration, with peak plasma concentrations reached in 2 hours.[23] However, diclofenac undergoes significant presystemic elimination (first-pass effect), resulting in a bioavailability of only 60%. Rectal administration of diclofenac appears to be equivalent to the oral route of administration in terms of rate and extent of absorption.[24] Synovial concentrations of diclofenac rapidly increase to significantly higher levels than in plasma within 4 hours following administration. Diclofenac is highly bound to plasma proteins and has a low volume of distribution. Diclofenac is largely eliminated by biotransformation, with urinary excretion of unchanged diclofenac less than 1% of the dose.

Alclofenac is more rapidly absorbed, with usual peak concentrations reached in 1–2 hours. However, absorption data are extremely variable, and bioavailability ranges from 36% to 90% of the dose.[25] Peak concentrations in synovial fluid are reached about 2 hours after a single dose of alclofenac. As with diclofenac, alclofenac concentrations in synovial fluid are higher than in plasma at 6 hours and are not significantly different after 9 hours. Alclofenac is highly bound to plasma proteins and has a very small volume of distribution. Urinary excretion of unchanged alclofenac is highly variable and ranges from 10% to 50%. The remainder of alclofenac dose undergoes extensive metabolism in the liver.

Fenclofenac has been studied even less. Peak concentrations following a 600-mg oral dose are achieved within 3–4 hours.[26] As with the other two drugs in this class, a low volume of distribution was found. Fenclofenac is metabolized in the liver and the metabolites are subsequently excreted via the kidneys. The terminal half-life of fenclofenac varies from 20 to 38 hours and appears to be dose independent. This property makes fenclofenac an excellent candidate for twice-daily dosing. In contrast, alclofenac has an elimination half-life of 3½ hours, while diclofenac has an elimination half-life of approximately 1 hour.

Diclofenac is the only member of this class that has been studied in the elderly. Similar disposition kinetics were observed in eight young and eight elderly females. Moreover, diclofenac is the only member of this group studied in rheumatoid arthritis patients. Again, similar elimination half-lives and areas under the plasma concentration-time curves were observed in the two study groups. Peak concentrations, however, were significantly reduced in the rheumatoid arthritis group.

Co-administration of diclofenac and aspirin results in an increased apparent volume of distribution and increased total plasma clearance for diclofenac. As suggested for many of the other nonsteroidal anti-inflammatory agents, possible mechanisms for this interaction include competition for plasma protein binding sites. Diclofenac was found to decrease lithium renal clearance by 23% and to increase lithium plasma concentrations by a corresponding 26%. Of the drug interactions reported between nonsteroidal anti-inflammatory drugs and other agents, this interaction may be clinically significant since it involves a risk of lithium intoxication in patients treated with lithium salts and diclofenac and possibly other nonsteroidal anti-inflammatory agents as well.

REFERENCES

1. Orme M. L'E.: Plasma concentrations and therapeutic effect of anti-inflammatory and anti-rheumatic drugs. *Pharmacol. Ther.* 16:167–180, 1982.
2. Verbeeck R.K., Blackburn J.L., Loewen G.R.: Clinical pharmacokinetics of nonsteroidal anti-inflammatory drugs. *Clin. Pharmacokinet.* 8:297–331, 1983.
3. Alvan G., Bertillson L., Ekstrand R., el al.: Pharmacokinetics of indomethacin. *Clin. Pharmacol. Ther.* 18:364–373, 1975.
4. Duggan D.E., Hogans A.F., Kwan C.E., et al.: The metabolism of indomethacin in man. *J. Pharmacol. Exp. Ther.* 181:563–575, 1972.
5. Helleberg L.: Clinical pharmacokinetics of indomethacin. *Clin. Pharmacokinet.* 6:245–258, 1981.
6. Emori H.W., Paulus H.E., Bluestone R., et al.: Indomethacin serum concentrations in man: Effects of dosage, food and antacid. *Ann. Rheum. Dis.* 35:333–338, 1976.
7. Kwan K.C., Breault G.O., Umbenhauer E.R., et el.: Kinetics of indomethacin absorption elimination and enterohepatic circulation in man. *J. Pharmacokinet. Biopharm.* 4:255–280, 1975.
8. Traeger A., Stein G., Kuntze M., et al.: Zur Pharmakokinetic von Indomethazin bei Nierengeschadigten Patienten. *Int. J. Clin. Pharmacol.* 6:237–242, 1972.
9. Kunze M., Stien G., Kunze E., et al.: Zur Pharmakokinetic von Indomethazin in Abhängigkeit von Lebensalter bei Patienten mit Gallenwegsverschluss: Nierenfunktionseinschrankung und Unvertaglichkeitserscheinungen. *Dtsch. Gesundheitw.* 29:351–353, 1974.
10. Jeremy R., Towson J.: Interaction of aspirin and indomethacin in the treatment of rheumatoid arthritis. *Med. J. Aus.* 2:127–129, 1970.
11. Kwan K.C., Breault G.O., Davis R.L., et al.: Effects of concomitant aspirin administration on the pharmacokinetics of indomethacin in man. *J. Pharmacokinet. Biopharm.* 6:451–476, 1978.
12. Duggan D.E., Hare L.E., Ditzler C.A., et al.: The disposition of sulindac. *Clin. Pharmacol. Ther.* 21:326–335, 1972.
13. Brogden R.N., Heel R.C., Speight T.M., et al.: Sulindac: A review of its pharmacological properties and therapeutic efficacy in rheumatic diseases. *Drugs* 16:97–114, 1978.
14. Triggs E.J., Nation R.L., Long A., et al.: Pharmacokinetics in the elderly. *Eur. J. Clin. Pharmacol.* 8:55–62, 1975.
15. Higham C., Aaron S.L., Holt P.J.L., et al.: A chronic dose-ranging study of the pharmacokinetics of phenylbutazone in rheumatoid arthritis patients. *Br. J. Clin. Pharmacol.* 12:123–129, 1981.
16. Ritch A.E.S., Perera W.N.R., Jones C.J.: Pharmacokinetics of azapropazone in the elderly. *Br. J. Clin. Pharmacol.* 14:116–119, 1982.
17. Mussche M.M., Belpaire F.M., Bogaert M.G.: Plasma protein binding of phenylbutazone during recovery from acute renal failure. *Eur. J. Clin. Pharmacol.* 9:69–71, 1975.
18. Held H., Enderle C.: Elimination and serum protein binding of phenylbutazone in patients with renal insufficiency. *Clin. Nephrol.* 6:388–393, 1976.
19. Breuning K.H., Gifrich H.J., Meinertz T., et al.: Disposition of azapropazone in chronic renal and hepatic failure. *Eur. J. Clin. Pharmacol.* 20:147–155, 1981.
20. Runkel R.A., Chaplin M., Boost G., et al.: Absorption, distribution metabolism and excretion of naproxen in various laboratory animals and human subjects. *J. Pharm. Sci.* 61:703–708, 1972.
21. Serge E.J., Chaplin M., Forchielli E., et al.: Naproxen-aspirin interactions in man. *Clin. Pharmacol. Ther.* 15:374–379, 1974.
22. Rogers H.J., Savitsky J.P., Glenn B., et al.: Kinetics of single doses of fenbufen in patients with renal insufficiency. *Clin. Pharmacol. Ther.* 29:74–80, 1981.
23. Willis J.V., Jack D.B., Kendall M.J., et al.: The influence of food on the absorption of diclofenac as determined by the urinary excretion of the unchanged drug and its major metabolites during chronic administration. *Eur. J. Clin. Pharmacol.* 19:39–44, 1981.
24. Riess W., Stierlin H., Degen P., et al.: Pharmacokinetics and metabolism of the antiinflammatory agent voltaren. *Scand. J. Rheumatol. Suppl.* 22:17–29, 1978.
25. Roncucci R., Simon M.J., Lambelin G., et al.: Kinetic studies on the absorption and excretion of 4-allyloxy-3-chlor-phenylacetic acid (alclofenac) in man. *Eur. J. Clin. Pharmacol.* 3:176–183, 1971.
26. Henson R., Lloyd-Jones J.G., Nichols J.D., et al.: Pharmacokinetics of fenclofenac following single and multiple doses. *Eur. J. Drug Metab. Pharmacokinet.* 5:217–223, 1980.

30 / Antidepressants and Adjunctive Psychotrophic Drugs

THOMAS OXMAN, M.D.
DONALD D. DENSON, Ph.D

TRICYCLIC ANTIDEPRESSANTS

Since their introduction nearly 30 years ago, the tricyclic antidepressants (TCAs) have become the most widely used medication in the treatment of depression. In selecting drugs for depressed patients, the clinician should be prepared to use a range of agents, depending on the presenting depressive syndrome. For example, if the symptoms are primarily anxiety and tension, treatment with antianxiety drugs may suffice. The use of antianxiety drugs in this circumstance would relieve not only the attendant symptoms but also the depression. On the other hand, symptoms of severe anxiety or agitation accompanying depression may require the use of an antipsychotic drug. The point is, not all depressed patients require antidepressants. The classic or retarded endogenous depression is a clear indication for the use of TCAs. This type of depression is most likely to respond well to these drugs.

Controlled studies of the tricyclics have concluded that each of the drugs in this group is of approximately equivalent value. While this finding may be true for groups of patients, it is not necessarily true for individual patients. For example, an individual patient may be far better on one drug than another. The reasons why are not clear. The matching of drug to patient is accomplished empirically at present. For example, some clinicians believe that the sedative TCAs such as amitriptyline or doxepin are the preferred drugs for patients with high levels of anxiety or agitation and with multiple somatic complaints, including sleep disorders. On the other hand, TCAs with low sedative action, such as di-

azepromen and protriptyline, may be preferred for patients with psychomotor retardation. These distinctions are based primarily on speculation rather than on scientific data.

Clinical Pharmacokinetics

Although ample blood concentration-time data are available for the TCAs that allow one to correlate plasma concentration with effect, detailed pharmacokinetic studies are lacking. All TCAs show marked differences in rate of elimination in individual patients. Thus, steady-state plasma concentrations can be expected to differ widely among individuals. There is a clear indication not only for individualization of dosage, but also for therapeutic drug monitoring. All of the TCAs are eliminated by extensive hepatic metabolism. A complicating factor is that the principal metabolities of the parent drugs are themselves potent TCAs, for example desipramine, the metabolite of imipramine, and nortriptyline the metabolite of amitriptyline. Dosing adjustments are particularly difficult because the antidepressant effects of the parent drug and its metabolite may well be additive (e.g., imipramine and desipramine).[1] The ratio between the parent drug and major active metabolite varies widely and has been reported to range from 0.3 to 15.0.[2] Different rates of formation of desipramine versus rates of retention of imipramine may be clinically important because of possible differences in the pharmacologic effects.

The elimination half-life for the TCAs varies widely among individuals. Table 30–1 summarizes

TABLE 30–1.—PHARMACOKINETIC PROPERTIES OF SELECTED TRICYCLIC ANTIDEPRESSANTS

	ELIMINATION HALF-LIFE* (hr)	VOLUME OF DISTRIBUTION* (L/kg)	TOTAL CLEARANCE† (L/kg/hr)	EXTENT OF PROTEIN BINDING (%)*
Amitriptyline	32–40	. . .	. . .	82–96
Desipramine	12–54	22–59	0.28–3.41	70–90
Doxepin	8–25	9–33	0.25–2.86	. . .
Imipramine	6–20	20–40	0.69–4.62	80–95
Nortriptyline	15–90	20–57	0.21–2.63	90–95
Protriptyline	54–92	15–31	0.11–0.40	92

*Compiled from Heel R.C., Avery G.S.: Appendix A: Drug data information, in Avery G.S. (ed.): *Drug Treatment*. New York, Adis Press, 1980, p. 1217.

†Calculated from volume of distribution and elimination half-life according to:

$$Cl = \frac{V_D \times 0.693}{t1/2}$$

the available pharmacokinetic parameters for the TCAs. In general, TCAs possess long half-lives, which makes steady-state plasma concentrations difficult to assess in less than 1–4 weeks. An additional consequence of the prolonged half-lives of these drugs is that there appears to be no difference in variability between once-daily and divided daily doses.[3] The tricyclic compounds are very lipid soluble and are readily absorbed from the gastrointestinal tract and diffuse readily in the tissues. The bioavailability of orally administered nortriptyline varies between 56% and 79%. Presumably, the low bioavailability is secondary to first-pass liver metabolism. Protein binding of the tricyclics is extremely high, and binding is thought to be primarily to α_1-acid glycoprotein. Thus, disease states such as stress or anxiety, which tend to change the α_1-acid glycoprotein concentration, would contribute to interindividual variation in protein binding. The TCAs as a whole exhibit extremely large volumes of distribution. This results in a hepatic extraction ratio that is intermediate to low.

Clinical Pharmacology

TCAs possess, to varying degrees, three primary pharmacologic actions: sedation, anticholinergic action, and block of the amine pump.

Basic Mechanisms

Recent evidence suggests that the acute effects of antidepressants on neurotransmitters do not explain their therapeutic action.[4] The biogenic amine hypothesis of depression theorizes that catecholamines and/or serotonin levels are reduced at relevant synapses in the brain. Antidepressants have been thought to relieve depression by making more neurotransmitters available at the synapse. Three major objections have been raised in rebuttal to this proposed mechanism of action of antidepressants. First, TCA inhibition of norepinephrine (NE) or serotonin (5-HT) reuptake is an immediate effect, yet antidepressant action takes 1–4 weeks. Second, amphetamine and cocaine are potent inhibitors of NE reuptake but are not useful antidepressants. Third, some clinically effective antidepressants such as iprindole and mianserin do not inhibit neuronal NE or 5-HT uptake.[4, 5, 97]

Current research on the therapeutic mechanisms of antidepressant drugs has changed from monitoring short-term effects on amine *metabolism* to assessing long-term adaptive changes in NE and 5-HT *functions*.[4, 6] Of particular research interest are (1) alterations in neuroendocrine responses on the dexamethasone suppression test and the growth hormone stimulation test, (2) disturbances in functions of neuroendocrine-regulated circadian rhythm (e.g., body temperature, rapid-eye-movement sleep, cortisol and prolactin secretion), and (3) reciprocal changes in α- and β-adrenergic receptor activity. Changes in NE and 5-HT postsynaptic function may prove to be a specific and shared mechanism of action of all somatic antidepressant therapy.[4]

Antidepressant Analgesia

TCAs were introduced for clinical use in depression in 1975. Their use in the control of rheumatic pain was reported as early as 1962.[7] There are now numerous reports involving over 1,000 patients in which these drugs were used to treat chronic pain.[8–25] The majority of these patients were suffering from headache. Over 50% of all patients reported at least some relief. Despite this record, the mechanism of TCA-induced analgesia is unclear, and further research in humans is needed to separate primary TCA analgesic effects from secondary effects due to antidepressant and sedative-hypnotic properties.

Numerous studies in animals have indicated some role for NE and 5-HT in pain modulation, separate from antidepressant activity. This modulation occurs in both brain stem descending and spinal cord ascending pathways. Electrical activation of central NE systems produces analgesia[26] as does pharmacologic stimulation of spinal NE receptors.[27] Anatomical studies have shown that NE neurons project to areas of the brain which modulate incoming pain,[28] and iontophoretic application of NE agonists to these regions suppresses pain transmission.[29] Conversely, destruction of central NE systems produces a hypersensitivity to pain.[27] Electrophysiologic, anatomical, and neurochemical research also supports the role of 5-HT in pain suppression. Electrical stimulation of 5-HT neurons produces analgesia,[30, 31] and this stimulation-produced analgesia is associated with increased 5-HT activity, as judged by increased 5-HT metabolism. Serotonin neurons preferentially project to areas of the brain known to modulate pain.[32] These pain-modulating areas contain neurons that relay pain centrally to the thalamus, and application of 5-HT agonists to these cells suppresses their response to noxious stimulation,[33] indicating that the 5-HT system can suppress pain as it enters the CNS as well as at a spinal level.[32] Furthermore, administration of analgesics is correlated with increased 5-HT and NE neural activity.[34–36]

Many human studies of pain relief with TCA have been conducted on patients with migraine headache. This raises difficulties in establishing the validity of an analgesic property of TCAs; other potential mechanisms of action of TCAs occur in migraine, such as alterations of platelet function and vasomotor receptors.[37] Furthermore, only two of the studies are double-blind and crossover in design.[8, 10]

In patients with back pain of varying etiology, Sternbach et al.[25] found that 150 mg of chlorimipramine was more effective in reducing pain than 150 mg of amitriptyline or placebo. Although the study was confounded by other concurrent therapies, it is of note because chlorimipramine is a more selective 5-HT reuptake inhibitor than amitriptyline. In addition, the subjects were not depressed according to the Zung self-rating depression scale. On the other hand, two studies of imipramine in low back pain were inconclusive in separating an analgesic mechanism from an affective mechanism for TCA. Jenkins et al.[21] found 4 weeks of low-dose imipramine (25 mg t.i.d.) to be no different than placebo. Alcoff et al.[24] found a positive effect on patient reports of pain and function after 8 weeks of imipramine, 150 mg/day, versus placebo. However, they found no difference in physician ratings of the patients, nor were they conclusive in separating modulation of affect from modulation of pain.

Studies of experimental pain in humans do not support TCA analgesia. Chapman and Butler[38] used sensory decision theory to study the effects of 150 mg of doxepin on experimental pain in healthy volunteers. They found that both drug and placebo lowered subjects' willingness to report pain but did not alter pain detection threshold or sensory sensitivity. Using a similar technique, Davis et al.[39] found that depressed male patients were significantly *more* analgesic to experimental pain than depressed females or controls. These studies raise the question of the relationship between experimental and clinical pain and emphasize the need for careful control of doctor-patient interaction (e.g., placebo effects), depressive illness, and the sex compostion of patient groups.

It is possible that the apparent analgesic effects of TCAs are the result of changes in sleep. Moldofsky[40] reviewed the relationship between sleep patterns and pain. He suggests that a decreased amount of stage IV sleep is associated with musculoskeletal pain. This sleep change may be either causative or the result of neurophysiologic arousal secondary to pain. NE and 5-HT may be a common link in sleep physiology, some pain syndromes, and antidepressants.[41]

In summary, both theoretical investigations and animal studies suggest a TCA analgesic action not due to alleviation of depression. Several double-blind crossover studies in different homogeneous pain populations with and without depression are indicated before TCAs can be recommended for use in humans as an analgesic. In such studies, careful attention must be given to placebo effects, sleep recording, other forms of concurrent therapy, and TCA blood levels, in addition to dose. Animal studies provide evidence of involvement of both NE and 5-HT. Most antidepressants have variable effects on both of these neurotransmitters due to metabolites and widely varying rates of metabolism. Although the reuptake inhibition of antidepressants may be useful for analgesia, there is increasing evidence for the importance of TCA effects other than reuptake inhibition.

Clinical Use of Antidepressants

The first step in the use of antidepressants is proper diagnosis. The clinician must first decide if the major objective is relief of depressive illness. If this is the case, adequate doses must be used to obtain clinical benefit. Lower doses may be tried initially if antidepressants are being used for their hypnotic effect or for their putative analgesic effects. In the discussion that follows, it will be assumed that they are being used for treatment of depression.

In a typical therapeutic course, the initial dose will be determined by the patient's size, age, and general health. It is prudent to begin with no more than 50 mg at bedtime and increase the dose by 50 mg every three days up to 150 mg for most antidepressants. Table 30–2 lists the most effective antidepressant drugs available in the United States. They are all TCAs except for maprotiline, which is a tetracyclic antidepressant, trazodone, which is a phenylpiperazine derivative of triazolopyridine, and nomifensine, which is a tetrahydroisoquinoline derivative. Amoxapine and trazodone are one-half as potent as other TCAs. Desipramine is slightly more potent, nortriptyline is three times as potent, and protriptyline is five times as potent as other TCAs. In a patient who somatizes, has a somatoform disorder, or is very sensitive to and observant of any bodily changes, compliance will be improved if the dose is set initially at 10 mg, to be taken at bedtime, and increased every 4–6 days up to 150 mg. Lower doses should be used in the elderly, with an initial limit of 100 mg. A controlled study in outpatients[42] did not show any benefit from a divided daily dosage compared to a single bedtime dose. Of crucial importance for compliance is explaining to the patient and family that these drugs do not achieve their full therapeutic potential for 1–4 weeks. Patients must be prepared to tolerate side effects without initial benefit. Since many chronic pain patients are already leery of medications, it is also useful to assure them that the antidepressants are not addicting drugs. If the patient reports suicidal ideation, it is best to prescribe no more than 1 week's supply at a time and in smaller forms (i.e., 25- or 50-mg/tablets), which may result in a patient not taking enough pills to achieve a lethal dose. More pills will

also have to be taken daily for a therapeutic effect.

Adequate doses must be used for an adequate length of time if benefit is to be obtained. In most cases this means at least 150 mg/day for a 4-week trial. If no response is obtained after 2 weeks, the dose of most antidepressants can be gradually increased to 300 mg, or if side effects are intolerable, an alternative antidepressant can be used. Once a therapeutic response is achieved, the same dose should be maintained for at least a month. Most patients should have maintenance therapy for at least 6 months to prevent a relapse. If the dexamethasone suppression test was used initially and did not show suppression, then it can be repeated at 6 months or sooner if a patient cannot tolerate continued TCAs. If suppression now occurs, relapse is unlikely. Rebound insomnia sometimes occurs when a TCA is discontinued. Tapering the dosage over several weeks may diminish this effect. Chronic pain patients may require maintenance therapy for years. In such cases, antidepressants may be periodically discontinued while both patient and physician remain alert for early signs of relapse. At least one study has shown no adverse effects from prolonged (1–10 years) TCA therapy.[43]

The selection of a particular antidepressant should be determined by side effects and the patient's response to any previous TCA therapy. No TCA has been demonstrated to be more effective than any other. In general, the physician should consider using only TCAs or related newer agents, such as tetracyclic antidepressants, or the second-generation antidepressants, such as trazodone. Monoamine oxidase inhibitors are not considered to be as effective as TCAs in the treatment of a major depressive disorder.[44–47]

Adverse side effects occur in approximately 15%–20% of individuals given antidepressants.[45, 48] Autonomic anticholinergic and adrenergic side effects are numerous. Dry mouth is probably the most common side effect. It can be relieved by increased fluid intake and the use of salivary stimulants such as sugarless candy. Cycloplegia is also common but usually not long-lasting. Patients must be cautioned about using dangerous machinery if blurred vision is severe. The main difficulty is usually with reading. Inexpensive, nonprescription magnifying glasses may be helpful. Urinary retention can be a problem, most commonly in males with prostate enlargement; bethanechol, 10–25 mg t.i.d., may help. Constipation may occur as a result of either depressive illness or TCA use. Bran cereals and bulk lax-

TABLE 30–2.—CHARACTERISTICS OF ANTIDEPRESSANTS*

ANTIDEPRESSANT	DOSE RANGE (mg)	RELATIVE SEDATION†	RELATIVE ANTICHOLINERGIC POTENCY†	SUGGESTED SERUM LEVELS‡ (ng/ml)
Protriptyline	15–60	0	2	70
Desipramine	100–250	1	1	125
Amoxapine	150–600	1	1–2	
Imipramine	75–300	1–2	2	180
Nortriptyline	20–150	2	2	>50, <150
Maprotiline	75–300	2	1–2	
Trazodone	150–600	3	0	
Doxepin	75–300	3	2	100
Amitriptyline	75–300	3	3	160
Trimipramine	75–300	3		
Nomifensine	100–300	0	1	

*Based on data from Snyder and Yamamura,[44] Perry et al.,[45] Baldesserini,[46, 47] Ayd,[94] Amsterdam et al.,[95] Freedman and Gershon,[96] APA Task Force.[98]
†Greatest is 3.
‡Best measured 12 hours after last dose and avoiding Vacutainer rubber tops, which may react with blood and result in false low values. Values are the sum of drug and active metabolite levels.

atives such as Metamucil are useful adjuncts. Patients should be questioned about narrow angle glaucoma, and, if it is present, antidepressants should be used only after consultation with an ophthalmologist.

Delirium secondary to central anticholinergic effects is an important side effect, particularly in the elderly. It is manifested by several or all of the following: perceptual disturbances (misinterpretations, illusions, or hallucinations); incoherent speech; further alterations of sleep and psychomotor activity; disorientation; recent memory impairment; dry flushed skin, tachycardia, and elevated temperature.

The cardiovascular effects of antidepressants are probably the most serious side effects and include primarily conduction abnormalities, tachycardia, and orthostatic hypotension. Approximately 20% of patients given TCAs will demonstrate electrocardiogram (ECG) changes, including T wave flattening and prolongation of the PR interval.[48] A pretreatment ECG is indicated in patients over 50 or with a history of cardiovascular disease. A dose-related increase in intraventricular condition time has been demonstrated with some antidepressants. Doxepin has been reported to be free of this effect; however, some authors have questioned whether the doses and blood levels used were really equipotent.[46, 48] Patients with preexisting intraventricular conduction abnormalities (first- or second-degree AV blocks, bundle-branch block) are at increased risk for exacerbation of these abnormalities by antidepressants. On the other hand, ventricular arrhythmias (premature ventricular contractions) may improve with imipramine, permitting a decrease in the dosage of drugs given concomitantly, particularly quinidine.[49] Two uncontrolled retrospective studies suggest that amitriptyline is associated with sudden death in patients with coronary artery disease.[50, 51] Another study failed to confirm this finding,[52] but, at present, it seems prudent to avoid amitriptyline in patients with cardiac disease or abnormal ECGs.[53]

TCA-induced tachycardia can be a problem in patients with angina or overt congestive heart failure. TCA use results in an average increase of 7 to 16 beats per minute, usually with a greater increase when there is a slower predrug rate. There may be some decrease after 4 weeks. Amitriptyline and nortriptyline may cause more of a tachycardia than desipramine and imipramine.[48] It is unclear whether TCAs have any effect on the mechanical function of the human heart; if so, it is of practical importance only when there is overt heart failure.

By far the most common and serious cardiovascular complication is orthostatic hypotension. As many as 20% of all individuals given TCA will develop postural decreases in systolic blood pressure of more than 35 mm Hg.[48] It may occur at subtherapeutic doses (e.g., 75 mg). Adverse effects of orthostatic hypotension are particularly serious in the elderly, of whom 49% will suffer fractures and lacerations and 10%–15% will require a change in treatment.[48] Nortriptyline appears to cause less symptomatic orthostatic hypotension than other antidepressants.[54, 55] In using nortriptyline it is important to remember that there is a therapeutic window.[56] Plasma levels must be maintained between 50 and 150 mg/ml.[57]

Table 30–3 lists some important adverse drug interactions of TCAs. These probably will be true for second-generation antidepressants such as maprotiline and trazodone. Other rare miscellaneous side effects include nightmares, sexual dysfunction, skin rashes, and weight gain.

Depending on a physician's experience in treating depressed patients, psychiatric consultation may be useful at any point in the course of antidepressant therapy. When there is no therapeutic response, consultation may be beneficial to reconsider the diagnosis, the choice of antidepressant, or whether potentiating adjuncts such as thyroid hormone[56] or lithium[58] should be given. Electroconvulsive therapy may also be recommended. Despite the social stigma, electroconvulsive therapy is the quickest and safest form of antidepressant therapy.[46, 48]

ADJUNCTIVE PSYCHOTROPIC DRUGS

Sedative-Hypnotics

Insomnia and agitation due to depressive illness usually respond to treatment with one of the initially sedating antidepressants. Occasionally a patient may require an additional hypnotic for the first few days, but generally not for more than 2 weeks.

Separate from depression, some patients have anxiety as a personality trait such that their habitual style of response is with anxiety. Sedatives are generally best avoided in these individuals except for transient periods of acute, exacerbating stress. Nonpharmacologic therapy such as self-relaxation is more appropriate to avoid psychological or physiologic addiction to drugs.

TABLE 30–3.—IMPORTANT DRUG INTERACTIONS
WITH TRICYCLIC ANTIDEPRESSANTS

DRUG	REACTION BY DRUG	REACTION BY TCA
Alcohol	Lowers blood levels	In initial week can potentiate CNS effects of alcohol
Antihypertensives		
Guanethidine		Decreases effectiveness
Clonidine		Decreases effectiveness (at least desipramine does)
Barbiturates	Lower blood levels	
Diphenylhydantoin	Increases blood levels	
Phenothiazines and related neuroleptics	Increase blood levels	
Sympathomimetic amines (especially IV epinephrine, norepinephrine, phenylephrine)		Increases pressor response

Anxiety may also present as a specific new state or disorder as the result of a patient's attempt to cope and adapt to the stresses of chronic pain. The stresses may be internal, external, or both. An anxiety state is considered a disorder or maladaptation when it causes impairment in social or occupational functioning and has symptoms in excess of a normal and expectable reaction to the stress of pain. The three psychiatric disorders most likely to be seen in the chronic pain patient are posttraumatic stress disorder (acute or chronic), adjustment disorder with anxious mood, and social phobia.[59] These disorders are often characterized by sleep disturbance and avoidance of activities that arouse recollection of the initial onset of pain or in which the individual has an unrealistic fear that he will suffer humiliation or embarrassment. Furthermore, there may be episodes of fear with concomitant somatic symptoms such as motor tension, autonomic hyperactivity, and hyper-alertness or vigilance. Such individuals may benefit from periodic courses of a sedative agent (approximately 2–3 months) in conjunction with supportive counseling or behavior therapy.

The sedative-hypnotics carry a potential for drug abuse. The risk in an individual patient is not easy to predict, but the following characteristics should raise suspicions of drug abuse potential: (1) over-emphasizing the need for drugs, (2) history of a depleted supply from another physician, (3) alcoholism or other drug abuse, (4) spontaneous dose increases by the patient in the first few weeks. Patients with a marked anxiety personality trait, when transiently treated, may require higher than average doses. Some individuals require the reassurance of having the drug with them at all times even though

they do not frequently use it. These two situations are not considered abuse.[60]

Table 30–4 lists the recommended sedative-hypnotics and their characteristics. Although many sedative-hypnotic agents are available, some are more toxic than others (e.g., short-acting barbiturates, propanediols, glutethimide, methyprylon, methaqualone). The benzodiazepines are generally the drugs of choice because of their demonstrated efficacy, low lethality, and lack of hepatic enzyme induction. Benzodiazepines appear to interfere less with rapid-eye-movement (REM) sleep and cause less or no withdrawal rebound insomnia, compared to other hypnotics.[61] Most of these drugs have long half-lives, especially those with active metabolites. Thus, there is no reason to prescribe these drugs in multiple doses for daily use.[62] If given 1–2 hours before bedtime in equipotent doses, most benzodiazepines act as hypnotics and provide anxio-

TABLE 30–4.—SEDATIVE-HYPNOTICS

AGENTS	DOSE RANGE (mg/day)	HALF-LIFE *(Range, hr)	ACTIVE METABOLITES
Benzodiazepine sedative-anxiolytics			
Alprazolam	0.5–4	12	
Chlordiazepoxide	15–100	5–30	Yes
Clorazepate	15–60	30–200	Yes
Diazepam	6–40	20–50	Yes
Lorazepam	2–6	10–15	No
Oxazepam	30–120	5–20	No
Prazepam	10–60	30–200	Yes
Benzodiazepine hypnotics			
Flurazepam	15–30	50–100	Yes
Temazepam	15–30	9–12	No
Triazolam	0.125–0.5	2–5	No
Others			
Phenobarbital	30–90	48–144	No
Chloral hydrate	500–2,000	7–10	Yes

*Including active metabolites.

lytic effects during the next day,[60, 63-65]

There appear to be two separate types of brain receptors specific for benzodiazepines. In animals the two receptors have differing anxiolytic and sedative properties and drug affinities.[66]

Flurazepam, temazepam and triazolam are marketed solely as hypnotics, partly because blood levels of these compounds reach peak levels quickly to drop to subhypnotic levels by the next day. Flurazepam, however, does result in the accumulation of active metabolites. In healthy males this drug impairs psychomotor performance the next day, although temazepam does not.[67] This may not be true in insomniacs.[68] Temazepam and triazolam have also been promoted as superior to flurazepam because they produce less REM sleep suppression. The significance of the amount of REM sleep, however, is still controversial.[69] Accumulation of metabolites can be a serious problem, especially in the elderly. For this reason, drugs without active metabolites are often recommended. Nevertheless, potent benzodiazepines without active metabolites may cause anterograde amnesia or result in rebound anxiety the following day if drug levels drop markedly.[70]

The most common side effect of all these drugs is daytime sedation with impairment of cognition and coordination. Cigarette smoking diminishes the incidence of drowsiness in people taking diazepam and chlordiazepoxide, while the elderly are more susceptible to sedative effects.[71] All benzodiazepines produce a dose-related decrease in the speed of psychomotor test performance which is not strictly related to half-life.[68] Anterograde amnesia for information presented during the night following bedtime administration of benzodiazepine has also been reported.[72] Potentiation of other psychotropic drugs is common. Ethanol increases diazepam absorption.[73] Benzodiazepines do not usually produce physiologic addiction when used at doses less than 40 mg/day.[72, 74] Overdoses are seldom lethal when taken alone, but they are much more hazardous in combination with ethanol.

Neuroleptics

Antipsychotic (neuroleptic) medications such as phenothiazines and butyrophenones have historically been used as adjunctive anesthetic/analgesic agents. Chlorpromazine was first used in 1951 as a preanesthetic sedative. Droperidol is now frequently used with fentanyl to induce apathy and psychomotor immobility as a supplement to general anesthesia.[75] In 1965 Janssen[76] developed haloperidol in the search for synthetic opiates. Bloomfield et al.[77] reported improvement of pain in 9 of 18 cancer and arthritis patients treated with levomepromazine. Subsequently, several others have described beneficial effects of other neuroleptics alone or in combination with antidepressants.[78–81]

With the discovery of the endogenous opiate-like system, investigators have measured the interaction of psychotropic drugs, including neuroleptics, with opiate receptors in neural tissue. Anticholinergics, antidepressants, and neuroleptics have been shown to inhibit the binding of radiolabeled enkephalins to opiate receptors.[82, 83] The functional significance and specificity of enkephalins is far from clear, but studies using neuroleptics with different properties is one important technique for investigating the specificity of the endogenous opiate-like system. For example, Somoza et al.[84] found that haloperidol and chlorpromazine inhibit met-enkephalin binding more than leu-enkephalin binding. Clay and Brougham[85] found that haloperidol displaces (3H)-naloxone with characteristics of a weak agonist. However, these in vitro kinetic analyses also indicated that several neuroleptics interact with the receptor by a multiprocess mode of action rather than by simple competitive or noncompetitive inhibition. Creese et al.[86] measured the opiate receptor interaction of numerous butyrophenones and phenothiazines. They found that benperidol and pimozide were nearly as potent opiate receptor binders as morphine and more potent opiate receptor binders than meperidine or propoxyphene. However, the binding of these two neuroleptics was characteristic of opiate antagonists since binding was not inhibited by 100 mM NaCl. Of the phenothiazines, thioridazine had a receptor affinity approximately equal to that of meperidine and seven times greater than that of fluphenazine. Nevertheless, thioridazine's affinity response to NaCl was that of an antagonist, while fluphenazine responded as a weak agonist. Differences in experimental methods, tissue preparation, and radioactive ligand used have led to conflicting results. For example, in contrast to Creese et al.,[86] Clay and Brougham[85] reported that pimozide did not inhibit naloxone binding and that haloperidol binding was greatly inhibited with 100 mM NaCl.

Opiate receptor affinity studies lend theoretical support to those studies using neuroleptics for the treatment of opiate withdrawal in animals and narcotic potentiation or substitution in man. As noted earlier, several collections of case reports have found neuroleptics to be beneficial in chronic pain. Unfortunately, few well-controlled studies substantiate the use of neuroleptics as analgesics, and Baldesserini has stated that antipsychotic drugs are not useful in opiate withdrawal in man.[47] Much of the literature regarding chronic pain and neuroleptics consists of collections of uncontrolled case reports. In several of the cases, psychosis was a prominent feature of the patient's condition.[79, 87] Furthermore, the effective dose has ranged from 1 mg of fluphenazine or haloperidol to 40 mg of haloperidol.[79] The latter dose is quite high and likely to result in a strong, often unpleasant degree of sedation as opposed to analgesia. It is also important to account for the different effects of neuroleptics on sleep.[88] As with the TCAs, the major benefit of neuroleptics in chronic pain may be due to changes in sleep patterns or nonspecific sedation rather than to direct analgesia. With respect to acute pain, McGee and Alexander[89] reviewed 16 available double-blind studies of phenothiazine analgesia or narcotic potentiation. Six of the studies were placebo-controlled crossover in design: three of these studies found no beneficial effect of promazine, promethazine, or propiomaxine, two found a beneficial effect of methotrimeprozine, and one found a beneficial effect of chlorpromazine. On the basis of their review, McGee and Alexander concluded that the risk of neuroleptic side effects (sedation, hypotension, extrapyramidal movement disorders) was greater than the possible benefit.

As with several other aspects of pain research, experimental and laboratory findings concerning neuroleptics have yet to be adequately tested clinically. Before neuroleptics can be recommended for regular use in chronic pain, further empirical research is necessary. Such research should include the use of a double-blind crossover design, patients with homogeneous pain etiologies, measurement of blood levels of neuroleptics, and monitoring of sleep and sedation.

Placebos

Approximately one third of the population will respond to placebos.[90] This response may be related to release of endorphin-like substances.[91] Accordingly, placebo response is a poor means of diagnosis, and the use of placebos is discouraged in the management of pain unless it is with the informed consent of the patient.[92, 93] If the patient discovers that the physician has been surreptitiously administering placebos, then trust in the doctor-patient relationship will be greatly if not irreparably damaged. On the other hand when informed in advance, some patients may desire to make use of their potential placebo response in order to reduce intake of active medications. Furthermore, the physician can use the power of positive suggestion to enhance active medication response in positive placebo responders.

REFERENCES

1. Graham L.F.: Plasma level monitoring of tricyclic antidepressant therapy. *Clin. Pharmacokinet.* 2:237–251, 1977.
2. Nagy A., Treiber L.: Quantitative determination of imipramine and desipramine in human blood by direct densitometry of thin-layer chromatography. *J. Pharm. Pharmacol.* 25:599–603, 1973.
3. Zeigler V.E., Meyer D.A., Rosen S.H., et al.: Amitriptyline dosage schedule sampling time and tricyclic plasma levels. *Br. J. Psychiatry* 131:168–173, 1977.
4. Charney D.S., Menkes D.B., Heninger G.R.: Receptor sensitivity and the mechanism of action of antidepressant treatment: Implications for the etiology and treatment of depression. *Arch. Gen. Psychiatry* 38:1160–1180, 1981.
5. Berger P.A., Barchas J.O.: Biochemical hypotheses of affective disorder, in Barchas J.D., Berger P.A., Ciaranello R.D., et al. (eds.): *Psychopharmacology: From Theory to Practice.* New York, Oxford University Press, 1977.
6. Charney D.S., Heninger G.R., Sternberg D.E., et al.: Presynoptic adrenergic receptor sensitivity in depression. *Arch. Gen. Psychiatry* 38:1334–1340, 1981.
7. Scott W.A.: The relief of pain with an antidepressant in arthritis. *Practitioner* 202:802–807, 1969.
8. Gringras M.: A clinical trial of Tofranil in rheumatic pain in general practice. *J. Int. Med. Res.* 4 (suppl.): 41–49, 1976.
9. Tyler G.S., McNeely H.E., Dick M.L.: Treatment of post-traumatic headache with amitriptyline. *Headache* 20:213–216, 1980.
10. Morland, T.J., Storli O.V., Mogstad T.E.: Doxepin in the prophylactic treatment of mixed vascular and tension headache. *Headache* 19:382–383, 1979.
11. Couch J.R., Hassanein R.S.: Amitriptyline in migraine prophylaxis. *Arch. Neurol.* 36:695–699, 1979.
12. Gomershall J.D., Stuart A.: Amitriptyline in migraine prophylaxis: Changes in pattern of attack during a controlled clinical trial. *J. Neurol. Neurosurg. Psychiatry* 36:684–690, 1973.
13. Couch J.R., Ziegler D.K., Hassanein R.S.: Evalua-

tion of amitriptyline in migraine prophylaxis. *Trans. Am. Neurol. Assoc.* 99:94–98, 1974.

14. Couch J.R., Hassanein R.S.: Migraine and depression: Effect of amitriptyline prophylaxis. *Trans. Am. Neurol. Assoc.* 101:234–237, 1976.

15. Diamond S., Baltes B.J.: Chronic tension headache treated with amitriptyline: A double blind study. *Headache* 11:110–116, 1971.

16. Okasha A., Ghaleb H.A., Sadek A.: A double blind trial for the clinical management of psychogenic headache. *Br. J. Psychiatry* 122:181–183, 1973.

17. Ellman S.J., Arkin A.M., Nelson W.T., et al.: Sleep-related periodic headache and imipramine. *Int. J. Neurosci.* 7:22–27, 1976.

18. Couch J.R., Ziegler D.K., Hassanein R.: Amitriptyline in the prophylaxis of migraine: Effectiveness and relationship of anti-migraine and antidepressant effects. *Neurology* 26:121–127, 1976.

19. Lance J.W., Curran D.A.: Treatment of chronic tension headache. *Lancet* 1:1236–1239, 1964.

20. Carrasso R.L., Yehuda S., Streifler M.: Chlormipramine and amitriptyline in the treatment of severe pain. *Int. J. Neurosc.* 9:191–194, 1979.

21. Jenkins D.G., Ebbutt A.F., Evans C.D.: Tofranil in the treatment of low back pain. *J. Int. Med. Res.* 4 (suppl.2):28–40, 1976.

22. Ward N.G., Bloom V.L., Friedel R.D.: The effectiveness of tricyclic antidepressants in the treatment of coexisting pain and depression. *Pain* 7:331–341, 1979.

23. Dalessio D.J.: Chronic pain syndromes and disordered cortical inhibition: Effects of tricyclic compounds. *Dis. Nerv. System* 28:325–328, 1967.

24. Alcoff J., Jones E., Rust P., et al.: Controlled trial of imipramine for chronic low back pain. *J. Fam. Pract.* 14:841–846, 1982.

25. Sternbach R.A., Janowsky D.S., Huey L.Y., et al.: Effect of altering brain serotonin activity on human chronic pain. *Adv. Pain Res. Ther.* 1:601–606, 1976.

26. Segal M., Sandberg D.: Analgesia produced by electrical stimulation of catecholamine nuclei in the rat brain. *Brain Res.* 123:369, 1977.

27. Zemlan F.P., Corrigan S.A., Pfaff D.W.: Noradrenergic and serotonergic medition of spinal analgesia mechanisms. *Eur. J. Pharmacol.* 61:111–124, 1980.

28. Bowker R.M., Coulter J.D.: Studies of descending projections from caudal medulla in the cat. *Soc. Neurosci. Abst.* 4:291, 1978.

29. Engberg I., Ryall R.W.: The inhibitory action of noradrenaline and other monoamines on spinal neurons. *J. Physiol. (Lond.)* 185:298–322, 1966.

30. Oleson T.D., Liebeskind J.C.: Relationship of neural activity in the raphe nuclei of the rat to brain stimulation-produced analgesia. *Physiologist* 18:338, 1975.

31. Oliveras J.L., Redjeini G., Guilbaud G., et al.: Analgesia induced by electrical stimulation of the inferior centralis nucleus of the raphe in the cat. *Pain* 1:139–145, 1975.

32. Basbaum A.I., Fields H.L.: The origin of descending pathways in the dorsolateral funiculus of the spinal cord of the cat and rat. *J. Comp. Neurol.* 187:413–432, 1979.

33. Jordan L.M., Kenshalo Jr. D.R., Martin R.F., et al.: Two populations of spinothalamic tract neurons with opposite responses to 5-hydroxytryptamine. *Brain Res.* 164:342–346, 1979.

34. Shiomi H., Takagi H.: Morphine analgesia and the bulbospinal noradrenergic system: Increase in the concentration of normetanephrine in the spinal cord of the rat caused by analgesics. *Br. J. Pharmacol.* 52:519–526, 1974.

35. Takagi H., Shiomi H., Kuraishi Y., et al.: Pain and the bulbospinal noradrenergic system: Pain-induced increase in normetanephrine content in the spinal cord and its modification by morphine. *Eur. J. Pharmacol.* 54:99–107, 1979.

36. Lee R., Spencer P.S.J.: Antidepressants and pain. *J. Int. Med. Res.* 5(suppl.):146–156, 1977.

37. Oxman T.E., Hitzemann R.J.: Serotonin and platelet membrane abnormalities in migraine, in Rose F.C. (ed.): *Progress in Migraine Research*, ed. 2. London, Pitman Books Ltd., 1984, pp. 186–193.

38. Chapman C.R., Butler S.H.: Effects of doxepin on perception of laboratory-induced pain in man. *Pain* 5:253–262, 1978.

39. Davis G.C., Buchsbaum M.S., Bunney W.E.: Analgesia to painful stimuli in affective illness. *Am. J. Psychiatry* 136:1148–1151, 1979.

40. Moldofsky H.: Rheumatic pain modulation syndrome: The interrelationships between sleep, central nervous system serotonin, and pain. *Adv. Neurol.* 33:51–57, 1982.

41. Kay D.C., Blackburn A.B., Buckingham J.A., et al.: Human pharmacology of sleep, in Williams R.L., Karacan I. (eds): *Pharmacology of Sleep*. New York, John Wiley & Sons, Inc., 1976, pp. 83–209.

42. Weise C.C., Stein M.K., Pereira-Ogan J., et al.: Amitriptyline once daily versus three times daily in depressed outpatients. *Arch. Gen. Psychiatry* 37:555–560, 1980.

43. Ayd F.: Continuation and maintenance of doxepin (Sinequan) therapy: Ten years experience. *Int. Drug Ther. Newsletter* 14:9–16, 1979.

44. Snyder S., Yamamura H.: Antidepressants and the muscarini acetylcholine receptor. *Arch. Gen. Psychiatry* 34:236–239, 1977.

45. Perry P.J., Alexander B., Liskow B.I.: *Psychotropic Drug Handbook,* ed. 3. Cincinnati, Harvey Whitney Books, 1981.

46. Baldesserini R.J.: *Chemotherapy in Psychiatry.* Cambridge, Mass., Harvard University Press, 1977.

47. Baldesserini R.J.: Drugs and the treatment of psychiatric disorders, in Gilman A.G., Goodman L.S., Gilman A. (eds.): *Goodman and Gilman's The Pharmacologic Basis of Therapeutics,* ed. 6. New York, Macmillan Publishing Co., Inc., 1980, pp. 391–447.

48. Glassman A.H., Bigger J.: Cardiovascular effects of therapeutic doses of tricyclic antidepressants: A review. *Arch. Gen. Psychiatry* 38:815–820, 1981.

49. Bigger J.T., Giarding E.G.V., Perel J.M., et al.: Cardiac antiarrhythmic effect of imipramine hydrochloride. *N. Engl. J. Med.* 296:206–208, 1977.

50. Coull D.C., Crooks J., Fordyce D.I., et al.: A method of monitoring drugs for adverse reactions: II. Amitriptyline and cardiac disease. *Eur. J. Clin. Pharmacol.* 3:51–53, 1970.

51. Moir D.C., Crooks J., Cornwell W.B., et al.: Cardiotoxicity of amitriptyline. *Lancet* 2:561–564, 1972.

52. Boston Collaborative Drug Surveillance Program Report: Adverse reactions to the tricyclic antidepressant drugs. *Lancet* 1:529–531, 1972.

53. Jefferson J.W.: A review of the cardiovascular effects and toxicity of tricyclic antidepressants. *Psychosom. Med.* 37:160–179, 1975.

54. Reed K., Smith R.C., Schoolar J.C., et al.: Cardiovascular effects of nortriptyline in geriatric patients. *Am. J. Psychiatry* 137:986–989, 1980.

55. Roose S.P., Glassman A.H., Siris S.G., et al.: Comparison of imipramine- and nortriptyline-induced orthostatic hypotension: A meaningful difference. *J. Clin. Psychopharmacol.* 1:316–319, 1981.

56. Whybrow P.C., Prange A.J.: A hypothesis of thyroid-catecholamine-receptor interaction: Its relevance to affective illness. *Arch. Gen. Psychiatry* 38:106–113, 1981.

57. Amsterdam J., Brunswick D., Mendels J.: The clinical application of tricyclic antidepressant pharmacolinetics and plasma levels. *Am. J. Psychiatry* 137:653–662.

58. DeMontigny C., Grunberg F., Mayer A., et al.: Lithium induces rapid relief of depression in tricyclic antidepressant drug non-responders. *Br. J. Psychiatry* 138:252–256, 1981.

59. Lee R., Spencer R.S.J.: Antidepressants and pain. *J. Int. Med. Res.* 5(suppl 10):146–156, 1977.

60. Hartmann E.: The effect of four drugs on sleep patterns in man. *Psychopharmacologia* 12:346–353, 1968.

61. Greenblatt D.J., Shader R.I.: Benzodiazepine (second of two parts). *N. Engl. J. Med.* 291:1239–1243, 1974.

62. Magnus R.V.: Once-a-day potassium chlorazepate in anxiety. *Br. J. Clin. Pract.* 27:449–452, 1973.

63. Kales A., Scharf M.B.: Sleep laboratory and clinical effects of benzodiazepines on sleep: Fluorozepam, diazepam, chlordiazepoxide, and RO 5-4200, in Garattini S., Mussini E., Randall L.O. (eds.): *The Benzodiazepines*. New York, Raven Press, 1973, pp. 577–598.

64. Itil T.M., Saletu B., Marasa J.: Digital computer analyzed sleep EEG in predicting the anxiolytic properties of chorazepate dipotassium (Tranxene). *Curr. Ther. Res.* 14:415–427, 1972.

65. Imlah N.W.: Clinical experience with lorazepam in hospital patients. *Curr. Med. Res. Opin.* 1:276–281, 1973.

66. Hoehn-Saric R.: Neurotransmitters in anxiety. *Arch. Gen. Psychiatry* 39:735–742, 1982.

67. Roth T., Piccione P., Salis P., et al.: Effects of temazepam, flurazepam, and quinalbaibitone on sleep: Psychomotor and cognitive function. *Br. J. Clin. Pharmacol.* 8(suppl. 1):47s–54s, 1979.

68. Johnson L.C., Chernik D.A.: Sedative-hypnotics and human performance. *Psychopharmacology* 76:101–113, 1982.

69. Feinberg I., Fein G., Walker J.M., et al.: Flurazepam effects on sleep EEG. *Arch. Gen. Psychiatry* 36:95–102, 1979.

70. Dundee J.W., Lilburn J.K., Nair S.G., et al.: Studies of drugs given before anesthesia: XXVI. Lorazepam. *Br. J. Anaesth.* 49:1047, 1977.

71. Boston Collaborative Drug Surveillance Program: Clinical depression of the central nervous system due to diazepam and chlordiazepoxide in relation to cigarette smoking and age. *N. Engl. J. Med.* 288:277–279, 1973.

72. Hollister L.E., Conley F.K., Britt R.H., et al.: Long-term use of diazepam. *JAMA* 246:1568–1570, 1981.

73. Hayes S.L., Pablo G., Radomski T., et al.: Ethanol and oral diazepam absorption. *N. Engl. J. Med.* 296:186–189, 1977.

74. Abernathy D.R., Greenblatt D.J., Shader R.I.: Treatment of diazepam withdrawal syndrome with propranolol. *Ann. Intern. Med.* 94:354–355, 1981.

75. High-dose fentanyl, editorial. *Lancet* 1:81–82, 1979.

76. Janssen P.A.J.: The butyrophenone story, in Ayd F.J., Blackwell B. (eds.): *Discoveries in Biological Psychiatry*. Philadelphia, J.B. Lippincott Co., 1970, pp. 165–179.

77. Bloomfield S., Simard-Savoie S., Bernier J., et al.: Comparative analgesic activity of levomepromazine and morphine in patients with chronic pain. *Can. Med. Assoc. J.* 90:1156–1159, 1964.

78. Kocher R.: The use of psychotropic drugs in the treatment of chronic, severe pains. *Eur. Neurol.* 14:458–464, 1976.

79. Maltbie A.A., Cavenar J.O., Sullivan J.L., et al.: Analgesia and haloperidol: A hypothesis. *J. Clin. Psychiatry* 40:323–326, 1979.

80. Davis J.L., Lewis S.B., Gerich J.E., et al.: Peripheral diabetic neuropathy treated with amitriptyline and fluphenazine *JAMA* 238:2291–2292, 1977.

81. Turkington R.W.: Depression masquerading as diabetic neuropathy. *JAMA* 243:1147, 1980.

82. Somoza E.: Influence of neuroleptics on the binding of met-enkephalin, morphine and dihydromorphine to synaptosome-enriched fractions of rat brain. *Neuropharmacology* 17:577–581, 1978.

83. Somoza E., Galindo A., Bazan E., et al.: Antidepressants inhibit enkephalin binding to synaptosome-enriched fractions of rat brain. *Neuropsychobiology* 7:297–301, 1981.

84. Somoza E., Bazan E., Galindo A.: Inhibition of leu-enkephalin binding by neuroleptics. *Neuropsychobiology* (in press).

85. Clay G.A., Brougham L.R.: Haloperidol binding to an opiate receptor site. *Biochem. Pharmacol.* 24:1363–1367, 1975.

86. Creese I., Feinberg A.P., Snyder S.H.: Butyrophenone influences on the opiate receptor. *Eur. J. Pharmacol.* 36:231–235, 1976.

87. Taub A.: Relief of posttherapeutic neuralgia with psychotropic drugs. *J. Neurosurg.* 39:235–239, 1973.

88. Hartmann E., Spinweber C.: The effects of psychotropic medication on sleep, in Usdin E., Forrest I.S. (eds.) *Psychotherapeutic Drugs. Part 1: Principles.* New York, Marcel Dekker, 1976, pp. 665–698.

89. McGee J.L., Alexander M.R.: Phenothiazine analgesia: Fact or fantasy? *Am. J. Hosp. Pharm.* 36:633–640, 1979.

90. Beecher H.K.: *Measurement of Subjective Responses.* New York, Oxford University Press, 1959, pp. 65–72.

91. Levine J.D., Gordon N.C., Fields H.L.: The mechanism of placebo analgesia. *Lancet* 2:654–657, 1978.

92. Silber T.J.: Placebo therapy. *JAMA* 242:245–246, 1979.

93. Pfefferbaum A.: The placebo, in Barchas J.D., Berger P.A., Ciarnello R.D., et al.: (eds.): *Psychopharmacology: From Theory to Practice.* New York, Oxford University Press, 1977, pp. 493–503.

94. Ayd F.: Continuation and maintenance of doxepin (Sinequan) therapy: Ten years' experience. *Int. Drug Ther. Newsletter* 14:9–16, 1979.

95. Amsterdam J., Brunswick D., Mendels J.: The clinical application of tricyclic antidepressant pharmacokinetics and plasma levels. *Am. J. Psychiatry* 137:653–662, 1980.

96. Freedman D.X. Gershon S.: Pharmacology, efficacy and safety of a new antidepressant. *J. Clin. Psychopharmacol.* 2(suppl.): 93, 1981.

97. Siever L.J., Davis K.L.: Overview: toward a dysregulation hypothesis of depression. *Am. J. Psychiatry* 142:1017–1031, 1985.

98. American Psychiatric Association Task Force on the Use of Laboratory Tests in Psychiatry: Tricyclic antidepressants: Blood level measurements and clinical outcome. *Am. J. Psychiatry* 142:155–162, 1985.

31 / Local Anesthetics

RUDOLPH H. de JONG, M.D.

THE MOLECULAR CHAIN that links the lipophilic aromatic portion of the local anesthetic molecule to the hydrophilic aliphatic amine portion determines many key properties. The two major linkage groups are the *ester* and the *amide* bonds. The former group has benzoic acid derivatives as its aromatic foundation, the latter is built up from derivatives of aniline. The subsequent synthesis of the local anesthetic molecule entails linking the aromatic foundation to an amino alcohol or amino acid, as shown in Fig 31–1.

Ester-linked local anesthetics such as procaine and tetracaine are readily hydrolyzed in aqueous surroundings to the parent aromatic acid and amino alcohol. Amide-linked anesthetics such as lidocaine and mepivacaine, on the other hand, are much more resistant to immediate hydrolysis and must undergo one or more preliminary degradation steps. Resistance of the amide bond to nonenzymatic hydrolysis is well shown by the ability of amide-linked anesthetics to withstand autoclaving without significant loss of potency.

ESTER-LINKED LOCAL ANESTHETICS

This important class of local anesthetics has in common ester-linkage to benzoic acid or benzoic acid derivatives (Fig 31–2). Cocaine (the first local anesthetic discovered) is an ester, and subsequently developed local anesthetics (e.g., procaine) all were esters too. Not till the middle of this century was a new class of local anesthetics, the amide-linked group, synthesized.

Cocaine

Cocaine, a rather complex alkaloid, is obtained from the leaves of the Peruvian coca shrub. Chem-ically, it is the benzoyl methyl ester of *ecgonine*, a 2-carboxy derivative of tropine. The latter, an amino alcohol, is in turn the major constituent of atropine. Cocaine is used as a topical anesthetic, especially of the nose and throat, where it causes local vasoconstriction by inhibiting reuptake of norepinephrine. Mood elevation is a much sought-after property, and cocaine is an ingredient of Brompton's cocktail, useful in treating terminally ill cancer patients. Addiction and high toxicity are the main drawbacks of cocaine use.

Since cocaine is a double ester, two routes of hydrolysis are available, one yielding the methyl, the other the benzoyl ester. The direction and rate of hydrolysis both are species dependent. In man, mainly dependent on nonenzymic hydrolysis, up to one fifth of the administered dose of cocaine is eliminated unchanged in the urine.

Procaine

Procaine (Novocaine), one of many synthetic para-aminobenzoic acid esters, has long been synonymous with local anesthesia. As more potent, longer acting, and more readily diffusible amide-linked anesthetics are available, it is little used in the United States.

The first step in procaine metabolism is hydrolysis—by plasma enzymes in man—to form para-aminobenzoic acid (PABA) and diethylaminoethanol. Little if any of the drug is metabolized in neural tissue or spinal fluid. In man, hydrolysis of procaine is complete, and only traces of the parent substance is found in urine.

The plasma enzyme originally designated as procainesterase has since been shown to be pseudocholinesterase. Low pseudocholinesterase levels, encountered in patients with advanced liver disease or

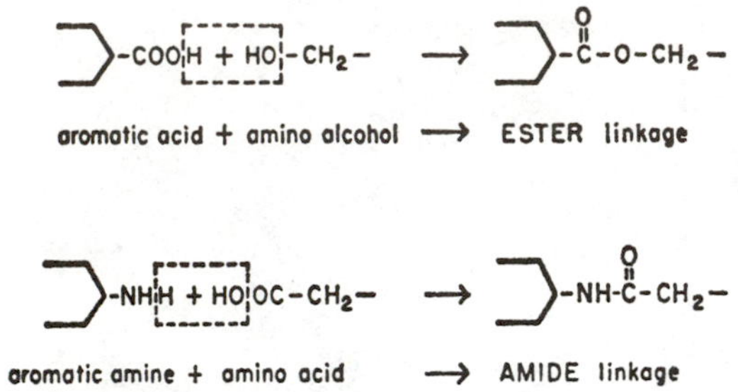

Fig 31–1.—Synthesis of the all-important linkage from basic aromatic building blocks. One molecule of water *(broken lines)* splits off. (From de Jong R.H.: *Local Anesthetics.* Springfield, Illinois, Charles C Thomas, Publishers, 1977. Reproduced by permission.)

an inherited defect, could give rise to persistently elevated procaine levels and protracted toxic symptoms. Where this condition is present or suspected, a local anesthetic metabolized in different fashion— lidocaine, for instance—would be the better choice.

Procaine Analogues

A fascinating aspect of local anesthetics is that minor alterations in the molecule produce major differences in biologic properties. For instance, 2-chloroprocaine hydrochloride (chloroprocaine, Nesacaine) is hydrolyzed about four times faster than

procaine in human plasma. Because of faster intravascular metabolism, chloroprocaine is less toxic than procaine. This property has made chloroprocaine a popular drug in obstetrics, all the more so because the fetus can metabolize any drug spilled over into the fetal circulation. In pain control, chloroprocaine has gained popularity because of its rapid onset, brief duration, and low systemic toxicity. Metabolism is similar to that of procaine, except that meta-chloro-PABA rather than PABA is formed.

Reports have appeared of prolonged neurologic deficits following unintended intrathecal placement of large volumes of chloroprocaine intended for extradural analgesia. The exact mechanism is unclear but may be related to the acid preservative in commercial solutions inhibiting chloroprocaine hydrolysis in spinal fluid. When injected extradurally, a test dose given prior to the full therapeutic dose will confirm placement outside the dural membrane.

Tetracaine

Substitution of the para-amino group on procaine's aromatic ring with a butyl-amino radical (and shortening the alkyl-amino tail) yields tetracaine (Pontocaine, Amethocaine). This fairly simple substitution spawns a radically different local anesthetic that is ten times more potent and about four times more slowly hydrolyzed than procaine. Unfor-

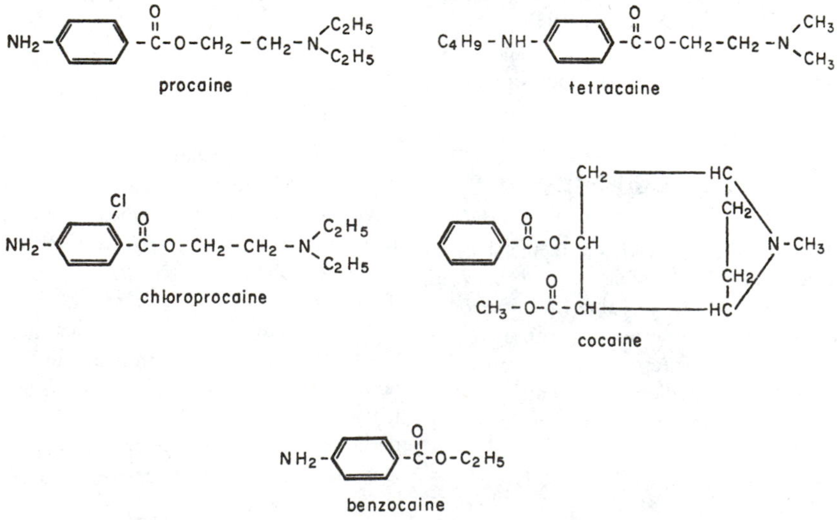

Fig 31–2.—Ester-linked local anesthetics in common use. Cocaine is the only naturally occurring anesthetic. (From de Jong R.H.: *Local Anesthetics.* Springfield, Illinois, Charles C Thomas, Publishers, 1977. Reproduced by permission.)

tunately, tetracaine is also about ten times more toxic than procaine, so its net therapeutic advantage resides mainly in longer duration of action. When used as the sole agent to block peripheral nerves, tetracaine has been disappointing in that diffusion is slow, causing an uncomfortably prolonged induction time. If tetracaine is mixed with faster-diffusing agents (e.g., lidocaine, mepivacaine), however, rapid induction and a long-lasting block can be achieved. Little is known about the fate of tetracaine other than that labeled drug appears in quantity in the bile.

Benzocaine

The ethyl ester of PABA lacks the hydrophilic amine tail characteristic of other local anesthetics, making it nearly insoluble in water (1 part in 2,500). Even so, benzocaine possesses the classic chemical configuration of a local anesthetic. Irritating on injection, it is used primarily as a surface anesthetic. With a pK_a well below physiologic range, benzocaine exists almost entirely as the undissociated base, producing anesthesia by membrane swelling rather than by specific receptor binding.

AMIDE-LINKED LOCAL ANESTHETICS

The amide-linked local anesthetics (Fig 31–3) are much more resistant to hydrolysis than their ester-linked cousins. In most cases, the molecule must be transformed into a simpler form before it can be cleaved at the linkage. Enzymatic mechanisms for reducing tertiary amines to secondary and primary amines by N-dealkylation facilitate subsequent hydrolysis of the amide linkage, presumably hastening elimination thereby. Nevertheless, the plasma half-life of lidocaine in man is 90 minutes, versus just a few minutes for procaine.

Lidocaine

In the 35 years since its discovery, lidocaine (Xylocaine, lignocaine) has supplanted procaine as *the* standard local anesthetic. Though its activity/toxicity ratio is not much different from that of procaine, lidocaine diffuses faster and yields a more solid block. In addition, anesthesia lasts longer than with procaine. Further, and again supplanting a procaine analogue (procainamide), lidocaine has found unexpected application in the treatment of cardiac arrhythmias. Small wonder, then, that more is known about lidocaine than about any other local anesthetic.

Where not contraindicated, addition of a vasoconstrictor such as epinephrine to the anesthetic solution is desirable to slow drug absorption, particularly when injecting into vascular regions. A bonus of this practice is prolongation of anesthesia, without incurring the penalty of slower induction. Little epinephrine is needed, with concentrations in the 4–5 µg/ml (1/200,000 to 1/250,000) range providing optimal conditions.

Lidocaine is metabolized in the liver by microsomes whose synthesis is potentially susceptible to

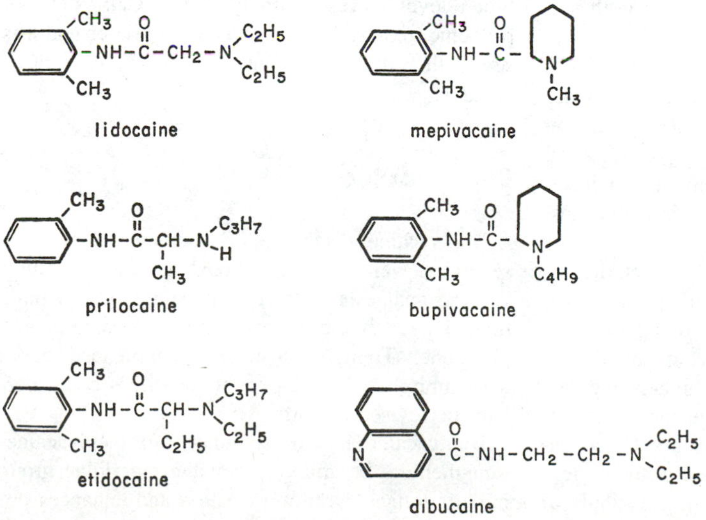

Fig 31–3.—Amide-linked local anesthetics in common use. With the exception of dibucaine, an amino-alkyl amide, all are amino-acyl amides. (From de Jong R.H.: *Local Anesthetics.* Springfield, Illinois, Charles C Thomas, Publishers, 1977. Reproduced by permission.)

drug-induced stimulation or inhibition. However, enzyme induction of lidocaine biotransformation affects blood levels in man only minimally. Conversion of the tertiary amine lidocaine molecule to a secondary amine is the important initial step in man. In the liver, lidocaine de-ethylation yields monoethylglycine xylidide (MEGX), and acetaldehyde. MEGX, a secondary amine, is much more readily hydrolyzed than lidocaine, forming xylidine and N-ethyl glycine. Nevertheless, the greater portion of MEGX is excreted unchanged as various conjugates. Some MEGX is degraded by further de-ethylation to glycine xylidide (GX), a process even slower than MEGX hydrolysis.

Lidocaine metabolites are excreted to a large extent by the biliary route, only to be reabsorbed along the intestinal tract for eventual renal clearance. Lidocaine metabolism is reasonably complete, less than 50% of unchanged anesthetic appearing in the urine. MEGX is the primary urinary metabolite, along with smaller quantities of xylidine and N-ethyl glycine, and even smaller amounts of GX.

Mepivacaine

Though it has a ringed piperidine rather than an alkyl-amino hydrophilic component, mepivacaine (Carbocaine) resembles lidocaine in most clinical respects. Its duration of action may be slightly longer than that of lidocaine, though the difference is not sufficiently pronounced to warrant selection of one agent over the other. Though a vasoconstrictor action has been attributed to mepivacaine, epinephrine still slows mepivacaine absorption, decreases the blood level, and prolongs anesthesia, much as it does for lidocaine.

Mepivacaine yields carbon dioxide as one of its breakdown products, suggesting oxidative N-demethylation of the piperidine portion. The formation of N-desmethyl mepivacaine (pipecolylxylidine) in man is less important than the formation of meta- and para-hydroxy derivatives and their conjugates, which form the chief urinary products. As in the case of lidocaine, the chief metabolic activity resides in the liver, with the resulting products appearing both unchanged and as conjugates with glucuronic acid in the bile. Mepivacaine and metabolites are also excreted via salivary glands and gastric mucosa. In adults, mepivacaine metabolism is quite complete, from 16% to only about 1% unchanged mepivacaine being identified in the urine.

Mepivacaine provides an interesting example of the body's attempts at lowering the toxicity of a xenobiotic. Desmethyl mepivacaine is about two-thirds as toxic as mepivacaine, while the para-hydroxy compound is only one-third as toxic. Subsequent breakdown or conjugation further lower toxicity. Mepivacaine's asymmetric carbon atom gives rise to stereoisomerism. Whether the d- and l-forms are metabolized by different pathways or at different rates is not yet known.

Prilocaine

Prilocaine (Citanest; propitocaine), one of many lidocaine homologues, is the only secondary amine local anesthetic in common use. When first introduced it received considerable attention as it is approximately as potent as lidocaine, yet has markedly lower intravenous (IV) toxicity.

The biotransformation of prilocaine is of interest as its amino-phenol end products oxidize hemoglobin to methemoglobin. While other local anesthetics (e.g., lidocaine) may cause minimal methemoglobinemia, prilocaine can decrease the oxygen-carrying capacity of the blood sufficiently to cause clinically detectable cyanosis. By limiting the total dose of prilocaine to 600 mg, cyanosis can be avoided. Fortunately, methemoglobinemia is readily reversed with 1–2 mg/kg of methylene blue.

Prilocaine metabolism differs in other respects because it is observed not only in liver but, to a lesser degree, also in kidney and lung tissue. Prilocaine is metabolized faster and more completely than lidocaine. Furthermore, it is taken up more rapidly than lidocaine by many organs, lowering the blood level correspondingly faster. CNS signs of prilocine toxicity in man indeed are briefer and less severe than those following the same IV dose of lidocaine.

Bupivacaine

Bupivacaine (Marcaine; Sensorcaine) is one of several newer long-acting local anesthetics. Bupivacaine analgesia lasts several hours, two to three times longer than that provided by lidocaine or mepivacaine. Though currently recommended upper dose limits are 2–3 mg/kg, these values could perhaps be revised upward.

Bupivacaine is closely related to mepivacaine. Lengthening the amino tail of the piperidine group imparts longer duration of action and enhances potency, albeit with a trade-off of greater toxicity than its homologue. The metabolism of bupivacaine is similar to that of mepivacaine, described above. The resultant pipecolylxylidine is only one-eighth as toxic as the parent compound.

Etidocaine

Etidocaine (Duranest), a long-acting derivative of lidocaine, is four times more potent and four times more toxic than lidocaine; however, its analgesic effects last considerably longer than those of lidocaine. Etidocaine differs from bupivacaine in that it produces motor block that sometimes is more profound than sensory block. This unusual feature is best explained by the great lipid solubility of etidocaine, which would tend to collect in the thick myelin sheaths of motor nerves. Little is known about the metabolism of etidocaine in man.

PRESERVATIVES AND ADDITIVES

Most of the commonly used local anesthetics, especially of the amide type, are extremely stable compounds and will remain unchanged in solution indefinitely. Thus, solutions do not require additives if they are stored in airtight ampules. Antimicrobial agents such as methylparaben are added to local anesthetics if distributed in multidose vials. In sealed ampules, antimicrobial additives are unnecessary. Methylparaben is effective against gram-positive organisms and fungi, less so against gram-negative bacteria. Methylparaben may have been responsible for some of the allergic reactions attributed to local anesthetics. This is because paraben drugs are derivatives of p-hydroxybenzoic acid, closely related to the PABA nucleus of procaine and related ester-linked drugs. PABA is an effective ultraviolet light–blocking agent widely used in sunscreen preparations. And a substantial number of users develop contact dermatitis to PABA with continued exposure. So sensitized, these patients could conceivably experience cross-reactions with procaine or with paraben preservative.

PHYSIOLOGY OF NERVE CONDUCTION

In the nerve membrane at rest, potassium ions pass freely back and forth through their specialized channels, whereas sodium ions are essentially barred passage through their special channels when the nerve membrane is at rest (Fig 31–4). Selective exclusion of positive sodium ions from the nerve interior ensures that the resting membrane's voltage is generated by the concentration gradient for potassium ions across the membrane—the so-called potassium battery.

Depolarization

When the membrane is triggered by an electrical impulse, the gates that locked the sodium channels at rest abruptly swing open. Positively charged sodium ions, driven by the combined forces of concentration gradient and electrostatic attraction, avalanche inward (Fig 31–5). The inward rush of sodium ions is so massive that the membrane poten-

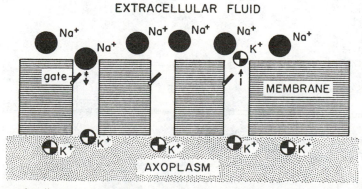

Fig 31–4.—Highly schematized figure to illustrate the generation of resting potential by a potassium battery. At rest, the membrane is impermeable to sodium ions (*solid circles*) because the sodium channel gates are closed; conversely, potassium ions (*checkered circles*) freely pass through their channels. Since the potassium ion concentration in the axoplasm is some 25 times greater than in the extraneural fluid, an electrochemical gradient—the resting potential—is generated. The membrane interior is negatively charged with respect to the exterior. (From de Jong R.H.: *Local Anesthetics.* Springfield, Illinois, Charles C Thomas, Publishers, 1977. Reproduced by permission.)

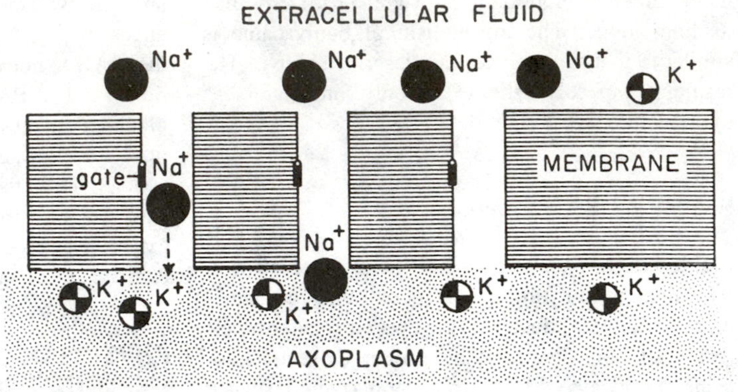

Fig 31–5.—Depolarization (compare with resting membrane in Fig 31–4). Electrical fields accompanying an impulse open the sodium channel's gate. Sodium ions are whipped inward by the push of the concentration gradient and the pull of electrostatic attraction. Potassium ions are not immediately affected. (From de Jong R.H.: *Local Anesthetics.* Springfield, Illinois, Charles C Thomas, Publishers, 1977. Reproduced by permission.)

tial overshoots, causing a brief swing to positivity (Fig 31–6).

Soon thereafter, potassium ions start to leave the axon down their outward concentration gradient, and the sodium channels begin to close, stopping the inrush of sodium ions and restoring the resting potential. The rapid change in membrane permeability to sodium ions, and the corresponding voltage change is called *depolarization;* the activity is manifested by an *action potential* or *impulse.*

The traveling voltage pulse (impulse) is the nerve's fundamental information unit. Plainly, if the process of depolarization is interrupted somewhere along the nerve fiber, an impulse can no longer be transmitted, and the nerve becomes inexcitable. That is to say, the nerve is blocked.

Each depolarization sequence dumps sodium into the nerve and bleeds potassium from it. Eventually, both the sodium and the potassium ionic gradient would be wiped out, rendering the nerve totally inexcitable. This potentially weak link is corrected by a continually active transport mechanism (the so-called sodium pump) that extrudes invading sodium ions from the axon and returns wayward potassium ions to the axoplasm. (Worth noting at this stage is that local anesthetics do not act on the sodium pump.)

Myelinated Nerve

The preceding description of impulse conduction by spreading electrical fields applies to nonmyelinated axons (C fibers). In these axons, impulse velocity is slow, though the thicker the axon, the faster the impulse travels. By depositing *myelin* (a lipid insulating material) around the axon, current wastage is reduced and electrical efficiency im-

Fig 31–6.—Action potential. Reoriented by electrical field changes induced by an appropriate stimulus, the gates of the sodium channels swing open. Sodium ions pour inward, attracted by the dual forces of concentration gradient and electrical charge. The massive influx of positively charged sodium ions reverses the normally negative charge on the nerve membrane interior, as shown by the voltmeter. (From de Jong R.H.: *Local Anesthetics.* Springfield, Illinois, Charles C Thomas, Publishers, 1977. Reproduced by permission.)

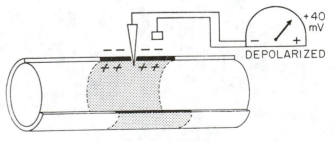

proved. At regular intervals, which are the farther apart the thicker the axon, the myelin is lacking. At these *nodes of Ranvier,* the membrane of myelinated axons contacts the extracellular fluid directly. These nodes, being more excitable than the rest of the membrane, permit an impulse to skip rapidly from node to node, instead of slowly crawling forward along the surface of unmyelinated nerve. Such *saltatory* (by jumps) impulse conduction notably speeds conduction (Fig 31–7). In humans, for example, fast alpha fibers conduct impulses at rates up to 100 m/sec, while our C fibers conduct at a bare 1 or 2 m/sec.

Mode of Action

Local anesthetics block impulse generation in nerve fibers. While other substances (phenol or alcohol, for example) share this property, local anesthetics are unique in that their action is completely reversible, blocking nerve without damaging it.

Local anesthetics impede sodium ion passage during depolarization by occluding the transmembrane sodium channels. That is, the nerve behaves as if the gates of the sodium channel were locked so that depolarization cannot take place: the axon thus remains polarized. A local anesthetic block is a *nondepolarization block,* resembling in some ways the action of curare at the neuromuscular junction.

Site of Action

Receptor Binding

The sodium channel's internal (axoplasmic) entry is the likely site of major local anesthetic action, with the local anesthetic molecule lodged in the mouth of the sodium channel somewhat like a lunar module docked in its mothership. Once inside the sodium channel's mouth, the local anesthetic molecule is held in place by physicochemical bonding forces. Of these, electrostatic attraction imparted by the positive charge on the cationic form of local anesthetic is the strongest, bonding to negatively charged phosphate tails in the sodium channel. To enter or leave the channel's mouth, the local anesthetic molecule must move past the opened gates. Hence, nerve actively involved in conducting impulse traffic is more readily blocked than inactive nerve because the gates are open longer in the for-

mer than in the latter state. This phenomenon is called *frequency-dependent block.*

Blocking action at the internal mouth of the sodium channel requires that the molecule reach that site by one means or another. Since local anesthetics are applied externally, their effectiveness can be explained only by diffusion through, or solution in, the membrane.

Membrane Expansion

Benzocaine, a simple local anesthetic ester, is a notorious exception to the above mechanism for it exists as virtually cation-free uncharged base species at normal tissue pH. The membrane expansion theory proposes that the uncharged local anesthetic base blocks impulse transmission when the lipid-soluble free base species dissolves in the nerve membrane. Physical entry of a large number of foreign molecules into the rigid membrane structure causes it to swell, with resultant partial collapse of unsupported ionic channels. External compression of their channel by the sideways-expanded membrane skeleton impedes passage of sodium ions and eventually closes the channel altogether. Some of the activity of commonly used local anesthetics with high lipid solubility (e.g., etidocaine) might be attributable in part to this mechanism, too.

Fiber Size and Membrane Function

The diameter of a nerve fiber has turned out to be a most important physical factor to which nerve function and modality—not to mention sensitivity to local anesthetics—are related. To simplify description, nerve fibers have been categorized into three major anatomical classes. Myelinated somatic nerves are called A fibers, myelinated preganglionic autonomic nerves are called B fibers, and nonmyelinated axons are called C fibers.

Since A fibers vary in diameter from 4–20 μ approximately, they are subdivided into four groups according to decreasing size: alpha, beta, gamma, and delta. Largest are the alpha fibers, related to motor function, proprioception, and reflex activity. Beta fibers also innervate muscle and transmit touch and pressure sensations, while gamma fibers control muscle spindle tone. The thinnest A fibers, the delta group, subserve pain and temperature functions and signal tissue damage.

The thinly myelinated B fibers are preganglionic

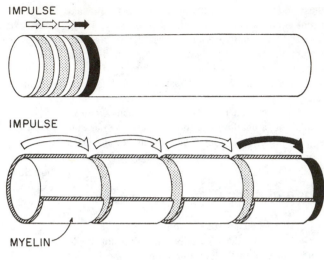

Fig 31–7.—Comparing impulse propagation in unmyelinated *(top)* and myelinated *(bottom)* axons of equal diameter. In the former, the impulse creeps forward by sequential depolarization of neighboring membrane slices. In the latter, the impulse leaps forward by skipping from one node to the next, jumping over the electrically insulated myelinated nerve sectors. Note how much farther ahead the impulse has moved after four depolarizations in the myelinated axon, as compared with the unmyelinated axon. (From Cousins M.J., Bridenbaugh P.O.: *Neural Blockade.* Philadelphia, J.B. Lippincott Co., 1980. Reproduced by permission.)

autonomic axons that innervate vascular and intestinal smooth muscle, among others; B fibers thus are extremely important during spinal or peridural anesthesia. The nonmyelinated C fibers, like the myelinated delta fibers, subserve pain and temperature transmission, as well as postganglionic autonomic functions. C fibers are thinner than myelinated fibers (about 1 μ) and have a much lower conduction velocity than even A delta fibers.

Fiber Size and Impulse Block

The diameter and myelinization of a nerve fiber determine not only its message-carrying function, but also its sensitivity to local anesthetics. In general, a thick nerve fiber is less readily blocked by local anesthetics than a thin fiber. In other words, the thicker a nerve fiber, the greater the concentration of local anesthetic required to block conduction. Preganglionic autonomic B fibers are an exception: although myelinated, they are more readily blocked than any other fiber group. Hence, sympathetic blockade after a spinal or epidural block extends several segments beyond the cutaneous dermatomal level.

The Minimum Blocking Concentration

The minimum concentration of a local anesthetic (C_m) is the lowest concentration of anesthetic that blocks impulse conduction. The concept is impor-

tant clinically, for only drug concentrations greater than C_m will solidly anesthetize a nerve. The pharmacologic potency of local anesthetics varies considerably, hence each agent has a unique C_m.

As a rule, the thicker a myelinated nerve fiber, the greater the concentration of local anesthetic required to block it: a thick axon has a greater C_m than a thin axon. As a yardstick, the C_m of alpha motor fibers is approximately twice that of delta sensory fibers. Preganglionic autonomic B fibers have the lowest C_m of mammalian axons, about one-third that of C fibers.

Differential Nerve Block

Since thick nerve fibers are less readily affected by local anesthetics than thin ones, one can tailor the anesthetic concentration so that the thin fibers in a nerve trunk are blocked, whereas the thicker fibers are not. Even unintended, as in a peripheral nerve block one often notes that pain is obtunded completely (A delta and C fibers are blocked) but that motor function, touch, and pressure (alpha and beta fibers) are little affected. This situation is called a *differential nerve block.*

Speed of Action

As local anesthetics generally are injected in the fluid medium surrounding a nerve or nerve endings, they must diffuse some distance before reaching the target area. Diffusion being a relatively slow process, the local anesthetic solution is steadily diluted with tissue fluid. At the same time, drug is constantly absorbed via vascular and lymphatic channels. Further, the local anesthetic is bound to tissue components along its diffusion path. Hence, the more lipid-soluble the agent, the slower the onset of the block.

SPECIAL PROPERTIES OF LOCAL ANESTHETICS

The pure synthetic local anesthetic is a weakly basic amine, soluble in lipids but poorly soluble in water and unstable. Salts of the local anesthetic base, in contrast, are readily soluble and stable in aqueous solution. The usual local anesthetic solution contains a salt (commonly the hydrochloride) of the local anesthetic base.

Ionization

Inclusion of a nitrogen-containing amino group in the structure of local anesthetics confers upon them the "split personality" of a weak base. This means that they exist in solution as a combination of the positively charged quaternary amine species of the local anesthetic (the *cation*) and the uncharged tertiary amine local anesthetic *base*. Simplifying the components of the equilibrium reaction, we shall represent it by:

$$R{\equiv}NH^+ \leftrightarrows R{\equiv}N + H^+$$
$$\text{(cation)} \qquad \text{(base)}$$

It can be seen that the relative concentrations of cation and base vary with the hydrogen ion concentration (pH) of the solution; the more acid the medium, the more the reaction shifts to the left. The ratio of base to cation form is determined by the dissocation constant (K_a) of the local anesthetic, and the hydrogen ion concentration (H^+) of the solution, as shown below:

$$K_a = \frac{[H^+]\,[base]}{[cation]}$$

where the brackets denote "concentration of." By taking negative logarithms of both sides, the familiar Henderson-Hasselbalch equation is obtained:

$$pK_a = pH - \log \frac{[base]}{[cation]}$$

where pK_a—analogous to the derivation of pH from hydrogen ion concentration—represents the negative logarithm of the dissociation constant. With just a bit more rearranging the equation becomes:

$$\log \frac{[cation]}{[base]} = pK_a - pH$$

Now we readily see that when the pH of a solution equals the pK_a, equal proportions of cation and base are present. Also, since the pK_a of injectable local anesthetics is in the 7.5 to 9 range, we see that at tissue pH of 7.4, more local anesthetic cation is present than base. Procaine has a high pK_a (8.9) and therefore dissociates only a small percentage of lipid-soluble, nonionized base at physiologic pH; this explains procaine's poor spreading qualities.

Ionization is important to the solubility, activity, and toxicity of local anesthetics and to their equilibrium distribution in various body compartments. Decreasing ionization, as by alkinization, effectively raises the initial concentration gradient of diffusible drug. The higher concentration of base increases the rate of drug transfer and decreases the latent period to nerve block, whereas a lowered pH, due to infection in tissues that surround a nerve, results in decreased concentration of nonionized diffusible anesthetic base, hence incomplete block.

pH and Blocking Action

The cation (i.e., the positively charged species) is the local anesthetic species that binds to oppositely charged membrane receptors and plugs the sodium channels, so rendering the nerve inexcitable. Hence, the cation concentration determines how effectively impulse conduction is blocked. The concentration of local anesthetic base, in contrast, determines drug penetration and thereby the quantity of local anesthetic to reach nerve membrane receptors. Hence, the base concentration determines how much drug eventually reaches the neural target.

The proportion of base is increased by raising the pH of the solution: alkalinizing a local anesthetic solution enhances drug penetrance. Conversely, an acidified solution is less effective, as fewer local anesthetic molecules diffuse to the neural target. One immediate corollary of local anesthetic dissociation is the common observation that local anesthetics are less effective when injected into an infected area. Because the pH of injected tissue is lowered by the formation of lactic and other acids, less local anesthetic base dissociates. Although more cation is formed, it is virtually useless, for, being electrically charged, it cannot by itself migrate through tissue barriers to the neural target.

Solubility

The partition coefficients of drugs determined in aqueous/organic solvent systems in vitro are often used to indicate their relative in vivo partition characteristics or degree of lipid solubility. The higher values for the long-acting agents tetracaine, bupivacaine, and etidocaine suggest more extensive entry into body membranes and tissues as a result of greater lipid solubility.

Also, aqueous solubility diminishes as lipid solubility increases. If a local anesthetic has a high lipid solubility, the correspondingly low aqueous solubility places an upper limit on the amount of drug available for transport and blocking activity.

Protein Binding

Besides being more lipid soluble, the long-acting local anesthetics also bind more strongly to plasma (and other) proteins, suggesting that the binding forces are predominantly hydrophobic. But, since a consistent relationship between partition coefficient and binding is not evident, little-known electrical or steric features must also contribute to differences in binding.

Binding of local anesthetic to plasma proteins on either side of a membrane affects the overall transfer and distribution of drug. The process is analogous to ionization, as only the unbound drug diffuses readily. The more tightly bound the drug, the lower will be the net drug transfer.

At equilibrium, the concentration of unbound nonionized local anesthetic will be the same on either side of the membrane. But total drug concentrations will differ, depending on the relative binding capacities and the pH values of the two aqueous phases.

TOXICITY OF LOCAL ANESTHETICS

Although local anesthetics are potentially toxic drugs, they have one great advantage over most other drugs: they are applied directly to the neural site of action. Direct application builds up a very high drug concentration around the target nerves to be blocked, with only a relatively low concentration in the bloodstream. Still, a considerable fraction of the drug will be absorbed directly into the bloodstream without ever having reached the target. When the drug concentration in the blood builds up beyond a certain level, local anesthetics may cause *systemic reactions*. These are manifested most dramatically in the CNS; their severity depends on drug concentration in the blood.

Particularly worrisome is unintended direct injection of local anesthetic into a blood vessel. By this means, a high concentration of local anesthetic is attained very quickly in the blood, and the drug is quickly carried to key responding organs such as brain and heart. In performing a stellate ganglion block, for instance, it is all too easy to slip past the protective abutment of the cervical vertebral transverse process into the vertebral artery. The resultant injection into the cerebral circulation could have disastrous results if not preceded by a test injection, for aspiration through a fine needle may not always yield immediate flashback of blood. Along the same line, radiopaque solution injected into terminal branches of the facial artery travels retrograde up the vascular tree to reach the carotid circulation, and so the brain. This may explain the puzzling observation that facial or intraoral injection of elsewhere innocuous quantities of local anesthetic can give rise to CNS reactions. Similarly, a catheter placed in the epidural space could easily slip into one of the many venules in that area. Aspiration in that case is notoriously uncertain, and only a test dose of local anesthetic (with added epinephrine) will provide a measure of certainty regarding extravascular placement.

The quantities of local anesthetics used in pain therapy ordinarily are well below the recommended upper limits for man, yet adverse reactions are seen on occasion, often when least expected. Particularly when a block is missed, when inflamed tissues are infiltrated, or when a wide field is to be anesthetized, large volumes of local anesthetic may have to be injected. Also to be considered, though not a complication of local anesthetic administration, some patients are so fearful of needles and anticipated discomfort that they become faint before even being touched. Such instances of vasovagal reflexes are not uncommon in anxious patients, and are exacerbated in the sitting position, for the heart must then pump blood to the brain against the gravity gradient.

Local Anesthetic Combinations

Astute clinicians often combine two local anesthetics to take advantage of the virtues of each. Thus, lidocaine provides rapid onset and profound block but suffers from a short duration of action. Long-acting agents such as bupivacaine, on the other hand, offset the advantage of prolonged blockade by slower onset of anesthesia. By combining lidocaine and bupivacaine (a mixture sometimes called "supercaine"), one obtains long-lasting block along with rapid onset. Also used commonly for injection of myoneural trigger points is a combination of bupivacaine and etidocaine—the former to provide intense sensory (afferent) block, the latter for its preferential blocking action on motor (efferent) nerves. Experimentally, the toxicity of such mixtures seems additive at most. That is, the total toxicity is the sum of toxicities of the component local anesthetics.

CENTRAL NERVOUS SYSTEM TOXICITY

Perineurally injected local anesthetic eventually appears in the bloodstream. Any local anesthetic injected unintentionally into a blood vessel peaks almost instantaneously in the bloodstream. Depending on the concentration of local anesthetic in the blood a spectrum of CNS symptoms and signs may be observed, varying from slight dizziness to grand mal convulsions and even respiratory arrest. In an ill-defined range between these extremes are blood levels that give rise to telltale symptoms proclaiming the presence of rising concentrations of local anesthetic in the brain. Moderate symptoms occur at blood levels of 5–6 μg/ml of lidocaine or mepivacaine, 1.6 μg/ml of bupivacaine, and 2 μg/ml of etidocaine. At higher blood levels, muscle twitching appears, and at about twice the acute blood levels specified above, convulsions occur. It is interesting to note here that the slope of the time-concentration curve appears to affect the brain's reaction. Thus, a tiny test dose injected directly into the vertebral artery can precipitate intense convulsions. Conversely, when local anesthetic is delivered slowly, as by continuous perineural or epidural infusion, far higher blood levels can be tolerated without any symptoms at all. At the University of Cincinnati, several patients with bupivacaine plasma levels of 5 μg/ml or higher were symptom-free.

The earliest known records of CNS responses to local anesthetics describe the euphoric and stimulant qualities of cocaine, a property still explored (illegally to be sure) these days. Such excitement may be seen with procaine, too. Chloroprocaine, given by direct IV infusion for certain intractable pain problems, has produced a curious "fear" reaction in some, a "high" in other patients. The newer amide-linked local anesthetics, on the other hand, induce sedation and amnesia rather than euphoria. Otherwise, local anesthetics, whether of the ester or amide family, evoke remarkably similar experiences in humans.

Commonly reported symptoms of a rising local anesthetic blood level may be any combination of headache, lightheadedness, numbness and tingling of lips or tongue, ringing in the ears, drowsiness, blurring of vision along with difficulty in focusing, and either a flushed or chilled sensation. Objectively, obtundation, confusion, slurred or hesitant speech, nystagmus, and muscle tremors or twitches may be observed. At subseizure blood levels, and when drug administration is slowed or halted, these signs and symptoms of early CNS toxicity soon fade. But, occasionally, these symptoms progress to the point of seizures. It is important, then, to recognize the above danger signals that could foreshadow an imminent convulsion (Fig 31–8).

Few electrical clues of imminent toxic disturbance are registered at the brain's cortical surface by standard electroencephalography (EEG). By contrast, profound alterations are recorded from neural structures buried deep within the brain. Components of the limbic system, such as the amygdala and hippocampus, develop self-sustaining spike or spike-and-wave spindle bursts that coincide with the onset of behavioral reactions in laboratory animals; such patterns are considered representative of a focal seizure generator. These focal limbic seizures have been recorded in humans, too.

Local Anesthetic Seizures

Certainly the most dramatic (and potentially the most hazardous) complication of local anesthetic administration is the sudden onset of generalized tonic-clonic convulsions. Local anesthetic–induced convulsions differ in several key aspects from organic convulsive disorders, even though the ultimate external manifestations of both are identical. The two react oppositely, for instance, to hyperventila-

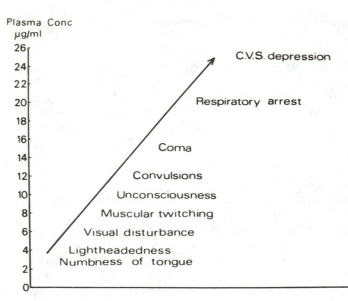

Fig 31–8.—Association between cerebral symptoms and plasma concentration of lidocaine. Respiratory arrest and cardiovascular system (C.V.S.) depression do not occur until at least twice the convulsant plasma level is reached. (From Cousins M.J., Bridenbaugh P.O.: *Neural Blockade.* Philadelphia, J.B. Lippincott Co., 1980. Reproduced by permission.)

tion. It is because of this fundamental difference that some aspects of prophylaxis and therapy of local anesthetic-induced convulsions differ from those of epilepsy.

Although total local anesthetic dosage is a convenient guide for use in most cases, rate, mode, and site of administration are important determinants of toxicity as well. This is, of course, because the brain reacts to the concentration of anesthetic delivered to it by the bloodstream, regardless of how the drug got there; the local anesthetic blood level is the ultimate guide to the toxic threshold (see Fig 31–8).

Clear evidence that patients have been adversely affected by seizures is difficult to find. However, the cardiovascular depression caused by the high anesthetic blood level, and the respiratory impediment caused by uncoordinated muscle spasms, may indirectly affect brain function through reduced cerebral blood flow and hypoxemia. Also, the violent muscle spasms of a seizure rapidly exhaust local oxygen reserves, leading to anaerobic metabolism. The consequent release of large quantities of lactic and other acids precipitates profound metabolic acidosis that may cause cardiovascular problems in older or debilitated patients.

Carbon Dioxide

Of practical interest are experimental observations that the threshold of the cerebral cortex to seizures induced by local anesthetics varies inversely with the arterial CO_2 tension. Put differently, when the CO_2 tension is high, even a small amount of local anesthetic in the blood may produce seizures. Conversely, when the CO_2 tension is low, far more local anesthetic can be given before seizures appear. Hyperventilation, by decreasing CO_2 tension, evidently heightens the brain's resistance to local anesthetic convulsions. Plasma hydrogen ion activity (pH) additionally modifies CNS toxicity, with acidemia lowering the seizure threshold. The combination of metabolic acidosis coexisting with hypercarbia further heightens the toxic potential of local anesthetics.

Anticonvulsants

In 1925 Tatum and colleagues discovered that barbiturates prevent cocaine-induced convulsions in monkeys. Ever since, barbiturates have been given prophylactically in hopes of averting convulsions from an overdose of local anesthetics. However, this practice appears to be little better than homeopathy; to double the median convulsant dose of lidocaine, for instance, a near-anesthetic dose of pentobarbital (10 mg/kg) must be given intramuscularly. Clinical impression bears out the relative impotence of routine barbiturate premedication. Other anticonvulsants, diphenylhydantoin (phenytoin) for instance, not only are ineffective but may even enhance the convulsant potency of local anesthetics in animal studies.

An interesting, albeit puzzling, observation is that lidocaine itself possesses anticonvulsant properties in man. In this context, it is worth noting that inhalation anesthetics, even nitrous oxide, have also been shown to prevent local anesthetic-induced seizures in laboratory animals.

With the discovery of a limbic seizure focus for local anesthetics, the search could be narrowed to anticonvulsants that specifically affect the limbic brain. Diazepam (Valium) proved to be particularly effective, having minimal undesirable side effects with maximal therapeutic efficiency in several animal models. In comparative studies with other common premedicant drugs, diazepam proved even more unique in that it decreased the overall mortality associated with local anesthetic–induced toxicity.

Controlled studies of the prophylactic efficacy of diazepam in man have not yet appeared, although the drug is now widely used as a premedicant for surgical procedures requiring major nerve blocks. Likewise, firm data are not yet available to show whether diazepam is as effective as thiopental in arresting ongoing convulsions, though clinical experience suggests it is. In one uncontrolled study, diazepam prophylaxis gave higher local anesthetic blood levels in control patients given the same dose of local anesthetic. Subsequent studies have failed to confirm this.

CLINICAL MANAGEMENT OF CNS REACTIONS

The two aspects to consider in the management of CNS reactions are how to prevent a reaction from occurring in the first place, and what to do when one unexpectedly occurs. Easily the most conspicuous clinical manifestation of local anesthetic toxicity is a generalized convulsion. During a convulsion, respiration is impaired or impossible because of violent and uncoordinated contractions of airway, chest, and abdominal muscles. A less conspicuous but equally vital consideration is impaired circulation owing to local anesthetic–induced cardiovascular depression and/or arrhythmias. Convulsions thus pose an immediate threat to brain and heart, a threat that becomes increasingly critical the longer the seizures last. The abrupt onset and the possibly serious consequences of local anesthetic seizures make it imperative that anyone who administers a local anesthetic know how to manage CNS reactions, and that local anesthetics be administered only where suitable equipment and drugs to manage adverse reactions are immediately at hand.

Prevention

Convulsions do not occur unless the blood level of the local anesthetic exceeds a certain lower threshold. Accordingly, the surest way of preventing seizures is to limit the total dose of local anesthetic. With local or infiltration anesthesia, a vasoconstrictor, such as epinephrine, often is incorporated into the anesthetic solution to slow vascular absorption; longer-lasting anesthesia is an added bonus. It is important, of course, to guard against inadvertent direct intravascular injection by repeated aspiration and slow injection. High blood levels may occur immediately after unintended intravascular injection, or up to 20–30 minutes following soft tissue injection. Thus it is essential to monitor and to maintain regular verbal contact with the patient during the first 20–30 minutes following injection.

Premonitory signs usually indicate an impending convulsion. The drug injection should be stopped and preventive measures instituted. The protective effect of hyperventilation, which raises the cortical seizure threshold to local anesthetics, may be used to advantage at this stage. Often, administering oxygen and asking the patient to breathe deeply suffice. Should a seizure develop later on, some nitrogen washout has been accomplished, and the replacement with oxygen safeguards cerebral and cardiac oxygenation.

A common hospital and office routine is to precede local anesthetic administration with a nondepressant dose of barbiturate (about 1–2 mg/kg) in hopes of minimizing CNS reactions. As discussed, this is a false hope: seizure protection is slight unless near-anesthetic doses of barbiturate are administered. Fortunately, if experimental work is any indication, effective prophylaxis is attainable with diazepam (Valium) and related benzodiazepines. The great advantage of the benzodiazepines over barbiturates is that they combine maximal seizure protection with minimal cardiovascular and respiratory disturbance. However, this feature should not be taken as justification for exceeding recommended safe dosages of local anesthetics. The sedative effect of benzodiazepines also becomes a consideration in the management of elderly or debilitated outpatients. Not yet known is whether long-standing therapy with a benzodiazepine (as is often the case in patients with chronic pain) blunts seizure prophylaxis by receptor saturation.

Without controlled clinical studies, it is difficult

to recommend dosage schedules for diazepam in man. Laboratory evidence suggests that as little diazepam as 0.1 mg/kg raises the seizure threshold, with additional drug providing increasingly more protection. This amount (7 mg for a 70/kg person) is well below the 10 mg (about 0.15 mg/kg) oral or intramuscular dose commonly employed as preanesthetic medication in many centers.

Treatment

Preventive measures notwithstanding, convulsions occasionally do result from accidental intravascular injection, unusually rapid absorption, or plain overdosing. Local anesthetic–induced seizures ordinarily do not last long because the blood level quickly falls during the early phases of rapid dilution and distribution in man (that is, assuming effective circulation). Rarely does a cluster of seizures last more than a minute. Because of that, local anesthetic seizures should not cause morbidity if appropriate resuscitation equipment is at hand, the patient is properly prepared, and the person administering the regional block is well versed in the treatment of seizures.

An important first step in treatment is protecting the patient from injury, such as falling from the treatment table, biting the tongue, or twisting the extremities. To increase blood flow to the brain, the head should be placed level with the heart and, if necessary, the legs elevated to return more blood to the heart. Oxygen administration is important, as convulsions increase muscular and cerebral oxygen demand yet at the same time impede respiration. If the patient is unresponsive, manual ventilation should be instituted to oxygenate the blood and to wash out carbon dioxide. If there are no mechanical devices immediately at hand, give mouth-to-mouth respiration. As a rule, spontaneous respiration resumes soon after seizures end.

Thiopental (Pentothal), 50–100 mg given IV, remains widely recommended as an effective anticonvulsant. Resist the temptation to use too much thiopental (or other rapidly acting barbiturate); respiratory, cardiovascular, and cerebral depression may ensue. Studies in primates have demonstrated the efficacy of small amounts (0.05–0.1 mg/kg) of IV diazepam. Clinical reports show that seizures can be arrested in humans with IV doses of diazepam as low as 2.5–5 mg. Controlled clinical studies comparing diazepam and thiopental treatment of local anesthetic convulsions remain to be done, however.

Whichever drug is chosen, both barbiturates and benzodiazepines are CNS depressants, and recovery of consciousness may be delayed if too much of the dose is given.

Rapid-acting neuromuscular blocking agents like succinylcholine have been advocated to stop the paroxysmal muscle spasms of a convulsion. While these paralyzing drugs may be perfectly safe in the hands of persons trained and equipped to perform tracheal intubation and mechanical ventilation, the hazards of this form of therapy are considerable when used by personnel unfamiliar with their actions. Equally important, the paralyzing agent does not affect the electrical seizure discharges from the brain; it merely arrests the external muscular manifestations, giving a false sense of therapeutic accomplishment. Also to be considered is that the cardiac toxicity of lipid-soluble amide-linked local anesthetics such as bupivacaine or etidocaine is enhanced by hyperkalemia, an occurrence common after administration of succinycholine.

On the other hand, when prolonged seizures threaten effective ventilation, muscle relaxants become the drugs of choice, especially as hyperventilation decreases the apparent CNS toxicity of a local anesthetic by raising the seizure threshold. In general terms, indications for paralyzing agents are inability to ventilate a convulsing patient adequately, and recurrent convulsions refractory to moderate incremental doses of a barbiturate or benzodiazepine.

Hypersensitivity

Another form of systemic response to local anesthetic is hypersensitivity or allergy, where a minute quantity of drug can give rise to a variety of major tissue reactions. Allergic manifestations to local anesthetics are infrequent and virtually limited to the ester-linked drugs. Procaine is a well-known offender, and contact dermatitis was not unknown in medical personnel. Administration of procaine to sensitized subjects may cause edema, hives, wheezing, bronchospasm, and other allergic manifestations. Painful injectable material (penicillin, for instance) commonly has procaine added to it to make the injection less uncomfortable. Some of the allergic reactions attributed to penicillin in the past might well have been due to the admixed procaine.

Susceptibility to procaine also implies hypersensitivity to other ester-linked local anesthetics derived from PABA. This can be demonstrated with techniques such as passive transfer, which, however, introduces the hazards of foreign serum administration. Simpler, albeit less sensitive, methods are preferable. Drugs such as tetracaine and chloroprocaine, which share the PABA nucleus with procaine, are probably best avoided in patients suspected of having a procaine allergy.

The situation is further confused by the fact that paraben preservative, widely used in multiple-dose vials, may itself induce hypersensitivity. Probably this is because the parabens are derived from para-hydroxybenzoic acid, a close relative of PABA. In testing a patient for presumed hypersensitivity to local anesthetics, one should therefore include a separate test for the paraben preservative. Being benzoic acid derivatives, the parabens are structurally related to procaine, so that cross-sensitivity between the two substances is not inconceivable. Also, many sunscreen lotions contain PABA as the active ingredient, and some patients develop allergy to the product. Although no direct link has been demonstrated, one might prudently select a local anesthetic other than procaine or its congeners in these patients.

The amide-linked local anesthetics (e.g., lidocaine or mepivacaine), conversely, are singularly free of documented hypersensitivity in man. Isolated case reports of an allergic response to lidocaine have appeared, mostly in the dental literature, but some of these might have been due to the preservative instead. One may well consider hypersensitivity to lidocaine and related amide-linked anesthetics to be so rare as to be virtually negligible.

Histotoxicity

Tissue damage might be expected whenever a xenobiotic comes into physical contact with living cells. Soft tissue effects might be unpleasant, but the consequences ordinarily would not be serious. However, potential damage to neural structures is of considerable significance because of the long-lasting effect.

White blood cells, an important part of the body's defense mechanisms, are inhibited by concentrated local anesthetic solutions. Lidocaine for instance, depresses phagocytosis, lymphocyte transformation, and oxygen uptake. The importance of the response of white blood cells to local anesthetics in decreasing the body's resistance to bacterial invasion remains to be seen. In view of the modest bactericidal properties of local anesthetics, a reasonable overall balance may well be struck. Red blood cells are

quite resistant to damage by local anesthetics, unless extremely high anesthetic concentrations are used. In that case, the cells are hemolyzed. Certainly therapeutic levels of lidocaine (in the microgram per milliliter range) do not adversely affect the cellular constituents of blood.

The majority of local anesthetics in common use are singularly free of tissue-irritating properties. Nevertheless, traumatic injection, high drug concentration, poor absorption, and other mechanical factors may cause microscopic and macroscopic tissue damage. Some studies have demonstrated profound destruction of muscle cells by local anesthetics injected directly into skeletal muscle. Longer-acting agents such as bupivacaine, and local anesthetics with added epinephrine or acid antioxidant (such as chloroprocaine), exert more profound myotoxicity than plain lidocaine. Fortunately, muscle regenerates quickly and completely following local anesthetic injection. Whether this new knowledge would alter the current practice of injecting myofascial trigger points with local anesthetic remains to be seen.

Neurotoxicity

The local anesthetics in clinical use today by and large appear to have minimal irritating effects on nerve tissue, at least in commonly recommended concentrations. Negligible neurotoxicity is demonstrated by complete recovery of function after regional nerve block, as well as by light microscopic studies. Neural damage may, however, be produced by non-drug-related physical actions. Thus, whereas extraneurally applied anesthetics cause neither short- nor long-term disturbances in nerve function, a high percentage of human subjects show electroneurographic signs of nerve damage after intentional intraneural injection of the ulnar nerve. Such damage is attributable to the increased intraneural pressure caused by injection into a closed space, with compression of, and consequent impairment of, blood supply.

Studies at the subcellular level, however, indicate that local anesthetics may exert a subtle neurotoxic effect after all. Electron micrographic examination of nerves exposed to local anesthetic solution in clinical strengths for half an hour or longer showed loss of neurotubules. Fast axonal transport likewise is slowed, and eventually halted, by prolonged in vitro exposure to lidocaine. The clinical importance of these observations probably is quite limited, since the local anesthetic is rapidly diluted by tissue fluids, and moved from the injection site by diffusion and vascular absorption.

Chloroprocaine Neurotoxicity

In 1979, four cases of prolonged neurologic deficit were reported following unintentional subarachnoid injection of a large dose of chloroprocaine. Animal studies on the neurotoxicity of chloroprocaine have yielded conflicting results. Barsa et al., using a rabbit vagus nerve preparation, showed that chloroprocaine 3%, but not lidocaine or bupivacaine, produced conduction defects, axonal degeneration, perineural fibrosis, and extraneural and perineural cellular infiltration and fibrosis. Ravindran et al., using a dog model, found that of 20 dogs receiving subarachnoid chloroprocaine 35% developed hind limb paralysis and 13 of 15 spinal cords examined showed subpial necrosis. While studies in sheep and monkeys have not shown chloroprocaine neurotoxicity, the issue remains undecided. Recent studies have suggested that sodium metabisulfite in high concentrations may be neurotoxic especially associated with low pH of the solution.

The commercial preparation of chloroprocaine, Nesacaine CE, contains 0.2% sodium metabisulfite and this may explain some of the reported complications that have occurred with Nesacaine.

Studying rabbits, Wang et al. injected subarachnoid either pure 2-chloroprocaine in lactated Ringers solution or 0.2% sodium bisulfate dissolved in lactated Ringer solution. Repeated 2–4 mg spinal anesthetic doses of pure 2-chloroprocaine did not produce chronic hind limb paralysis even though accumulated doses reached 50 mg. However, 1.2–2.4 mg of sodium bisulfite, resulted in irreversible hind limb paralysis in 12 out of 14 animals.

Gissen et al., studying isolated desheathed rabbit vagus nerves, found that 3% Nesacaine CE produced irreversible nerve block. Chloroprocaine without bisulfite did not produce an irreversible block. Subsequent studies showed that a nerve perfused with 0.2% sodium bisulfite solution alone is blocked irreversibly at a pH below 5.0, and shows no block at a pH above 7.0. A 0.05% bisulfite solution allowed normal nerve conduction at pH 4.5 or greater, but blocked the nerve at pH 3.5 or less. Their explanation for the neurotoxicity of bisulfite is that at low pH bisulfite does not act as an antioxidant but rather as a reducing agent, first being reduced to sulfurous acid and then molecular SO_2.

This uncharged molecule readily migrates through the cell membrane, hydrates to sulfurous acid, which then ionizes to bisulfite and hydrogen ion. The marked acidification of the nerve axoplasm causes the damage.

Despite potential neurotoxicity, chloroprocaine has a number of useful properties which make it very popular in obstetrics. Rapid onset, short duration of action, and low systematic toxicity, under certain clinical circumstances, make chloroprocaine the preferred local anesthetic.

CARDIOVASCULAR EFFECTS

Local anesthetics exert a suppressant effect on vascular smooth muscle. Applied directly to a muscular vessel such as an artery, local anesthetics relax the vessel wall. In fact, infusing large quantities of local anesthetic causes widespread vasodilation and consequent hypotension. Cocaine is an exception; by preventing norepinephrine reuptake, it mimics the actions of a vasopressor agent, thus causing intense vasoconstriction. Good use of this property is made when anesthetizing the nasal passages.

Not unexpectedly, in view of their powerful impulse-blocking properties, local anesthetics also block transmission in the conducting system of the heart and decrease myocardial excitability. These properties have been applied therapeutically. As procaine is metabolized so quickly, its amide-linked congener procainamide (Pronestyl) has been widely used instead. One drawback of procainamide is the rather high incidence of hypotension. Increasingly, lidocaine has been used to treat cardiac arrhythmias, those of ventricular origin in particular. One should note nevertheless that bizarre ventricular complexes and even electrical asystole may accompany gross lidocaine overdosage.

Long-lasting local anesthetics—bupivacaine, tetracaine, and etidocaine, for example—alter cardiac conduction much more profoundly than equitoxic doses of less lipid-soluble local anesthetics such as lidocaine.

Bupivacaine Cardiotoxicity

Bupivacaine precipitates nodal and ventricular arrhythmias, and blocks intraventricular conduction in IV doses well below the convulsant level. Lidocaine given to ventilated cats under comparable conditions only rarely gave rise to arrhythmias. These findings might well explain the impression that cardiovascular collapse after bupivacaine is rather resistant to resuscitation. An unusual observation is that bupivacaine-induced cardiac arrhythmias can be reverted to sinus rhythm by the administration of lidocaine. Indeed, a case report of resuscitation from a massive overdose of bupivacaine pointed to successful cardiac conversion with electroshock and lidocaine.

Since 1973 bupivacaine-induced seizures followed by cardiac arrest have been associated with at least 15 maternal deaths and 4 cases of permanent brain damage. It has been estimated by some that cardiac arrest following regional anesthesia with etidocaine or bupivacaine may be relatively more cardiotoxic than the shorter-acting local anesthetics such as lidocaine. Others have maintained that the occurrence of cardiac arrest following seizures caused by local anesthetics was due to delay in the proper treatment of the seizures. Initial animal studies supported this latter theory.

Liu and colleagues, in a study using anesthetized and ventilated dogs, showed deterioration of hemodynamic parameters with increasing cumulative drug dose of all local anesthetics. The same group has also reported that the acute cardiovascular toxicity of all amide local anesthetics is similar and proportional to their in vivo anesthetic potency. They concluded that if animals are ventilated to prevent hypoxia and acidosis following seizures, the cardiovascular/CNS toxicity ratio of highly protein-bound and lipid-soluble agents such as bupivacaine was similar to that of lidocaine.

Recent studies in sheep and rabbits, however, indicate the bupivacaine is far more cardiotoxic than lidocaine. Awake unanesthetized sheep were given either 5.7 mg/kg of lidocaine or 2.1 mg/kg of bupivacaine intravenously over ten seconds. These doses were based on the clinical experience that the usual dose of local anesthetic needed to establish a T_4 sensory level in a 70 kg pregnant patient undergoing epidural anesthesia for cesarean delivery is approximately 20 ml of 2.0% lidocaine (5.7 mg/kg) or 20 ml of 0.75% bupivacaine (2.1 mg/kg). On separate days some animals received twice these doses in order to exaggerate the cardiac effect. All animals seized within 30 seconds of injection and all had significant increases in heart rate, and systemic and pulmonary arterial blood pressures. Sheep receiving intravenous lidocaine did not develop arrhythmias other than mild sinus tachycardia. In contrast, all sheep receiving intravenous bupivacaine had EKG abnormalities including widened QRS complexes and multifocal PVCs.

The most likely mechanism for the bupivacaine cardiotoxicity relates to its action on cardiac sodium channels. This was recently elucidated by Clarkson et al. in a series of studies on guinea pig papillary muscle. Lidocaine and bupivacaine both block sodium channels to the nerve and heart. Sodium channels open briefly during the upstroke of the action potential and are responsible for the fast conduction. Blockade of sodium channels will slow or stop conduction. The latter action at the level of the nerve membrane is considered the primary mechanism of action of local anesthetics.

Clarkson et al. found that although lidocaine and bupivacaine are similar, in that they both cause a fast development of block of cardiac sodium channels upon depolarization, they differ markedly in their recovery from block. Whereas a lidocaine block is complete within less than a second, recovery from bupivacaine requires about 5 times as long. As a result of the slow recovery in the presence of bupivacaine, frequency-dependent block accumulates even at slow heart rates. At normal heart rates, bupivacaine is more than 16 times as potent as lidocaine. Lidocaine gets into the sodium channel quickly but also leaves quickly, while bupivacaine is a "fast in, slow out" agent. As a result, it is a "potentially dangerous cardiac poison." When comparing the effects of lidocaine and bupivacaine upon contractility, it has been observed that bupivacaine is 16 times more potent than lidocaine in reducing isometric contraction by 33%.

Despite its potential cardiotoxicity, bupivacaine is still a very useful agent in regional anesthesia. When used for epidurals it produces high quality analgesia with minimal motor block and has a relatively long duration of action. It is effective in dilutions down to 0.125%.

Correct administration of any local anesthetic requires meticulous technique to avoid systemic toxicity: using the smallest effective dose, cautiously aspirating through the epidural catheter or needle, using adequate size test doses, and slowly administering the dose in fractional amounts. Aspiration that does not produce CSF or blood does not preclude intravascular or subarachnoid injection. Therefore, the anesthesiologist must administer an effective test dose and monitor results before giving the full dose. When using a continuous catheter technique, test doses should be given prior to the original dose and all reinforcing doses because plastic tubing in the epidural space can migrate. A test dose containing 10 to 15 μg of epinephrine, if injected into a blood vessel, will produce an "epinephrine response" within 45 seconds (i.e., an increase in pulse and blood pressure, circumoral pallor, palpitations, and nervousness). The sedated patient may exhibit only increased pulse rate of 20 or more beats per minute for 15 or more seconds on the electrocardioscope. Patients taking beta-adrenergic blocking drugs may not respond to this amount of epinephrine with increased heart rate but will usually have increased blood pressure. Oxygenation and the early termination of seizures are critical, not only to facilitate ventilation, but also to minimize the incidence of metabolic acidosis.

BIBLIOGRAPHY

1. Albright G.A.: Cardiac arrest following regional anesthesia with etidocaine or bupivacaine (editorial). *Anesthesiology* 51:285, 1979.
2. Barsa J., Batra M., Fink B.R., et al.: Local neurotoxicity of local anesthetics. *Anesthesiology* 55:A161, 1981.
3. Clarkson C.W., Thigpen J.W., Schnider S.M., et al.: Bupivacaine toxicity: Fast inactivation block and slow diastolic recovery. *Circulation* 68(suppl. 3):296, 1983.
4. Covino B.G., Vassallo G.H.: *Local Anesthetics: Mechanism of Action and Clinical Use*. New York, Grune & Stratton, 1976.
5. de Jong R.H.: *Local Anesthetics*. Springfield, Ill., Charles C Thomas, Publisher, 1977.
6. de Jong R.H., Ronfeld R.A., DeRosa R.A.: Cardiovascular effects of convulsant and supraconvulsant doses of amide local anesthetics. *Anesth. Analg.* 61:3–9, 1982.
7. DePace N.L., Betesh J.S., Kotler M.N.: "Postmortem" cesarean section with recovery of both mother and offspring. *JAMA* 248:971–973, 1982.
8. Incaudo G., Schatz M., Patterson R., et al.: Administration of local anesthetics to patients with a history of prior adverse reaction. *J. Allergy Clin. Immunol.* 61:339–345, 1978.
9. Kotelko D.M., Schnider S.M., Dailey P.A., et al.: Bupivacaine induced cardiac arrhythmias in sheep. *Anesthesiology* 60:10, 1984.
10. Marx G.F.: Cardiopulmonary resuscitation of late-pregnant women. *Anesthesiology* 56:156, 1982.
11. Moore D.C., Batra M.S.: The components of an effective test dose prior to epidural block. *Anesthesiology* 55:693–696, 1981.
12. Moore D.C., Crawford R.D., Scurlock J.E.: Severe hypoxia and acidosis following local anesthetic-induced convulsions. *Anesthesiology* 53:259–260, 1980.
13. Ravindran R.S., Bond V.K., Tasch M.D., et al.: Prolonged neural blockade following regional analgesia with 2-chloroprocaine. *Anesth. Analg.* 59:447–451, 1980.
14. Ravindran R.S., Turner M.S., Muller J.: Neurologic effects of subarachnoid administration of 2-chloroprocain-CE, bupivacaine, and low pH normal saline in dogs. *Anesth. Analg.* 61:279–283, 1982.
15. Reisner L.S., Hockman B.N., Plumer M.N.: Persistent neurologic deficit and adhesive arachnoiditis following intrathecal 2-chloroprocain injection. *Anesth. Analg.* 59:452–454, 1980.
16. Scott D.B.: Evaluation of the toxicity of local anaesthetic agents in man. *Br. J. Anaesth.* 49:121–125, 1977.
17. Thigpen J.W., Kotelko D.M., Schnider S.M., et al.: Bupivacaine cardiotoxicity in hypoxic-acidotic sheep. *Anesthesiology* 59:A204, 1983.
18. Wang B.C., Hillman D.E., Spielholz N.I., et al.: Chronic neurological deficits and Nesacaine CE. An effect of the anesthetic, 2-chloroprocaine, or the antioxidant, sodium bisulfate? *Anesth. Analg.* 63:445, 1984.
19. Gissen A.J., Dalta S., Lambert D., et al.: Is chloroprocaine (2 cp) neurotoxic? *Reg. Anesth.* 9:37, 1984.
20. Liu P., Feldman H.S., Covino B.M., et al.: Acute cardiovascular toxicity of intravenous amide local anesthetics in anesthetised ventilated dogs. *Anesth. Analg.* 61:317–322, 1982.

32 / Neurolytic Agents

P. PRITHVI RAJ, M.D.
DONALD D. DENSON, PH.D.

THE INJECTION OF neurolytic agents to interrupt pain pathways for a prolonged period of time has been practiced for many years. The object of such injections is to destroy the nerve fibers and thus produce a prolonged and sometimes permanent nerve block, with resulting effects resembling those of nerve section. Nerve blocking with these agents is employed in patients with severe intractable pain and in whom neurosurgical procedures are contraindicated, owing to poor physical condition or other circumstances.

Over the years, a variety of agents and combinations of agents have undergone clinical trials, with varying results. Many techniques, such as intrathecal injection of distilled water or hypertonic ice-cold saline, have fallen by the wayside. Serapin or pitcher plant distillate and ammonium salt solutions showed some promise but for the most part have been deleted from the list of useful neurolytics. Ethyl alcohol and phenol have received considerable clinical attention and, based on reasonable, long-term results, have remained the neurolytics of choice. Even though some pharmacologic and pathologic studies have been reported, there remains a paucity of scientific information with which the physician managing intractable pain can make rational choices.

ALCOHOL

The effect of alcohol on somatic nerves was studied by Schlosser,[1] who noted and recorded that alcoholization was followed by degeneration and absorption of all the components of the nerve except the neurolemma. There is general agreement that with 95% and absolute alcohol, the destruction involves sympathetic, sensory, and motor components of a mixed somatic nerve, and therefore it is undesirable to block a mixed nerve with such concentrations of alcohol. However, there is a great discrepancy in the conclusions concerning the effect of alcohol in concentrations below 80% on motor fibers (Table 32–1 and Fig 32–1).

Finkelburg studied this problem by injecting 0.5–1.5 cc of 60%–80% alcohol into the exposed sciatic nerve of dogs and rabbits.[2] Persistent paralysis resulted with these concentrations. May found that injection of 0.5 cc of alcohol (76%) into the exposed sciatic nerve of the cat was followed by motor paralysis, the duration of which varied considerably, irrespective of the strength of alcohol used, provided it was above 60%.[3] With 80% alcohol he observed motor paralysis lasting 91 days in one case and 19 days in another; with 90% alcohol paralysis lasted 64 days in one case and 88 in another. The paralysis was always followed by recovery. In some cases there was no microscopic evidence of nerve degeneration after recovery; in other cases there was evidence of nerve degeneration and regeneration after recovery. With absolute alcohol, however, May always found considerable fibrosis at the site of injection of normal nerve, with some regenerative process above and intermingled degeneration and regeneration below the fibrous zone. He also found that 50% alcohol produced no motor weakness. Gordon,[4] using 80% alcohol, found that by the ninth day there was less evidence of motor involvement than on the 29th day, when he observed partial degeneration in some cases and complete degeneration in others. Nevertheless, no animal was completely paralyzed. Nasaroff,[5] using 70% alcohol, never observed complete paralysis, only the onset of temporary paresis at the end of the second week, at which time he found progressive and simultaneous

557

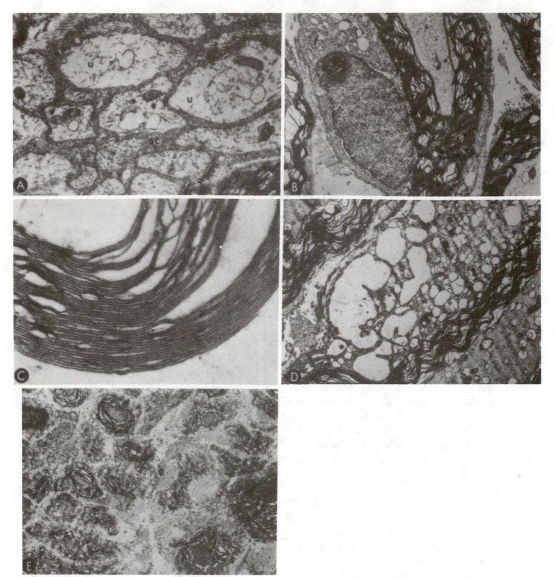

Fig 32–1.—A, effects of alcohol on the peripheral nerve, 15 seconds after application. Electron micrograph shows the sciatic nerve of a mouse after topical application of 100% alcohol. *Arrows* denote swelling of unmyelinated nerve fibers; *sc* indicates Schwann cell cytoplasm that is clumped and granular—Schwann cell destruction (×5000). **B,** effect of alcohol on the peripheral nerve, 15 seconds after application. Electron micrograph shows the Schwann cell after exposure to 100% alcohol. Note splitting of the myelin sheath *(MS)* and dilated endoplasmic reticulum *(ER),* indicating acute injury to the Schwann cell and myelin sheath (×4300). **C,** effect of alcohol on the peripheral nerve, 1 minute after application. Electron micrograph shows splitting of the myelin sheath after exposure to 100% alcohol (×9600). **D,** effect of alcohol on the peripheral nerve, 24 hours after a 15-second exposure to 100% alcohol. Note degenerating axons *(A),* splitting myelin lamellae *(M),* and beginning of connective tissue reaction (CR; ×2200). **E,** effect of alcohol on the peripheral nerve, 4 hours after 15-second exposure. Electron micrograph shows vacuolization *(V)* in the Schwann cell after exposure to 100% alcohol. (From Woolsey R.M., Taylor J.J., Nagel J.H.: Acute effects of topical ethyl alcohol on the sciatic nerve of the mouse. *Arch. Phys. Med. Rehabil.* 53:410, 1972. Reproduced by permission.)

TABLE 32–1.—CONCENTRATION, NERVE FIBER EFFECT, AND EFFICACY OF COMMONLY USED NEUROLYTIC AGENTS

AGENT	CONCENTRATION (%)	NERVE FIBER AFFECTED	% SUCCESS (APPROXIMATE)
Alcohol	100	All fibers	58
	75	Sensory and C fibers	
	50	C fibers	
Phenol in glycerin or	6–12	Motor, sensory, and C fibers	60
Renografin or			
metrizamide	3	C fibers	
Ammonium sulfate	10	C fibers	40
Cold saline	Hypertonic	C fibers	30

degenerative and regenerative processes. These findings seem to indicate that 70% alcohol does not cause irremediable damage to somatic nerves. Labat[6] extensively studied this subject, using 48% (equal parts of 95% alcohol and 1% procaine) and 95% alcohol. He observed temporary paralysis with both concentrations in all animals. The period of time required to recover from the paralysis varied, and was inconsistent with the concentration of the alcohol. Thus, in one case 48% alcohol caused paralysis for 50 days, the same duration of paralysis as in another case in which 95% alcohol had been used. On microscopic examination performed after recovery, no demonstrable nerve changes could be seen.

Labat and Greene[7] reported quite satisfactory clinical results in the management of painful disorders by employing 33⅓% alcohol without any resulting muscular paralysis or even paresis.

Ethyl Alcohol

Ethyl alcohol is a potent neurolytic agent that can nonselectively destroy spinal and peripheral nerves. The neuronal action of ethanol involves the extraction of phospholipid cholesterol and cerebroside. Precipitation of mucoproteins and lipoproteins is also noted. In peripheral nerves, these actions result in a separation of the myelin sheath and edematous Schwann cell and axon. Following subarachnoid injection, myelin sheath and beating of the axis cylinder are seen. Following subarachnoid injection, alcohol disappears from the CSF extremely rapidly,[8] declining from an initial concentration of 25.6% to 3.1% after only 10 minutes. After 30 minutes, the alcohol concentration was 0.9%. Unfortunately, no plasma concentrations were measured, and the absolute neural uptake could not be accurately assessed.

The minimum concentration of alcohol required

for neurolysis has not been definitely established. It has been stated that 30% ethanol in the subarachnoid space temporarily destroys sensory but not motor fibers, and that 80% ethanol causes only a reversible sensory block. In vitro studies on rabbit sciatic nerves showed equivalent suppression and action potential of large- and small-diameter nerve fibers when exposed to 35% ethanol.[9] Fisher et al. concluded there was no evidence of discrimination according to either fiber diameter or conduction velocity.

For subarachnoid block, concentrations between 50% and 100% are generally selected (Fig 32–2). The reported volumes required for neurolysis have ranged from 0.3 ml per segment to a maximum of 0.7 ml of absolute alcohol[8] to 0.5–1 ml per segment to a maximum of 1.5 ml per segment.[10] For celiac plexus block, volumes of 10–20 ml of absolute alcohol bilaterally may be used.[10] Similar volumes have been reported for lumbar sympathetic block. Often, 100% alcohol is diluted 1:1 with a local anesthetic prior to injection.

Complications of Alcohol Nerve Block

Neuritis

The use of alcohol to effect prolonged nerve block presents one great disadvantage—the possible occurrence of alcoholic neuritis. This complication, when it occurs, is so objectionable and so serious that many clinicians have rejected this method of nerve blocking.

It has been postulated that alcoholic neuritis is due to incomplete destruction of somatic nerves. This is probably so, because alcoholic neuritis has not been observed following the intraneural injection of a cranial or somatic nerve that produces a

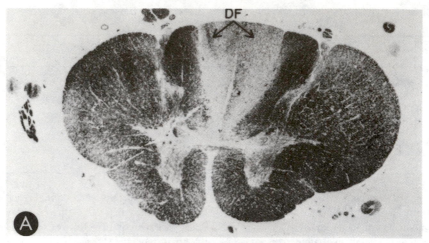

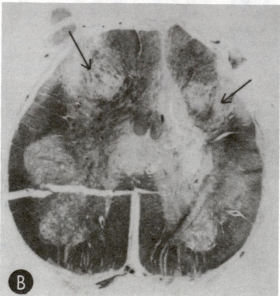

Fig 32–2.—A, effect of alcohol on the spinal cord, 4 days after neurolytic block. Cross section through the spinal cord at T-4 shows degeneration of the dorsal fascicularis *(DF)* after injection of 100% alcohol several interspaces lower. **B,** effect of alcohol on the spinal cord, 50 days after direct cord injection. Note necrosis and degeneration (arrows) following accidental injection of 100% alcohol into the spinal cord. (From Gallagher H.S., Yonezawa T., Hay R.C., et al.: Subarachnoid alcohol block: II. Histologic changes in the central nervous system. *Am. J. Pathol.* 35:679, 1961. Reproduced by permission.)

complete block. Alcoholic neuritis occurs most frequently following paravertebral block of the thoracic sympathetics, because here the sympathetic ganglia lie so close to the intercostal nerves that the alcohol, intended for the ganglion, also bathes and partially destroys the somatic nerve. During the period of regeneration, hyperesthesia and intense burning pain with occasional sharp shooting pain occur.

These pains are sometimes so severe that they are worse than the original pain. Fortunately, in most instances these symptoms subside within a few weeks or a month. Occasionally, however, this complication persists for many months, requiring sedation, and in some instances it is necessary to perform a subsequent rhizotomy or sympathectomy.

PROPHYLAXIS OF ALCOHOLIC NEURITIS.—In the thoracic region it is most difficult to avoid this complication, because the somatic nerves lie so close to the sympathetics that alcohol intended for the latter usually involves the former. Mandl recommends, as a prophylactic measure against this complication, the injection of a local anesthetic–procaine mixture during the insertion of the needle, at the site of injection before the alcohol is injected, and on withdrawing the needle. With this technique he has observed only two instances of alcoholic neuritis.

TREATMENT.—Mild cases of alcoholic neuritis are treated conservatively with mild analgesics such as aspirin or with small doses of codeine.

Moderate cases of alcoholic neuritis may require more active therapy. One can employ intravenous histamine, 2.75 mg dissolved in 500 cc of 5% glucose in distilled water, administered twice daily, with some success. Several patients have been helped by the intravenous administration of local anesthetics. Bonica has found pontocaine, 250 mg dissolved in 500 cc of fluid, superior to procaine.[11] In one case in which IV procaine had been administered several times with only transient relief of pain, one infusion of tetracaine effected prolonged relief. In some cases daily sympathetic blocks have been employed, with excellent results. In the case of lumbar nerve neuritis following lumbar sympathetic blocks, serial caudal blocks done at regular intervals can effect complete relief of pain.

Severe cases of alcoholic neuritis that do not respond to these conservative methods may require sympathectomy or rhizotomy. De Takats[12] reported three such cases in which sympathectomy was required.

Benzyl Alcohol

Benzyl alcohol has been advocated as a neurolytic agent for prolonged nerve blocking with the claim that it does not cause irritative phenomena like those caused by ethyl alcohol. Duncan and Jarvis[13] have demonstrated that the prolonged effects of the anesthetic mixtures in oil were caused almost entirely by the benzyl alcohol content, and that this substance in 10% concentrations will destroy all the small nerve fibers and in 5% concentrations will destroy a considerable number of them. This action is exerted without any concomitant neuritis. Irritant phenomena are rare following the use of oil mixtures.

Bromsalizol

Lee, Macht, and Pierpont[14] reported the use of monobromohydroxybenzyl alcohol, more familiarly known as bromsalizol, to prolong sympathetic block. Because of its low solubility in water, peanut oil was used as a vehicle. A 4% solution of the alcohol in oil was employed by these authors for paravertebral sympathetic blocks in 103 patients presenting with a great variety of peripheral circulatory disorders.[15] They observed sympathetic interruption for as long as 8 days following a single injection without the occurrence of irritative phenomena or motor paralysis.

Subsequently Harmel, Vandam, and Lamont[15] employed 4% bromsalizol, and although they observed blocking effects for a longer period of time than one would expect with procaine, there was great variation in the length of time. This difficulty in obtaining consistently prolonged effects, which they attributed to the low diffusibility of the peanut oil solution, led them to use a more concentrated and more diffusible solution. They chose 20% bromsalizol in polyethylene glycol-400. They soon observed, however, that following injection of this solution patients had fever, pain, and other signs of tissue irritation. They therefore concluded that 20% bromsalizol in polyethylene glycol-400 is too irritating for clinical use.

PHENOL

That phenol could destroy tissue has been known since its first discovery. Apparently its first deliberate use to destroy nervous tissue was by Doppler in Germany in 1925.[16] After trying it in rabbits, he painted it on ovarian vessels and noted downstream vasodilation and flush. Later Doppler reported treating peripheral vascular disease in the lower extremity by exposing and painting the femoral arteries with a 7% aqueous solution. He reported improvement in 12 patients, but did not give a failure or complication rate. In 1933 Binet[16] in France reported painting ovarian vessels with 7% phenol. Both workers attributed their good results to destruction of perivascular sympathetic fibers.

The first use of phenol by injection for the purpose of neurolysis was reported by Putnam and Hampton in 1936 for neurolysis of the gasserian ganglion.[17] The use of phenol as a local anesthetic had already been reported by Nechaev in the Russian literature in 1933.[18]

Mandl in 1947 suggested the injection of phenol to obtain permanent sympathectomy.[19] In 1950 he reported its use in 15 patients without complications, suggesting that it was preferable to alcohol.[20] In 1949 Haxton[21] and Boyd et al.[22] also reported on the paravertebral injection of phenol for peripheral vascular disease. In 1955 Maher introduced it as a hyperbaric solution for intrathecal use in intractable cancer pain, with the famous remark that "it is easier to lay a carpet than to paper a ceiling."[23] Thereafter he reported its epidural use as well.

By 1959 phenol was established as a neurolytic agent for the relief of chronic pain. Then Kelly and Gautier-Smith[24] and Nathan[25] simultaneously reported on the intrathecal injection of phenol in hyperbaric solution with positioning to fix it on anterior nerve roots, thus relieving spasticity caused by upper motor neuron lesions. Since then phenol has been widely used for neurolysis in the treatment of both pain and spasticity (Fig 32–3).

Phenol is not available as a ready-to-use pharmaceutical preparation. It must be prepared from an analytical grade phenol in sterile ampules by a hospital pharmacist. When it is to be mixed with glycerin, great care must be taken that both phenol and glycerin are free of water, or the necrotizing effect of the supposed phenol-glycerin mixture will be much greater than anticipated. Phenol is highly soluble in glycerin and diffuses from it slowly, an advantage in intrathecal injection that allows for limited spread and highly localized tissue fixation. Phenol has been prepared in sterile water, normal saline, Renografin and metrizamide. We prefer 6%–12% phenol in Renografin for extraspinal injections and phenol in metrizamide for epidural or intrathecal use.

Its mode of action when used as a neurolytic agent has been extensively studied, and was reviewed by Felsenthal in 1974.[26] Maher, seeking the ideal strength solution, tried concentrations of phenol in glycerin varying from 10% to 3.3% in the subarachnoid space.[24] The stronger concentration produced motor damage, and there was gradation of block according to the concentration, with pain sensation being blocked at lower concentrations (5%) than were touch and proprioception. The 3.3% concentration was ineffective. Iggo and Walsh followed with a study of action potentials in cat spinal rootlets and concluded that 5% phenol in either Ringer's solution or oil contrast medium produced selective block of smaller nerve fibers.[27] Simultaneously, Nathan and Sears, using the same preparation, arrived at the same conclusion.[28] For a long time

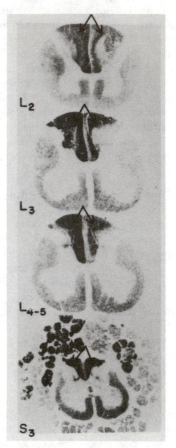

Fig 32–3.—Effect of phenol on the spinal cord. Micrographs of transverse sections at levels L–2, L–3, L4–5, and S–3. They show degeneration of the posterior column following subarachnoid injection of phenol at L3–4. (From Smith M.C.: Histological findings following intrathecal injections of phenol solutions for relief of pain. *Br. J. Anaesth.* 36:387, 1964. Reproduced by permission.)

thereafter the idea prevailed that phenol caused selective destruction of smaller nerve fibers with slower conduction rates, the C afferents carrying slow pain, the A delta afferents carrying fast pain, and the A gamma efferents controlling muscle tone.

These observations led to the histopathologic studies. Stewart and Lourie in 1963 saw nonselective degeneration in cat rootlets, the severity being parallel to the concentration.[29] Nathan et al. repeated their action potential studies and then looked at the histopathology.[30] This time they found evidence of A alpha and A beta damage in the electrophysiologic experiments and confirmed the nonselectivity of damage by histologic examination. They pointed out that phenol in low concentrations is a local anesthetic and when acting as such has a selective effect, as do other local anesthetics. However, when time of exposure and concentration are adequate, protein denaturating results, and this effect is nonselective.

Since this report the overall destructive effect of phenol has been confirmed by various authors. Knott et al.[31] noted nerve damage from phenol in saline or in dimethylsulfoxide; Møller et al.,[32] after comparing low concentrations of phenol with low concentrations of alcohol, concluded that 3% phenol was similar to 40% alcohol. Schaumberg et al.[33] performed a meticulous combined electrophysiologic and histologic study, while Burkel et al.[34] included electron microscopic observations and noted severe damage to the perineural vascular elements, maximum degeneration at 2 weeks, maximum recovery at 14 weeks, and no identifiable binding site for tritium-labeled phenol.

The block produced by phenol tends to be less profound and of shorter duration than that produced by alcohol. Axons of all sizes are affected by therapeutic concentrations and, as described for ethyl alcohol, appear edematous. Importantly, the posterior root ganglia are unaffected by phenol. Similar pathologic changes occur in peripheral nerves when exposed to phenol. The composition of phenol solutions determine the neurolytic potency. That is, aqueous solutions of phenol are far more potent than those prepared in glycerin. Solutions of phenol are subject to oxidative degradation on prolonged storage. While concentrations of 3%–10% have been evaluated, the most commonly selected concentrations are between 6 and 8% (Fig 32–4, Plate 12). Recent studies[53] of 6%, 9%, and 12% phenol in calsaphenous nerves show 12% phenol in renograffin to be a better neurolytic agent than lesser concentrations. Figure 32–4 shows ulceration of the skin with 6% phenol infiltration subcutaneously. The clinician is cautioned not to inject too superficially under the skin for this reason.

No pharmacokinetic data are available to describe the systemic absorption and disposition following neurolytic administration. Phenol is efficiently metabolized by liver enzymes. The principal pathways are conjugation to the glucuronides and oxidation to quinol compounds or to carbon dioxide and water, and excretion as a variety of conjugates via the kidneys.

AMMONIUM SALTS

In 1935 Judavich used pitcher plant distillate for long-term analgesia. It was later reported that the active component of pitcher plant distillate was in fact ammonium sulfate, ammonium chloride, or ammonium hydroxide, depending on the acid used to neutralize the distillate and on the pH.[35] Limited pathologic studies suggested that ammonium salts in concentrations of greater than 10% caused acute degenerative neuropathy. This degeneration is nonselective, affecting all types of nerve fibers. More recent in vitro studies with pitcher plant distillate attributed the effects to benzyl alcohol contained in the vehicle.[36] Associated complications such as nausea and vomiting, headache, paresthesia, and spinal cord injury have led to the clinical abandonment of ammonium salt solutions, including pitcher plant distillate.

The action of ammonium salts on nerve impulses produces obliteration of C fiber potentials with only a small effect on A fibers.[37, 38] Limited pathologic studies suggest that injection of ammonium salts around a peripheral nerve causes an acute degenerative neuropathy affecting all fibers.

Hand has reported the use of subarachnoid ammonium salts in 50 patients.[39] Transient complications were nausea, retching, and headache, while parethesias or burning sensation occurred in 30% of patients at doses of 500 mg of ammonium salt and lasted 2–14 days.

HYPERTONIC AND HYPOTONIC SOLUTIONS

A simple method for achieving neurolysis is by the subarachnoid injection of either distilled water or hypertonic salt solutions.[40]

The intrathecal injection of cold 0.9% NaCL (2°–4° C) is supposed to have a specific action on the pain carrying C fibers, sparing the larger fibers that subserve sensory, motor, and autonomic functions.[41] The technique requires the spinal fluid to be withdrawn and replaced with cold saline as rapidly as possible. Up to 40–60 ml of saline has been injected. The procedure is very distressing without the concomitant use of a local anesthetic. The pain relief is usually short-lived.

A variety of complications have been reported following intrathecal administration of hypertonic saline.[42] Some degree of complications occurred in

11% and significant morbidity in 1% of patients. Two deaths have been reported secondary to myocardial infarction. During saline injection, sinus tachycardia or premature ventricular contraction have been seen,[43] and localized paresis lasting for many hours and paresthesia extending for weeks has been observed.[44] Other complications reported include hemiplegia, pulmonary edema, pain in the ear, vestibular disturbances, and loss of sphincter control with sacral anesthesia.[45-48]

Pathologic changes due to hypertonic and hypotonic solutions have been extensively studied.[49-52] Microscopic changes seen on the peripheral nerves do not correlate with clinical effects of differential C fiber block.[46, 52] However, application of distilled water on the dorsal root ganglia for 5 minutes produced a differential C fiber block similar to that seen with in vitro hypertonic saline. The mechanism of action seems to be the intracellular shifts of water with extracellular change in osmolarity.

REFERENCES

1. Schlosser H.: Erfahrungen in der Neuralgiebehandlung mit Alkoholeinspritzungen. *Verh. Dtsch. Ges. Inn. Med.* 24:49, 1907.
2. Finkelburg R.: Experimentelle Untersuchungen über den Einfluss von Alkoholinjektionen und periferische Nerven. *Verh. Dtsch. Ges. Inn. Med.* 24:75, 1907.
3. May O.: Functional and histological effects of intraneural and intraganglionic injections of alcohol. *Br. Med. J.* 2:365, 1912.
4. Gordon A.: Experimental study of intraneural injections of alcohol. *J. Nerv. Ment. Dis.* 41:81, 1914.
5. Nasaroff N.N.: Über Alkoholinjektionen in Nervenstamine. *Zentralbl. Chir.* 52:2777, 1925.
6. Labat G.: Action of alcohol on the living nerve. *Curr. Res. Anesth. Analg.* 12:190, 1933.
7. Labat G., Greene M.B.: Contribution to the modern method of diagnosis and treatment of so-called sciatic neuralgias. *Am. J. Surg.* 11:435, 1931.
8. Matsuki M., Kato Y., Ichiyangi L.: Progressive changes in the concentrations of ethyl alcohol in the human and canine subarachnoid space. *Anesthesiology* 36:617, 1972.
9. Fisher E., Cress R.H., Haines G., et al.: Evoked nerve conduction after nerve block by chemical means. *Am. J. Phys. Med.* 49:333–334, 1970.
10. Dwyer B., Gibb D.: Chronic pain and neurolytic neural blockade, in Cousins M.J., Bridenbaugh P.O. (eds.): *Neural Blockade Clinical Anesthesia and Management of Pain.* Philadelphia, J.B. Lippincott, Co., 1980.
11. Bonica J.J.: Regional anesthesia with tetracaine. *Anesthesiology* 11:606, 716, 1950.
12. De Takats G.: Discussion of paper by H.S. Ruth: Diagnostic, prognostic and therapeutic nerve blocks. *JAMA* 102:419, 1934.
13. Duncan D., Jarvis W.H.: A comparison of the actions of nerve fibers of certain anesthetic mixtures and substances in oil. *Anesthesiology* 4:465, 1943.
14. Lee F.C., Macht D.I., Pierpont R.Z.: The use of bromsalizol in lengthening the effect of a sympathetic nerve block. *Am. J. Med. Sci.* 209:314, 1945.
15. Harmel M.H., Vandam L.D., Lamont A.: An attempt to prolong sympathetic block with bromsalizol in polyethylene glycol. *Anesthesiology* 8:266, 1947.
16. Binet A.: Valeur de la sympathectomie chimique en gynecologie. *Gynecol. Obstet.* 27:393–415, 1933.
17. Putnam T.J., Hampton A.O.: A technique of injection into the Gasserian ganglion under roentgenographic control. *Arch. Neurol. Psychiatry* 35:92–98, 1936.
18. Nechaev V.A.: Solutions of phenol in local anesthesia. *Soviet Khir.* 5:203, 1933.
19. Mandl F.: *Paravertebral Block.* New York, Grune & Stratton, 1947.
20. Mandl F.: Aqueous solution of phenol as a substitute for alcohol in sympathetic block. *J. Int. Coll. Surg.* 13:566–568, 1950.
21. Haxton H.A.: Chemical sympathectomy. *Br. Med J.* 1:1026, 1949.
22. Boyd A.M., Ratcliff A.H., Jepson R.P., et al.: Intermittent claudication. *J. Bone Joint Surg.* 3B:325, 1949.
23. Maher R.M.: Phenol for pain and spasticity, in *Pain: Henry Ford Hospital International Symposium.* Boston, Little, Brown & Co., 1966.
24. Kelly R.E., Gautier-Smith P.C.: Intrathecal phenol in the treatment of reflex spasms and spasticity. *Lancet* 2:1102–1105, 1959.
25. Nathan P.W.: Intrathecal phenol to relieve spasticity in paraplegia. *Lancet* 2:1099–1102, 1959.
26. Felsenthal G.: Pharmacology of phenol in peripheral nerve blocks: A review. *Arch. Phys. Med. Rehabil.* 55:13–16, 1974.
27. Iggo A., Walsh E.G.: Selective block of small fibres in the spinal roots by phenol. *Brain* 83:701–708, 1960.
28. Nathan P.W., Sears T.A.: Effects of phenol on nervous conduction. *J. Physiol. (London)* 150:565–580, 1960.
29. Stewart W.A., Lourie H.: An experimental evaluation of the effects of subarachnoid injection of phenol-pantopaque in cats. *J. Neurosurg.* 20:64–72, 1963.
30. Nathan P.W., Sers T.A., Smith M.C.: Effects of phenol solutions on the nerve roots of the cat: An electrophysiologic and histological study. *J. Neurol. Sci.* 2:7–29, 1965.
31. Knott L.W., Katz J., Rubenstein L.J.: Separate and combined effects of phenol, hyaluronidase, and dimethyl sulfoxide on the sciatic nerve of the rat. *Arch. Phys. Med. Rehabil.* 49:100–104, 1968.
32. Møller J.E., Helweg-Larson J., Jacobsen E.: Histo-

pathological lesions in the sciatic nerve of the rat following perineural application of phenol and alcohol solutions. *Dan. Med. Bull.* 16:116–119, 1969.

33. Schaumberg H.N., Byck R., Weller R.O.: The effect of phenol on peripheral nerves: A histological and electrophysiological study. *J. Neuropathol. Exp. Neurol.* 29:615–630, 1970.

34. Burkel W.E., McPhee M.: Effect of phenol injection into peripheral nerve of rat: Electron microscope studies. *Arch. Phys. Med. Rehabil.* 51:391, 1970.

35. Walti A.: Determination of the nature of the volatile base from the rhizome of the pitcher plant, *Sarracenia purpurea. J. Am. Chem. Soc.* 67:22–71, 1945.

36. Ford D.J., Phero J.C., Denson D.: Effect of pitcher plant distillate on frog sciatic nerve. *Reg. Anaesth.* 5(1):16–18, 1980.

37. Davies J.I., Steward P.B., Fink P.: Prolonged sensory block using ammonium salts. *Anesthesiology* 28:244, 1967.

38. Judovich B.D., Bates W., Bishop K.: Intraspinal ammonium salts for the intractable pain of malignancy. *Anesthesiology* 5:341, 1944.

39. Hand L.V.: Subarachnoid ammonium sulfate therapy for intractable pain. *Anesthesiology* 5:354, 1944.

40. Hitchcock E.: Osmolytic neurolysis for intractable facial pain. *Lancet* 1:434, 1969.

41. Lund P.C.: *Principles and Practice of Spinal Anesthesia.* Springfield, Ill., Charles C Thomas, Publisher, 1971.

42. Lucas J.T., Ducker T.B., Perok P.L.: Adverse reactions to intrathecal saline injection for control of pain. *J. Neurosurg.* 42:557, 1975.

43. McKean M.C., Hitchcock E.: Electro-cardiographic changes after intrathecal hypertonic saline solution. *Lancet* 2:1083, 1968.

44. Ventrafridda V., Spreafico R.: Subarachnoid saline perfusion. *Adv. Neurol.* 4:477, 1974.

45. O'Higgins J.W., Padfield A., Clapp H.: Possible complication of hypothermic saline subarachnoid injection. *Lancet* 1:567, 1970.

46. Thompson G.E.: Pulmonary edema complicating intrathecal hypertonic saline injection for intractable pain. *Anesthesiology* 35:425, 1971.

47. Hitchcock E.: Osmotic neurolysis for intractable facial pain. *Lancet* 1:434, 1969.

48. Booth A.E.: Intrathecal hypertonic saline. *Proc. R. Soc. Med.* 67:772, 1974.

49. Hewett D.L., King J.S.: Conduction block of monkey dorsal rootlets by water and hypertonic solutions. *Exp. Neurol.* 33:225, 1971.

50. King J.S., Jewett D.L., Phil D., et al.: Differential blockade of cat dorsal root C fibers by various chloride solutions. *J. Neurosurg.* 36:569, 1972.

51. Robertson J.D.: Structural alterations in nerve fibres produced by hypotonic and hypertonic solutions. *J. Biophys. Biochem. Cytol.* 4:349, 1958.

52. Nicholson M.F., Roberts F.W.: Relief of pain by intrathecal injection of hypothermic saline. *Med. J. Aust.* 1:61, 1968.

53. Gregg R.V., Constantini C.H., Ford D.J., et al.: Electrophysiologic and histopathologic investigation of phenol in renografin as a neurolytic agent. *Anesthesiology* 63:A239, 1985.

PART VI

Techniques of Pain Management

33 / Myofascial Trigger Point Injection

P. PRITHVI RAJ, M.D.

SKELETAL MUSCLE is the largest single organ of the human body and accounts for 40% of the body weight. Since the contractile muscle tissues are extremely subject to the wear and tear of daily activities, any one of these muscles can develop myofascial trigger points that can cause pain and muscle spasm.

Trigger points are extremely common. Latent trigger points are more common than active trigger points. Sola et al. found latent trigger points in 54% of the females and 45% of the males in a normal young adult population.[1] In patients hospitalized for myofascial pain, the incidence of active trigger points is highest in those between the ages of 31 and 50 years.[2] With advancing age and reduced physical activity, latent trigger points become more prominent.

A major difficulty in understanding myofascial pain has been the multiplicity of names given to this syndrome. Good used the term ''muscular rheumatism'' in 1938.[4] Later the same author used ''nonarticular rheumatism,'' ''myalgic spots,'' ''idiopathic myalgia,'' and ''muscular sciatica'' for the syndrome of myofascial pain.[4] Kelly used the term ''fibrositis,'' and Travell initially used ''idiopathic myalgia,'' changing it to ''myofascial trigger points'' in her later publications.[5-7] Other names given to this syndrome include rheumatic myositis, myofasciitis, nodular fibromyositis, and fibropathic syndrome.[8-11]

PATHOPHYSIOLOGY OF A TRIGGER POINT

Many workers believe that a myofascial trigger point starts as a neuromuscular dysfunction[12] and evolves into a histologically distinct lesion.[13]

Miehlke et al. reported biopsy findings that supported the existence of an initial dysfunction phase, followed by a dystrophic phase.[13]

An acute muscle strain may overload the muscle fibrils in one region of the muscle, causing tissue damage that includes damage to the sarcoplastic reticulum and release of stored calcium, with loss of ability in that region to remove the calcium ions. The presence of normal adenosine triphosphate (ATP) and excess calcium will initiate and maintain a sustained contracture of the fibers exposed to the calcium (Fig 33–1). This produces a region of uncontrolled metabolism within the muscle, to which the body responds with local vasoconstriction. This could be a local response or a trigger point–mediated reflex response involving the CNS and the sympathetic nervous system. There is now a region of increased metabolism with decreased circulation and shortened muscle fibers. This group of taut fibers is palpable as a band in the muscle (Tables 33–1 and 33–2).

A second mechanism may then take over. The total depletion of ATP could lead to conditions similar to others that are known to cause muscle contracture with electrical silence, as in McArdle's disease, carnitine deficiency, and rigor mortis. Without ATP the myosin heads do not release actin filaments and the sarcomeres become rigid.

Nerve-sensitizing substances such as histamine, serotonin, kinins, and prostaglandins may be released in the trigger point zone by several mechanisms. With the tissue injury, some blood would extravasate, forming a large source for serotonin due to increased platelets.[14] This could cause further local ischemia. Mast cells are also seen to increase in number at the site of muscle injury, causing a release of histamine.[14] The initial phase of increased metabolism with reduced circulation would result in

569

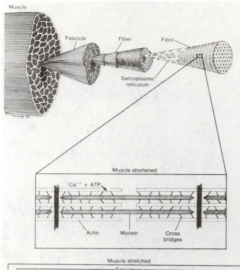

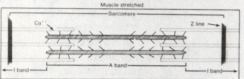

Fig 33–1.—Subunits of a skeletal muscle with the microanatomy of the myofibril, showing the relationship between Ca^{++} and ATP during muscle contraction and relaxation. (From Travell and Simons.[45] Reproduced by permission.)

accumulation of local metabolic products, which may result in the release of additional sensitizing agents such as prostaglandins.[13, 15]

DIFFERENTIAL DIAGNOSIS

To diagnose an active myofascial trigger point, one should look for a history of muscle injury or muscle overactivity, a characteristic trigger point and its referred pattern of pain, weakness and limitation of stretching in the affected muscle, a taut palpable band with exquisite local tenderness, and pain reproducible by digital pressure on the tender spot. Nonmyofascial trigger points are found in the skin and scar tissue, fascia and ligaments, and periosteum. They usually are circumscribed and do not have zones of referred pain in the muscles.

Three major musculoskeletal diseases must be distinguished from the syndrome of myofascial trigger points: myopathies, arthritis, and inflammatory musculoskeletal disorders (e.g., tendinitis, bursitis).

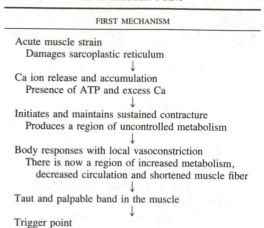

TABLE 33–1.—PATHOPHYSIOLOGY OF A TRIGGER POINT

FIRST MECHANISM
Acute muscle strain   Damages sarcoplastic reticulum ↓
Ca ion release and accumulation   Presence of ATP and excess Ca ↓
Initiates and maintains sustained contracture   Produces a region of uncontrolled metabolism ↓

Body responses with local vasoconstriction
   There is now a region of increased metabolism,
      decreased circulation and shortened muscle fiber
↓

Taut and palpable band in the muscle ↓
Trigger point

SYMPTOMS

The myofascial pain may begin acutely with muscle strain or may begin insidiously due to chronic muscular fatigue. Pain may continue for months or years.[16] Regardless of the mode of onset, characteristically pain due to myofascial trigger point is steady, deep, and aching. Rarely is it burning. Myofascial trigger point pain can be augmented by the following: strenuous use of the involved muscle, passive stretch of the muscle, pressure on the trigger point, cold or damp weather, viral infections, stress, and fatigue.

Even though pain may not be the main complaint, there is usually a limited range of motion and weak-

TABLE 33–2.—PATHOPHYSIOLOGY OF A TRIGGER POINT

SECOND MECHANISM
Tissue injury ↓
Releases histamine Serotonin Kinins Prostaglandins ↓
Further ischemia Increased metabolism with reduced circulation ↓
Accumulates metabolic products ↓
Increases further sensitizing products ↓
Active trigger point

ness. Limitation of motion and increased stiffness are worse in the morning and recur after periods of overactivity or immobilization during the day. Patients may report symptoms of autonomic dysfunction, e.g., excessive lacrimation, pilomotor activity, and changes in sweat patterns. The involved extremity may feel cold due to reflex vasoconstriction. Patients may have signs of depression and sleep disturbances, which in turn may lower the pain threshold.

CLINICAL CHARACTERISTICS

A myofascial trigger point is a hyperirritable locus within the taut band of skeletal muscle, located in the muscle or its associated fascia.[17] The trigger point is painful on compression and can evoke a characteristic referred pain and an autonomic response. A myofascial trigger point must be distinguished from tender spots in skin, ligaments, and periosteum.

Trigger points can be either active or latent. An active trigger point causes pain, while a latent trigger point may restrict movement and weaken the affected muscle. The latent trigger point persists for years after recovering from injury and predisposes to acute exacerbations of pain. The usual precipitating factors are jerky motion involving that muscle, fatigue, cold and damp surroundings, and emotional upset.

Normal muscles do not have trigger points or taut muscle bands. They are not tender on firm palpation. Sedimentary middle-aged women are more prone to develop trigger points and myofascial pain syndromes.[1] Infants and children can also develop trigger points. Myofascial trigger points are a common source of pain in musculoskeletal disorders in children.[18]

PHYSICAL EXAMINATION

To palpate a taut band, the muscle is stretched until the fibers of the taut band are under tension. The stretch should evoke local discomfort but not referred pain. This is usually at two thirds of the muscle's normal range of stretch. The examiner palpates along the taut band to locate the point of maximum tenderness and then maintains pressure firmly on that spot to elicit the referred pain pattern. Flat palpation is used when the muscle can be pressed against underlying bony surface (Fig 33–2). Pincer

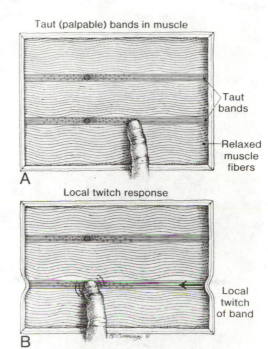

Taut (palpable) bands in muscle

Taut bands

Relaxed muscle fibers

A

Local twitch response

Local twitch of band

B

Fig 33–2.—Method of palpating a flat muscle to elicit a taut band in the muscle **(A)** or a local twitch **(B)**. (From Travell and Simons.[45] Reproduced by permission.)

palpation is used when the opposite sides of the muscle are accessible to grasping between the digits (Fig 33–3). This applies to the sternomastoid, lattissimus dorsi, biceps brachii, and pectoralis major and minor muscles, among others.

There can be a local twitch response when the trigger point is rolled between the fingers or touched by a needle.[5, 19] Exploratory palpation for an active trigger point can elicit simultaneously a local twitch response, a jump sign, and a referred pain pattern. When a nerve passes through a muscle between taut bands or between a taut band and a bone, the patient may have two kinds of referred pain: aching pain from the trigger point, and numbness, tingling, hyperesthesia, or hypoesthesia due to nerve compression (Table 33–3). Partial neuropraxia may be relieved within minutes after inactivation of responsible trigger points and muscle relaxation. Severe compression may require weeks for full recovery. The following should be noted on physical examination:

With an active trigger point, stretching of the involved muscle increases the pain,[20] and the muscle spasm is initiated. This further increases the tension

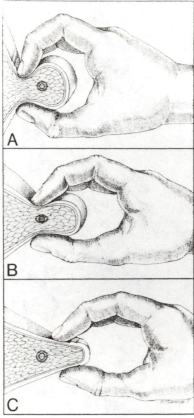

Fig 33–3.—Method of palpating the trigger point in a long thin muscle when the muscle can be grasped between the fingers and rolled through them. **A,** muscle fibers surrounded by the thumb and fingers in a pincer grip. **B,** hardness of the taut band felt. **C,** edge of the taut band sharply defined with a local twitch response. (From Travell and Simons.[45] Reproduced by permission.)

in the muscle and intensifies the pain. The painful spasm precludes further lengthening of the muscle unless therapeutic steps are taken to prevent the spasm.

• The range of the motion is restricted due to taut muscle bands and pain.
• Pain is increased on further contraction of the muscle in spasm.
• The muscle strength is diminished on examination and is not associated with muscle atrophy.
• Referred pain is elicited by deep palpation of the active trigger point.

Autonomic hyperactivity is noticed in the reference zone of the myofascial trigger point.[21] This hy-

TABLE 33–3.—COMMON MYOFASCIAL NERVE ENTRAPMENTS

MUSCLE	NERVE ENTRAPPED
Frontalis	Supraorbital
Semispinalis capitis	Greater occipital
Scaleni	Brachial plexus
Brachialis	Radial (sensory)
Triceps	Radial
Supinator	Deep radial
Flexor carpi ulnaris	Ulnar
Interossei (hand)	Digital (palmar)
Pectoralis minor	Brachial plexus
Paraspinal muscle	Posterior primary rami
Piriformis	Sciatic
Peroneus longus	Common peroneal
Tarsal tunnel	Tibial
Interossei (foot)	Digital (plantar)

peractivity includes increased vasomotor activity, lacrimation, and increased sudomotor and pilomotor activity. The electromyogram (EMG) shows increased motor unit activity, and thermography shows a decreased temperature in the reference zone.[22]

The involved muscle is extremely tense on palpation. The circumscribed hardening has been variously described as "fibrositic nodules," "myogeloses," "ropiness," or "palpable bands."[2, 23, 24] These nodules immediately disappear after effective treatment of the trigger points.

The trigger point is found on palpation as a circumscribed spot of exquisite tenderness. There is usually diminished tenderness for a few millimeters on either side of the trigger point. The patient may jump, out of proportion to the pressure applied to the trigger point; this is called "the jump sign."[2, 25]

The skin may show dermographia[2, 26] over the underlying trigger point. This is most commonly seen in the back.

INVESTIGATIONS

Routine laboratory tests shows no significant abnormalities in patients with a myofascial pain syndrome. The erythrocyte sedimentation rate, SMA, blood count, and serum muscle enzymes are all normal. Radiographs and CT scans are normal. EMG may show insertion potential, an increased number of polyphasic potentials in muscles with trigger points. Thermograms of skin overlying active trigger points may show areas of increased skin temperature.[27] Conversely, some workers have found decreased skin temperature in the same areas.[28, 29] Sola and Williams observed low skin resistance over the trigger point.[30]

MANAGEMENT

The goals of treatment are to decrease pain to tolerable levels, improve function, and prevent permanent disability. These goals can be achieved by muscle relaxation by spray-and-stretch techniques or trigger point injection, an exercise program, and stimulation analgesia.

Stretch-and-Spray Technique

The stretch-and-spray procedure is the workhorse of myofascial therapy. It inactivates myofascial trigger points quickly with less patient discomfort than local myoneural injection. A recent onset of muscle spasm responds with full return of pain-free function when the vapocoolant spray is applied while the muscle is passively stretched.[31] When more than one muscle is involved, a stretch-and-spray procedure is a practical means of covering a large area to make significant progress toward pain relief. The technique does not require precise localization of the trigger point. However, considerable skill is required to coordinate the course of spray so that it covers fibers that are being placed on maximum tension by passive stretch.

The patient must be positioned comfortably to permit voluntary relaxation (Fig 33–4). One end of the muscle must be anchored so that pressure can be applied to the other end to passively stretch it. With the patient in the position to stretch, the first sweep of spray is applied before any stretch pressure is applied. The vapocoolant spray is applied in one direction only. The spray is swept over the entire length of the affected muscle and then over the referred pain pattern. The stretch-and-spray steps are repeated until full muscle length is achieved. Time must be allowed after a series of two or three sprays to rewarm the skin. After the skin is rewarmed, the stretch-and-spray procedure can be repeated with several cycles of full active range of motion.

Detailed descriptions of the vapocoolant stretch and spray technique have been published elsewhere.[31-37] Both ethyl chloride and Fluorimethane can be used and are commercially available. Ethylchloride is a local anesthetic, flammable and explosive, and is too cold when applied. It can also

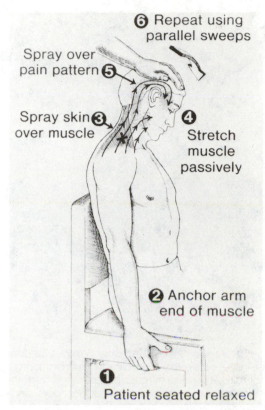

Fig 33–4.—The stretch-and-spray technique. (From Travell and Simons.[45] Reproduced by permission.)

be inhaled and can cause unconsciousness. Fire hazards must be eliminated during its use. Fluorimethane is nonflammable and nonexplosive and a good alternative. It is made up of a mixture of 85% trichloromonofluoromethane and 15% dichlorodifluoromethane. The fluorocarbon (Freon) has been tested for toxicity.[38] It had no effect on pulmonary function and did not change tracheal mucociliary transport.

The spring cap, which seals the nozzle of the bottle, permits on-off application. The bottle must be held inverted so that the fluid will flow from it (Fig 33–5). After adequate instructions patients may be given Fluorimethane spray for home use.

The jet stream of vapocoolant is directed at an acute angle (30°) to the skin and is swept parallel over the affected muscle. The sweeps move in one direction only. The bottle is held about 18 inches from the skin. Slow, even sweeps that progress over the skin at about 4 inches per second are spaced to provide a slight overlap of paths. Two or three

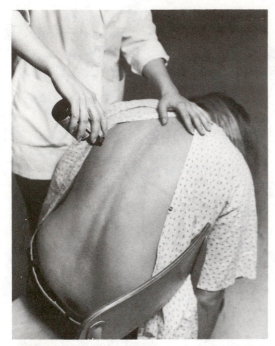

Fig 33–5.—Fluori-Methane Spray-n-Stretch being used on the thoracic and lumbar paraspinals while these muscles are stretched to increase the length of the muscle fibers and deactivate trigger points. The bottle is held 12–16 inches away from the surface to be treated and is sprayed at a 45° angle to the skin in unidirectional sweeps.

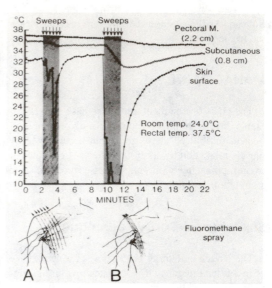

Fig 33–6.—Temperature changes that occur in skin, subcutaneous structures, or muscle with the stretch-and-spray technique. **A** shows results of first sweep of the spray; **B** shows results of second sweep (2 minutes' sweep each time). (From Travell and Simons.[45] Reproduced by permission.)

Responses to Stretch-and-Spray Treatment

The patient is seen for follow-up several days after treatment. The patient may have good or poor response to the treatment. When pain relief is adequate on follow-up, the patient is encouraged to pay more attention to the muscles and to avoid reactivating the trigger points. If within a few hours the patient experiences severe cramping pain in the general region of the treatment, then the stretch-and-spray procedure has produced shortening activation of an antagonist muscle. This phenomenon is avoided by systematically treating both the agonist and antagonist group of muscles. When active trigger points do not subside after stretch-and-spray treatments, one should look for perpetuating factors. These may be inadequate spraying of all trigger points, a nervous patient, inadequate technique, or chronicity of trigger points.[42, 34]

Trigger Point Injection

Trigger point injection is helpful when a few trigger points are present and the muscle cannot stretch because of excessive pain or its attachments.

sweeps are usually maximum. The skin must be rewarmed. Frosting of the skin can cause ulceration.[39] When the spray is applied for the first time over very irritable trigger points, the skin may be hypersensitive to the cold. However, after several passes of the spray the hypersensitivity usually abates (Fig 33–6).

The vapocoolant spray can be used for joint sprains,[39] thermal burns,[40, 41] calf cramps,[39] and bee stings.[39]

The patient benefits by soaking in a hot bath soon after returning home after stretch-and-spray treatments. Strenuous swimming should be avoided, but unstrained stretch and range of motion activities without pain are desirable.

The precise mechanism by which the vapocoolant spray exerts its effect has not been determined. It may act indirectly via skin afferent nerves rather than by direct cooling of the muscle. The stimulation of skin afferent nerves may procduce trigger point inhibition, spinal inhibition, or supraspinal inhibition.

An aseptic technique is required for injection of the trigger points. The solutions, needles, and syringes should be properly sterilized prior to use. Localization of a trigger point is done mainly by the sense of feel. The trigger point is the most sensitive spot in the palpable band. The muscle is placed on sufficient stretch that one can palpate the tight band and hold the trigger point in position.

With flat palpation the trigger point can be localized by feeling the band roll back and forth between the fingers (Fig 33–7). The trigger point is then fixed by keeping it between the fingers. The needle is inserted perpendicular to the skin and slowly advanced to the depth of the trigger point. The patient is asked to say when he feels the worst pain. At that site the needle will usually impale the trigger point.

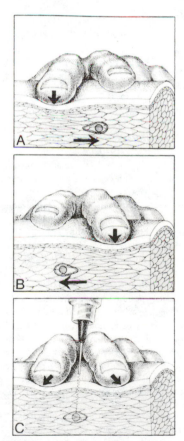

Fig 33–7.—Method of palpating and fixing the trigger point in the muscle with two fingers prior to inserting the needle tip in the trigger point for injection. *A,* fixation of trigger point by the proximal finger; *B,* fixation of trigger point by the distal finger; *C,* needle on the trigger point. (From Travell and Simons.[45] Reproduced by permission.)

With pincer palpation, the trigger point is rolled between the digits. When located, the trigger point is held tightly between the thumb and fingertips for injection. This technique is useful for muscles like the pectoralis major and minor, the lattisimus dorsi, the sternomastoid, and the trapezius at the shoulder region (Fig 33–8).

Dry needling of trigger points without injecting any solution may be effective but does not equal the therapeutic effectiveness of injecting a local anesthetic. Kraus noted that postinjection pain follows dry needling.[43] Sola and Kuitert treated a series of 100 patients with isotonic saline injected in the trigger points.[44] They found saline to be effective in relieving the pain. Hameroff et al., on the other hand, found long-acting local anesthetics–bupivacaine and etidocaine—to provide better and longer pain relief for up to 7 days after injection. Travell and Simons advocate use of procaine for trigger point injections.[45] They argue that procaine has less systemic and local toxicity, in addition to its vasodilator effect and curare-like action at the myoneural junction. I have used a mixture of 0.5% etidocaine and 0.375% bupivacaine and achieved a long-lasting effect without systemic toxicites or myotoxicity. In my experience, this mixture has produced better relief than dry needling, saline, or lidocaine.

Corticosteroids

Travell and Simons advocate mixing corticosteroid with a local anesthetic for trigger point injection[45] only for two groups of patients: those with soft tissue inflammation (adhesive capsulitis) and those with postinjection muscle soreness. They prefer oral steroids and believe that long-acting steroids are contraindicated because of their myotoxic properties[46] and delayed sequelae (Cushing's syndrome). I have used dexamethasone (4 mg/10 ml of local anesthetic solution) mixed it with bupivacaine and etidocaine in more than 10,000 patients, without sequelae from its use. It is true that a steroid may cause a burning sensation in the area of injection 24–48 hours after injection. But this subsides, and patients continue to have prolonged pain relief 7–10 days later. If patients are informed at the outset about the burning and its duration, they tolerate it better.

Postinjection Maneuvers

Stretch following trigger point injections is important.[37, 43] Vapocoolant spray or heat may also be

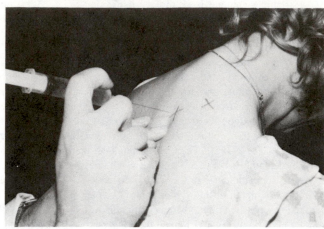

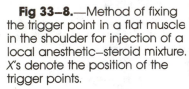

Fig 33–8.—Method of fixing the trigger point in a flat muscle in the shoulder for injection of a local anesthetic–steroid mixture. X's denote the position of the trigger points.

applied after injection during stretching of the muscle to full length.

Alternative techniques to stretch-and-spray and trigger point injections have also been practiced for myofascial pain. They include ischemic compression techniques, massage, deep heat, TENS, biofeedback, acupuncture, and central modulation.[47-49] A combination of some or all may be required in patients with chronic intractable trigger point pain. Commonly, however, the techniques employed are stretch-and-spray, trigger point injection, and TENS therapy, in conjunction with muscle relaxants, nonsteroidal anti-inflammatory agents, and exercises. It is useful to know that the earlier the patient is treated, the more effective and long-lasting is the treatment. Generally for a trigger point pain which is chronic (6–12 months) a series of six injections at weekly intervals must be completed, in conjunction with other therapy, before appreciable improvement in pain relief is noticed by the patient or the physician. The management plan should be evaluated periodically and different modalities tried if the one used is not effective.

REFERENCES

1. Sola A.E., Rodenberger M.L., Gettys B.B.: Incidence of hypersensitive areas in posterior shoulder muscles. *Am. J. Phys. Med.* 34:585–590, 1950.
2. Kraft G.H., Johnson E.W., LaBan M.M.: The fibrositis syndrome. *Arch. Phys. Med. Rehabil.* 49:155–162, 1968.
3. Gutstein M.: Diagnosis and treatment of muscular rheumatism. *Br. J. Phys. Med.* 1:302–321, 1938.
4. Good M.G.: Objective diagnosis and curability of nonarticular rheumatism. *Br. J. Phys. Med.* 14:1–7, 1951.
5. Kelly M.: The treatment of fibrositis and allied disorders by local anesthesia. *Med. J. Aust.* 1:294–298, 1941.
6. Travell J., Rinzler S., Herman M.: Pain and disability of the shoulder and arm: Treatment by intramuscular infiltration with procaine hydrochloride. *JAMA* 120:417–422, 1942.
7. Travell J.: Myofascial trigger points: Clinical view, in Bonica J.J., Albe-Fessard D. (eds.): *Advances in Pain Research and Therapy.* New York, Raven Press, 1976, vol. 1, pp. 919–926.
8. Yawger N.S.: Chronic ''rheumatic'' myositis (Muskelschwielen), with cases showing some common errors in diagnosis. *Lancet* 2:292–293, 1909.
9. Telling W.H.: ''Nodular'' fibromyositis, an everyday affliction, and its identity with so-called muscular rheumatism. *Lancet* 1:154–158, 1911.
10. Sola A.E., Kuitert J.H.: Quadratus lumborum myofascitis. *Northwest Med.* 53:1003–1005, 1954.
11. Neufeld I.: Pathogenetic concepts of ''fibrositis.'' *Arch. Phys. Med. Rehabil.* 33:363–369, 1952.
12. Popelianskii Ia. Iu., Zaslavskii E.S., Veselovskii V.P.: (Medicosocial significance, etiology, pathogenesis, and diagnosis of nonarticular disease of soft tissues of the limbs and back) (Russian). *Vopr. Revm.* 3:38–43, 1976.
13. Miehlke K., Schulze G., Eger W.: Klinische und experimentelle Untersuchungen zum Fibrositis-syndrome. *Z. Rheumaforsch.* 19:310–330, 1960.
14. Awad E.A.: Interstitial myofibrositis: Hypothesis of the mechanism. *Arch. Phys. Med. Rehabil.* 54:440–453, 1973.
15. Stenger R.J., Spiro D., Scully R.E., et al.: Ultrastructural and physiologic alterations in ischemic skeletal muscle. *Am. J. Pathol.* 40:1–20, 1962.
16. Ingle J.I., Beveridge E.E.: *Endodontics,* ed. 2. Philadelphia, Lea & Febiger, 1976.
17. Travell J.: Basis for the multiple uses of local block of somatic trigger areas (procaine infiltration and ethyl

chloride spray). *Miss. Valley Med. J.* 71:13–22, 1949.

18. Bates T., Grunwaldt E.: Myofascial pain in childhood. *J. Pediatr.* 53:198–209, 1958.

19. Lenman J.A.R., Ritchie A.E.: *Clinical Electromyography,* ed. 2. Philadelphia, J.B. Lippincott Co., 1977, pp. 86, 87.

20. Macdonald A.J.R.: Abnormally tender muscle regions and associated painful movements. *Pain* 8:197–205, 1980.

21. Travell J.: Pain mechanisms in connective tissue, in Ragan C. (ed.): *Connective Tissues: Transactions of the Second Conference, 1951.* New York, Josiah Macy, Jr. Foundation, 1952, pp. 96–102, 105–109, 111.

22. Travell J., Berry C., Bigelow N.: Effects of referred somatic pain on structures in the reference zone. *Fed. Proc.* 3:49, 1944.

23. Llewellyn L.J., Jones A.B.: *Fibrositis.* New York, Rebman, 1915.

24. Lange M.: *Die Muskelharten* (Myogelosen). Munchen, J.F. Lehmann Verlag, 1931.

25. Koenig W.C., Powers J.J., Johnson E.W.: Does allergy play a role in fibrositis? *Arch. Phys. Med. Rehabil.* 58:80–83, 1977.

26. Galletti R., Procacci P.: The role of the sympathetic system in the control of pain and of some associated phenomena. *Acta Neurovegetativa* 28:495–500, 1966.

27. Fischer A.A.: Thermography and pain. *Arch. Phys. Med. Rehabil.* 62:542, 1981.

28. Kohlrausch W.: Die sportbehindernden Wirkungen muskularer Erkrankungen. *Med. Klin.* 32:1420–1423, 1936.

29. Ruhmann W.: Muskelrheuma und Tastmassage: 2. Muskelrheumatische Disposition. *Med. Klin.* 27:1242–1245, 1279–1283, 1931.

30. Sola A.E., Williams R.L.: Myofascial pain syndromes. *Neurology* 6:91–95, 1956.

31. Travell J.: Rapid relief of acute "stiff neck" by ethyl chloride spray. *J. Am. Med. Women's Assoc.* 4:89–95, 1959.

32. Gardner D.A.: The use of ethyl chloride spray to relieve somatic pain. *J. Am. Osteopath. Assoc.* 49:525–528, 1950.

33. Mennell J.: Spray-stretch for relief of pain from muscle spasm and myofascial trigger points. *J. Am. Podiatry Assoc.* 66:873–876, 1976.

34. Travell J.: Ethyl chloride spray for painful muscle spasm. *Arch. Phys. Med. Rehabil.* 33:291–298, 1952.

35. Travell J.: Myofascial trigger points: Clinical view, in Bonica J.J., Albe-Fessard D. (eds.): *Advances in Pain Research and Therapy.* New York, Raven Press, 1976, vol. 1, pp. 919–926.

36. Travell J.: Identification of myofascial trigger point syndromes: A case of atypical facial neuralgia. *Arch. Phys. Med. Rehabil.* 62:100–106, 1981.

37. Zohn D.A., Mennell J. McM: *Musculoskeletal Pain: Diagnosis and Physical Treatment.* Boston, Little, Brown & Co., 1976, pp. 126–129, 190–193.

38. Friedman M., Dougherty R., Nelson S.R., et al.: Acute effects of an aerosol hair spray on tracheal mucociliary transport. *Am. Rev. Respir. Dis.* 116:281–286, 1977.

39. Modell W., Travell J., Kraus H., et al.: Relief of pain by ethyl chloride spray. *NY State J. Med.* 52:1550–1558, 1952.

40. Travell J.: Pain mechanisms in connective tissue, in Ragan C. (ed.): *Connective Tissues: Transactions of the Second Conference, 1951.* New York, Josiah Macy, Jr. Foundation, 1952, pp. 90, 92–94, 105, 119, 121.

41. Travell J., Koprowska I., Hirsch B.B., et al.: Effect of ethyl chloride spray on thermal burns. *J. Pharmacol. Exp. Ther.* 101:36, 1951.

42. Mennell J.M.: The therapeutic use of cold. *J. Am. Osteopath. Assoc.* 74:1146–1157, 1975.

43. Kraus H.: *Clinical Treatment of Back and Neck Pain.* New York, McGraw-Hill Book Co., 1970.

44. Sola A.E., Kuitert J.H.: Myofascial trigger point pain in the neck and shoulder girdle. *Northwest Med.* 54:980–984, 1955.

45. Travell J., Simon: Myofascial pain and dysfunction in *The Trigger Point Manual.* Baltimore, Williams & Wilkins Co., 1983, chaps. 2 and 3.

46. Pizzolato P., Mannheimer W.: *Histopathologic Effects of Local Anesthetic Drugs and Related Substances.* Springfield, Ill., Charles C Thomas, 1961, pp. 40, 41, 60, 71.

47. Prudden B.: *Pain Erasure: The Bonnie Prudden Way.* New York, M. Evans & Co., 1980, pp. 18, 19.

48. Williams H.L., Elkins E.C.: Myalgia of the head. *Arch. Phys. Ther.* 23:14–22, 1942.

49. Modell W., Travell J., et al.: Treatment of painful disorders of skeletal muscle. *NY State J. Med.* 48:2050–2059, 1948.

34 / Nerve Blocks

P. PRITHVI RAJ, M.D.
KATHY S. JOHNSON, R.N.
TERENCE M. MURPHY, M.D.
MICHAEL STANTON-HICKS, M.D.
STEPHEN E. ABRAM, M.D.
HANS NOLTE, M.D., D.A.

Introduction

NERVE BLOCKS, whereby a local anesthetic is injected into a nerve, have been used in the treatment of pain for over a century. Skillfully administered, they are among the most effective methods of relieving acute or chronic pain. Despite the long use of this technique, there is still some misconception about its role in managing chronic pain.

The basis for the efficacy of nerve blocks in chronic pain patients is the interruption of *sensory* and *nociceptive* pathways. Sensory nerve blocks relieve pain and interrupt the afferent limbs of an abnormal reflex mechanism. By using low concentrations of local anesthetic agents, it is possible to block the unmyelinated C fibers and small A delta fibers without significant impairment of motor function. In many instances, blocks with short-acting local anesthetic agents produce pain relief that outlasts the pharmacologic action of the drug by weeks. The exact mechanism of this long-lasting effect is not yet known. Alcohol and phenol produce prolonged pain relief by *destruction of nociceptive pathways*.

Nerve blocks may be used as a *diagnostic procedure* to ascertain the specific pain pathway and to aid in the differential diagnosis of the site of pain. *Prognostic blocks* are useful to predict the effects from prolonged interruption. They also afford the patient an opportunity to experience the numbness and other side effects that follow prolonged or permanent blocks. *Therapeutic blocks* can be achieved with either a local anesthetic agent or a neurolytic agent.

Local anesthetic blocks are useful for relieving severe pain in the head and neck, chest, abdomen, pelvis, and extremities. Continuous pain relief for prolonged periods in terminally ill cancer patients can be achieved by a continuous segmental epidural or peripheral nerve block with local anesthetics or narcotics. To obtain optimal results, it is essential to adhere to certain basic principles, as outlined by Bonica:[1] the physician must be willing to devote the necessary time to evaluate the patient thoroughly; the physician must diagnose the etiology, mechanism, and distribution of pain; the physician must be skilled in the procedure; and the physician makes sure that the patient and the patient's family have been informed about the procedure and its consequences.

TYPES OF NERVE BLOCKS USEFUL FOR PAIN RELIEF

Nerve blocks useful for chronic pain include somatic peripheral nerve blocks, intravertebral central neural blocks, and sympathetic blocks. They can be spectacularly effective in acute pain relief as witnessed daily in operative procedures in medical and dental practice where they are used to interrupt the transmission of nociceptive stimuli from the peripheral to the central nervous system. Because the mechanisms of chronic pain are frequently different from those of acute pain, nerve blocks may be less effective in chronic pain states. Nevertheless, they still have an important part to play in the diagnosis, prognosis, and sometimes therapy of chronic pain.

INDICATIONS FOR NERVE BLOCKS IN ACUTE PAIN

Nerve blocks effectively control acute pain by temporarily denervating the nociceptive pain source from conscious levels, as may occur, for example, in an intercostal block for broken ribs, a mandibular nerve block for a fractured mandible, a sciatic nerve block for a broken ankle, and so forth. In acute pain the diagnosis is usually less problematic, and nerve blocks are used as therapy. The limiting factor is usually a satisfactory delivery system whereby continuous regional analgesia can be provided around the clock in the postoperative and postinjury phase. Although the new long-acting local anesthetics have been of help in this area, there is still great need for an agent that will produce a reversible sensory nerve block for days rather than hours.

INDICATIONS FOR NERVE BLOCKS IN CHRONIC PAIN

Nerve blocks may be used for the diagnosis, prognosis, and therapy of chronic pain. They can be used to ascertain whether nociception is contributing to the patient's pain complaint, and, if so, diagnostic blocks can help elucidate the afferent nerve pathway of such nociception. The information obtained can often be useful diagnostically, although the nerve blocks of themselves may have little therapeutic application.

If neurosurgical ablative procedures (rhizotomy, sympathectomy) are being considered for relief of pain, nerve blocks can be used prognostically to let the patient experience the effects of such denervation and perhaps help him decide whether to proceed with surgical trespass or not. It is critically important that all parties concerned appreciate the fact that although the immediate numbness experienced followed a prognostic block may be a welcome relief, over time the numbness itself can become distressing, and that denervation dysesthetic sensations that follow chronic deafferentation can often become as distressing as the original nociception. Therefore, although prognostic blocks are useful in helping patients and surgeons make decisions, they do not guarantee the long-term satisfaction of neurodestructive procedures.

There is a small but appropriate subgroup of chronic pain patients who can and do benefit from therapeutic nerve blocks.

These therapeutic nerve blocks may involve such simple procedures as repeated trigger point injections (see Chap. 33) or profound and extensive chemical neurodestructive blocks of major afferent nerves.

34A / Patient Preparation

KATHY S. JOHNSON, R.N.
P. PRITHVI RAJ, M.D.

FACILITIES

FOR INVASIVE PROCEDURES SUCH AS nerve blocks, the facilities of a pain control center should promote an atmosphere of comfort and relaxation for the patient. Adequate space and equipment are imperative to ensure proper preparation and care of the patient undergoing such procedures.

Large major treatment rooms are necessary to perform the more invasive procedures such as epidural blocks, celiac plexus blocks, lumbar sympathetic blocks, and stellate ganglion blocks. They should be equipped to accommodate emergencies that may arise. Following is a list of equipment that is essential for such invasive procedures.

- Locking stretcher or surgical table that can be easily and quickly placed into many different positions.
- Anesthesia machine ready for use during emergency situations.
- Oxygen tank with ambu bag, oxygen mask, and nasal cannula available for emergencies.
- Suction machine and catheter.
- Cardiac monitor with defibrillator.
- Emergency crash cart with medication and intubation equipment.
- Intravenous tray which can be easily carried into an examination room should the need arise.
- Intravenous pole.
- 2 Mayo stands.
- Large supply cabinets and counters to store medication, procedure trays, gloves, extra supplies, etc.
- X-ray view box.

Figure 34A–1, shows many of these items in the procedure room at the University of Cincinnati Pain Control Center.

ROLE OF THE NURSE

The nurse plays an extremely important role in patient preparation and education prior to a procedure. This aids in allaying fears and apprehension experienced by the patient.

It is the responsibility of both the physician and the nurse to inform the patient of the purpose of the procedure, how the procedure is done, what the expected outcome is, and what the side effects and risks are. Unless the procedure is urgent, this is done on the visit prior to that of the procedure. In addition to a verbal explanation, an information sheet with a simple explanation of the procedure should be given to the patient. This reinforces the verbal explanation. Patients are told to bring an escort to accompany them home after the procedure. Written consent must be obtained. Although this is the responsibility of the physician, the nurse should verify that written consent has been obtained.

Commonly the chronic pain patient, when first seen at the pain control center, has already seen many professionals in various hospitals and has undergone many tests and procedures. This experience makes the patient fearful and apprehensive of seeing another new set of medical professionals. Nerve blocks are often foreign to patients and can be a source of apprehension. The patient must be reassured that nerve blocks are a standard form of therapy and are performed by experts at the pain control center.

Function During the Procedure

During the procedure the nurse not only sets up equipment, positions the patient, monitors vital signs, and assists as required during the procedure, but also helps the patient relax and anticipates the

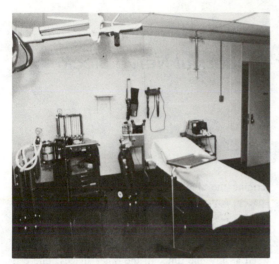

Fig 34A–1.—Equipment and facilities of the procedure room at the University of Cincinnati Pain Control Center.

needs of the patient and the problems that may arise.

The nurse can help the patient relax by employing techniques of relaxation, distraction, or guided imagery. Making sure the patient knows what to expect is important. The patient should continue to be informed of each step of the procedure. If the patient has a good idea of what is to happen, sudden unexpected movement could be avoided. All measures for comfort the nurse can provide should be offered as needed. These include proper positioning of extremities with pillows, and premedication if necessary.

The nurse must have a thorough knowledge of the anatomy and physiology of the region of the procedure as well as the pharmacology of the drugs to be used. Knowledge of the complications and side effects expected is imperative in anticipating problems and dealing with emergencies as they arise.

Discharge teaching

Following the procedure, patients are closely monitored as long as necessary, usually 30 minutes to 1 hour. Postblock monitoring is done to evaluate success of the block and its sequlae.

Verbal and written instructions are given to the patient prior to discharge. This includes a list of side effects that commonly occur with the block and the time when they should disappear. Patients are also informed how and when to call the personnel in the pain control center for any problems.

Function During Fluoroscopy Procedure

Many procedures that involve placement of a catheter for continuous infusion or a neurolytic block are done under fluoroscopy. Because of the nature of the block and the potential risks involved, it is imperative that a nurse accompany the physician. Essentially, the nurse provides the same assistance during this type of procedure as during any other nerve block.

A mobile cart is essential, stocked with supplies necessary for the procedure. They include IV supplies, procedure trays, appropriate needles and catheters, temperature probes, syringes, medication to be used, emergency drugs, and intubation equipment.

Prior to the procedure, a thorough explanation is given to the patient and written consent is obtained. An IV line is started in all patients.

The nurse's role during the procedure in the x-ray unit is critical. Tha nature of these blocks, and the presence of large pieces of x-ray apparatus, increase patients' apprehension. The nurse can provide relaxation techniques and medications to lessen this apprehension. Diazepam, although often used, may cause a generalized peripheral vasodilation that may make evaluation of the degree of sympathetic block more difficult.

After the procedure, the patient is monitored as necessary and reminded of what to expect. A postblock pain assessment is done to evaluate the success of the block, and arrangements are made for the safe transfer of the patient either to a hospital bed or to the pain control center before the patient is discharged home.

34B / Adjuvant Techniques for Successful Nerve Block

P. PRITHVI RAJ, M.D.

THE SUCCESS OF nerve blocks in producing regional anesthesia depends on the accurate placement of a local or neurolytic anesthetic solution in close proximity to the nerves to be blocked. In most peripheral somatic nerve blocks, this has depended on paraesthesia elicited by the physician and reported by the patient and on the experience of the physician performing the block. The success of the blocks may be poor because of inappropriate responses from the patient. This may be due to apprehension, oversedation, or disorientation, especially at the extremes of age, or because of the pain itself. Mechanical aids such as fluoroscopy or a peripheral nerve stimulator can help to confirm that the needle is in close proximity to the nerve and improve the success of the nerve block (Figs 34B–1 and 34B–2).

FLUOROSCOPY

In surgical anesthesia, the common regional blocks performed do not require confirmation by radiography prior to administration of a local anesthetic. However, this may not be the case in patients with chronic pain and who are obese, or who have anatomical anomalies. For example, in the morbidly obese patient, anteroposterior and/or lateral fluoroscopic views may be the only technique by which one could confirm the correct placement of the needle in the extradural space.[1] In uncommon blocks, such as blocks of the obturator nerve, celiac plexus, or lumbar sympathetic chain, fluoroscopy may be necessary to place the needle at the correct locations. For example, Magora et al. found radiographic localization more successful in obturator nerve blocks than a blind anatomical approach.[2]

The radiographs shown in Figures 34B–3 through 34B–6 illustrate needle position and spread of contrast material, in different views and for different procedures. Contrast material has been administered through the needle under fluoroscopic control to de-

termine the spread of solutions. In the extradural space, Amipaque (metrizamide, reconstituted to contain 250 mg of iodine per milliliter) is the material of choice because of its water solubility and absorption. Not more than 5 ml should be administered at any one time. In the other spaces, one can use 15–20 ml of Hypaque, or Angio Conray (meglumine diatrizoate) without any sequelae. The spread of contrast material helps localize the nerves.

Radiographic localization is indicated when difficulty is anticipated because of poor landmarks or anatomical anomalies; when deep nerves or plexuses are to be blocked; and when neurolytic procedures are planned.

Contrast materials should not be injected if the patient has a history of allergy to iodine-containing solutions. Metrizamide may inadvertently be injected into the subarachnoid space during the procedure. Even though this is usually innocuous, generalized muscle twitchings may be seen, due to the action of metrizamide on the spinal cord. Repeated doses of diazepam (0.1 mg/kg IV) may be needed for 24 hours before the muscle twitchings subside. However, in general, intravascular injection of any contrast material has not been deleterious.

PERIPHERAL NERVE STIMULATION[3, 4]

Another mechanical aid for nerve blocks is the nerve stimulator. Certain characteristics on the nerve stimulator are necessary to provide adequate stimulation: voltage range from 1 to 10 V or ampere range from 0.5 to 10 mamp, with 1–2 pulse/second (pps) capability. It is helpful if the instrument is pocket-sized, easily stabilized on an IV pole or the needle itself, battery operated, and sterilizable.

There are many peripheral nerve stimulators currently in use. Some do not have the essential characterisics required for nerve stimulation. Nerve stimulators manufactured by Professional Instru-

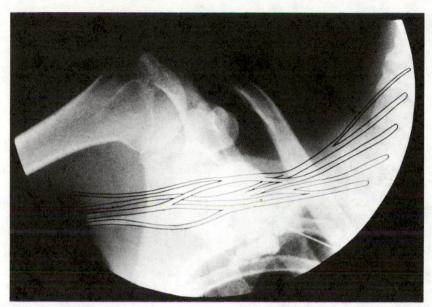

Fig 34B–1.—Radiograph showing the correct dispersal of contrast material with a needle on the brachial plexus.

ments, Dupaco, Neuro-Tech, Bard, and Regional Master Corporation are satisfactory.

Needles

Standard unsheathed needles are all that are necessary for peripheral nerve stimulation. However, sheathed and coated needles are more efficacious and require much less current to stimulate the nerve.

A kit is available which has sheathed needles of different lengths and sizes connected with an extension set and an alligator clamp.

Technique of Nerve Stimulation; Interscalene Block

Figures 34B–7 through 34B–10 illustrate different steps in an interscalene block performed with the

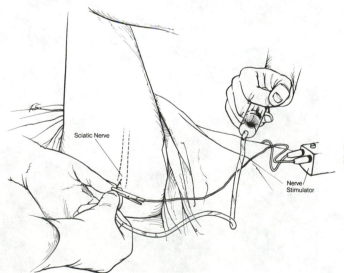

Sciatic Nerve

Nerve/Stimulator

Fig 34B–2.—Nerve stimulator in use during a sciatic nerve block.

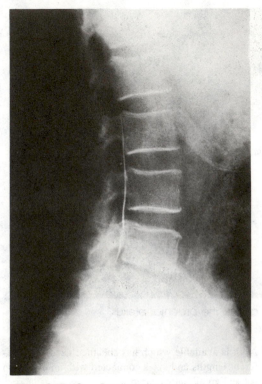

Fig 34B–3.—Radiograph, lateral view, demonstrating spread of 2 ml of Amipaque in the epidural space.

aid of a nerve stimulator. The ground electrode is attached to the ECG pad placed on the opposite shoulder. The syringe containing the anesthetic solution is attached to an extension set filled with anesthetic solution. The end of the extension set is connected to a 22-guage, 1½-inch needle. The needle is inserted through the skin, and the exploring electrode is affixed to the hub of the needle with the alligator clamp. The ampere control is set so that the current is flowing at 4 or 5 mamp at a frequency of 1 pulse per second.

The needle is advanced slowly while the patient's forearm and hand are observed carefully for muscle movements. Flexion or extension of the elbow, wrist, or digits confirms that the needle is in close proximity to nerve fibers of the brachial plexus. The best results are obtained if movements are observed as distally as possible—for example, with the brachial plexus block, in the hand or fingers.

The current is then reduced and the needle is moved deeper to find the point of maximum contraction. The current is further reduced and the needle moved deeper until there is maximal stimulation with lowest current (0.5–1 mamp). After careful aspiration, 1–2 ml of the anesthetic solution is injected through the needle, which should result in abolition of muscle movement within a few seconds. If a reduction in muscle movement does not occur, the stimulation is probably coming from the side of the needle, in which case the needle should be repositioned and the procedure repeated. When muscle movement has been abolished, the remaining an-

Fig 34B–4.—Obturator nerve block. Radiograph demonstrates catheter placement and location of contrast material, confirming that the catheter has passed through the obturator foramen.

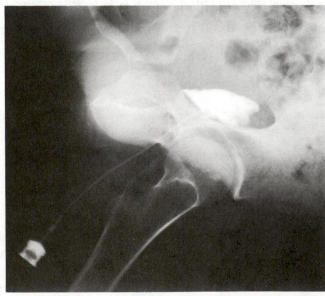

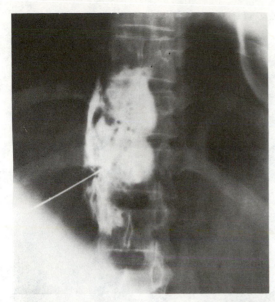

Fig 34B–5.—Celiac plexus block. Radiograph (AP view) demonstrates needle position and spread of contrast material.

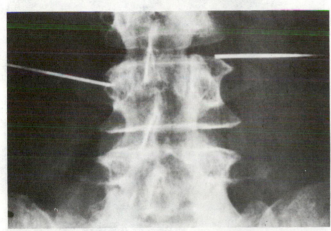

Fig 34B–6.—Lumbar sympathetic chain block. Radiograph, AP view, demonstrates bilateral catheter placement.

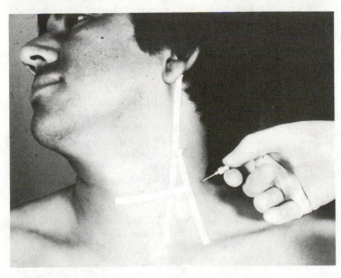

Fig 34B–7.—Patient ready for interscalene block. Landmarks have been identified and the needle is in position.

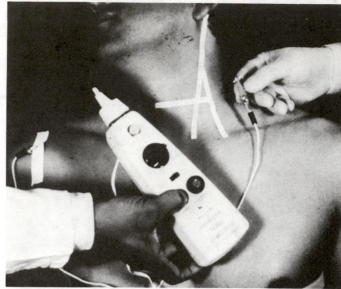

Fig 34B–8.—Interscalene block. The needle is attached to the exploring electrode and the ground electrode is attached to the opposite shoulder. The nerve stimulator is turned on to 4–5 mamp for initial stimulation as the needle penetrates deeper toward the brachial plexus.

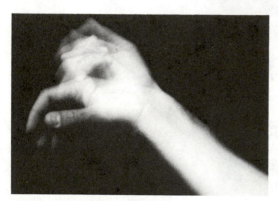

Fig 34B–9.—Interscalene block. Movements at the wrist (pronation and supination) confirm stimulation of the median and radial nerves, respectively, with the nerve stimulator.

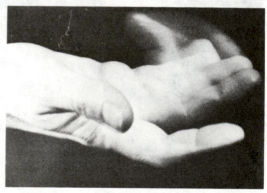

Fig 34B–10.—Interscalene block. Brachial plexus stimulation confirms placement of the needle on the ulnar nerve.

esthetic solution should be injected through the needle.

One to two minutes later, further testing should show no muscle movement except at very high current. The percentage change in amperes required for this movement usually reflects the percent change in nerve conduction of the nerves being blocked. The needle is withdrawn and routine testing is performed to confirm the nerve block.

The use of a nerve stimulator for nerve block is easily mastered and may shorten the time required to produce nerve block by providing more accurate localization of the peripheral nerves.

REFERENCES

1. Gelman S., Vitek J.J.: Thoracic epidural catheter placement under fluoroscopic control in morbidly obese patients. *Reg. Anaesth.* 5:4, 1980.
2. Magora E., Rozin R., Ben-Menachem Y., et al.: Obturator nerve block: an evaluation of technique. *Br. J. Anaesth.* 41:695, 1969.
3. Raj P.P., Rosenblatt R., Montgomery S.J.: Use of the nerve stimulator for peripheral blocks. *Reg. Anaesth.* 5:19, 1980.
4. Pither C.E., Raj P.P.: The use of peripheral nerve stimulators for regional anesthesia: A review of experimental characteristics, techniques, and clinical applications. *Reg. Anaesth.* 10:2, 1985.

34C / Techniques of Nerve Blocks—Cranial Nerves

TERENCE M. MURPHY, M.B., Ch.B.

TRIGEMINAL GANGLION

The trigeminal (gasserian) ganglion is situated in the middle cranial fossa and transmits sensation from the brow, orbital contents, and derivatives of the upper and lower jaws (Fig 34C–1).

Indications

Nerve blocks of the trigeminal ganglion are used in the treatment of tic douloureux, but the price of pain relief is hemifacial numbness—a significant burden. With modern therapies of carbamazepine (Tegretol) and the more innovative thermogangliolysis, there is less need for gasserian ganglion nerve blocks in pain therapy. This block is still occasionally used as a diagnostic technique, in patients in whom regional anesthetic techniques would be desirable for intraoperative or postoperative pain control, and in individuals with terminal cancer pain in the face. A catheter may be placed on the ganglion if pain relief must be evaluated prior to gangliolysis (Fig 34C–2).

Technique

An 8- or 10-cm, 22-gauge needle with a security bead is inserted 1–2 cm lateral to the angle of the mouth and directed medially and cephalad through the tissues of the cheek toward the infratemporal fossa. The index finger of the operator's other hand is placed intraorally to ensure that the needle does not enter the oral cavity and contaminate deeper structures.

The needle is introduced at such an angle that it is aimed toward the pupil (with the patient looking forward when viewed in the frontal plane) and toward the midpoint of the zygoma (when the patient is viewed laterally) (Figs 34C–3,A and B). With this approach, the needle should impinge on the foramen ovale in the roof of the infratemporal fossa or strike the surrounding bony plate. This procedure should be done under fluoroscopic control. The needle can thus be manipulated into the foramen ovale (Figs 34C–3,C and D). Success is usually indicated by paresthesia over the distribution of the mandibular division of the trigeminal nerve (lower lip and lower jaw, cheek, ear, or temple). After it enters the foramen ovale, the needle should not be advanced more than 1 cm; the 1-cm advance will usually be associated with paresthesia into the second and/or first division of the trigeminal nerve. For therapeutic purposes, particularly thermogangliolysis, it is necessary for paresthesia to be achieved in the affected painful part of the face. Because of the proximity of cerebrospinal fluid (CSF) in Meckel's cave, aspiration tests are mandatory.

Difficulties in Trigeminal Ganglion Block

When the needle is introduced in edentulous patients (many patients with tic douloureux are old and edentulous), the point of introduction of the needle may have to be a little more caudad than in patients with a full set of teeth; otherwise the needle will strike the foramen ovale at too acute an angle to reach the gasserian ganglion in the middle cranial fossa.

This is an uncomfortable procedure and, particularly with the introduction of large thermogangliolysis probes, some form of IV sedation such as .05 mg of fentanyl given immediately before the procedure often affords satisfactory analgesia without obtunding the patient's cooperation and necessary feedback.

Once the needle has been correctly positioned, aspiration tests are mandatory. Aspiration tests are particularly necessary in this situation because the

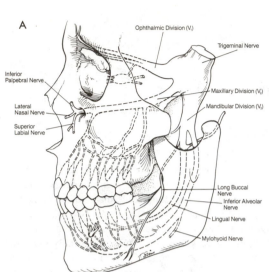

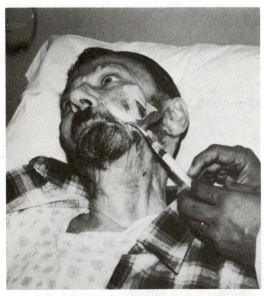

Fig 34C–1.—A, anatomy of the trigeminal ganglion and its branches coursing from the intracranial region to terminate in the face. **B,** sensory distribution of the ophthalmic maxillary and mandibular divisions of the trigeminal nerve. (From Gesund P.: Rationale and choice of regional anesthesia techniques, in Raj P.P. (ed.): *Handbook of Regional Anesthesia Technique.* New York, Churchill Livingstone, Inc., 1985. Reproduced by permission.)

Fig 34C–2.—The catheter has been inserted on the trigeminal ganglion under fluoroscopic control. A local anesthetic was injected through the catheter for initial pain relief, then alcohol was injected into the ganglion.

gasserian ganglion, over its posterior part, is surrounded by Meckel's cave, an invagination of cranial dura containing CSF, and inadvertent injection of therapeutic agents into this cul-de-sac can cause spread to other intracranial structures, producing profound and rapid loss of consciousness and collapse. The situation is eminently reversible when local anesthetic agents are used, but when neurolytic agents are used inadvertent neurolysis of adjacent cranial nerves could occur. With the advent of thermogangliolysis there has been little need to perform neurolytic gasserian ganglion blocks. Chemical neurolysis of a gasserian ganglion may result in hemifacial numbness, a distressing sensation for patients to experience. Because of the subsequent analgesia of the conjuctiva, the eye must be protected from chronic inflammatory process that would go undetected because of the analgesia. Therefore, ophthalmologic help is regularly needed to surgically approximate the upper and lower eyelid and thereby reduce the amount of conjunctiva exposed to environmental dust and other debris. Also, protective spectacles with side shields can help prevent the introduction of foreign bodies into the numb eye.

Another difficulty with long-term hemifacial an-

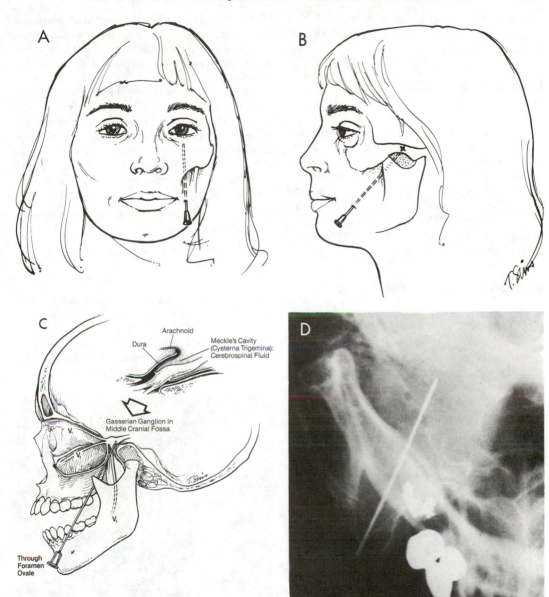

Fig 34C–3.—**A,** AP view showing position of the needle, directed toward the pupil. **B,** lateral view showing position during the first insertion; needle is directed toward the middle of the zygoma. **C,** needle entering the foramen ovale and touching the trigeminal ganglion. *Inset* shows the relationship of the ganglion to the reflections of the dura mater and cerebrospinal fluid. **D,** radiograph, AP view, demonstrating correct placement of the needle on the trigeminal ganglion through the foramen ovale. (Parts A, B, and C from Raj P.P.: Chronic pain, in Raj P.P. (ed.): *Handbook of Regional Anesthesia.* New York, Churchill Livingstone, Inc., 1985. Reprinted by permission.)

algesia is saliva dribbling from the anesthetic half of the mouth. Sometimes an antisialogogue will help (Benadryl, 25 mg t.i.d.).

Drug Dosages for Trigeminal Ganglion Block

Only small quantities—1 ml—of either local anesthetic or neurolytic agent are needed here. Incremental injection of 0.25-ml aliquots of the selected agent with testing performed after every injection is usually necessary. For local anesthetic use, bupivacaine 0.5% or lidocaine 1%, depending on the desired duration of the block, is an appropriate agent. For neurolytic purposes, absolute alcohol is the agent of choice.

TRIGEMINAL NERVE BRANCHES

First Division

Retrobulbar block of the first division is often used in ophthalmic surgery but rarely used in pain control. More commonly the peripheral branches, especially the supraorbital and supratrochlear terminal branches of the first division, are blocked above the eyebrow, providing analgesia of the brow (Fig 34C–4,A).

A skin wheal is raised over the medial aspect and rostral to the eyebrow. A 25-gauge, 1½-inch needle is inserted through the skin wheal and a local anesthetic is infiltrated above the medial half of the eyebrow, blocking both the supratrochlear and supraorbital nerves and producing analgesia of the ipsilateral forehead from eyebrow to vertex and from the midline to the temporal region (Fig 34C–4,B).

Indications for First Division Trigeminal Block

A first division trigeminal block is indicated when regional anesthesia of the affected area is required for minor surgery or postoperative or posttraumatic analgesia. This block was frequently used as a means of temporarily controlling the pain of frontal headaches of extracranial etiology, such as muscle

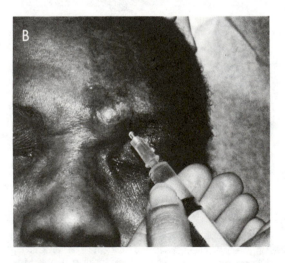

Fig 34C–4.—A, peripheral branches of the trigeminal nerve that are frequently blocked. The supraorbital and supratrochlear branches of the first division are blocked above the medial half of the eyebrow, resulting in analgesia over the area *1A* on the ipsilateral side of the face. The infraorbital terminal branch of the maxillary nerve is anesthetized 1 cm below the intraorbital margin in the same vertical plane as the pupil resulting in analgesia over the area *2A* on the same side. The terminal mental branch of the mandibular nerve is located in the same vertical plane and blocked resulting in ipsilateral analgesia of area *3A*. **B,** technique of supraorbital nerve block.

tension headaches. It was rarely a long-term solution but, in the days before biofeedback, did provide some pain control in these patients.

Difficulties of Supraorbital and Supratrochlear Nerve Block

This block is usually a very simple procedure and is not associated with major complications.

If the block is attempted inferior to the level of the eyebrow, i.e., in the roof of the orbit, it is feasible to produce regional anesthesia, but because of a highly vascular supply and the loose areolar tissue of the orbit, periorbital hematoma (black eye) is a possibility.

Second Division

The second division of the trigeminal nerve (maxillary nerve) can be anesthetized as the parent nerve in the pterygopalatine fossa, its branches can be anesthetized at the posterior and lateral borders of the maxilla, and its terminal branch can be anesthetized as it emerges through the infraorbital foramen on the front of the face 1 cm below the orbital margin and in the same vertical plane as the pupil.

Block of the Maxillary Nerve in the Pterygopalatine Fossa

As it lies in the pterygopalatine fossa, the second division of the trigeminal nerve can be approached either via the infratemporal fossa or via the infralateral wall of the orbit. The former approach is most frequently used. The needle is inserted through the coronoid notch of the mandible, which can usually be palpated under the midpoint of the zygoma. The needle is inserted at a right angle to the skin and advanced medially through the infratemporal fossa until it impinges on the bony medial wall of this compartment (Fig 34C–5). This is the lateral pterygoid plate. The depth of the needle is noted and the needle is "walked" anteriorly off the anterior border of the lateral pterygoid plate. Further advancement of the needle will carry it into the pterygopalatine fossa (a small bony compartment containing mostly emissary veins from the orbit and the five terminal branches of the maxillary artery). The needle is advanced into this fossa approximately 1 cm. It is not essential to elicit paresthesia, as the small

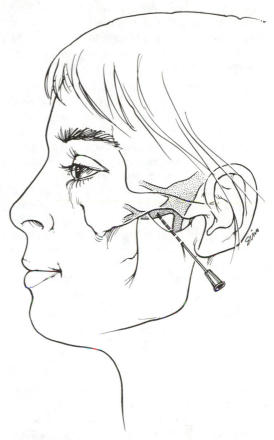

Fig 34C–5.—Maxillary nerve block. A 22-gauge, 2½-inch needle is introduced below the midpoint of the zygoma, passing medially through the coronoid notch of the mandible, and impinging on the lateral pterygoid plate. The needle is then "walked" anteriorly off the lateral pterygoid plate into the pterygopalatine fossa and advanced into the fossa approximately another 0.5–1 cm. (From Phero J., Robins G.: Eyes, ear, nose, and throat surgery, in Raj P.P. (ed.): *Handbook of Regional Anesthesia*. New York, Churchill Livingstone, Inc., 1985. Reproduced by permission.)

confined space usually ensures that the injected bolus of local anesthetic bathes the maxillary nerve.

Indications for Maxillary Nerve Block

Maxillary nerve block is usually performed for regional analgesia of the upper jaw and its derivatives. It can be used for acute intraoperative pain during maxillofacial surgery. Maxillary block provides excellent postoperative pain relief for such surgical maneuvers. It is most often used in chronic pain for diagnostic and therapeutic blocks involving painful tumors of the maxillary antrum unresponsive to more conventional methods of treatment.

DIFFICULTIES ASSOCIATED WITH THE MAXILLARY BLOCK.—It is essential that the needle be introduced in a horizontal fashion; certainly the needle should not enter the pterygomaxillary fissure in a cephalad direction or advance too deeply, as anesthetic injections here rapidly spread to the posterior aspect of the orbit and the optic nerve, producing temporary blindness with reversible agents or more catastrophic permanent blindness with neurolytic agents.

Because of the exceedingly vascular nature of the compartment in which it lies—the pterygomaxillary fissure is a veritable network of emissary orbital veins and the five terminal branches of the maxillary artery—intravascular injection is quite possible, and meticulous aspiration tests are essential.

TECHNIQUE OF BLOCKING PERIPHERAL BRANCHES OF THE MAXILLARY NERVE.—The infraorbital branch is usually blocked. The infraorbital branch supplies sensation to those derivatives of the maxillary arch which form the face, including the nerves of the lower eyelid, the cheek, the lateral aspect of the nose, the upper lip, and part of the temple. The infraorbital nerve emerges through the foramen of the same name in the same vertical plane as the pupil with the eye looking straightforward. The nerve can be blocked at this site with a small-gauge needle introduced either through the cheek over the foramen, or via an intraoral approach between lip and upper jaw. In the latter approach, the finger of the physician's nondominant hand is placed over the foramen externally and the needle is guided to the foramen. Paresthesia of the upper lip or ipsilateral cheek or nose is usually obtained, and 2 cc of local anesthetic will provide satisfactory analgesia of the area.

The intermediate branches of the second division, such as the zygomaticofacial and zygomaticotemporal branches and the posterior alveolar branches, are rarely blocked in either acute or chronic pain situations. The posterior alveolar nerves are frequently blocked for dental anesthesia, however.

Third Division

The third division of the trigeminal nerve (mandibular nerve) emerges through the foramen ovale in the floor of the middle cranial fossa and enters the infratemporal fossa at the posterior border of the pterygoid plate.

The approach for blocking this nerve is identical to that for blocking the second division: the needle introduced through the coronoid notch of the mandible, traverses the infratemporal fossa; the lateral pterygoid plate is used as a bony end point. However, in this instance the needle is "walked" backward off the lateral pterygoid plate at the depth of the plate until paresthesia of the lower lip, lower jaw, ipsilateral tongue, or ear is obtained (Fig 34C–6).

INDICATIONS FOR MANDIBULAR NERVE BLOCK.—A mandibular nerve block is excellent for intraoperative or postoperative pain control during the surgical reduction of fractured mandibles. It is also useful for patients with chronic pain states, such as carcinoma of the tongue, lower jaw, or floor of the mouth, which involve these nociceptive pathways.

DIFFICULTIES.—The mandibular block can be performed in a relatively straightforward fashion with a high degree of success. There is always the risk of complications. As the needle is walked posteriorly off the lateral pterygoid plate, it comes to lie on the muscle that is attached to that border, namely, the superior constrictor muscle of the pharynx. If the needle is advanced deeper at this stage, it may enter the pharynx. A very close posterolateral relation of the mandibular nerve at this site is the middle meningeal artery, which enter the cranial cavity through the foramen spinosum; therefore, meticulous aspiration tests are necessary.

Blocks of Branches of the Mandibular Nerve

The only branch that is blocked with any degree of frequency is the terminal mental branch. This branch is found in the face in the same vertical plane as the pupil. The foramen through which the mental nerve emerges from the mandible varies in its vertical position with age. It is more caudad in infancy and more cephalad on the mandibular ramus with advancing years, so that in the edentulous older individual, alveolar resorption often results in the mental foramen being virtually on the superior border of the mandibular ramus where it can often be seen glistening under the mucous membrane. At this site it is readily blocked via an intraoral approach.

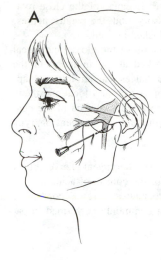

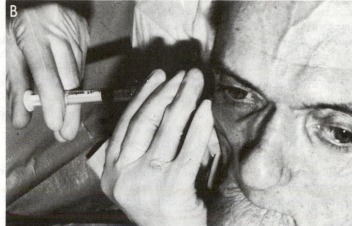

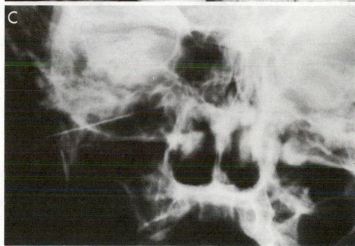

Fig 34C–6.—Mandibular nerve block. The needle is "walked" posteriorly off the lateral pterygoid plate at the same depth. Mandibular nerve paresthesia of the lower jaw or lower lip is usually obtained immediately posterior to the posterior border of the lateral pterygoid plate. (From Phero J., Robins G.: Eyes, ears, nose, and throat surgery, in Raj P.P.: *Handbook of Regional Anesthesia.* New York, Churchill Livingstone, Inc., 1985. Reproduced by permission.) **B,** alcohol is injected on the mandibular nerve for pain in the mandible. **C,** AP radiograph demonstrating needle placement on the mandibular nerve. An extraoral approach was used.

MENTAL NERVE BLOCK.—The mental nerve is usually blocked for acute surgical trespass on the lower lip. Mental nerve block is rarely, if ever, used for chronic pain states.

The other terminal branches of the mandibular nerve, such as the auriculotemporal and buccal nerves, are rarely blocked for pain states. The other ipsilateral branches are blocked for dental and oral surgical procedures.

Glossopharyngeal Nerve Block

The glossopharyngeal nerve is the sensory nerve that supplies the posterior third of the tongue and the pharynx from the level of the soft palate down to the laryngeal opening. A block of the glossopharyngeal nerve can produce analgesia in this distribution.

TECHNIQUE.—The nerve leaves the cranium through the middle compartment of the jugular foramen along with the accessory nerve but rapidly parts company with this nerve as it follows the course of the styloid process prior to curving forward into the pharynx. The styloid process is used as a bony landmark for this nerve and is located as described below.

A 5-cm, 22-gauge needle is inserted at the midpoint of the line joining the tip of the mastoid process to the angle of the mandible. The needle passes through the substance of the sternomastoid muscle, and at a depth of approximately 3 cm, contact is sought with the bony styloid process. The needle is walked off the posterior border of the styloid process. A small bolus of 1–2 cc of local anesthetic injected at this point will produce anesthesia of the glossopharyngeal nerve. Because of the close relationship of the accessory and the vagus nerves, these are frequently blocked as well.

The terminal distribution of the glossopharyngeal nerve can also be blocked at the midpoint of the posterior pillar of the fauces via an intraoral approach. An injection of 1–2 cc of a local anesthetic at this site will produce rapid analgesia of the posterior third of the tongue and the adjacent pharynx (Fig 34C–7).

INDICATIONS.—Glossopharyngeal nerve block is usually performed for the control of acute pain in peroral endoscopy procedures. In the control of chronic pain it is most commonly performed in pa-

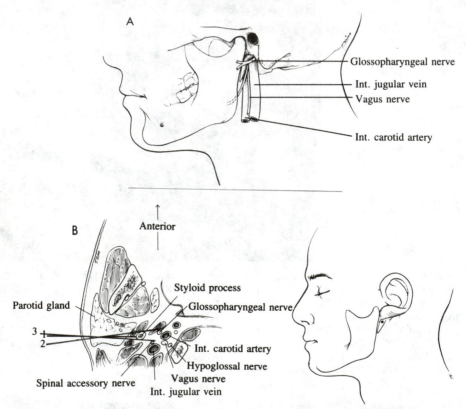

Fig 34C–7.—Glossopharyngeal nerve block. **A,** the 5-cm, 22-gauge needle is inserted halfway between the mastoid process and the angle of the mandible, seeking the styloid process. When this bony end point has been located, the needle is "walked" off the anterior aspect of the styloid process at the same depth (usually about 3 cm). A glossopharyngeal paresthesia should be obtained. A small bolus of 1–2 cc of either a local anesthetic or neurolytic agent is sufficient for block at this site. Note the proximity of the underlying internal carotid artery and internal jugular vein, necessitating meticulous attention to aspiration testing. **B,** point of entry of needle for glossopharyngeal and vagal nerve block. 1, the needle inserted at the point of entry perpendicularly to the skin until it touches the styloid process. 2, the needle tip is slipped anteriorly and seeks paresthesia of the glossopharyngeal nerve. 3, for vagal nerve block the needle tip is slipped posteriorly to the same depth ($\approx$ 3 cm).

tients with invading carcinomas of the posterior third of the tongue or pharynx that are unresponsive to other therapies. Because extraoral blocks of the glossopharyngeal can readily spread to the vagus and accessory nerves, neurolytic blocks often produce analgesia of the hemilarynx and/or trapezius muscle, and sternomastoid paralysis on the ipsilateral side. Both these complications may be well tolerated by patients with terminal cancer pain. Glossopharyngeal nerve block is occasionally used in the exceedingly rare condition of idiopathic glossopharyngeal neuralgia.

Often patients with pharyngeal cancer will have undergone a radical neck dissection and the sternomastoid muscle will have been removed, which makes identification of the styloid process much easier since this particular bony landmark is now almost subcutaneous and these blocks can be easily performed.

Because of the proximity of the large vascular conduits of the internal carotid artery and the internal jugular vein, the risks of intravascular injection are always significant, demanding meticulous aspiration tests. With the temporary and perhaps permanent analgesia that comes with these blocks, a degree of incoordination of swallowing with its accompanying potential risk of aspiration must be appreciated by patient and attendants alike. With numbness of half of the pharynx and the larynx, ingestion and swallowing are often severely compromised.

Vagus Nerve Block

The vagus nerve is rarely blocked except inadvertently as a complication of glossopharyngeal block. However, branches of the vagus nerve to the larynx can be easily blocked to produce very effective local anesthesia of the larynx and trachea for both endoscopic procedure and more permanent analgesia for invasive tumors of this region.

Superior Laryngeal Nerve Block

This branch of the vagus supplies sensation to the inferior surface of the epiglottis and the laryngeal inlet down to the level of the vocal cords, and also supplies motor nerve to the cricothyroid muscle. It is easily blocked as it passes below the greater cornu of the hyoid bone. This bone is readily palpable cephalad to the thyroid cartilage, and if the hyoid bone is displaced by pressure exerted on the con-

tralateral cornu, a short 2.5-cm, 25-guage needle can be inserted over the greater cornu and then walked off its inferior border. A small bolus of 3 cc of local anesthetic injected at this site will produce analgesia of the distribution described above. Bilateral block of this nerve will produce analgesia of the whole laryngeal inlet (Fig 34C–8).

The recurrent laryngeal nerves enter the larynx by

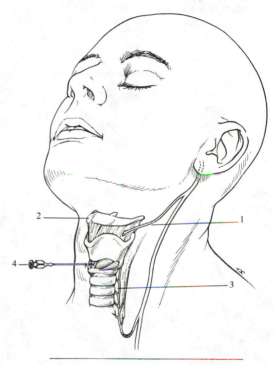

Fig 34C–8.—Superior laryngeal nerve block. The superior laryngeal nerve is blocked just below the greater cornu of the hyoid bone *(2)*. This bone is palpated and a small gauge 2½-cm needle is walked off the inferior border of the hyoid bone. A small bolus of 2 cc of local anesthetic is usually sufficient to anesthetize the ipsilateral laryngeal inlet *(1)*. If the hyoid bone is difficult to palpate, pressure on the contralateral side of the neck will frequently push the hyoid out towards the examiner's finger and make it easier to identify. The recurrent laryngeal nerve is shown curving up from within the thorax *(3)* and distributing its terminal branches to the trachea and larynx below the level of the vocal cords. It is anesthetized by introducing the needle through the cricothyroid membrane *(4)*. When the larynx is entered, as evidenced by loss of resistance and aspiration of air, a small bolus of 2 cc of 4% lidocaine will produce effective surface analgesia.

ascending from below the thoracic inlet in the groove between the trachea and the esophagus. Their terminal branches are usually anesthetized by either transtracheal injection or transoral and laryngeal spray.

Indications for laryngeal nerve blocks.—These nerves are most frequently blocked to facilitate endoscopic procedures on the larynx or trachea, or intubation. Laryngeal nerve blocks are rarely used for chronic pain states but could be used in patients with invasive carcinomas or tumors of this area.

Difficulties of laryngeal block.—When sensory analgesia of the larynx is produced, protective reflexes are abolished and aspiration is a risk if the patient ingests liquids or solids. If the main trunk of the recurrent laryngeal nerve is blocked by spread of drug, speech facility is profoundly impaired. If the injection is bilateral, speech is severely compromised.

34D / Techniques of Nerve Blocks—Spinal Nerves

TERENCE M. MURPHY, M.B., Ch.B.
P. PRITHVI RAJ, M.D.
MICHAEL STANTON-HICKS, M.D.

CERVICAL PLEXUS

The cervical plexus is formed by the roots of the upper four cervical nerves (Fig 34D–1). The first cervical nerve does not innervate the skin but it supplies the muscles of the suboccipital triangle.

After emerging from the intervertebral foramina, the cervical roots lie on the grooved superior surface of the transverse processes, behind the vertebral artery.

The posterior primary division separates from the anterior primary division at the articular pillar to reach the dorsal aspect of the vertebrae. Here it divides into lateral and medial branches. The lateral branch supplies the muscles of the back of the neck; the medial branch supplies the skin. The medial branch of the second cervical nerve forms the greater occipital nerve and the medial branch of the third cervical nerve forms the third occipital nerve. These two nerves supply the upper part of the back of the neck and head up to the vertex.

The anterior primary divisions form the cervical plexus. These nerves lie in the groove between the scalenus medius posteriorly and scalenus anterior and longus colli muscles anteriorly. The plexus is enclosed in the fascial sheath derived from the prevertebral fascia. This fascial compartment is the interscalene space of the brachial plexus.

The cervical plexus gives rise to deep branches, which are primarily muscular, and forms the phrenic nerve (C-3, C-4, and C-5). The superficial cervical plexus is formed by the superficial branches of the second, third, and fourth cervical nerves. These branches pierce the deep fascia close to the midpoint of the posterior border of the sternocleidomastoid muscle, to enter the subcutaneous tissue.

The branches that make up the great auricular, lesser occipital, and supraclavicular nerves supply the skin over the neck, the lower border of the mandible, the lobe of the ear, the tip of the shoulder, the chest up to the second rib, and over the back up to the spine of the scapula.

Superficial Cervical Plexus Block

This block is done with patient's head turned to the opposite side. The midpoint of the posterior border of the sternocleidomastoid muscle is identified by asking the patient to elevate his head. A skin wheal is made and a 22-guage, 8-cm needle is advanced slowly in a caudal direction from the midpoint of the posterior border of the sternocleidomastoid muscle until the deep fascia is entered. After aspiration, 5 ml of a local anesthetic solution is deposited and the needle is gradually withdrawn as another 5 ml is injected. The needle is reinserted in the cephalad direction and the procedure is repeated, using another 10 ml of the local anesthetic solution. This block results in analgesia of the cutaneous branches of the second, third, and fourth cervical nerves. The muscular branches and the phrenic nerve are not anesthetized by this block.

Accidental intravasular injection is the only complication. It can be avoided with frequent aspiration.

Deep Cervical Plexus Block

The cervical plexus can be blocked by blocking the roots at the tips of the transverse process. This

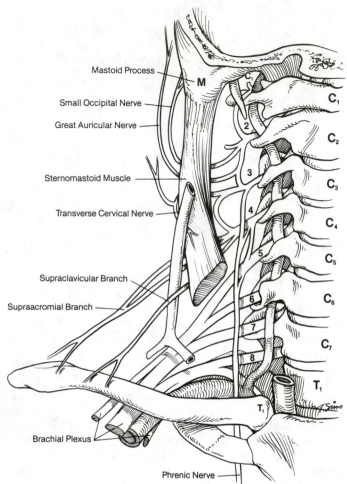

Fig 34D–1.—Anatomy of the cervical plexus and its relationship to the brachial plexus. (From Raj P.P., Pai U.: Techniques of nerve blocking, in Raj P.P. (ed.): *Handbook of Regional Anesthesia.* New York, Churchill Livingstone, Inc., 1985. Reproduced by permission.)

Labels in figure: Mastoid Process; M; Small Occipital Nerve; Great Auricular Nerve; Sternomastoid Muscle; Transverse Cervical Nerve; Supraclavicular Branch; Supraacromial Branch; Brachial Plexus; Phrenic Nerve; C₁; C₂; C₃; C₄; C₅; C₆; C₇; T₁

block can be accomplished by two methods: by blocking the roots at the groove between the anterior and posterior tubercles individually, and by blocking the roots collectively with a single injection at any one site or by the interscalene approach (Fig 34D–2).

Traditional Approach

The tip of the mastoid process and Chassaignac's tubercle, the prominent anterior tubercle of the sixth cervical transverse process, are marked and a line is drawn between them (Fig 34D–3). The second cervical root is blocked by inserting a 22-guage, 5-cm needle 1.5 cm caudal and 1 cm dorsal to the tip of the mastoid process. The needle is advanced in a slightly caudal direction until the tip of the transverse process is contacted at approximately 3 cm. If

the needle is withdrawn and reinserted in a slightly more caudal direction, the transverse process is contacted.

This procedure is repeated 1.5 cm lower, on the line drawn to contact the third cervical transverse process (level of hyoid bone), and again 1.5 cm below that point to contact the fourth cervical transverse process (upper border of the thyroid cartilage).

The needle is held in position if paresthesias are encountered. Second cervical nerve root produces paresthesia in the ear or back of the head, third cervical nerve root produces paresthesia over the neck, and fourth cervical nerve root produces paresthesia over the shoulder or the chest. Five milliliters of the local anesthetic solution is injected through each needle. If a single-needle approach is used, 10 ml of the solution is injected at any of these sites, with the operator firmly pressing a finger at the C-5 level to contain the solution at the cervical plexus alone.

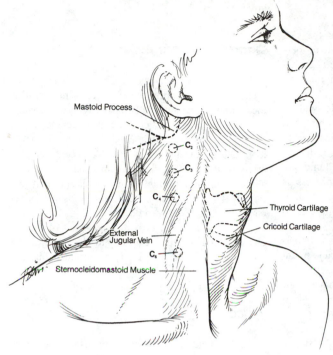

Fig 34D–2.—Landmarks for superficial and deep cervical plexus blocks. (From Raj P.P., Pai U.: Techniques of nerve blocking, in Raj P.P. (ed.): *Handbook of Regional Anesthesia.* New York, Churchill Livingstone, Inc., 1985. Reproduced by permission.)

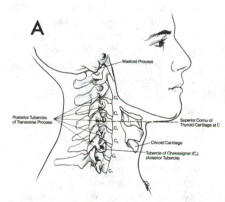

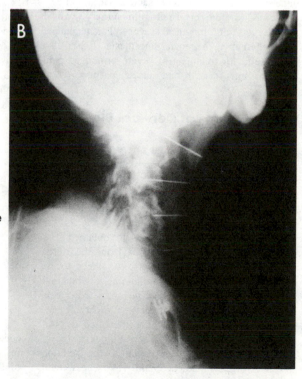

Fig 34D–3.—**A,** bony landmarks that must be palpated prior to performing the deep cervical plexus block. The anterior tubercle of the C-4 transverse process is at the level of the thyroid cartilage. (From Raj P.P., Pai U.: Techniques of nerve blocking, in Raj P.P. (ed.): *Handbook of Regional Anesthesia.* New York, Churchill Livingstone, Inc., 1985. Reproduced by permission.) **B,** x-ray film (oblique view) showing needle placement on the C–1 to C–4 transverse processes for a neurolytic cervical plexus block.

Interscalene Approach[1]

The interscalene groove is palpated at the C-6 level and traced cephalad. The block can be performed at any level, but it is usually done at the C-4 level (level of the upper border of the thyroid cartilage).

A 22-gauge, 5-cm short-bevel needle with a translucent hub, attached to an extension tubing and a 20-ml syringe, is used. The needle is inserted in the skin slightly above the C-4 level in a slightly caudal and dorsal direction and is advanced until paresthesia is obtained. If the transverse process is contacted, the needle is "walked" slightly anteriorly into the groove onto the transverse process to obtain paresthesia.

Ten milliliters of the local anesthetic solution is injected after frequent aspiration. This results in analgesia in the distribution of C-2, C-3, and C-4. Larger volumes may anesthetize upper roots of the brachial plexus.

Indications for Cervical Plexus Block

A cervical plexus block is indicated for patients undergoing cervical surgery, such as carotid endarterectomy, thyroid or parathyroid surgery, radical neck surgery, and laryngeal surgery. This technique is an alternative to general anesthesia. It has also been useful for treatment of severe prolonged pain due to arthritis, cancer, and muscle spasms.

Complications of Cervical Block

Injection into the vertebral artery, subarachnoid space, or epidural space is a possible complication if the needle is advanced deeper in a horizontal position between the transverse processes. This can be avoided by having a slightly caudal direction to the needle. Then the needle is likely to contact the transverse process if paresthesia is not obtained. The phrenic nerve, which is derived from the third, fourth, and fifth cervical roots, is likely to be blocked. Even though a unilateral or bilateral phrenic nerve block may have no untoward effects in healthy individuals, patients with chronic obstructive lung disease may have increased respiratory difficulty following a unilateral block.

Horner's syndrome can occur if the solution spreads to the sympathetic chain. Hoarseness could result from block of the vagus nerve or its recurrent laryngeal branch.

Occipital Nerve Block

The greater occipital nerve is the cervical plexus branch most frequently anesthetized. This nerve is located approximately halfway between the mastoid process and the greater occipital protuberance at the crest of the occipital bone (Fig 34D–4,A). It can be identified by the pulsation of the adjacent occipital artery at this site. A short, 2-cm needle is inserted and paresthesia is sought in the occipital region (Fig 34D–4,B). A nerve stimulator may be useful for accurate localization. An injection of 3–5 ml of local anesthetic at this site provides analgesia of the occipital region of the scalp up to the vertex. The block can be done bilaterally to produce bilateral occipital analgesia.

Indications

Occipital nerve block has been used extensively for the treatment of occipital muscle tension headaches and can afford temporary relief. But in patients with refractory chronic headaches, it is rarely curative, and biofeedback has now more or less replaced this strategy as an ongoing means of controlling recurrent tension headaches. The block can still be used for crisis intervention if it is not counterproductive to long-term management goals, which usually include decreasing the patient's reliance on medical technology.

The occipital nerve block has been useful in early occipital nerve entrapment syndromes, where inflammation plays a large part. Injection of a local anesthetic–corticosteroid mixture has produced dramatic and even permanent relief. In post-occipital neurectomy syndrome, an occipital nerve block can be tried as a means of controlling severe intractable pain when other alternatives have been exhausted.

Difficulties Associated With the Occipital Nerve Block

The occipital nerve block is a very simple and easily accomplished procedure. If the block is done cephalad to the insertion of the cervical paraspinal musculature into the occipital crest, the bony end point of the cranium will prohibit further progress

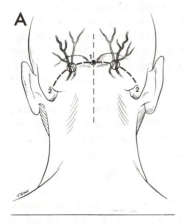

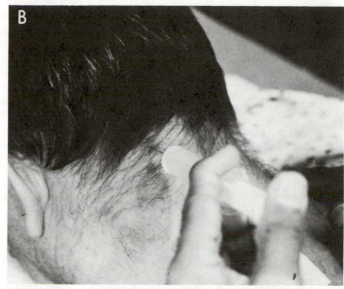

Fig 34D–4.—Greater occipital nerve block. **A,** the nerve is blocked as it crosses the superior nuchal line approximately halfway between the external occipital protuberance *(1)* and the mastoid process *(2)*. **B,** technique of performing the occipital nerve block.

of the needle. The only noteworthy complication is accidental intravascular injection of the drug into the occipital artery or vein, which, because of the small quantities of drug needed for this block, is unlikely to cause much damage.

SPINAL ACCESSORY NERVE BLOCK

The accessory nerve is the 11th cranial nerve. It emerges from the jugular foramen. The cranial portion separates and joins the vagus. The spinal accessory portion continues into the upper part of the sternocleidomastoid muscle and emerges from its posterior border at the junction of the lower and middle thirds. There it crosses the neck to supply the trapezius muscle. The nerve can be blocked in the substance of the sternocleidomastoid muscle.

A 23-gauge, 2.5-cm needle is inserted into the sternocleidomastoid muscle 2 cm below the tip of the mastoid process. The patient's head should be turned to the opposite side to make the muscle prominent. Five milliliters of the local anesthetic will block the branches to the sternocleidomastoid and the trapezius muscles (Fig 34D–5). A neurolytic block can be done using 3 ml of 50% alcohol or 3%–6% phenol. Use of a nerve stimulator and looking for trapezius contractions will increase the accuracy of the injection.

A spinal accessory nerve block results in weakness of the sternocleidomastoid and trapezius muscles. The patient has difficulty lifting the head off the bed, turning the head, or raising an arm above the head. No serious complications should be encounted if the local anesthetic is placed in the substance of the muscle. A lesser occipital nerve block may result in numbness behind the ear.

A successful block is recognized by the absence of contraction of the sternocleidomastoid muscle when the patient turns the head to the opposite side, and weakness of the trapezius muscle when the patient attempts to shrug the shoulders.

Indications

The spinal accessory nerve block has been useful as an adjunct to cervical plexus block for carotid surgery. It may be helpful for acute and chronic torticollis.

SPINAL NERVE ROOTS

Cervical

The cervical roots can be blocked by a lateral approach or by a posterior approach.

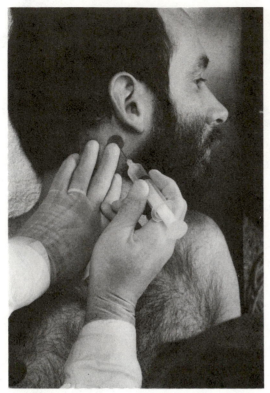

Fig 34D–5.—Spinal accessory nerve block. Figure shows injection of 5 ml of local anesthetic in the substance of the sternocleidomastoid muscle.

LATERAL APPROACH.—This method is useful for blocking the second through sixth cervical roots. Landmarks are the tip of the mastoid process and the anterior tubercle of the sixth cervical transverse process (Chassaignac's tubercle) at the level of the cricoid. The second cervical root is blocked 1.5 cm below and 1 cm behind the tip of the mastoid, the third cervical root is blocked at the level of the hyoid, the fourth cervical root is blocked at the level of the top of the thyroid cartilage, the fifth cervical root is blocked 1.5 cm below the fourth, and the sixth cervical root is blocked at the level of Chassaignac's tubercle. The dome of the pleural interferes with a block of the seventh and eighth roots when a lateral approach is used.

A 5-cm, 22-gauge needle is inserted at a level slightly above the level of the root to be blocked. The needle is directed slightly caudally and is advanced to contact the transverse process, at which point 3–5 ml of local anesthetic is injected. Paresthesias should be elicited by ''walking'' the needle on the tip of the transverse process. For a neurolytic block, fluoroscopy is recommended. Phenol 6% or absolute alcohol 0.5–1 ml per nerve root is recommended. Injection should be done after fluoroscopy has confirmed that the needle is in the correct position and an aspiration test is negative for CSF or blood.

If the needle is advanced in a horizontal direction, injection into the vertebral artery or epidural or subarachnoid space is possible. A slightly caudal direction usually avoids these complications.

POSTERIOR APPROACH.—This method is suitable when the lateral approach cannot be used because of carcinoma or infection. It is a technically more difficult approach. Since the cervical spines are difficult to feel above the level of C-6, the lines that correspond to the transverse processes are extended to the posterior aspect to serve as landmarks.

An 8-cm, 22-gauge needle is inserted perpendicularly through the skin wheal and 3 cm lateral to the midline. The needle is advanced until the transverse process or articular pillar is contacted or paresthesias are obtained. The needle can be walked off the lateral edge and advanced 0.5 cm beyond; then 3–5 ml of local anesthetic is injected. A successful block should result in hypoesthesia in the distribution of the root.

Indications

Indications for a cervical nerve root block are similar to those for a cervical plexus block.

Complications

Vertebral artery injection is possible if the needle is advanced between the transverse processes. Epidural and subarachnoid block can occur due to retrograde movement of the local anesthetic in the root sleeve. At lower cervical nerve roots, pneumothorax is a possibility. Vagal and laryngeal nerve and stellate ganglion blocks can occur if the needle is placed too far medially and anteriorly.

Thoracic

The 12 pairs of thoracic nerve roots can be blocked as they emerge from the thoracic intervertebral foramina. The spine of the thoracic vertebrae inclines downward, especially in the midthoracic area; therefore the tip of the vertebral spine in the thoracic region could be opposite the intervertebral foramen, two levels below. However, from T-1 to T-3 and from T-9 to T-12 this overlap does not exceed one level below.

A thoracic nerve root block can be done with the patient prone or in the lateral position with the affected side up. Vertebrae can be counted from C-7 down and checked again by counting from L-4 up. Fluoroscopy is essential.

A 22-gauge, 8-cm needle is advanced perpendicularly through a skin wheal 3 cm lateral to the level of the cephalad edge of the vertebrae to contact the transverse process. The needle is then withdrawn and advanced slightly medially (25°) and caudally (20°). If paresthesias are obtained, 5 ml of a local anesthetic is injected. If paresthesias are not obtained, the needle is advanced 2.5 cm deeper than the transverse process or until it contacts the posterolateral aspect of the vertebra, where the local anesthetic is injected.

The development of cutaneous analgesia in the appropriate dermatome indicates a successful block. It is hard to confirm analgesia of one dermatome because of the overlap of dermatomes. Three roots may have to be blocked to provide good analgesia in one dermatome.

Indications

A thoracic nerve root block is useful for diagnostic, prognostic, and therapeutic purposes, and for pain secondary to nerve root irritation or compression at the foramina level or distally. It can be used for treatment of intercostal neuralgia secondary to herpes zoster, fractured ribs, tumors, or metastasis.

Complications

Pneumothorax is possible but unlikely. If the patient has a coughing spasm or if air is aspirated, the pleura has been punctured. The patient should be observed for development of a pneumothorax.

Epidural or subarachnoid spread of the injection solution can occur, especially if there is a long dural sleeve. Segmental sympathetic block can result from the block of the sympathetic fibers which accompany the root.

If the volume is increased, solution can spread paravertebrally or epidurally up and down, and more roots may be anesthetized. It is important to use small volumes (1–3 ml) of local anesthetic when performing a neurolytic block. In addition, use of a small volume will define the contribution of the individual nerve root to the patient's pain.

Lumbar

A lumbar nerve root block is similar to a thoracic nerve root block. The spine of the lumbar vertebrae is straight and has a rectangular surface under the skin. The upper edge of the spine corresponds to the transverse process of the same vertebra. The line joining the highest part of iliac crest corresponds to the L-4 vertebra or the L4–5 interspace.

A 22-gauge, 8-cm needle is advanced perpendicularly through a skin wheal 4 cm lateral to the cephalad edge of the lumbar spine (Fig 34D–6). The needle is advanced until it impinges on the transverse process. It is then withdrawn and reinserted caudally and medially. If paresthesia is obtained, 5 ml of a local anesthetic solution is injected. If no paresthesia is obtained and if the posterolateral aspect of the vertebra is encountered, the needle is withdrawn 1 cm and the solution is injected.

A successful block is recognized by hypoesthesia in the appropriate dermatome. All lumbar nerves innervate postural muscles. A lumbar root block may result in weakness and inability to stand or walk.

Indications

A lumbar nerve root block is indicated for acute or chronic pain relief for radiculopathies secondary to disk prolapse or tumor.

Complications

Epidural or subarachnoid injection can result if the anesthetic solution is injected through the intervertebral foramen or into a long dural sleeve.

BRANCHES OF SPINAL NERVE ROOTS

Intercostal Nerves

The thoracic spinal nerves in the paravertebral region divide into a dorsal branch which innervates the muscle and skin of the posterior third of the back, and a ventral branch, which forms intercostal

B

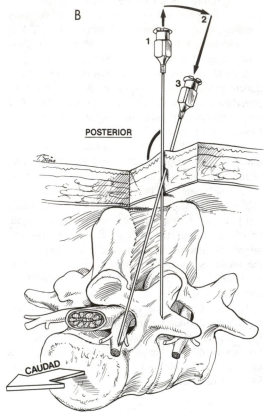

A

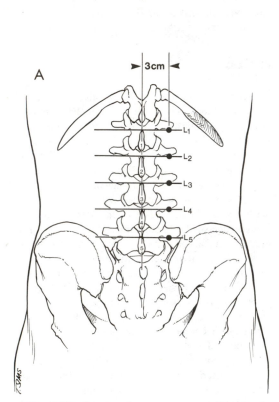

Fig 34D–6.—Lumbar nerve root block. **A,** needle inserted 3 cm lateral to the tip of the spinous processes of the lumbar vertebrae perpendicularly until it touches the transverse process. **B,** 8-cm, 22-gauge needle touching the transverse process (position 1). Positions 2 and 3 show the needle directed caudally to touch the nerve root at a deeper level. (From Raj P.P.: Chronic pain, in Raj P.P. (ed.): *Handbook of Regional Anesthesia.* New York, Churchill Livingstone, Inc., 1985. Reproduced by permission.)

nerves for the 11 intercostal spaces and the subcostal nerve below the 12th rib (Fig 34D–7).

The thoracic ventral branches of T-1 and T-2 also contribute to the formation of the lower trunk of the brachial plexus. Only a small part of T-1 continues first as the intercostal nerve. The second intercostal nerve gives rise to the lateral cutaneous branch, called the intercostobrachial nerve, which innervates the medial side of the upper arm. Each of the other intercostal nerves gives rise to a lateral branch that innervates the skin of the lateral body wall and an anterior cutaneous branch that innervates the anterior body wall; the upper six intercostal nerves innervate up to the xiphisternum, the lower six intercostal nerves innervate from the xiphisternum to the umbilicus.

The upper six intercostal nerves innervate the muscle in the intercostal space. The lower five intercostal nerves and the subcostal nerves innervate the abdominal muscles, in addition to the intercostal muscles. The nerve runs in the neurovascular plane between internal intercostal muscle, and the innermost layer (subcostal, sternocostal, innermost intercostal) is protected by the costal groove in the intermediate part of the rib where the innermost layer of muscle is deficient.

Indications

An intercostal nerve root block is indicated for patients undergoing surgery of the upper abdominal region (in conjunction with a celiac plexus block) and for patients with pain following thoracoabdom-

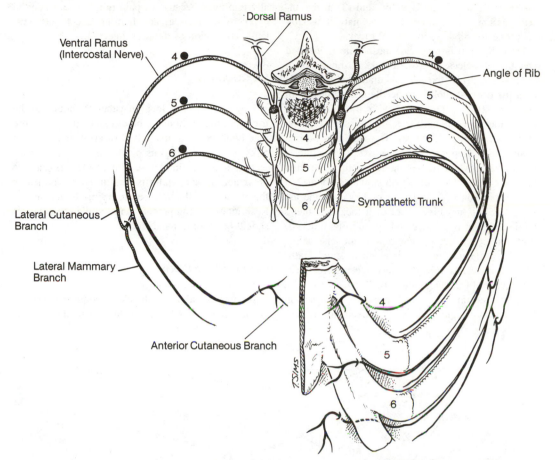

Fig 34D–7.—Anatomy of the intercostal nerves. (From Raj P.P., Pai U.: Techniques of nerve blocking, in Raj P.P. (ed.): *Handbook of* *Regional Anesthesia*. New York, Churchill Livingstone, Inc., 1985. Reproduced by permission.)

inal surgery. It is also useful for patients who have incurred trauma to the chest wall, especially fracture of the ribs, and for neurolytic blocks for cancer.

Equipment

22-gauge, 1½-inch needle.
23-gauge, 1/2-inch needle.
10-ml syringes.
Usual preparation tray.

Drugs

The volume of injectate is 3–5 ml per intercostal nerve. For a short-duration block, 1%–1.5% lidocaine is used; for a long duration block, 0.5% bu-

pivacaine or 1% etidocaine is used. For a neurolytic block 6%–8% phenol in Renografin is used.

Technique

For bilateral intercostal blocks, the patient is positioned prone with the arms hanging or elevated above the head. For a unilateral block at the posterior or midaxillary line, the patient lies in a lateral position with an arm over the head. For an anterior block to cover the paresternal region, the patient lies supine.

Procedure

The intercostal block can be done (1) at the angle of the rib posteriorly, (2) at the posterior axillary line or midaxillary line laterally, and (3) at the anterior axillary line anteriorly. The patient usually lies prone for bilateral intercostal blocks.

After the skin is prepared, the needle is inserted over the rib selected for the block. It should touch the lower half of the rib subcutaneously. At this point the operator holds the needle and syringe with one hand (Fig 34D–8) and with the other hand moves the skin caudally over the rib such that the needle point slips off the rib. The needle is pushed about 3 mm deeper until a click is felt. The hub is now turned downward and the needle tip is directed under the lower edge of the rib cephalad about 2–3 mm. Aspiration is done for air or blood. If the aspiration test is negative, 3 ml of a local anesthetic is injected. For one intercostal space to be blocked, three intercostal nerves, one above and one below the nerve selected, must be injected. A single catheter technique has been described recently for postoperative and trauma pain relief.

An intercostal nerve block provides analgesia in the intercostal region. Respiratory excursion is usu-ally improved because of pain relief. There may be hypotension, nausea, and fainting due to fast systemic absorption of the drug injected.

Precautions

Large volumes of local anesthetics should not be used for intercostal nerve blocks since they are more readily absorbed at this site than at other sites. The risks associated with this block are intravascular injection and pneumothorax. Pneumothorax can be prevented if the operator is careful, slow, and learns the anatomy of the area before trying the technique. Resuscitative equipment and skilled personnel should be close at hand.

Contraindications

An intercostal nerve block is contraindicated if pneumothorax would be deleterious to the patient,

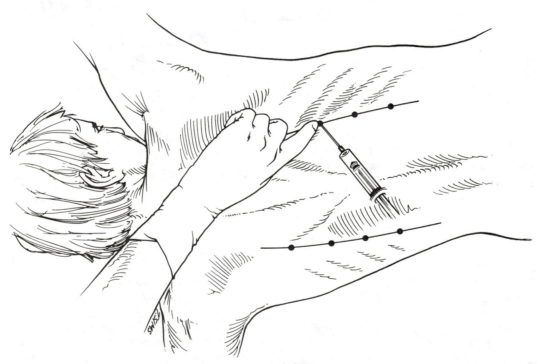

Fig 34D–8.—Intercostal block. Figure shows correct placement of the anesthetist's finger on the inferior edge of the patient's rib. Note that the needle with the syringe touches the rib before slipping under it to touch the intercostal nerve. The needle should be in-serted obliquely under the rib to prevent the development of a pneumothorax. (From Raj P.P., Pai U.: Techniques of nerve blocking, in Raj P.P. (ed.): *Handbook of Regional Anesthesia.* New York, Churchill Livingstone, Inc., 1985. Reproduced by permission.)

if there is infection at the site of the injection, if the patient is on anticoagulant therapy, if the patient is allergic to local anesthetics, and in a patient in shock.

Complications

PNEUMOTHORAX.—Careful performance of the block will reduce the risk of pneumothorax developing. If it does develop, it should be recognized and treated as necessary. The patient must be reassured.

SUBARACHNOID BLOCK.—An inadvertent subarachnoid block should be treated as a spinal block. This complication has been reported and actually proved with dye studies. Because the dura occasionally extends out along the intercostal nerve a variable distance before it adheres to the nerve as the neurilemma or nerve sheath, an anesthetic drug deposited in this potential space can dissect back into the subarachnoid space and result in spinal anesthesia (Fig 34D–9). Therefore, all of the devices necessary to support the patient should be present (airway equipment, breathing bag, IV fluids, vasopressors).

INTRAVASCULAR INJECTION LEADING TO SYSTEMIC TOXICITY.—Treat the toxicity. Intravascular absorption is much more problematic. Since the intercostal space is supplied by a rich network of vascular anastomoses because of the high metabolic activity of the intercostal muscles, there is a much greater absorption of the local anesthetic, leading to high plasma levels. Blood anesthetic levels are higher here and peak sooner than when the same amount of local anesthetic is injected elsewhere, such as axillary sheath or other nerve blocks. This may lead to toxic reactions. Careful attention must be paid to the maximum dosage allowed and a vasoconstrictor should be added in small concentrations—a 1:200,000 to 1:400,000 concentration is useful.

THE BRACHIAL PLEXUS AND ITS BRANCHES

The brachial plexus is formed by ventral rami of C-5, C-6, C-7, C-8, and T-1, with minor contributions from C-4 and T-2. From above as it traverses distally, the brachial plexus divides into roots, trunks, divisions, cords, and branches (Fig 34D–10).

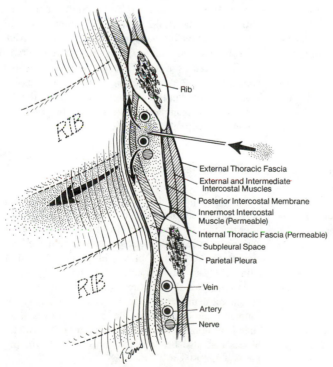

Fig 34D–9.—Intercostal block. Figure shows potential spaces which the injected solution can traverse. (From Raj P.P., Pai U.: Techniques of nerve blocking, in Raj P.P. (ed.): *Handbook of Regional Anesthesia.* New York, Churchill Livingstone, Inc., 1985. Reproduced by permission.)

Rib

External Thoracic Fascia
External and Intermediate Intercostal Muscles
Posterior Intercostal Membrane
Innermost Intercostal Muscle (Permeable)
Internal Thoracic Fascia (Permeable)
Subpleural Space
Parietal Pleura

Vein

Artery

Nerve

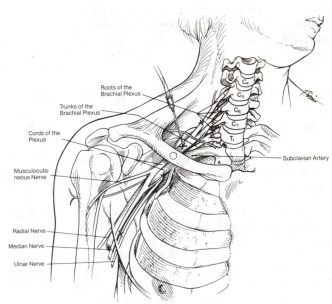

Fig 34D–10.—Anatomy of the brachial plexus and the four sites at which the brachial plexus block can be performed. (From Raj P.P., Pai U.: Techniques of nerve blocking, in Raj P.P. (ed.): *Handbook of Regional Anesthesia.* New York, Churchill Livingstone, Inc., 1985. Reproduced by permission.)

The roots enter the interscalene groove between the scalenus anterior and the scalenus medius muscles. C-5 and C-6 nerve roots form the upper trunk. The C-7 nerve root continues as the middle trunk, and the C-8 and T-1 nerve roots unite to form the lower trunk at the lateral part of the scalenus anterior muscle. The lower trunk is ensheathed by the prevertebral fascia and lies in the same plane as the subclavian artery. The upper and middle trunks lie above the subclavian artery; the lower trunk lies posterior to the subclavian artery close to the first rib.

Each trunk divides into anterior and posterior divisions. The posterior divisions of all the trunks unite to form the posterior cord. The anterior divisions of the upper and middle trunks form the lateral cord, and the anterior division of the lower trunk forms the medial cord. The cords are designated as posterior, lateral, or medial according to their relationship to the second part of the axillary artery, behind the pectoralis minor muscle.

Branches of the brachial plexus given at the roots are: (1) C-5 contribution to the phrenic nerve; (2) C-5, 6, 7 nerve to the seratus anterior; and (3) nerve to rhomboids and levator scapulae (C-5). The branches given at the trunks are at the upper trunk: (1) nerve to subclavicus; and (2) suprascapular nerve to supraspinatus and infraspinatus. The branches given at the cords are the: (1) lateral cord (lateral pectoral nerve, musculocutaneous nerve, and lateral head of the median nerve; (2) medial cord (medial pectoral nerve, medial cutaneous nerve

of the arm and forearm, medial head of the median curve, and ulnar nerve; and (3) posterior cord (upper and lower subscapular nerve, nerve to latissimus dorsi, axillary nerve to shoulder joint and to deltoid and terus minor, and radial nerve.

Except for the innervation of the skin over the upper part of the shoulder (C3–4) and the upper part of the medial arm (T-2), all of the motor and sensory innervation of the upper extremity is derived from the brachial plexus. The sympathetic innervation is derived from the T-1 to T-5 spinal segments. The T-1 to T-2 postganglionic fibers traverse the brachial plexus via the stellate ganglion, and the T-3 to T-5 postganglionic fibers join the vascular branches of the subclavian artery to the arm.

Indications

A brachial plexus block is indicated for anesthesia of the upper extremity during surgery, for pain relief after trauma, for relief of postoperative pain, and for chronic pain relief in patients with certain medical conditions. A brachial plexus block is indicated if pain relief is not adequate after stellate ganglion blocks for causalgia, reflex sympathetic dystrophy, peripheral neuropathies, or Raynaud's phenomenon. Catheters can be placed on the brachial plexus at all sites if prolonged pain relief is required. Neurolytic blocks can also be done for cancer pain involving the brachial plexus.

Ten milliliters of a local anesthetic will produce a consistently good block of each trunk, division, or the mixed peripheral nerve. Since the brachial plexus block involves four major nerves, a total of 40 ml is required for surgical anesthesia. Lesser volumes of 10–20 ml are required for pain relief. The site of needle entry does not change the volume requirement. A higher needle entry in the brachial plexus sheath, such as that used for the interscalene, supraclavicular, or infraclavicular blocks, causes the motor block to appear earlier than the sensory block. A more distal needle entry, such as that used for an axillary block, is associated with greater sensory block and poorer motor block.

For a consistent brachial plexus motor block, the recommended agents are 0.5% bupivacaine, 3% chloroprocaine, 1% etidocaine, 1.5% lidocaine, 1.5% mepivacaine, or 2% prilocaine. For a sensory block alone, lesser concentrations of a local anesthetic such as 2% chloroprocaine or 1% lidocaine may be used. For brachial plexalgia involving the nerve trunks, divisions, or cords secondary to cancer, neurolytic blocks can be tried. Phenol 6% to 10% may be injected, up to a maximum volume of 10 ml at any one time.

Interscalene Approach[2]

The brachial plexus in the interscalene region consists of roots and trunks covered by the prevertebral fascia and enclosed between the fasciae of the anterior and middle scalene muscles (Fig 34D–11).

EQUIPMENT
Two 20-ml syringes.
Extension set.
22-gauge, 1½-inch needle.
27-gauge local infiltration needle with a 2-ml syringe.
Nerve stimulator with alligator clips and ECG pad, if this is used.

DRUGS.—For a procedure of short duration (< 1 hour), 40 ml of 2%–3% 2-chloroprocaine is appropriate. For a procedure of medium duration (2 hours), 40 ml of 1%–1½% lidocaine, with or without 1:200,000 ephinephrine, is appropriate. For a procedure of long duration (> 3 hours), 40 ml of 0.5% or 0.75% bupivacaine or 1% may be used, or 20 ml of 2% lidocaine plus 20 ml of 0.5% bupivacine.

TECHNIQUE.—The patient lies supine with the head turned to the opposite direction. One arm rests

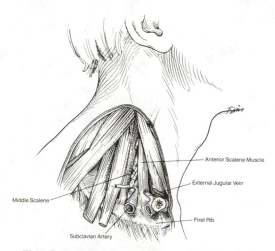

Fig 34D–11.—Regional anatomy of the brachial plexus in the interscalene groove. (From Raj P.P., Pai U.: Techniques of nerve blocking, in Raj P.P. (ed.): *Handbook of Regional Anesthesia.* New York, Churchill Livingstone, Inc., 1985. Reproduced by permission.)

on the side, extending to the knee. The physician stands on the side to be blocked at the level of the neck.

Landmarks.—To identify landmarks, the operator palpates the cricoid cartilage (C-6 level) and the posterior border of sternocleidomastoid muscle. Then he rolls his fingers posteriorly to the posterior border of the sternomastoid and onto the interscalene groove. The interscalene groove can be accentuated if the patient raises the head against resistance. The point of entry of the needle is where the external jugular vein crosses the sternomastoid (C-6 level) (Fig 34D–12).

PROCEDURE.—After a sterile preparation, the physician stands on the side to be blocked at the level of the neck and palpates the interscalene groove at the C-6 level. Any local anesthetic is infiltrated intracutaneously with a 27-gauge needle. The operator then takes in hand a 20-ml syringe attached to an extension set and a 22-gauge needle. The needle is inserted through the landmark, perpendicular to the skin and in a caudal direction. At this point a nerve stimulator could be attached to the needle, with the ground electrode in the opposite shoulder. As the needle enters the interscalene groove, a paresthesia should be elicited in the shoulder, elbow, or thumb. When paresthesia of the elbow or thumb is obtained, the needle advancement should be stopped. As the nerve stimulator current

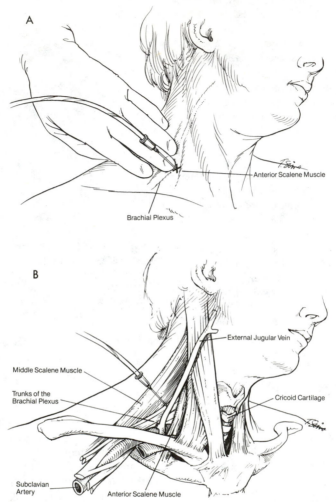

Fig 34D–12.—A and **B,** superficial landmarks, site of entry, and position of the needle for the interscalene approach to the brachial plexus block. Note that in **B** the needle usually contacts the upper trunk. (From Raj P.P., Pai U.: Techniques of nerve blocking, in Raj P.P. (ed.): *Handbook of Regional Anesthesia.* New York, Churchill Livingstone, Inc., 1985. Reproduced by permission.)

is applied, the biceps, forearm muscles, or wrist and hand muscles will contract. The needle is in a correct position if the paresthesia is in the thumb or contractions are seen in the wrist or fingers. If paresthesia of the shoulder or elbow is present or the biceps are contracting, the needle may be at the C5–6 nerve root. If the diaphragm is contracting unilaterally, the phrenic nerve has been stimulated; the needle is too anterior and medial.

A brachial plexus block performed via the intersalene approach provides anesthesia of the shoulder, elbow, forearm, and hand; usually there is no anes-

thesia of the inner aspect of the upper arm and the elbow. The ulnar nerve is blocked in about half the cases.

PRECAUTIONS.—Prior to injection the aspiration test is done to prevent vascular or CSF spread. A test dose of 1–3 ml of local anesthetic solution should be administered to test for CNS toxicity or total spinal block. The injection should be stopped as soon as signs of toxicity appear.

COMPLICATIONS.—A total spinal block may be prevented by performing the aspiration test prior to injection. A high epidural block is managed by airway control, oxygen administration, and maintenance of blood pressure.

CNS toxic reactions causing unconsciousness are managed with oxygen administration and the maintenance of respiratory, cardiac, and CNS functions. Cardiac toxic reactions causing cardiac arrhythmias are managed with oxygen administration and the maintenance of respiratory, cardiac, and CNS functions.

An inadvertent stellate ganglion block requires no treatment. Similarly, an inadvertent laryngeal nerve block requires no treatment; however, there should be no oral intake until the patient can sip water. An inadvertent phrenic nerve block is managed by maintaining adequate ventilation.

The treatment of a pneumothorax depends on the size of the pneumothorax. A chest x-ray film must be made and a pulmonary physician consulted for further management.

Supraclavicular Approach[3]

ANATOMY.—The trunks of the brachial plexus form divisions and cords at this level. The medial cord lies posterior to the third part of the subclavian artery. The lateral and posterior cords lie posterolateral to the artery.

EQUIPMENT
Same as for infraclavicular and axillary and interscalene approaches.
23-gauge, 1/2-inch needle for skin infiltration.
Extension set for immobile needle technique.
Two 20-ml syringes.
Nerve stimulator with its accessories, if used.

DRUGS.—For a procedure of short duration (< 1 hour), 40 ml of 2%–3% 2-chloroprocaine, is appropriate. For a procedure of medium duration (2 hours) 40 ml of 1%–1½% lidocaine is appropriate. For a procedure of long duration (> 3 hours), 40 ml of 0.5% or 0.75% bupivacaine or 1% etidocaine may be used, or 20 ml of 2% lidocaine plus 20 ml of 0.5% bupivacaine. For neurolytic procedures, 6% in Renografin is recommended.

TECHNIQUE.—The patient is positioned supine with a roll between the scapulae. The arms rest on the side, extended toward the knee. The patient's head is turned to the opposite side. For accentuation of the sternomastoid and scalene muscles, the head may be lifted 30° off the table.

Landmark.—The landmark is the midpoint of the clavicle midway between the prominence of the top of the shoulder (acromial end of the clavicle) and the sternal end of the clavicle. The point of needle entry is on the lateral border of the anterior scalene muscle at the midpoint of the clavicle.

Alternative technique.—For a perivascular subclavian approach,[4] the needle entry site is at the C-7 level in the interscalene groove, with the needle directed caudad and the needle hub in line with the ear (Fig 34D-13).

PROCEDURE.—After a sterile preparation of the region, the needle is inserted at the point of entry above the midpoint of the clavicle in the backward, inward, and downward direction. The needle appears to be at right angles to all planes at this level of the neck (Fig 34D-14). Even though the needle is directed toward the first rib, it need not touch the rib. Paresthesia of the digits of the hand or wrist is sought. If it is obtained, and an aspiration test is negative for air or blood, 1–3 ml of local anesthetic is injected, as a test dose followed by injection of the total calculated volume of the local anesthetic after 5 minutes if there are no systemic effects. If paresthesia is not obtained and the needle touches the first rib, it usually touches it at the subclavian groove. The needle is walked posteriorly to elicit paresthesia. If paresthesia is not obtained, contact with the rib will be lost. Contact with the rib is again made and the needle is walked toward the ver-

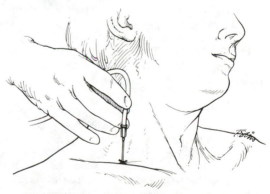

Fig 34D–13.—Subclavian perivascular approach of the brachial plexus. Note the point of entry is at the interscalene groove, where the subclavian artery pulsation is felt. (From Raj P.P., Pai U.: Techniques of nerve blocking, in Raj P.P.: (ed.): *Handbook of Regional Anesthesia.* New York, Churchill Livingstone, Inc., 1985. Reproduced by permission.)

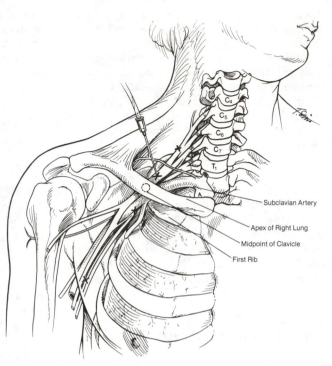

Fig 34D–14.—Direction of the needle (backward, inward, and downward) for the supraclavicular approach to the brachial plexus block. The point of entry is at 1 cm superior to the upper border of the clavicle at its midpoint. (From Raj P.P., Pai U.: *Techniques of nerve blocking,* in Raj P.P. (ed.): *Handbook of Regional Anesthesia.* New York, Churchill Livingstone, Inc., 1985. Reproduced by permission.)

Subclavian Artery

Apex of Right Lung

Midpoint of Clavicle

First Rib

tebra. If no paresthesia is obtained at this point, the procedure is repeated. The nerve stimulator can be used as described earlier in this section to aid in location of the brachial plexus.

A brachial plexus block by the supraclavicular approach provides anesthesia of the whole arm up to the shoulder, except the inside of the upper third of the upper arm. A sympathetic block is also produced in the same regions.

PRECAUTIONS.—The operator should avoid puncturing the subclavian artery or the lung and should avoid entering the epidural or subarachnoid space.

The stellate ganglion may be blocked, especially with large volumes. The vagus nerve and its branches in the neck may also be blocked.

COMPLICATIONS.—Possible complications include a hematoma in the neck, and pneumothorax. A hematoma in the neck is treated by reassuring the patient, watching, and aspirating or evacuating the hematoma, if necessary. The hematoma will disappear spontaneously in 2–3 weeks.

A pneumothorax of less than 10% may be treated conservatively; a pneumothorax of more than 20% requires chest tube placement.

Infraclavicular Approach[5]

ANATOMY.—The axilla occupies the pyramid-shaped infraclavicular space between the upper lateral part of the chest and the medial side of the arm. It consists of an apex, base, and four walls. The apex faces the root of the neck and is limited by the outer border of the first rib, the superior border of the scapula, and the posterior surface of the clavicle. The base is formed by the skin and the axillary fascia. The pectoralis major and minor muscles form the anterior wall. The subcapularis teres major and the latissimus dorsi complete the posterior wall. The medial wall is formed by the first four ribs, and the lateral wall is formed by the medial side of the arm. The contents of the axilla include the axillary vessels, the brachial plexus with its branches, some branches of the intercostal nerves, a large number of lymph glands, fat, and loose areolar tissue.

INDICATIONS.—Deposition of a local anesthetic solution inside the brachial plexus sheath in the infraclavicular region blocks the cords and branches of the brachial plexus above and below the level of formation of the musculocutaneous and axillary nerves. Thus, an infraclavicular approach is useful when anesthesia from hand to shoulder is desired. In addition, this technique allows easy blocking of the ulnar segment of the medial cord and the intercostobrachial nerve, which helps to prevent tourniquet pain without requiring additional infiltration.

The infraclavicular approach to the brachial plexus block provides adequate anesthesia of the entire arm. Although the danger of penetrating blood vessels is the same as in other approaches, the risk of pneumothorax is less, because the needle is directed laterally from the midpoint of the clavicle. The lung lies behind the medial third of the clavicle and hence escapes potential damage from the needle tip.

For consistently good results with the infraclavicular approach, it is necessary to use a peripheral nerve stimulator. The neurostimulator technique simplifies the process of locating the brachial plexus, which is deeper in the infraclavicular region than at other sites, and improves the success rate of the infraclavicular block.

EQUIPMENT
- One 3-ml syringe for skin infiltration.
- One 22-gauge, unsheathed, standard 3½-inch spinal needle.
- Extension set.
- Two 20-ml plastic syringes.
- Peripheral nerve stimulator.
- Anesthetic solution.

TECHNIQUE.—The patient lies supine and the physician stands opposite the arm to be blocked. Although the patient's arm is usually abducted 90° and the head is turned away from the arm, the block can be performed with the patient's arm and head in any position.

Landmarks.—A line drawn from the C-6 tubercle to the brachial artery in the arm and which crosses the midpoint of the clavicle provides the surface marking of the brachial plexus in the infraclavicular region.

Prior to cleansing, the whole length of the clavicle and the subclavian artery where it dips under the clavicle should be identified by palpation and marked. If the artery cannot be felt, the midpoint of the clavicle should be identified. The point of needle entry is 1 inch below the midpoint of the clavicle (Fig 34D–15).

PROCEDURE.—After the field has been sterilized and draped, the stimulator and the leads should be tested and the ground electrode attached to the patient's shoulder opposite the site of needle entry. The skin is infiltrated with a small amount of local anesthetic 1 inch below the inferior border of the clavicle at its midpoint. A 22-gauge, unsheathed standard 3½-inch spinal needle is introduced through the skin wheal with the needle point directed laterally toward the brachial artery (Fig 34D–16). When the needle has just penetrated the skin, the exploring electrode should be attached to either the stem or the metal hub of the needle with a sterile alligator clip. The voltage control of the peripheral nerve stimulator should be set to deliver 6–8 V at 1 or 2 impulses per second, and the needle should be advanced at an angle of 45° to the skin. The pectoralis group of muscles will contract and adduct the shoulder. When that occurs, the voltage should be reduced until the patient is comfortable. When the needle tip is past the muscles, the contraction should stop.

As the needle approaches the fibers of the brachial plexus, the muscles supplied by the musculocutaneous, median, ulnar, and radial nerves will move. The forearm and hand should be observed carefully for these movements. When flexion or extension of the elbow, wrist, or digits is observed, the needle point is close to nerve fibers of the brachial plexus. At this point, voltage should be decreased to the lowest level (2–4 V) that still allows muscle movement to be observed. The needle should again be advanced until maximum muscle movements are seen and then begin to diminish. The diminution in muscle movement signals that the needle tip has passed the nerve. The needle should then be withdrawn slowly until maximum muscle movements are again observed at the lowest voltage. The needle should be held in that position for the injection. It is preferable to use extension tubing so that the needle is not displaced when the syringe is attached.

After negative aspiration for blood, 2 ml of local anesthetic solution should be injected. If the needle is correctly located, within 0.5 cm of the nerve fibers, muscle movements will cease within 30 seconds. If muscle movement continues, the needle tip may have passed the nerve; in this case, the needle should be withdrawn until best muscle movements are seen and then the test dose should be repeated.

When the needle is in position on the nerve fibers, an adequate volume and concentration of local anesthetic solution should be injected.

If another nearby nerve is to be located, the nee-

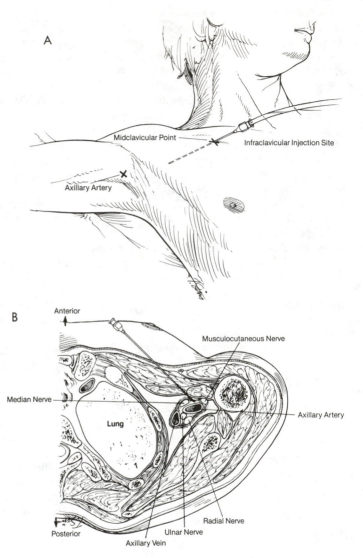

Fig 34D–15.—A, technique of brachial plexus block by the infraclavicular approach. A 22-gauge, 3½-inch needle is directed from 1 inch below the midpoint of the clavicle toward the brachial artery in the upper arm. The needle is at a 45° angle to the skin. **B,** horizontal section of the axillary space showing the relationship of the axilla and the direction of the needle laterally from the point of entry. (From Raj P.P., Pai U.: Techniques of nerve blocking, in Raj P.P. (ed.): *Handbook of Regional Anesthesia.* New York, Churchill Livingstone, Inc., 1985. Reproduced by permission.)

dle should be withdrawn and immediately advanced toward it. A delay may result in the disappearance of helpful muscular movement, since the first injection may block adjacent nerves. If that occurs, the procedure is repeated at a higher voltage to locate and block the second nerve.

After successful injection, anesthesia and weakness spread from the shoulder to the wrist. The outer fibers are anesthetized first. The anesthetic takes longer to reach the core bundles, which supply the distal parts, so the hand is anesthetized last.

The block should be confirmed by clinical examination and by using the peripheral nerve stimulator to confirm that no muscle movements appear at higher voltages.

CONTRAINDICATIONS.—This technique is not indicated if there is an infection in the skin, chest wall, or axilla.

Axillary Approach[6]

ANATOMY.—In the axilla, the nerves from the brachial plexus and the axillary artery are enclosed in a fibrous neuromuscular fascial sheath. The median and musculocutaneous nerves are anterior or anterolateral, i.e., above and beyond the artery. The ulnar nerve is medial. The radial nerve is posterolateral, or below and behind the vessel.

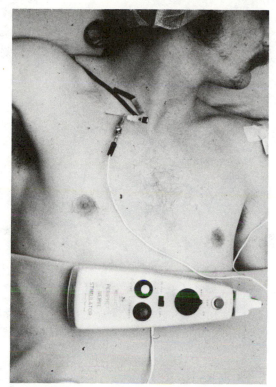

Fig 34D–16.—Infraclavicular approach to the brachial plexus block. A 3½-inch, 22-gauge needle has been inserted in a lateral direction. A nerve stimulator is used for performing this block. (From Raj P.P., Pai U.: Techniques of nerve blocking, in Raj P.P. (ed.): *Handbook of Regional Anesthesia.* New York, Churchill Livingstone, Inc., 1985. Reproduced by permission.)

EQUIPMENT
- One 3-ml syringe for skin infiltration.
- One 23- or 25-gauge 1-inch needle.
- Extension set, if used.
- Peripheral nerve stimulator, if used.
- Anesthetic solution.

TECHNIQUE.—The patient should be supine with the arm abducted 90° at the shoulder joint; the forearm should be placed in the supine position. Some prefer to hyperabduct the arm at the shoulder joint with external rotation and flexion at the elbow joint; this position should be avoided, because abduction beyond 90° will impede the proximal spread of local anesthetic to the origin of the musculocutaneous nerve. However, hyperabduction may be necessary to palpate the artery in a difficult case.

Landmarks.—The axillary artery at the border of the anterior axillary wall and the upper arm should be palpated and marked up to a distance of 2 cm.

PROCEDURE.—After the area has been sterilized and draped, the physician stands on the side of the arm to be blocked and palpates the axillary artery, with the palm of one hand lying comfortably over the upper arm. Next, the needle is inserted just proximal to the palpating finger and within the borders of the finger (the envisioned size of the brachial sheath at that level) (Fig 34D–17).

As the needle is inserted, three different methods can be used to confirm the needle's position in the brachial plexus sheath: (1) when or if the needle penetrates the axillary artery, the needle should be withdrawn until the needle pulsates over the artery and blood can no longer be aspirated; (2) paresthesia can be elicited in the distribution of the ulnar, median, or radial nerve; (3) with the use of a peripheral nerve stimulator, muscular movements of the hand will be seen at the lowest voltage (2 V) and will be abolished by injection of 2 ml of a local anesthetic solution.

Once the needle position is confirmed, the axillary artery should be compressed and an adequate volume and concentration of anesthetic solution should be injected. Compression of the axillary artery during injection facilitates the proximal spread of the anesthetic solution to block the musculocutaneous nerves.

If signs of toxicity are seen after injection, indicating that inadvertent intravascular injection has occurred, it is essential to stop the injection, withdraw the needle, and stabilize the patient. If the axillary block must be done, the procedure should be repeated when the patient is stable.

After injection, the needle should be removed, the area massaged, and the arm brought down to the side while the operator continues to compress the axilla for a few minutes.

LIMITATIONS.—Although the axillary approach is the approach most commonly used today, it has several limitations. It can be performed only when the arm is abducted to 90° or more. Anesthesia proximal to the elbow progresses slowly and may not reach the mid to upper arm. Furthermore, an axillary approach makes it difficult to block the musculocutaneous and axillary nerves, which supply the shoulder and the lateral arm region. When a tourniquet is used, additional infiltration is necessary to block the intercostobrachial nerve.

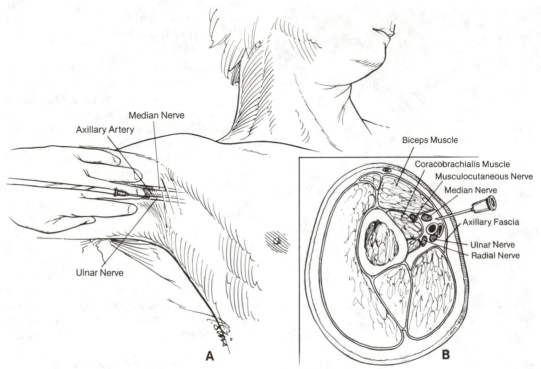

Fig 34D–17.—Axillary approach to the brachial plexus block. The middle finger of the anesthetist's nondominant hand is on the axillary artery. The 25-gauge, 1-inch needle is directed toward the axilla. *Inset* shows the needle in the neurovascular bundle close to the brachial artery. The musculocutaneous nerve lies in the coracobrachialis muscle, outside the brachial plexus sheath at this site. (From Raj P.P., Pai U.: Techniques of nerve blocking, in Raj P.P. (ed.): *Handbook of Regional Anesthesia.* New York, Churchill Livingstone, Inc., 1985. Reproduced by permission.)

CONTRAINDICATIONS.—Axillary block is contraindicated if the patient has infected glands or the arm cannot be abducted to 90° at the shoulder joint.

Complications of the Brachial Plexus Block

Since most major nerves occupy a neurovascular bundle, inadvertent intra-arterial injection is always a risk. Even an extremely low dose of local anesthetic, e.g., a "test" dose, may precipitate a seizure if injected into an artery under high pressure and if reverse flow occurs.

Although direct IV injection is more likely to occur than intra-arterial injection, the volume or total dose of local anesthetic required to produce a seizure is much greater. This provides the opportunity for the clinician to observe preseizure symptoms such as dizziness.

Because a toxic response to intravascular injection occurs immediately, resuscitation equipment and drugs (including IV diazepam and barbiturates) must be available before the block is begun. Injections resulting in CNS toxicity are treated the same way.

Hematoma may occur after any nerve block. Although most hematomas are not serious, they may cause complications. The early effect of a hematoma is to compress the neurovascular bundle, rendering ischemic the area distal to the hematoma. The hematoma should be decompressed before irreversible neurologic damage occurs. Calcification of a hematoma is a theoretical and late complication.

Nerve Blocks at the Elbow

A single nerve or a combination of nerves can be blocked to reinforce the brachial plexus block or for diagnostic or therapeutic purposes. Nerve blocks at the elbow by themselves can produce anesthesia of the hand and wrist and are indicated for surgery at those sites when a tourniquet is not required or the procedure is short. Neurolytic blocks can be done for cancer patients if pain relief has been provided by previous local anesthetic diagnostic blocks.

ANATOMY.—The median nerve is situated on the medial side of the brachial artery and on the biceps tendon, underneath the deep fascia. The radial nerve is located between the brachioradialis and brachialis muscles, lateral to the tendon of the biceps. It lies in front of the lateral condyle of the humerus. The ulnar nerve lies in the groove posterior to the medial condyle of the humerus, midway between the olecranon and the medial epicondyle. The musculocutaneous nerve lies superficially lateral to the biceps tendon at the crease of the elbow. At this point it lies superficial to the deep fascia (Fig 34D–18).

EQUIPMENT
• 5-ml syringe.
• 22-gauge, 1½-inch needle.
• 27-gauge local infiltration needle.

DRUGS.—For each nerve, 5 ml of a local anesthetic and 1–2 ml of 6% phenol in Renografin are required. For a short procedure (up to 1½ hours), 1%–1.5% Xylocaine with or without 1:200,000 epinephrine may be used. For a long procedure (3–3½ hours), 0.5% or 0.75% of bupivacaine, or 1% etidocaine may be used. For prolonged anesthesia, 6% phenol in Renografin is appropriate.

TECHNIQUE.—For a block of the median, radial, or musculocutaneous nerves, the patient lies supine with the arm in slight flexion at the elbow to accentuate the crease. Flexion also will make the biceps tendon and brachioradialis muscle prominent. For a block of the ulnar nerve, the elbow should be flexed a little more than 90° with the hand angled toward the contralateral shoulder.

Landmarks.—For a block of the median nerve, the biceps tendon at its insertion is located by the pulsation of brachial artery. The point of needle entry is medial to the brachial artery. For a block of the radial nerve, a point 1 cm lateral to the biceps tendon is located medial to the brachioradialis. For a block of the ulnar nerve, a point is located between the medial epicondyle and the olecranon process in the ulnar groove. For a block of the musculo-

cutaneous nerve, a point is located 1 cm lateral to the biceps tendon.

PROCEDURE.—After a sterile preparation, the 22-gauge needles are inserted at each nerve. Paresthesia of the ulnar, median, and radial nerves is obtained. A nerve stimulator can be attached and appropriate muscle contractions identified.

COMPLICATIONS.—Possible complications include infection, bruising, and post-block dysthesia. One should avoid too many paresthesias. Post-block dysthesia is treated by a stellate ganglion block. It usually subsides in 3 weeks.

Wrist Block

ANATOMY.—The median nerve is situated medial to the flexor carpi radialis tendon deep to the palmaris longus tendon under the deep fascia at the palmar crease of the wrist. The ulnar nerve is situated lateral to the flexor carpi ulnaris tendon and medial to the ulnar artery under the deep fascia at the palmar crease of the wrist. A superficial branch of the radial nerve is situated as branches in the superficial fascia at the lateral aspect of the distal end of the radius.

INDICATIONS.—A wrist block is indicated for surgery or to provide analgesia distal to the metacarpophalangeal joint. It is useful for suture of a laceration or fracture of the digits, and for incision of paronychia or abscesses of the digits.

EQUIPMENT
• 5-ml syringe.
• 22-gauge, 1½-inch needle.
• 27-gauge local infiltration needle.

DRUGS.—For each nerve, 5 ml of a local anesthetic is injected, as follows. For a short procedure (up to 1½ hours), Xylocaine is injected with or without 1:200,000 epinephrine. For a long procedure, 0.5%–0.75% of bupivacaine or etidocaine is injected. For neurolytic procedures, 1–2 ml of 6% phenol in Renografin is recommended.

TECHNIQUE.—The patient is positioned supine with the hand resting on the table for the block of the median and ulnar nerves. For a block of the radial nerve the patient's hand should be in a midprone position.

Landmarks.—The ulnar nerve is located by identifying the flexor carpi ulnaris tendon, pisiform

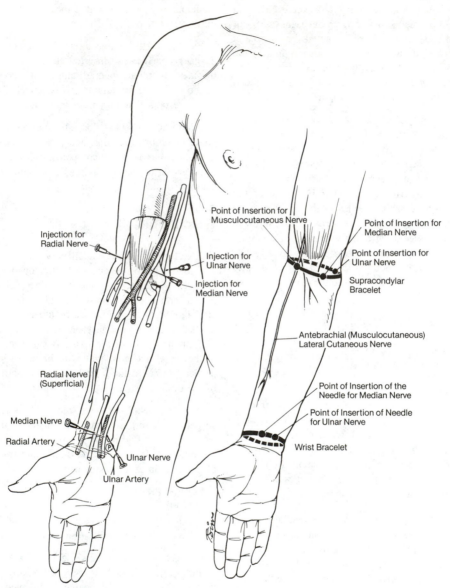

Labels in figure:
Injection for Radial Nerve
Point of Insertion for Musculocutaneous Nerve
Injection for Ulnar Nerve
Injection for Median Nerve
Point of Insertion for Median Nerve
Point of Insertion for Ulnar Nerve
Supracondylar Bracelet
Antebrachial (Musculocutaneous) Lateral Cutaneous Nerve
Radial Nerve (Superficial)
Median Nerve
Radial Artery
Ulnar Nerve
Ulnar Artery
Point of Insertion of the Needle for Median Nerve
Point of Insertion of Needle for Ulnar Nerve
Wrist Bracelet

Fig 34D–18.—Anatomy of the median, ulnar, radial, and musculocutaneous nerves at the elbow and the wrists. Note the landmarks at the wrist and elbow for blocks of these nerves. (From Raj P.P., Pai U.: Techniques of nerve blocking, in Raj P.P. (ed.): *Handbook of Regional Anesthesia.* New York, Churchill Livingstone, Inc., 1985. Reproduced by permission.)

bone, and ulnar artery. The median nerve is located by identifying the palmaris longus tendon and the flexor carpi radialis tendon with the wrist flexed. The radial nerve transverses the anatomical snuffbox at the lateral aspect of the wrist, bounded by abductor pollicis longus, extons or pollicis brevis, and extensor pollicis longus overlying the styloid process of the radius.

PROCEDURE.—After a sterile preparation, the 22-gauge needles are inserted at each nerve, as shown in Figures 34D-19, and 34D-20. Paresthesia

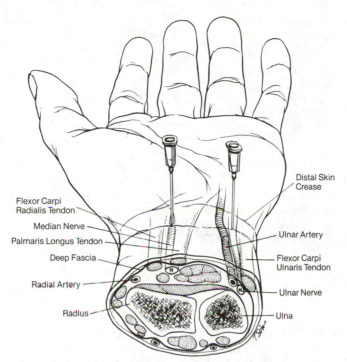

Flexor Carpi
Radialis Tendon

Median Nerve

Palmaris Longus Tendon

Deep Fascia

Radial Artery

Radius

Distal Skin
Crease

Ulnar Artery

Flexor Carpi
Ulnaris Tendon

Ulnar Nerve

Ulna

Fig 34D–19.—Technique of blocking the median and ulnar nerves at the wrists. (From Raj P.P., Pai U.: Techniques of nerve blocking, in Raj P.P. (ed.): *Handbook of Regional Anesthesia.* New York, Churchill Livingstone, Inc., 1985. Reproduced by permission.)

of the ulnar, median, and radial nerves is obtained. A nerve stimulator can be attached and appropriate muscle contractions identified.

COMPLICATIONS.—Possible complications include infection, bruising, and post-block dysesthesia. Post-block dysesthesia is treated by stellate ganglion block. It usually subsides in 3 weeks.

In addition, because of the close proximity of the synovial sheaths of the space of the hand and forearm, special precautions must be taken to prevent sepsis. Epinephrine should *not* be used.

Digital Block

ANATOMY.—Palmar digital nerves are the branches of the median nerve for the thumb, index, middle, and one half of the ring fingers and the ulnar nerve supplies the little finger and the medial side of the ring finger. Dorsal digital nerves arise from radial nerve to the lateral supply of the thumb, index, and middle fingers and the ulnar nerve supplies one half of the ring and little fingers.

Common digital nerves in the palm are located proximal to the metacarpal heads and deep to the palmar aponeurosis.

INDICATION.—A digital block is indicated for minor procedures on the finger and for neurolysis of a digital nerve for pain relief.

EQUIPMENT
• 27-gauge local infiltration needle.
• 5-ml syringe.

DRUGS.—The block is achieved with 1% Carbocaine or Xylocaine or 6% phenol in Renografin.

TECHNIQUE.—The hand and fingers are extended.

Landmarks.—Landmarks are the heads of the metacarpal bones and the bases of the proximal phalanx.

PROCEDURE.—The patient's fingers are extended and abducted from each other. A skin wheal is raised on the dorsal surface of the intermetacarpal space of the hand at the level of the head of the

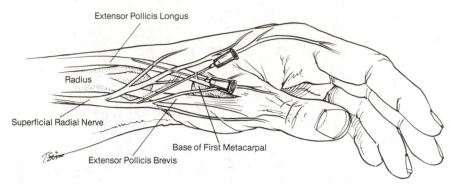

Extensor Pollicis Longus

Radius

Superficial Radial Nerve

Base of First Metacarpal

Extensor Pollicis Brevis

Fig 34D–20.—Technique of blocking the superficial branches of the radial nerve at the wrist. (From Raj P.P., Pai U.: Techniques of nerve blocking, in Raj P.P. (ed.): *Handbook of* *Regional Anesthesia.* New York, Churchill Livingstone, Inc., 1985. Reproduced by permission.)

metacarpal bone. A No. 23 1½-inch needle is introduced deep into the hand along the axis of the fingers until the resistance of the palmar aponeurosis is felt. Local anesthetic, 1–2 ml, is injected as the needle is withdrawn. Through the same skin wheal subcutaneous infiltration at the bases of fingers on either side is done to block the dorsal digital branches.

COMPLICATIONS.—Injection of a large volume of the local anesthetic is to be avoided as it may cause pressure on the blood vessels and ischemia of the digit. Epinephrine is contraindicated as the vasoconstriction may jeopardize the blood supply to the digit.

Suprascapular Nerve Block

ANATOMY.—The suprascapular nerve is a branch at the level of the trunk of the brachial plexus from the fifth and sixth cervical nerves. After leaving the brachial plexus it enters the scapular region through the suprascapular notch on the cephalic border of the scapula and then is distributed to the suprascapular and infrascapular muscles. It supplies a large sensory component to the shoulder joint, with a variable cutaneous branch to the cephalic and lateral aspects of the upper extremity just below the deltoid insertion.

LANDMARKS.—The operator identifies the spine of the scapula and then draws a line vertically through the midpoint of the spine and parallel to the vertebral column. The upper and outer quadrant so

formed is bissected and a needle is inserted at a distance of 2 cm along this line (Fig 34D–21). The needle is inserted at a right angle to the skin and advanced until the dorsal surface of the scapula is located. The needle is then walked along this dorsal surface until the suprascapula notch is identified. If a nerve stimulator is used, contractions of the supraspinatus and infraspinatus muscles will confirm placement. At this location, 5 cc of local anesthetic is injected. It is not always possible to ascertain any dermal analgesia as a result of this block. The success of block can be determined if motor blocking concentrations of drug are used, when abduction of the arm will be compromised for the first 15° before the deltoid muscle takes over (Fig 34D–22).

INDICATIONS.—The suprascapular nerve is blocked diagnostically for pains around the shoulder in an attempt to see if the pain is arising from within the shoulder joint. Therapeutically, repeated blocks can be performed for arthritic shoulder pain, although this is usually not a satisfactory long-term solution.

DIFFICULTIES.—The main concern with this block is the risk of pneumothorax if the needle, during its initial advancement, passes over the superior border of the scapula and enters the thoracic cavity between the ribs. Also, if and when the needle is walked into the suprascapular notch, it should not be advanced because pleural puncture with subsequent pheumothorax could occur. The nerve is accompanied by the corresponding suprascapular vessels, and intravascular injection is a risk.

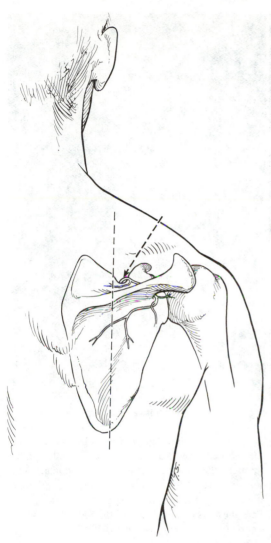

Fig 34D–21.—Suprascapular nerve block. The nerve is blocked in the suprascapular fossa. The spine of the scapula is divided by a vertical line, and the upper and outer quadrant so formed is bisected and a needle introduced 2 cm along this line and advanced to a depth of approximately 5–6 cm, at which point the dorsal surface of the scapula should be located. If this end point is not reached at this depth, the needle should be withdrawn and repositioned. When osseous contact is achieved, the needle is "walked" until the suprascapular notch is located, or, if an electrical stimulator is used, needle placement is confirmed by movements of the suprascapular and infrascapular muscles. At this point 5 cc of local anesthetic is injected.

THE LUMBOSACRAL PLEXUS AND ITS BRANCHES

For chronic pain relief or for operations on the lower extremity, the subarachnoid block and the epidural block are still the most common nerve block procedures performed. Although conduction anesthesia has a high success rate and is relatively easy to perform, spinal or epidural procedures may not be indicated in certain groups of patients, including the elderly, debilitated, arthritic, obese, or critically ill, or those for neurolysis of the nerves. In these patients branches of the lumbosacral plexus can be blocked. The common branches of the lumbosacral plexus include the sciatic nerve, the femoral nerve, the obturator nerve, and the lateral femoral cutaneous nerves (Fig 34D–23,A).

Sciatic Nerve

Anatomy

The sciatic nerve (L4–5, S1–3), the largest nerve in the body, measures 1.5–2 cm in width and 0.3–0.9 cm in thickness as it leaves the pelvis. After leaving the pelvis it passes through a tunnel between the greater trochanter and the ischial tuberosity. At this point the greater sciatic nerve passes posterior to the gamelli, obturator internus, and quadriceps femoris and anterior to the gluteus maximus muscles (Fig 34D–23,B).

The posterior femoral cutaneous branch (S1–3), which innervates the posterior aspect of the thigh, varies in proximity to the sciatic nerve and may either travel with it or separate from it cephalad. Blood vessels accompanying the sciatic nerve at this point of blocking are the sciatic artery, a branch of the inferior gluteal artery, and the inferior gluteal veins. However, in this region, both arteries and veins are relatively small.

EQUIPMENT
- 23-gauge, ½-inch needle for infiltration.
- 22-gauge, 3½-inch needle.
- 20-ml syringe with extension set.
- Nerve stimulator with accessories, if used.

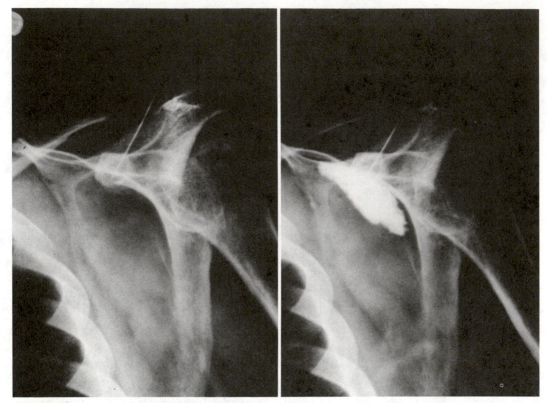

Fig 34D–22.—Needle placement on the suprascapular nerve and the radiographic spread.

Drugs

For a procedure of short duration, 1%–1.5% lidocaine or its equivalent is used. For a procedure of long duration, 0.5% bupivacaine or 1% etidocaine is used.

Technique

In the posterior approach of labat,[7] the patient is placed in the Sim's position. The superior iliac spine and the greater trochanter are identified. A line is drawn between the two, and a second perpendicular line is dropped at its midpoint. The point of entry is 1–1½ inches along this line. This point should lie on a line drawn from the sacral hiatus to the greater trochanter (Fig 34D–24).

Procedure

POSTERIOR APPROACH (LABAT).—After preparation and infiltration of the skin, a 3½-inch, 22-gauge needle is inserted perpendicular to the skin at the chosen landmark. After the needle passes through the muscle (piriformis) it contacts the sciatic nerve (2½ inches deep), which at this point is traversing the leg from the greater sciatic notch. Paresthesia is obtained toward the foot, or dorsiflexion or plantar flexion is noted with the nerve stimulator.

ANTERIOR APPROACH (BECK)[8].—With the patient supine, a line is drawn from the anterior superior iliac spine to the pubic tubercle. It is divided into three parts: a parallel line is drawn to the above at the level of the greater trochanter; a perpendicular line is dropped from the top line to the bottom at the junction of the medial and middle one third; and the point of entry is at the bottom line where the perpendicular line meets the lesser trochanter (Fig 34D–25).

A 6-inch, 22-gauge needle is inserted through the landmark perpendicularly until bone is contacted (lesser trochanter). The depth of needle entry is noted. A marker is placed 1 inch proximally and the needle is slipped past the bone medially until either

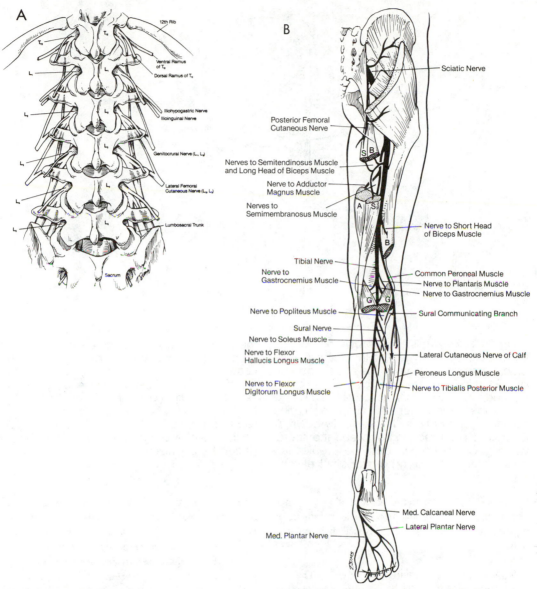

Fig 34D–23.—**A,** formation of the lumbosacral plexus and its branches. The important branches of the plexus include the sciatic nerve, the femoral nerve, the obturator nerve, and the lateral femoral cutaneous nerves. **B,** anatomy of the lower extremity and course of the sciatic nerve and its branches. (From Raj P.P., Pai U.: Techniques of nerve blocking, in Raj P.P. (ed.): *Handbook of Regional Anesthesia.* New York, Churchill Livingstone, Inc., 1985. Reproduced by permission.)

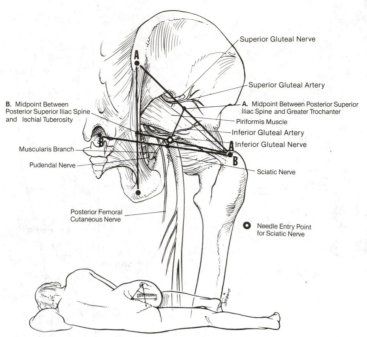

Superior Gluteal Nerve

Superior Gluteal Artery

A. Midpoint Between Posterior Superior Iliac Spine and Greater Trochanter

Piriformis Muscle

Inferior Gluteal Artery

Inferior Gluteal Nerve

Sciatic Nerve

B. Midpoint Between Posterior Superior Iliac Spine and Ischial Tuberosity

Muscularis Branch

Pudendal Nerve

Posterior Femoral Cutaneous Nerve

○ Needle Entry Point for Sciatic Nerve

Fig 34D–24.—This figure shows the position for the Labat technique of the sciatic nerve block. The point of entry of the needle can be arrived at in various ways: *A,* by drawing a line between the posterior superior iliac spine and the greater trochanter and dropping a line from its midpoint 1½ inches vertically down; *B,* by taking a midposition between the sacral coccygeal membrane and the greater trochanter; or *C,* by taking a midpoint between the posterosuperior iliac spine and the ischial tuberosity. The point of entry is where a line drawn from this point horizontally meets the line dropped between the posterior iliac spine and the greater trochanter. (From Raj P.P., Pai U.: Techniques of nerve blocking, in Raj P.P. (ed.): *Handbook of Regional Anesthesia.* New York, Churchill Livingstone, Inc., 1985. Reproduced by permission.)

it touches the sciatic nerve or until it goes 1 inch deeper than the first insertion. Local anesthetic is injected in the neurovascular space between the muscles.

SUPINE SCIATIC APPROACH (RAJ)[9].—The patient is placed supine. The extremity to be blocked is flexed at the hip as far as possible (90°–120°) (Fig 34D–26). The extremity may be supported by the use of a Mayo table, an assistant, the patient himself, or by placing it in lithotomy position. In this position, the sciatic nerve is stretched tightly in the hollow between the greater trochanter and the ischial tuberosity and the gluteus maximus muscles are thinned, making the sciatic nerve more superficial (Fig 34D–27).

The midpoint of a line drawn between the greater trochanter and the ischial tuberosity is located. A skin wheal is raised and 1% lidocaine is injected through a 25-gauge, 1.588-cm needle. A 22-gauge, 8.89-cm spinal needle, attached to a peripheral nerve stimulator, is used as a probing electrode.[10] The needle is inserted perpendicular to the skin and the nerve stimulator is activated after the needle has penetrated the skin. The needle is advanced slowly until the best plantar flexion or dorsiflexion of the foot is noted (Fig 34D–28). A 2-ml test dose of 2% lidocaine is injected and should abolish this movement. An additional 18–20 ml of anesthetic solution is deposited if the test is positive, that is, if the movements previously noted disappear.

This supine approach is practical for repeat blocks, for moribund patients, and for patients with multiple trauma who cannot be positioned otherwise. If the patient has had a hip prosthesis, so that the greater trochanter may be absent, probing by the nerve stimulator allows identification of the sciatic nerve without difficulty.

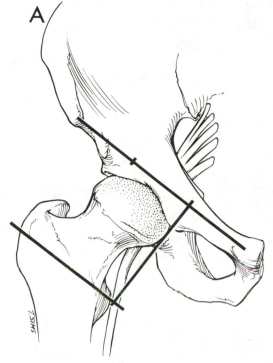

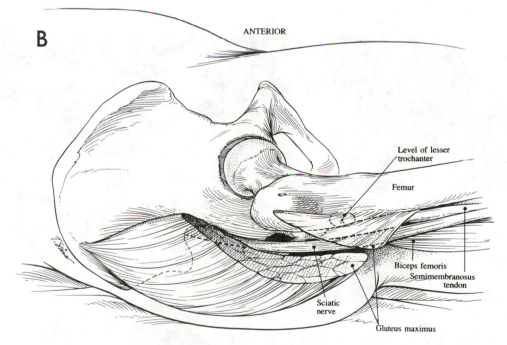

Fig 34D–25.—A, anterior approach to the sciatic nerve as described by Beck. **B,** anatomy of the sciatic nerve with patient in the supine position as viewed from the side. Note the course of the sciatic nerve behind the femur and anterior to the gluteus maximus muscle.

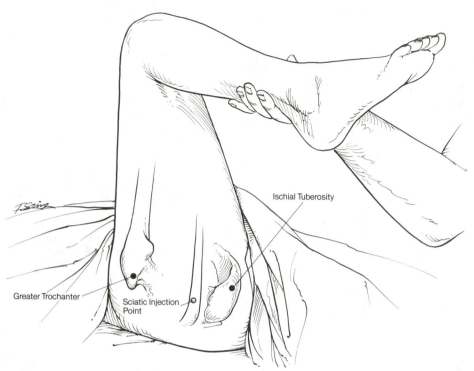

Ischial Tuberosity

Greater Trochanter

Sciatic Injection
Point

Fig 34D–26.—Position of the patient and the landmark for the supine approach to the sciatic nerve. (From Raj P.P., Pai U.: Techniques of nerve blocking, in Raj P.P. (ed.): *Handbook of Regional Anesthesia.* New York, Churchill Livingstone, Inc., 1985. Reproduced by permission.)

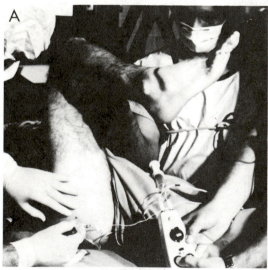

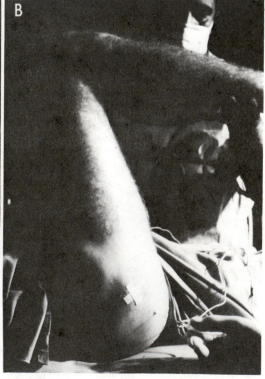

Fig 34D–27.—**A** and **B,** approach to the sciatic nerve block with the patient supine. The needle is at an angle of 90° to the skin.

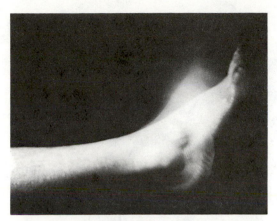

Fig 34D–28.—Dorsiflexion with nerve stimulation of the sciatic nerve. A 2-ml test dose of the local anesthetic abolishes this movement if the needle has been correctly placed on the nerve. The rest of the calculated solution is injected if this test is positive.

Indications and Contraindications

A sciatic nerve block provides analgesia and anesthesia in the lower extremity in the area of the sciatic nerve distribution. It also provides sympathetic block in the same distribution. It is indicated for surgical procedures of leg and foot and for diagnostic and therapeutic nerve blocks for acute or chronic pain in the leg and foot. It has been useful for poor healing ulcers due to poor peripheral circulation, for treating traumatic pain, and for providing pain relief for exercises during rehabilitation of limb trauma.

Contraindications are relative and include local infection and recent injury at the site of injection to the nerve.

Femoral Nerve[11]

Anatomy

The femoral nerve (L-2, L-3, L-4) arises from the lumbar plexus and runs downward between the psoas major and iliacus muscles, covered by the iliopsoas fascia. The psoas fascia separates the nerve from the femoral artery. The femoral nerve lies lateral to the artery and deep to the inguinal ligament. About 1 inch below the inguinal ligament, the nerve divides into muscular and cutaneous branches. Muscular branches supply the muscles of the front of the

thigh. The cutaneous branches are the medial and intermediate cutaneous nerves of the thigh, which supply the skin of the front of the thigh, and the saphenous nerve. The saphenous nerve innervates the medial side of the leg up to the middle of the medial border of the foot (Fig 34D–29).

Indications

A femoral nerve block is indicated for superficial surgery on the anterior aspect of the thigh such as skin grafting, saphenous vein stripping, and saphenous vein harvesting. It is also included as one of the multiple lower extremity blocks used for arthroscopy, knee surgery, amputations, and ankle surgery. For the relief of postoperative knee pain, a

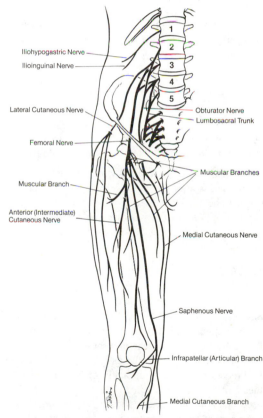

Iliohypogastric Nerve
Ilioinguinal Nerve
Lateral Cutaneous Nerve
Femoral Nerve
Muscular Branch
Anterior (Intermediate) Cutaneous Nerve
Obturator Nerve
Lumbosacral Trunk
Muscular Branches
Medial Cutaneous Nerve
Saphenous Nerve
Infrapatellar (Articular) Branch
Medial Cutaneous Branch

Fig 34D–29.—Anatomy of the lumbar plexus and its branches. Note especially the formation of the femoral nerve, obturator nerve, and lateral femoral cutaneous nerve. (From Raj P.P., Pai U.: Techniques of nerve blocking, in Raj P.P. (ed.): *Handbook of Regional Anesthesia.* New York, Churchill Livingstone, Inc., 1985. Reproduced by permission.)

catheter can be placed on the femoral nerve for prolonged analgesia and for healing of ischemic ulcers on the medial aspect of the leg.

Equipment

- No. 22 1½-inch needle with extension set.
- No. 27 local infiltration needle.
- Nerve stimulator.
- Alligator clamps.
- ECG pad.
- 20-cc syringe.
- Sterile drapes.
- B.D. 4-inch catheter for continuous infusion.

Drugs

The drugs used are 15–30 cc of 0.5% Marcaine or a mixture of 2% lidocaine and 0.75% Marcaine (50:50).

Technique

The patient is positioned supine with the thigh on the flat surface, slightly abducted from midline (see Fig 34D–30).

LANDMARKS.—Landmarks are the anterior superior iliac spine, the pubic symphysis, the pulsation of the femoral artery, and the inguinal ligament. The point of entry is one fingerbreadth lateral to the femoral artery at the midinguinal point.

Procedure

After local infiltration at the point of entry, the physician places his nondominant hand on the front of the patient's thigh with the middle finger on the femoral artery. The needle is inserted on a line with the finger and lateral to the artery (Fig 34D–30). It is directed cephalad at an angle of 30° until paresthesia of the knee is elicited. If a nerve stimulator is used, patellar movement should be elicited. Once the position of the needle has been confirmed, an aspiration test for blood is performed, then the calculated volume of the local anesthetic is injected.

A femoral nerve block provides sensory anesthesia of the anteromedial thigh, the medial aspect of the leg, and the proximal foot. There is loss of extension of the knee and some loss of the flexion at the hip joint.

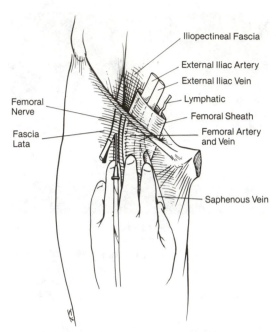

Fig 34D–30.—Femoral nerve block technique. Note that the femoral nerve is separated from the femoral artery by a sheath. (From Raj P.P., Pai U.: Techniques of nerve blocking, in Raj P.P. (ed.): *Handbook of Regional Anesthesia.* New York, Churchill Livingstone, Inc., 1985. Reproduced by permission.)

CONTRAINDICATIONS.—Contraindications include ulceration in the groin, glandular infection, and septicemia.

COMPLICATIONS.—Complications include infection, hematoma, femoral neuritis, and prolonged block.

Obturator Nerve

Anatomy

The obturator nerve (L-2, L-3, L-4) is the motor nerve to the adductor muscles of the thigh. It innervates a small segment of the medial side of the thigh in the lower third. It also gives articular branches to the hip and knee joint. The obturator nerves arise from the lumbar plexus in common with the femoral nerve and within the substance of psoas major muscle. The nerve emerges out at the medial border, runs along the lateral pelvic wall, exits through the obturator foramen, and reaches the medial thigh (Fig 34D–31).

The obturator nerve has a variable sensory contribution to the medial part of the thigh, about a handbreadth below the perineum. It can, however, extend down the medial thigh to the level of the knee. Its main distribution is motor to the adductor muscles of the thigh and it does supply a geniculate branch to the knee joint. Because of its large motor supply, this nerve is readily identifiable when a nerve stimulator is used: contractions in the adductor muscle mass of the thigh are readily seen.

Indications

Along with the femoral and lateral femoral cutaneous nerves, the obturator nerve is blocked for

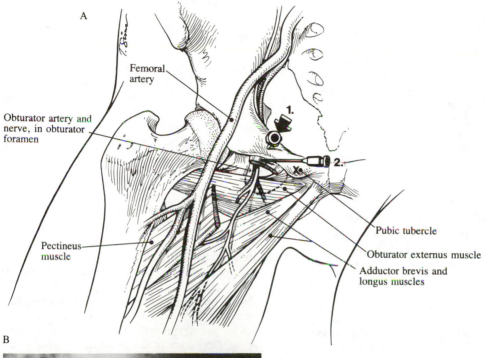

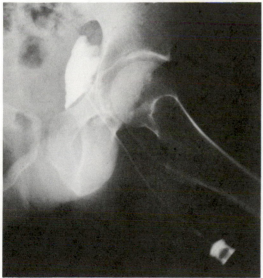

Fig 34D–31.—A, anatomy of the technique of the obturator nerve block. The obturator nerve is shown to exit from the obturator foramen. *1* shows the needle position on the superior ramus. *2* shows the needle position in the obturator foramen. **B,** radiograph shows a catheter in position in the obturator foramen with spread of contrast material from the obturator nerve block.

acute pain control intraoperatively and for postoperative pain in this area. The main indication for nonoperative blockade is a spastic condition associated with spinal cord damage in which adductor spasm interferes with rehabilitation or personal toilet and hygiene. Neurolytic blockade of this particular nerve is often indicated, and diagnostic nerve blocks ahead of time can be used to ascertain how much of the persistent adduction is due to muscle tension, as opposed to contractures, which would require surgical tenotomy for relief. Blockade of this nerve is effected with 5–10 ml of a local anesthetic or neurolytic agent.

Equipment

- No. 27 local infiltration needle.
- No. 22 2-inch needle.
- No. 22 3½-inch spinal needle in obese patients.
- 10-cc syringe.

Drugs

For a short-duration block, 1% Xylocaine or Carbocaine is used. For a block of longer duration, 0.5% bupivacaine is used. For a neurolytic block, 6% phenol is used.

Procedure

The patient is placed in a supine position with the thigh abducted to make the adductor longus tendon prominent at its attachment to the pubic bone. The physician-anesthesiologist stands on the opposite side to be blocked, facing the patient.

A skin wheal is made 1 cm lateral and inferior to the pubic tubercle. A 22-gauge 3½-inch needle is introduced through the wheal in a direction perpendicular to the skin until the inferior pubic ramus is contacted. The needle is withdrawn and directed laterally 2.5 cm deeper in a slightly superior and posterior direction. After the needle placement is confirmed by fluoroscopy or by a nerve stimulator situated in the obturator foramen, 10 ml of the analgesic solution is injected. Paresthesia is not usually obtained. An effective block will result in loss of adduction and external rotation of the thigh.

DIFFICULTIES.—It is often difficult to locate the obturator nerve because of its deep location. Because the block is often performed on individuals with spinal cord injury, spasticity, and contractures, it is not feasible to place the thigh in the optimal laterally rotated position for this block.

COMPLICATIONS.—Intravascular injection or hematoma may occur because of the close proximity of the obturator vessels to the nerve.

Lateral Femoral Cutaneous Nerve Block

Anatomy

The lateral femoral cutaneous nerve arises from L-2 and L-3 and lies on the iliac muscle at the lateral border of the psoas major muscle. After running on the medial side of anterosuperior iliac spine, it pierces the fascia lata 1½–2 inches below the inguinal ligament to innervate the lateral side of the skin of the thigh.

Indications for Lateral Femoral Cutaneous Nerve Block

The lateral femoral cutaneous block is indicated primarily for the control of acute pain in operative procedures involving this anatomical distribution. It has been used for the diagnosis and treatment of chronic painful states. The chronic pain state most often associated with this particular nerve distribution is "meralgia paresthetica," a neuritic-type pain in the distribution of this nerve that is usually due to ongoing trauma to the nerve such as that caused by a heavy belt riding low on the hip. A temporary nerve block can be diagnostic in this condition. The permanent solution is usually correction of the precipitating cause.

Equipment

- No. 27 needle.
- No. 22 1½-inch needle.
- 10-cc syringe.

Drugs

For a short-duration block, 1% Carbocaine or 1% Xylocaine is used. For a block of longer duration, 0.25% bupivacine is used.

Technique

The patient is positioned supine with the thigh in a neutral position on the bed (Fig 34D–32,A).

LANDMARKS.—Landmarks are the anterosuperior iliac spine and the inguinal ligament.

PROCEDURE.—A skin wheal is made at a point 2–3 cm below and medial to the anterosuperior iliac spine with a No. 27 needle. A No. 22 1½-inch needle attached to a 10-ml syringe is introduced upward and laterally through the skin wheal and toward the iliac crest just posterior to the anterosuperior iliac spine until it touches the inner side of the shelving iliac crest (Fig 34D–32,B). Local anesthetic, 5 ml, is injected as the needle is withdrawn (Fig 34D–32,C). The process is repeated at another angle and another 5 ml of local anesthetic is injected.

The lateral femoral cutaneous nerve can also be blocked in conjunction with the femoral nerve component of the lumbar plexus by injecting a large volume in a cephalad direction when doing a femoral nerve block.

DIFFICULTIES.—Because this nerve is strictly a sensory nerve, blockade is not associated with any motor weakness and is well tolerated, although the

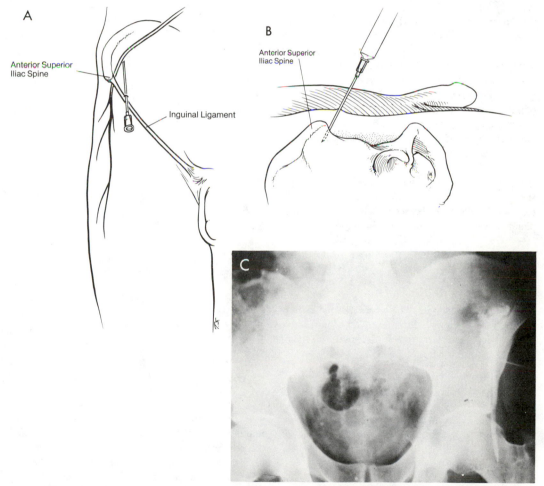

Fig 34D–32.—**A,** approach to lateral femoral cutaneous nerve block. **B,** direction of the needle in the lateral view. **C,** radiograph showing spread of the local anesthetic on the lateral femoral cutaneous nerve. (From Raj P.P., Pai U.: Techniques of nerve blocking, in Raj P.P. (ed.): *Handbook of Regional Anesthesia.* New York, Churchill Livingstone, Inc., 1985. Reproduced by permission.)

permanent numbness that can follow both trauma and/or permanent blocks to this nerve can become a source of chronic pain.

Because this nerve is not in immediate relation to any important structures at the injection site described above, there are no significant complications.

Tibial Nerve Block at the Knee

Anatomy

The tibial nerve is the medial of the two terminal branches of the sciatic nerve that are given off in the upper part of the popliteal fossa. It descends vertically in the middle of the popliteal fossa from the upper angle to the lower angle. The popliteal artery is related medially to the nerve in the upper part, laterally to the nerve in the lower part, and deep to the nerve in the middle. Pulsation of the popliteal artery at the joint line of the knee is a good landmark for the nerve. The tibial nerve descends down the back of the leg to innervate the muscles of the posterior compartment of the leg. At the medial side of the ankle it divides into medial and lateral plantar branches, which traverse toward the respective sides of the foot. The tibial nerve gives off the medial calcanean branches before dividing into plantar nerves at the ankle (Fig 34D–33).

Indications

This block can be useful for pain in the ankle and the foot, during surgery or postoperatively. It may also be used to relieve the severe pain of intractable reflex sympathetic dystrophy, decubitus ulcers of the heel, and trauma.

Equipment

- No. 27 local infiltration needle.
- No. 23 1½-inch needle.

Technique

The patient may be positioned either prone, with the knee extended, or laterally, with the leg extended.

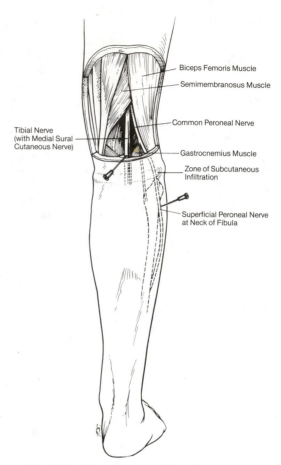

Fig 34D–33.—Course of the tibial and the common peroneal nerves at the knee and the technique of blocking them. (From Raj P.P., Pai U.: Techniques of nerve blocking, in Raj P.P. (ed.): *Handbook of Regional Anesthesia*. New York, Churchill Livingstone, Inc., 1985. Reproduced by permission.)

LANDMARKS.—Landmarks are the pulsation of the popliteal artery at the bend of the knee, and the vertical line in the middle of the popliteal fossa.

PROCEDURE.—A skin wheal is raised in the middle of the popliteal fossa over the midline and the needle is inserted vertically toward the popliteal artery. Paresthesia of the leg and the sole of the foot is sought. A nerve stimulator can be used to objectively confirm placement of the needle on the nerve, as there will be visible plantar flexion of the foot. Analgesic solution, 5–10 ml, is injected at the appropriate site.

COMPLICATIONS.—Vascular injection is possible due to proximity of the popliteal artery to the tibial nerve.

Ankle Block

Indications

An ankle block is indicated for surgery or relief of pain in the sole or the dorsum of the foot.

Anatomy

An ankle block involves five nerves that innervate below the ankle. These are described below.

1. *Tibial nerve.* Continuing from the leg, the tibial nerve runs about the midpoint between the medial malleolus and calcaneous muscles on the medial side of the ankle under the flexor retinaculum. It lies posterior to the pulsation of the posterior tibial artery. It innervates the skin and the muscle of the plantar aspect of the foot.

2. *Deep peroneal nerve.* As a continuation of the nerve in the front of the leg, the deep peroneal nerve lies deep to the extensor retinaculum with the anterior tibial artery on the anterior surface of the distal end of the tibia. It lies lateral to the tendon of the extensor hallucis longus. It innervates the extensor hallucis muscle, some neighboring joints and skin, and the adjacent sides of the great toe and second toe (Fig 34D–34).

3. *Sural nerve.* The sural nerve is formed at the back of the calf muscles in the midline by contributions from the tibial and common peroneal nerves. It runs on the lateral aspect of the ankle midway between the lateral malleolus and calcaneous muscles toward the lateral side of the little toe.

4. *Saphenous nerve.* The only branch of the femoral nerve below the knee, the saphenous nerve runs

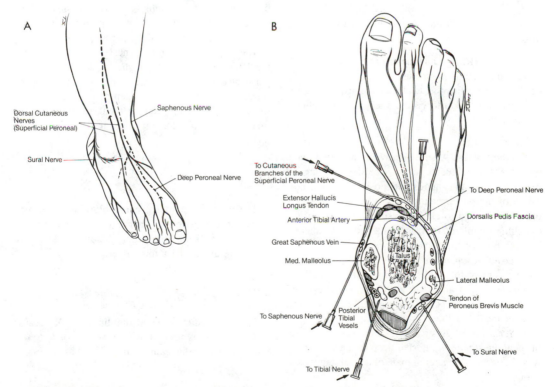

A

Dorsal Cutaneous Nerves (Superficial Peroneal)

Saphenous Nerve

Sural Nerve

Deep Peroneal Nerve

B

To Cutaneous Branches of the Superficial Peroneal Nerve

To Deep Peroneal Nerve

Extensor Hallucis Longus Tendon

Dorsalis Pedis Fascia

Anterior Tibial Artery

Great Saphenous Vein

Talus

Med. Malleolus

Lateral Malleolus

Tendon of Peroneus Brevis Muscle

To Saphenous Nerve

Posterior Tibial Vesels

To Sural Nerve

To Tibial Nerve

Fig 34D–34.—A, anatomy of the tibial and peroneal nerves and their branches at the ankle. **B,** sites of block. (From Raj P.P., Pai U.: Techniques of nerve blocking, in Raj P.P. (ed.): *Handbook of Regional Anesthesia.* New York, Churchill Livingstone, Inc., 1985. Reproduced by permission.)

in the superficial fascia in front of the medial malleolus with the great saphenous vein. It innervates up to the middle of the medial side of the foot.

5. *Superficial peroneal nerve.* The superficial peroneal nerve pierces the deep fascia in the lower third of the lateral aspect of the leg, then lies in the superficial fascia to divide into branches to supply the dorsum of the foot and the toes not innervated by the sural and deep peroneal nerves.

Drugs

One of the local anesthetics listed below is injected, 5 ml per nerve. For a procedure of short duration, 1%–1.5% Xylocaine with or without 1:20,000 epinephrine is injected. For a procedure of longer duration (3–3½ hours), 0.5%–0.75% bupivacaine or 1% etidocaine is injected.

Technique

The foot is placed on the bed with the knee flexed.

LANDMARKS.—Landmarks are the medial malleolus, the lateral malleolus, the posterior tubercle of the calcaneous, the tendocalcaneous, the pulsation of the tibial artery, and the extensor hallucis longus tendon.

PROCEDURE

1. *Tibial block.* After a skin wheal has been made with a 27-gauge needle midway between the medial malleolus and calcaneous and posterior to the pulsation of the posterior tibial artery, a 23-gauge needle is introduced to elicit paresthesia in the foot (or twitching of sole of foot, with the nerve stimulator). Then 5–6 cc of local anesthetic is injected.

2. *Deep peroneal nerve.* A skin wheal is raised on the front of the ankle lateral to extensor hallucis longus tendon at about the anterior tibial artery and a 23-gauge needle is inserted to hit the bone. Then 5 ml of local anesthetic is injected.

3. *Sural nerve.* After a skin wheal is raised, 5 ml of local anesthetic is injected deep to the point midway between the lateral malleolus and the calcaneous.

4. *Saphenous nerve.* Five milliliters of local anesthetic are injected around the great saphenous vein in front of the medial malleolus.

5. *Superficial peroneal nerve.* A skin wheal is raised on the lower third of the leg just lateral to the anterior border of the tibia at the upper part of the lateral malleolus. The subcutaneous tissue just superficial to the deep fascia is infiltrated. The depth of needle insertion depends on the amount of subcutaneous fat. It is done as a field block over an area 2–3 inches wide and lateral to the anterior border of the tibia to block all the branches of the superficial peroneal nerve as they go on to the dorsum of the foot.

COMPLICATIONS.—Complications include neuropathy, prolonged block, infection, and hematoma.

Common Peroneal Nerve Block

Anatomy

The common peroneal nerve usually arises about the upper part of the back of the thigh as one of the two terminal branches of the sciatic nerve. After descending obliquely downward and laterally across the lateral angle of popliteal fossa, it runs toward the lateral aspect of the neck of the fibula to divide into the superficial and deep peroneal nerves.

The superficial peroneal nerve traverses toward the lateral compartment of the leg to innervate the perineal muscles and then becomes cutaneous at the lower third of the leg. The deep peroneal nerve goes toward the anterior compartment of the leg and finally ends at the dorsum of the foot (see Fig 34D–33).

Indication

The common peroneal nerve block is performed in conjunction with tibial nerve and saphenous nerve blocks at the knee for surgery below the knee not involving the use of a tourniquet.

Drugs

For a procedure of short duration, 1% Xylocaine or Carbocaine is used. For a procedure of long duration, 0.5% bupivacaine is used.

Technique

The common peroneal nerve block may be performed with the patient in one of two positions: supine, with the thigh flexed at the hip joint and the leg flexed at the knee, the foot flat on the bed, or in the lateral position, with the down leg extended and the upper leg flexed at the knee.

LANDMARK.—The landmark is the head of the fibula below the lateral condyle of the tibia in the posterior part. The neck of the fibula lies below the head, where the common peroneal nerve can be felt on deep pressure.

PROCEDURE.—After a skin wheal has been made at a point in the region of the anterior part of the neck of the fibula (below the head), a 23-gauge needle is inserted posteriorly and medially to touch the bone. Paresthesia can be elicited, or nerve stimulation will cause twitching of the leg muscles and dorsiflexion of the ankle. Then 5–6 ml of local anesthetic is injected.

COMPLICATION.—Neuritis of the common peroneal nerve can be produced if the anesthetic is injected into the nerve, as the nerve lies directly against the neck of the fibula.

Pudendal Nerve Block

Anatomy

The pudendal nerve (S-2, S-3, S-4) arises from the sacral plexus. After crossing the ischial spine and the sacrospinous ligament it enters the lesser sciatic foramen and runs on the medial side of the ischium with the pudendal vessels in the pudendal canal (Alcock canal). At the anterior end of the canal it sends branches to the perineal region. The inferior hemorrhoidal nerve innervates the anal region, and other anterior branches innervate the urogenital region.

Indications

A pudendal nerve block is indicated for obstetric vaginal procedures, e.g., vaginal delivery and forceps delivery, and for somatic perineal pain.

Equipment

- Iowa trumpet.
- 12- to 14-cm, 20-gauge needle.

Technique

The patient is placed in the lithotomy position.

LANDMARKS.—Landmarks are the ischial spine sacrospinous ligament and the ischial tuberosity.

PROCEDURE.—In the transvaginal approach the needle is guided within the Iowa trumpet along the operator's index and middle finger; the needle progresses transvaginally toward the ischial spine after piercing the sacrospinous ligament. Local anesthetic is injected in the pudendal canal.

In the perineal route approach, a skin wheal is

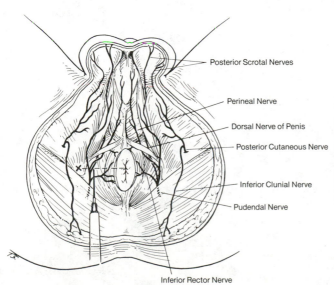

Posterior Scrotal Nerves

Perineal Nerve

Dorsal Nerve of Penis

Posterior Cutaneous Nerve

Inferior Clunial Nerve

Pudendal Nerve

Inferior Rector Nerve

Fig 34D–35.—Anatomy and technique of pudendal block (perineal route). (From Raj P.P., Pai U.: Techniques of nerve blocking, in Raj P.P. (ed.): *Handbook of Regional Anesthesia.* New York, Churchill Livingstone, Inc., 1985. Reproduced by permission.)

raised 2–3 cm posteromedially to the ischial tuberosity. A 12- to 15-cm, 22-gauge needle is introduced through the skin wheal in a posterior and lateral direction (Fig 34D–35); it is guided by the operator's finger in the rectum or vagina toward the ischial spine. After the needle pierces the sacrospinous ligament, 10–15 ml of local anesthetic is injected around the ligament.

REFERENCES

1. Winnie A.P., et al.: Interscalene cervical plexus block. *Anesth. Analg.* 54:370, 1975.
2. Winnie A.P.: Interscalene brachial plexus block. *Anesth. Analg.* 49:455–466, 1970.
3. Kulenkampff D.: Anesthesia of the brachial plexus (German). *Zentralbl. Chir.* 38:1337–1350, 1911.
4. Winnie A.P., Collins V.J.: The subclavian perivascular technique of brachial plexus anesthesia. *Anesthesiology* 25:353–363, 1964.
5. Raj P.P., Montgomery S.J., Nettles D., et al.: Infraclavicular brachial plexus block: A new approach. *Anesth. Analg.* 52:897–904, 1973.
6. deJong R.H.: Axillary block of the brachial plexus. *Anesthesiology* 22:215–225, 1961.
7. Labat G.: *Regional Anesthesia.* Philadelphia, W.B. Saunders Co., 1930.
8. Beck G.P.: Anterior approach to sciatic nerve block. *Anesthesiology* 24:222–224, 1963.
9. Raj P.P., Parks R.I., Watson T.D., et al.: New single position supine approach to sciatic femoral nerve block. *Anesth. Analg.* 54:489, 1975.
10. Raj P.P., Rosenblatt R., Montgomery S.J.: Use of the nerve stimulator for peripheral blocks. *Reg. Anesth.* 5:19, 1980.
11. Winnie A.P., Ramamurthy S., Durrani Z.: The inguinal paravascular technic of lumbar plexus anesthesia: The "3-in-1 block." *Anesth. Analg.* 52:989–996, 1973.

34E / Conduction Blocks

MICHAEL STANTON-HICKS, M.D.

ANATOMY OF THE SPINAL COLUMN

There are 33 vertebral bodies joined together as 7 cervical, 12 thoracic, 5 lumbar, 5 sacral, and 4 coccygeal vertebrae. A typical vertebra consists of two essential parts, the *anterior vertebral body* and the *posterior vertebral arch*. The vertebral bodies along with the intervertebral disks form a strong column for the support of the head and trunk, and the vertebral arch protects the spinal cord. The vertebral column presents two primary curves in the thoracic and sacrococcygeal regions and two compensatory curves in the cervical and lumbar regions (Figs 34E–1 and 34E–2).

In the midline of the dorsal surface of the vertebral column, one can identify and feel the spinous processes. In the cervical region they are short and horizontal, in the thoracic region they are vertical, and in the lumbar region they again are nearly horizontal. The interval between the spinous processes is wide in the lumbar region compared to the thoracic region, where the spinous processes are closely approximated.

On either side of the spinous process, a vertebral groove is formed by the laminae in the cervical and lumbar region. Next to the laminae are the articular processes and the transverse processes. The transverse processes are ventral to the articular processes, lateral to the pedicles, and between the intervertebral foramina.

The vertebral canal follows the different curves of the column. It is triangular in the regions where there is greater movement—the cervical and lumbar regions—and smaller and round in the thoracic region, where there is the least movement.

The sacrum is a large triangular bone situated below the fifth lumbar vertebra (Fig 34E–3). Its apex articulates with the coccyx. Its anterior surface is concave. Anteriorly its median part is crossed by four transverse ridges. The portions of the bone be-tween the ridges are the bodies of the sacrum. There are four anterior sacral foramina through which the sacral nerves exit and the lateral sacral arteries enter. The posterior surface of the sacrum is convex. There are rudimentary spinous processes from the first three or four sacral segments in the midline. The laminae unite to form a sacral groove. The laminae of the fifth sacral vertebra fail to unite posteriorly to form a sacral hiatus. The tubercles which represent the inferior articular processes are the sacral cornua and are connected inferiorly to the coccygeal cornua. Laterally one can identify four dorsal sacral foramina. They transmit the posterior divisions of the sacral nerves. The sacrum may have many variations. The bodies of the first and second may fail to unite, or the sacral canal may be open throughout.

Meninges of the Spinal Cord

In the vertebral canal, the spinal cord is covered by three membranes: (1) the dura mater, an outer tough, protective membrane, (2) the pia mater, the inner, delicate, fibrous membrane which contains the blood vessels to the spinal cord, and (3) the arachnoid membrane, the intermediate spider web-like structure which contains the cerebrospinal fluid. The spinal dura mater forms a loose sheath around the spinal cord and corresponds to the meningeal layer of the cranial dura. The outer or periosteal layer is interrupted at the foramen magnum and reappears below as the periosteum of the vertebrae.

The epidural space is found between the spinal dura and the vertebral canal. It contains loose areolar tissue and a plexus of veins. The dura mater is attached to the foramen magnum and by a fibrous slip to the posterior longitudinal ligament. The subarachnoid space occupies most of the tubular space of the dura mater. It ends at the level of the second

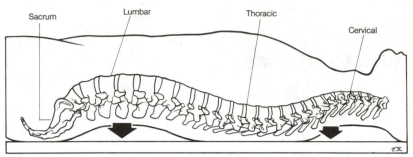

Fig 34E–1.—Primary and secondary curvatures of the spine. Note that in the supine position the cervical and lumbar curvature decreases. (From Raj P.P., Pai U.: Techniques of nerve blocking, in Raj P.P. (ed.): *Handbook of Regional Anesthesia.* New York, Churchill Livingstone, Inc., 1985. Reproduced by permission.)

sacral vertebra and continues as the filum terminale, attached to the back of the coccyx. The lower part of the subarachnoid space from the second lumbar vertebra to the second sacral vertebra is occupied by the cauda equina. The dura mater covers the spinal nerves as they pass from the cauda equina to the intervertebral foramina (Fig 34E–4).

The spinal arachnoid membrane loosely invests the spinal cord. It is continuous with the cranial arachnoid membrane and caudally encloses the cauda equina and ends at second sacral vertebra.

EPIDURAL BLOCK

The spectacular increase in the use of epidural block during the past 30 years is a direct consequence of the introduction of the amide class of local anesthetics and of research by a few dedicated anesthesiologists who explored the physiology and potential clinical applications of this technique for relieving acute and chronic pain.

Initially the caudal route was favored, but once

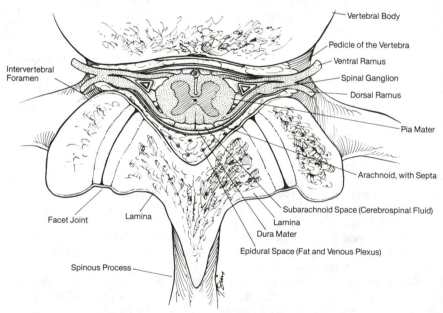

Fig 34E–2.—Cross section of the anterior vertebral body and the dorsal vertebral arch, enclosing the spinal cord and its nerve roots and vascular network. (From Raj P.P., Pai U.: Techniques of nerve blocking, in Raj P.P. (ed.): *Handbook of Regional Anesthesia.* New York, Churchill Livingstone, Inc., 1985. Reproduced by permission.)

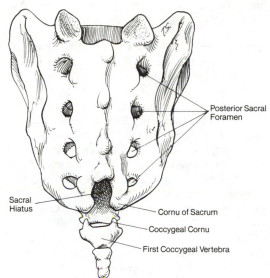

Fig 34E–3.—Dorsal surface of the sacrum. (From Raj P.P., Pai U.: Techniques of nerve blocking, in Raj P.P. (ed.): *Handbook of Regional Anesthesia.* New York, Churchill Livingstone, Inc., 1985. Reproduced by permission.)

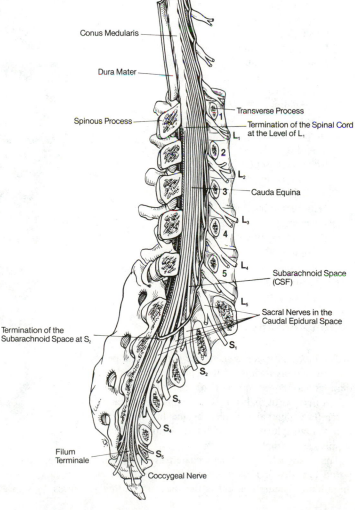

Fig 34E–4.—Relationship of the cauda equina to other structures in the lumbosacral region. (From Raj P.P., Pai U.: Techniques of nerve blocking, in Raj P.P. (ed.): *Handbook of Regional Anesthesia.* New York, Churchill Livingstone, Inc., 1985. Reproduced by permission.)

Dogliotti introduced his loss-of-resistance technique for identifying the epidural space in the lumbar region in 1939, interest in this form of major conduction block grew.[1]

The next major innovation was the adoption of the Huber tipped Tuohy needle, originally designed to introduce ureteric catheters into the subarachnoid space for continuous epidural block. The groundwork had now been laid for the exploration of different ways of utilizing this technique for managing postoperative pain, obstetric pain, nonsurgical pain, and intractable pain.

Indications

The indications for epidural block are listed below.

Acute pain
  Surgery
  Obstetrics
  Postoperative pain
  Nonsurgical pain
  Trauma
  Fractured ribs
  Pancreatitis
  Frostbite
  Herpes zoster
  Shingles
  Ischemic vascular pain
  Ureteric colic
Chronic pain
  Neurogenic back pain
  Postherpetic neuralgia
  Reflex sympathetic dystrophy
  Malignancy
  Phantom limb
Diagnostic and prognostic blocks

Functional Anatomy

The epidural space is the space between the periosteum and ligaments of the spinal canal and the dura covering the spinal cord and the segmental spinal nerves. In reality it is not a space, but rather a capillary interval occupied by the internal vertebral venous plexus, epidural fat, segmental blood supply, and lymphatics.

The veins, which form an arcuate pattern, are disposed laterally and anteriorly. This is fortunate, as an epidural needle that enters the space in the mid-line is therefore less likely to puncture a vein. Another aspect of these veins which is also of great importance to epidural block is that they are valveless and connect inferiorly with the pelvic veins, superiorly with the intracerebral veins, and laterally with the azygos and hemiazygos systems; therefore they provide an alternate route for venous return (Fig 34E–5). This feature, which has been emphasized in another context by Batson, means that their volume will change when the flow of venous traffic in the inferior cava is impeded, for example by pregnancy or an abdominal tumor.[2] This has a direct effect on the dose of local anesthetic that is injected into the epidural space. In addition, drugs or air injected into an epidural vein have direct access to the brain.

The epidural space varies in size, being largest in the midlumbar region. The distance between the ligamentum flavum and lamina and the dura in the midline is about 1.5–2 mm in the cervical and upper thoracic regions, 3–5 mm in the mid and lower tho-

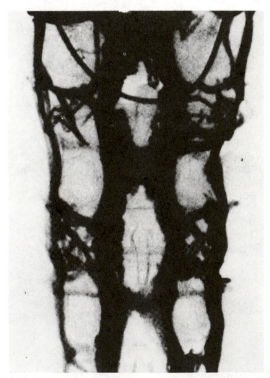

Fig 34E–5.—Disposition of the internal vertebral venous plexus within the epidural space. (From Stanton-Hicks M., Boas R.A.: *Chronic Low Back Pain.* New York, Raven Press, 1982. Reproduced by permission.)

racic regions, and 5–6 mm in the lumbar region. Structures related to the epidural space are, superiorly, the foramen magnum, where the meningeal dura fuses with the endosteal dura; inferiorly, the sacrococcygeal membrane; anteriorly, the posterolongitudinal ligament overlying the vertebral bodies and intervertebral disks; posteriorly, the arches of the laminae and intervening ligamenta flava; and laterally, the pedicles and intervertebral foramina.

The physiologic changes that follow an epidural block will depend on the level at which the procedure is performed and the number of spinal segments involved. The following discussion of the physiologic effects of epidural block is limited to observations on respiratory effects, cardiovascular effects, and neuroendocrine effects. These effects are considered separately for each of four regions.

Cervical Epidural Block

Normally it is not possible to restrict a cervical epidural block to these segments, principally because the negative intrathoracic pressure communicating through the thoracic intervertebral foramina sucks the local anesthetic solution into the upper thoracic epidural region.

Respiratory Effects

Normally, no effect on respiration will be seen when the usual short- and long-acting local anesthetic solutions are used for blocks in this region. The possibility of a block of the phrenic nerves, however, must always be borne in mind, although in a large series of cervical blocks with 2% lidocaine and mepivacaine, we have not seen any clinical effects on respiration, an agent such as etidocaine, which is both very lipid soluble and has powerful motor blocking properties, should not be used in this region in a strength greater than 1%. Prolonged analgesia with a continuous infusion of 0.25% bupivacaine at a rate of 5 ml/hour has not affected respiration.

Cardiovascular Effects

The principal cardiovascular effects are those due to sympathetic block. The preganglionic sympathetic outflow may reach up to C-2, and therefore a block extending to T-4, for example, will block most if not all of the cardiac sympathetic plexus.

McLean et al.[3] and Bonica et al.[4] have independently studied these effects in patients and volunteers. The principal effects observed were a 20% reduction in the mean arterial pressure and an 8% increase in the total peripheral resistance. A rise in the central venous pressure with no change in stroke volume also occurred, indicating a negative, although small, inotropic effect on the myocardium.

Thoracic Epidural Block

Respiratory Effects

Epidural anesthesia in the thorax has measurable effects on respiration due to interruption of the autonomic, somatosensory, and somatomotor fibers. However, it is now established that even if the entire thoracic motor outflow is blocked, the respiratory capacity will be reduced by only 20%, and the expiratory reserve volume will fall to zero. When thoracic or abdominal pain limits the capacity to breathe, epidural anesthesia clearly improves the vital capacity, functional residual capacity, and the Pa_{O_2}. Block of the autonomic nerves does not cause bronchoconstriction, as might be expected, but rather brings about the converse by preventing reflex activity. The main respiratory effects of thoracic sympathetic block arise from hemodynamic changes. The lowered pulmonary arterial pressure, reduced cardiac output, and consequent increase in alveolar dead space would cause an increase in the dead space to tidal volume ratio. Nevertheless, in spite of these changes, hyperventilation prevents any rise in the Pa_{CO_2}.

Cardiovascular Effects

The cardiovascular effects seen with a thoracic epidural block will depend on the number of segments blocked. Basically, they can be discussed under the following headings:

Influence of sympathectomy
Loss of cardiac sympathetics when blocks exceed T-5 level
Effects of absorbed local anesthetics
Effects of absorbed vasoconstrictors
Endocrine and metabolic effects

INFLUENCE OF SYMPATHECTOMY.—When only the lower sympathetic outflow is blocked with an anesthetic level no higher than T-5, little change in cardiovascular parmeters is seen in normovolemic subjects. A 5%–16% decrease in mean arterial pressure will occur, and an increase of about 5% in the cardiac output will follow as a consequence.

LOSS OF CARDIAC SYMPATHETICS.—Blocks involving the entire thoracic chain, that is, including also the cardiac sympathetics, will be associated with average falls in all of the cardiac measurements of 8%–30% in normovolemic unmedicated subjects. Because of a compensatory vasoconstriction in the upper extremities, the peripheral resistance falls by about 6%. These changes are associated with bradycardia.

EFFECT OF LOCAL ANESTHETICS.—Harrison et al.[5] have reported excellent cardiovascular stability with lidocaine plasma concentration of 3–5 μg/ml. When these levels are increased to 4–7 μg/ml, evidence of cardiovascular stimulation is seen. The underlying mechanism for this stimulation must have a peripheral origin, because at this concentration the cardioaccelerator nerves are blocked and the remaining thoracic sympathetics are also obtunded. Local anesthetics do have biphasic effects on smooth muscle, although it is unclear whether this is the mechanism in this case.

Normal blood levels of the long-acting agents bupivacaine and etidocaine associated with epidural block do not exert any significant effects on cardiovascular parameters. However, toxic doses of local anesthetics, such as might be seen after an accidental IV injection of the therapeutic dose, are almost always associated with cardiovascular depression.

The local anesthetics commonly used for an epidural block are listed in Table 34E–1.

EFFECTS OF VASOPRESSORS.—When epinephrine is added to the local anesthetic, both β- and α-adrenergic effects are seen. In general there is a slightly greater fall in the total peripheral resistance than occurs with plain solutions, since with blocks in the thoracic region, compensatory vasoconstriction is already prevented by the sympathectomy involving the upper limbs.

ENDOCRINE AND METABOLIC EFFECTS.—A thoracic epidural block involving the lower six thoracic segments will block both efferent fibers to the adrenal glands and the afferent pathways of visceral pain, as well as many fibers mediating reflex responses. As a result, inhibition of catecholamine release prevents the normal hyperglycemic response to surgery in the lower abdomen and pelvis. Also, renin activity, which is normally activated during surgery, is depressed. Plasma cortisol levels during labor and lower abdominal surgery are suppressed.

TABLE 34E–1.—LOCAL ANESTHETIC DRUGS USED FOR EPIDURAL BLOCK

INDICATION AND CONCENTRATION	CHARACTERISTICS
SURGICAL ANESTHESIA	
2% lidocaine HC1 and epinephrine	Short latency, medium duration, moderate motor block
0.75% bupivacaine HC1	Long latency, long duration, good motor block
1.5% etidocaine HC1 and epinephrine	Short latency, long duration, excellent motor block
OBSTETRIC ANESTHESIA	
Caesarian section, instrumental delivery	
3% chloroprocaine and epinephrine	Short latency, short duration, good motor block
2% lidocaine HC1 and epinephrine	Short latency, medium duration, good motor block
0.5% bupivacaine HC1	Long latency, long duration, adequate motor block
Normal labor	
0.125%–0.25% bupivacaine HC1	Long latency, medium duration, weak to absent motor block
Postoperative pain and trauma	
0.25%–0.5% bupivacaine HC1	Long latency, long duration, weak motor block
Diagnostic and therapeutic blocks	
Sympathectomy: 0.5% lidocaine HC1	Latency longer with weakest solutions
Sensory block: 1% lidocaine HC1	
Motor block: 2% lidocaine HC1	

Lumbar Epidural Block

If an epidural block is restricted to the lumbar region and remains below T-4, the principal physiologic effects will be limited to a sympathetic block of the lower limbs. However, as long as no epinephrine is used, reflex compensatory vasoconstriction occurs in the upper limbs and thorax in response to the fall in total peripheral resistance. In addition, because the cardiac sympathetic nerves escape block, the heart responds with up to a 20% increase in rate and cardiac output in unmedicated volunteers. The situation in premedicated patients, however, is quite different. Although the peripheral resistance decreases and the heart rate and cardiac output remain unchanged, there is only a 10% fall in mean arterial pressure. This increased sympathetic activity in the unblocked upper parts of the body prevents the vascular resistance from falling more than 25%.

Caudal (Sacral Epidural) Block

The principal failure of caudal anesthesia is failure to identify the sacrococcygeal hiatus due to anatomical abnormalities of the sacrum. In most instances the sacral hiatus is at S-5, the cornua, while somewhat variable, do give a clue to its location.

It should be remembered that the dural sac extends to S-2 in the adult and therefore the caudal needle should not be advanced more than 1.5 cm through the sacrococcygeal membrane. Physiologic effects associated with caudal anesthesia restricted to L-5 are minimal and do not require elaboration. The reader should refer to the earlier discussion of the cardiovascular effects of an absorbed local anesthetic under thoracic epidural block.

Technique

Cervical Epidural Block

A cervical epidural block may be performed using either a midline approach, in which case the patient should be sitting up or lying in a lateral position with a steep head-up tilt, or a paramedian approach, in which case the patient must be lying in a lateral position.

MIDLINE APPROACH.—The "hanging-drop" sign of Gutierrez is most commonly employed to identify the epidural space.

The patient is positioned as shown in Figure 34E–6, with an assistant steadying the shoulders, while the head and neck are flexed. Illumination must be good, because the operator is totally dependent on seeing a good light reflex from the meniscus on the drop of fluid in the needle hub.

The most satisfactory space is C7–T1, where the vertebra prominens (C-7) can be easily palpated and the posterior foramen is also large (Fig 34E–7). A skin wheal is made midway between the spinous processes and a 22-gauge spinal needle is used to explore the subcutaneous tissues down to the base of the spinous process and to infiltrate the tissues with local anesthetic. A winged or spool-type Huber tipped epidural needle is introduced to a depth of about 2 cm, the stylet is withdrawn, and a drop of fluid is placed in the needle hub. With the hands gripping the needle as shown, and with the hypothenar eminences of each hand braced against the patient's back, the operator firmly and carefully advances the needle during the patient's inspirations while constantly watching for any movement of the drop of fluid (Fig 34E–8). Precisely as the needle tip enters the epidural space, the drop is sucked in, and a feeling of release is transmitted to the holding hands. Further movement must cease immediately to prevent puncture of the dura. Confirmation of the correct position may be obtained by squirting a stream of local anesthetic from a syringe into the

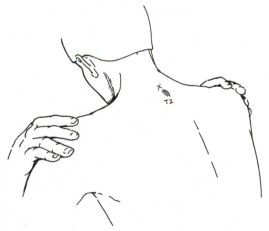

Fig 34E–6.—Optimal patient position for the midline approach for a cervical epidural puncture.

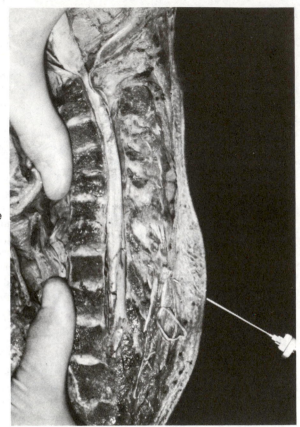

Fig 34E–7.—The cervical region in the cadaver showing anatomy and relations of cervical canal, with needle positioned in the epidural space. (Longitudinal section.)

needle hub. The persistent subatmospheric pressure within the spinal canal will cause this fluid to disappear rapidly.

PARAMEDIAN APPROACH.—The patient is placed in a left or right lateral position with the head

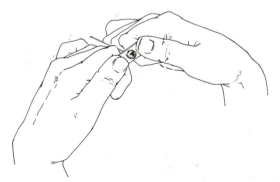

Fig 34E–8.—Proper position of the hands for performing a midline cervical epidural puncture using the hanging drop technique. Note the drop of fluid in the needle hub.

and neck well flexed (Fig 34E–9). The same interspace, C7–T1 or C6–7, is identified and a skin wheal is made 1.5 cm lateral to the midline. A 22-gauge spinal needle is then used to infiltrate the subcutaneous tissues and to plumb the depth of the lamina. The needle is withdrawn to the skin and reinserted at an angle of 15° to the sagittal plane and angled so as to contact the lamina at its ipsilateral superomedial margin. A track of local anesthetic is infiltrated, a skin puncture is made with a 22-gauge needle, and an 18-gauge Crawford needle is inserted. The bevel of the Crawford needle should point caudad throughout its insertion. Once the lamina is contacted, the stylet is withdrawn, and a syringe containing saline or air is attached. After making a small adjustment to ensure engagement of the needle tip with the ligamentum flavum, the operator carefully advances the needle while maintaining constant unremitting pressure in the case of fluid, or a tremolo percussion if air is to be used. Loss of resistance will be immediately transmitted to the thumb by the plunger, and further advance of the

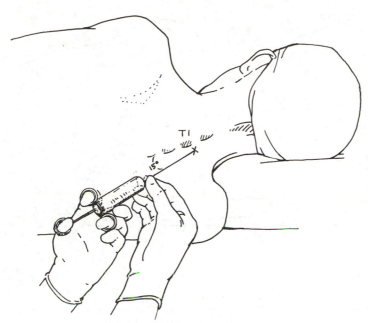

Fig 34E–9.—Position of needle and correct grip for a paramedian approach to the cervical epidural space. The hands are held in the same manner for the same approach in the thoracic region.

needle must cease. The shallow inclination of the needle with this approach makes it very easy to insert a catheter when desired.

Thoracic Epidural Block

A paramedian approach is preferred, although a midline technique which utilizes the hanging-drop sign can be employed in the upper four thoracic interspaces. The same technique is used as for the cervical epidural block.

A skin wheal is raised 1.5 cm lateral to the caudal tip of the spinous process, denoting the interspace. A 22-gauge spinal needle is introduced at a right angle to the plane of the back and local anesthetic is infiltrated as the needle is advanced until it contacts the lamina. The needle is withdrawn to the skin and redirected at an angle of 15° to the sagittal plane. It is again carefully advanced, infiltrating the tissues with local anesthetic, until it contacts the superomedial aspect of the ipsilateral lamina or the ligamentum flavum. The depth is noted, a skin hole is made with a 22-gauge needle, and the Crawford epidural needle is introduced with its bevel directed caudad (Fig 34E–10). As soon as the resistance of the ligamentum flavum or lamina is felt, the stylet is removed and a syringe containing saline or air is attached. While maintaining constant unremitting pressure (in the case of fluid) or a tremolo percus-

sion (in the case of air), the operator advances the needle until a sudden release of the plunger signals entry of the needle point in the epidural space. Movement is halted immediately. Injection is made through the needle, or a catheter is introduced if a continuous technique is to be used.

Lumbar Epidural Block

MIDLINE APPROACH.—The patient may be either sitting up or lying in a lateral position. Unless the clinical status precludes it, the sitting position should always be used in the obese patient as it facilitates identification of the midline, often extremely difficult to determine. In addition, one has a better chance of abolishing the lumbar lordosis in such patients. Unless a specific preferential block of the L5–S1 segments is required, in which case entry should be made at this level, it is simpler to select either the L2–3 interspace, the most superficial, or the L3–4 interspaces, both of which are below the termination of the spinal medulla at L-1 in the adult. If the sitting position is utilized, the patient must be steadied by an assistant.

For the lateral approach one should attempt to gain as much flexion as possible by flexing the patient's head and neck forward and bringing the knees up toward the abdomen. Unlike the joints in the thoracic region, which allow only lateral rotary

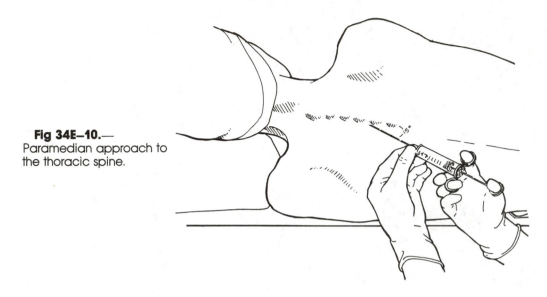

Fig 34E–10.— Paramedian approach to the thoracic spine.

movements, the facet joints in the lumbar region allow anteroposterior motion, and considerable widening of the posterior foramina can be achieved by this maneuver (Fig 34E–11).

A skin wheal is made midway between the chosen spinous processes. Deeper infiltration can be carried out with a 22-gauge spinal needle, which at

the same time is used to determine the depth of the ligamentum flavum from the skin.

A Tuohy needle with its bevel pointing cephalad is introduced almost at a right angle in all planes, down to the ligamentum flavum (Fig 34E–12). This structure in the lumbar region offers considerably greater resistance than in the thoracic region, and

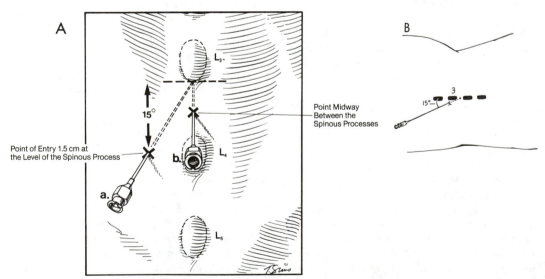

Fig 34E–11.—A, point of entry for the median and paramedian approaches in the lumbar region for an epidural or spinal block. **B,** paramedian approach for spinal and epidural blocks. Note angle and direction of the needle. (From Raj P.P., Pai U.: Techniques of nerve blocking, in Raj P.P. (ed.): *Handbook of Regional Anesthesia*. New York, Churchill Livingstone, Inc, 1985. Reproduced by permission.)

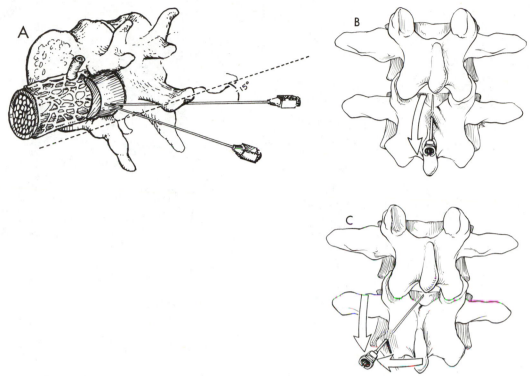

Fig 34E–12.—A, position of Tuohy and Crawford needles and their relationship to bony structures. **B** and **C,** bony relationship in the median and paramedian approaches to an epidural and/or spinal block. (From Raj P.P., Pai U.: Techniques of nerve blocking, in Raj P.P. (ed.): *Handbook of Regional Anesthesia.* New York, Churchill Livingstone, Inc, 1985. Reproduced by permission.)

resistance here can be readily distinguished from the resistance offered by the interspinous ligament. The stylet is withdrawn and a 5- or 10-ml syringe filled with saline or air is attached. With the hands held as shown, the operator applies constant unremitting pressure to the plunger, in the case of fluid, or rapid tremolo percussion, if air is used, while at the same time firmly advancing the needle with the other hand. As the needle point enters the epidural space the plunger will suddenly release, signifying its position by the loss of resistance (Fig 34E–13).

PARAMEDIAN APPROACH.—The paramedian approach is essentially a paraspinous approach, the needle making the same 15° angle to the sagittal plane as it does in the cervical or thoracic spine. However, its point of entry in the skin is different. Because the lumbar spinous processes do not overlap one another, as do the thoracic spines, the skin puncture must be lateral to the interspace below that in which the epidural puncture is to be made (see

Fig 34E–11,B). As described by Bonica, the wheal is made 1.5 cm lateral to the caudal edge of the spinous process below the space in which epidural puncture is to be made.[6] Some leeway has to be acknowledged with this rule because in the extremely obese patient, the needle might not be long enough to reach the ligamentum flavum from this point, in which case it must be moved cephalad alongside the adjacent spinous process.

As before, the use of a 22-gauge spinal needle is advocated, first to plumb the lamina below the skin wheal and then to lay a track of local anesthetic down to the ligamentum flavum. With a knowledge of the local anatomy assured by this maneuver, a 22-gauge needle makes a hole in the skin and the very blunt Crawford needle, with its point caudad, is advanced down to the ligamentum flavum (or superomedial aspect of the ipsilateral lamina), the stylet is removed, and a 5- or 10-ml syringe containing saline or air is attached.

The operator maintains constant pressure, when

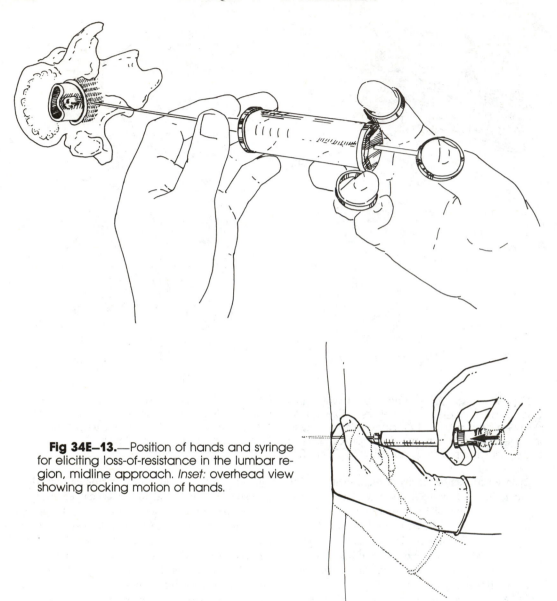

Fig 34E–13.—Position of hands and syringe for eliciting loss-of-resistance in the lumbar region, midline approach. *Inset:* overhead view showing rocking motion of hands.

fluid is used, or rapid tremolo percussion, when air is used, and firmly advances the needle until the perceived loss of resistance confirms entry of the needle point into the epidural space.

The very shallow attitude and greater distance traveled by the needle in the paramedian approach as compared to the midline approach will mean that in many cases, the entire needle length may lie beneath the skin. This position facilitates catheter insertion and was one of the reasons Bonica recom-

mended the paramedian approach over the midline approach.

Caudal Block

The sacral hiatus is most easily identified with the patient lying prone over a pillow placed under the pelvis (Fig 34E–14). With the feet internally rotated so as to relax the gluteal muscles, the surface anat-

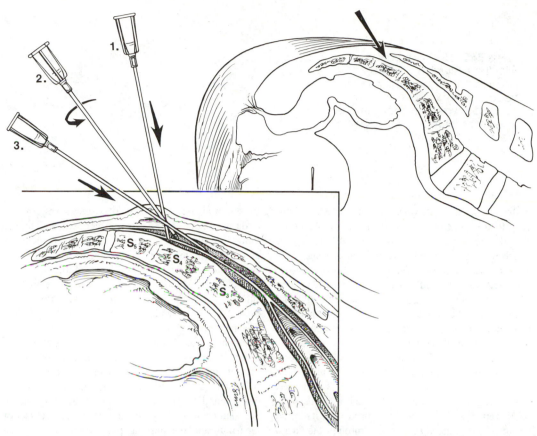

Fig 34E–14.—Technique of caudal block with the patient prone. As shown in the *inset*, the needle is first inserted through the sacrococcygeal membrane at a 90° angle to the skin (needle position *1*). Position *2* shows the rotation of the needle such that the bevel is turned dorsally before the needle is inserted deeper, with the hub down toward the feet (needle position *3*). (From Raj P.P., Pai U.: Techniques of nerve blocking, in Raj P.P. (ed.): *Handbook of Regional Anesthesia*. New York, Churchill Livingstone, Inc, 1985. Reproduced by permission.)

omy can be identified by palpation, and insertion of the needle will be rewarded with the greatest success. However, it may be impossible for some patients to assume this position, in which case the procedure must be performed with the patient in the lateral position (Fig 34E–15).

The sacral cornua are often visible in thin patients, making identification of the sacral hiatus comparatively easy, but this is certainly not the rule. If the operator's left forefinger is laid over the coccyx such that its tip palpates the apex, then the second interphalangeal joint will lie approximately over the sacrococcygeal membrane in most adults. Some authorities recommend marking the posterior superior iliac spine and then drawing lines to each cornu

to form a triangle, the apex of which lies over the sacrococcygeal membrane. Prior to the usual skin preparation, a swab should be placed in the natal cleft to prevent cleaning solution from passing anteriorly onto the sensitive perineal skin.

A skin wheal is made over the sacral hiatus. With the same needle, a small amount of local anesthetic is infiltrated down to the sacrococcygeal membrane. The interstitial swelling caused by the local anesthetic and/or any edema present can be dispersed by maintaining pressure for 30 seconds or so with the thumb.

A 21-gauge short-bevel needle can be used for single shot injections and an 18-gauge caudal needle is used for continuous techniques. The needle is in-

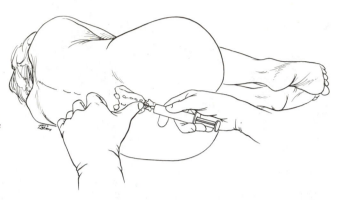

Fig 34E–15.—Caudal block with the patient in a lateral position. Note penetration of the needle through the sacrococcygeal membrane. The operator's thumb is at the shelf of the sacral hiatus.

troduced through the wheal at an angle of about 120° to the back. The tip will pierce the sacrococcygeal membrane (see Fig 34E–14) with a snap, at which point it is rotated about 60° while at the same time the needle shaft is depressed to prevent disengagement of the needle point. The needle is then advanced about 1.5 cm. If the needle lies within the canal, it can be moved from side to side without resistance, the shaft of the needle being held by the sacrococcygeal membrane.

The dural sac ends at S-2 in the adult and therefore the needle should not be advanced more than 1.5 cm. In small children and infants it is lower. Therefore, a small-gauge needle such as a 23-gauge or 25-gauge × 2 cm should be used, and it should be introduced only up to 0.5 cm through the sacral hiatus. Fortunately, in this age group the anatomy is readily visualized and palpated and it is more constant, unlike the changes brought by age and disease in the adult. A catheter can be placed for prolonged analgesia, as shown in Figure 34E–16.

Epidural Neurolysis

Although the epidural route avoids the risk of meningeal irritation and allows good localization of the neurolytic solution, the method is not widely used for relief of intractable pain. Morever, there does not appear to be increased use of epidural neurolysis paralleling the contemporary popularity of epidural block for both surgical and obstetric analgesia. One reason may be that at the time of injection, it is not as easy to gauge the response and effectiveness as with subarachnoid injection. Some studies have claimed good results with extradural alcohol, but the injection is often painful and may be followed by postinjection neuropathy with neuralgia.[7] Phenol appears to be a more promising agent

for epidural use. A number of workers employ extradural phenol for pain in the cervical and higher thoracic segments to avoid the risk of subarachnoid neurolysis at this level. Louri and Vanasupa claim pain relief lasting more than 9 months with 6% phenol,[8] but Madrid, although finding the method successful, could not achieve relief lasting more than 2–4 weeks with 7.5% phenol and glycerin.[9] For neck and shoulder pain of malignancy, 7%–10% phenol has been very satisfactory. Raftery has reported the use of intermittent small doses of 6% phenol with an epidural catheter.[10] The technique was used at all levels of the spinal cord and was often found to give good relief. Extradural phenol has also been used by Doughty to relieve attacks of tenesmus and the burning pain which occurs with rectal cancer.[11] Continuous epidural analgesia can be used to provide useful pain relief in terminally ill patients.[12] In patients who have widespread pain and are too ill for more major pain-relieving procedures, and in whom analgesic drugs are unsatisfactory, good relief can be achieved by the intermittent injection of a diluted local anesthetic solution through an appropriately positioned epidural catheter. Such a catheter can be retained for several weeks and can even be used in patients at home. Recently some progress has been made in the permanent placement of epidural catheters and connecting them either to reservoirs or to continuous in vivo infusion pumps.[13, 14]

Epidural neurolysis does not offer the same scope or precision as the spinal block for the same purpose. However, it is useful in two types of pain: the pain of malignancy, and nonmalignant intractable pain affecting the thoracic segments. Swerdlow has considerable experience[15] with the latter application.

Absolute alcohol has been shown to diffuse into the subarachnoid space in significant concentration

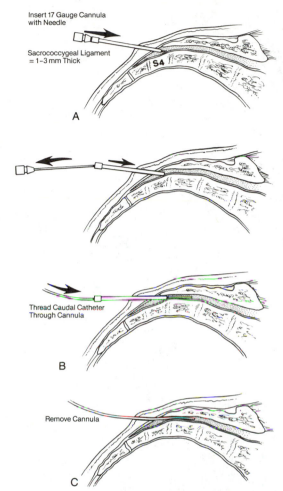

Insert 17 Gauge Cannula with Needle

Sacrococcygeal Ligament = 1–3 mm Thick

S4

A

Thread Caudal Catheter Through Cannula

B

Remove Cannula

C

Fig 34E–16.—Catheter placement for continuous analgesia by the caudal approach. *A*, large cannula or Tuohy needle is inserted in the caudal canal. *B*, epidural catheter is threaded through the needle. *C*, needle is removed and catheter is anchored. (From Raj P.P., Pai U.: Techniques of nerve blocking, in Raj P.P. (ed.): *Handbook of Regional Anesthesia.* New York, Churchill Livingstone, Inc., 1985. Reproduced by permission.)

(0.2%–0.9% 30 minutes after injection of 10 ml of 30% alcohol), so considerably higher levels can be expected after injection of absolute alcohol.[16]

Phenol 6% in aqueous solution is probably the most satisfactory agent for this procedure, and because it is nephrotoxic, it should be limited to about 15 mg/kg, or 15 ml of a 6% solution in a 60-kg adult.

Epidural Neurolytic Blocks with a Catheter

A catheter is placed, and local anesthetic injection is used to provide pain relief. This will determine the volume required to provide analgesia and also allow the patient a chance to evaluate the degree of numbness, weakness, and pain relief.

After the volume required has been determined (usually 4–5 ml), 6% aqueous phenol is slowly injected through the catheter. There is an initial burning sensation, followed by hypesthesia. The catheter is left in place (Fig 34E–17) because it may be necessary to reinject in a day or two to achieve adequate analgesia. Injection of large volumes may result in extensive spread.

Complications

All technical procedures performed in patients carry a certain risk; epidural analgesia is no exception, although the incidence of the most serious complication, permanent neurologic injury, is less than 1:26,000 in the best hands, which attests to the safety of the technique.

Potential complications may develop immediately or some time after the procedure. In the following discussion complications are grouped as minor and major and subgrouped by early and late occurrences.

Minor Complications

DURAL PUNCTURE.—The dura is usually punctured by needle, although it can also be perforated by a catheter. If dural puncture is recognized at the time, or on subsequent aspiration of the catheter, the worst that can befall the patient is a "spinal" headache. This is serious enough for the patient, but if the puncture goes unrecognized, it may result in a massive spinal injection of local anesthetic being made.

MASSIVE SUBARACHNOID INJECTION.—Massive subarachnoid injection is manifested by rapid, complete spinal analgesia, hypotension, apnea, and unconsciousness. Treatment is supportive and is aimed at maintaining circulation, providing ventilation, and continuing sedation until the block has worn off.

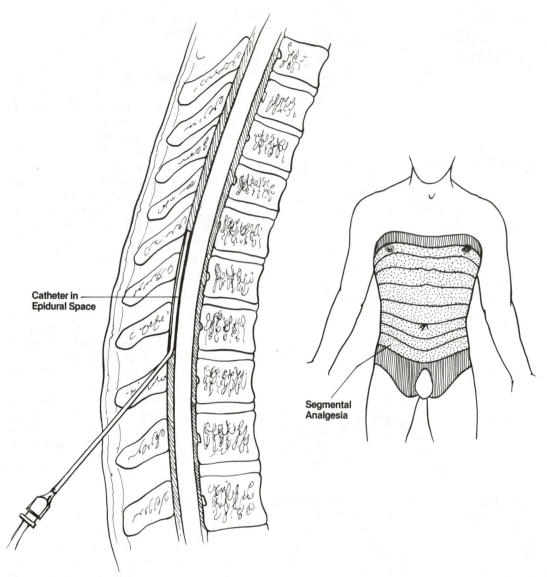

Catheter in Epidural Space

Segmental Analgesia

Fig 34E–17.—Catheter placement, in the epidural space for segmental analgesia. This technique can be used for neurolytic blocks in the epidural space. (From Raj P.P., Pai U.: Techniques of nerve blocking, in Raj P.P. (ed.): *Handbook of Regional Anesthesia.* New York, Churchill Livingstone, Inc., 1985. Reproduced by permission.)

MASSIVE SUBDURAL INJECTION.—A massive subdural injection, although rare, is possible. Local anesthetic travels great distances in this space.

INTRAVENOUS INJECTION.—Not infrequently the epidural veins are damaged either by the needle or by the catheter. Bleeding usually stops quickly unless there is a coagulation defect. Puncture of these veins has been reported by Bromage to occur in 1% of cases, mostly pregnant women at term.[16] If this goes unnoticed, the therapuetic dose of local anesthetic may be injected IV, in which case the systemic local anesthetic toxicity may be manifested by convulsions and/or cardiovascular collapse. The convulsions should be treated with IV barbiturates or diazepam. Circulatory support with a vasopressor may be necessary to counteract hypotension, should this occur.

HEADACHE.—This complication has an incidence of about 70%–80% following dural puncture with a large-bore epidural needle. Treatment is aimed at increasing CSF production with a high fluid intake. The patient should remain in bed and be given analgesics. If after 24 hours the headache persists, an autologous blood patch should be performed.

BROKEN EPIDURAL CATHETER.—The catheter may shear off at the needle tip. This accident was more common with the older polyvinyl catheters. Teflon or nylon catheters are more pliable, and if such an event should occur, the sequestered portion, being inert, should be left in situ, unless the end is readily accessible from the subcutaneous tissues. The morbidity associated with laminectomy is far greater than the morbidity associated with a sequestered foreign body. If the foreign body should cause a problem at a later date, it can be removed by laminectomy.

Major Complications

NEUROLOGIC TRAUMA.—Neurologic trauma to the nerve roots and spinal cord is a grave sequel of epidural block. Most instances of neural damage result from the operator's ignorance of anatomy or from carelessness; some instances occur during training. However, some cases have resulted from an anomalous anatomical situation such as a spinal tumor which was unknown at the time the epidural puncture was made.

Any paraesthesia elicited during the performance of epidural block is a warning that the needle must be adjusted, or if the paresthesia is elicited during catheter insertion, further introduction should cease, the needle reintroduced in a new position, and the procedure again attempted. To persist in the face of paresthesia is folly and risks causing temporary or permanent neural injury.

EPIDURAL HEMATOMA.—This may occur spontaneously or in association with anticoagulant therapy. Spinal cord compression can develop rapidly from an expanding hematoma such that recognition of the symptoms of pain in the back and weakness of the legs requires urgent confirmation of the diagnosis so that emergency laminectomy can be performed to avoid permanent neurologic damage.

ANTERIOR SPINAL ARTERY SYNDROME.—This syndrome is characterized by painless motor weakness or paralysis of the legs. The lesion may be due to failure of the segmental supply—in particular the radicularis magna artery of Adamkiewicz—to reinforce the anterior spinal artery because of atheroma, low flow states, surgical interference with the segmental blood supplies, or other unknown causes. The ischemia affects the lower cord and then predominantly its anterior two thirds. Unfortunately, there is little one can do for this syndrome. The differential diagnosis from epidural hematoma abscess is obviously extremely important since the latter two conditions are both amenable to surgery.

EPIDURAL ABSCESS.—Infection in the epidural space can take the form of meningitis or an abscess. The source is usually hematogenous, particularly from a source in the pelvis, and only rarely is it introduced from outside the body. The organism is commonly *Staphylococcus aureus*. Symptoms are usually pain in the back, motor weakness, and sensory disturbance followed by paraplegia unless the diagnosis is made and an urgent laminectomy carried out. Its development may take up to 2 weeks in some cases. It is important in the differential diagnosis that unlike hematoma, there is typically a change in the character of pain from severe back pain to a radicular pain over a period of 3 days. Motor symptoms will appear 24–48 hours later. However, once weakness is evident, paraplegia may require only 24 hours to develop.

ARACHNOIDITIS.—This condition, rarely associated with epidural anesthesia, may have some foreign material, bleeding, or infection as its genesis.

Subarachnoid Block

Functional Anatomy

The subarachnoid space extends to the level of S-2 and the enclosed spinal cord usually extends down to L-1. A needle inserted below L-2 should not encounter the substance of the spinal cord but may encounter cauda equina. In the midline the spinal needle traverses the skin, the supraspinous ligament, the interspinous ligament, the ligamentum flavum, and the epidural space before entering the subarachnoid space. In the lateral approach, the needle passes through the skin, subcutaneous fat, lumbar aponeurosis, paravertebral muscles, ligmentum flavum, and the epidural space prior to entering the subarachnoid space (Fig 34E–18).

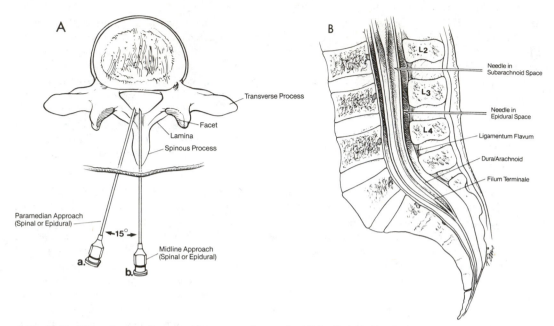

Fig 34E–18.—**A,** median and paramedian approach for a subarachnoid block. **B,** sagittal section showing needle placement in the subarachnoid and the epidural space. (From Raj P.P., Pai U.: Techniques of nerve blocking, in Raj P.P. (ed.): *Handbook of Regional Anesthesia.* New York, Churchill Livingstone, Inc, 1985. Reproduced by permission.)

Equipment

There are many disposable trays available on the market. The reusable trays should be sterilized and checked prior to use.

Anesthesiologists have their own idea of what is essential in a block tray. It is important that the smallest-gauge spinal needle be used to decrease the incidence of post-dural puncture headache.

Technique

The *lateral decubitus position,* the *sitting position,* and the *jackknife position* are the positions most frequently used for spinal anesthesia.

If the patient is placed in the lateral position, the line of the spinous processes should be parallel to the table. To open up the vertebral interspaces, the patient is asked to flex the back by drawing the knees up toward the chest and flexing the neck so that the chin touches the chest. The head should be supported by a small pillow. An assistant should support and calm the patient.

In the sitting position, the patient sits on the edge of the table with the feet resting on a stool. The neck is flexed so that the chin touches the chest, with the arms folded across the upper thighs on a pillow or on a Mayo tray, or on the shoulders of the assistant who is supporting the patient from the front.

The jackknife position is used mainly for anorectal surgery with a hypobaric solution. Care must be taken to avoid pressure points on the pelvis, thighs, or lower legs from the position during the procedure.

Procedure

The gloved anesthetist prepares the skin of the lumbar area with a bactericidal preparation, wiping off the excess solution. The field is draped with sterile towels. The appropriate interspace is located. Depending on the special anatomical features of the patient, the second, third, or fourth lumbar interspace may be most suitable. After locating the most prominent point of the right and left iliac crests the operator draws an imaginary line between the two points that usually crosses the L-4 spinous process of the L-4 interspace (the interspace between the L-4 and L-5 vertebrae).

In the lateral position, the line of the spinous processes must be parallel to the table and the surface of the patient's back must be vertical. This will align the spinous processes in the horizontal plane. The elected entry point is infiltrated with a small amount of local anesthetic using a 25-gauge needle. In addition, a small amount (1–2 ml) of local anesthetic may be injected into the subcutaneous tissue and the interspinous ligament. When satisfactory analgesia of the entry point has been achieved, an 18-gauge needle is used as an introducer and is inserted through the skin wheal. The index and the middle fingers of the operator's free hand straddle the interspace to fix the tissues of the underlying structures. The introducer is used for passage of the fine spinal needle and, theoretically, prevents a plug of skin or fat from being carried into the subarachnoid space. However, some prefer not to use an introducer. An improperly inserted introducer makes it impossible to point the needle in the correct direction. It is preferable to select a thin-gauge (No. 25 or 26) spinal needle for the spinal anesthesia. However, a 22-gauge spinal needle can also be used without an introducer.

The needle must first be examined for any imperfections. It should be noted that the bevel of the needle is on the same side as the key notch for the stylet in its hub. Once the physician is satisfied with the needle, he should insert it in such a fashion that the bevel does not cut across the longitudinal fibers of the dura. Therefore, the bevel should face laterally during its passage through the dura.

The spinal needle is held between the index and middle fingers by the thumb and is inserted through the introducer. The thumb exerts pressure on the stylet to prevent its displacement as the needle is pushed through the tissues. The ring and little fingers rest on the patient's back and support the anesthetist's hand. The spinal needle is then slowly advanced. Its progress through the tissues is followed by noting the variations in resistance as the various structures are crossed. First, the firm resistance of the interspinous ligament and the ligamentum flavum is felt. After this a lessening of resistance is observed as the needle crosses the epidural space. This is followed by the characteristic "pop"—an abrupt disappearance of resistance as the needle pierces the dura to enter the subarachnoid space. The anesthetist now should check his needle position by withdrawing the stylet to see if CSF appears at the hub of the needle. When a 25-gauge needle is used, aspiration with a 2-ml syringe may be needed.

If CSF does not appear at the hub of the needle, one should consider the following:

1. A nerve root or the dura may block the bevel of the needle. After withdrawing the stylet, the anesthetist should rotate the needle 90°–180° to see if the bevel can be freed of this obstruction.

2. The CSF pressure may be too low to push the fluid through the needle. The anesthetist can confirm the needle position by aspirating CSF with a syringe.

3. A tissue plug may be blocking the bevel. This also may be dislodged by an aspiration attempt.

4. The bevel may still be in the epidural space, at least partially. Therefore, the anesthetist should replace the stylet in the needle and then slowly advance the needle. Then the above maneuvers are repeated.

If contact with bone has been made, stop. The needle must not be forced against this resistance because the lumen of the needle can be easily blocked and the needle point can become "barbed." If one feels that the needle lumen is plugged, the needle should be taken out and flushed with normal saline or local anesthetic solution. Contact with bone usually means that the vertebral lamina has been encountered. This necessitates a small change in the direction of the spinal needle. To do this effectively, the needle point is withdrawn completely into the introducer and then a fresh attempt is made for a puncture in a different direction. Success is indicated by the appearance of CSF in the hub of the spinal needle. When this is achieved, the hub of the spinal needle is held firmly between the index finger and thumb of one hand to prevent any displacement of the needle from its proper location. The back of the anesthetist's hand is steadied against the patient's back. A syringe filled with the appropriate dose of local anesthetic solution is attached to the spinal needle (Tables 34E–2 and 34E–3).

Negative pressure is applied to the syringe to draw up a small amount of CSF to ascertain that the proper position of the needle bevel has been maintained. Then local anesthetic solution in the syringe is injected slowly. This is to prevent a jet effect in the subarachnoid space. Some prefer a small amount of aspiration and reinjection in the middle after the local anesthetic has been injected, to rule out inadvertent movement of the needle during instillation of the drug. The patient is turned gently after the needle is removed. Vital signs are monitored continuously at this point. Verbal contact with the patient is essential. Early signs of hypotension will appear during the change in position and should be prevented or treated as early as possible.

TABLE 34E–2.—LOCAL ANESTHETIC DRUGS AND DOSAGES FOR HYPERBARIC SUBARACHNOID BLOCK FOR GENERAL SURGERY*

LOCAL ANESTHETIC	DESIRED LEVEL	DOSE (MG) BY PATIENT HEIGHT			ONSET OF ACTION (min)	DURATION OF ACTION (min)
		60 in.	66 in.	72 in.		
Lidocaine 5% in 7.5% dextrose, in water	T-10	50	55	60	1–3	60–90†
(premixed)	T-4	70	75	80		
Tetracaine 1% and equal volume of 10%	T-10	10	12	14	3–5	120–180†
dextrose in water	T-4	14	16	18		

*After Osthiemer: ASRA Workshop. Philadelphia, 1979.
†The addition of epinephrine, 0.2–0.5 ml (1 mg/ml), will extend the duration of action up to 50% longer.

With the patient resting comfortably, the spread of anesthesia is frequently checked by gentle repeated pinpricks or by a cotton swab moistened with alcohol. Since pain and temperature sensation are lost simultaneously, the use of alcohol to check the spread of anesthesia is more pleasant for the patient. Repeated pinpricks may not accurately differentiate the area of complete loss of pain sensation from an area of partial analgesia.

When the anesthesia reaches the desired segmental level, the patient is positioned so as to prevent any further spread of the anesthetic. The local anesthetic drug "fixes" to the neuronal elements, so that usually no further spread of anesthetic effect is seen after a "fixation time" of approximately 20 minutes.

The spread of the local anesthetic depends on specific gravity and the baricity between the local anesthetic solution used and the CSF.

A hyperbaric solution has a higher specific gravity than CSF, so that it will move to low-lying parts of the subarachnoid space. This technique is recommended for surgical and obstetric procedures performed on a patient in the supine or sitting position.

A hypobaric solution has a specific gravity lower than CSF and therefore will spread to higher-lying areas within the subarachnoid space. However, some believe that the block is effected by displacement of the CSF from the superior part of the subarachnoid space by the hypobaric solution. This technique is primarily used for pelvic, perineal, and lower extremity procedures performed with the patient in the lateral, prone, or jackknife positions. One advantage of using a hypobaric technique is that the patient is placed in the position in which the operation will be performed, so that after the block is established, no further movement of the patient is necessary. One needs to keep the operative site uppermost and the table in 20° head-down position.

An isobaric solution, with a specific gravity matching that of CSF, tends to remain at the injection point, even during the fixation time. Although this technique is rarely used at present, it is gaining popularity with the introduction of bupivacaine as a spinal agent.

With hyperbaric solutions, it is possible to attempt to block one leg (the dependent extremity). When the patient resumes the supine or prone posi-

TABLE 34E–3.—LOCAL ANESTHETIC DRUG AND DOSAGE FOR HYPOBARIC SUBARACHNOID BLOCK FOR GENERAL SURGERY (PELVIS AND LOWER EXTREMITIES)

LOCAL ANESTHETIC	DOSE DEPENDS ON PT. HEIGHT	ONSET OF ACTION (min)	DURATION OF ACTION (min)
Tetracaine 0.1%*	Site of operation and level needed: 6–20 ml (6–20 mg), most commonly 6–15 ml	3–5	90–120

*Tetracaine 0.1% can be prepared by dissolving 20 mg of crystalline tetracaine in 20 ml of distilled water, or 1 ml (10 mg) of tetracaine 1% can be diluted by 9 ml of distilled water.

tion, there is sufficient mixing to obtain a bilateral block, although it may be less intense in the superior extremity.

Prevention of Deleterious Effects

To ensure safety and success of spinal anesthesia, several precautions should be taken. The entry point for the needle should be below the level of L-2 to avoid injury to the spinal cord.

The spinal needle on occasion may puncture one of the epidural vessels, resulting in a blood-tinged return of CSF at the hub of the needle. If this occurs, one should wait until the return clears completely. If the CSF return fails to clear, an attempt is made to repeat the block through another interspace. The vital signs must be monitored continuously, especially in the initial 10 minutes during fixation of the block, with close attention paid to any fall in blood pressure.

Contraindications

Circumstances that make spinal anesthesia inadvisable include conditions that may potentiate bleeding into the CNS (blood dyscrasias, coagulopathies), that may cause infection of the meninges of the spinal cord (septicemia, local cutaneous infections at the puncture site), or in which preexisting CNS pathology may be aggravated by the pharmacologic action of the local anesthetic (poliomyelitis, amyotrophic lateral sclerosis, etc).

Deformities of the lumbosacral spine may make spinal anesthesia technically difficult. In these patients the potential for trauma may be unacceptably high.

Continuous (Intermittent) Spinal Anesthesia

Continuous spinal block is rarely used with the increased use of continuous epidural anesthesia. The incidence of spinal headache after this block can be expected to be unacceptably high because it may cause clinically significant loss of CSF. The spinal needle inevitably must be of a large gauge and therefore will produce a relatively large dural defect. The presence of the catheter inserted through the dura also potentiates the loss of CSF by capillary action.

SPINAL NEUROLYTIC BLOCK

Subarachnoid Neurolysis

When properly employed, subarachnoid neurolysis provides good-quality pain relief in a reasonable proportion of patients.[7] It could easily be made available to all patients with cancer pain. It requires only brief hospitalization, provides an adequate duration of relief for many patients, and can be repeated if necessary. It can be applied to the old and very ill, and complications are usually slight. Pathologic studies have shown that neurolytic solutions injected intrathecally affect large and small fibers indiscriminantly. The degree of block produced depends on the number rather than the type of fibers destroyed, and this in turn is related to the quantity and concentration of solution employed. In the early years, phenol was often used dissolved in iophendylate (Pantopaque). It has subsequently been shown that phenol solution in iophendylate is less active than in glycerin, and there is now a consensus that iophendylate is only indicated when it is necessary to have radiologic control of the injection. Nathan et al.[18] considered that phenol has a biphasic action, an almost immediate but temporary local anesthetic action and a permanent destructive action of the blocked fibers. The destructive effects of alcohol are more intense and less localized than those of phenol.

The technique of intrathecal neurolytic injection is now well established. For injection of hyperbaric solutions, the patient is positioned with the painful site lowermost and the spinal puncture is made at a level such that the neurolytic solution will fall onto the appropriate posterior nerve roots. When alcohol is to be injected, the patient is placed with the painful side uppermost. The patient should be kept in the same position for about 45 minutes to allow the neurolytic agent to become fixed to the nerve roots. Sub-arachnoid neurolysis is particularly appropriate in patients with fairly localized pain. In patients with widespread pain, and especially in those whose pain arises early in the disease, a percutaneous cordotomy or, in appropriate cases, pituitary adenolysis would offer a better chance of long-term relief. In patients with bilateral multifocal pain, however, many workers consider that the serious risks of bilateral cordotomy should be avoided by performing cordotomy only on the worst side and applying subarachnoid neurolysis on the other side. In patients who are unfit, unwilling, or unable to have a cordotomy, intrathecal neurolysis is usually the best therapy. There is little to choose between the results of alcohol and phenol in expert hands. The choice usually depends on the operator's training and experience, but sometimes the patient's state will dictate whether hypobaric and hyperbaric solution is used. In our opinion, phenol injection is the choice for blocks in the lumbosacral segments and alcohol injection is the choice for blocks at higher spinal levels. An analysis of pooled data on more than 1,000 patients treated at many institutions showed that subarachnoid neurolysis resulted in good relief in about 56% of patients, fair relief in 27%, and no change in 17%.[7]

Neurolytic blocks are done above the level of cauda equina. These nerves are separated from each other sufficiently to be blocked individually. Below L-1 it is difficult to block the individual nerves, and there is the ever-present danger of bladder and/or bowel denervation.

Before performing a subarachnoid neurolytic block, the operater should consult a chart to determine the origin of the nerve from the spinal cord. Neurolysis is better accomplished at this level because the nerve fibers are in rootlets rather than a single large nerve.

Prior local anesthetic blocks and placebo blocks should be utilized to ascertain which root carries the pain and to give the patient an opportunity to assess the degree of numbness, weakness, and pain relief.

Procedure for Intrathecal Phenol Neurolysis

Phenol 5% or 6% in glycerin is a hyperbaric solution. The patient is placed in a position with the painful side dependent and the level of the root to be blocked most dependent. The back is angled 45°, with the unaffected side more posterior (Fig 34E–19). This will help concentrate the solution closer to the dorsal root.

The dural puncture is performed at the level where the root is attached to the spinal cord. This may be two to four interspaces superior to the exit of the root from the intervertebral foramen. It is important to establish clear flow in all quadrants to avoid injection into the cord.

Phenol, 0.1–0.2 ml, injected slowly at first produces a burning sensation. This will help localize the root that is to be blocked. If the desired root is different, a separate dural puncture should be performed. When the burning sensation is elicited over the painful dermatome, the solution is injected in 0.1-ml increments after the sensation ceases. Phenol has some local anesthetic action. If many roots are to be blocked, injection should start in the middle, and not more than 1 ml should be injected through one needle. A separate dural puncture is needed if more than 1 ml is to be used. Injection of larger volume through one needle may cause uncontrolled spread of the solution. Injection of more than 2–3 ml in one section is to be avoided for the same reason.

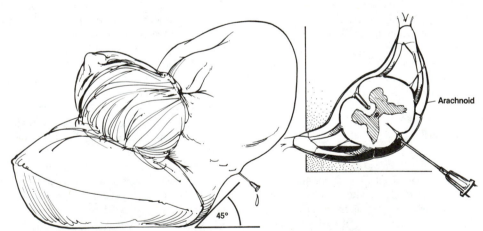

Fig 34E–19.—Position of the patient for a neurolytic block with phenol in the subarachnoid space. Note in *inset* the 45° rotation of the body to isolate the posterior nerve root for chemical rhizotomy. (From Raj P.P., Pai U.: Techniques of nerve blocking, in Raj P.P. (ed.): *Handbook of Regional Anesthesia.* New York, Churchill Livingstone, Inc., 1985. Reproduced by permission.)

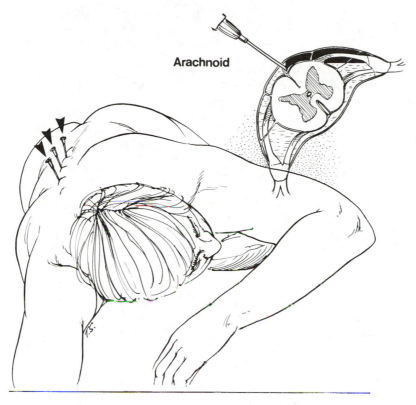

Arachnoid

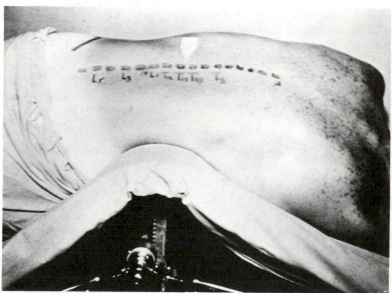

Fig 34E–20.—**Top,** position of the patient for a neurolytic block with alcohol in the subarachnoid space. Note the relation of the body to 45° in the inset. (From Raj P.P., Pai U.: Techniques of nerve blocking, in Raj P.P. (ed.): *Handbook of Regional Anesthesia.* New York, Churchill Livingstone, Inc, 1985. Reproduced by permission.) **Bottom,** note the break in the operating room table and placement of the region for alcohol rhizotomy in the higher position in relation to the rest of the body. (Courtesy of Jordan Katz, M.D.)

Procedure for Intrathecal Alcohol Injection

Alcohol is a hypobaric solution. The patient is positioned in the lateral position with the painful side up, and a chart is consulted to determine the level at which the root exits from the spinal cord. The position of the patient and the position of the table are adjusted so that the interspace to be entered is at the highest point (Fig 34E–20). This increases the chance of alcohol coming into contact with the desired root.

The patient's back is tilted forward to make a 45° angle to the table. This position is important to predominantly affect the dorsal root. For both anterior and posterior nerve root block on the same side, the patient stays on the lateral position at 90° to the table. For bilateral dorsal root block the patient is placed in the prone position. If more than two sites are to be injected, it is better to do them on separate sessions. A 2- to 3-day waiting period is necessary to evaluate the extent of neurolysis.

The subarachnoid space is entered using a 22- or 25-gauge needle and free flow of fluid is confirmed in all quadrants. Injection of 0.1 ml of alcohol produces a burning sensation in the dermatomal distribution of the root that is to be blocked. If this is not the correct level, the appropriate space above or below the previous needle is entered after the patient has been repositioned. After it is confirmed that a burning sensation has been produced in the area of pain, 0.1-ml increments are injected after the burning stops, to a total of 0.8–1 ml. This is usually adequate to block one to two roots. If more extensive block is needed, it is preferable to enter the subarachnoid space at a different level. Injection of larger volumes of alcohol may result in uncontrollable spread of the drug.

Cauda Equina Block

Patients in whom sacral or lower lumbar root block is necessary and who already have impaired bladder or bowel function (colostomy, indwelling withdrawal catheter) may derive pain relief from an alcohol block of the cauda equina. The subarachnoid space is entered at the L4–5 or L5–S1 level with the patient in the jackknife position. After removal of 5 ml of spinal fluid, 4–5 ml of absolute alcohol is slowly injected. The patient is kept in the jackknife position for 40 minutes and thereafter in the supine head-down position for 12 hours.

After completion of the injection, the patient is kept in the jackknife position for 20 minutes to prevent the spread of alcohol, and thereafter in the supine head-down position for 12 hours.

REFERENCES

1. Dogliotti A.M.: A new method of block anesthesia: Segmental peridural spinal anesthesia. *Am. J. Surg.* 23:107, 1933.
2. Batson O.V.: The function of the vertebral veins and their role in the spread of metastases. *Am. Surg.* 112:138, 1940.
3. McLean A.P.H., Mulligan G.W., Otton P., et al.: Haemodynamic alterations associated with epidural anesthesia. *Surgery* 62:79, 1967.
4. Bonica J.J., Berges P.V., Morikawa K.: Circulatory effects of peridural block: 1. Influence of level of analgesia and dose of lidocaine. *Anesthesioloy* 33:619, 1970.
5. Harrison D.C., Sprouse H., Morrow A.G.: The antiarrhythmic properties of lidocaine and procaine amide. *Circulation* 28:486, 1963.
6. Bonica J.J.: Continuous peridural block. *Anesthesiology* 17:626, 1956.
7. Swerdlow M.: Subarachnoid and extradural neurolytic blocks, in Bonica J.J., Ventrafridda V. (eds.): *Advances in Pain Research and Pain Therapy.* New York, Raven Press, 1979, vol. 2, p. 325.
8. Louri H., Vanasupa P.: Comments on the use of intraspinal phenol Pantopaque for relief of pain and spasticity. *J. Neurosurg.* 20:60, 1963.
9. Madrid J.: *Proceedings of a Symposium on Cancer Pain.* Florecne, Italy, 1975.
10. Raftery H.: *Proceedings of the Intractable Pain Society of Great Britain,* 1977.
11. Doughty A.: *A Practice of Anaesthesia.* Wylie W.D., Churchill-Davidson H. (eds.). London, Lloyd Luke, 1972.
12. Raj P.P.: Epidural narcotics for out-patients. *Pain Workshop,* ASA Annual Meeting, New Orleans, 1984.
13. Pilon R.N., Baker A.R.: Chronic pain control by means of an epidural catheter. *Cancer* 37:903, 1976.
14. Coombes D.W., Saunders R.L., Gaylor M., et al.: Epidural narcotic infusion reservoir: Implantation technique and efficacy. *Anesthesiology* 56:469, 1982.
15. Swerdlow M.: *Relief of Intractable Pain,* ed. 2. Amsterdam, Excerpta Medica, 1978.
16. Groenendijk H.J.: *De Peridural Anaesthesie.* Amsterdam, J.H. DeBussy, 1954, pp. 110–118.
17. Bromage P.R.: *Epidural Analgesia.* Philadelphia, W.B. Saunders Co., 1978.
18. Nathan P.W., Sears T.A.: Effects of phenol on nervous conduction. *J. Physiol.* 150:565, 1960.

34F / Sympathetic Blocks

MICHAEL STANTON-HICKS, M.D.
STEPHEN E. ABRAM, M.D.
HANS NOLTE, M.D., D.A.

STELLATE GANGLION BLOCK

ALTHOUGH MANY APPROACHES to the stellate ganglion have been described in this century, Leriche and Fontain in 1934 were the first to show that an anterior approach would provide a safe, simple, and reproducible method of blocking the sympathetics at this level.[1]

Although the use of neurolytic solutions for this block have been described, they are not recommended and should be reserved for selective thoracic ganglion block.

Patients with the following clinical conditions may benefit from this block:

Pain
  Posttraumatic syndrome, reflex sympathetic dystrophy
  Herpes zoster (shingles)
  Paget's disease
  Phantom limb (questionable)
Vascular insufficiency
  Thrombosis (arterial)
  Embolic vascular occlusion
  Raynaud's disease
  Scleroderma
  Occlusive vascular disease (questionable)
  Frostbite
Miscellaneous
  Ménière's disease (questionable)
  Hyperhidrosis
  Shoulder-hand syndrome
  Sudden blindness or deafness
  The differential diagnosis of vascular headaches
  Stroke (pain in the arm)

Anatomy

The cell bodies of preganglionic sympathetic fibers to the upper extremities are located in the intermediolateral columns of the spinal cord from T-2 through T-8. The preganglionic fibers exit through the ventral horn, passing through the white rami communicantes to the sympathetic chain. The postganglionic fibers to the arm leave the sympathetic chain via the T-3 (in some patients), T-2, stellate (fusion of the inferior cervical and first thoracic), and middle cervical ganglia (Fig 34F–1). To block all of the sympathetic outflow to the arm, therefore, enough volume must be injected to allow spread of the drug downward to the T-3 level of the chain. Most postganglionic fibers pass through the gray rami communicantes to the nerve roots of C-5 through T-2, although some fibers pass directly from sympathetic ganglia to the subclavian perivascular plexus.

The cervical portion of the sympathetic chain lies anterior to the transverse processes (anterior tubercles) of the cervical vertebrae. At the C-7 level, the chain lies just anterior and in close proximity to the vertebral artery. The artery passes through a foramen posterior to the C-6 anterior tubercle and, at the C-6 level and above, is separated from the chain by bone and longus colli muscle. The C-7 anterior tubercle is a vestigial structure which lies deep to the sympathetic chain and can rarely be palpated, whereas the prominent C-6 anterior tubercle (Chassaignac's tubercle) lies directly behind the chain, is fairly large, and is easily palpable in all but the very obese or muscular individual. The dome of the pleura generally lies in front of the T-1 transverse process and neck of the first rib, but may extend somewhat higher in tall thin individuals. Because of these anatomical relationships, the paratracheal ap-

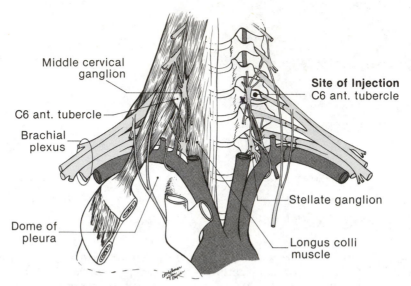

Fig 34F–1.—Anatomy of the stellate ganglion.

proach to the sympathetic chain at C-6 is the easiest and safest technique, with less risk of pneumothorax and vertebral artery injection than lower approaches.

Technique

A stellate ganglion block may be performed with 10 ml 1% lidocaine or mepivacaine, or a mixture of 1% lidocaine with 0.25% bupivacaine.

The equipment used consists of a 10-ml control ring syringe and a 22-gauge, 1½-inch needle.

The area should be antiseptically prepared prior to the block. Because of the proximity of the palpating fingertips to the needle during this block, it is recommended that sterile gloves be worn.

Technique for Needle Placement at the C-6 Transverse Process

1. The patient is positioned supine with the neck slightly extended, but not supported by a pillow. A folded sheet under the shoulders facilitates palpation of the C-6 anterior tubercle in some patients (Figs 34F–2,A and B).

2. The cricoid cartilage is palpated.

3. At the level of the cricoid cartilage, the examiner palpates for the C-6 anterior tubercle at the anterior border of the sternocleidomastoid muscle with the index finger.

4. While retracting the sternocleidomastoid and carotid sheath laterally, the operator positions his index finger firmly on the tip of the C-6 transverse process.

5. The needle is inserted just medial to the tip of the index finger and inserted straight downward (directly posteriorly) until contact is made with the anterior tubercle (about 0.5 cm depth, if firm pressure is maintained with the index finger).

4a. An alternative method involves palpation of the anterior tubercle with both the index and third fingers. The operator retracts the sternocleidomastoid muscle and carotid sheath laterally, with both fingers exerting downward pressure. The tip of the transverse process should be felt between the fingertips.

5a. The needle is introduced between the fingertips and inserted straight downward (posteriorly) until it contacts the anterior tubercle (Figs 34F–2,C and D).

6. The operator aspirates and begins the injection. If resistance to the injection is felt, the needle tip is brought slightly off the tubercle, aspiration is performed, and injection is begun. The patient will usually report shoulder pain during injection. If paresthesia of the arm or hand is elicited, the needle is deep to the anterior tubercle, adjacent to the C-6 or C-7 nerve root, and should be repositioned.

7. The patient sits up for 1–2 minutes after injection to facilitate spread of the drug downward to the upper thoracic ganglia.

Technique for Needle Placement at the C-7 Transverse Process

The technique described utilizes an anterior approach which is paratracheal and requires identification of the C-7 transverse process rather than the classic C-6 (Chassaignac's tubercle) as a bony landmark.

The patient is placed in a semi-Fowler's position (supine with the back raised about 15°). A pillow is placed under the shoulders to allow increased flexion of the head, making the trachea more prominent and the anatomy of the anterior neck more easily discernible.

Chassaignac's tubercle is identified, and a fingerbreadth below it, the index and middle fingers of the palpating hand are inserted between the trachea and carotid sheath, separating these two structures and bringing the skin in closer proximity to the transverse process of C-7 (Fig 34F–3,A, B, and C, Plate 12). It is unnecessary to raise a skin wheal if the 22-gauge short bevel needle is introduced through the skin with a quick sure movement. This elicits no more discomfort than does the skin wheal, and the needle is positioned ready for further advancement to the transverse process.

The needle described is attached to a control syringe containing 8 ml of local anesthetic. The needle is held in a strictly parasagittal plane and advanced slowly for 1–2 cm until the transverse process has been contacted. Advancement of any greater distance probably means that the needle is passing between adjacent transverse processes. The needle is now withdrawn 2 mm and an attempt at aspiration is made to ensure that the tip is not within the vertebral artery. Without movement of the syringe, the entire contents are rapidly injected. If as the injection is commenced a high resistance is encountered, the injection should not proceed, as such resistance probably indicates a periosteal location of the needle tip. The bone should be reengaged, the needle withdrawn 2 mm, aspiration performed, and with the syringe again immobilized, injection is recommenced.

The principal advantages of this lower approach to the stellate ganglion are that a much lower volume of local anesthetic is required, an improved sympathectomy is achieved, and there is a lower incidence of recurrent laryngeal nerve block.

Documentation of Efficacy of Block

In patients with Horner's syndrome, efficacy of the block is indicated by ptosis, pupillary constriction, and enophthalmos (Fig 34F–3,C, Plate 12). Additional facial changes are conjunctival injection, nasal congestion, facial anhidrosis.

In patients with other conditions, efficacy of the block is indicated by an increased skin temperature of the hand on the side of the block (little or no change will be seen if the temperature was above 33° C before the block) and by decreased skin conductivity and abolished sympathogalvanic reflex on the side of the block.

Apart from these general indications of the effects of sympathetic block, the most immediate evidence of a successful block is the patient's subjective experience of a decrease in the pain or other symptoms that warranted the procedure in the first place. These subjective signs are usually immediate or occur within 15–20 minutes of the time the block is initiated. Objective signs include changes in skin color, evidence of arterial pulsation where previously there was none, and absence of sweating on the affected side. The therapeutic effect of stellate ganglion block is high when it is used for the conditions indicated. In conditions such as traumatic reflex sympathetic dystrophy, the sooner the procedure is performed after injury, the higher will be the incidence of complete success. Depending on the chronicity of the condition, some cases may require numerous blocks. There is practically no limit to the number of times stellate ganglion blocks can be performed, which attests to the comparative safety of the procedure.

Complications

The possible complications of stellate ganglion block include vertebral artery injection (manifested by loss of consciousness, possible seizures, hypotension, and apnea), total spinal anesthesia, partial brachial plexus block, pneumothorax (rare with the C-6 approach), recurrent laryngeal nerve block, phrenic nerve block, hematoma, and neuritis.

THORACIC SYMPATHETIC BLOCK

Of all the sympathetic blocks, the thoracic sympathetic block has the most limited application; nev-

Fig 34F–2.—A, surface landmarks and needle position for a stellate ganglion block. Note that the head is well extended. The anesthetist's fingers retract the carotid sheath laterally with the needle at the C-6 level in the paratracheal space. **B,** anterior approach to the stellate ganglion block. Needle is on the transverse process anterior to the prevertebral fascia. Note the lateral displacement of the carotid sheath. **C** and **D,** landmarks and technique of stellate ganglion block at the C-6 level. (From Raj P.P.: Chronic pain, in Raj P.P. (ed.): *Handbook of Regional Anesthesia.* New York, Churchill Livingstone, Inc, 1985. Reproduced by permission.)

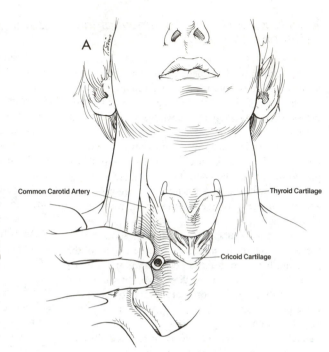

ertheless it has a definite place in the management of certain pain states. It is well described by Adriani[2] and Labat[3] and several accounts appear in the German literature, a notable one being that by Kappis.[8]

Clinically, the procedure is used to control pain in patients with posttraumatic syndrome (T2–3), for reflex sympathetic dystrophy, and for hyperhidrosis (probably the main nonsurgical indication).

While the possibility of prognostic procedures in this region would presuppose the use of a local anesthetic, except in an intractable condition such as reflex sympathetic dystrophy, there is practically no indication for using a local anesthetic block in this region when such procedures can be performed with less hazard by using the less specific thoracic epidural block. The thoracic sympathetic block is therefore limited to conditions where permanent interruption of a specific sympathetic distribution is desired, such as hyperhidrosis affecting the upper extremities.

Anatomy

The sympathetic chain in the thoracic region lies posterolateral to the vertebral bodies and anterior to the necks of the ribs (Fig 34F–4,A, Plate 13). Un-

like the sympathetic chain in the cervical and lumbar regions, which is separated from the roots of the segmental nerves by the longus colli and psoas muscles, respectively, no such effective barrier exists in the thoracic region. Therefore, one must be extremely precise with both needle position and the amount of neurolytic agent used when performing such blocks. Additionally, the immediate lateral relation to the sympathetic chain is the pleura, which poses yet another hazard to the exploring needle.

Technique

The safety of both thoracic and lumbar sympathetic blocks is increased by such a wide margin with the use of an image intensifier that it can be categorically stated, when such equipment is available, these procedures should not be performed without it.

The patient is positioned prone on a radiolucent table (Fig 34F–4,B, Plate 13). The spinous process of T-2 or T-3 is identified, a wheal is made 6 cm from the midline, and a 10-cm needle is introduced in a parasagittal plane until it strikes the transverse process on the same side (Fig 34F–4,C, Plate 13). The needle is withdrawn 0.5–1 cm and angled so as to pass just below the inferior edge of the rib. With

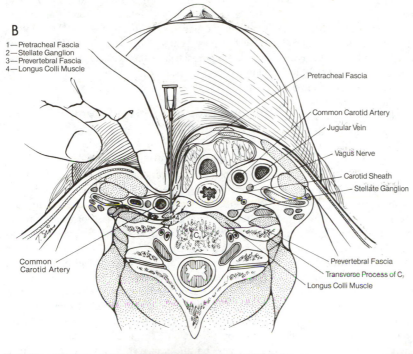

B

1—Pretracheal Fascia
2—Stellate Ganglion
3—Prevertebral Fascia
4—Longus Colli Muscle

Pretracheal Fascia

Common Carotid Artery

Jugular Vein

Vagus Nerve

Carotid Sheath

Stellate Ganglion

Common Carotid Artery

Prevertebral Fascia

Transverse Process of C$_7$

Longus Colli Muscle

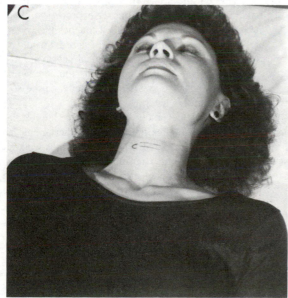

C

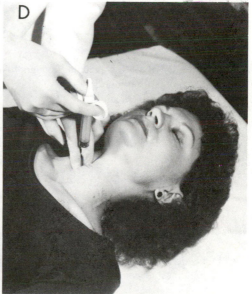

D

the needle maintained in a strict sagittal plane, the vertebral body is contacted about 1 cm deeper. The needle is then redirected slightly to pass by the body, at which point further advancement should be arrested. The image intensifier is positioned laterally and a small amount of Renografin or Conray-420 is injected through the needle. The position of the needle tip is confirmed, and following rotation of the image intensifier through 90°, the tissue plane in which the contrast is situated is identified. Small adjustments of the needle can be made, but only after the position of the tip has been identified with tiny amounts of contrast in each instance.

Phenol is the most satisfactory neurolytic agent to use. It can be prepared with Renografin, in which case the total amount of contrast material required can be kept to a minimum. One should be careful not to use too much contrast or it will distort the tissues and make identification more difficult.

No more than 2 ml of neurolytic agent is required, and it is possible to denervate the ganglion with 1.5 ml. The patient should remain prone for about 30 minutes after the injection. This will minimize posterior spread of the neurolytic solution onto the corresponding spinal nerve root.

Drugs Used

Phenol 6% or 10% dissolved in Renografin or Conray-420 are the most satisfactory solutions for neurolytic blocks in this region.

In the case of intractable reflex sympathetic dystrophy or hyperhidrosis, immediate remission of symptoms will follow injection. However, no neurolytic procedure should be performed without first ascertaining the effects with a prognostic local anesthetic block.

Complications

Complications include somatic nerve block, causalgia, intradural injection, and pneumothorax.

Prognosis

Hyperhidrosis responds particularly well to a thoracic sympathetic block, with the symptoms remitting for more than 3 years. In bilateral conditions such as hyperhidrosis, the effects of a unilateral procedure must be assessed over a 2-month period be-

fore a block on the other side is attempted. With the aid of the image intensifier, and particularly in younger patients, a thoracic sympathetic block is a far more benign procedure to perform than an axillary approach to a thoracic surgical sympathectomy.

Technique of Thoracic Sympathetic Chain Block

The thoracic sympathetic chain lies much more posteriorly on the vertebral bodies than its lumbar sympathetic component. It is difficult if not impossible to selectively produce sympathetic blockade without risking spillover onto the corresponding somatic nerves emerging from the paravertebral foramen (Fig 34F–5). The needle is inserted 2.5 cm from the midline at the vertebral level required. The classic technique is to introduce the needle at a right angle to the skin and lateral to the spine at the vertebral level above the one to be blocked, or two vertebral levels above the one to be blocked in the midthoracic region. The needle is inserted until it impinges on the transverse process and then is walked caudally off the transverse process with a medial angle and dropped until it touches the vertebral body at an additional depth of approximately 1 cm. A small bolus of 2–3 cc of local anesthetic injected at this site will anesthetize the thoracic sympathetic chain, but may well spill over onto the somatic nerve at this level.

An alternative technique is to introduce the needle in the paramedian area until it strikes the lamina of the vertebra level desired. Then the needle is walked laterally off the lamina into the paravertebral space and advanced until contact with the vertebral body is achieved. The block proceeds as above.

Indications

The thoracic sympathetic chain block is done for pain conditions in the thorax, and especially for the recent onset of herpes zoster pain, both as a means of acute pain relief and prophylactically to prevent the appearance of postherpetic neuralgia.

A sympathetic nerve block in this area can also afford analgesia of the intrathoracic viscera that may be involved in neoplastic or other painful processes. Although it can afford pain relief in chronic postherpetic neuralgia, it is rarely curative when the disease has progressed to this stage.

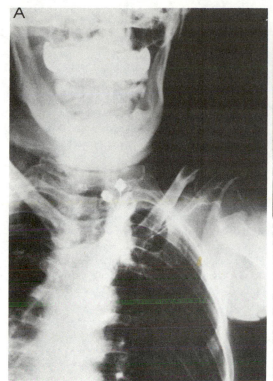
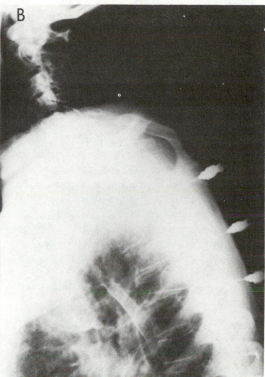

Fig 34F–5.—Anteroposterior **(A)** and lateral **(B)** views of needles on the thoracic sympathetic chain. In the lateral view the tips of the spinal needles are posterior to the anterior edge of the vertebrae. The AP view shows the spread of contrast material through the needles on the thoracic sympathetic chain.

Difficulties

The main problem with this block is the possibility of pneumothorax because of the close proximity of the pleural reflections to the needle target zone. Even when the block is performed by experienced personnel, a 4% incidence of pneumothorax can be expected. Because of proximity to the paravertebral nerve and paravertebral foramen, spread to that nerve and even misplacement of the needle into the paravertebral foramen with subsequent epidural and/or subarachnoid spread of injectate is possible.

SPLANCHNIC NERVE AND CELIAC PLEXUS BLOCK

The main visceral sympathetic innervation can be interrupted either above or below the diaphragm. Both routes of denervation have been described during the past 70 years. Most recently Boas[5] has re-emphasized the splanchnic approach, which was first described in part by Bonica,[6] while Moore[7] has promoted the use of the celiac plexus block, originally described by Kappis in 1919.[8]

While both techniques have their applications, splanchnic nerve block is probably the most suitable block for visceral pain states, particularly when a degree of lateralization can be obtained by the technique, whereas with celiac plexus block the spread of neurolytic solution is not limited to one side or the other, and the result is less discriminate.

Indications

DIAGNOSTIC.—A splanchnic nerve block or a celiac plexus block may be performed to distinguish sympathetic from somatic pain components, or, with a local anesthetic, to determine whether a satisfactory response will follow a permanent neurolytic block.

THERAPEUTIC.—These blocks may be performed as treatment for intractable visceral pain states, such as chronic pancreatic pain or visceral malignancy.

Anatomy

The sympathetic rami of T5–12 run a long course down the lateral aspect of the vertebral bodies to form the greater, lesser, and least splanchnic nerves. At the upper border of T-12 they are both superior and posterior to the diaphragmatic crura when they pass forward in this supracrural space and abruptly enter the right and left crura of the diaphragm to enter the abdomen, where they divide to become components of the celiac plexus (Fig 34F–6). These nerves can be blocked in the left and right supracrural compartments from behind, or by passing a needle forward to block the celiac plexus below the diaphragm.

Technique

The patient is placed prone on a radiolucent table. The point of needle insertion is at the lower margin of the 12th rib, where a line through the transverse process of L-1 is drawn (Fig 34F–7). This point should be 8 cm from the midline. Unless a unilateral splanchnic nerve block is to be performed, after adequate infiltration with local anesthetic, two 15-cm, 20-gauge parasympathectomy needles are inserted, both cephalad and medially below the 12th rib on each side. For a splanchnic block the needle is aimed at the body of T-12, whereas for a celiac plexus block the needle is directed toward the body of L-1. The projection of the image intensifier should initially be in an anteroposterior direction to confirm the correct vertebral level, after which the final adjustments for both blocks should be made from a lateral projection to ensure the proper relationship between the needle tips and the vertebral bodies.

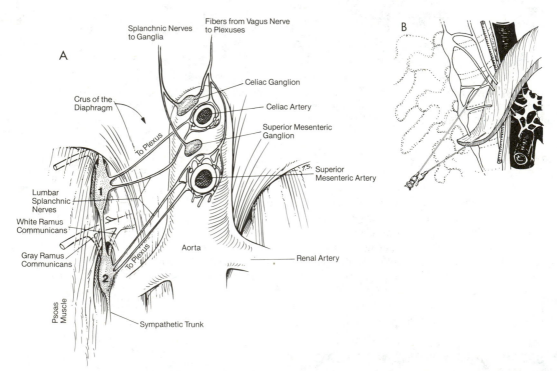

Fig 34F–6.—A, formation of the celiac plexus. (From Raj P.P.: Chronic pain, in Raj P.P. (ed.): *Handbook of Regional Anesthesia.* New York, Churchill Livingstone, Inc, 1985. Reproduced by permission.) *Inset* shows periaortic and preaortic relationship of the celiac plexus to the celiac artery, indicating connection to the sympathetic ganglion and vagus. **B,** needle positions for splanchnic and celiac plexus blocks.

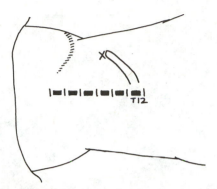

Fig 34F–7.—Landmarks for the technique of celiac plexus block by the Kappis method. The patient is prone and the point of entry is along the 12th rib, 8 cm lateral to the L-1 spinous process.

For a splanchnic nerve block, the needle tip should appear 0.5 cm dorsal from the anterior margin of the vertebral body. For a celiac plexus block, the needle tip should lie 2 cm anterior to the anterior margin of the vertebral body.

A small amount of contrast material should be injected through each needle and its dispersion observed radiographically (Fig 34F–8). Alternatively, if a neurolytic block is performed, a pre-prepared solution of phenol dissolved in Renografin or Conray can be used, in which case not only is the location of the injection confirmed, but also its ultimate dispersion in the correct compartment is monitored during injection.

Although alcohol has long been a standard solution for block of the celiac plexus, it precludes the concomitant use of radiographic contrast media because it is not compatible with these substances, and in addition it elicits so much pain that it is frequently necessary to anesthetize the patient beforehand.

The other advantage of using a phenol contrast medium solution is that a permanent roentgenogram can be taken in each case.

Drugs Used

For diagnostic blocks, 10 ml of 0.5% lidocaine injected on each side will block visceral pain afferents in splanchnic blocks. This agent is satisfactory for use when the procedure is to be immediately followed by a neurolytic block. If, however, a longer block is desired so that the patient may experience the effects of pain relief for an extended period, a 1% etidocaine or 0.5% bupivacaine solution should be substituted. For blocks of the celiac plexus, 25 ml of solution is required on each side. Phenol 10% in Renografin 76 is a stable mixture and is recommended as the agent of choice.

Complications

Hypotension is more common with celiac block. Hypotension can be avoided if a fluid load with lactated Ringer's solution is given prior to injection. A tendency for hypotension may last 2–3 years in ambulant patients.

Pleuritic pain may occur and last 2–3 days, but it is self-limiting. Increased gut motility may produce frequent stools during the first week after the block.

Neurovascular or intrathecal injection is possible but can always be avoided if an image intensifier and contrast-containing solutions are used.

LUMBAR SYMPATHETIC BLOCK

Sympathectomy in this region has been performed ever since Hunter and Royle[9] showed that the skin temperature of the extremity could be increased by surgical sympathectomy. The first description of a percutaneous sympathectomy by Mandl in 1926 followed a similar approach to the celiac ganglion reported by Kappis 12 years earlier.[10, 11]

Anatomy

In the lumbar region the sympathetic chain lies on the anterolateral side of the vertebral bodies and is separated from the somatic nerve roots by the psoas muscle. The inferior vena cava lies just anterior to the right sympathetic chain, while the aorta lies anterior and slightly medial to the chain on the left. Several small lumbar arteries and veins lie adjacent to the sympathetics (Fig 34F–9).

The preganglionic fibers that supply the lower extremities arise from cell bodies located in the T-10 through L-2 levels of the spinal cord. Nearly all of the postganglionic fibers to the leg leave the sympathetic chain at or below L-2. A small volume of local anesthetic deposited at the L-2 level of the lumbar chain should therefore totally block the sympathetic outflow to the lower extremity.

The rami communicantes have a long course to run from the ganglion and lie between the perios-

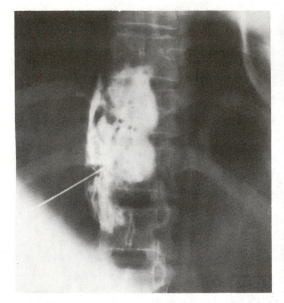

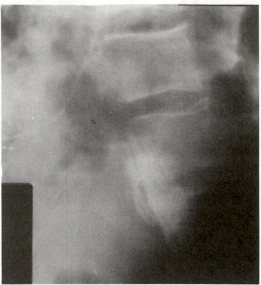

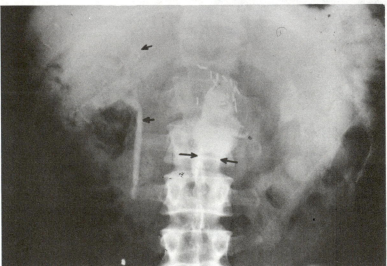

Fig 34F–8.—AP (*top left*) and lateral (*top right*) views of needle positions for celiac plexus block. Note the spread of dye in the AP view—up and down toward the 11th vertebra. In the lateral view the needles lie 1–1½ cm anterior to the anterior edge of the vertebral body. *Bottom*, note the contrast material injected in the vascular space during the celiac plexus block. This radiograph, taken 5 minutes after the injection, lights up the renal pelvis, which confirms the vascular injection.

teum of the vertebral bodies and the fibrous arch on the side of each body which gives rise to the origin of the psoas muscle. This tunnel is a possible route for the posterior migration of neurolytic solutions to the somatic nerve root, causing neuritis. Anteriorly, the visceral peritoneum and the great vessels form important adjacent structures.

Indications and Prognosis

Sympathetic blocks in the lumbar region benefit the following conditions: sympathetic dystrophies, peripheral vascular disease, pelvic and lower abdominal malignancy, and miscellaneous conditions.

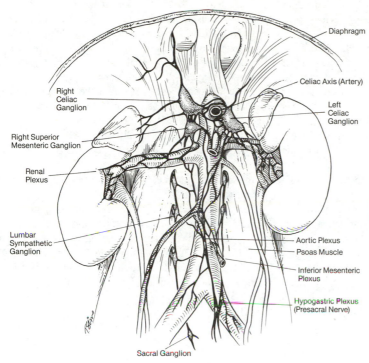

- Diaphragm
- Celiac Axis (Artery)
- Right Celiac Ganglion
- Left Celiac Ganglion
- Right Superior Mesenteric Ganglion
- Renal Plexus
- Lumbar Sympathetic Ganglion
- Aortic Plexus
- Psoas Muscle
- Inferior Mesenteric Plexus
- Hypogastric Plexus (Presacral Nerve)
- Sacral Ganglion

Fig 34F—9.—Formation of the lumbar sympathetic chain and its connections to the preaortic and periaortic plexus by the postganglionic fibers.

SYMPATHETIC DYSTROPHIES.—Complete remission of symptoms can be obtained in most of these disorders.

VASCULAR INSUFFICIENCY.—The ischemic pain of vascular insufficiency disappears as soon as the sympathetic block is performed. The local ischemic changes are arrested, and development of a collateral circulation soon follows.

PELVIC AND LOWER ABDOMINAL MALIGNANCY.—Patients with these conditions may benefit from sympathectomy both because of relief of any vasospastic or ischemic element and because of interruption of visceral pain afferents traveling with the sympathetic fibres. The principal advantage of sympathetic blocks over epidural or spinal neurolytic procedures is the preservation of somatic function.

MISCELLANEOUS.—Patients with the postherpetic syndrome or phantom limb pain sometimes benefit from sympathetic blocks. There is nothing to lose in doing the procedure when such conditions have proved refractory to other treatment. In fact, both conditions have elements of reflex sympathetic dystrophy, and these components often respond to sympathetic block. Intractable neurogenic back pain also has associated elements of sympathetic dys-

function which can be relieved by lumbar sympathetic blocks. The normalization of this function often makes the difference between an ambulatory and an inert existence.

Drugs and Equipment

The requisite equipment includes a 5-inch (6-inch for large or obese patients), 20-gauge needle with a security bead, or a 20-gauge BD longdwell catheter, and a 10-cc syringe.

The block is performed with a 1% lidocaine or mepivacaine solution containing Renografin 76, or with 0.5% marcaine.

Technique

Two techniques are described, the classic technique of Mandl, and a lateral approach similar to that described by Reid et al.[10, 12]

Classic Approach

The patient is placed prone over a firm bolster or cushion on a radiolucent table. The spinous processes of L-2, L-3, and L-4 are identified. Skin wheals are raised 4 cm lateral to these spinous processes.

Starting at L-2, a 22-gauge spinal needle is used to infiltrate a track of local anesthetic between the skin and transverse process. The needle is then walked off the inferior border and advanced until it contacts the body of the vertebra (Fig 34F–10). This procedure allows relatively pain-free introduction of the 20-gauge sympathectomy needle, which is put through the same motions before it contacts the body of the vertebra.

The same procedure is repeated for the other two needles at L-3 and L-4.

The image intensifier should be used to verify the depth and relationship of each needle to the vertebral bodies. Both lateral and anteroposterior projections must be used. If the position of each needle is satisfactory, it is in turn redirected to pass lateral to the vertebral body. A small 2-ml syringe full of air is attached and the loss-of-resistance test is carried out while the needle is advanced through the body

of the psoas muscle. As soon as the needle tip escapes the muscle, a positive test should identify the plane in which the sympathetic chain is lying. With each needle tip observed from a lateral projection of the large intensifier, a small amount of radiopaque material is injected through each needle. Whether the injection has been made into the correct retroperitoneal place can be readily confirmed. Only small adjustments will be necessary to ensure optimal positioning of the needle. Both AP and lateral projections are necessary to ensure a correct depth of the needle, its lateral relationship to the vertebral body, and the correct spread of injectate through each needle (Fig 34F–11).

The lateral view should be used during therapeutic injection. The contrast material appears as a linear opacity along the anterolateral aspect of the vertebral bodies. It is possible to achieve a three-vertebral-body spread through one needle when it is correctly placed. An AP projection will show the solution spreading along the line of the psoas muscle (Fig 34F–12).

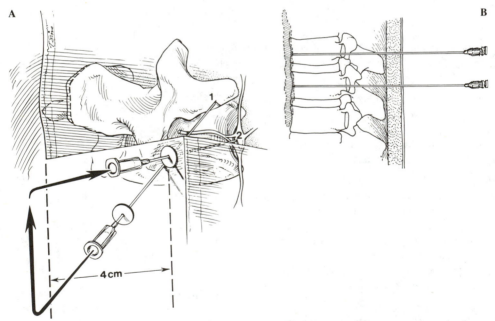

Fig 34F–10.—Lumbar sympathetic block: classic or paramedian approach. **A,** *1,* the needle touches the transverse process. An equal distance is measured on the needle before it is withdrawn to the subcutaneous tissue. *2,* it is then inserted deep to the transverse process to the measured distance, until it slips off the vertebral body. **B,** lateral view of the needle position for lumbar sympathetic block with spread of the solution anterior to the vertebral bodies. (From Raj P.P.: Chronic pain, in Raj P.P. (ed.): *Handbook of Regional Anesthesia.* New York, Churchill Livingstone, Inc., 1985. Reproduced by permission.)

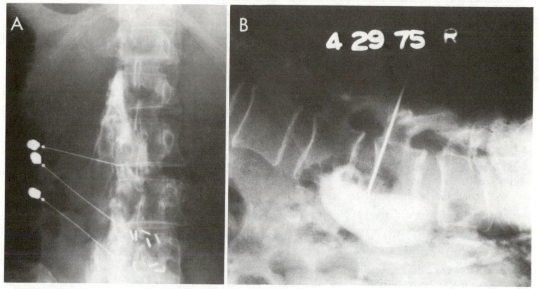

Fig 34F–11.—A, radiograph, AP view, demonstrating multiple needle placements on the lumbar sympathetic chain and the spread of contrast material from each needle. **B,** lateral view demonstrating spread of 10 mls of contrast material with a single needle during the performance of the lumbar sympathetic block.

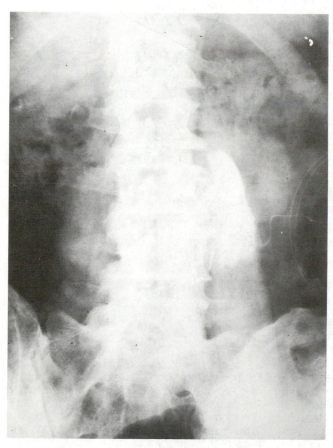

Fig 34F–12.—Anteroposterior view of the contrast material spreading from the lumbar sympathetic chain over the psoas muscle.

673

Reid Technique (recommended)

Single Needle Technique

1. The patient is placed supine, with the table flexed slightly or with a pillow under the patient's abdomen to place the spine in a position of flexion.

2. A line is drawn along the lower border of the 12th rib on the side to be blocked.

3. A second line is drawn 10 cm lateral to the middle of the spine and parallel to the spine, to intersect the first line. The point of intersection will be directly lateral to the L-2 spinous process (Fig 34F–13).

4. A point 8 cm from the midline at the level of the L-2 vertebral body is marked (as described above). This is the point through which the needle is introduced. Introduction of the needle more laterally at the L-2 or L-3 level may result in renal trauma.

5. The skin is prepared with antiseptic solution.

6. A skin wheal is raised at the point described in step 4.

7. The needle is introduced at a 45° angle from the sagittal plane and advanced medially. At a depth of approximately 3½ inches, the vertebral body will be encountered. The transverse process may be encountered more superficially (e.g., 2–2½ inch depth), in which case the needle should be introduced at a slightly lower level. If the intervertebral disk is encountered, the needle is withdrawn and readvanced in a slightly cephalad direction.

8. The needle is retracted to the subcutaneous tissue and advanced at a slightly steeper angle. If the

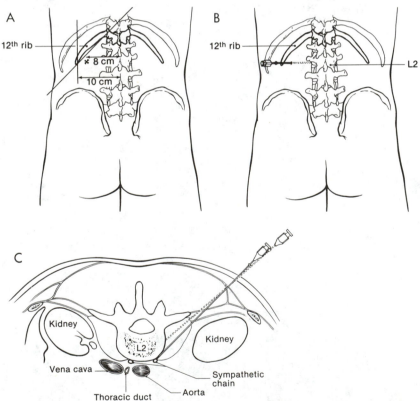

Fig 34F–13.—Reid's technique of lumbar sympathetic block. **A,** with the patient prone, a line is drawn along the lower border of the 12th rib. A second line is dropped 10 cm lateral and parallel to the middle of the spine. The lines will intersect at the L-2 spine. The point of entry of the needle is 8 cm from the L-2 spine at this level. **B,** needle in position. **C,** initially the needle is advanced anteriorly at a 45° angle. It will touch the vertebral body. The needle is withdrawn to the skin and reinserted more acutely 1 inch deeper than the initial insertion to lie at the anterior lateral surface of the vertebral body.

body is still encountered, the needle is retracted and advanced at still steeper angle.

9. When the proper needle angle is achieved, the tip of the needle will be felt to slide with some resistance along the anterolateral surface of the vertebral body. As the tip passes just anterior to the body, a decreased resistance to its movement will be felt. Advancement should be stopped at that point. In most patients the needle tip will be at a depth of 4–4½ inches (Fig 34F–14).

10. The operator aspirates carefully, injects 1 ml of local anesthetic to clear the needle of possible clots or debris, and aspirates again. Then 10 ml of 1% lidocaine or 1% mepivacaine is injected. If a more prolonged block is desired, 0.5% bupivacaine may be substituted.

Two Needle Technique

With the patient lying prone on a radiolucent table, as described for the Reid technique, surface markings are made opposite the L-3 and L-4 vertebrae approximately 10 cm from the midline. Local anesthetic is infiltrated through the fascial layers at these two points. Two 20-gauge sympathectomy needles are passed at an angle of 60° to the parasagittal plane toward and until in contact with the anterolateral aspect of each vertebral body. By using the image intensifier, this can be accomplished rapidly and almost painlessly. An AP view is now required to ensure that the needles lie 0.5 cm medial from the outer edge of the vertebral bodies. A lateral view is used for final adjustments to ensure alignment of the needle tips with the anterior margin

of each body. Catheters can be placed unilaterally or bilaterally for diagnostic and therapeutic indications. These may allow longer periods of monitoring prior to neurolytic blocks (Fig 34F–15).

Documentation of Efficacy of Block

INCREASED SKIN TEMPERATURE OF THE FOOT.—The plantar aspect of the big toe is a convenient site to monitor skin temperature. If the needle is correctly positioned, there will be a dramatic rise in skin temperature, beginning within 3 minutes of the time of injection. A final skin temperature of 34°–35° C signifies complete sympathetic denervation (such temperatures are rarely achieved in patients with peripheral vascular disease).

DECREASED SKIN CONDUCTIVITY AND LOSS OF SYMPATHOGALVANIC REFLEX.—If evidence of sympathetic denervation does not occur within 5 minutes, the needle should be repositioned and the injection repeated. If only partial sympathetic denervation occurs, injection of additional volume will usually produce complete blockade. If not, the block should be repeated at the L-3 level.

Comment on Drugs Used

Lidocaine 1% is a suitable local anesthetic to use for diagnostic purposes. However, if a more prolonged block is needed or if one is attempting to break the cycle of pain, i.e., the procedure is not so much a pharmacologic one but rather one that aims

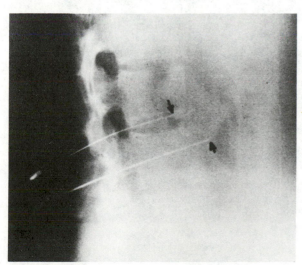

Fig 34F–14.—Upper needle lies just short of a correct position on the lumbar sympathetic chain. Injection of a local anesthetic or contrast material would most likely be in the psoas muscle. The lower needle is in the correct position in the retroperitoneal space.

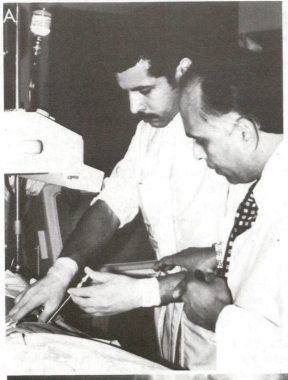

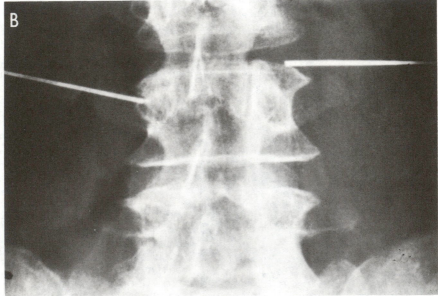

Fig 34F–15.—A, placement of a 6-inch extracatheter (longdwell BD) on the lumbar sympathetic chain. **B,** correct placement of catheters on the lumbar sympathetic chain bilaterally for prolonged analgesia.

to interrupt a neurophysiologic process by pharmacologic means, then an agent such as 1% etidocaine or 0.5% bupivacaine should be used.

When a semipermanent block is to be used in the treatment of intractable pain from cancer or vascular insufficiency, a neurolytic solution is indicated.

Phenol, either 6% in water or 10% in glycerin, is satisfactory. A very stable solution of phenol in Renografin 76 allows both visualization and therapeutic injection to be carried out with one solution.

Complications

Complications of a lumbar sympathetic block include intravascular injection, subarachnoid injection, lumbar somatic nerve block, thoracic duct puncture, renal trauma, and orthostatic hypotension (more likely with bilateral block).

The most common problem immediately following sympathectomy (subfascial or chemical) is a dysesthetic pain, usually in the L1–2 distribution. The pain manifests as a cutaneous hypersensitivity over the inner thigh and groin. It is exacerbated by heat or cold, and most often resolves within 6 weeks. When protracted, it can be treated by a further local anesthetic sympathetic block or by a lidocaine infusion, 150–200 mg given over a 5-minute period, which will produce either a permanent remission or one lasting hours or days, when the therapeutic procedure should be repeated. Retroperitoneal hemorrhage can occur and is commonly associated with anticoagulation therapy that is started after the neurolytic block.

Neurolytic Lumbar Sympathetic Block

If chemical sympathectomy is to be performed, the procedure described for a local anesthetic block should be followed as outlined above. After injection of local anesthetic, the following steps should be undertaken.

1. The efficacy of the block (a rise in skin temperature) should be documented.

2. After at least 20 minutes with the needle still in place, the operator should make sure no sensory or motor block has occurred (local anesthetic will occasionally spread posteriorly to the upper lumbar nerve roots).

3. The needle position is checked radiographically. A lateral view is used to ensure that the needle tip is anterior to the L-2 vertebral body (1 or 2 ml of contrast material may be injected. This should spread in a thin layer along the anterior surface of the vertebral bodies.)

4. Five milliliters of 6% aqueous phenol is injected.

5. The needle is flushed with 1 ml of normal saline or local anesthetic before it is withdrawn.

The catheter placement technique is described in chapter 36.

Intravenous Regional Guanethidine Injection[13]

1. A pneumatic tourniquet is placed on the thigh or upper arm.

2. An IV catheter is inserted into a distal vein. An obturator is inserted into the catheter and taped in place (Fig 34F–16).

3. The extremity is elevated and wrapped in an Esmarch bandage (the limb may be elevated, unwrapped, for 2 minutes if it is extremely sensitive).

4. The tourniquet is inflated and the Esmarch bandage removed.

5. The operator injects 10 mg of guanethidine and 500 IU of heparin in 25 ml of normal saline for the upper extremity, or 20 mg of guanethidine and 1,000 IU of heparin in 50 ml of normal saline for the lower extremity.

6. The tourniquet is deflated after 10 minutes.

7. Blood pressure is checked immediately after cuff deflation and at 30-second intervals for several minutes. Transient hypertension may occur, but a slight fall in blood pressure is usually seen. Significant hypotension should be treated with IV fluids and the patient should be placed in the Trendelenburg position. If a vasopressor is needed, one that acts directly should be selected, as norepinephrine depletion at the adrenergic nerve terminal occurs. Severe burning pain may occur soon after injection, and patients should be aware of the possibility. The pain usually subsides within 2–3 minutes.

Intravenous Regional Reserpine Injection[14]

Essentially the same procedure is followed as described for guanethidine, except that 1 mg of reserpine is used for the upper extremity and 1.5 mg is used for the lower extremity, instead of the guanethidine. Higher doses have been reported, but we have

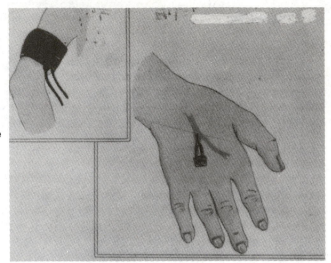

Fig 34F–16.—Technique of IV regional anesthesia for reserpine and guanethidine injections.

seen two cases of delayed orthostatic syncope develop even with the lower doses. Hypotension should be treated as described for hypotension following guanethidine injection.

Intra-arterial Reserpine Injection[15, 16]

A 23- or 25-gauge needle and a 5-ml syringe are required. For injection into an upper extremity, 1 mg of reserpine is diluted to 5 ml in normal saline. For injection into a lower extremity, 1.5 mg of reserpine is diluted to 5 ml in normal saline.

The total dose of reserpine is injected into the axillary, brachial, or femoral artery.

A venous tourniquet inflated to slightly below diastolic pressure may be applied above the painful portion of the limb and kept inflated for 5 minutes. Heparin (500 IU) should be added to the injectate if the tourniquet is used. As with IV regional reserpine injection, hypotension may occur, but its onset may be delayed by several hours.

EVALUATION OF EFFECTIVENESS OF SYMPATHETIC BLOCKADE

For a precise evaluation of diagnostic, prognostic, and therapeutic blockade, it is important to decide precisely and objectively if the sympathetic nerve system really has been blocked. The performance of some tests certifying this effect is advisable. Several ways may be used. One can, for example, measure changes in muscle blood flow, changes in tempera-

ture of the skin, oscillometric and rheographic changes, changes in sweating, and the sympathogalvanic reflex. In clinical situations, the anesthesiologist is for practical purposes limited to tests that require minimal time and the smallest possible apparatus to perform. Some methods that have proved useful and practicable are mentioned below.

Verification of the effectiveness of a block is done by combined measurement of the skin temperature and the sympathogalvanic reflex. Obviously, both tests must be done before and after the block. For correct evaluation, testing of both extremities is mandatory. This is the best way to get reliable and reproducible results.

Measurement of skin temperature is possible by using any electric thermometer if an appropriate skin electrode is applied. This apparatus measures superficial skin temperature rather than percutaneous temperature. In anticipation of such measurement, the patient's extremities should be exposed to an environment where a constant air temperature is established. All measurements must be done on the same spots of the extremity.

On the upper extremity the skin temperature should be measured at the shoulder, on the flexor side of the forearm, on the back of the hand, and on the thumb. On the lower extremity the temperature is measured on the thigh (10–15 cm above the knee), on the medial side of the leg, on the back of the foot, and on the big toe. To ensure that the skin temperature before and after the sympathetic block is always measured in the same area, these areas should be marked beforehand. Because modern electrothermometers can measure the skin temperature within 10–20 seconds, the time necessary for a comparative measurement of the skin temperature is not more than 1–2 minutes.

The sympathogalvanic reflex reflects electrical activity in the skin. Other names for this reflex include the galvanic skin reaction, the electrodermal reaction, the psychogalvanic reflex, and skin conductance.

In 1955 Lewis described the sympathogalvanic reflex as follows:

1. The reflex reaction is conducted by efferent fibers of the sympathetic chain.

2. All sensory stimuli (e.g., noise, pinprick or bright light), physiologic factors (e.g., Valsalva maneuver), or emotional stimuli (e.g., loud noise or swear words) are capable of initiating this reflex. The reflex can be provoked only as long as nerve conduction in the sympathetic chain is intact.

3. Special cells surrounding the sweat glands in the skin are responsible for the changes in electrical activity of the skin. This is more or less a sudden change in skin resistance.

To measure the sympathogalvanic reflex, a two-channel ECG recorder with unipolar electrodes is necessary. Instead of using normal ECG electrodes it is advisable to use special electrodes, which can be produced by every technician. With the special electrodes, it is much easier for the paramedical personnel to adapt the technical performance.

For registration of the sympathogalvanic reflex, either on the upper or lower extremity, two electrodes are applied on the back or plantar region of the hand or foot, respectively. The patient should close his eyes and rest for several minutes during absolute silence in the room.

By whistling or clapping his hands, or, in "difficult" cases, by using pinprick, examiner can easily provoke the sympathogalvanic reflex. On the ECG recorder one can see the typical wave form of the reflex. The changes from the baseline are in the range of 1–3 m V. For practical reasons, the transportation velocity of the ECG paper should be 10 or 12.5 mm/sec. At higher speeds, evaluation of the sympathogalvanic reflex seems to be more difficult.

Before lumbar or cervical sympathetic blockade the sympathogalvanic reflex should be recorded on the side to be blocked as well as on the side which remains unblocked. In many cases the sympathogalvanic reflex cannot be provoked by different stimuli. In these cases certain drugs, especially depressive drugs, should be omitted. In a high percentage of cases the sympathogalvanic reflex cannot be recorded following the intake of barbiturates, opiates,

or other centrally depressive drugs. If patients can tolerate a drug-free period of at least 48 hours before the sympathogalvanic reflex is measured, this should always be aimed at. In addition, the reflex is often negative in diabetic patients. In many cases only a weak response (1 mV) of the sympathogalvanic reflex can be recorded.

After blockade of the sympathetic nerve the examiner should wait at least 20–30 minutes before measuring the sympathogalvanic reflex. At the same time the skin temperature should be measured. A negative reflex on the blocked side is an indication that conduction of the sympathetic chain has been interrupted.

Simultaneous recording of skin temperature and sympathogalvanic reflex allows an evaluation of the effectiveness of sympathetic blockades. One can decide if one should apply a series of sympathetic blockades, use neurolytic agents, or even perform surgery on the sympathetic chain. Thus, the simultaneous measurement of skin temperature and sympathogalvanic reflex allows one not only to confirm the technical application of the block, but also to ascertain the effectiveness of a temporary or long-term sympathetic block.

A difference in skin temperature of 2° C or more between the blocked and unblocked side and a negative reflex are the important criteria (Figs 34F–17 through 34F–19).

1. If the skin temperature on the blocked side increases and the sympathogalvanic reflex becomes negative, a positive effect for the patient following interruption of the sympathetic function can be expected.

2. If the reflex becomes negative and the difference in skin temperature does not change, sympathetic interruption cannot be expected.

3. An increasing skin temperature and a positive remaining reflex indicate that a part of the sympathetic chain is blocked and the skin blood flow is increased. In the lumbar area a positive reflex with an increasing difference in skin temperature may be caused by a bypass of the sympathetic chain in this area. The remaining sympathetic activity is caused by accessory ganglia in the psoas muscles.

4. If the skin temperature does not change and the sympathogalvanic reflex remains positive, the only decision which can be made is that the block is ineffective because of technical failures. In these cases the block should be repeated, and a new determination of changes in skin temperature and sympathogalvanic reflex should be made.

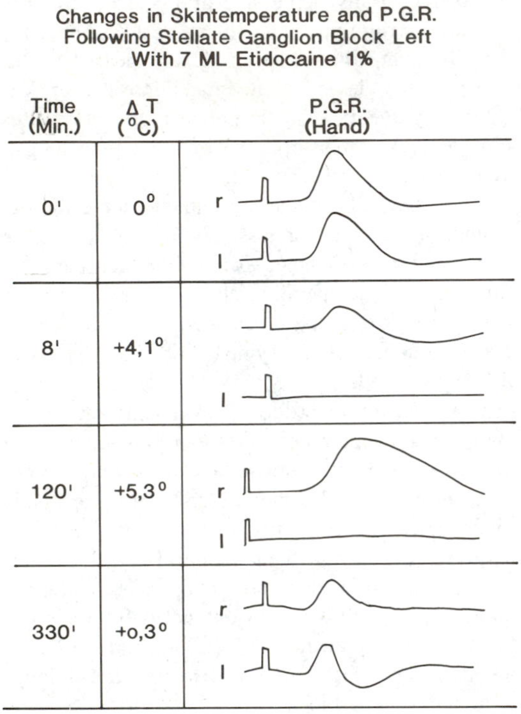

Changes in Skintemperature and P.G.R.
Following Stellate Ganglion Block Left
With 7 ML Etidocaine 1%

Time (Min.)	Δ T (°C)	P.G.R. (Hand)
0'	0°	r ⌐ l ⌐
8'	+4,1°	l
120'	+5,3°	r l
330'	+0,3°	r l

Fig 34F–17.—Changes in skin temperature and sympathogalvanic reflex *(PGR)* following stellate ganglion block with 7 ml of 1% etidocaine. *r,* right; *l,* left.

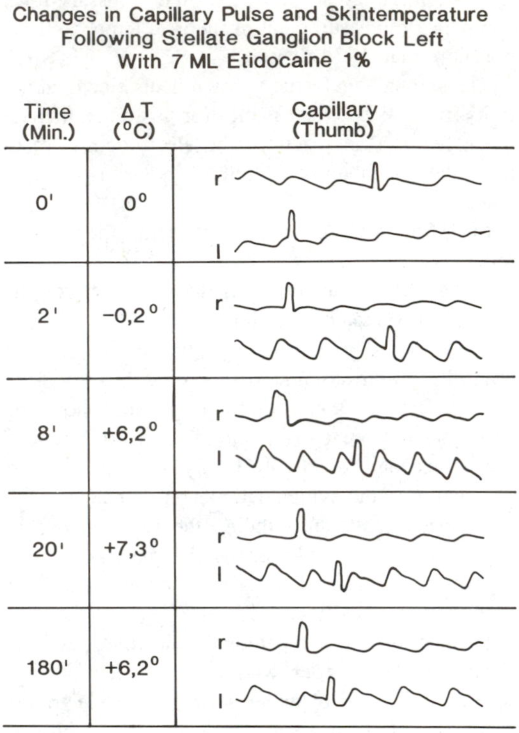

For better understanding of the evaluation of sympathetic blockade, Figure 34E–19 surveys the different possibilities of a change in skin temperature with respect to a change in sympathogalvanic reflex.

If a determination of the skin temperature or the sympathogalvanic reflex is not possible, one could use changes in capillary pulsation instead as an alternative to the measurement of skin temperature differences (see Fig 34–18).

Finally, these measurements could be used for prognostic purposes before surgical or chemical sympathectomy is performed.

Other Methods of Assessment

Sweat Test

NINHIDRIN TEST.—This test relies on the change of color to yellow as the chemical reacts with the protein in sweat. It is very accurate and can

Changes in Capillary Pulse and Skintemperature
Following Stellate Ganglion Block Left
With 7 ML Etidocaine 1%

Time (Min.)	Δ T (°C)	Capillary (Thumb)
0'	0°	r l
2'	-0,2°	r l
8'	+6,2°	r l
20'	+7,3°	r l
180'	+6,2°	r l

Fig 34F–18.—Changes in capillary pulse and skin temperature following stellate ganglion block with 7 ml of 1% etidocaine.

be used to determine the segments blocked on the trunk.

COBALT BLUE.—Filter papers soaked in cobalt blue are dried and kept in a dessicator prior to use. The color changes from blue to pink in the presence of sweat.

Evaluation of Sympathetic Nerve Block

Δ Skintemp.	P.G.R.	Effect
↑	∅	+ + +
=	∅	∅
↑	+	+ ("Psoas Ganglion")
=	+	No Block

↑ Increase ∅ Negative
= Unchanged + Positive

Fig 34F–19.—Techniques of evaluating efficacy of sympathetic nerve block.

Blood Flow Measurements

Indirect Doppler measurements of blood pressure by occlusion of blood flow in upper and lower limbs can be used to determine reactivity of blood vessels to sympathetic block. Cuffs are placed on upper limb and ankle. The ankle to brachial blood pressure index is calculated as follows:

$$\text{Ankle} \quad \frac{\text{Syst.}}{\text{Diast.}}$$

$$\text{Brachial} \quad \frac{\text{Syst.}}{\text{Diast.}}$$

before and after sympathetic block.

Impedance plethysmography is a useful and reproducible procedure that correlates changes in electrical impedance with flow changes.

Electromagnetic flow probes can be placed directly on blood vessels during surgery. The ultrasound probes are extremely small and can be left in situ for days. The effects of sympathectomy can be very accurately monitored by this means.

Venous occlusion plethysmography using Whitney mercury in Silastic strain gauges can be used to determine blood flow in muscle in both forearm and leg.

Clearance techniques utilizing xenon can be used to determine skin blood flow.

Small skin thermistors are probably the most widely used device for monitoring the success of sympathetic blocks. The apparatus is comparatively cheap and little interpretation is required, although the observer is cautioned to make sure that measurements are made in a room of a temperature of at least 25° C; otherwise environmental temperature extremes will negate the accuracy and interpretation of the readings.

Pain Assessment

A number of tests, mostly subjective, have been designed to determine the nature and intensity of pain. Psychological screening tests may be employed in an attempt to establish the patient's personality and behavioral reaction to a chronic pain state. However, a measure of the pain relative to a ''standard'' pain such as that obtained by a tourniquet can be used for comparison and expressed as a ratio, the so-called tourniquet ratio.

The pain estimate is a simple test and merely relies on the patient's subjective assessment of pain by asking the patient to assign a number from 0–100 expressing the severity of the pain. On this scale 0 indicates no pain, and 100 indicates the worst possible pain the patient can experience. Both psychological screening tests and pain scales can be used before and after a diagnostic or therapeutic block to determine the efficacy of the block.

REFERENCES

1. Leriche R., Fontain R.: L'anesthesie isolee du ganglion etoile: Sa technique, ses indications, ses resultatas. *Presse Med.* 42:849, 1953.
2. Bonica J.J.: *Management of Pain.* Philadelphia, Lea & Febiger, 1953.
3. Labat G.: *Regional Anesthesia: Its Technique and Clinical Application.* Philadelphia, W.B. Saunders Co., 1924.
4. McLean A.P.H., Mulligan G.W., Otton P., et al.: Hemodynamic alterations associated with epidural anesthesia. *Surgery* 62:79, 1967.
5. Boas R.A.: Sympathetic block in clinical practice. *Int. Anesthesiol. Clin.,* vol. 16, No. 4, 1978.
6. Bonica J.J.: *Clinical Applications of Diagnostic and Therapeutic Nerve Blocks.* Springfield, Ill., Charles C Thomas, Publisher, 1959.
7. Moore D.C.: Celiac (splanchnic) plexus block with alcohol for cancer pain of the upper intra-abdominal viscera, in Bonica J.J., Ventafridda V. (eds.): *Advances in Pain Research and Therapy.* New York, Raven Press, 1979, vol. 2.
8. Kappis M.: Sensibilität and local anästhesie in chirurgischen gebiet der bauchhohle mit besonderen berücksichtigung der Splanchnicus-anästhesie. *Bruns. Beitr. Klin. Cher.* 15:161, 1919.
9. Cousins M.J., Wright C.J.: Graft muscle skin blood flow after epidural block in vascular surgery procedures. *Surg. Gynecol. Obstet.* 133:62, 1971.
10. Mandl F.: *Die paravertebral Injection.* Vienna, Springer Verlag, 1926.
11. Kappis M.: Erfahrungen mit lokal Anästhesie bei Bauchoperationen. *Verh. Dtsch. Ges. Chir.* 43:87, 1914.
12. Reid W., Watt J.K., Gray T.G.: Phenol injection of the sympathetic chain. *Br. J. Surg.* 57:45, 1970.
13. Hannington-Kiff J.G.: Intravenous regional sympathetic block with guanethidine. *Lancet* 1:1019–1020, 1970.
14. Bengon H.T., Chomka C.M., Brenner E.A.: Treatment of reflex sympathetic dystrophy with regional intravenous reserpine. *Anesth. Analg.* 59:500–502, 1980.
15. Abram S.E.: Intra-arterial reserpine. *Anesth. Analg.* 59:889–890, 1980.
16. Romeo S.G., Whalen R.E., Tindall J.P.: Intra-arterial administration of reserpine: Its use in patients with Raynaud's disease or Raynaud's phenomenon. *Arch. Intern. Med.* 125:825, 1970.

35 / Epidural Steroids

P. PRITHVI RAJ, M.D.

LIEVRE in 1957 first introduced hydrocortisone into the epidural space.[1] Since then, caudal, lumbar epidural, spinal, and nerve root injections of local anesthetic–steroid mixtures have become popular for the conservative management of lumbosacral and cervical radiculopathy due to diskogenic disease.[2–4]

PATHOPHYSIOLOGY OF DISKOGENIC PAIN

Many workers have studied the mechanisms by which the pain is caused by the disk protrusion. Mixter and Barr felt that disk-initiated radicular pain was caused by mechanical pressure. However, Hiteselberger and Wilson found that 37% of protruded disks confirmed by myelography did not produce any pain. Smyth and Wright also were not able to produce pain by pulling a thread passing through the annulus of the disk. However, touching the inflamed spinal root produced sciatica. It is now generally accepted that disk narrowing, spur formation, and facet joint sclerosis are not reliable predictors of pain.

Neural inflammation is considered to play a major role in pain production. At surgery, neural tissue is seen to be swollen, hyperemic, and is adjacent to disk prolapse. Myelographically, when root edema is seen, it is symptomatic. The prolapsed disk produces local irritation of nerve root, which then becomes edematous and releases nociceptive agents. The rationale for epidural steroid administration is to reduce inflammation and inhibit the action of nociceptive agents.

MODE OF ACTION OF EXTRADURAL INJECTIONS

Some workers believe the extradural injection causes counterirritation which then stimulates resolution.[5] The use of local anesthetic in the mixture is believed to break the vicious pain cycle, produce muscle relaxation, and promote breakdown of adhesions.[6–8] Large volumes of saline, local anesthetic, and steroid solutions, when injected in the epidural space, have the combined effect of increasing hydrostatic pressure to break adhesions, anesthetizing the involved nerve root, and permitting painless lumbar movement. The painless lumbar movement permits relaxation of back muscles and prolongs pain relief.[9] Steroids reduce edema of the inflamed nerve root.[10]

CLINICAL INDICATIONS

The most effective use of epidural steroid therapy is for the treatment of nerve root entrapment and irritation secondary to diskogenic disease. The diskogenic disease is characterized by radicular pain, with an increase in the pain on coughing, sneezing, straining, or acute flexion of the lumbosacral spine.

Some workers have extended this technique to back pain of multiple etiologies, often with equivocal results. Use of epidural steroids for spondylolisthesis, degenerative arthritis, or pain due to posterior primary rami may give temporary relief, sufficient to permit institution of exercise programs and other alternative physical methods. However, when the initial block does not provide adequate relief, alternative therapy should be considered.

Carron and Toomey believe that every patient with low back pain and sciatica, except those with bladder and bowel dysfunction, should be placed on a trial of at least 2 weeks of anti-inflammatory agents and bed rest. Epidural steroid injection is performed if the condition does not improve with enforced bed rest.[11] Even though some workers claim improved results with subarachnoid injection, most believe epidural steroids are safer and produce equally good results. Since the nerve root compression is extradural in diskogenic disease, it is rational to introduce the steroid epidurally at the site of compression rather than intradurally, where it will be subject to dilution, dispersion, and precipitation.

TECHNIQUE

Epidural puncture should be done at the site of the nerve root lesion, with the painful side down in the lateral decubitus position. When the epidural space has been identified by standard techniques, 80 mg of methylprednisolone acetate or 50 mg of triamcinolone diacetate is suspended in 10 ml of 0.25% or 0.125% bupivacaine and injected slowly in the epidural space. In patients with previous back surgery, identification of the epidural space may be difficult. Initial administration of a local anesthetic will make identification of the epidural space easier under these circumstances (Fig 35–1).

Following epidural steroid injection, a catheter can be introduced to inject another dose of steroid and local anesthetic, if needed to reach the appropriate nerve root. This is determined by objectively measuring improvement on the straight-leg-raising test and absence of radicular pain during performance of the test.

The patient is kept in the lateral position for 10 minutes to keep the injected solution on the dependent side.

Two weeks after the epidural steroid injection the patient is reevaluated. If there is significant improvement in function and subjective pain relief, no further epidural injection is administered. However, if after the first injection the initial improvement is not maintained, another injection can be repeated, to a maximum of three injections. Similarly, if there is no change in the patient's condition after the first injection, alternative measures are sought.

COMPLICATIONS

Undesirable side effects can be due to the technique, the steroid used, the vehicle or a combination of all of them. The most common technical complication consists of inadvertent spinal tap. This has been thought to be of little importance, as intrathecal steroid has been advocated.[3] However, meningitis and CSF fistula have been linked to spinal tap.[12, 13] Other reported complications include aseptic meningitis, torula meningitis, tuberculous meningitis, transient bladder paralysis, conus medullaris syndrome, arachnoiditis, and sclerosing pachymeningitis. Thus it seems prudent to postpone the procedure when inadvertent spinal tap has occurred.

Wood et al. have shown patchy degenerative changes, including demyelinization, axonal disorganization, and endoneural collagen formation, in nerves treated with the methylprednisolone suspension or the vehicle, which consists of polyethylene glycol and myristyl-gamma-picolinium chloride (Fig 35–2). The clinical significance of this finding was uncertain, since the animals showed no neurologic deficit.[14]

Delaney et al. tested the effects of triamcinolone diacetate suspended in a solution containing polyethylene glycol and benzyl alcohol. Microscopic ex-

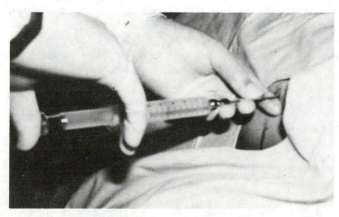

Fig 35–1.—The lateral decubitus position facilitates administration of epidural steroids. Note technique for placement of the needle in the epidural space.

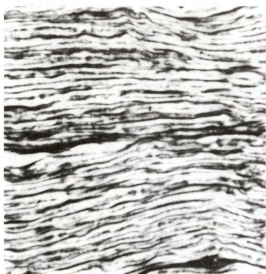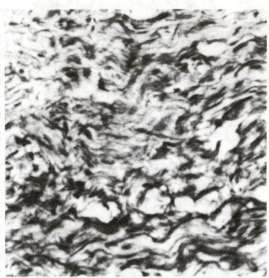

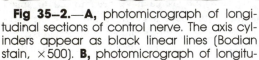

Fig 35–2.—A, photomicrograph of longitudinal sections of control nerve. The axis cylinders appear as black linear lines (Bodian stain, ×500). **B,** photomicrograph of longitudinal section of experimental nerve after injection of methylprednisolone acetate suspension (Bodian stain, ×500). (From Wood et al.[14] reproduced by permission.)

amination at 30 days showed minimal localized mononuclear cell meningeal infiltration with no clinical significance.[15]

RESULTS

Many workers have reported impressive results with epidural steroid injections (Table 35–1)[2, 3, 15–18] Winnie et al. reported subjective total relief of symptoms in 80% of patients after either epidural or subarachnoid injections.[2] Brown reported "excellent to good" results in 100% of patients with acute diskogenic disease of less than 3 months' duration, but in only 14% of those with pain of more than 3 months' duration.[17]

Arnhoff and co-workers reported a significant reduction in pain and improvement in function in their patients.[19] Toomey et al. extended their study to 5 years and found that gains noted at 1–2 years after epidural steroid injection were maintained at 5–6 years.[20]

Erdemir et al. studied 122 patients with postlaminectomy syndrome after treatment with intradural and extradural steroids. Fifty-three percent of patients reported satisfactory results, i.e., 75%–100% pain relief.[21]

When one considers epidural steroid administration, the following points should be kept in mind:

1. Histologic and biochemical evidence supports its use in the 30- to 50-year-old age group with low back or cervical pain with radiculopathy, when the pain is primarily diskogenic.

2. Features of this pain are shooting pain in brachial plexus, sciatic, or femoral distribution with sensory and/or motor deficits, reflex changes, and impaired straight leg raising above 30°.

3. There are proponents for both epidural and subarachnoid injection.

4. Meningitis or arachnoiditis may occur after intrathecal use, and there is no appreciable advantage to this route of administration compared with the extradural route. This makes the subarachnoid technique risky.

5. Bupivacaine 0.125% or 0.25% with either Depo-Medrol, 80 mg, or Aristocort, 50 mg, in 8–10 ml is commonly used.

6. Three injections are recommended as a maximum, performed 2 weeks apart in a 1-year period.

7. Complications arise due to excessive or frequent use.

8. Two thirds of patients with acute diskogenic disease will benefit from epidural steroids.

9. Only one third will benefit after 6 months.

TABLE 35–1.—EFFECT OF EPIDURAL INJECTIONS ON CHRONIC BACK PAIN*

STUDY	NO. OF PTS. INJECTED	STEROID INJECTED	LOCAL ANESTHETIC INJECTED	VOLUME INJECTED (ml)	% IMPROVED
SALINE ONLY					
Davidson and Robin[25]	28	No	No	72	57
LOCAL ANESTHETIC ONLY					
Swerdlow and Sayle-Creer[4]	208	No	Yes	50	47
Coomes[9]	20	No	Yes	50	60
Kelman[6]	116	No	Yes	50–100	81
Brevik et al.[24]†	19§	No§	Yes	100	26
STEROIDS ONLY					
Swerdlow and Sayle-Creer[4]	117	Yes	No	5	65
Ito[23]	142	Yes	No	2	63
Winnie et al.[2]‡	20	Yes	No	2	95
Dilke et al.[26]	35	Yes	No	10	60
BOTH LOCAL ANESTHETICS AND STEROIDS					
Warr[27]	500	Yes	Yes	40	63
Cho[22]	16	Yes	Yes	20–30	88
Goebert et al.[18]	113	Yes	Yes	30	73
Ito[23]	136	Yes	Yes	10	72
Brevik et al.[24]†	16	Yes	Yes	20	56
Arnhoff[19]	140	Yes	Yes	10	39

*Adapted from Miller R.D., Munger W.L., Powell P.E.: Chronic pain and local anesthesia neural blockade, in Cousins M.J., Bridenbaugh P.O. (eds.): *Neural Blockade*. Philadelphia, J.B. Lippincott, Co., 1980.
†Caudal block.
‡Ten with epidural and ten with subarachnoid block.
§Of the 14 patients who did not receive relief, 11 did get relief with the steroid.

10. Initial improvement is usually maintained. However, there seems to be no tendency for continued improvement.

11. Finally, epidural steroid injection is only one modality to treat low back pain.

REFERENCES

1. Lievre J.A., Bloch-Michel H., Attali P.: L'injection trans-sacree: Etude clinique et radiologique. *Bull. Mem. Soc. Med. Hôp. Paris* 73:1110–1118, 1957.

2. Winnie A.P., Hartman J.T., Meyers H.L., et al.: Pain clinic: II: Intradural and extradural corticosteroids for sciatica. *Anesth. Analg.* 51:990–999, 1972.

3. Sehgal A.D., Gardner W.J.: Place of intrathecal methylprednisolone acetate in neurological disorders. *Trans. Am Neurol. Assoc.* 88:275–276, 1963.

4. Swerdlow M., Sayle-Creer W.: The use of extradural injections in the relief of lumbosciatic pain. *Anaesthesia* 25:128, 1970.

5. Viner N.: Intractable sciatica: The sacral epidural injection. An effective method of giving relief. *Can. Med. Assoc. J.* 15:630–634, 1925.

6. Kelman H.: Epidural injection therapy for sciatic pain. *Am. J. Surg.* 64:183–190, 1944.

7. Cyriax J.: *Textbook of Orthopaedic Medicine*, ed. 3. London, Cassell, 1957.

8. Greenwood J.J., McGuire T.A., Kimbell F.: A study of the causes of failure in the herniated intervertebral disc operation. *J. Neurosurg.* 9:15–20, 1952.

9. Coomes E.N.: A comparison between epidural anaesthesia and bed rest in sciatica. *Bri. Med. J.* 1:20, 1961.

10. Lindhal O., Rexed B.: Histological changes in the spinal nerve roots of operated cases of sciatica. *Act Orthop. Scand.* 20:215, 1951.

11. Carron H., Toomey T.C.: Epidural steroid therapy for low back pain, in Stanton-Hicks M., Boas R. (eds.): *Chronic Low Back Pain*. New York, Raven Press, 1982, pp. 193–198.

12. Ball C.G., D'Alessandro F.T., Rosenthal J., et al.: Case history number 86: An unusual complication of lumbar puncture. A CSF cutaneous fistula. *Anesth. Analg.* 54:691–694, 1975.

13. Dougherty J.H., Fraser R.A.R.: Complications following intraspinal injections of steroids. *J. Neurosurg.* 48:1023–1025, 1978.

14. Wood K.M., Arguelles J., Norenberg M.D.: Degenerative lesions in rat sciatic nerves after local injections on methylprednisolone in sterile aqueous suspension. *Reg. Anaesth.* 5:13–15, 1980.

15. Delaney T.J., Rowlingson J.C., Carron H., et al.: The effects of steroids on nerves and meninges. *Anesth. Analg.* 59:610–614, 1980.

16. Abram S.E.: Subarachnoid corticosteroid injection following inadequate response to epidural steroids for sciatica. *Anesth. Analg.* 57:313–315, 1978.

17. Brown F.W.: Management of diskogenic pain using epidural and intrathecal steroids. *Clin. Orthop.* 129:72–78, 1977.

18. Goebert H.W., Jallo S.J., Gardner W.J., et al.: Sciatica: Treatment with epidural injections of procaine and hydrocortisone. *Cleve. Clin. Q.* 27:191–197, 1960.

19. Arnhoff F.N., Triplet H.B., Pokorney B.: Follow-up status of patients treated with nerve blocks for low back pain. *Anesthesiology* 46:170–178, 1977.

20. Toomey T.C., Taylor A.G., Skelton M.A., Carron H.: Five-year follow-up status of chronic low back pain patients. *Pain* 11:272, 1982.

21. Erdemir H., Karamvir M., Gelman, S.: Intradural and extradural corticosteroids for postlaminectomy syndrome. *Ala. J. Med. Sci.* 19:137–138, 1982.

22. Cho K.O.: Therapeutic epidural block with a combination of a weak local anesthetic and steroids in managenent of complicated low back pain. *Am. Surg.* 36:303, 1970.

23. Ito R.: The treatment of low back pain and sciatica with epidural corticosteroids injection and its pathophysiological basis. *Nippon Seikeigeka Gakkai Zasshi* 45:67, 1971.

24. Brevik H., et al.: Treatment of low back pain and sciatica: Comparison of caudal epidural injections of bupivacaine and methylprednisolone with pubivacaine followed by saline, in Bonica J.J., Albe-Fessard D. (eds.): *Advances in Pain Research and Therapy.* New York, Raven Press, vol. 1, pp. 927–932, 1976.

25. Davidson J.T., Robin G.C.: Epidural injections in the lumbosciatic syndrome. *Br. J. Anaesth.* 33:595, 1961.

26. Dilke T.F.W., Burry H.C., Grahame R.: Extradural nerve root compression. *Br. Med. J.* 2:635, 1973.

27. Warr A.C., et al.: Chronic lumbosciatic syndrome treated by epidural injection and manipulation. *Practitioner* 209:53, 1972.

36 / Prolonged Analgesia Technique With Local Anesthetics

P. PRITHVI RAJ, M.D.
DONALD D. DENSON, Ph.D.

PROLONGED ANALGESIA can be maintained with an intermittent injection or a continuous infusion of a local anesthetic in the epidural space or on any part of the peripheral nervous system. In patients with postoperative pain, labor pain, or chronic pain, there is an indication for prolonged analgesia.

The first continuous caudal anesthetic in North America was administered through a malleable lemmon spinal needle with extension tubing attached.[1] Later, smaller catheters and thinner needles were developed to promote safer techniques of prolonged analgesia.[2] Curbelo was the first to use the Tuohy needle for insertion of a catheter in the epidural space.[3]

Various types of catheters have been used. Originally, lacquered gum elastic ureteric catheters were readily available, but since the 1940s, a wide variety of materials have been introduced. These include polyethylene, polyvinylchloride, nylon, and polytetrafluoroethylene (Teflon). Catheters with radiolucency or radiopacity are also available.

The following properties are essential for a catheter to be used for prolonged analgesia according to Bromage:[4]

1. The catheter material should be inert and flexible.

2. The catheter material should be soft, but durable.

3. A sudden jerk or slow traction should not break the catheter.

4. The external diameter should pass through a 17-gauge Tuohy needle for the epidural space with ease.

5. The bore of the catheter should be large enough for fluids to flow through without resistance when injected with a 10-ml syringe.

6. Kinking and obstruction should not occur when the catheter is bent sharply.

7. Graduations marked at the distal end should be clear and indicate the distance of the catheter tip past the needle.

Sterility must be maintained during the introduction of the catheter in the perineural space and as long as continuous analgesia is maintained. Bacterial filters should be incorporated between the delivery system and the catheter mount.[5] The catheter should be securely anchored and kept sterile during the period of analgesia. There should be enough length in the delivery system for the patient to be mobile. For intermittent injection, the site of injection should be kept sterile. For the continuous infusion technique, a volumetric pump should be inserted between the local anesthetic reservoir and the catheter.

TOP-UP TECHNIQUE

By repeating the injection of local anesthetic agent through an indwelling catheter, one can keep the segmental level of analgesia constant. The repeat dose required is one-half of the initial dose or less. The "top-up" needs to be given prior to two-segment regression or by patient demand.

Bromage has calculated the two segment regression curves for all the common local anesthetic agents used today.[4] He advocates the timing of the repeat injection to be duration of two-segment regression - 1.5 × standard deviation. The following table shows the two-segment regression and the timing of repeat injections of various local anesthetic agents (Table 36–1).

687

TABLE 36–1.—DURATION OF LUMBAR EPIDURAL ANALGESIA
FOR CHLOROPROCAINE, LIDOCAINE, PRILOCAINE, TETRACAINE,
BUPIVACAINE AND ETIDOCAINE WITH 1/200,000 EPINEPHRINE*

DRUG	DURATION† (2-SEGMENT RECESSION) (mins)	S.D.	DURATION (1.5 × S.D.) (mins)
3% Chloroprocaine	57	7	47
2% Lidocaine	97.5	19	70
2% Prilocaine	97	10	82
3% Prilocaine	99	17	74
0.4% Tetracaine	135	23	100
0.5% Tetracaine	146	22	113
0.5% Bupivacaine	196	31	150
0.75% Bupivacaine	201	40	141
1% Etidocaine	170	57	85

*From Bromage P.R.[4] Used by permission.
†Duration is measured from the moment of complete spread until analgesia
has regressed two spinal segments.

Indications

Analgesia for Acute Pain and Trauma

Perineural analgesia with "top-up" technique can
be used to provide analgesia for prolonged hours or
days. The object is to replace systemically prescribed narcotics with regionally applied local anesthetics. As far as possible, motor sensory function
should be retained. Bupivacaine is the drug of

choice for such patients. This technique has been
used extensively to provide analgesia for postoperative pain and trauma. Initially, its use was restricted to upper abdominal operations and chest
wall trauma. Recently, its use has been extended to
postoperative pain due to hip and knee surgery,
urological or gynecological surgery, and trauma to
the extremities.

TECHNIQUE.—The local anesthetic agent is administered when the patient complains of returning

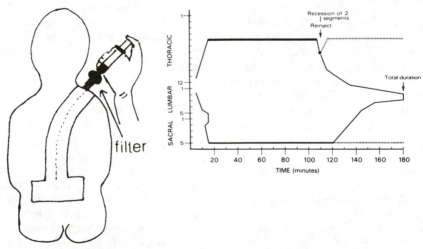

Fig 36–1.—*Left,* final anchoring of the epidural catheter with the attachment of the micropore filter for top-up injections. *Right,* timing
of top-up dose in conscious patients. Seg-
ment-time diagram showing spread and
regression of analgesia. A stable upper level

of analgesia is maintained by injecting one
half of the induction dose when the upper
level of analgesia has regressed two spinal
segments. (From Bromage P.[4] Reproduced by
permission.)

pain or at a predetermined frequency, as described in Table 36–1. The second method is preferable to spare the patient the intervals of pain that might occur between doses (Fig 36–1).

The patient is placed in a supine position. Blood pressure, respirations, pulse, and CNS status are monitored during the "top-up" doses. The chosen local anesthetic is administered with strict sterile precautions. After the injection, the patient is kept supine for 30 minutes. Vital signs are checked every 5 minutes to cover the period of sympathetic block and the systemic effect of the peak concentration of drug in plasma. If they are satisfactory, the patient is then placed in any desired position.

Analgesia for Chronic Pain

The object of producing prolonged analgesia for chronic pain is to have a prognostic and therapeutic effect. The initial volume and concentration of the local anesthetic agent is determined by how many segments need to be blocked. The "top-up" doses then maintain that quality of analgesia for a period of time, usually days, for the physician to evaluate the beneficial effect of pain relief and its side effects. For the patient, this state of prolonged analgesia allows him to experience the feeling of numb-

ness or weakness that accompanies the analgesia. The patient can then determine if a proposed neurolytic block in that region would be tolerable. When prolonged analgesia is used for a therapeutic regimen, one evaluates the benefits of prolonged sympathetic block, an exercise program during the pain-free period, and the benefits of reducing the nociceptive impulses on the reflex mechanisms.

TECHNIQUE—The "top-up" technique is similar to that used for post-operative or trauma patients. The same precautions are necessary. Since the duration of prolonged analgesia is longest in patients with chronic pain, tachyphylaxis is common. Bromage et al. studied epidural tachyphylaxis in man.[4] They state that tachyphylaxis will appear if intervals between injections are long enough to allow analgesia to wear off completely. On the other hand, augmentation of analgesia is seen when injections are given too closely. Long-acting local anesthetic agents tend to postpone the occurrence of tachyphylaxis because of reducing the need for frequent "top-ups."

DRUGS.—It is possible to administer any local anesthetic agent for "top-up" continuous perineural analgesia. However, some agents are more efficacious than others. Table 36–2 shows the local anesthetic agents used in various "top-up" tech-

TABLE 36–2.—TOP-UP TECHNIQUE*

CATHETER SITE	SOURCE OF PAIN	DRUG INJECTED	VOL. FOR TOP-UP (ml)	TIMING OF "TOP-UP" DOSE (min)
CAUDAL				
Cleland 1949	Abdomen	1. Tetracaine 0.15% + epinephrine 1:200,000 2. Dibucaine 0.2% + epinephrine 1:200,000	6–15	Not known
LUMBAR				
Stanton-Hicks 1971	Hip	Bupivacaine 0.5% + epinephrine 1:200,000	6.4	180–360
Renck 1969	Perineum		1–12	240
Abel, Salem and Scott 1975	Lower abdomen	Bupivacaine 0.5% or etidocaine 1.0%	10	160
THORACIC				
Miller et al. 1976	Upper abdomen	Lidocaine 1–2%	Not known	60–120
Ellis et al. 1968	Upper abdomen	Lidocaine 1.5% or Prilocaine 1.5% or bupivacaine 0.375%	5–7 3–6 5–6	60 67 125
Spence and Smith 1971	Upper abdomen	Bupivacaine 0.5% + epinephrine 1:200,000	5–7	120
Renck 1976	Upper abdomen	Etidocaine 1%	4–5	300

*From Buckley F.P., Simpson B.R.[18] Used by permission.

niques. The longer-acting local anesthetic agents are preferred to shorter-acting local anesthetic agents. Bupivacaine is the drug of choice because of its prolonged analgesic effect and minimal motor effect.

Duration of analgesia in continuous intermittent epidural technique is shorter than for surgical anesthesia. The addition of epinephrine does not appear to produce the prolongation of analgesia one sees during surgery. Adequate analgesia is produced by 0.25% bupivacaine in most of the patients. However, if the duration of the analgesia is short, it can be increased by using 0.375% or 0.5% bupivacaine. It should be cautioned that higher concentrations increase the chances of toxicity.

The volume of local anesthetic agent needed is determined by the region at which it is administered and the number of segments that need to be blocked. The largest volume is injected in the caudal region and the least in the cervical region. The following are the maximum "top up" injection volumes at various sites: caudal, 20–25 ml, lumbar 15–20 ml, thoracic 5–10 ml, and cervical 2–5 ml.

With "top up" injections, plasma concentrations of the drug will peak 15–20 minutes after each "top up." This may produce a "saw-toothed" pattern, and if the injection is given at short intervals, toxic concentrations may be reached. This has been shown to occur rapidly with lidocaine and slowly with etidocaine.[6] Bupivacaine pharmacokinetics have not been studied in postoperative analgesia "top up" technique.

At our institution, we have had unsatisfactory experiences with intermittent injections of either lidocaine or bupivacaine via an indwelling catheter. The following example typifies such unsatisfactory experience.

A 45-year-old male with a history of pain in the left hand and arm was seen at the Pain Control Center. He gave the history of laceration of the left hypothenar eminence with injury to the ulnar nerve and primary nerve repair one year previously. Burning pain started in the hand soon after the operation and was present at examination in the Pain Control Center. Diagnosis of causalgia was made, and the patient was initially managed with a series of left stellate ganglion blocks and TENS. The pain was not relieved completely, and then only temporarily. To provide the patient with prolonged and adequate pain relief, it was decided to insert an indwelling catheter on the left brachial plexus and inject intermittent injection of 0.5% bupivacaine on "patient demand." Prolonged analgesia was anticipated to be for a period of a week to allow for the intensive physical therapy necessary for the rehabilitation of the hand.

After the placement of an indwelling catheter in the left infraclavicular region of the brachial plexus, 10 ml of 0.5% bupivacaine were injected. Further bolus injections were given on "patient demand" during the day. Within 24 hours the volume of the 0.5% bupivacaine had to be increased to 20 ml. The pain relief lasted only 2–3 hours after each bolus injection, and even after 40 ml or 0.5% bupivacaine. Figure 36–2 shows the frequency of injection of bupivacaine and the period of pain relief associated with each injection. It is obvious that analgesia was short-lived with this technique, and had we persisted in increasing the frequency of injections, cumulative toxicity may have occurred. Serum bupivacaine concentrations taken at random over 48

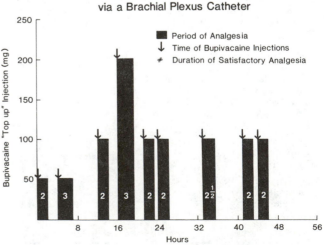

Analgesia with Intermittent Injection of Bupivacaine via a Brachial Plexus Catheter

Fig 36–2.—The inadequacy of analgesia with the top-up technique in a patient with severe pain in the right arm due to causalgia. Duration of analgesia with top-up injection of bupivacaine is shown in *black*. The *numbers* denote the hours of analgesia. *Arrows* denote the time of top-up injection.

hours ranged from as low as 0.14 μg/ml to 1.58 μg/ml. The technique had to be abandoned after 48 hours because of inadequate periods of analgesia and appearance of minor symptoms of CNS toxicity (dizziness, ringing in ears) in the 60-minute period following bolus injections.

INFUSION TECHNIQUE

This method was developed to provide continuous analgesia between "top up" injections. It provides continuous infusion into a perineural space that equals the rate it is removed from it.[7] There are two techniques of infusion: (1) gravity-feed infusion; or (2) with infusion pumps.[8, 9]

Gravity-Feed Drip

The local anesthetic agent is infused via an infusion set into the perineural space. The high resistance offered by the catheter does not allow for high infusion rates. It seems to be a simple and practical method, if the local anesthetic solution is not concentrated. For example, 0.4% to 0.8% lidocaine has been used successfully by this method.[10] It is, however, very difficult to adjust by gravity the exact rate of local anesthetic to be delivered per unit time. Cox and Spoerel modified the gravity drip technique by replacing it with a large syringe containing the local anesthetic agent and attaching to it a power driven pump.[11] The pump was timed to drive a preset volume in the syringe at different time intervals (top up technique), or continuously (constant infusion technique). A newer Autosyringe is presently available and used at some centers in the United States.

Infusion Pump Technique

Recently infusion pumps have been popularized for prolonged analgesia.[10, 11] Volumetric pumps are preferable.

Continuous bupivacaine infusion is instituted in the epidural space if the patient has pain in the trunk or lower extremity; on the brachial plexus for pain in the upper extremity; and on the celiac plexus and lumbar sympathetic chain for pain of sympathetic origin in the viscera or in the lower extremity. Other peripheral nerves (cervical plexus, femoral, sciatic nerves, and stellate ganglion) have also been cathertized for prolonged infusion at our institution (Fig 36–3).

If needed, 0.15 mg/kg of diazepam is administered intravenously for sedation one hour before the block. The catheter is inserted either in the procedure room or in the x-ray unit under strict sterile conditions. After confirmation of the proper placement of the catheter, a loading dose of 1.5% lidocaine or 3% 2-chloroprocaine is injected to obtain the objective evidence of the block. Bupivacaine infusion is started at a chosen concentration and rate of infusion, using either an Abbott Lifecare or IVAC or a similar volumetric infusion pump. Each patient's pain pathway determines the initial bupivacaine concentration. Bupivacaine concentration of 0.125% is chosen for C-fiber pain, 0.25% for C and A-delta fiber pain, and 0.5% for C, A-delta, and A-alpha fiber pain.

The appropriate concentration of bupivacaine is prepared by the hospital pharmacy in a 300- or 500-ml bottle containing NaCl under sterile conditions. The bottle and the infusion set are changed every 24 hours. Monitoring is done by the physicians and the

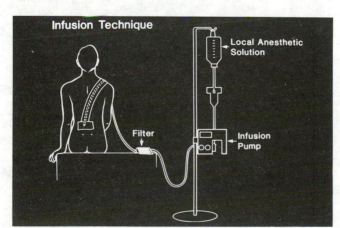

Fig 36–3.—Arrangement used for continuous epidural analgesia. Similar arrangement can be used at any other perineural site. (From Pither C., Hartick C.: Postoperative pain, in Raj P.P. (ed.): *Handbook of Regional Anesthesia.* New York, Churchill Livingstone, Inc., 1985. Reproduced by permission.)

nurses as a team to evaluate the continuous infusion technique for (1) efficacy, (2) technical problems, and (3) side effects. The protocol for the nurses is specially designed and approved by the nursing service to monitor physiological and systemic effects of the block (see Appendix, this chapter). The patients are followed for three months for any sequelae secondary to the infusion technique.

Blood samples can be taken before the start of the infusion, at 3–5 hours after the start of infusion, and at 12-hour intervals during the infusion. Blood samples can be obtained at termination and at 2-hour intervals for 8 hours to 12 hours to determine the pharmacokinetics of the continuous bupivacaine infusion.

Techniques of Catherization and Infusion

EPIDURAL SPACE.—A 19-gauge Teflon catheter is placed either in the lumbar or in the thoracic space via a 17-gauge Tuohy needle using a loss-of-resistance technique. The catheter tip is placed at the midpoint of the pain segments. Where there is doubt, the placement is confirmed with x-ray (AP and lateral views) after injecting the catheter with 1 ml of metrizimide, reconstituted to contain 250 mg I/ml. Special care is taken to secure the catheter in the following manner. Two 1″ Steri-strips are firmly adhered to the skin (which is previously sprayed with tincture of benzoin) to half their length. The other halves of the Steri-strips were put over the skin in a crisscross fashion to reinforce it. Op-site is

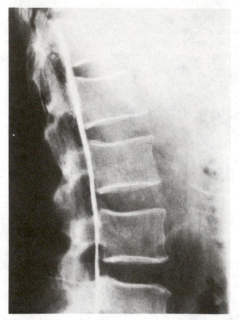

Fig 36–4.—Lateral view of the epidural space and catheter with merrizamide confirming the catheter placement.

then used to keep the area transparent and sterile (Figures 36–4 through 36–7)

After a 3-ml test dose of either 2-chloroprocaine or 1.5% lidocaine, a loading dose of either drug is administered for objective evidence of the block. For the thoracic region 5 to 10 ml are used and for the lumbar region 15 to 20 ml are used. The pain

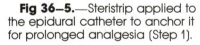
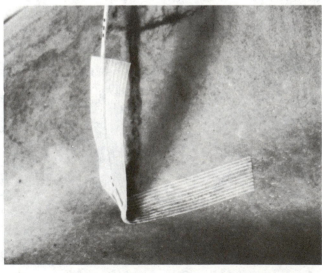

Fig 36–5.—Steristrip applied to the epidural catheter to anchor it for prolonged analgesia (Step 1).

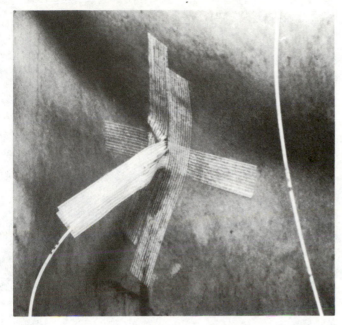

Fig 36–6.—Steristrips applied crisscross to firmly anchor the catheter (Step 2).

pathway is assessed by the retrograde method.[12] The pain is considered to be in the C-fiber pathway if the relief persists after the return of motor and sensory function. If the pain appears with the return of sensation, it is considered to be in the A-delta and C fibers, and if the pain returns with recovery of motor function, it is considered to be in all pain pathways (A-alpha, A-delta, and C fibers). The appropriate concentration of bupivacaine is then infused via a 300- or 500-ml bottle attached to the distal end of the catheter with an infusion pump containing a 0.22 micropore filter in the infusion set.

BRACHIAL PLEXUS.—Any site can be chosen for brachial plexus catheterization, e.g., axillary space, infraclavicular region, or interscalene space. Usually an 18-gauge 4″ or 6″ BD Longdwell catheter is used for the axillary and infraclavicular regions, and a 20-gauge 1-½ angiocath is used for the interscalene space. Sometimes a 19-gauge epidural catheter inserted through a Tuohy needle at all these spaces is used if the extracaths are considered too big. All catheters are placed with the aid of a peripheral nerve stimulator according to the technique of Raj et al. and confirmed by x-ray[13] (Fig 36–8). To visualize the spread of the solution on the bra-

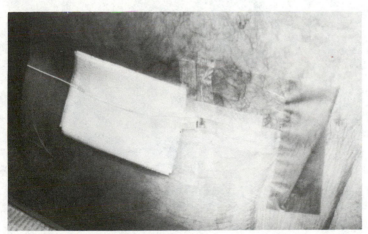

Fig 36–7.—Steristrips reinforced with op-site (Step 3).

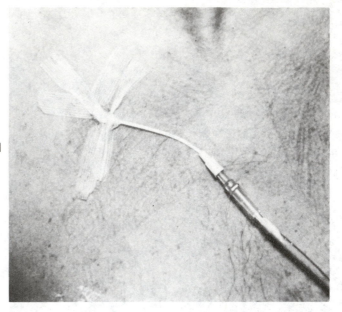

Fig 36–8.—Infraclavicular brachial plexus catheter inserted with nerve stimulator, and anchored with steristrips.

chial plexus (Fig 36–9) 20–30 ml of a 50:50 mixture of either 3% 2-chloroprocaine or 2% lidocaine with meglumine diatrizoate is used. When confirmed by the x-ray and by objective evidence of block, the infusion assembly with a pump and filter are attached to the catheter (see Fig 36–3) for the epidural space. The appropriate bupivacaine concentration is started for pain relief.

LUMBAR SYMPATHETIC AND CELIAC PLEXUS.—For these techniques 18-gauge 6″–8″ BD Longdwell extracaths are used. All catheters are inserted under fluoroscopy and confirmed by injecting 10 ml of 50:50 mixture of meglumine diatrizoate with either 3% 2-chloroprocaine or 2% lidocaine. Lumbar sympathetic chain catheterization is done by the method of Reid, and celiac plexus catheterization by

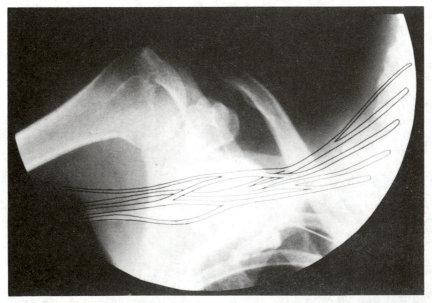

Fig 36–9.—Infraclavicular catheter in place on Brachial plexus with x-ray confirmation.

the method of Kappis[14, 15] (see chapter 34F). Once confirmed, the infusion assembly is similar to that in Figure 36–3.

EFFICACY

Patients (n = 50) undergoing continuous infusions were evaluated at the University of Cincinnati. There were 29 infusions in the epidural space, 13 infusions on the brachial plexus, and 14 infusions on the sympathetic chain (celiac plexus or lumbar regions).

Overall, the intial concentration of bupivacaine was 0.5% in 4 infusions (A-alpha, A-delta, and C fiber pain), 0.25% in 34 infusions (A-delta and C fiber pain), and 0.125% in 18 infusions (C fiber pain). All patients had at least 48 hours of infusion; 73% of the infusions continued for 4 days and 52% for 5 days.

In patients with adequate analgesia, the concentration or rate of infusion of bupivacaine was changed only if spreading numbness, motor weakness, or urinary retention was present. Sixty-nine percent of the patients with an initial concentration of 0.25% had the concentration decreased to 0.125% to treat the above side effects.

Adequate pain relief was obtained in 75% of the infusions (N = 38). In the remaining 25% (N = 12), inadequate analgesia was reinforced with "top-up" doses or 5 ml to 10 ml of 1% lidocaine once or twice a day. This provided satisfactory analgesia.

Tachyphylaxis

In the epidural group, 30 mg/hr was the maximum initial rate of infusion required to provide adequate analgesia. Figure 36–10 shows the time course of three groups of patients with varying initial rates of infusion. On subsequent days, the rate of infusion for the group receiving more than 25 mg/hr on day one was decreased to a mean of 20 mg/hr. In the group with 15–25 mg/hr, the mean rate was decreased to 18 mg/hr on the third day. However, there was essentially no difference in the group with the initial infusion rate of less than 15 mg/hr over the course of infusion.

In the brachial plexus and sympathetic chain groups, the infusion rates usually remained constant. Once adequate analgesia was obtained, there was no increase in the rate of infusion in any patient to provide the same analgesia.

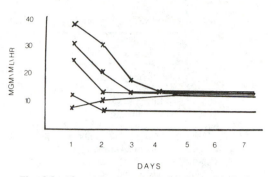

Fig 36–10.—Varying initial rates of infusion in 5 patients. On subsequent days, the rate of infusion for the group greater than 25 mg/hr decreased to a mean of 20 mg/hr; for the group starting with 15–25 mg/hr decreased to 18 mg/hr; there was no difference in the group below 15 mg/hr.

Side Effects

There were no convulsions observed in patients in this study. Some patients complained of minor CNS toxicity, which was recorded as either tinnitus, dizziness, circumoral numbness, nausea, vomiting, or diaphoresis. The majority of the patients with minor CNS toxicity complained of dizziness, usually on the first or second day, while the infusion rates were being minimized to maintain adequate analgesia. Table 36–3 shows the details of side effects.

Bradycardia was observed in one patient with a cutaneous sensory loss extending up to T2 with a thoracic epidural infusion. This patient was managed by discontinuing the infusion until the analgesic level receded below T6 and the cardiac rate returned to normal. No further sequelae occurred in this patient with resumption of the infusion. One patient had hypotension, which was managed by having the patient lie supine from a sitting position and stopping the infusion until the patient's blood pressure returned to his normal. Upon resumption, the rate of infusion was decreased to maintain normotension while providing adequate analgesia.

There were 6 incidences of urinary retention in 29 epidural infusions. These usually occurred when the rate was adjusted during the first two days or when the quality of block increased on the later days of the infusion. In either case, the rate of infusion was adjusted to eliminate these side effects while providing adequate analgesia.

Three patients had infection, either at the entry site of the catheter in the skin or from the catheter

TABLE 36–3.—SIDE EFFECTS OF CONTINUOUS INFUSION

	1	2	3	DAYS 4	5	6	7
CNS toxicity							
Major	—	—	—	—	—	—	—
Minor (42%)							
Tinnitus (8%)	2%	4%	—	—	—	—	—
Dizziness (22%)	2%	8%	6%	—	4%	2%	—
Circumoral numbness (2%)	2%	—	—	—	—	—	—
Nausea/vomiting (4%)	—	4%	—	—	—	—	—
Diaphoresis (6%)	—	2%	—	2%	2%	—	—
CVS toxicity (4%)	—	2%	2%	—	—	—	—
Respiratory	—	—	—	—	—	—	—
Urinary retention (16%)	4%	6%	—	2%	2%	—	2%
Immobilization due to numbness or paresis (18%)	2%	10%	2%	2%	—	2%	—

tip. Two patients had Staphylococcus aureus and one patient had E. coli. One of these patients (E. coli) had signs and symptoms of meningitis. Adequate antibiotic therapy, usually a cephalosporin, was sufficient to treat these infections.

Mobilization was not possible in 9 out of 29 patients during the first two days while the rate of infusion was still being adjusted.

Technical Problems

Leaking, kinking, and filter resistance in the delivery system was seen in some patients. These complications usually occurred on the second, third, and fourth days, during the period of mobilization. The catheter was reinserted in 7 infusions. There were no problems in reinserting the catheters or maintaining the infusion after reinsertion (Table 36–4).

Two catheters broke, one in the lumbar sympathetic region and one in the thoracic sympathetic region. These catheters were soft and kinked. The break occurred at the kinked site as the catheters were pulled out. Some catheters are better than others in this regard. The break seems to be a function of catheter type rather than the technique.

COMMENT

Successful prolonged analgesia has been obtained by previous workers in postoperative periods and for labor and delivery.[16, 17] They reported that the technique of intermittent injection is preferable to continuous infusion because of its simplicity and the impossibility of accidentally injecting large doses of the local anesthetic.[18] The authors, however, did not find the intermittent injection technique for prolonged analgesia adequate.

All patients in their study had satisfactory analgesia within 48 hours with continuous bupivacaine infusion, even though clinical adjustment of the rate of infusion was needed in this early period. The rates of infusion were constant only in a minority of the patients.

TABLE 36–4.—TECHNICAL PROBLEMS IN CONTINUOUS INFUSIONS

	1	2	3	DAYS 4	5	6	7
Catheter (18%)							
Leaking							
Kinking	—	6%	4%	6%	2%	—	—
Filter							
Inc. resistance							
Leak							
Catheter reinsertion (14%)	—	8%	2%	4%	—	—	—
Infection (3%)	—	1%	—	—	—	—	2%

Once analgesia was adequate with a certain rate of infusion, it was interesting to note that the quality of the block was increased if the same rate was maintained. This shows that tachyphylaxis was not a problem with the continuous infusion technique.

It is reported that cumulative toxicity may result if the intermittent injection or continuous infusion technique is continued for longer than 48 hours.[6] Significant systemic toxicity with infusions longer than 48 hours is not observed.

Patients treated with continuous infusions are not prevented from being mobilized and rehabilitated during the period of analgesia. Patients are usually sent to the physical therapy department for exercise (see Fig 36–11). Perhaps this is due to the very low doses of bupivacaine infused. The rehabilitation and exercise program is the essential part of the prolonged analgesia in postoperative and chronic pain patients.

Infusion pumps are satisfactory in infusing through catheters placed at the different perineural sites. Some of the catheters and infusion tubing have a high resistance, usually in the lumbar sympathetic and celiac plexus regions.

The catheters presently available are not ideal for the continuous perineural infusion. Perhaps the new Teflon epidural catheters being tested will be more suitable. Some of the catheters tend to become soft and kink during body movements. The softness may be due to the effect of the body temperature. Once the catheters do become soft and kinked, they are more likely to break when pulled. The catheters may also pull out during mobilization. This can be prevented by taking proper care to anchor them firmly. Experience at the University of Cincinnati shows that this can be done successfully with the Steri-strip technique. Long tubing also helps in preventing the catheter pull out during the patient's mobilization.

Close monitoring of the patient with continuous infusion is necessary by the team of physicians and nurses. Daily communication among the responsible physician and the nurse is mandatory to maintain adequate monitoring of the patient with the continuous bupivacaine infusion. The nurse should be fully knowledgeable of the technique and follow the nursing protocol (see Appendix, this chapter). The physician can initially start the infusion and then monitor these patients at routine intervals without jeopardizing the care and safety of such patients. When side effects are seen, they appear gradually (dizziness, hypotension, increasing numbness, etc.). The primary nurse is able to monitor these changes and inform the physician in ample time to treat these minor symptoms and prevent any serious sequelae.

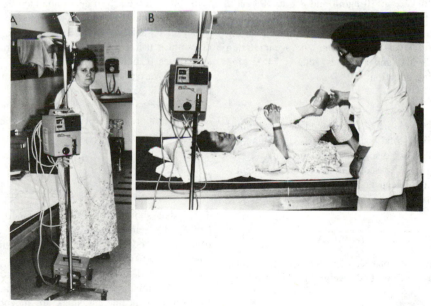

Fig 36–11.—Patient with chronic low back pain treated with continuous bupivacaine infusion. **A,** photograph shows the patient mobilized for physical therapy within 48 hours. **B,** the same patient undergoing physical therapy with continuous infusion of bupivacaine in the epidural space.

KINETICS OF CONTINUOUS PERINEURAL INFUSIONS

Kinetics of continuous perineural infusion in patients (n = 50) with chronic pain were studied by Raj, Denson et al.[19] After placement of the catheter at either the lumbar sympathetic chain, in the epidural space, or on the brachial plexus, a 2-ml test dose followed by 15–20 ml of 1.5% lidocaine or 3% 2-chloroprocaine was injected to obtain initial pain relief. The catheters were then connected within one hour to the infusion pump. Bupivacaine concentrations were either 0.125%, 0.25%, or 0.5%, and R_o (initial rate of infusion) varied from 5 to 30 mg/h. The bupivacaine solutions were prepared in the pharmacy and were changed daily. Peripheral venous blood samples were obtained at 0, at 3 to 5 hours, and then every 12 hours until termination. In 37 of the 50 patients, a sample was obtained every 2 hours for 6–12 hours and at the time of termination of the infusion. Termination sampling was not possible for every patient, since some were discharged soon after the infusion was terminated. Accumulation samples were obtained for 42 patients. Serum bupivacaine concentrations were determined by a modification of the method of Mather and Tucker.[19] The coefficient of variation was 10% to 12% at 10 ng/ml and 8% to 10% at 2 μg/ml. Estimation of pharmacokinetic parameters for a given patient was accomplished by measuring serum blood levels taken during the accumulation phase (t = 3–5H) and at steady state (t 24h) using the following equation:[20]

$$Vz = CL/\lambda_z \qquad \text{eq. 1}$$

(V_z, average volume of distribution in the elimination phase; CL, total body clearance; λ_z, elimination of terminal (slow) disposition rate constant)
Estimations of C^{ss} based on initial R_o and a patient's body weight or lean body mass was accomplished using equation 2:

$$C^{ss} = \frac{R_o}{\lambda_z \times Vz \times (BW/LBM)} \qquad \text{eq. 2}$$

(C^{ss}, steady state plasma concentration; R_o, initial rate of infusion; BW, body weight; LBM, lean body mass)

Vz is the average volume of distribution in the elimination phase adjusted for either body weight or lean body mass and λ_z is the average value for λ_z. Actual pharmacokinetic parameters were calculated from the blood level data at the termination of infusion using standard equations for an open one-compartment model to calculate λ_z. Vz was calculated from the following equation:

$$\frac{R_o}{V_z \cdot \lambda_z} \times \frac{(1 - 3^{\lambda_z \times t(i)})(1 - e^{\lambda_z \times tp(i)})}{(C_{max} - C_{min})}$$

$$\text{eq. 3}$$

where C_{max} is the blood concentration at the termination of the infusion and C_{min} is the last blood concentration measured. t(i) is the total time of infusion and tp(i) corresponds to the time after termination of the infusion when the last sample was taken.

CL was then calculated as the product of λ_z and Vz.

Infusion rate (R_o) adjustments required to achieve a desired clinical effect were calculated by substituting the estimated clearance and the desired steady state blood concentration (C^{ss}) into eq. 4:

$$CL = \frac{R_o}{C^{ss}} \qquad \text{eq. 4}$$

Estimated serum concentrations were compared with actual blood concentrations measured after steady state had been established (i.e., 5 × elimination half-life for a given patient). Similarly, the patient's body weight (BW) was lean body mass (LBM) were substituted into eq. 3 to determine the effect of both of these parameters on C^{ss} estimations.

Serum α_1-acid glycoprotein concentrations were determined using monospecific radial immunodiffusion plates (Calbiochem-Behring Corp.). The coefficient of variation of this assay technique ranges between 2.5% and 6%.

Data were analyzed by paired 't' and Student's 't' test where appropriate for intragroup and intergroup comparisons.

Discussion

The data show that the pharmacokinetic parameters λ_z, CL, and Vz can be accurately estimated from two blood samples drawn three to five hours after the start of infusion and at steady state (Fig 36–12). The data also demonstrate that the steady state and elimination kinetics of continuous extravascular bupivacaine infusions are independent of the site of infusion (Table 36–5).

The results of this study suggest that continuous perineural infusions of bupivacaine exhibit a wide margin of systemic safety and can be continued for

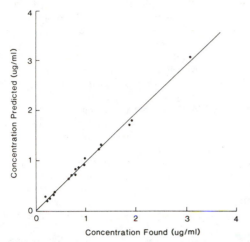

Fig 36–12.—The comparison of predicted bupivacaine concentration using the rapid two-point method with concentrations actually measured. (From Denson D.D., et al.[21] Reproduced by permission.)

five or more days at rates less than 30 mg/h in normal patients. Such patients do not require routine monitoring of their serum bupivacaine concentrations. Infusion rates of up to 30 mg/h do not appear to produce systemic toxicity even when CL is reduced by 60%. Minor toxicity was observed in patients with renal and hepatic disease at 30 mg/hr. Infusion rates to achieve a desired C^{ss} can be accurately predicted based solely on a patient's body weight or lean body mass. However, C^{ss} cannot be accurately predicted when an estimated CL is deter-

mined for each individual from two blood samples.[21] Although a full description of bupivacaine kinetics requires a multi-exponential function, a mono-exponential function suffices to produce the elimination half-life ($t_{1/2}$) and Vz during the post-infusion period.[22] However, prior knowledge of $t_{1/2}$ and Vz are not necessary to predict safe infusion rates since it only depends upon knowing the clearance.

Clearance was shown to be inversely related to serum α_1-acid glycoprotein concentrations. This suggests caution in interpreting *total* serum drug concentrations in relationship to those recorded through accompanying systemic toxicity. Ideally, unbound drug concentrations should be related to effects. This is particularly true in cancer patients, where higher than normal steady state concentrations of bupivacaine were found. However, no evidence of systemic toxicity was observed in any of these patients. Concomitantly, the patients had elevated α_1-acid glycoprotein levels. The higher C^{ss} levels of bupivacaine in these patients are consistent with the finding reported here that bupivacaine CL decreases with increases in α_1-acid glycoprotein concentrations. A decrease in CL should, however, produce a higher incidence of systemic toxicity. This was not observed, and the safety may be due to increased protein binding of bupivacaine to α_1-acid glycoprotein.

Summary

When epidural analgesia is adequate for the source of pain, there is no doubt that this method of

TABLE 36–5.—Comparison of the Mean Pharmacokinetic Values for Continuous Epidural, Sympathetic, and Brachial Plexus Infusions*†

		λ_z (L/h)	CL (L/h)	Vz (L)	Vz (ml/g) (BW)	Vz (ml/g) (LBM)
Brachial plexus	Estimated	0.169 ±0.019	28.5 ±4.2	174.9 ±23.3	2.51 ±0.40	2.78 ±0.44
	Actual	0.165 ±0.018	26.0 ±4.4	155.3 ±14.6	2.58 ±0.24	2.80 ±0.38
Sympathetic	Estimated	0.181 ±0.021	30.4 ±2.5	177.9 ±14.5	3.02 ±0.42	2.80 ±0.31
	Actual	0.204 ±0.028	29.2 ±2.8	151.8 ±10.8	2.47 ±0.25	2.45 ±0.25
Epidural	Estimated	0.179 ±0.010	33.2 ±2.4	195.7 ±14.5	2.94 ±0.30	2.82 ±0.23
	Actual	0.176 ±0.010	29.6 ±2.8	173.7 ±18.2	2.36 ±0.33	2.61 ±0.28

*Mean ± standard error of mean.
†From Denson D.D., Thompson G.A., Raj P.P.: *Int. J. Clin. Pharmacol. Ther. Toxicol.* 21:596, 1983. Used by permission.

pain relief is excellent. However, not all clinicians have been enthusiastic about its success. The criteria for which the infusion is used is different with different authors and this makes the comparisons difficult. The top-up technique is certainly easier to set up and simpler to use. Drug accumulation and tachyphylaxis is a serious problem with this technique. Hypotension is seen anywhere from 6% to 34%. The incidence of urinary retention is reported up to 20% in the literature.

The infusion technique has been criticized for providing inadequate analgesia. Cumulative toxicity and tachyphylaxis is another reason given for its inefficacy.[23] The authors' experience of 500 patients has found the infusion technique to be safe, adequate and with minor problems. No tachyphylaxis or cumulative toxicity is observed. This is significant because the duration of infusion is usually up to 7 days at this institution. Pharmacokinetic data correlate well with the clinical results obtained except for those patients with abnormal α_1-acid glycoprotein. The addition of volumetric pump to the infusion set has allowed the infusion to be continued accurately and uninterrupted without the presence of the physician. This makes the infusion technique superior to the top-up technique.

REFERENCES

1. Hingson R.A., Southworth J.L.: Continuous caudal anesthesia. *Am. J. Surg.* 58:93, 1942.
2. Adams R.C., Lundy J.S., Seldon T.H.: Continuous caudal anesthesia or analgesia: A consideration of the technic, various uses and some possible dangers. *JAMA* 122:152, 1943.
3. Curbelo M.M.: Continuous peridural segmental anesthesia by means of a ureteral catheter. *Curr. Res. Anesth.* 28:13, 1949.
4. Bromage P.R.: *Continuous Epidural Analgesia,* Chapter 7. Philadelphia, W.B. Saunders, Co., 1979, p.239.
5. Crawford J.S., Williams M.E., Veales S.: Particulate matter in the extradural space. *Brit. J. Anaesth.* 47:807, 1975.
6. Tucker G.T., et al.: Observed and predicted accumulation of local anaesthetic agents during continuous extradural analgesia. *Brit. J. Anaesth.* 49:237, 1977.
7. Green R., Dawkins C.J.M.: Postoperative analgesia: The use of a continuous drip epidural block. *Anaesthesia* 21:372, 1967.
8. Pflug A.E., Murphy T.M., Butler S.H., et al.: The effects of postoperative peridural analgesia on pulmonary therapy and pulmonary complications. *Anesthesiology* 41:8, 1974.
9. Spoerel W.E., Thomas A., Gerula G.R.: Continuous epidural analgesia: Experience with mechanical injection devices. *Canad. Anaesth. Soc. J.* 17:37, 1970.
10. Buckley F.P.: Acute traumatic and postoperative pain management; in Bridenbaugh P.O., Cousins M.J. (eds.): *Neural Blockade in Clinical Anesthesia and Management of Pain.* Philadelphia, J.B. Lippincott, Co., 1980, p. 599.
11. Cox J.M.R., Spoerel W.E.: Continuous epidural analgesia: The use of an intermittent injection device. *Can. Med. Assoc. J.* 11:72, 1964.
12. Raj P.P., McLennan J.E., Phero J.C.: Assessment and management planning of chronic low back pain, Stanton-Hicks M., Boas R. (eds.): *Low Back Pain.* New York, Raven Press, 1982, pp. 70–99.
13. Raj P.P., Rosenblatt R.M., Montgomery S.J.: The use of the nerve stimulator for peripheral blocks. *Regional Anaesth.* 5:2, 1980.
14. Reid W., Watt J.K., Gray T.G.: Phenol injection of the sympathetic chain. *Br. J. Surg.* 57:45, 1970.
15. Kappis M.: Erfahrungen mit local anasthesie bei bauchoperationen. *Verh. Dtsch Ges. Chir.* 1914; 43:1 teil 87.
16. Abdel-Salem A., Scott D.B.: Bupivacaine and etidocaine in epidural block for postoperative relief of pain. *Acta Anaesthesiol. Scand.* 60 (suppl.): 80, 1975.
17. Renck H., Edstrom H., Kinneberger B., et al.: Thoracic epidural analgesia. II. Prolongation in the early postoperative period by continuous injection of 1.0% bupivacaine. *Acta Anaesth. Scand.* 20:476, 1976.
18. Buckley F.P., Simpson B.R.: Acute traumatic and postoperative pain management. Neural blockade, in Cousins M.J., Bridenbaugh P.O., (eds.): *Clinical Anesthesia and Management of Pain.* Philadelphia, J.B. Lippincott, Co., 1980, p. 601.
19. Denson D.D., Raj P.P., Saldahna F., et al.: Perineural infusions of bupivacaine for prolonged analgesia: Pharmacokinetic considerations. *Int. J. Clin. Pharmacol. Ther. Toxicol.* 21:591–597, 1983.
20. Denson D.D., Raj P.P., Finnsson R.: Continuous epidural infusions of bupivacaine for management of terminal cancer pain: Pharmacolinetic considerations. *Anesthesiology* 57:A215, 1982.
21. Denson D.D., Thompson G.A., Raj P.P., et al.: Continuous perineural infusions of bupivacaine for prolonged analgesia: A rapid two-point method for estimating individual pharmacokinetic parameters. *Int. J. Pharmacol. Ther. Toxicol.* 22:552–556, 1984.
22. Ball W.D.: Unstructured two-point estimation of one-compartment linear pharmacokinetic parameters. *J. Clin. Pharmacol.* 22:326, 1982.
23. Tucker G.T., Mather L.E.: Clinical pharmacokinetics of local anesthetics. *Clin. Pharmacokinet.* 4:241–278, 1979.

Appendix 1: Nursing Protocol for Prolonged Infusion of Analgesic Solutions

Procedure:

Continuous perineural infusion of local anesthetic or analgesic solution

Purpose:

Insertion of a catheter into the epidural space, brachial or lumbar plexus, paravertebral sympathetic chain or caudal canal to provide continuous infusion of local anesthetic or narcotics for the removal of pain.

Policies Governing Procedure:

1. Nursing Care Policy F 13.0, "Intravenous Infusion Devices."
2. Nursing Care Procedure A 29.1, "Central Venous Catheter Dressing Change."
3. Nursing Care Procedure F 1.1, "Setting up an IV."

Precautions:

1. Frequent nursing observations and recordings of patient's subjective response to neural blockage is necessary to evaluate:
   A. Placement of catheter—if catheter is displaced patient will have partial or total return of pain.
   B. Signs and symptoms of systemic toxicity—central nervous system depression, convulsions, respiratory depression, dizziness, blurred vision, tremors, tinnitus, circumoral numbness, metallic taste, hypotension, or hypertension. If these signs are exhibited, the nurse should stop the infusion and notify physician.
2. Strict aseptic technique must be observed during insertion, dressing change, and removal of catheter. Each time dressing is changed check for signs of infection (redness, swelling, drainage).
3. Displacement of epidural and caudal catheters may be prevented by maintaining the patient on bedrest. However, there are indications for ambulation. Follow activity orders written by physician. Patients with axillary catheters should limit abduction of the affected arms. Dressings must be very secure.
4. Urinary retention or fecal incontinence may result with epidural or caudal blocks. The nurse must assess adequate output every eight hours and notify physician of questionable decreased output.
5. No other solutions or medications may be infused through this line.

Responsibility:

1. Registered Nurse.
2. Licensed Practical Nurse as trained.

Equipment:

1. Infusion pump (IVAC or Abbott/Shaw Life Care).
2. 0.22 micron in-line filter.
3. Extension tubing.
4. 500 ml of local anesthetic or analgesic solution (i.e., bupivacaine, morphine, or meperidine) from pharmacy.
   a. Provided in standard concentrations of:

Bupivacaine	Morphine	Meperidine
1. 0.5% (rarely used)	0.05%	0.1%
2. 0.25%		
3. 0.125%		

      Other analgesics and concentrations by special request to pharmacy.
   b. The amount of solution sent to the floor by pharmacy will be appropriate for a 24-hour period.

General remarks:

1. The order for local anesthetic solution will be written the night before by a physician to be ready when patient returns from the Pain Control Center the next day.
2. Analgesic solutions must be reordered every 24 hours.
3. The new bottle will be hung at 2:00 p.m. each day unless the physician orders a concentration change, then this change should be done immediately.

701

STEPS

On return to unit:

1. Obtain local anesthetic or analgesic solution from pharmacy.
2. Assemble infusion set-up (to be the responsibility of RN only).

3. Make initial neurovascular assessment and reevaluate:
   a. Every 4 hours with vital signs for bupivacaine infusion.
   b. Every 15 min in the first 2 hours, every 30 min in the next 6 hours, and every 1 hour for 12 hours for spinal narcotic infusion.
4. Instruct patient to notify the nurse if he/she experiences metallic taste, numbness of tongue or lips, tinnitus or dizziness, or difficulty in breathing.
5. Instruct patient to notify nurse if pain in affected area returns. Nurse should describe area as precisely as possible.

Maintenance

6. Check dressing every 4 hours for fluid leakage or bleeding. If either is present, notify physician. Change wet gauze only.

7. If the catheter appears to be causing the patient a problem, observe site for redness, edema, drainage, and note steri-strips or Op-Site security. Replace 4 × 4.
8. Change solution, tubing and filter to catheter hub every 24 hours. If concentration is changed prior to 2 p.m., change tubing with the new bottle or bag. *Tape all connections.*
9. Blood samples must be drawn until catheter is removed, for determination of serum anesthetic levels, per physician's orders.

POINTS OF EMPHASIS

Infusion must be started within one hour to maintain adequate analgesia.

A. Regulate infusion device according to physician's orders.
B. Tape all connections to avoid leakage or disconnection.
A. Assess degree of block by patient's subjective perception of pain.
B. Observe for color, temperature, strength and movement of the involved extremity (or extremities).
C. Check peripheral pulses.

These are early signs of toxicity. The nurse should stop the infusion and notify the physician if these symptoms occur.

Notify physician if pain returns but do not stop infusion. Concentration of local anesthetic may not be high enough to maintain sensory block. Catheter may also be displaced.

Epidural catheters—observe for CSF leakage. CSF Fluid will show a positive glucose using a Dextrostix.

Epidural and caudal catheters: Secure catheter length up the back and over the shoulder with 3-inch paper tape.
Any signs and symptoms of infection or loose steri-strips or Op-Site should be reported to the physician immediately. *Only physician* may change Op-Site or steri-strips.
Routine time for the complete change is 2 p.m.

Blood samples will be drawn by laboratory personnel every day. Order is written by physician every day.

Removal of Catheter

10. Catheter is removed by physician (after approximately 5 days). Catheter tip is sent for culture. The site is also cultured.

A. Culture catheter insertion site:
   1. Remove swabs from culturette tube and obtain culture.
   2. Place swabs in culturette tube.
   3. Crush end of tube to release media.
   4. Label tube and send to Bacteriology laboratory.
B. Cleanse catheter insertion site with betadine paint and allow to dry.
C. Note catheter length and condition of tip.
D. For culturing tip:
   1. Place tip of cannula into a dry sterile container.
   2. Snip cannula with sterile scissors and allow it to fall freely into sterile container.
   3. Label and send to Bacteriology lab.
E. Apply dry sterile dressing to site.

Charting guidelines:

To be entered on the Data Flow Sheet or Progress Notes.
   1. Note neurovascular assessments, catheter location and integrity of infusion system each shift.
   2. Record condition of extremity (or extremities) and dressing each shift.
   3. Note when catheter is removed, culture taken, and by whom.
   4. Chart any problems and course of action taken to resolve them.

Reviewed by:

Nursing Care Policies and Procedures Committee

37 / Analgesia With Intravenous Local Anesthetics

JAMES C. PHERO, D.M.D.
JOHN S. McDONALD, D.D.S.

SINCE 1908, MANY reports describing the analgesic effect of intravenous (IV) local anesthetics have been published. This technique has been beneficial in managing such painful conditions as burns, post-surgical pain, central pain, deafferentation syndrome, Raynaud's disease, phantom limb pain, causalgia, neuritis, and myofascial pain.

Although the classic local anesthetic agent utilized has been procaine, the choice of drug has varied from chloroprocaine to tetracaine. When employed for pain management, these anesthetics have been historically administered in large, incremental dosages. However, techniques of administration have also utilized the flowmeter and the IV pump in an attempt to control the infusion rate of the local anesthetic agents.

MECHANISM OF ACTION

Various theories have been proposed to describe the pharmacodynamics of local anesthetics. In 1938, Leriche proposed that injury to tissue caused reflex vasoconstriction, resulting in anoxia, capillary dysfunction, and increased permeability.[1, 2] This process would lead to the accumulation of nociceptive metabolites and to the irritation of peripheral nerve endings. Leriche believed that procaine, by acting directly on the arteriolar, meta-arteriolar, and capillary endothelia, produced widespread vasodilation, thereby anesthetizing the irritated endothelial nerve endings and breaking the reflex arc.

Lundy observed 4 hours of analgesia in several jaundiced patients with pruritus after the slow injection of 20 cc of 0.1% procaine solution.[3] His reported results supported Leriche's theory that peripheral irritation is accompanied by capillary hyperpermeability, allowing transudation of procaine into the tissues, anesthetizing the nerve endings.

Gordon in 1943 produced analgesia in burn patients, but only in the burned area and tissues affected by edema.[4] One year later, Bigelow and Harrison subcutaneously injected 5–40 cc of 2.0% procaine solution into the arm of normal subjects.[5] They noted a marked increase in the pain threshold in the forehead and therefore asserted that the change resulted from a systemic action of procaine following circulatory absorption rather than from a direct action of the agent.

In 1946 Allen et al. discovered six to eight times more procaine in the transudate of the injured area than in normal tissue.[6] Using the work of Gordon, Bigelow, and Harrison, they postulated that analgesia resulted both from procaine's local anesthetic action in the inflamed and traumatized tissue and from central action in the nervous system, partially blocking the sympathetic nervous system and neutralizing the abnormal vasoconstriction from the pain.

Graubard and Peterson combined these theories in 1950 and attributed the resulting relief of pain to the direct anesthetic action on irritated nerve fibers and to the indirect action of the procaine metabolite, diethylaminoethanol, on the vascular endothelium.[7]

Rowlingson et al. used IV lidocaine in normal volunteers and observed that blood levels below 3.0 μg/ml did not produce analgesia to ischemic pain produced by a tourniquet.[8]

Boas et al. used IV lidocaine (1.5–2 μg/ml, serum level) in patients with neuralgia and deafferentation syndrome to produce pain relief.[9] Anderson et al.[10] and Loeser et al.[11] hypothesized that pain associated with neurologic deafferentation may have a spinal electrogram pattern characterized by spontaneous high-frequency burst-discharge activity in the CNS.

CHOICE OF DRUG

Procaine has been the classic local anesthetic agent for IV administration because of its potency and low toxicity; however, its short action, even at maximum dosages, has been its major disadvantage. Since the mid-1940s, other local anesthetics have been utilized in an attempt to increase analgesic effects without compromising potency and low toxicity; such anesthetic agents as tetracaine, lidocaine, and chloroprocaine have been administered IV.

Bonica advocated IV tetracaine as particularly beneficial "in painful states, pruritus, and any other conditions in which a reflex pattern must be broken" because of its potency and longer duration.[12] Horan reported that 80%–90% of patients receiving IV tetracaine indicated pain relief lasting two to three times longer than that achieved with procaine; he advocated its use in cases of muscle spasm pain. However, because of its high toxicity potential, the recommended dosage was 3 mg/kg (not exceeding 250 mg of tetracaine) of 0.025%–0.05% tetracaine solution, to be infused over 2–3 hours.

Interest has also arisen in the efficacy of IV lidocaine in managing such painful conditions as neuralgia, deafferentation syndrome, and paroxysmal attacks associated with postherpetic neuralgia. For the latter pain problems, Hatangdi et al. used IV lidocaine, 1.0–1.5 mg/kg.[14] In general, there was complete relief of lancinating pain within seconds after injection. In addition, the degree of success with IV lidocaine often indicated patient response to oral antiepileptic drugs. Boas et al. used this local anesthetic agent in patients with deafferentation syndrome and noted significant pain relief within 15–20 minutes of starting the infusion.[9] In 1982, Atkinson advocated IV lidocaine for the management of intractable pain of adiposis dolorosa, administering a 0.1% solution of lidocaine IV until a total dose of 200 mg had been delivered over a 35-minute period.[15] Significant pain relief lasted for 2 to over 12 months.

Since 1952, focus has been placed on the IV administration of 2-chloroprocaine, the ortho-chloro derivative of procaine. Foldes and McNall found chloroprocaine to be two times more potent and to be hydrolyzed four times faster than procaine.[16] They recommended its use in poor-risk patients because of its low toxicity and high potency. In 1981, Parris et al. successfully used a 60-ml bolus of IV 3% chloroprocaine solution to control pain associated with partial splenic embolization.[17]

Schnapp et al. used IV chloroprocaine to treat chronic intractable pain.[18] Forty-three percent of the patients reported more than 50% relief, lasting longer than 30 days. Phero et al. consider IV chloroprocaine to be safe and efficacious in managing certain chronic intractable pain problems, particularly in patients with musculoskeletal pain.[19]

TECHNIQUE OF ADMINISTRATION

Two techniques have been used to administer IV local anesthetics in pain management, either as a single-dose or with continuous infusion. Leriche was the first to use a single dose of 5–10 cc of 1% procaine solution. Lundy used a 0.1% solution of procaine infused over several hours for pruritus.[3] Graubard and Peterson devised the procaine unit, defined as 4 mg/kg of 0.1% procaine infused over 20 minutes via flowmeter.[7] Half of this dose was initially given as a bolus, then the rest of the dose was adjusted according to the incidence of side effects. In 500 patients, Bonica used one-tenth Graubard's procaine unit of pontocaine, delivering a total dose of 3.0 mg/kg (not exceeding 250 mg) over 2–3 hours.[12] The onset of analgesic effect was noted within one-half hour and was reported to last longer than with procaine.

Boas et al. administered lidocaine at a rate of 4 mg/minute using a Harvard pump for 1 hour in patients with deafferentation syndrome; these patients reported pain relief with serum lidocaine levels of 1.5–2.0 μg/ml.[9]

Foldes and McNall compared four local anesthetic agents (procaine, chloroprocaine, tetracaine, and lidocaine) in the conventional concentration ratios used in regional anesthesia for toxicity in man.[16] They observed no significant difference in the time of onset of signs and symptoms of toxicity in these agents. However, the signs and symptoms disappeared faster with 2-chloroprocaine, which was hydrolyzed four times faster than procaine. On the other hand, tetracaine hydrochloride was hydrolyzed 3.5 times slower than procaine. Investigators noted that the more rapidly an agent was hydrolyzed in the serum, the larger was the quantity of that agent required to maintain toxicity. Conversely, the slower an agent was hydrolyzed, the smaller was the dosage required to produce a toxic blood level.

In 1981, Schnapp et al. used 3% 2-chloroprocaine without preservatives delivered via a 30-ml syringe at a rate of 30–120 mg/minute until either the pain had subsided or 900 mg had been injected.[18] In that study, 44 patients were given a series of four IV 2-chloroprocaine injections 1 to 14 days apart. Forty-three percent of the patients had pain relief lasting more than 30 days. Patients with allodynia and/or chronic pain responded favorably to this treatment.

From 1981 to 1984, the University of Cincinnati Pain Control Center has administered IV chloroprocaine via IV pump to control the incidence of side effects. All patients exhibit chronic pain problems refractory to conventional therapeutic modalities (surgery, nerve blocks, physical therapy, analgesics, etc.). They were ASA I or II status, had no known allergy to ester compounds, and had normal serum pseudocholinesterase levels.

A 1% chloroprocaine solution was administered at a rate of 1–1.5 mg/kg/minute until a total dose of 10–20 mg/kg had been delivered. All infusions were conducted in a controlled environment where resuscitative equipment and drugs were immediately available. In addition, the patient's vital signs (ECG, blood pressure, heart rate, and mentation) were monitored. If evidence of CNS toxicity except for mild symptoms (tinnitus, metallic taste, lightheadedness) occurred, the rate of infusion was decreased by one half, or, if the symptoms persisted or worsened the infusion was discontinued. Patients were required to rest for 1 hour after conclusion of the treatment, and then, if in satisfactory condition, were discharged home, in the company of an escort.

MONITORING

Monitoring of the patient during IV infusion of a local anesthetic is essential. The patient's vital signs (ECG, blood pressure, heart rate, and mentation) are evaluated every 5 minutes. In over 108 treatments at the University of Cincinnati, patients did not have any deleterious sequalae.

EVALUATION

Patients receive a series of four or five IV chloroprocaine infusions to evaluate efficacy of the modality. Pain relief scores are obtained prior to, during, and after the infusion. For the period between treatments in the diagnostic series, usually 1–3 weeks, patients are required to evaluate pain relief, function and psychological scores on a visual analogue scale four times daily (morning, afternoon, evening, and night). In addition the amount of oral medication consumed per day are documented.

SIDE EFFECTS

The side effects of IV local anesthetics have long been documented and are associated with CNS toxicity.[20–23] Early signs and symptoms include metallic taste, tinnitus, lightheadedness, agitation, and drowsiness. Moderate signs of CNS toxicity include difficulty with ocular focusing, nystagmus, slurred speech, dysarthria, numbness in the lips and tongue, and tingling or a heavy feeling in the extremities. Untoward effects of late CNS toxicity include hypotension or hypertension, bradycardia or tachycardia, seizure, anaphylaxis, and unconsciousness. Cardiac and respiratory failure, coma, and death may occur in the very late stages of CNS toxicity.

PROGNOSIS

Patients with certain types of chronic intractable pain problems refractory to conservative modalities may respond well to this type of therapy. Thirty-eight patients received 178 IV chloroprocaine treatments over a 30-month period, an average of 4.7 treatments per patient. The time between treatments ranged from 3 days to 18 weeks, averaging 2.4 weeks per treatment. Of the 27 patients seen in the last 18 months, 15 (56%) completed the diagnostic series of four to five IV chloroprocaine infusions; 12 of the 15 (80%) continued to receive additional treatments for continued pain relief. Fifty-eight percent of these patients (7/12) returned to usual conservative therapeutic modalities or were maintained on IV chloroprocaine infusions at a 3- to 6-month interval. Five of the 7 patients (72%) with chronic intractable musculoskeletal pain had at least 30% pain relief for more than 11 months.

CASE REPORTS

CASE 1.—A 42-year-old woman presented with a 1½-year history of chronic right-sided headaches, common over the temples. She had previously been seen by at least five different medical practitioners who had prescribed at least 19 different pain medications. Chronic muscle contraction headache was diagnosed and the patient was initially treated with myoneuronal blocks, physical therapy, TENS, and behavioral medicine. Not until IV 2-chloroprocaine infusions were added to the treatment regimen did the pain remit. The photograph shown in Figure 37–1 was made 5 minutes following the completion of a session of IV 2-chloroprocaine therapy.

CASE 2.—A 25-year-old man presented with a 4-year-history of disabling headaches, for which he had consulted more than five health professionals. At the Pain Control Center, no pathology was detected. The patient did have a mild depressive disorder with mixed anxiety, and the diagnosis of chronic muscle contraction headaches was made. Pain control modalities attempted prior to IV 2-chloroprocaine administration included physical therapy, TENS, meditation, behavioral medicine, myoneural injections, and diagnostic somatic blocks. The patient was treated for 3 months at the Pain Control Center, with minimum response to conservative management.

Intravenous 2-chloroprocaine therapy initiated after an initial normal saline control test injection. The treatment schedule was as follows:

Treatment	Rate	Total Dose
1. 1 mg/kg/min	15 mg/kg	990 mg
2. 1 mg/kg/min	15 mg/kg	1,010 mg
3. 1 mg/kg/min	15 mg/kg	1,010 mg
4. 1 mg/kg/min	20 mg/kg	1,220 mg
5. 1 mg/kg/min	15 mg/kg	990 mg
6. 1 mg/kg/min	20 mg/kg	1,320 mg
7. 1.5 mg/kg/min	20 mg/kg	1,320 mg

SUMMARY

Because most patients receive further IV chloroprocaine infusions, the average pain relief tends to approach and remain at 50% and lasts for longer periods of time. All patients exhibited signs and symptoms of mild CNS toxicity, primarily due to an increase in blood levels of 2-chloroprocaine and its metabolites. Rapid recovery from CNS effects was due to the hydrolysis of chloroprocaine, its half-life being 23 seconds in the average adult. The results suggest that the appropriate patient who undergoes a series as described might experience enough pain cycle disruption to have conventional therapy reinstituted, the frequency of oral analgesics decreased, and eventually receive only IV 2-chloroprocaine maintenance treatments for pain exacerbation. Furthermore, the technique of controlled IV chloropro-

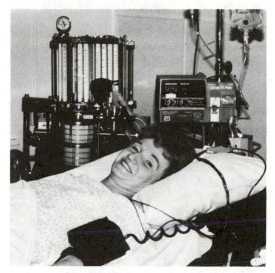

Fig 37–1.—Case 1. See text.

caine administration has the advantage of increased patient safety when compared to multiple large incremental injections because of the reduced risk of convulsions, respiratory failure, coma, and cardiac failure because of the ability to regulate steady-state therapeutic levels of 2-chloroprocaine. It is not recommended that patients with atypical quantitative and/or qualitative assessments of cholinesterase levels receive this treatment.

REFERENCES

1. Leriche R.: Intra-arterial therapy of infections and other diseases. *Mem. Acad. Chir.* 64:220, 1938.
2. Leriche R.: Simple methods of easing pain in the extremities in arterial diseases and in certain vasomotor disorders. *Presse Med.* 49:799, 1941.
3. Lundy J.S.: *Clinical Anesthesia.* Philadelphia, W.B. Saunders Co., 1941.
4. Gordon R.A.: Intravenous Novocaine for analgesia in burns. *Can. Med. Assoc. J.* 49:478, 1943.
5. Bigelow N., Harrison I.: General analgesic effects of procaine. *J. Pharmacol. Exp. Ther.* 81:368, 1944.
6. Allen F.M., Grossman L.W., Lyons L.V.: Intravenous procaine analgesia. *Anesth. Analg.* 25:1, 1946.
7. Graubard D.J., Peterson M.C.: *Clinical Uses of Intravenous Procaine.* Springfield, Charles C Thomas, 1950.
8. Rowlingson J.C., DiFazio C.A., Foster J., et al.: Lidocaine as an analgesic for experimental pain. *Anesthesiology* 52:20, 1980.
9. Boas R.A., Covino B.G., Shahnarian A.: Analgesic responses to IV lignocaine. *Br. J. Anaesth.* 54:501, 1982.

10. Anderson L.S., Black R.G., Abraham J., et al.: Deafferentiation neuronal hyperactivity: A possible etiology of paresthesias following retrogasserian rhizotomy. *J. Neurosurg.* 35:444, 1971.

11. Loeser J.D., Ward A.A., White D.E.: Chronic deafferentiation of human spinal cord neurons. *J. Neurosurg.* 29:48, 1968.

12. Bonica J.J.: Regional anesthesia with tetracaine. *Anesthesiology* 11:606–716, 1950.

13. Horan J.S.: The intravenous administration of local anesthetic agents in the management of pain, in Bonica J.J.: *The Management of Pain.* Philadelphia, Lea & Febiger, 1953, pp. 522–564.

14. Hatangdi V.S., Boas R.A., Richards E.G.: Post-herpetic neuralgia: Management with anti-epileptic and tricyclic drugs, in Bonica J.J., et al. (eds.): *Advances in Pain Research and Therapy.* New York, Raven Press, 1976, vol. 1, pp. 583–587.

15. Atkinson R.L.: Intravenous lidocaine for the treatment of intractable pain of adiposis dolorosa. *Int. J. Obes.* 6:351, 1982.

16. Foldes F.F., McNall P.G.: 2-chloroprocaine: A new local anesthetic agent. *Anesthesiology* 13:287–296, 1981.

17. Parris W.C.V., Gerlock A.J., MacDonnell R.C.: Intra-arterial chloroprocaine for the control of pain associated with partial splenic embolization. *Anesth. Analg.* 60:112–115, 1981.

18. Schnapp M., Mays K.S., North W.C.: Intravenous chloroprocaine in the treatment of pain. *Anesth. Analg.* 60:844–845, 1981.

19. Phero J.C., McDonald J.S., Raj P.P., et al.: Controlled intravenous administration of chloroprocaine for intractable management. *Reg. Anaesth.* 9:50–51, 1984.

20. Covino B.G., Vassallo H.G.: *Local Anesthetics: Mechanism of Action and Clinical Use.* New York, Grune & Stratton, Inc., 1976.

21. De Jong R.H.: *Local Anesthetics,* ed. 2., Springfield, Ill., Charles C Thomas, Publisher, 1977.

22. Cousins M.J., Scott D.B.: Clinical pharmacology of local anesthetic agents, in Cousins M.J., Bridenbaugh P.O. (eds.): *Neural Blockade in Clinical Anesthesia and Management of Pain.* Philadelphia, J.B. Lippincott Co., 1980, pp. 86–121.

23. Savarese J.J., Covino G.B.: Pharmacology of local anesthetic drugs, in Miller R.D. (ed.): *Anesthesia.* New York, Churchill Livingstone, Inc., 1981, pp. 583–591.

38 / Spinal Opiates

LAURENCE E. MATHER, Ph.D.
P. PRITHVI RAJ, M.D.

ENDOGENOUS OPIATE

IT NOW APPEARS certain that there are at least three different synthetic pathways in the very complex endogenous opiate peptide systems in the CNS and elsewhere in the body. They are:

1. The β-lipotropin to β-endorphin family.—This occurs predominately in the pituitary. β-lipotropin and ACTH both arrive from a common pro-hormone known as pre-pro-opiomelanocortin and stressful stimuli which increases ACTH outflow also appear to cause increased outflow of β-endorphin. β-lipotropin also gives rise α-, γ-, and δ-endorphins. β-endorphin administered intracerebroventricularly may produce profound analgesia with a molar potency ratio of about 50 times that of morphine. It is active if administered intravenously, but the molar potency ratio is diminished to about 3 to 4 times that of morphine.

2. The pentapeptides.—The pro-hormone pre-pro-enkephalin A can be cleaved to multiple copies of both methionine (met-) and leucine (leu-) enkephalins. Pentapeptide sequences extended by one or two amino acids have also been found along with the pentapeptides in hormone granules. These compounds also have opiate activity and are more resistant to metabolic degradation than the pentapeptides themselves. The enkephalins are attacked by both N-peptidases and carboxy peptidases in blood and tissues. Therefore, the duration of analgesia is exceedingly brief, irrespective of the route of administration. Potentially useful derivatives for clinical work have required a balance between the desired properties of chemical stability, lipid solubility, and receptor fit. While it is difficult to demonstrate tolerance to the naturally occurring enkephalins due to the rapidity of their metabolism, tolerance to stable synthetic enkephalins can be demonstrated. Furthermore, naloxone can precipitate withdrawal effects after enkephalin use and the enkephalins can substitute for morphine in morphine withdrawal.

3. Dynorphin.—This is a more recently discovered 17 amino acid peptide which is derived from pre-pro-enkephalin B (also called pre-pro-dynorphin). This peptide contains the 1–5 sequence of leu enkephalin and its NH_2 terminus. It is also differently distributed from β-endorphin and met- and leu-enkephalin in the brain.

Although these and related peptides may all be classified as opiates, there are several differences in their effects, in particular, in their potency ratios to other opiates. This would require the possibility of multiple types of opiate receptors and, indeed, there is a growing body of evidence to suggest that they do exist.

CLASSIFICATION OF OPIATE RECEPTORS

Five categories of different receptors have been postulated to date, and the concept has taken hold in the clinical use of opiates. The receptors have been given the Greek letter which corresponds to the first letter in their primary putative agonists: μ for morphine, δ for DADL (D-ala^2-D-leu^{5}enkephalin, a synthetic compound which is resistant to metabolism), κ for EKC (ethyl ketocyclazocine), ε for beta-endorphin, and σ for SKF 10007 (also known as N-allyl cyclazocine). The strongest evidence for multiple receptor types have come from:

1. Differential responses of bioassays to different opiate agonists.

2. Some neuroeffective functions may be resistant to one drug but responsive to another.

3. Tolerance induced by one drug may not be transferred as tolerance to another.

4. Radioreceptor binding studies.

Unfortunately, claims for both receptor selectivity and primary putative agonists have to be somewhat tempered. There is a great deal of cross-reactivity, so either the receptors are not specific, or, more likely, the agonists tested are able to activate more than one receptor type. In the brain and spinal cord the three main types of receptors are μ, δ, and κ.

Do these receptors interact, and if so, how? μ and δ receptors appear to have a positive interaction in the modulation of pain in the spinal cord. κ agonists are potent spinal analgesics but do not appear to be inhibitory or additive with μ and δ receptors. μ and δ agonists produce analgesia when injected directly into the periaqueductal gray, κ agonists do not. The μ, κ, and δ receptors in the brain all appear to mediate behavioral effects. The κ receptors are less sensitive than μ receptors to naloxone, and the σ receptors are not sensitive to naloxone. In the spinal cord, the κ receptors are the most sensitive to naloxone and the δ receptors are the least sensitive. Two subclasses of μ receptors have been suggested—a higher affinity $\mu1$ receptor which modulates analgesic response, and a lower affinity $\mu2$ receptor which modulates respiratory effects.

The ϵ receptors are probably true opiate receptors that respond primarily to endorphin, β-endorphin, α-, γ-, and δ-endorphin. These receptors may be the active site for the neuroregulatory action of the endorphins. The σ receptors, on the other hand, are probably not true opiate receptors. σ agonists do not produce analgesia; they have only neurobehavioral effects and compete with phencyclidine rather than with naloxone for the active site.

Using the increasing knowledge of the location of the specific opiate receptor types, it may be possible to utilize, for example, a κ agonist to produce spinal analgesia with a reduced incidence of respiratory depression. However, this may be at the cost of increased euphoria or sedation. One could propose the use of an agent which is a κ and δ agonist but a μ antagonist, e.g., pentazocine. Future work in clinical trials should address new pharmacologic agonists or agonist-antagonist combinations. One may be able to achieve the differential action of analgesia alone as a distinct opiate agonist effect.

CLINICAL APPLICATIONS

One of the most important recent advances in opiate physiology and pharmacology, undoubtedly is recognition of their usefulness in intraspinal administration for acute and chronic pain. The rationale for this use is simple: high concentrations of opiate receptors present in the dorsal horn may be reached readily and stimulated so that analgesia occurs from opiate agonists administered in such small doses that their systemic effects would be negligible if administered systemically. Intraspinal opiates produce analgesia without altering autonomic or neuromuscular function, proprioception, or light touch. This allows patients to ambulate without orthostatic hypotension or incoordination.

Following the discovery of spinal opiate receptors, animal studies soon documented the effectiveness of intraspinal opiates. Yaksh demonstrated in unanesthetized rats that intrathecal opiates produced profound segmental analgesia which was dose dependent and naloxone reversible.[1] Although analgesia was profound and segmental after 40–60 minutes, cephalad spread was evident, especially at higher doses. Following the reports of animal studies, a flurry of brief clinical reports appeared in the literature. The majority described profound and prolonged analgesia from epidural and intrathecal morphine without side effects and without motor or autonomic blockade. However, many of these early studies were not controlled, and there was no agreement as to a minimally effective dose, even for the commonly used opiates such as morphine, meperidine, and fentanyl.

Further evidence was based on animal studies that there is a multiplicative relationship between opiates applied spinally and centrally.[2] This is, whereas analgesia can be obtained by stimulating either spinal or central receptors with an opiate agonist more profound analgesia can be obtained by stimulating both spinal and central receptors simultaneously. The clinical correlate of this observation is that systemically absorbed opiate can enhance the analgesia obtained by local spinal application. Although some have even suggested that the systemically absorbed fraction is *the primary determinant* of analgesia,[3] others have collected evidence which clearly demonstrates that after the epidural administration of morphine, patients have analgesia in the presence or absence of a morphine plasma concentrations known to produce analgesia when administered intravenously (IV).[4] Furthermore, the amount of drug administered intrathecally in many cases and which produces analgesia would be totally without effect even if injected as an IV bolus (Fig 38–1).

DIFFUSION OF OPIATES THROUGH DURA MATER

Before considering the epidural and intrathecal dose-response relationship appropriate to clinical practice, we will examine the role of physicochemical properties of the opiate in determining the nature of the response. An innovative study by Moore and co-workers determined permeability constants for the diffusion of a variety of substances across isolated sections of human dura.[5] Their studies indicate that when the concentration gradient to spinal cord is high—for instance, immediately after epidural injection—the primary determinant of the permeability constant is the molecular weight of the substance. As a consequence, morphine and methadone diffuse across the dura mater at the same rate, since their molecular weights are almost the same. The increased lipid solubility derived from acetylating morphine to produce heroin is offset by the increased molecular weight so that heroin too diffuses through the dura at the same rate as morphine. According to these authors, fentanyl, having a "long thin" molecular shape, diffuses faster than the "globular" morphine analogues. However, this model fails to take into account direct transport into the spinal cord of substances absorbed into the local blood supply, in particular, the radicular artery.

Countering the direct effect of the permeability constant, the rate of systemic absorption competes with the rate of dural penetration by reducing the concentration of drug available to penetrate the dura. Other physical factors are potentially important also. The rate of dural penetration is directly related to the surface area in contact with the drug solution and inversely related to the local apparent and real volume of distribution of the drug. Thus it would be expected that both the volume of injectate as well as any local binding factors and fat solubility of lipid-soluble agents would play roles in regulating the time-course of analgesia. The model also predicts that the rate of dural penetration of common opiates, and therefore the rate of onset of effects, should not show marked differences, since for a given volume injected, many effects offset each other. By and large this is observed clinically, although the analgesia from morphine does take slightly longer to develop fully than the analgesia from more lipid-soluble agents (Table 38–1).

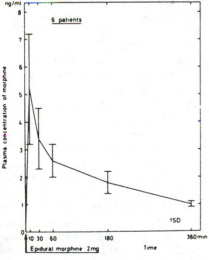

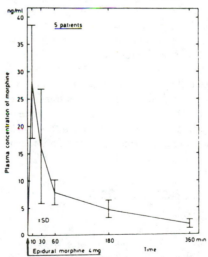

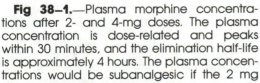

Fig 38–1.—Plasma morphine concentrations after 2- and 4-mg doses. The plasma concentration is dose-related and peaks within 30 minutes, and the elimination half-life is approximately 4 hours. The plasma concentrations would be subanalgesic if the 2 mg dose was given systemically. Since the patients have profound analgesia with these doses epidurally, one must infer that the intraspinal concentration is analgesic at the receptor site. (From Rawal et al.[11] Reproduced by permission.)

TABLE 38–1.—EPIDURAL OPIOIDS: LATENCY AND DURATION OF POSTOPERATIVE ANALGESIA

DRUG	DOSE (mg)	DETECTABLE ONSET* (min)	COMPLETE PAIN RELIEF* (min)	DURATION* (hr)
Meperidine	30–100	5–10	12–30	6 (median) 4–20 (6.6 ± 3.3)
Morphine	5–10		60	20
	5	23.5 ± 6	37 ± 6	18.1 ± 6.8
			60–90	12.3 ± 7.7
Methadone	5	12.5 ± 2	17 ± 3	7.2 ± 4.6
				8.7 ± 5.9
Hydromorphone	1	13 ± 4	23 ± 8	11.4 ± 5.5
Fentanyl	0.1			5.7 ± 3.7
	0.1	4–10	20	2.6–4
Diamorphine	5		9	12.4 ± 6.5
	6	5	15	2–21

*Values are in means ± SD or range.

DURATION OF ACTION

When the extradural to intradural concentration gradient has ceased to exert a dominating influence, the duration of action will be regulated by the rate of systemic absorption and the rate of receptor dissociation. Thus, duration will be governed by penetration rate across capillary endothelium: i.e., the more lipid soluble the agent, the faster its removal. This is further modulated by receptor dissociation so that a slowly dissociating agonist agent like buprenorphine can outlast a pure agonist like methadone, despite a much lower clearance of methadone than buprenorphine from the blood. The high water solubility and low lipid solubility of morphine also produce prolonged duration due to retarded escape from the spinal fluid. The consequence is that morphine dissolved in spinal fluid becomes transmitted cephalad with bulk flow of CSF and has the propensity to produce effects by direct combination with central opiate receptors from within the CNS rather than by delivery via the blood.

PLASMA CONCENTRATION OF OPIATES

Pharmacokinetic data for epidurally administered opiates reveal that rapid vascular uptake of opiates from the epidural venous plexus gives rise to plasma concentrations similar to those achieved with an equivalent intramuscular (IM) dose. To some degree, vascular uptake may contribute to the onset of epidural opiate analgesia; however, analgesic effects more closely correlate with CSF opiate concentrations than with plasma concentrations. Cousins and co-workers studied the pharmacokinetics of 100 mg of epidural meperidine and found that the onset of analgesia at 5 minutes correlated with high CSF meperidine concentrations (>2 ug/ml) rather than with plasma concentrations, which were subanalgesic (Fig 38–2).[6]

Jorgensen et al. studied simultaneous plasma and CSF morphine concentrations after epidural and intrathecal administration of morphine.[7] After 10 minutes, CSF concentrations exceeded plasma concentrations in the patients receiving epidural administration. Peak CSF concentrations occurred at 2 hours, and, after 6 hours, the CSF concentrations remained significantly higher than those in plasma. Jorgensen et al. suggested that the onset of pain relief after epidural injection may be due to combined systemic and spinal effects, but that the continued analgesia was due to spinal effects alone. Extremely high CSF concentrations were noted after administration of 1 mg of intrathecal morphine, which indicates that even smaller doses should be used.

Nordberg et al. studied the pharmacokinetics of epidural morphine in postthoracotomy patients and found that both the duration of analgesia and the peak concentrations of morphine in plasma and CSF were dose dependent.[8] Again, plasma concentrations were in proportion to those obtained by doses for IM injection and did not correlate with onset or duration of analgesia. The plasma and CSF elimination half-lives of morphine were similar (mean = 4.3 hr), suggesting that the long duration of analgesia from epidural morphine was due to the high CSF concentrations attained. These authors also found that the lumbar and thoracic approaches to

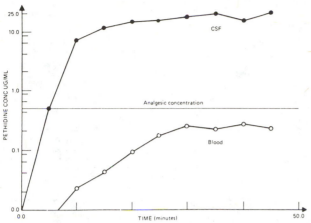

Fig 38–2.—CSF and blood meperidine concentrations after epidural injection of 100 mg. Onset of analgesia (5 minutes) coincided with a very high CSF meperidine concentration. (Adapted from Cousins et al.[6] Reproduced by permission.)

thoracic pain resulted in an equivalent duration of analgesia.

Youngstrom et al. compared 4 mg of morphine delivered IM or epidurally in a double-blind, randomized study of postcesarean analgesia.[9] They found that 4 mg of epidural morphine resulted in better analgesia, compared to 4 mg delivered IM. The onset of epidural analgesia was delayed up to 2 hours and lasted 20 hours. At 10 minutes the mean peak plasma morphine concentrations after epidural injection were 50% lower than after IM administration. These investigators suggest that the onset of analgesia, which was delayed in these patients up to 2 hours, was entirely secondary to selective spinal action. Their data suggested that epidural morphine gives rise to similar peak plasma concentrations as achieved with IM injections, so that vascular uptake may contribute to the onset of analgesia, but analgesic effects, especially duration, correlate more closely with CSF concentrations.

SIDE EFFECTS OF SPINAL OPIATE ANALGESIA

Although there is no effect on motor or sympathetic function, side effects can develop in several organ systems. These include pruritis, nausea and vomiting, urinary retention, and respiratory depression.

About 5%–15% of patients given intraspinal opiates develop pruritis. Perhaps it is less frequent with preservative-free morphine, but is not related to histamine release, so antihistamines are ineffective. It is often segmentally limited, but it can be widespread and most often affects the head and neck and may be related to the cephalad spread of opiate. This complication is antagonized with 0.2–0.4 mg of naloxone administered intravenously.

Nausea and vomiting are common with all routes of opiate administration and occur secondary to altered modulation of afferent input at the area postrema and nucleus solitarius. Some 15%–30% of patients given intraspinal opiates experience nausea and vomiting, which can occur early after epidural administration secondary to vascular uptake and late secondary to rostral spread. Nausea and vomiting can be treated with droperidol, promethazine, or 0.2–0.4 mg of naloxone administered systemically.

Urinary retention occurs in 15%–20% of patients, mostly men. The underlying mechanism is not clear but may be related to decreased bladder sensation and increased sphincter tone. Bromage et al. have shown that all ten young males given 10 mg of epidural morphine developed urinary retention. Whereas this was unresponsive to 5 mg of bethanecol it was responsive to naloxone, 0.4 mg IV.[10] Rawal et al. observed evidence of increased bladder capacity and relaxation of the detrusor muscle in a urodynamic study of 30 volunteers given morphine epidurally. The intensity of detrusor muscle relaxation was similar for 2 mg, 4 mg, or 10 mg of epidural morphine (Fig 38–3).[11] Urinary retention is not a serious clinical problem, but it should be remembered that catheterization can cause urinary tract infection and bacteremia.

Respiratory depression is the most distressing of all the complications because it is life-threatening. It occurs more frequently after intrathecal (4%–7%) than after epidural (0.1%–0.4%) administration, and after the administration of as little as 1 mg intrathecally. Both early and late respiratory depres-

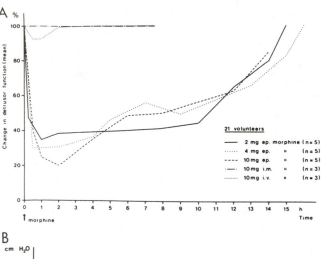

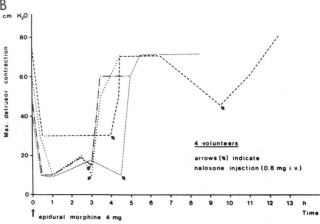

Fig 38–3.—A, effects of systemic and epidural morphine injection on detrusor function. IM and IV injections of 10 mg of morphine do not result in a significant change in detrusor function. Epidural morphine (all doses), on the other hand, results in a 60%–80% difference from control detrusor function within 30 minutes. Recovery takes 14–15 hours. **B,** effect of 0.8 mg of IV naloxone on detrusor contraction in four volunteers. Dose was given after the effect of epidural morphine had been established. Bladder function returned to normal within minutes. (From Rawal N., Mollefors K., Axelsson G., et al.: An experimental study of urodynamic effects of epidural morphine and of naloxone reversal. *Anesth. Analg.* 62:641–647, 1983. Reproduced by permission.)

sion are seen. Early respiratory depression results from vascular uptake of the opiate, and late respiratory depression is the result of rostral spread of opiate-laden CSF to the medullary respiratory centers. Late respiratory depression is especially insidious since it may occur at a time when the patient is less well monitored and may seem unrelated to the dose of the opiate. With the less lipid soluble opiates (principally morphine), the rate of vascular uptake of opiate is slow so that late respiratory depression occurs by slow CSF redistribution. Respiratory depression has been reported occurring 6–11 hours after injection (Fig 38–4). With intrathecal injection, early respiratory depression is rare, but with the epidural route, early and late respiratory depression occur as the result of vascular uptake and CSF redistribution, respectively. Kafer et al.[12] have demonstrated two discrete nadirs in CO_2 sensitivity after 0.1 mg/kg of epidural morphine: the first at 1–2 hours from vascular uptake and the second at 8 hours, when the segmental level of analgesia had

risen to upper thoracic and cervical segments. Rising levels of hypalgesia to pinprick and temperature differences can be helpful as a warning sign of impending late respiratory depression.

When respiratory depression occurs, it is often prolonged and requires repeated doses of naloxone. It should be remembered that naloxone is a high clearance drug. Morphine's low lipid solubility, which contributes to its prolonged analgesia, also contributes to prolonged respiratory depression. Naloxone reversal of respiratory depression leaves analgesia unaffected, probably because CSF opiate concentrations at the region of injection are many times larger than those at the floor of the fourth ventricle. Furthermore, the relative blood flows to the brain and spinal cord favor transport of antagonist to the brain more than the spinal receptors.

In a study by Bromage et al. comparing 10 mg of epidural and IV morphine, early respiratory depression at 1–2 hours was equivalent by the two routes; however, at 3–22 hours, CO_2 responsiveness was

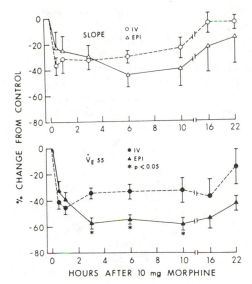

Fig 38–4.—CO_2 response curves after epidural or IV administration of 10 mg of morphine in a crossover study. Mean values ± SEM percentage changes in slope and ventilation at end-tidal Pco_2 of 55 mm Hg are indicated. (From Neilson C.H., Camporesi E.M., Bromage P.R., et al.: CO_2 sensitivity after epidural and IV morphine. *Anesthesiology* 55:A372, 1981. Reproduced by permission.)

significantly lower after epidural administration and reached its nadir at 6–10 hours.[13]

In 9,300 patients with respiratory depression after intraspinal opiates, Gustafsson et al. identified the following risk factors for the development of respiratory depression:[14]

Age ≥ 70

Impaired respiratory function

Thoracic epidural approach

Concomitant parenteral administration of opiates

Each of these is logical and emphasize the need for a cautious approach in deciding to use this method.

DOSING OF SPINAL OPIATES

What are the appropriate doses for intrathecal or epidural opiates? There are few controlled studies demonstrating standardized responses, and even fewer studies that used the same protocol to study response as a function of dose in order to determine optimal dose. Original studies on intrathecal morphine used 0.5–1 mg in patients with cancer.[15] Oth-

ers have reported that doses on this order also are effective in producing analgesia after abdominal surgery.[16] Samii and co-workers examined two dosages, 0.2 and 0.02 mg/kg of morphine sulfate, and concluded that although the larger dose provided slightly longer analgesia, the associated incidence of side effects, including late onset of sedation, outweighed its benefits.[17] Consequently they recommended the lower dose. Barrow and String have suggested that doses should be related to age: morphine sulfate, 1.5 mg, for ages 18–55 years; 1 mg for ages 65–75 years; and 0.5 for those older than 75 years.[18] This schedule seems to make sense, in view of the age-related sensitivity that is known generally for opiates.[19]

Intrathecal meperidine has been used as the sole medication for patients undergoing surgery of the abdomen and lower limbs. Mirceau and colleagues used an average dose of 1 mg/kg injected as a 50 mg/ml solution and reported a remarkable success rate (90%–95%), with a duration of analgesia of 90–120 minutes in a series of more than 700 patients.[20] Adverse effects occurred in only 0.5% of the patients and consisted of hypotension and bradycardia, which were readily corrected with ephedrine, and of hypoxemia, which responded to ventilation. Analgesia was inadequate in 5% of the patients. Intuitively, the choice of meperidine makes sense, since it is known to have a potent local anesthetic activity along with its opiate activity.

For the reasons given above, many authorities prefer to use the epidural route. Optimum doses have been debated extensively, and a variety of studies with morphine in volunteers have demonstrated the folly of using any but the minimum doses necessary.[13,21] The optimum dose of epidural morphine appears to be 2–6 mg.[12,22] Although 8 or 10 will give a longer duration of action, the incidence of adverse effects is disproportionately higher.[13] Systemic uptake occurs at a similar rate as after IM injection.[23]

Epidural injections of meperidine, 50–100 mg, have been used in postsurgical patients, and these larger doses appear to afford analgesia without undue adverse effects.[24] Systemic uptake has been studied in cases where both epidural and intravenous administration was performed in the same patient. From these it has been estimated the absorption half-life of meperidine is approximately 15–30 minutes.[25] In patients with chronic pain, lower doses (25–50 mg) of meperidine may be adequate, and this is consistent with such patients having a lower MEAC than postsurgical patients. Both methadone

(5 mg) and hydromorphone (1-mg) produce analgesia characterized by a faster onset but shorter duration than an "equianalgesic" (5-mg) dose of morphine.[12] However, what constitutes an "equianalgesic" dose given intraspinally, compared to IV or IM, may require reevaluation.

Torda and Pybus pointed out that morphine, 6 mg, and methadone, 6 mg, both outlasted meperidine, 60 mg, and fentanyl, 60 μg, when studied in a Latin square design.[26] While subjects preferred the drugs in the order listed, they preferred whatever drug was given last, so that carryover effects may be important factors in assessing multiple drug trials. However, Houlton observed that repeat doses of fentanyl or diamorphine last longer than first doses, so these observations might reflect accumulation in the epidural space "depot."[27]

The low doses of opiates potentially useful when given epidurally would seem to make these routes attractive for obstetric analgesia. However, with few exceptions, the results have been dismal.[28,29] The probable reason is related to the favored systemic uptake over dural penetration, due to central venous engorgement, since intrathecal administration meets with considerably more success.[30] In confirmation of this hypothesis, fentanyl given epidurally provides excellent analgesia during labor.[31,32]

It would seem rational, therefore, to use a vasconstrictor such as epinephrine to decrease the rate of systemic absorption and thereby enhance analgesia. The approach too has been largely unsuccessful for both morphine and meperidine.[9,13,34] It appears that successful obstetric analgesia can be achieved with these agents only by increasing the dose.[35,30] Under these circumstances, the choice of agent should be restricted to the more lipid-soluble agents to avoid late-onset respiratory complications, which are more frequent with morphine. Other side effects, notably somnolence and pruritus, are not differentiated by agents.

LONG-TERM ANALGESIA WITH SPINAL OPIATES

Repeated epidural injections of opiates can provide continuous analgesia in patients with cancer for several months and apparently without tolerance affecting their usefulness.[36] A logical extension of this technique is to use a method of continuously infusing opiate solution via a catheter in the epidural space. Coombs and co-workers described an implantable drug delivery system (Infusaid) which can be refilled percutaneously and which delivers flow rates of 2–3 ml/day for 15–20 days.[37] Pilot studies in patients with cancer-related pain indicated that six of the seven patients treated benefited.* The continuous infusion techniques avoid the peak and trough blood concentration pattern arising from repeated injections. At dose rates ranging from 2 to 30 mg of morphine sulfate per day, there was no evidence of respiratory depression, pruritus, nausea, or urinary retention in the small group of patients studied.

In analyzing the usefulness of the intraspinal route of administration, several points are pertinent. The choice of opiate is important. Preservative-free solutions are essential, although the use of sodium metabisulfite does not appear to be contraindicated.[26] Morphine, a water-soluble pure agonist, may not be the most appropriate choice. Its prolonged sojourn in the CSF increases the duration of action, but the duration of action is unpredictably variable, both between patients and between doses.[27,38] Thus the propensity for late onset and prolonged side effects parallels the analgesic action.[13] In contrast, the more lipid-soluble agents are more rapidly removed from CSF but are less likely to cause late-onset adverse effects. In terms of "patient preference" for lipid-soluble agents given epidurally, a decreasing progression from methadone, meperidine, to fentanyl was reported.[27] While each of these agents has merits, it should be realized that methadone clearance from plasma is slow, and while this can augment the spinally mediated analgesia, it may lead to centrally mediated adverse effects after several days of continuous or repeated dosing. Meperidine, like morphine, is rapidly absorbed systemically and may also produce peripheral vascular effects, possibly mediated via histamine release. Fentanyl is less likely to produce peripheral effects and does not cause histamine release.[39] The duration of action is not necessarily a problem, since epidural catheter techniques can be used to control this. The partial agonist buprenorphine was reported to cause fewer side effects than morphine.[30] Plainly, this observation needs to be confirmed by others because of its potential value to clinical practice. Lofentanil has also shown promise in early reports for effective prolonged analgesia but may be limited by a relatively high incidence of nausea and vomiting.

---

*This device, however, is very expensive. Other simpler devices based on silastic reservoirs (e.g., Port-a-Cath) and costing less also have been successful clinically.

TECHNIQUES OF DELIVERY OF SPINAL OPIATES

Three basic approaches have been in use: (1) implantation of an intraspinal catheter exiting percutaneously, (2) implantation of a subcutaneous reservoir with or without a valve mechanism in series with a intraspinal catheter, (3) implantation of a continuous infusion device in series with a intraspinal catheter.

Technique of Catheter Placement

For all three approaches, the intraspinal catheter placement involves standard percutaneous techniques. Tunneling the catheter to reduce the hazard of infection is essential for prolonged use. Optimal kits and materials have not been identified as yet. Long experience and study in lumbo- and ventriculoperitoneal shunts confirm the essential acceptability of Silastic catheters. For intrathecal placement, an 0.40- to 0.47-mm outer diameter catheter (Dow Corning) can be used with a 14- or 16-gauge epidural needle. A lubricated 0.18-inch-wire-wound cardiovascular guide wire can be used to stiffen the catheter to facilitate placement. A radiopaque catheter of this type may be available for such use. This same catheter may be acceptable for epidural use, although we prefer a large bore, 0.60-mm outer diameter catheter (Dow Corning medical grade Silastic tubing) stabilized by an 0.25 inch cardiovascular guide wire. The needles for this purpose are custom manufactured and are not yet commerically available. An alternate approach is to utilize a wire wound RACZ® catheter (Arrow, Inc.) or the Krames® intraspinal kit (Cook, Inc.). A polyurethane radiopaque catheter is included in the latter kit.

Prior to any such procedure, preparations for a surgical aseptic procedure should be complete. Prophylactic antibiotics such as Cephadyl should be administered. Anesthesia can be provided with general anesthesia or with regional anesthesia in the operative site. The procedure should be done in the operating room and under fluoroscopy. The patients are prepared and draped in the lateral position with the lower back and flank areas exposed.

As an alternative, 17–19 gauge nylon catheters such as Porlex or Daval epidural catheters can be inserted percutaneously and tunnelled without a large skin incision under local anesthesia. The catheter is brought out of the skin in the iliac fossa and anchored there for long-term injections on infusion.

Intraspinal Cannulation

Actual intrathecal or epidural cannulation is performed with a modified epidural needle and using standard techniques, except that a small incision must be made (Figs 38–5 and 38–10). Intrathecal puncture is performed in the midline below the level of the conust medullaris if possible. When morphine is used, the craniospinal gradient CSF concentration is minimal at steady-state, usually at 4–5 days of infusion. Therefore, no regional advantage obtains from advancing the catheter rostrally, and some risk of chronic spinal cord irritation may exist, manifested as myoclonus, muscle spasms, or spinal cord injury. One should implant at L2–3, 3–4, or 4–5, wherever is anatomically easiest. Once spinal fluid is returned through the needle, the catheter–guide wire combination is carefully advanced. Some paresthesia is common but usually does not persist. Fluoroscopy can help one direct the guide wire caudally, along with and facing the epidural needle, bevel turned downward. Ideally, a 3–4-inch length of catheter is threaded intrathecally from an 8- to 10-inch catheter. Shorter catheter lengths facilitate guide wire removal. If Silastic is used and lateral tunneling is planned, a second length catheter and connector will be required, whether the conduit is intrathecal or epidural. After the catheter and sheath have been fastened to the ligament with a silk ligature, 2-0 silk suture passed through the preformed tunnel is tied to the end of the catheter. Subsequently the catheter is carefully pulled through the tunnel. Some may want to incorporate a Dacron cuff (Broviac cuff) to reduce bacterial migration along the catheter. Use Betadine liberally throughout the procedure with an intrathecal catheter. Chronic spinal headache may ensue and/or a CSF pseudomeningocele (hygroma) may develop unless the needle used is small. As a further precaution, a circumferential dressing may be applied for several days, with constant posterior wound pressure applied.

Epidural placement is accomplished using a standard loss-of-resistance technique. Again, if morphine is used, thoracic or cervical epidural cannulation may be avoided. For more lipid-soluble drugs demonstrating regional localization, such as fentanyl, however, placement adjacent to the afferent input may be required. Again, catheter placement is

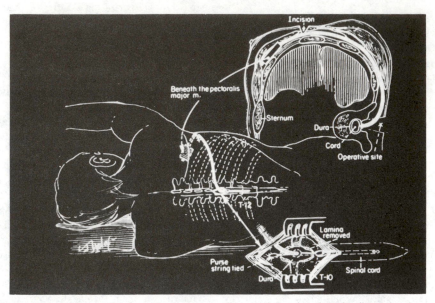

Fig 38–5.—Technique of intraspinal cannulation for long-term opioid analgesia. Procedure entails surgical laminotomy and placement of a catheter subcutaneously from the vertebral spine to the chest wall. (From Onofrio B.M., Yaksh T.L., Arnold P.G.: *Mayo Clin. Proc.* 56:516, 1981. Used by permission.)

guided by fluoroscopy. The final position of either intrathecal or epidural catheters is best defined by water-soluble radiopaque contrast injection if possible (5–7 ml of 190–200 mg/dl of metrizamide). Conduit fixation and tunneling are accomplished as with an intrathecal conduit (see Fig 38–7).

Tunneling

In order to tunnel the catheters laterally from the intraspinal area, a small incision about 1 inch long is made down to the posterior spinous ligament prior to needle insertion. The catheter must be anchored to prevent dislodgment. Placement of the stitch is best accomplished at this point prior to needle insertion. A single stitch of 2-0 silk is placed in the rigid lumbar fascia and supraspinous ligament and set aside with a snap. Actual lateral tunneling will be done through the incision following intraspinal cannulation by passing a shunt tunneling instrument or blunt clamp laterally from the incision. An alternative way to fix the catheter over the spine is to run the catheter through a Heyer-Schulte sheath, which is then incorporated into the stitch prior to lateral tunneling. If an infusion device or reservoir is to be connected to the intraspinal catheter, this is accomplished at this point over a straight metal titanium or stainless steel connector. Both ends are trimmed,

advanced onto the connector, and anchored with free ties of 2-0 silk. A fluorocarbon solution (Infusaid Corp., Norwood, Mass.) can be used to soften and dilate Silastic catheters for joining over connectors. Sterile Silastic cement is useful to cement such junctions and stabilize catheters.

Intraspinal Catheters With Reservoir, Shunt Pump, External Pump

Once an intraspinal catheter is implanted and tunneled, it is a simple matter to convert the procedure from a percutaneously exiting lateral flank catheter to an implanted reservoir (see Figs 38–9 through 38–10). The Ommaya reservoir and the Selker reservoir have been modified for this purpose. Infusoport and Porto-a-Cath are the currently used reservoirs. Unfortunately, in some cases three to four injections per day are required. Incorporating a one-way valve pump into this system and expanding the reservoir volume accomplishes two things: patient-activated control, and a reduced frequency of injection and thus a reduced risk of infection. The salient part of the procedure, in addition to the foregoing description, is the choice of a site for implantation of the auxiliary equipment. The reservoir or refill part must be easily delineated for percutaneous injection (i.e.,

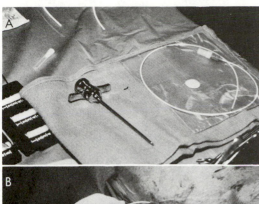

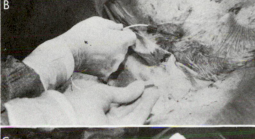

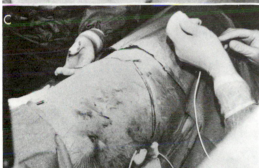

Fig 38–6.—A, equipment needed for intraspinal cannulation. The catheter setup consists of a 16-gauge Silastic cannula, a 12- or 14-gauge bone marrow biopsy needle, and an extra-long Silastic catheter with a connector to allow subcutaneous cannulations from the vertebral spine to the chest wall or abdominal wall. **B,** needle in place in the epidural space, as confirmed by fluoroscopy. The Silastic catheter is introduced through the needle. **C,** technique of subcutaneous cannulation of the epidural catheter.

chest wall or iliac fossa). Also, the one-way valve must be easily found and compressed. Several such systems are under development and testing. External pumps such as the Cormed and the Autosyringe have also been used to deliver opiates intraspinally (Figs 38–11 and 38–12). After the catheter is tunneled and brought out of the skin, it is connected to the pump for continuous infusion of the calculated amount of drug. Compared to implanted infusion

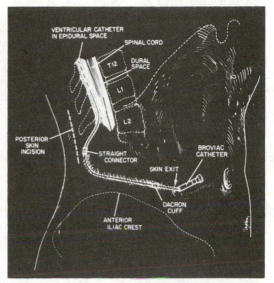

Fig 38–7.—Placement of Broviac catheter in the epidural space. (From PoleHi C.E., et al.: *J. Neurosurg.* 55:581–584, 1981. Used by permission.)

devices, external pumps are inexpensive and easier for the patient, nurse, and family to manage.

Implanted Infusion Devices

Elegant but expensive, such a device as the Infusaid 400 can be attached to an intraspinal conduit to deliver 1.5–4 ml/day. The only such device available for morphine use is the Infusaid 400. Driven by a fluorocarbon generating 428 mm Hg of pressure at body temperature, the device reliably deliv-

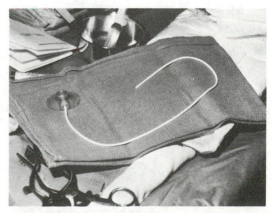

Fig 38–8.—Infusoport device for subcutaneous injection through an epidural catheter.

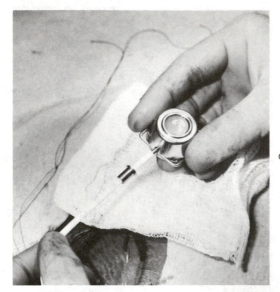

Fig 38–9.—Porto-A-Cath assembly for epidural injection.

Fig 38–10.—Porto-A-Cath placed subcutaneously in the left iliac fossa through a small incision. Later it will be connected to the epidural catheter.

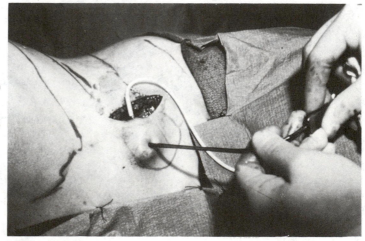

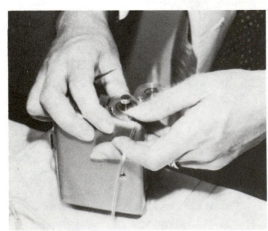

Fig 38–11.—Cormed external pump.

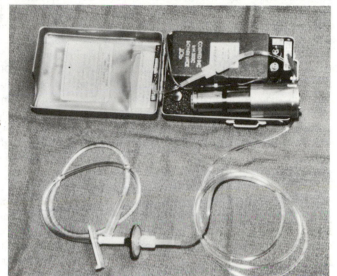

Fig 38–12.—Inside of the Cormed pump. The plastic bag is connected via the tubing to the pump before the pump is connected to the epidural catheter.

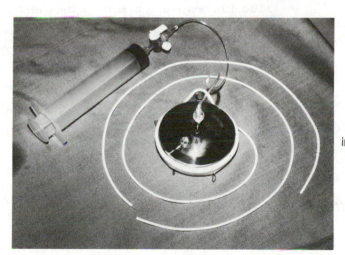

Fig 38–13.—Infusaid 400 internal pump.

Fig 38–14.—Cross section of Infusaid 400 device showing the pump mechanism, which is driven by a fluorocarbon generating 426 mm Hg of pressure at body temperature.

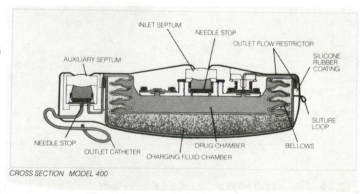

ers a fixed flow of agent from a bellows drug chamber (Figs 38–13 and 38–14). Refill of the 30- or 50-ml reservoir is accomplished by percutaneous injection. The refill cycle is dependent on the flow rate. Flow rates vary with temperature, viscosity, and barometric pressure. The device is implanted on the abdominal wall or on the chest wall through a 3- to 4-inch incision. A subcutaneous pocket is formed by blunt dissection, with cautery used to prevent hematoma formation. The device is anchored to the bed of the wound (fascia) with four-quadrant single proline ligatures. Connection to the intraspinal conduit was described earlier. The initial dosage range is 0.5–2 mg/day intrathecally or 4–10 mg/day epidurally. A model with a side port allows bolus injection of a local anesthetic or opiate. This system has been used also for continuous epidural bupivacaine administration, with equivocal results.

Efficacy of Route

To date, no data are available that demonstrate the superior efficacy of either the intrathecal or the epidural route. The risk of meningitis, spinal headache, and hygroma with the intrathacal route is counterbalanced by the ease of checking CSF opiate drug concentrations, for assessing intrathecal potency, the ability to give lipid-insoluble agents (e.g., DADL, endorphin) and the use of lower doses necessary to achieve a given CSF opiate concentration. The epidural route is free of spinal headache and hygroma. Meningitis is likely to be a late complication, with epidural abscess perhaps occurring sooner. Higher doses are required to achieve a given CSF opiate concentration. There is some risk of inadvertently placing the catheter in an epidural vein.

Zenz et al. have reported chronic percutaneous epidural opiate administration for more than 360 days in some patients with two cases of meningitis with tunneled catheters existing percutaneously. In both cases the condition improved with antibiotics and catheter removal.[36] While dosage escalation occurs during certain phases of tumor growth, true tolerance is not a problem if the dosage is constantly adjusted up or down to meet the patient's need. Clearly, for the majority of cancer pain patients, this is the simpler technique with intraspinal agents.

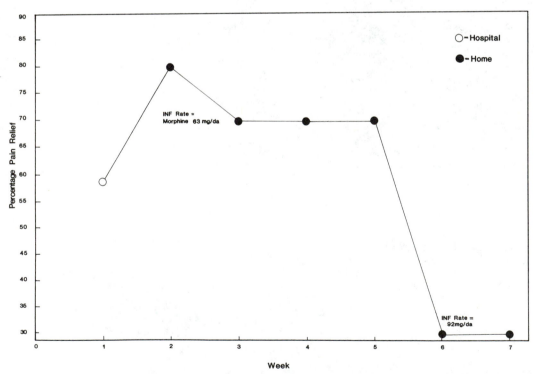

Pain Relief
ID=656554

Fig 38–15.—Long-term morphine infusion with the Cormed pump in a pain patient (case 1).

CASE STUDIES: SPINAL NARCOTICS

CASE 1.—A woman, aged 35 years, underwent a modified radical mastectomy in 1981 for carcinoma of the right breast. In March 1984 local recurrence with metastases to the right lung and chest wall was treated with chemotherapy. In April the patient was referred to the University of Cincinnati Pain Control Center for treatment of right thoracic pain. In May she was admitted to the hospital for insertion of a thoracic epidural catheter for continuous infusion of bupivacaine. Opiate was added to the infusion and the rate was increased as needed to control pain. Twenty-four days later the patient was discharged home with a thoracic catheter in place and a Cormed battery-operated external pump supplying 1% morphine in 60 ml of 0.25% bupivacaine. The infusion rate of morphine was set at 2.2 mg/hour (55 mg/day). Good pain relief (70%–80%) was sustained with this dose for approximately 1 month. In late June, however, increased pain and muscle spasms in the right posterior thoracic area necessitated increasing the rate of infusion of morphine to 92 mg/day. Two small papules, closed and indurated, were

noted on the posterior thoracic area adjacent to the site of catheter insertion. Culture of the papules revealed *Staphylococcus epidermidis*.

On July 9 the patient returned to the Pain Control Center with increased pain and muscle spasms of the right posterior thoracic area. The epidural catheter was removed and pus was expressed from the catheter tract. She was admitted to the hospital for treatment of the back abscess and antibiotic therapy. Pain relief was maintained with the continuous IV infusion of morphine (4.5 mg/hour). On July 18 the patient was discharged home; the continuous IV infusion rate of morphine was increased to 19 mg/hour.

On July 25 the patient was readmitted to the hospital for placement of a Port-a-Cath for continuous IV morphine administration at home. On August 1 she was discharged home; the continuous IV morphine infusion rate with the Cormed pump was 19.8 mg/hour (477 mg/day). On August 8 the infusion rate was increased to 23.3 mg/hour, and 3 weeks later it was increased to 25.7 mg/hour.

Comment.—The thoracic epidural catheter was left in place for approximately 2 months. Until the week prior to catheter removal, the patient experi-

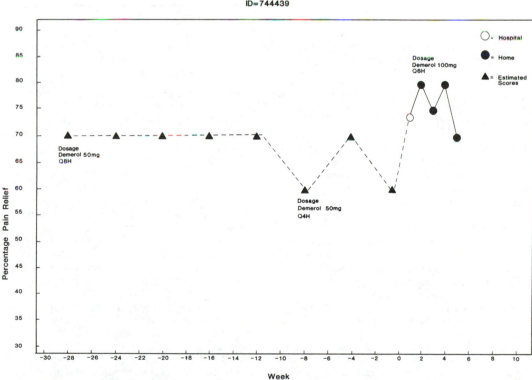

Fig 38–16.—Long-term intermittent injection of meperidine hydrochloride (Demerol) in a pain patient (case 2).

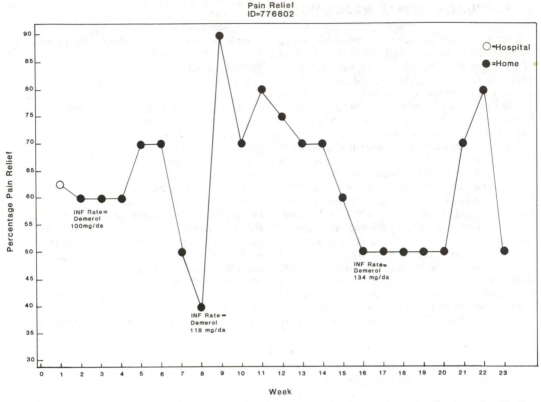

Fig 38–17.—Long-term continuous infusion of meperidine hydrochloride (Demerol) with the Cormed pump in a pain patient (case 3).

enced fairly good pain relief (70%–80%). One problem encountered during this period of infusion was the acute onset of torticollis and weakness in the neck and upper extremity; these were treated with physical therapy and postural changes. Because of increased pain at the catheter insertion site, the catheter was removed and purulent material was expressed from the catheter tract. Two small indurated areas on the posterior thoracic area were found to be tumor. Some of the tumor was surgically removed, resulting in increased pain relief.

With the beginning of continuous IV administration of morphine, pain relief was less consistent, and frequent increases in the infusion rate were necessary to maintain relatively good pain relief (50%–70%) (Fig 38–15). Visiting nurses assisted with the patient's home care. Weekly visits were made to add new medication to the pump and to maintain the Port-a-Cath system.

CASE 2.—In October 1982 a 28-year-old woman was referred to the University of Cincinnati Pain Control Center for the relief of pain of a sarcoma of the left buttock and metastases to the lung (original diagnosis had been made in May 1981). A continu-

ous lumbar epidural infusion of bupivacaine was started for pain relief, followed by S-1 and S-2 nerve root blocks. Good pain relief was achieved, and the patient was discharged home on a regimen of amitriptyline hydrochloride (Elavil), q.h.s., and methadone, 20–40 mg t.i.d., as needed.

In early January 1983 the patient reported new onset of pain in the right buttock. Continuous lumbar epidural infusion of bupivacaine was started, with great relief of pain. The patient's opioid requirement was reduced to an occasional oral dose of 20–40 mg of methadone. The bupivacaine infusion was changed to meperidine, 5–7.5 mg/hour, and then to intermittent boluses of meperidine, 50 mg q8h, with good pain relief (Fig 38–16).

In late January a permanent epidural catheter was placed with an Infusaport for percutaneous injections. The patient did not like the pain of the needle insertions, so a stopper was placed over the catheter hub for injection. Good pain relief continued, with little oral or IM analgesic supplementation required. In February the patient was readmitted to the hospital because of repeated problems with the catheter

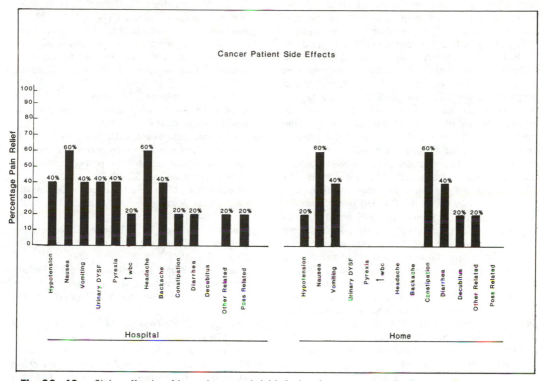

Fig 38–18.—Side effects of long-term opioid infusion in cancer patients, hospitalized and at home.

coming out of the Infusaport. The catheter system was externalized surgically.

In March the patient reported lethargy and disorientation. Ativan was discontinued and meperidine was changed to a b.i.d. schedule, then, with return of pain, to a t.i.d. schedule. The patient was then alert and oriented and reported good pain relief.

In April good pain relief continued. Once-daily supplementation with methadone was required. In June the pain increased and the patient used methadone more often. The meperidine schedule was changed to 50 mg q4h, with good pain relief.

In August the patient reported increased pain and was readmitted for adjustment of the dose schedule. Meperidine levels were measured to establish a new narcotic regimen. The schedule was changed to 100 mg of meperidine q6h, which provided good pain relief (70%–80%). The patient remained on this schedule until her sudden death on October 1, believed to be due to a ruptured lung tumor. In the final weeks of her life good pain relief was maintained with little supplementary analgesia.

Comment.—The lumbar epidural catheter was in place for approximately 8 months. Throughout that time fairly good pain relief was maintained, with little need for supplementary analgesics. No major problems with the catheter were encountered.

CASE 3.—In 1982 a 70-year-old woman was diagnosed to have small cell cancer of the lung with metastases to the liver. Treatment was with chemotherapy. Later acute herpes zoster (T1–2) developed. The patient's initial treatment for pain consisted of a series of stellate ganglion blocks. Her initial response was good, but eventually pain returned and her opiate requirements increased. In February 1984 she was referred to the University of Cincinnati Pain Control Center and admitted to the hospital for epidural catheterization. On February 24 she was discharged home with a permanent indwelling catheter and a Cormed battery-operated external pump supplying a 2% meperidine solution in 60 ml of 0.25% bupivacaine. The meperidine infusion rate was 4 mg/hour (100 mg/day). The patient had 50%–70% pain relief on this dose schedule for approximately 1½ months.

On April 12 the patient reported increased pain and the meperidine infusion rate was changed to 4.9 mg/hour (118/day). Thereafter 50%–70% pain relief was again maintained for approximately 1½ months.

On June 7 the patient reported increased pain and the infusion rate was increased to 5.5 mg/hour (134 mg/day). At this time she was hospitalized for 5 weeks with generalized edema and abdominal ascites secondary to the liver disease. During the hospitalization 50%–70% pain relief was maintained, but supplementary Tylox II, three or four times a day, was needed, as was occasional IM meperidine.

On July 13 the patient was discharged home to be cared for by her family. Pain relief at this time was about 70% with continuous epidural meperidine and supplementary Tylox I, two to three times a day. A week later the patient was admitted to a nursing home, as her family was unable to care for her. One week after admission she died. Pain relief prior to death had been maintained at 40%–60%.

Comment.—The duration of continuous epidural tranfusion was approximately 5½ months (Fig 38–17). Throughout the home care process, there was no major problem with the Cormed pump. Initially there was a kink in the catheter and air in the tubing, but both problems were easily corrected. No major side effects of narcotic infusion were encountered. The patient did have intermittent nausea and vomiting and constipation, managed with Compazine, stool softeners, and laxatives. Edema and abdominal ascites increased as the disease progressed.

With the assistance of the patient's private physician and hospice home care nurses, the infusion was maintained. Nurses visited the patient weekly to add new medication to the pump and maintain the dressing around the catheter.

Figure 38–18 compares the incidence of side effects from permanently placed catheters in patients in the hospital or at home. Note the overall reduced incidence of side effects, especially hypotension, urinary dysfunction, elevated WBC count, headache, and diarrhea, in patients at home. Patients at home did have an increased incidence of constipation or diarrhea.

REFERENCES

1. Yaksh T.L.: Spinal opiate analgesia: Characteristics and principles of action. *Pain* 11:293–346, 1981.
2. Yeung J.C., Rudy T.A.: Multiplicative interaction between narcotic agonisms expressed at spinal and supraspinal sites of antinociceptive action as revealed by concurrent intrathecal and intracerebroventricular injections of morphine. *J. Pharm. Exp. Ther.* 215:633–642, 1980.
3. Crawford J.S.: Site of action of intrathecal morphine. *Br. Med J.* 281:1144, 1980.
4. Dahlstrom B., Tamsen A., Paalzow L., et al.: Patient-controlled analgesic therapy: IV: Pharmacokinetics and analgesic plasma concentrations of morphine. *Clin. Pharmacokinet.* 7:285–311, 1982.
5. Moore R.A., Bullingham R.S.J., McQuay H.G., et al.: Dual permeability to narcotics: In vitro determination and application to extradural administration. *Br. J Anaesth.* 54:1117–1128, 1982.
6. Cousins M.J., Mather L.E., Glynn C.J., et al.: Selective spinal analgesia. *Lancet* 1:1141–1142, 1979.
7. Jorgensen B.G., Andersen H.B., Engkuist A.: Influence of epidural morphine on postoperative pain, endocrine-metabolic and renal responses to surgery: A controlled study. *Acta Anaesthesiol. Scand.* 26:63–68, 1982.
8. Nordberg G., Hedner T., Mellstrand T., et al.: Pharmacokinetic aspects of epidural morphine analgesia. *Anesthesiology* 58:545–551, 1983.
9. Youngstrom P.C., Cowan R.I., Sutheimer C., et al.: Pain relief and plasma concentrations from epidural and intramuscular morphine in post-cesarean-section patients. *Anesthesiology* 57:404–409, 1982.
10. Bromage P.R., Camporesi E., Chestnut D.: Epidural narcotics for postoperative analgesia. *Anesth. Analg.* 59:473–480, 1980.
11. Rawal N., Sjostrand U., Dahlstrom B.: Postoperative pain relief by epidural morphine. *Anesth. Analg.* 60:726–731, 1981.
12. Kafer E.R., Brown J.T., Scott D., et al.: Biphasic depression of ventilatory responses to CO_2 following epidural morphine. *Anesthesiology* 58:418–427, 1983.
13. Bromage P.R., Camporesi E.M., Durant P.A.C., et al.: Rostral spread of epidural morphine. *Anesthesiology* 56:431–436, 1982.
14. Gustafsson L.L., Ackerman S., Adamson H., et al.: Disposition of morphine in cerebrospinal fluid after epidural administration. *Lancet* 3:1982.
15. Wang J.K., Nauss L.A., Thomas J.E.: Pain relief by intrathecally applied morphine in man. *Anesthesiology* 50:149–151, 1979.
16. Katz J., Nelson W.: Intrathecal morphine for postoperative pain relief. *Reg. Anesth.* 6:1–3, 1981.
17. Samii K.: Postoperative spinal analgesia with morphine. *Br. J. Anaesth.* 53:817, 1981.
18. Barrow D.W., String J.E.: Postoperative analgesia in major orthopaedic surgery: Epidural and intrathecal opiates. *Anaesthesia* 36:937–941, 1981.
19. Kaiko R.F.: Age and morphine analgesia in cancer patients with postoperative pain. *Clin. Pharmacol. Ther.* 28:823–826, 1980.
20. Mirceau N., Constantinescu C., Jianu C., et al.: Anesthesie sous-arachnoidienne par la pethidine. *Ann. Fr. Anesth. Reanim.* 1:167–171, 1982.
21. Knill R.L., Clement J.L., Thompson W.R.: Epidural morphine causes delayed and prolonged ventilatory depression. *Can. Anaesth. Soc. J.* 6:537–543, 1981.
22. Martin R., Salbaing J., Gilbert, et al.: Epidural morphine for postoperative pain relief: A dose-response curve. *Anesthesiology* 56:423–426, 1982.
23. Chauvin M., Samii K., Schermann J.M., Sandouk P. et al.: Plasma morphine concentration after intrathecal administration of low doses of morphine. *Br. J. Anaesth.* 53:1065–1067, 1981.
24. Glynn C.J., Mather L.E., Cousins M.J., et al.: Peridural meperidine in humans: Analgetic response,

pharmacokinetics, and transmission into CSF. *Anesthesiology* 55:520–526, 1981.

25. Huesemeyer R.P., Cummings A.J., Rosankiewicz J.R., et al.: A study of pethidine kinetics and analgesia in women in labour following intravenous, intramuscular and epidural administration. *Br. J. Clin. Pharmacol.* 13:171–176, 1982.

26. Torda T., Pybus D.A.: Comparison of four narcotic analgesics for extradural analgesia. *Br. J. Anaesth.* 54:291–294, 1982.

27. Houlton P.G.: Epidural diamorphine and fentanyl for postoperative pain. *Anesthesia* 36:1144–1147, 1981.

28. Chayen M.S., Ruaick V., Borvine A.: Pain control with epidural injection of morphine. *Anesthesiology* 53:338–339, 1980.

29. Writer W.D.R., James F.M., Wheeler A.S.: Double blind comparison of morphine and bupivacaine for continuous epidural analgesia in labor. *Anesthesiology*. 54:215–219, 1981.

30. Baraka A., Noueihid R., Hajj S.: Epidural meperidine-bupivacaine for obstetric analgesia. *Anesth. Analg.* 61:652–656, 1982.

31. Nalda M.A.: Obstetric analgesia with fentanyl administered by the extradural route. *Br. J. Anaesth.* 3:113P, 1981.

32. Justins D.M., Francis D., Houlton P.G., et al.: A controlled trial of extradural fentanyl in labour. *Br. J. Anaesth.* 54:409–414, 1982.

33. Bullingham R.E.S., McQuay J., Dwyer D., et al.: Sublingual buprenorphine used postoperatively: Clinical observations and preliminary pharmacokinetic analysis. *Br. J. Clin. Pharmacol.* 12:117–122, 1981.

34. Skjolderbrand A., Garle M., Gustafsson L.L., et al.: Extradural pethidine with and without adrenaline during labour: Wide variation in effect. *Br. J. Anesth.* 54:415–420, 1982.

35. Perriss B.W.: Epidural pethidine in labour. *Anaesthesia* 35:380–382, 1980.

36. Zenz M., Piepenbrock S., Husch M., et al.: Experience with long-term peridural catheters: Peridural morphine analgesia in cancer pain. *Anaesthetist: Reg. Anaesth.* 4:26–28, 1981.

37. Coombs D.W., Saunders R.L., Gaylor M., et al.: Epidural narcotic infusion reservoir: Implantation technique and efficacy. *Anesthesiology* 56:496–473, 1982.

38. Chambers W.A., Sinclair C.J., Scott D.B.: Extradural morphine for pain after surgery. *Br. J. Anaesth.* 53:921–924, 1981.

39. Rosow C.E., Moss J., Philbin D.M., et al.: Histamine release during morphine and fentanyl anesthesia. *Anesthesiology* 56:93–96, 1982.

39 / Neurosurgical Procedures

ELIZABETH BULLITT, M.D.
ALLAN FRIEDMAN, M.D.
LALIGAM N. SEKHAR, M.D.

39A / Benign Pain

ELIZABETH BULLITT, M.D.
ALLAN FRIEDMAN, M.D.

THE TREATMENT OF pain of nonmalignant origin is often more difficult than the treatment of cancer pain. In cancer patients with short life expectancies, destruction of a pain pathway will often bring good symptomatic relief. Unfortunately, the CNS has a remarkable capacity to circumvent lesions placed within its pain conduction systems. Many destructive operations for pain relief are initially effective but become ineffective with the passage of time, as pain signals stubbornly find their way to the level of conscious perception. Patients with long life expectancies will therefore often outlive the benefits of operation. In addition, deafferentation pain may develop in skin areas rendered anesthetic or analgesic from a previous destructive procedure. The risks of a destructive procedure often outweigh its benefits when the patient is likely to outlive the period of transient pain relief provided by operation.

To treat the patient with nonmalignant disease, the cause of the pain and the site of pathology must be known. Certain well-defined syndromes respond to specific modes of therapy. Destructive, decompressive, or stimulation procedures are of benefit in certain conditions.

DESTRUCTIVE PROCEDURES

Peripheral Nerve and Nerve Roots

Peripheral Nerve Division

Peripheral nerve division is not commonly employed as a means of pain control. The receptive fields of neighboring sensory nerves tend to overlap, and if even a few fibers enter the painful area from an adjacent peripheral nerve, the patient's pain will persist unabated. The success of peripheral nerve section for pain control is also limited by the propensity of peripheral nerves to regenerate and form painful neuromas. It is also frequently impossible to interrupt the desired sensory fibers in a peripheral nerve without also sacrificing motor function. The indications for peripheral nerve section have therefore been limited largely to the treatment of peripheral nerve tumors or of painful neuromas.

The diagnosis of a neuroma or peripheral nerve tumor is usually based on the history and physical examination findings. Tapping over the injured nerve segment will often produce painful paresthesias. Occasionally a mass may be palpated. Nerve damage may be confirmed by electromyographic (EMG) and nerve conduction studies. The diagnosis is sometimes made only at the time of surgical exploration.

Some patients may achieve excellent pain relief with excision of the tumor or neuroma (Fig 39A–1). In general, the procedure is justified when local blockade of the sensory nerve brings total pain relief. Exploration is also indicated if the diagnosis is in question. The difficulty with neuroma resection is that regeneration of the sectioned nerve often produces a new neuroma. The likelihood of continued pain relief at 1 year is less than 50%.[37] A number of methods have been proposed to reduce the chance of recurrent neuroma formation, including Silastic capping of the sectioned nerve, burying the nerve in bone, and cutting the nerve with a laser to seal the individual fascicles.[6, 13, 37] None of these approaches has proved definitely effective. If a neuroma reforms after initial excision, a second operation is unlikely to be successful. When the affected nerve carries useful motor function, neuroma resection is usually not advisable.

Dorsal Rhizotomy

The technique of dorsal rhizotomy is discussed in detail in chapter 39C. The procedure is not often indicated in the treatment of benign disease. Dorsal rhizotomy is not useful in treating arachnoiditis, but a few neurosurgeons do believe it to be of benefit in the patient with scarring around a particular nerve root. It may also be useful in the small number of patients with postherpetic pain who experience good pain relief with local anesthetic infiltration of the painful region. Paraplegic patients with painful spasticity benefit temporarily from rhizotomy, but the spasticity tends to recur with time. Dorsal rhizotomy is of no benefit in the patient with deafferentation pain and should not be attempted in patients with syndromes such as postcordotomy dysesthesia or pain following spinal cord injury. Visceral pain may be treated by bilateral denervation, but the loss of visceral sensation may cause a delay in the diagnosis of intra-abdominal pathology, such as duodenal ulcer.[37]

Sympathectomy

Sympathectomy is of value in two distinct pain syndromes: causalgia and visceral pain of the upper abdomen. The treatment of visceral pain is discussed in chapter 20.

Causalgia was first described by Weir Mitchell during the American Civil War. It is a pain syndrome that classically involves the hand or the foot and follows a high-velocity missile injury to the proximal portion of a major nerve trunk with partial disruption of the nerve. The pain is intense and burning. Characteristically, the pain is exacerbated by stress, loud noise, or vibration, as well as by any touch of the affected area. It is not uncommon for the patient with causalgia to protect the affected extremity with a plastic bag or a cool, moist cloth to prevent any unexpected stimulation of the sensitive region. The extremity itself may be abnormally warm or abnormally cool, and the skin becomes glossy and smooth. Profuse sweating is common. Osteoporosis may occur. The pain is excruciating, and Weir Mitchell wrote that "under such torments the temper changes, the most amiable grow irritable, the soldier becomes a coward, and the strongest man is scarcely less nervous than the most hysterical girl."[16]

The diagnosis is generally implied by the history and physical examination findings. EMG studies may help in pinpointing the region of peripheral nerve damage, but an abnormal electrical study is not diagnostic of causalgia.

The exact mechanism of pain production is unclear but is thought by most researchers to be related to cross-stimulation between sympathetic and afferent sensory fibers.[25] Whatever the cause of the painful signals, sympathectomy is almost invariably effective in the treatment of true causalgia. White and Sweet have cautioned that the results of sympathectomy can be counted on only when the patient's clinical picture includes burning pain, glossy skin, trophic changes, and exacerbation of symptoms with increased sympathetic activity. Patients with an incomplete clinical syndrome tend to respond less well to sympathetic denervation.[37]

A trial of sympathetic blocks should always be undertaken prior to the definitive surgical procedure. Patients who do not respond to temporary blockade will not improve with surgical sympathectomy. Of additional importance, a few patients may experience permanent relief of symptoms after a series of temporary blocks.

Surgical sympathectomy is done as an open procedure. The lumbar sympathetic chain is interrupted when pain is in the foot, and the cervical chain is divided when the pain is in the upper extremity. The operation is always performed ipsilateral to the side

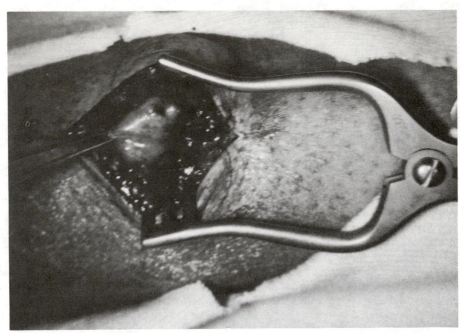

Fig 39A–1.—Subcutaneous neurofibroma in a patient with peripheral neurofibromatosis. Four painful tumors were resected, and the patient remained free of pain 2 years later.

of the pain. Horner's syndrome or the development of a pneumothorax may complicate a cervical sympathectomy, and impotence will result in males if a lumbar sympathectomy is performed bilaterally.

The patient with atypical causalgia is more difficult to treat. Oral phenoxybenzamine[39] or guanethidine administered orally[42] or intravenously[40] has been successful in relieving symptoms in some patients. Sympathetic blocks also may be helpful in some cases. If the range of motion of a joint is reduced, vigorous physical therapy is indicated once the patient's pain has been controlled by pharmacologic means. Placement of a peripheral nerve stimulator may be considered. No single approach has been uniformly successful in the treatment of atypical causalgia.

Spinal Cord

Cordotomy

The technique of cordotomy is discussed in chapter 39C. The operation is occasionally useful in treating elderly patients with unilateral pain of benign origin. The technique is not appropriate in patients with life expectancies of more than 2 years because of the likelihood of pain recurrence.

Dorsal Root Entry Zone Lesions

DREZ lesions were initially advocated by Nashold as a form of treatment for brachial plexus avulsion injury. The indications for the operation have now been extended to include a variety of patients who suffer from deafferentation pain refractory to other treatment modalities. DREZ lesions are the procedure of choice in patients with intractable pain following brachial plexus avulsion injuries and in the patient with central pain and paraplegia. They should also be considered in patients with intractable postherpetic pain and in patients with phantom limb pain.[19–21]

DREZ lesions involve the production of a longitudinal series of lesions, by means of radiofrequency current, in the dorsal root entry zone of the spinal cord on the side ipsilateral to the patient's pain (Fig 39A–2). The lesions destroy the tract of Lissauer, the substantia gelatinosa, and a superficial portion of the dorsal horn over the area operated on. A profound ipsilateral sensory deficit is created over the affected dermatomes. Why DREZ lesions alle-

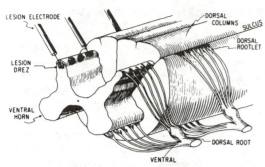

Fig 39A–2.—Schematic drawing of cross section of spinal cord showing areas of lesions in dorsal root entry zone. (From Nashold B.S. Jr., Ostdahl R.H., Bullitt E.[21] Reproduced by permission.)

viate pain is unclear but may involve the interruption of accessory ascending pain pathways, the destruction of disinhibited pain-mediating cells within the spinal cord, or the rebalancing of excitatory and inhibitory inputs within a damaged sensory network.

Approximately two thirds of patients with brachial plexus avulsion injuries or with central pain and paraplegia have received good relief from DREZ lesions, with follow-up periods of up to 5 years. Approximately 50% of patients with postherpetic pain experience good relief, with follow-up periods of up to 2 years. Results in patients with phantom limb pain without root avulsion have been disappointing.

The risks of DREZ lesions include the development of denervation pain and the production of motor weakness, sensory deficits, or ataxia in the ipsilateral lower extremity. In the earlier series, approximately 50% of patients showed some degree of ipsilateral motor weakness immediately following operation. The risk of producing motor weakness has been reduced through the use of a thermocouple electrode that produces a temperature-controlled lesion. Some centers have used the laser to produce DREZ lesions,[12] but it is too soon to tell if the laser will prove superior to the radiofrequency electrode.

DREZ lesions seem to be of benefit in patients with intractable pain from brachial plexus avulsion injuries or from spinal cord injury. In patients with postherpetic pain, the long-term success of the operation has not yet been proved. As no other procedure is of clear benefit, DREZ lesions may be offered to these patients. Transcutaneous stimulation and a trial of antidepressant medication should be offered first. Operation should be delayed for 6–12

months in patients with postherpetic pain, as the pain resolves spontaneously in many patients.

Cranial Nerve and Intracranial Procedures

Intracranial destructive procedures are almost never beneficial in the treatment of benign pain because of the risks inherent to operation and because of the likelihood of pain recurrence. One major exception to this rule is the treatment of trigeminal neuralgia.

Cranial Nerve Division

Trigeminal neuralgia is characterized by sharp lancinating pains confined to one or more divisions of the trigeminal nerve on one side of the face. Pain is commonly provoked by facial touch. The neurologic examination is normal. Tegretol should be given in increasing doses of up to 1 gm/day before one commits a patient to any operative procedure.

Trigeminal neuralgia is unusual in that it can be treated by either a destructive or a decompressive operation. Many different destructive procedures have been employed in the past, and division of the trigeminal root within the middle fossa, temporary compression of the trigeminal root, and injection of alcohol into the gasserian ganglion have all enjoyed periods of popularity. At present, however, the two most commonly employed operations are percutaneous trigeminal rhizotomy and decompression of the trigeminal nerve within the posterior fossa.

Percutaneous trigeminal rhizotomy is the procedure of choice in the elderly, poor-risk surgical patient. Percutaneous rhizotomy was discussed in detail in chapter 20. The results in trigeminal neuralgia are good, and 99% of patients experience pain relief. The disadvantage of percutaneous trigeminal rhizotomy is that ipsilateral facial analgesia is produced. Approximately 20% of patients will complain of numbness or associated dysesthesias. The facial analgesia may wane with time, and as sensation returns the pain may recur. In a series of 700 trigeminal neuralgia patients treated by percutaneous rhizotomy, van Loveren et al. reported a 20% pain recurrence rate at 6 years. Coagulation may be repeated if sensation and pain recur. Risks include a small chance of meningitis, carotid artery injury, or transient diplopia.[36] Patients whose corneas are rendered anesthetic must be taught to use eye drops to prevent keratitis.

Glycerol injection of the gasserian ganglion may be used as an alternative to trigeminal rhizotomy in trigeminal neuralgia patients. A needle is inserted percutaneously into the gasserian ganglion and 0.2–0.4 ml of sterile glycerol is injected.[7, 31] Proponents of the procedure believe that glycerol is able to relieve the pain of trigeminal neuralgia without producing major facial numbness. Significant sensory deficits do occur in some patients, however, and the likelihood of pain recurrence is higher than that following radiofrequency coagulation.[32]

In younger healthy patients, intracranial decompression of the fifth nerve may be preferable to a destructive procedure. Trigeminal decompression does not usually cause facial sensory deficits. Many trigeminal neuralgia patients have an artery compressing the fifth nerve at the dorsal root entry zone within the posterior fossa. Insertion of a small pad to separate the artery from the nerve will result in relief of symptoms in the majority of patients. If no compressing artery is found, a partial division of the trigeminal root will usually result in loss of pain with less sensory deficit than occurs following percutaneous rhizotomy. The disadvantage of this approach is that a major operation is required. Risks include a 5%–10% chance of temporary or permanent injury to adjacent cranial nerves. Hematoma development or stroke may also follow operation, although such complications are rare.[2, 36]

Patients with atypical facial pain do not respond well to any kind of operative procedure. Postherpetic pain also responds poorly to rhizotomy, except in the rare case in which symptoms are relieved by subcutaneous infiltration of local anesthetics. Posttraumatic neuralgia and anesthesia dolorosa are often made worse by further denervation procedures. The pain of chronic sinusitis or of dental neuralgia is best treated by nonoperative means.

DECOMPRESSIVE PROCEDURES

Acute pressure on a nerve or nerve root will generally produce pain and paresthesias in the sensory distribution of that nerve. More severe or prolonged pressure will also cause motor weakness. Decompressive operations on nerves or nerve roots are among the most common of neurosurgical procedures, and in properly selected patients, decompression may produce excellent results.

Peripheral Nerve and Nerve Root

Peripheral nerve entrapment neuropathies may occur in either the upper or lower extremities. These are primarily benign conditions that are caused by pressure on a nerve by a fibrous band or a thickened ligament, by angulation of the nerve over a fascial layer, or by compression of the nerve between bone and soft tissue. Symptoms are generally those of pain and paresthesias in the affected nerve, sometimes accompanied by motor weakness. It is beyond the scope of this chapter to provide detailed descriptions of the multiple syndromes that may occur, but a number of excellent reviews are available.[9, 17, 33] Relief of symptoms by decompression of the affected nerve is often gratifying.

Disk herniation can produce focal pressure on a nerve root and is a common cause of back and leg or neck and arm pain. Pain generally begins in the spine and radiates down the extremity along the path of the affected nerve root. Motor weakness, sensory changes, and reflex abnormalities may occur. In the absence of major motor weakness or bladder disturbance, conservative treatment consisting of bed rest for lower extremity pain and cervical traction for upper extremity pain should be continued for at least 2 weeks. Indications for surgical removal of the ruptured disk include intractable pain or significant motor weakness. The development of bladder dysfunction constitutes a neurosurgical emergency. The diagnosis is made by physical examination and should be confirmed by computerized tomography (CT) or myelography (Fig 39A–3 and 39A–4). Disk operations for nonradiating spinal pain produce disappointing results.

Surgical decompression of the nerve root produces good pain relief in 80%–90% of properly selected patients. A second or third operation is less likely to be successful,[10] and if pain is due to compression by scar, a decompressive operation, which itself may produce more scar, is generally futile.

Chymopapain injection may be an alternative to surgical decompression in patients with bulging disks. The advantage of chymopapain injection is that it is a relatively brief and safe procedure that does not require general anesthesia and may reduce the chance of postoperative scar formation. The disadvantage of the procedure is that it may take a number of weeks for disk dissolution to occur and for the symptoms to abate. One third of patients de-

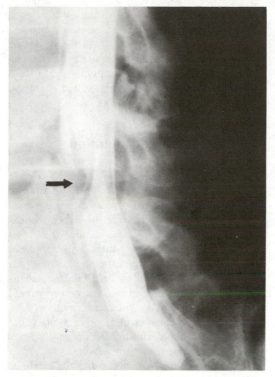

Fig 39A–3.—Metrizamide lumbar myelogram, oblique projection, showing a ruptured disk at L4–5 *(arrow)*. Note the nerve root deviation around the focal defect.

velop severe spasms of the lumbar paraspinal muscles. The enzyme is injected directly into the disk space and so will not relieve symptoms produced by an extruded fragment. The procedure is contraindicated in women with high erythrocyte sedimentation rates because of the incidence of anaphylaxis. The long-term results of chymopapain injection are still unknown, and the procedure is still under investigation.

Spondylosis involves the overgrowth of bone which may compress the spinal cord, cauda equina, or an individual nerve root at its exit foramen. Neurologic symptoms may include myelopathy or radiculopathy. Compression of the lumbar dural sac sometimes produces a syndrome strikingly similar to vascular claudication, with pain that occurs during ambulation and is relieved by rest. The diagnosis of spondylosis must be confirmed by CT or myelography (Fig 39A–5). Decompression of the lumbar sac by laminectomy, or of an affected nerve root by foraminotomy, may bring gratifying relief.

Cranial Nerves

Trigeminal neuralgia may be treated successfully by decompression of the fifth cranial nerve. The treatment of trigeminal neuralgia was discussed earlier in this chapter.

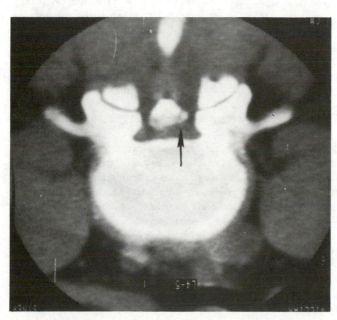

Fig 39A–4.—CT scan of L4–5 following metrizamide myelography (same patient as in Fig 39A–3). One side of the dural sac is elevated by the free disk fragment *(arrow)*.

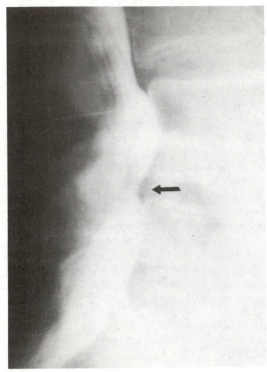

Fig 39A–5.—Lateral myelogram showing spinal stenosis at L4–5. A disk bulge is present at L4–5 *(arrow)*. The facets at this level are markedly hypertrophied, compressing the dural sac. Symptoms resolved following laminectomy without disk removal.

STIMULATION PROCEDURES

In 1965, when Melzack and Wall proposed their gate theory of pain perception,[15] the theoretical ground was established for an entirely new approach to the treatment of painful conditions. Rather than achieving pain relief through the destruction of neural pathways, it now seemed possible to alleviate pain through the stimulation of low threshold primary afferent fibers whose activation caused central inhibition of pain signals. Electrodes were designed for the stimulation of peripheral nerves, of the spinal cord, and of the brain itself. However, when it became apparent that the long-term results were less spectacular than early reports had suggested, enthusiasm for stimulation procedures waned. The results of stimulation are best in selected patients with a few specific problems.

All stimulation procedures require the surgical placement of electrodes at the desired target site. The electrode is attached by lead wires to a subcutaneously placed receiver. The patient carries a pocket stimulator connected to a plastic antenna which can be taped to the skin over the implanted receiver. When stimulation is desired, the antenna is taped into place and the patient turns on the stimulator. Electrical signals are transmitted along the system to the desired target area.

Peripheral Nerve Stimulation

Peripheral nerve stimulators are most effective in the treatment of chronic pain following peripheral nerve injury. The reported success rates have been variable, although there is some suggestion that patients with median or ulnar nerve injuries respond better to stimulation than do patients with peripheral nerve injuries of the lower extremity. Long et al. report an 88% long-term success rate in patients with pain following median or ulnar nerve injury.[14] Nashold et al. found good long-term results in 53% of patients with median or ulnar nerve injuries, but only 31% of patients with lower extremity injuries responded to sciatic nerve stimulation.[41]

Stimulation is most effective when the electrode is implanted proximal to the site of injury, and sciatic nerve stimulation has therefore proved ineffective in controlling chronic leg pain in the patient with arachnoiditis or epidural scarring. The results of brachial plexus stimulation have been disappointing. Cancer pain and phantom limb pain respond poorly to peripheral nerve stimulation.[3, 14]

Placement of a peripheral nerve stimulator involves an open operation in which the electrode is wrapped around the target nerve. Complications include infection, peripheral nerve damage, scarring at the electrode site resulting in loss of stimulation, and breakage or migration of the electrode or wires.[13, 14, 18, 23]

In general, peripheral nerve stimulation may be helpful in patients with pain of peripheral nerve injury when the electrode can be inserted on the damaged nerve proximal to the injured area. The success of peripheral nerve stimulation in the treatment of other disorders has been limited. The specific syndrome of causalgia is better treated by sympathectomy.

Dorsal Column Stimulation

Early dorsal column stimulator electrodes were inserted into the spinal epidural or subarachnoid space during an open operation. The majority of electrodes presently used are long, thin wires that can be inserted into the epidural space through an epidural needle. Some neurosurgeons have used a temporary system in which the electrode wires are inserted percutaneously into the epidural space and the externalized ends are attached to an externalized receiver. If the patient responds to stimulation, the receiver can then be implanted subcutaneously.

Dorsal column stimulation is employed primarily in patients with chronic back and leg pain. Some patients with multiple sclerosis, diabetic pain, or stump neuromas may also benefit from stimulation.[5, 28] The longer-term success rate of dorsal stimulation is, however, disappointingly low. While some groups have reported long-term pain relief in about a third of patients, [28, 30, 35] other groups have found that after 4 years few if any patients experience symptomatic relief.[4, 14, 38] Long et al. stress the importance of psychological evaluation in patient selection,[14] but it is not clear that careful psychological screening always improves the results.[4] Electrode migration, wire breakage, and infection are not uncommon. At least one reoperation is necessary in 10%–70% of patients.[28, 30, 35, 38] The recent development of flocked electrodes, which are less likely to migrate, and of single electrodes with multiple contact points may reduce the technical failure rate. Cancer pain is not relieved by dorsal column stimulation.

Deep Brain Stimulation

Deep brain stimulation is a relatively new technique, and the long-term success rate is not known. At present, however, it may be the procedure of choice in some patients with difficult pain problems refractory to standard forms of therapy.

Deep brain electrodes are inserted stereotactically using stimulation techniques to confirm electrode position. Two different target areas have been used, and the mechanism of pain relief seems to be different at each site.

One target area lies in the region of the medial posterior thalamus and periventricular gray. Stimulation at this site is associated with the release of endogenous opiates into the third ventricle. Tolerance occurs with prolonged stimulation but can sometimes be reversed through the use of disulfiram, tryptophan, or tricyclic compounds. Pain relief is blocked by naloxone. The effects of stimulation are commonly bilateral, although the effect is most

pronounced contralateral to the side of electrode placement.

Stimulation of the posterior internal capsule or sensory thalamus produces pain relief by a different mechanism. The pain relief achieved through stimulation of these primary sensory pathways is unaffected by naloxone, is not associated with the appearance of endogenous opiates within the ventricular system, does not exhibit tolerance, and produces effects that are strictly contralateral to the side of stimulation. The mechanism of pain relief following stimulation of the sensory pathways is unclear but may involve increasing the sensory input into partially deafferented areas of the somatosensory cortex.[22]

The results of deep brain stimulation are still under investigation. Deafferentation pain has been treated primarily with the stimulation of the internal capsule, and some good preliminary results have been reported in patients with postherpetic pain,[29] anesthesia dolorosa,[8] and pain associated with various lesions of the CNS.[1, 8] Chronic back and leg pain has been treated by stimulation of either the sensory pathways or the periventricular gray,[24, 26, 27, 34] although it still remains to be seen if the long-term results surpass those of dorsal column stimulation. Cancer pain has been treated successfully with periventricular gray stimulation, although tolerance may become a problem in some cases.[11, 27]

Two primary advantages of deep brain stimulation are that pain in the head and neck can be treated as easily as pain elsewhere in the body, and the procedure carries a lower morbidity rate than many intracranial destructive procedures. In addition, the operation may be of value in the treatment of conditions such as the thalamic syndrome, which is extraordinarily difficult to treat.

Disadvantages of deep brain stimulation include the high incidence of mechanical malfunction common to all stimulation procedures, the development of tolerance in patients undergoing periventricular gray stimulation, and the fact that at the present time the operation is performed in only a few centers in the United States. Risks include infection, a small chance of hemorrhage, and the possibility of inadvertent brain damage during passage of the electrode to the target site.

At present, there is no single, generally recognized surgical treatment for patients with some kinds of pain such as the thalamic syndrome or postherpetic pain. Deep brain stimulation, despite its uncertainties, may provide a reasonable option for some of these patients. The cancer patient with facial pain and a long life expectancy may also be a good candidate for operation, although the development of tolerance may limit the usefulness of the procedure. The cost of the stimulator and the complexities of its use may make it inappropriate for the severely debilitated cancer patient with a limited life expectancy. Such cancer patients may be better treated by a destructive procedure such as cordotomy, mesencephalotomy, or thalmotomy.

CONCLUSIONS

The management of pain of benign origin is often difficult. Some specific conditions, such as causalgia or trigeminal neuralgia, respond extremely well to surgical therapy. The operative treatment of many other kinds of pain is less gratifying. The transmission of pain signals within the CNS is a complex process. At present, the network of excitatory and inhibitory circuits is only poorly understood. As we learn more about the nature of pain transmission, it is probable that new and more effective modalities will be found to treat chronic pain patients. Until then, it is likely that the successful treatment of many painful conditions will continue to elude the clinician's best efforts.

REFERENCES

1. Adams J.E., Hosobuchi Y., Fields H.E.: Stimulation of internal capsule for relief of chronic pain *J. Neurosurg*. 41:740–744, 1974.
2. Apfelbaum R.I.: Surgical management of disorders of the lower cranial nerves, in Schmidek H.H., Sweet W.H. (eds.): *Operative Neurosurgical Techniques*. New York, Grune & Stratton, 1982, pp. 1063–1082.
3. Campbell J.N., Long D.M.: Peripheral nerve stimulation in the treatment of intractable pain. *J. Neurosurg*, 45:692–699, 1976.
4. Erickson D.L., Long D.M.: Ten year follow up of dorsal column stimulation. *Adv. Pain Res. Ther.* 5:583–589, 1983.
5. Feeney D.M., Gold G.N.: Chronic dorsal column stimulation: Effects on H reflex and symptoms in a patient with multiple sclerosis. *Neurosurgery* 6:564–566, 1980.
6. Fischer D.W., Beggs J.L., Shetter A.G., et al.: Comparative study of neuroma formation in the rat sciatic nerve after CO_2 laser and scalpel neurectomy. *Neurosurgery* 13:287–294, 1983.
7. Hakanson S.: Trigeminal neuralgia treated by the injection of glycerol into the trigeminal cistern. *Neurosurgery* 9:638–646, 1981.
8. Hosobuchi Y., Adams J.E., Fields H.L.: Chronic thalamic and internal capsular stimulation for the control of facial anesthesia dolorosa and dysesthesia of thalamic syndrome. *Adv. Neurol.* 4:783–787, 1974.
9. Kopell H.P., Thompson W.A.L.: Peripheral entrapment neuropathies of the lower extremity. *N. Engl. J. Med.* 262: 56–60, 1960.
10. Law J.D., Lehman R.A.W., Kirsch W.M.: Reoperation after lumbar intervertebral disc surgery. *J. Neurosurg.* 48:259–262, 1978.
11. Lazorthes Y., Siegfried J., Gouarderes C., et al.: Periventricular grey matter stimulation versus chronic intrathecal morphine in cancer pain. *Adv. Pain Res. Ther.* 5:467–475, 1983.
12. Levy W., Nutkiewicz A., Ditmore G., et al.: Laser-induced dorsal root entry zone lesions for pain control: Report of three cases. *J. Neurosurg.* 59:884–886, 1983.
13. Long D.M.: Pain of peripheral nerve injury, in Youmans J.R. (ed.): *Neurological Surgery*. Philadephia, W.B. Saunders, 1982, vol. 6, pp. 3634–3643.
14. Long D.M., Erickson D., Campbell J., et al.: Electrical stimulation of the spinal cord and peripheral nerves for pain control: A 10-year experience. *Appl. Neurophysiol.* 44:207–217, 1981.
15. Melzack R., Wall P.D.: Pain mechanisms: A new theory. *Science* 150:971–979, 1965.
16. Mitchell W.: Injuries of nerves and their consequences: Neurosurgical Classics XXVII. *Arch. Neurol.* 22:89–94, 1970.
17. Nakano K.K.: Selective upper limb entrapment syndromes: Neurological aspects. *J. Neurol. Orthop. Surg.* 1:109–120, 1980.
18. Nashold B.S., Goldner J.L., Bright D.S.: Electrical stimulation of peripheral nerves with micro-electircal implants for pain relief, in Omer G.E., Spinner M. (eds.): *Management of Peripheral Nerve Problems*. Philadelphia, W.B. Saunders, 1982, pp. 3702–3716.
19. Nashold B.S., Ostdahl R.H.: Dorsal root entry zone lesions for pain relief. *J. Neurosurg.* 51:59–69, 1979.
20. Nashold B.S., Bullitt E.: Dorsal root entry zone lesions to control central pain in paraplegics. *J. Neurosurg.* 55:414–419, 1981.
21. Nashold B.S., Ostdahl R.H., Bullitt E., et al.: Dorsal root entry zone lesions: A new neurosurgical therapy for deafferentation pain. *Adv. Pain Res. Ther.* 5:739–750, 1983.
22. Ojeman G.A., Loeser J.D.: Brain stimulators for pain. *Contemp. Neurosurg.* 2(20):1, 1980.
23. Picaza J.A., Cannon B.W., Hunter S.E., et al.: Pain suppression by peipheral nerve stimulation: Part II. Observations with implanted devices. *Surg. Neurol.* 4:115–126, 1975.
24. Ray C.D., Burton C.V.: Deep brain stimulation for severe, chronic pain. *Acta Neurochir. Suppl.* 30:289–293, 1980.
25. Richards R.L.: Causalgia: A centennial review. *Arch. Neurol.* 16:339–350, 1967.
26. Richardson D.E., Akil H.: Pain reduction by electrical brain stimulation in man: Part I. Acute administration

in periaqueductal and periventricular sites. *J. Neurosurg.* 47:178–183, 1977.

27. Richardson D.E., Akil H.: Pain reduction by electrical brain stimulation in man: Part I. Acute administration in periaqueductal and periventricular sites. *J. Neurosurg.* 47:184–194, 1977.

28. Richardson R.R., Siqueira E.B., Cerullo L.J.: Spinal epidural stimulation for treatment of acute and chronic intractable pain: Initial and long-term results. *Neurosurgery* 5:344–348, 1979.

29. Siegfried J.: Monopolar electrical stimulation of nucleus ventroposteromedialis thalami for postherpetic facial pain. *Appl. Neurophysiol.* 45:179–184, 1982.

30. Siegfried J., Lazorthes Y.: Long term follow up of dorsal cord stimulation for chronic pain syndromes after multiple lumbar operations. *Appl. Neurophysiol.* 45:201–204, 1982.

31. Sweet W.H., Poletti C.E., Macon J.B.: Treatment of trigeminal neuralgia and other facial pain by retrogasserian injection of glycerol. *Neurosurgery* 9:647–653, 1981.

32. Sweet W.H., Poletti C.E.: Retrogasserian glycerol injection as treatment for trigeminal neuralgia, in Schmidek H.H., Sweet W.H. (eds.): *Operative Neurosurgical Techniques.* New York, Grune & Stratton, 1982, pp. 1107–1118.

33. Thompson W.A.L., Kopell H.P.: Peripheral entrapment neuropathies of the upper extremity. *N. Engl. J. Med.* 260:1261–1265, 1958.

34. Turnbull I.M., Shulman R., Woodhurst W.B.: Thalamic stimulation for neuropathic pain. *J. Neurosurg.* 52:486–493, 1980.

35. Urban B.J., Nashold B.S.: Percutaneous epidural stimulation of the spinal cord for relief of pain: Long term results. *J. Neurosurg.* 48:323–328, 1978.

36. van Loveren H., Tew J.M., Keller J.T.: A 10 year experience in the treatment of trigeminal neuralgia: Comparison of percutaneous stereotaxic rhizotomy and posterior fossa decompression. *J. Neurosurg.* 57:757–764, 1982.

37. White J.C., Sweet W.H. *Pain and the Neurosurgeon: A Forty Year Experience.* Springfield, Ill., Charles C Thomas, 1969.

38. Young R.F.: Evaluation of dorsal column stimulation in the treatment of chronic pain. *Neurosurgery* 3:373–379, 1978.

39. DeSaussure R.L.: Causalgia. *Clin. Neurosurg.* 25:626–636, 1978.

40. Loh L., Nathan P.W.: Painful peripheral states and sympathetic blocks. *J. Neurol. Neurosurg. Psychiatry* 41:664–671, 1978.

41. Nashold B.S., Goldner L., Mullen J.B., et al.: Long-term pain control by direct peripheral nerve stimulation. *J. Bone Joint Surg.* 64A:1–10, 1982.

42. Tabira T., Shibasaki H., Kuroiwa Y.: Reflex sympathetic dystrophy (causalgia) treatment with guanethidine. *Arch. Neurol.* 40:430–432, 1983.

39B / Surgical Management of Pain Due to Peripheral Nerve Lesions

LALIGAM N. SEKHAR, M.D.

PERIPHERAL NERVE lesions are a common cause of intractable pain encountered in clinical practice. In the past decade, advances in microsurgical techniques and the availability of neurophysiologic stimulation and ablation methods have greatly improved the outlook for patients with such pain. However, as in other areas of medicine, diagnosis of the source of pain and appropriate referral of the patient for treatment are of paramount importance for relieving the patients' problem. Although a causal relationship is easily established in cases of pain relating to peripheral nerve injuires, the diagnosis of an entrapment neuropathy, which may result from a variety of natural and iatrogenic causes, may be difficult to make. This chapter briefly discusses the etiology, pathogenesis, and methods of managing such pain problems.

ETIOLOGY AND CLASSIFICATION OF PERIPHERAL NERVE LESIONS

A number of acute and chronic nerve lesions may be responsible for the production of nerve injuries (Table 39B–1). In practice, nerve lesions may have multiple causes.

It is useful to classify nerve lesions on the basis of the extent of damage to neural elements. The anatomy of a normal peripheral nerve is as follows.[1] The nerve is surrounded by adventitia, sometimes termed the *mesoneurium*. The *epineurium* is the thick outer layer which ensheaths the whole nerve. Within this sheath lie varying amounts of loose connective tissue and the nerve fascicles. The nerve fascicles are surrounded by a very elastic and organized sheath termed the *perineurium*, which is primarily responsible for the tensile strength of the nerve. The amount of interfunicular connective tissue is variable, and where the amount of interfuni-

TABLE 39B–1.—CAUSATIVE AGENTS IN PERIPHERAL NERVE LESIONS

ACUTE NERVE LESIONS
High-velocity missile injuries
Lacerations caused by sharp objects
Injuries caused by fracture dislocations
Acute nerve compression by blunt objects
Nerve injury due to prolonged compression (e.g. "Saturday night palsy")
Severe traction injuries
Iatrogenic lesions due to surgical anesthesia or operations
Injuries due to injection of drugs into and around the nerve
Thermal injuries due to freezing or burns
CHRONIC NERVE LESIONS
Radiation-induced nerve damage
Entrapment neuropathy
Compression of nerve within an enclosed space
Entrapment due to perineural and intraneural fibrosis
Neoplasms
Nerve and nerve sheath tumors
Adjacent tumors compressing or invading nerves

cular connective tissue is increased, fascicles have a tendency to occur in groups. The size of nerve fascicles varies. Each contains up to 10,000 myelinated and nonmyelinated axons. Each axon in turn is surrounded by a thin layer of connective tissue termed the *endoneurium*. An axon is ensheathed by several Schwann cells, which produce the myelin sheath of myelinated axons. These cells are essential for the functional integrity of the axon and also play an important role in the regeneration of nerves after injury. The nerve receives its blood supply from nutrient arteries that occur at intervals. The nutrient arteries join an important longitudinal plexus of blood vessels in the epineurium, which in turn communicates with a rich plexus of arteries and arterioles between the fascicles. These vessels eventually feed into a rich network of capillaries in the endoneurium. The capillaries eventually drain into venules and thence into epineurial veins. The veins leaving the nerve often run alongside the nutrient arteries but may also run independently.

Nerve injuries have been classified by Sunderland[1] and Seddon[2] on the basis of the extent of damage. The Seddon classification is simpler and uses three categories—neurapraxia, axonotmesis, and neurotmesis. The Sunderland classification is more comprehensive and differentiates five degrees of nerve injury. *Neurapraxia* is transient conduction block and corresponds to the first-degree injury of the Sunderland classification. Neurapraxia is pathologically due to segmental demyelination without any damage to the axon. Complete recovery of muscle function occurs often within days or a few weeks. Since there is no wallerian degeneration distal to the area of demyelination, recovery of muscle function occurs independently of the distance of the muscle from the site of the lesion. *Axonotmesis* corresponds to the second-degree injury of the Sunderland classification. It is caused by damage to the axon and the Schwann cells, but without interruption of the endoneurial sheath. Wallerian degeneration occurs distal to the lesion. Recovery occurs by axonal growth at a rate of 1–3 mm/day, and therefore the proximal muscles recover first. The quality of recovery is excellent since there is no loss or misdirection of axonal sprouts. *Neurotmesis* implies nerve injury with interruption of the endoneurium. Sunderland further classifies neurotmesis into three grades: third-degree injuries are accompanied by an interruption of the endoneurium but the fascicular structure is preserved by an intact perineurium; in fourth-degree injuries the perineurium is interrupted as well, but continuity of the nerve trunk is preserved bacause of an intact epineurium; in fifth-degree injuries there is a total interruption of all elements of the nerve. After neurometic lesions, there is total loss of function distally, and wallerian degeneration follows. Recovery is incomplete or absent and occurs by axonal sprouting and growth.

Neurotmetic injuries may result in the formation of artificial synapses and traumatic neuromas, which are important in the production of intractable pain.[1] When the insulating property of the myelin and the endoneurium is lost by injury, axons can be excited by activity in neighbouring fibers; this is termed an artificial synapse. The formation of artificial synapses between sympathetic and pain-sensitive sensory fibers has been implicated in the genesis of causalgic pain. A similar mechanism may also be responsible for noncausalgic pain. Neuromas may occur on nerves in continuity or at the ends of sev-

ered nerves. Neuromas in continuity may occur because of repeated pathologic friction, recurrent trauma, or involvement of the nerve in an adjacent fibrotic process. More commonly, such neuromas are the result of nerve injury in which the endoneurium and/or the perineurium is injured, but the nerve is in continuity because other fascicles are intact or because the epineurium is intact. Pathologically such neuromas consist of excessive proliferation of fibrous tissue in and around the epineurium, in the damaged fascicles, and even between the normal fascicles. The proliferative fibrous tissue strangles the nerves and reduces their vascularity, further impairing conduction through the nerve. Neuromas that occur at the end of completely severed nerves consist of a bizzare mixture of proliferated axons and fibrous tissue. The part of the nerve proximal to the neuroma often exhibits a fair amount of epineurial and intraneural fibrosis as well.

TYPES OF CHRONIC PAIN DUE TO PERIPHERAL NERVE INJURY

Intractable and persistent pain following peripheral nerve injuries is uncommon, if one considers the number of peripheral lesions which occur without any accompanying pain. Such pain is primarily of two types: causalgic pain and noncausalgic pain.[2]

Causalgic Pain

Causalgia is relatively uncommon, and its incidence has been estimated at 2%–16% of all traumatic peripheral nerve lesions.[1] It often follows injuries associated with emotional trauma, such as missile injuries. The nerves most frequently affected have been found to be the median, the lower trunk and the medial cord of the brachial plexus, and the tibial division of the sciatic nerve. Causalgia usually follows incomplete or partial lesions of the nerve. The pain has the following characteristics: (1) It is spontaneous, severe, and persistent, lasting more than 5 weeks after the trauma. (2) It can be related to injury to a nerve trunk and is unrelated to involvement of nonneural tissues. (3) The pain is usually described as burning but may also be described as crushing, tearing, throbbing, or clamping. (4) The pain often spreads beyond the territory of the injured nerve or nerves. (5) The pain is invariably affected by both emotional and physical stimuli. (6) The extremity is usually held very stiffly and the affected skin is hyperesthetic. (7) Trophic changes are prominent. The area affected may be pink or cyanotic and the skin thin and shiny, nails may be prominent and growth of hair excessive, sweating may be excessive, and the patient generally prefers moisture to dryness. (8) The pain is usually although not invariably relieved by sympathetic blocks and/or sympathectomy.

The pathogenesis of causalgia is controversial. Because of the response to sympathectomy, the formation of artificial synapses between injured sympathetic efferent fibers and somatic afferent pain fibers has been implicated. Another suggested mechanism is the peripheral release of pain-producing vasodilator substances. Central mechanisms may also be responsible.

Noncausalgic Pain

Noncausalgic pain is commoner after peripheral nerve lesions. The pain does not have the previously described characteristics of causalgia. Trophic changes are less marked, and emotional and physical factors do not aggravate the pain as much.

It is sometimes difficult to distinguish between causalgic and noncausalgic pain, and both components may be present in a patient. The pain that follows brachial plexus avulsion injuries and phantom limb pain following amputation are also distinct and are easily distinguished from the other types.

PATHOGENESIS OF PERIPHERAL NERVE PAIN

The genesis of peripheral nerve pain may be explained on the basis of peripheral and central mechanisms.[1, 2] Although all theories have pitfalls, they form a basis for the rational management of patients with peripheral nerve pain syndromes.

Peripheral Mechanisms

Peripheral mechanisms include the following: (1) The formation of artificial synapses between injured nerves. This was already alluded to with respect to causalgia, and may also play a role in noncausalgic pain.[5, 6] (2) The release of pain-producing vasodilator substances at the site where pain is felt. The release of such substances may be triggered by the spontaneous hyperactivity of the fine unmyelinated axons at the site of the nerve injury, or by activity through the artificial synapses. (3) An imbalance between fast conducting and slow conducting fibers. This theory has its origin in the protopathic and epicritic concept of Head and has been subsequently elaborated upon by Noordenbos[7] and by Melzack and Wall.[8] Melzack and Wall's gate control hypothesis envisages facilatory and inhibitory influences on the cells of the substantia gelatinosa (SG) of the spinal cord. The effect of the large-diameter fast conducting touch fibers is to suppress the central output of the cells of the SG, while the effect of the smaller diameter slower conducting pain fibers is to increase the central output from the SG cells. Since most nerve lesions shift the balance in favor of smaller fibers, overactivity of the SG results. The gate control hypothesis explains many but not all features of causalgic and noncausalgic pain. (4) Intraneural and epineurial scar formation at the site of nerve injury causes chronic nerve irritation, venous congestion, ischemia, and resulting intrafunicular edema, all of which increases the excitability of the nerve at the site of the lesion.

Central Mechanisms

Central mechanisms involved in pain are more complex. A hyperactive state of the internuncial neuron pool in the SG may result from chronic discharge from the periphery. Descending central tracts, which are predominantly inhibitory to the SG cells, have been demonstrated. Such a mechanism has been exploited in central stimulation procedures for the relief of pain.

EVALUATION OF A PATIENT WITH PERIPHERAL NERVE PAIN

When one evaluates a patient for pain resulting from a peripheral nerve lesion, other sources of pain must be excluded. Such sources include pain resulting from joint, muscular, or fibrous tissues which may be referred to the extremity and pain resulting from ischemia to the extremity. Besides the clinical examination, electromyography (EMG), nerve conduction studies, and evoked potentials are useful in evaluating these patients. In addition, local anesthetic blocks of the injured segment of the nerve and sympathetic blocks are extremely useful in evaluating the source of the pain and the expected response to treatment. In some cases, repeated blocks may alleviate the pain permanently, especially in the causalgic states.

MANAGEMENT OF PERIPHERAL NERVE PAIN

A trial of medical management is worthwhile in those with peripheral nerve pain from recent trauma and in those in whom pain is unassociated with progressive motor or sensory deficits (Table 39B–2). However, prolonged, severe, and intractable pain of any cause produces adverse psychological and social changes in the patient which accentuate the pain problem. Perpetuation of the peripheral nerve pain state also activates central pain mechanisms which may not revert after treatment of the peripheral nerve problem.

While medical treatment is being tried, both the physician and the patient must be aware of the dangers of addiction. Strong narcotic medications must be avoided. A combination antidepressant drug such as Triavil may be effective in relieving pain. Nerve blocks and sympathetic blocks may also give temporary and occasionally lasting pain relief.

SURGICAL PROCEDURES

Peripheral Nerve

In the surgical management of all peripheral nerve pain problems, peripheral nerve procedures should be tried first. Such procedures are simpler, attempt to correct the problem at the source, and are often effective. In the past decade, the application of microsurgical techniques to peripheral nerve surgery has greatly improved the prospects for the patient with peripheral nerve pain.[3, 4, 9–13] This has been greatly aided by the intraoperative recording of nerve action potentials. Recording of nerve action potentials is performed above and below the injured segment by bipolar electrodes and summated by computer. This technique allows evaluation of neuromas in continuity. Electrical conduction across a neuroma indicates the presence of viable original or regenerated nerve fibers.[14] When the nerve can be dissected into its fascicular components at the site of the neuroma, nerve action potentials can be recorded individually from the fascicles. This reveals which of the fascicles are not in functional continuity and therefore need resection and suture or graft-

TABLE 39B–2. MANAGEMENT OF PERIPHERAL NERVE PAIN

MEDICAL
  Reassurance
  Avoid narcotics
  Antidepressants (e.g., Elavil-Prolixin, Deseril)
  Nerve blocks and sympathetic blocks
SURGICAL
  Peripheral nerve procedures
    Release of entrapment
    Neurolysis: epineurial, fascicular
    Nerve suture (epineurial, fascicular, group fascicular)
    Nerve grafting
    Neuronal trap
  Sympathectomy
  Central procedures
    Stimulation
      Transcutaneous electrical nerve stimulation (TENS)
      Direct peripheral nerve stimulation
      Dorsal column stimulation
      Deep brain stimulation
    Ablation
      Dorsal root entry zone lesion

ing.[15] In addition, we have recently used continuous audio monitoring of electrical activity from the muscles innervated by the nerve during an operation. Such a technique is particularly useful in preventing injury to nerve fascicles during their dissection.

When a peripheral nerve is explored surgically, one may encounter entrapment of the nerve by ligamentous, muscular, or bony structures; involvement of the nerve in an adjacent fibrotic process with epineurial fibrosis; a neuroma in continuity, as the result of a previous injury to some of the fascicles only or as the result of regeneration following previous nerve suture; or a neuroma at the end of a completely divided nerve, with a corresponding glioma at the end of the distal severed segment. One of the following procedures may be performed to correct the pathology.

Release of Entrapment

Accurate preoperative diagnosis and a good familiarity with the anatomy are essential prior to undertaking such an operation.[16] The nerve is traced from a normal area through the abnormal area. Fibrous or ligamentous constricting tissues are divided. When the entrapment is caused by a bony structure such as a cervical rib, the structure is resected. The optimal treatment for some entrapment lesions such as entrapment of the ulnar nerve at the elbow varies from patient to patient and, to some extent, with the surgeon's preference. After release of entrapment, an epineurial neurolysis usually must be performed to release constricting scar around the nerve.

Neurolysis

Neurolysis is the release of scar tissue constricting the nerve. It is best performed under magnification afforded by the operation microscope. As a first step, the thickened epineurium is slit open and the fascicles are dissected free of it until normal epineurium is reached on either side. Care must be taken to preserve branches of the nerve. After the performance of epineurial neurolysis, the fascicles are inspected (Fig 39B–1). When a significant amount of fibrous tissue is present in the interfascicular tissues, a fascicular neurolysis (Fig 39B–2) is performed.[3] The fascicles are carefully freed from surrounding fibrous tissue, with care taken to preserve interfascicular bridges. Such dissection must be performed sharply and under high magnification of the microscope, and preferably with continuous audio monitoring of muscle electrical activity, since there is a great risk of injuring the fascicles.

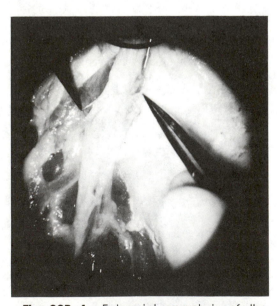

Fig 39B–1.—Epineurial neurolysis of the common peroneal nerve. The epineurium has been removed and the fascicles are distinctly visible, with minimal interfascicular scarring. No fascicular neurolysis was necessary.

Management of Neuroma in continuity by fascicular neurolysis

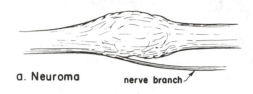

a. Neuroma   nerve branch

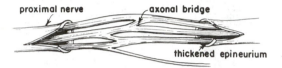

b. After fascicular neurolysis

Fig 39B–2.—Technique of fascicular neurolysis for management of a neuroma in continuity. After removal of the epineurium and dissection of the fascicles, no nerve resection is performed if conduction is present through all the fascicles.

Nerve Suture and Grafting

In case of neuromas in continuity, electrical evaluation will reveal whether there is any conduction across the segment. When electrical conduction is absent, the abnormal segment must be resected and sutured primarily, or grafted. When electrical conduction is present, the individual fascicles are dissected. Evaluation of the fascicles under the operative microscope and with nerve action potential recording will reveal the abnormal segment. The fibrotic segment is then excised and nerve continuity is established by suture or a nerve graft (Fig 39B–3).

In the past few years, there has been some controversy regarding the value of epineurial versus fascicular suture and regarding the extent of nerve gap before cable grafting is employed.[9–13, 18–21] Based on experimental studies in animals, Kline et al. concluded that fascicular suture with or without grafting was not better than epineurial suture, when tension was avoided at the suture line.[19, 20] They advocate nerve mobilization and joint flexion as much as possible to appose the nerve ends primarily, and epineurial suture, without magnification, whenever

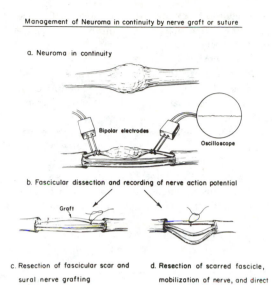

Management of Neuroma in continuity by nerve graft or suture

a. Neuroma in continuity

Bipolar electrodes

Oscilloscope

b. Fascicular dissection and recording of nerve action potential

Graft

c. Resection of fascicular scar and sural nerve grafting

d. Resection of scarred fascicle, mobilization of nerve, and direct suture

Fig 39B–3.—Technique of nerve graft or suture for management of a neuroma. After fascicular neurolysis, one fascicle is seen to be involved in scar. When intraoperative recording of nerve and muscle action potentials reveals no physiologic continuity, resection of the scarred segment is performed, followed by direct fascicular suture or nerve grafting.

possible. Millesi, Samii, and others, on the other hand, on the basis of clinical experience and other experimental studies, advocate a fascicular or a group fascicular suture whenever possible. To avoid any tension at the suture line, they advocate cable grafting when the gap exceeds 2.5 cm or when the nerve ends cannot be brought together without tension.[3, 9–13, 21] It is difficult to establish clinical guidelines because of the conflicting results of experimental studies. Furthermore, since the peripheral nerves of most experimental animals, including primates, are much smaller than human peripheral nerves, with a correspondingly lesser amount of interfunicular fibroconnective tissue, such experimental studies may not accurately represent the human situation. Thus, one must rely on clinical experience even though no randomized controlled studies have been performed.

I avoid extensive neural mobilization and excessive joint flexion. Epineural suture is performed only for small-diameter cutaneous and motor nerves. A fascicular or group fascicular suture is performed under the microscope with 9–0 or 10–0 nylon sutures for most nerves, whenever this is pos-

sible without tension. When the nerve gap cannot be bridged by minimal mobilization of nerves, transposition in the case of the ulnar nerve, or minimal joint flexion, nerve grafting is employed. The nerve most frequently used for grafting is the sural nerve; when it is not available, other nerves such as the medial cutaneous nerve of the forearm or the superficial radial nerve are used. The scar tissue is excised from the proximal and distal segments of the nerve until healthy fascicles with nervous tissue bulging from the perineurial sheath are identified. The bulging axons are then trimmed down to the perineurial sheath, and the previously prepared graft is united with two 9–0 or 10–0 nylon sutures. When there is a disparity between the size of the fascicles and the graft, a group of fascicles may have to be united with a single graft, or a large fascicle may have to be united with more than one graft.

Reconstruction of nerves using the above-mentioned techniques reestablishes the balance between the small- and large-diameter fiber neurons in time, with resolution or remission of the pain problem.

Neuronal Trap

In the case of amputation neuromas, or if the small distal segment of a divided cutaneous nerve cannot be found, the neuronal trap technique first advocated by Samii is employed.[3, 17] The proximal segment of the nerve is dissected into its component fascicles, which are then reanastomosed to each other (Fig 39B–4). Among many techniques which have been advocated to prevent the redevelopment of a painful neuroma, this appears to be the most effective.[1] The proximal end of the nerve should also be moved to an area devoid of constant pressure and friction.

Sympathectomy

For patients with causalgic pain, peripheral nerve procedures should be tried first if a local anesthetic block of the area is effective in temporarily relieving the pain. In the majority of patients, however, sympathectomy is essential for relief. In some patients repeated sympathetic blocks alone provide permanent pain relief. When the pain relief remains temporary, preganglionic sympathectomy will provide permanent relief. Even in patients who do not have the features of causalgia, and in whom peripheral nerve procedures have been ineffective or have ex-

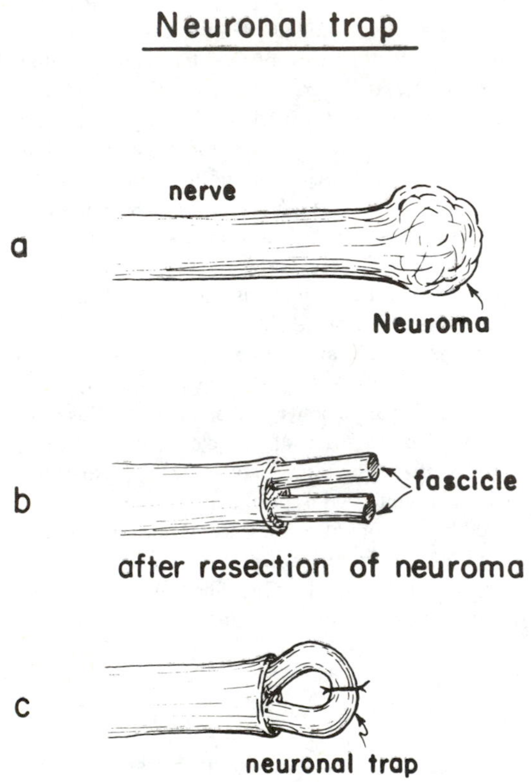

Neuronal trap

Fig 39B–4.—Neuronal trap. This is the ideal method of managing a neuroma when the distal end cannot be identified or is absent due to amputation. The nerve is split into its component fascicles, which are then sutured to each other.

acerbated the pain, sympathetic blockade should be tried. In our experience, the two types of procedures (peripheral nerve and sympathetic nerve blockade) have to be combined to provide relief in some patients with intractable pain.

Central Procedures

Central procedures for pain relief are usually utilized as an adjuvant to pain control when peripheral nerve procedures and sympathectomy are not effective in relieving the pain.[23] *Stimulation* proceudres are much more useful in this regard; destructive procedures should be generally avoided for pain problems not caused by cancer. Transcutaneous electrical nerve stimulation (TENS) of the nerve above the area of injury is based on the gate control hypothesis. The large-diameter fast conducting fibers are stimulated to block the effect of the smaller diameter, slow conducting fibers. This is the technique most frequently employed as an adjuvant to pain control. Direct stimulation of the nerve by electrodes sutured to the nerve has been successfully employed by Nashold in patients with intractable peripheral nerve pain.[22] Dorsal column stimulation utilizes the same principle. The electrodes are positioned in the epidural space under fluoroscopy and are connected to a radioreceiver implanted subcutaneously. Stimulation is then performed by portable battery-powered equipment. There is a high failure rate with this technique with the passage of time. Deep brain stimulation of the periventricular gray, the thalamus, or the internal capsule is rarely needed for peripheral nerve pain problems. These methods presumbably stimulate descending inhibitory pain pathways.

Of the variety of destructive procedures available, the one worth mentioning is the radiofrequency current lesioning of the dorsal root entry zone (the substantia gelatinosa) in the spinal cord, for the treatment of pain caused by nerve root avulsion. Developed by Nashold and others, this technique appears to be extremely effective for pain following brachial plexus avulsion, although long-term follow-up is not available in a large number of patients.

CASE REPORTS

The following case reports are presented to illustrate the management of some peripheral nerve pain problems.

CASE 1.—A 35-year-old woman underwent biopsy of lymph nodes in the posterior cervical triangle. Postoperatively she noticed some weakness of the right shoulder and eventually atrophy of the muscle overlying the right shoulder. She also developed a steady dull pain with an intermittent component shooting down the right neck, shoulder, and retroauricular area. Seven months after the initial procedure she was evaluated by us. Atrophy of the right trapezius muscle and numbness behind the right ear were noted. EMG revealed a complete denervation of the trapezius muscle. To restore continuity of the nerves, the posterior cervical triangle was explored under magnification provided by the operating microscope. The accessory nerve and lesser occipital nerve were found to be divided, and the transverse cervical and the greater auricular nerve were involved in scar. Epineurial neurolysis of the latter two nerves was performed. The distal end of the accessory nerve was identified and a 4-cm gap was bridged with a sural nerve graft (Fig 39B–5). Since the distal end of the lesser occipital nerve could not be found, the neuroma was excised, the proximal stump was split into two fascicular groups, and the fascicles were anastomosed to each other (a neuronal trap). On follow-up 6 months later, the patient reported total relief of pain. There was excellent regeneration of her accessory nerve, and the trapezius muscle had almost regained its normal strength.

Comment.—This case illustrates the genesis of a pain syndrome due to scar involvement of intact nerves and due to neuroma formation in a divided nerve.

CASE 2 (Hand pain following median and ulnar nerve scarring).—A 32-year-old man had sustained a shrapnel injury to the medial aspect of the forearm 10 years earlier. Exact details of the operative exploration were not available, but the patient stated that the ulnar nerve had been injured. He recovered a significant amount of function in the ulnar distribution, but not completely. In the immediately previous year he had noticed an increasing amount of numbness involving all the fingers of his hand, weakness of the hand, and intermittent sharp shooting pain involving all the fingers.

On examination there was impaired sensation over the palmar aspect of the entire hand and all the fingers, but more marked in the ulnar distribution. The function of the thenar muscles was normal but the hypothenar and interosseous muscles were somewhat atrophic. A linear scar was present along the medial aspect of the upper arm. EMG and nerve conduction studies suggested an ulnar and median neuropathy in the mid-upper arm.

The median and ulnar nerves were explored from the axilla to the elbow. The ulnar nerve exhibited a neuroma in continuity, with no evidence of a previous reconstruction. Epineurial and fascicular neurolysis of this nerve was performed (Fig 39B–6). Since all of the fascicles were conducting, none was resected. The median nerve was also involved in surrounding scar.

Postoperatively, the patient noticed total relief of pain in the median distribution and 75% remission of pain in the ulnar distribution. The function of the hand muscles was somewhat improved but did not return to normal. He has intermittently used a TENS unit to control the residual ulnar pain, which worsens with excessive activity and in cold weather. He has been followed up for 2 years with no worsening of his problem.

CASE 3 (Sciatic nerve causalgia following a gunshot injury).—A 63-year-old man underwent exploration about 6 months earlier by a general surgeon following a low-velocity gunshot wound to his thigh. At the initial exploration, the sciatic nerve was found to be transected with a 5-cm gap. The nerve was not repaired. Wound healing was delayed because of infection. About 3 months after the injury, the patient developed severe, crushing, and constant pain involving the right foot and leg. The pain was exacerbated by cold weather and emotional distress. It was relieved somewhat by back massage, but unchanged with transcutaneous stimulation. The patient was using only mild narcotic medication (Tylenol with codeine) because of religious convic-

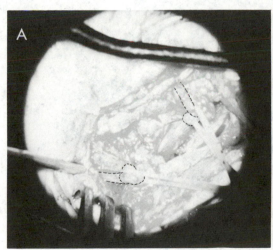
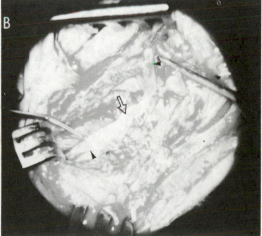

Fig 39B–5.—Case 1. **A,** note the upper and lower ends of the spinal accessory nerve with the attached neuroma and glioma *(outlined).* **B,** appearance after resection of the neuroma and distal glioma and sural nerve grafting. *Arrowheads* point to the anastamoses; *open arrow* points to the graft.

tions concerning the use of drugs. A trial of Elavil-Prolixin failed to relieve the pain.

On examination, the muscles innervated by the sciatic nerve below the knee were totally paralyzed. There was total loss of touch and pinprick sensation in the foot and leg, except for the part supplied by the saphenous nerve. Trophic changes were very prominent in the foot, including redness and thinning of the skin and excessive nail growth. Thus the patient had several but not all features of causalgia.

Puckered and scarred entrance and exit wounds were present in the upper thigh. Tinel's sign could not be elicited on tapping along the course of the sciatic nerve.

At operative exploration, the proximal end of the sciatic nerve was found just below the edge of the gluteus maximus muscle. After resection of the neuroma and the distal glioma, the nerve gap was about 8 cm. The medial popliteal portion of the sciatic nerve was reconstructed with five grafts from the opposite sural nerve (Fig 39B–7). A neuronal trap was performed for the lateral popliteal portion.

On follow-up for 2 years, the patient's pain has been relieved about 90%. Functional recovery in the calf muscles has been confirmed electromyographically. Relieved of the pain problem, the patient made a better emotional and social adjustment to his disability. He now uses a foot drop brace. Further recovery of sensation is expected in the leg and foot.

CASE 4 (Neuronal trap for superficial peroneal nerve neuroma).—A 60-year-old man had presented 6 months previously with radiating pain in the distal peroneal nerve distribution. On examination, a 0.5 × 0.5-cm nodule had been found along the course of the superficial peroneal nerve about 6 cm above the ankle. It had been explored under local anesthesia. A neuroma in continuity had been found and was resected by another surgeon. The proximal stump of the nerve had been ligated to prevent the recurrence of the neuroma. The patient's pain, however, recurred after 3 months, with similar characteristics. Tapping the location of the proximal stump elicited Tinel's sign. There was sensory loss to touch and pinprick on the dorsum of the foot and toes.

An operation was undertaken to reconstruct the superficial peroneal nerve. Since the distal end was extremely atrophic and scarred, the neuroma was excised from the proximal end and a neuronal trap was performed, after splitting the nerve into two fascicular groups. The patient has been pain free for 1 year, on follow-up.

CASE 5 (Upper limb causalgia).—A 56-year-old man reported an intractable pain syndrome involving the medial aspect of the forearm, hand, and ring and little finger for 2 years. The pain had been of relatively acute onset and had failed to respond to mild narcotics or to Triavil. The patient could not use his hand on account of extreme hyperesthesia.

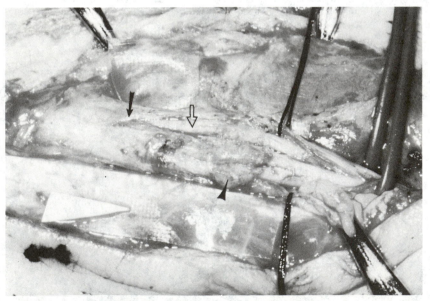

Fig 39B–6.—Case 2. Surgical appearance during performance of epineurial and fascicular neurolysis of the ulnar nerve. Note the epineurium *(closed arrow)*, fascicles *(open arrow)*, and neuromas in continuity with the fascicles *(arrowhead)*. Since all fascicles were conducting across the neuromas, no nerve resection was performed but the scar tissue was removed.

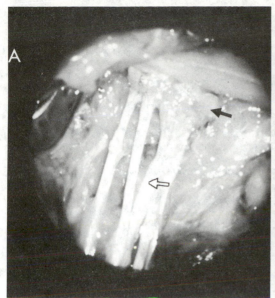

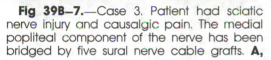

Fig 39B–7.—Case 3. Patient had sciatic nerve injury and causalgic pain. The medial popliteal component of the nerve has been bridged by five sural nerve cable grafts. **A,** upper end of nerve. **B,** lower end of the nerve. *Closed arrow* indicates nerve; *open arrow* indicates graft.

Repeated EMG and nerve conduction studies had failed to demonstrate a lesion of the brachial plexus, and studies for a thoracic outlet syndrome, ulnar neuropathy, and a cervical disk herniation were negative.

On examination, the medial two fingers and the medial aspect of the hand were flushed, hyperhydrotic, and demonstrated prominent trophic changes. The medial two fingers were held curled and stiff. Diminished light touch and extreme hyperpathia were present in the involved area. Motor testing was difficult because of the hyperesthesia.

A diagnosis of brachial plexus causalgia was made. Because repeated sympathetic blocks provided temporary pain relief, a cervicothoracic sympathectomy was performed by a supraclavicular approach. Immediately after the procedure, the patient noticed a resolution of pain and return of the skin color to normal. He has been able to use his hand well, on follow-up for 6 months.

REFERENCES

1. Sunderland S.: *Nerves and Nerve Injuries,* ed. 2. New York, Churchill Livingstone, 1978, p. 1046.
2. Seddon H.: *Surgical Disorders of the Peripheral Nerves,* ed. 2. New York, Churchill Livingstone, 1975, p. 336.
3. Samii M.: Modern aspects of peripheral and cranial nerve surgery, in Krayenbuhl H. (ed.): *Advances and Technical Standards in Neurosurgery.* New York, Springer-Verlag, 1975, vol. 2, pp. 34–85.
4. Sekhar L.H., Alemo-Hammad S.: Saphenous neuropathy and subsartorial canal syndrome. Unpublished manuscript.
5. Granit R., Leksell L., Skoglund C.R.: Fiber interaction in injured or compressed region of nerve. *Brain* 67:125–140, 1944.
6. Skoglund C.R.: Transsynaptic and direct stimulation of post-fibers in the artificial synapse formed by severed mammalian nerve. *J. Neurophysiol.* 8:365–376, 1945.
7. Noordenbos W.: Pathologic aspects of central pain states. *Adv. Neurol.* 4:333, 1974.
8. Melzack R., Wall P.D.: Pain mechanisms: A new theory. *Science* 150:971–979, 1965.
9. Millesi H., Meissl G., Berger A.: The interfascicular nerve grafting of the median and ulnar nerves. *J. Bone Joint Surg.* [Am.] 54:727–750, 1950.
10. Millesi H.: Nerve grafts: Indications, techniques, and prognosis, in Omer G.E., Jr., Spinner M. (eds.): *Management of Peripheral Nerve Problems.* Philadelphia, W.B. Saunders Co., 1980, pp. 410–431.
11. Millesi H.: Trauma involving the brachial plexus, in Omer G.E. Jr., Spinner M. (eds.): *Management of Peripheral Nerve Problems.* Philadelphia, W.B. Saunders Co., 1980, pp. 548–568.
12. Beek A.V., Kleinert H.E.: Peripheral nerve injuries and repair, in Rand R.W. (ed.): *Microneurosurgery.* St. Louis, C.V. Mosby, 1978, pp. 415–440.

13. Smith J.W., Gillen F.J.: Current techniques in peripheral nerve repair, in Rand R.W. (ed.): *Microneurosurgery*. St. Louis, C.V. Mosby, 1978, pp. 399–414.

14. Kline D.G.: Evaluation of the neuroma in continuity, in Omer G.E. Jr., Spinner M. (eds.): *Management of Peripheral Nerve Problems*. Philadelphia, W.B. Saunders Co., 1980, pp. 450–461.

15. Terzis J.K., Daniel R.K., Williams H.B.: Intraoperative assessment of nerve lesions with fascicular dissection and electrophysiological recordings, in Omer G.E. Jr., Spinner M. (eds.): *Management of Peripheral Nerve Problems*. Philadelphia, W.B. Saunders Co., 1980, pp. 462–472.

16. Kopell H.P., Thompson W.A.Z.: *Peripheral Entrapment Neuropathies*. Huntington, New York, R.E. Krieger, 1976.

17. Lagarrique J., Chavoin J.P., Belahouari L., et al.: Treatment of painful neuromas with "neuronal trap." *Neurochirurgie* 28:91–92, 1982.

18. Kline D.G., Judice D.J.: Operative management of selected brachial plexus lesions. *J. Neurosurg.* 58:631–649, 1983.

19. Bratton B.R., Kline D.G., Coleman W., et al.: Experimental interfascicular nerve grafting. *J. Neurosurg.* 51:323–332, 1979.

20. Hudson A.R., Hunter D., Kline D.G., et al.: Histological studies of experimental interfascicular graft repairs. *J. Neurosurg.* 51:333–340, 1979.

21. Terzis J.K., Orgel M.G.: Epineurial vs perineurial repair: An ultrastructural and electrophysiological study of nerve regeneration. *J. Plast. Reconstr. Surg.* 60:80–91, 1977.

22. Nashold B.S. Jr.: Electrical stimulation of peripheral nerves with microelectrical implants for pain relief, in Omer G.E. Jr., Spinner M. (eds.): *Management of Peripheral Nerve Problems*. Philadelphia, W.B. Saunders Co., 1980, pp. 303–315.

23. Gildenberg P.L.: Central surgical procedures for pain of peripheral nerve origin, in Omer G.E. Jr., Spinner H. (eds.): *Management of Peripheral Nerve Problems*. Philadelphia, W.B. Saunders Co., 1980, pp. 303–313.

39C / Neurosurgical Treatment of Cancer Pain

ELIZABETH BULLITT, M.D.
ALLAN FRIEDMAN, M.D.

THE GOAL OF ANY procedure for pain relief should be to provide complete and long-lasting relief of symptoms with minimal side effects. Unfortunately, this goal is not always achieved. Our understanding of pain and of the anatomical pathways involved is as yet imperfect. The very word "pain" actually refers to a variety of unpleasant symptoms which may respond differently to any given form of treatment. The differences in the pain pathways involved and the factors that make a particular kind of pain respond to one therapeutic modality and not to another are not always clear.

This chapter provides an overview of the standard neurosurgical procedures available for the treatment of cancer pain. In general, neurosurgical operations for pain relief can be divided into four categories. Destructive procedures, which entail the surgical interruption of pain pathways, are extremely useful in the treatment of cancer pain. Decompressive and stimulation procedures are most commonly employed in the treatment of pain of benign origin but also may benefit selected cancer patients. The application of pharmacologic agents to the CNS is a fourth and newer approach that seems to offer great promise in the treatment of cancer patients. This chapter is therefore divided into sections according to the approach used and the anatomical level chosen for surgical intervention. Within each section an attempt has been made to delineate which problems are most likely to benefit from a particular therapeutic approach.

DESTRUCTIVE PROCEDURES

Peripheral Nerves and Nerve Roots

Pain signals are transmitted centrally by unmyelinated and thinly myelinated fibers that enter the dorsal surface of the spinal cord as a series of rootlets. Theoretically, therefore, pain signals originating peripherally could be interrupted by division of the dorsal roots supplying the painful area.

The sympathetic nervous system also plays some role in the transmission of pain signals. Interruption of the celiac plexus can provide gratifying pain relief in the patient with visceral pain in the upper abdomen.

Dorsal Rhizotomy

The purpose of dorsal rhizotomy is to interrupt all sensory input from a painful area. Rhizotomy can be performed by a variety of methods. Most commonly, the procedure is performed as an open operation under general anesthesia. Following a laminectomy and dural opening, the desired nerve roots are identified and divided under direct vision. Some neurosurgeons have found preoperative nerve blocks to be helpful in identifying the nerve roots to be sacrificed,[1] whereas others have found preoperative nerve blocks to be unreliable indicators of the final result.[2, 3] In any case, because of the extensive overlap of sensory dermatomes, it is necessary to render a large area anesthetic. Most neurosurgeons recommend the additional division of dorsal roots at least one and often two levels above and below the nerve roots supplying the painful area (Fig 39C–1, Plate 14).

Rhizotomy may also be performed chemically, by injecting alcohol or phenol into the subarachnoid space. This approach is particularly useful in the paraplegic patient with painful spasticity. Intrathecal phenol should not be administered to patients with normal bladder function.[4] Percutaneous radiofrequency rhizotomy is also sometimes performed as an alternative to open operation. This technique involves the insertion of radiofrequency electrodes percutaneously into the desired neural foramina under fluoroscopic control. As motor roots may be affected by coagulation, the procedure is most often used in patients with preexisting motor impairment. Coagulation of a major radicular artery may cause infarction of the spinal cord.

One disadvantage of dorsal rhizotomy is that extensive denervation is required in order to relieve pain in a small area. As many as five roots must be coagulated in order to obtain anesthesia over one dermatome. Another disadvantage is that all sensory modalities are interrupted in the denervated area. The production of anesthesia may be of little importance in the thoracic region, but an arm or leg deprived of all sensory input becomes a useless extremity. If bowel and bladder function are present preoperatively, a bilateral sacral rhizotomy for pelvic pain will result in loss of these functions. Bladder function may sometimes be preserved when a single S-2 root is left intact.[5]

The long-term success rate of dorsal rhizotomy is open to question. Although some neurosurgeons have reported significant pain relief in up to 70% of patients,[5, 6] the results of other series have been discouraging.[1] Indeed, Onofrio and Campa concluded at the end of their review of 286 patients operated on at the Mayo Clinic that spinal rhizotomy for pain relief had only a "poor to fair chance of succeeding."[2] The reason for the failure rate is not clear, but may include section of an insufficient number of nerve roots or transmission of pain signals via alternate pathways such as the ventral roots.

King and Hodge have demonstrated that the area of sensory alteration produced by either cordotomy or rhizotomy can be modified pharmacologically. Postoperative oral administration of levodopa will decrease the region of analgesia or anesthesia and cause pain recurrence. In patients with late postoperative pain recurrence and contraction of the analgesic area, oral tryptophan or methyldopa may cause expansion of the analgesic region and produce remission of symptoms.[7, 8] These studies suggest that pain recurrence following an initially successful operation may result from alterations in the central processing of pain signals. The mechanisms involved are unclear.

In general, dorsal rhizotomy may be considered in the patient with cancer pain in the cervical region or torso, or in the patient with cancer pain in the arm or leg when the extremity is already functionally useless. Sacral rhizotomy is effective in treating those with pelvic pain, but should be employed with caution when bowel and bladder function are intact. The long-term results of rhizotomy are disappointing.

Sympathetic Denervation

Sympathectomy is most commonly associated with the treatment of causalgia, a benign form of pain. However, sympathectomy can also be of significant benefit in the treatment of malignant pain arising from the upper abdominal viscera. The celiac plexus and splanchnic nerves contain fibers which innervate the liver, stomach, and pancreas. Interruption of the sympathetic supply to those organs can result in gratifying pain relief in the patient with cancer pain.

Although the celiac plexus may be approached by open operation, denervation is most commonly performed percutaneously. Gorbitz and Leavins have described the procedure in detail.[9] Bilateral needles are introduced under radiographic control so as to lie just anterior to the body of L-1. After aspiration and injection of a test dose of local anesthetic, absolute alcohol is injected to provide a permanent block.

The major complication of the procedure has been the development of postoperative postural hypotension. A potential risk is the inadvertent puncture of a major vessel, an abdominal viscus, or the spinal canal. Although some neurosurgeons have employed sympathetic denervation in the treatment of benign disease,[3] others have preferred to reserve the treatment for patients suffering from cancer because of the potential operative risks.

The procedure is generally effective as long as the disease process does not involve the abdominal wall, the intercostal nerves, or the lumbar plexus. In these cases somatic pain will persist after interruption of the sympathetic pathways. Abdominal computerized tomography may be of use in determining the extent of tumor involvement. When the disease process does involve somatic nerves, other procedures such as dorsal rhizotomy, percutaneous cordotomy, midline myelotomy, or the use of intraspinal morphine should be considered. Cervical or lumbar sympathectomy will not relieve cancer pain in an extremity.

Spinal Cord

Within the spinal cord, pain-carrying fibers synapse within the dorsal horn. Painful impulses are transmitted centrally largely by neurons whose cell bodies lie in laminae I, II, and V and whose processes cross in the anterior commissure over several cord segments before ascending in the contralateral spinothalamic tract. This segregation of pain-carrying fibers within the spinal cord allows the surgical destruction of pain pathways without destruction of other tracts. The role of the spinoreticular formation in the transmission of pain signals is less clear, but the passage of pain signals over such alternate pathways is sometimes offered as an explanation for pain recurring after cordotomy.

Cordotomy

Cordotomy, or interruption of the lateral spinothalamic tract within the spinal cord, is the procedure of choice in the treatment of many patients with cancer pain. It is an extremely effective technique that produces pain relief in 80%–90% of cases. In addition, cordotomy interferes only with pain and temperature sensation and therefore does not result in the disabling loss of touch and position sense entailed by dorsal rhizotomy. Unfortunately, the usefulness of the procedure is limited by the tendency of pain to recur with time. Cordotomy has therefore proved most effective in the treatment of cancer patients with limited life expectancies.

Percutaneous cordotomy has largely replaced cordotomy by open operative techniques. A number of excellent procedure descriptions are available.[10–12] In brief, the operation involves the insertion of a radiofrequency electrode laterally into the spinal cord through the C1–2 interspace and the subsequent production of radiofrequency lesions within the anterolateral quadrant of the spinal cord (Figs 39C–2 and 39C–3.) The patient is awake during the procedure, which allows continuous monitoring of neurologic function.

A unilateral cordotomy produces contralateral loss of temperature and pain sensation. Patients with bilateral or midline pain must undergo bilateral cordotomies staged at least a week apart. The procedure is most effective when the patient complains of sharp or aching pain but is much less advantageous in treating burning, crawling, dysesthetic pain. It is difficult to attain levels of analgesia above C-4, and patients with pain in the upper neck or head are best treated by other means.

The risks of cordotomy include a small risk of permanent bladder dysfunction and approximately an 8% risk of ipsilateral paresis. Difficulty with respiration may also occur in about 8% of cases. The risks of serious pulmonary dysfunction are greater when there is preexisting pulmonary disease, such as may occur in the patient with advanced lung cancer. In this situation, cordotomy may eliminate pain but may also impair control of the healthy lung.

Bilateral cordotomies are more likely to result in

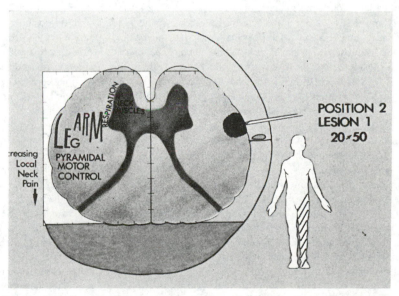

Fig 39C–2.—Position for creating a lesion in the spinothalamic tract. (Courtesy of James E. McLennan, M.D.)

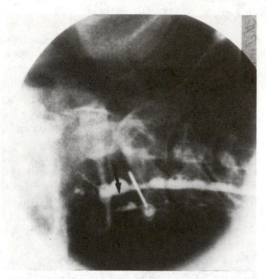

Fig 39C–3.—Cervical cordotomy: lateral cervical spine film showing a spinal needle inserted at C1–2. The thick line of Pantopaque outlines the dentate ligaments *(arrow)* and the thinner line of Pantopaque delineates the posterior margin of the spinal canal. The spinothalamic tract lies a few millimeters anterior to the dentate ligament, so the spinal needle was positioned more posteriorly before the electrode was inserted.

respiratory complications or urinary retention than are unilateral lesions. Sleep-induced apnea sometimes occurs in patients following bilateral high cervical cordotomy and may be lethal.[13] Because of the potential pulmonary complications of bilateral high cordotomy, some neurosurgeons have preferred to make the second lesion below the C-4 level of the phrenic outflow, via a more difficult anterior approach.[14, 15] An open operation may be done at any desired spinal level, but the risks of producing weakness or sphincter dysfunction are higher than in the percutaneous procedure. Approximately 1% of patients will develop postoperative dysesthesias throughout the analgesic area.

A major drawback to cordotomy is that while it is initially effective in relieving pain in the majority of patients, the level of analgesia may drop over time. Rosomoff estimates that 90% of patients are pain free immediately following the procedure, but that at 1 year the success rate drops to 60%. By 2 years, only 40% show continued pain relief.[12]

In general, cordotomy is the procedure of choice in patients with adequate pulmonary function and unilateral cancer pain below the level of the neck.

Cordotomy may also be considered in the patient with bilateral cancer pain or severe pulmonary disease, but the relative risks and benefits of the procedure must be considered. In some of these patients commissural myelotomy, hypophysectomy, or intraspinal morphine may provide a preferable therapeutic approach. Cordotomy is almost never indicated in the treatment of the younger patient with benign disease.

Commissural Myelotomy

The goal of commissural myelotomy is interruption of secondary pain-carrying fibers as they cross in the anterior commissure of the spinal cord. Proponents of commissural myelotomy believe it to be effective in treating bilateral or midline cancer pain, with a lower complication rate than bilateral cordotomy.

Commissural myelotomy is performed as an open operation. Following laminectomy and dural opening, a midline incision is made between the dorsal columns over approximately three vertebral body segments and the commissures are divided. The operative level depends on the level of entry of the spinal roots involved, and on the knowledge that decussation of secondary pain fibers occurs about two segments rostral to the site of entry of the involved spinal roots. There is a normal anatomical variation in the number of spinal segments required for decussation.[3] It is therefore not surprising that a number of patients fail to exhibit postoperative analgesia over the desired area. What is surprising is that many patients do show postoperative pain relief even without the production of analgesia. The success of the operation therefore may not depend solely on the interruption of decussating fibers bound for the spinothalamic tract.[16]

The operation is initially successful in 60%–70% of patients[16–18] with one series reporting a 90% success rate.[7] As with cordotomy, pain relief wanes with time. The procedure is not appropriate in patients with benign disease and normal life expectancies. Lippert et al. found the procedure to be most effective in patients with hip or leg pain.[19] Cook and Kawakami report excellent pain relief in patients with bilateral metastases, except in the case of intrapelvic metastases.[18]

Disadvantages of the procedure include the necessity of a major operation, the development of transient but severe dysesthesias following surgery, the production of posterior column dysfunction in some cases, and, as in cordotomy, the loss of pain relief with time. Postoperative bladder dysfunction or motor weakness is uncommon.

Our experience with this technique is limited, but in our single patient with carcinoma and sacral pain there was no pain relief following midline myelotomy. Intraspinal morphine may prove to be a more effective and benign technique than either midline myelotomy or bilateral cordotomy in the patient with pelvic or bilateral lower extremity pain.

Cranial Nerve and Intracranial Operations

A number of different therapeutic alternatives are available to treat pain in the torso or extremities. Cephalic pain, however, can only be treated by the interruption of intracranial nerves or by an intracranial operation. The risks of intracranial surgery tend to be higher than the risks of spinal or peripheral nerve surgery. With only a few exceptions, intracranial operations have therefore been used primarily to treat cancer pain extending into the head and neck.

Division of Cranial Nerves

Pain sensation in the face is conducted centrally through the fifth cranial nerve. The ninth and tenth nerves supply the throat and nasopharynx, and the angle of the jaw is innervated by C-2. When pain is confined to the trigeminal distribution, interruption of the fifth cranial nerve may produce good pain relief. When the pain extends beyond the territory of the fifth nerve, more extensive procedures are required.

Division of the fifth nerve may be performed percutaneously. Percutaneous rhizotomy involves the insertion of a radiofrequency electrode through the skin of the cheek lateral to the corner of the mouth. The needle is passed through the foramen ovale and into the gasserian ganglion (Fig 39C–4). Stimulation is used to ensure proper needle placement within the desired trigeminal nerve division, and a radiofrequency lesion is created within the ganglion.

If pain extends into the throat, the ninth and tenth cranial nerves may also be coagulated percutaneously. The technique used is similar to that of trigeminal rhizotomy, except that the needle is inserted into the jugular foramen.

The advantage of percutaneous rhizotomy is the relative ease and safety of the procedure. No general anesthetic is required. However, coagulation of the trigeminal nerve is usually effective only if analgesia is produced. The operation is therefore impractical in the treatment of bilateral facial pain because of the consequent difficulty with eating. If the cornea is rendered analgesic, special eye care is required to prevent keratitis. Vocal cord paralysis oc-

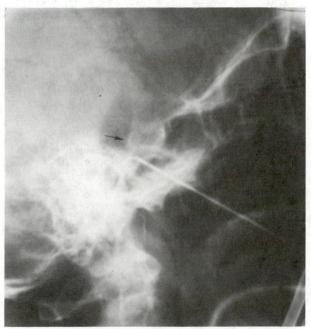

Fig 39C–4.—Percutaneous trigeminal rhizotomy: lateral skull film. A curved electrode has been inserted through the foramen ovale so as to lie at the level of the clivus 4–5 mm posterior to the dorsum sella (arrow). The curve of the electrode is directed posteriorly so as to lie within the V_2 and V_3 fibers. A V_1 lesion can be produced by directing the curve of the electrode anteriorly.

curs commonly following coagulation of the ninth and tenth nerves.[20] Syncope and seizures have been reported in association with glossopharyngeal and vagal coagulation.[21] Additional risks of percutaneous rhizotomy include a small chance of meningitis, of carotid artery injury, or of diplopia.[22]

One disadvantage of the percutaneous operation is that tumor of the skull base may distort the cranial nerves, making adequate lesion placement impossible. Another disadvantage of the percutaneous approach is that it will not relieve pain extending caudally into the neck. If adequate lesion placement is impossible, or if pain extends beyond the fifth and ninth nerve territories, a posterior fossa approach may be the procedure of choice. It is possible to divide the fifth, ninth, and tenth cranial nerves and to perform posterior cervical rhizotomies through the same skin incision. If pain extends into the ear, the nervus intermedius should also be interrupted. The disadvantage of the posterior fossa approach is that a major operation under general anesthesia is required. As with percutaneous rhizotomy, bilateral nerve sections should be avoided. Risks include a 5%–10% chance of injury to adjacent cranial nerves, resulting in diplopia, facial weakness, or deafness. Hematoma or infarction may also complicate the operation.[22, 23]

Patients with bilateral facial pain are particularly difficult to treat. In some cases, it may be advisable to perform rhizotomies on one side and to treat the contralateral pain with a different procedure such as thalamotomy or a midbrain lesion.

Brain Stem Lesions

MEDULLA.—Specific pain pathways may be interrupted not only within the spinal cord, but at various brain stem levels as well. Pain fibers from the face and throat descend ipsilaterally into the upper cervical cord before decussating to ascend in the contralateral quintothalamic tract. The descending pain fibers can be divided in the medulla just below the level of the obex, producing ipsilateral facial analgesia without total sensory loss. The procedure may be performed as an open operation, but the risk of morbidity has led most neurosurgeons to rely on other techniques. Stereotactic trigeminal tractotomy has been performed at a few centers, using an electrode inserted between the occiput and C-1. We have little experience with this technique, but Nashold and Crue have reported good pain relief in 9 of 11 cancer patients, with no morbidity and no deaths.[24]

MIDBRAIN.—The mesencephalon has proved to be an important area in the surgical treatment of pain. Lesions of the spinothalamic tract within the human midbrain were first performed by Dogliotti in 1938. This lesion was made by cutting the tegmentum of the midbrain under the temporal lobe. Although this method of pain relief was occasionally utilized, high operative mortality and morbidity rates discouraged most neurosurgeons from employing the procedure.

In 1948, Spiegel and Wycis first performed a stereotactic lesion of the spinothalamic tract within the midbrain. Six years later the same physicians reported a remarkable finding. They noted that a lesion within the reticular activating system adjacent to the periaqueductal gray matter within the midbrain tegmentum would also result in pain relief. Thus there appear to be two distinct fiber tracts which conduct pain sensation through the midbrain.

The first tract is composed of neospinothalamic and quintothalamic fibers and lies in the lateral tegmentum. The fibers in this tract are topographically arranged with the fibers from the head lying medially and the fibers from the foot lying laterally. Most of these fibers synapse in the ventral lateral thalamic nucleus, although some terminate in the posterior thalamus. Electrical stimulation of this tract at the time of surgery frequently results in the production of a warm or cold sensation. Painful sensations are evoked only rarely. A lesion of this pathway results in the same neurologic deficit seen following lesions of the anterolateral quadrant of the spinal cord. Postoperatively, patients note a diminution of contralateral pain and temperature sensation.

The second mesencephalic pathway implicated in the transmission of pain lies in the reticular formation just lateral to the periaqueductal gray matter.[25] This pain pathway is much less clearly demarcated and is thought to be polysnaptic in character. The tract conveys paleospinothalamaic fibers to the posterior thalamus, intralaminar nuclei, subthalamus, and hypothalamus. Intraoperative single cell recordings performed in this area demonstrate delayed neuronal firing in response to cutaneous pinprick stimulation within a large receptive field.[25] Electrical stimulation of the pathway is perceived by the patient as an extremely unpleasant sensation within the central portion of the body.[26] Following lesion placement, patients have minimal hypesthesia. Most stereotactic midbrain lesions for the obliteration of pain are aimed at this pathway.

Recent reports have noted encouraging results from stereotactic mesencephalotomies for pain.

Amano et al. reported that of 15 patients treated for pain by mesencephalotomy, 11 patients remained relieved of symptoms at follow-up 3 months to 5 years later.[27] Unfortunately the cause of pain is not described. Frank et al. reported the results of mesencephalotomy performed on 18 patients with face, neck, or arm pain secondary to cancer. Short-term follow-up showed that 14 patients had satisfactory pain relief an average of 4.9 months following surgery.[28] These results corroborate those reported earlier by Nashold.[29]

Undesirable effects which may accompany lesion placement within the mesencephalon include limitation of upward gaze, downward gaze, and ocular convergence.[29] These side effects have been reduced by moving the lesion to a position 5 mm behind the posterior commissure. As with cordotomy, pain relief diminishes in effectiveness with the passage of time. A mesencephalotomy is therefore rarely performed for the treatment of pain that is not the result of malignant disease. As with cordotomy, annoying dysesthesias sometimes follow operation.[29] Contralateral motor weakness is rare, and perioperative mortality is less than 3%.[30]

In summary, stereotactic mesencephalotomy is a relatively safe operation which is best suited for patients suffering from pain associated with malignancies of the head and neck.

THALAMOTOMY.—Thalamic lesions may also be of significant benefit in the patient with cancer pain of the head and neck. The procedure is done stereotactically. As with midbrain lesions, electrode placement is confirmed by intraoperative stimulation. Patient cooperation is required during the procedure.

Three primary target areas have been used.[3, 31–33] Initially, lesions were placed within the ventral posterior thalamus, destroying the specific sensory relay nuclei. Although this procedure was sometimes effective in relieving pain, a major disadvantage was the production of a marked contralateral sensory loss. Severe dysesthetic pain sometimes developed postoperatively as well. Lesion production in this area of the thalamus has therefore been abandoned in favor of other sites.

Intrathalamic lesions may also be placed within the intralaminar nuclei. Destruction of this area interrupts pain fibers ascending in the reticular system without affecting the specific sensory fibers terminating in the ventral posterior nuclei. No major sensory loss occurs with proper lesion placement. The intralaminar nuclei are the most common thalamic targets in the treatment of pain.

A third target area is the dorsomedian or anterior nuclear group. The dorsomedian nucleus projects fibers to the frontal lobe, and the anterior nuclei project to the cingulate gyrus. Destruction of either of these areas does not affect primary pain sensation but will reduce the suffering and emotional distress that often accompany cancer pain. Dorsomedian or anterior nuclear lesions are usually not used in isolation but are combined with destruction of the intralaminar nuclei.

A unilateral thalamotomy relieves pain in the contralateral face and body. If bilateral or midline pain is present, bilateral lesions are necessary and should be staged 3–6 weeks apart. The initial results are good, and 80%–90% of cancer patients experience pain relief. The results wane with time, however, and pain often recurs by 6 months. The risks of thalamotomy are relatively low but include a small chance of hemorrhage or infection. If lesion placement is inaccurate, sensory disturbance or motor weakness may occur.

Thalamotomy is therefore a procedure that is best limited to the patient with cancer pain. It may be the procedure of choice in some debilitated patients with short life expectancies and pain in the head and neck. Thalamotomy should not be used in the patient with pain of benign origin.

CINGULUMOTOMY.—Cingulumotomy involves the placement of bilateral lesions within the cingulate gyrus. The effect is similar to that of lesion placement within the anterior thalamic nuclei. Pain sensation is not interrupted directly, but suffering and anxiety may be reduced. The operation can be done under local anesthesia, does not require patient cooperation, and may be performed with or without a stereotactic frame. The direct operative risks are low.

Hurt and Ballantine reported moderate, marked, or complete pain relief in 56% of cancer patients immediately after operation. By 3 months, however, no cancer patient reported complete pain relief, and only 22% showed moderate or marked symptomatic improvement. In patients with pain of nonmalignant origin, 45% showed initial pain relief of moderate degree or better, and these statistics remained stable over 3 months.[34]

Foltz followed up his pain patients for 3–15 years after cingulumotomy and reported good or excellent results in 13 of 16 cancer patients and in 13 of 18 patients with nonneoplastic disease. He believes that the patient's premorbid personality type should be a major criterion in patient selection for this procedure. Those with a tendency to respond to small insults with a vigorous emotional response are likely to benefit from cingulumotomy.[35]

Cingulumotomy may be the procedure of choice in the moribund, uncooperative patient with widespread, intractable pain. Patients whose pain problem is compounded by anxiety and depression may be more likely to benefit from the operation. Although cingulumotomy has been used successfully to treat some patients with psychiatric disease, the procedure is only rarely indicated in the treatment of benign pain. Pain relief does not always occur, and the operation may result in a blunting of emotional responses. The ethical and legal complexities entailed often contraindicate the procedure in the patient with pain of nonmalignant origin.

HYPOPHYSECTOMY.—Destruction of the pituitary gland may be of significant benefit in relieving the pain of bony metastases in patients with carcinoma of the breast and prostate. Since the pioneering work of Higgins and Hodges, the manipulation of certain endogenous hormones has been used to induce regression of metastatic breast and prostate tumors.[36] Hypophysectomy was shown to further palliate symptoms in many patients who demonstrated an initial response to other forms of endocrine manipulation. As experience was gained with this procedure it was noted that a high percentage of patients reported good pain relief without objective evidence of tumor regression.

Because many patients with metastatic disease are not suitable candidates for craniotomy, less invasive methods of hypophysectomy were sought (Fig 39C–5). Stereotactic cryosurgery and radiofrequency pituitary coagulation frequently failed to obliterate the gland. Destruction of the pituitary gland with yttrium implants had an unacceptably high incidence of parasellar nerve damage and cerebrospinal fluid (CSF) rhinorrhea. Transphenoidal hypophysectomy, however, was well tolerated by patients debilitated by metastatic tumor and resulted in few complications. Tindall et al. reported satisfactory pain relief

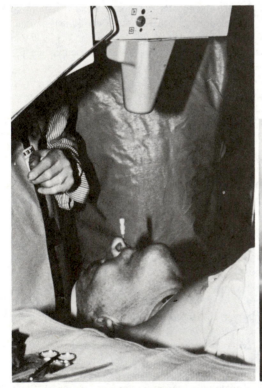

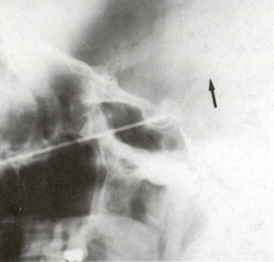

Fig 39C–5.—A, the needle in position for pituitary adenolysis under fluoroscopic control. **B,** stereotactic hypophysectomy: lateral skull film. A spinal needle has been inserted through the sphenoid sinus and lies within the sella turcica. Metrizamide has been injected with the alcohol. The third ventricle is faintly opacified. The arrow points to the floor of the third ventricle. (Courtesy of James E. McLennan, M.D.).

in 75% of patients with metastatic breast or prostatic carcinoma treated by this method.[37] Their results in treating pain associated with metastatic tumor of other origin were less clear.[38]

In 1963, Moricca found that severely debilitated patients with metastatic cancer could obtain satisfactory pain relief if alcohol was injected transnasally into the pituitary fossa. Of 813 patients treated by this technique, 709 had tumors known to be potentially sensitive to hormonal manipulation. Eight hundred nine patients reported immediate relief of their tumor pain, although the relief was transient in 101 cases.[39] Unfortunately, Moricca does not provide enough follow-up data to assess the long-term results of this technique.

Levin et al. reported the results of chemical hypophysectomy in 29 patients who were more closely followed up postoperatively. Good results were found in 10 of 17 patients with metastatic prostatic carcinoma and in 10 of 12 patients with other types of metastatic tumors.[40] These authors noted that the procedure was not effective in treating patients with pain secondary to direct invasion of the peripheral nervous system.

Although chemical hypophysectomy has been performed under local anesthesia, light general anesthesia is often necessary to avoid the pain generated by the sensitive parasellar dura. After the mucosa is injected with a dilute solution of epinephrine to ensure hemostasis, an 18-gauge spinal needle is positioned in the sella turcica under fluoroscopic control. Absolute alcohol, 1–2 ml, is injected into the sella in 0.1-ml increments over 30 minutes. During the procedure the patient's pupillary light reflex is lost. Some neurosurgeons routinely inject ethyl α-cyanoacrylate through the spinal needle as it is being withdrawn from the sella in order to avoid CSF rhinorrhea.

Headaches frequently persist for 2–3 days postoperatively. Neurologic complications are rare and consist of occasional oculomotor or optic nerve dysfunction. Diabetes insipidus commonly occurs postoperatively, and hypothyroidism or hypoadrenalism may also develop.

Because the pain of metastatic disease usually abates within 48 hours of operation, it is unlikely that the diminution of pain is the direct result of tumor regression. Although it is likely that pain relief is a response to endocrine manipulation, the exact mechanism by which this occurs remains poorly understood. It is known that the administration of levodopa, an inhibitor of prolactin release, diminishes pain associated with metastatic breast carcinoma, and that the administration of growth hormone to hypophysectomized patients with metastatic tumor will cause pain recurrence. Levin et al. noted a strong correlation between pain relief and the development of postoperative diabetes insipidus, but found no correlation between pain relief and levels of circulating pituitary hormone.[40] A similarly poor correlation between pain relief and the completeness of hypophysectomy as determined by postoperative endocrine testing was noted by La Rossa et al. when assessing 15 patients with metastatic breast carcinoma.[41]

Although the pituitary contains a high concentration of endogenous opiates, no connection can be made between these opiates and pain relief. Naloxone does not reverse the pain relief following hypophysectomy.

Alcohol injected into the pituitary has been noted to travel up the pituitary stalk into the third ventricle. Of interest is that postmortem examination of hypophysectomized patients demonstrates degeneration of the supraoptic and paraventricular nuclei of the hypothalamus. Although these observations have led to considerable speculation, the mechanism by which pain relief is achieved remains unknown.

In summary, transphenoidal hypophysectomy is a good palliative procedure to relieve the pain of bony metastases in patients with breast or prostatic cancer. Its role in the treatment of pain associated with other tumors is less clear. The procedure has a low complication rate and is tolerated well by patients who are debilitated by their disease. The mechanism of pain relief is unknown.

DECOMPRESSIVE PROCEDURES

Decompressive procedures are employed far more commonly in the treatment of benign pain than in the treatment of cancer pain. It is worth noting, however, that some patients with spinal metastatic disease and pain from nerve root compression will benefit from a decompressive laminectomy, even when motor function fails to improve.

STIMULATION PROCEDURES

Stimulation procedures are discussed in detail in chapter 40. Deep brain stimulation has been used to treat some cancer patients. The results of operation are still under investigation.

INTRASPINAL NARCOTICS

Within the last 5 years, a new approach to pain has evolved in which pharmacologic agents are applied directly to the CNS. The substantia gelatinosa and dorsal horns of the spinal cord contain opiate receptors, and application of a low narcotic dose to the dorsal periphery of the spinal cord may produce profound segmental pain relief. The use of intraspinal narcotics may therefore be the procedure of choice in some patients with malignant disease and intractable abdominal, pelvic, or lower extremity pain. A detailed description of spinal narcotics is given in Chapter 38.

A number of different pharmacologic agents have been used. Local anesthetics may provide good pain relief, but the problem of systemic toxicity and the difficulty in adjusting the dose to provide pain relief without also producing paraplegia make these drugs less than ideal for long-term use. Narcotics will provide pain relief without concurrent motor weakness and are currently the drugs of choice. Morphine, with its strong receptor binding and low lipid solubility, has a prolonged duration of action. The pain relief provided by a single dose of morphine may last from 12 to over 24 hours. Other narcotics such as meperidine or fentanyl have been used, but may show a shorter duration of action. When morphine is employed, a preservative-free solution should be used (DuraMorph).[42] Meperidine is already commercially available in preservative-free solution.

Narcotics may be employed either intrathecally or epidurally. The effects are primarily segmental.[43] Therefore, when an epidural catheter is inserted, it is best placed over the cord segment receiving pain signals. When an intrathecal catheter is used, it is usually placed high within the lumbar thecal sac. Some narcotic will spread rostrally, particularly when large fluid volumes are injected. After several hours, analgesia may rise to the high cervical or thoracic levels, and an occasional patient develops respiratory arrest 10 or more hours after narcotic administration.[44]

Prior to implantation of a permanent delivery system, a series of test injections should be given to assess the patient's therapeutic response. Morphine, 4–6 mg in 6–10 cc of normal saline, may be used as an epidural test dose, or 0.5–2 mg of morphine in 1 cc of normal saline may be given intrathecally. All patients should be monitored carefully for respiratory depression and should be kept in a semisitting position for 12 hours. Coombs et al. define a successful response as one that results in greater than 50% pain relief persisting for more than 8 hours.[45]

A number of different implantable systems are available for long-term morphine delivery.[46, 47] One option is to insert an implantable pump beneath the skin and muscle of the chest and to connect the pump to an epidural or intrathecal catheter. The pump must be refilled under sterile conditions every 3–4 weeks. Between refills, the pump delivers a continuous low-dose narcotic infusion. Pain relief can be achieved through the delivery of as little as 0.5 mg of morphine daily with intrathecal administration, or 4 mg daily with an epidural infusion.[45]

An alternative delivery system involves the placement of a Broviac catheter externalized through the skin of the abdomen. The patient may then inject a narcotic solution through the catheter into the spinal canal once or twice a day. Even in debilitated and immunosuppressed patients the infection rate is reported as only 8%.[47]

The use of intraspinal morphine carries a number of significant advantages. Pain relief occurs within 30–60 minutes after the initial injection, is bilateral, and is unassociated with motor weakness or sensory deficits. However, as with all operations, a number of limitations and potential risks are involved.

The most dangerous complication of morphine administration is respiratory depression. Although narcotics have been instilled into the ventricular system without complication,[42] most investigators have been reluctant to treat pain rostral to the midthoracic area. Even when pain is located in the lower extremities and narcotics have been injected caudally, delayed respiratory depression may occur. During the initial evaluation period, all patients should be monitored continuously. If ventilatory embarrassment occurs, the effect of the narcotic can be reversed with IV naloxone.

A major drawback to the use of intraspinal narcotics is the development of tolerance. In the series of Lazorthes et al., patients were followed up for up to 10 months with little increase in narcotic requirements.[46] On the other hand, Greenberg et al. described a patient whose pain was initially relieved with 1 mg of intrathecal morphine daily, but who needed 150 mg/day by the time of her death 3 months later.[48] The rate at which tolerance develops is variable, and many patients will fall between these two extremes. Chayen et al. suggest that a single dose of epidural lidocaine may restore the sensitivity of the opiate receptors.[49] However, in our experience, a limited number of local anesthetic injections has not succeeded in reducing narcotic requirements in the patient who has developed tolerance.

The indications for intraspinal morphine in the treatment of benign pain are limited. Quite apart from the problem of tachyphylaxis, patients with chronic benign pain respond less well to narcotic administration than do patients with cancer pain. Coombs and colleagues report disappointing results in five patients with chronic benign pain evaluated at 12 weeks.[45] Short-term intraspinal narcotics have been administered successfully in the treatment of incisional pain following abdominal or thoracic surgery.[50]

In summary, intraspinal narcotics may be the treatment of choice in the patient with malignant disease and intractable pelvic, abdominal, or bilateral lower extremity pain. Although the risk of respiratory depression is unclear, intraspinal narcotics are not generally employed at this time to treat pain rostral to the midthoracic level. Patients with chronic pain of benign origin are best treated by other means.

CONCLUSIONS

The selection of a particular operative approach in the treatment of intractable cancer pain is often a complex process that depends on a variety of factors. It is essential to know the exact location of the pain and the patient's life expectancy. The general condition of the patient must be assessed, as this may determine the choice between a stereotactic procedure and an open operation under general anesthesia. Finally, the neurosurgeon's own experience with and preference for a particular procedure will affect the final decision.

Our success in treating cancer pain varies greatly with the location of the pain. As our understanding of the anatomy and pharmacology of the CNS grows, it is probable that many of the operations now in use will be supplanted by less invasive procedures, and that safer and more effective forms of treatment will be found to treat the most difficult problems, such as bilateral pain in the head and neck.

REFERENCES

1. Loeser J.D.: Dorsal rhizotomy, in Youmans J.R. (ed.): *Neurological Surgery,* ed 2. Philadelphia, W.B. Saunders Co., 1982, pp. 3664–3671.
2. Onofrio B.M., Campa H.K.: Evaluation of rhizotomy: Review of 12 years experience. *J. Neurosurg.* 36:751–755, 1972.
3. White J.C., Sweet W.H.: *Pain and the Neurosurgeon: A Forty Year Experience.* Springfield, Ill., Charles C Thomas, 1969.
4. Pederson E., Juul-Jensen P.: Intrathecal phenol in the treatment of spasticity. *Acta Neurol. Scand.* 38(Suppl. 3):69–77, 1962.
5. Felsoory A., Crue B.L.: Results of 19 years experience with sacral rhizotomy for perineal and perianal cancer pain. *Pain* 2:431–433, 1976.
6. Barrash J.M., Leavens M.E.: Dorsal rhizotomy for relief of intractable pain of malignant tumor origin. *J. Neurosurg.* 38:755–757, 1973.
7. Hodge C.J., King R.B.: Medical modification of sensation. *J. Neurosurg.* 44:21–28, 1976.
8. King R.B.: Pain and tryptophan. *J. Neurosurg.* 53:44–52, 1980.
9. Gorbitz C., Leavens M.E.: Alcohol block of the celiac plexus for control of upper abdominal pain caused by cancer and pancreatitis. *J. Neurosurg.* 34:575–579, 1971.
10. Lorenz R.: Methods of percutaneous spino-thalamic tract section. *Adv. Tech. Standards Neurosurg.* 3:124–145, 1976.
11. Mullan S.: Percutaneous cordotomy. *J. Neurosurg.* 35:360–366, 1971.
12. Rosomoff H.L.: Stereotaxic cordotomy, in Youmans J.R. (ed.): *Neurological Surgery,* ed. 2, Philadelphia, W.B. Saunders Co., 1982, pp. 3672–3685.
13. Krieger A.J., Rosomoff H.L.: Sleep induced apnea: Part I. A respiratory and autonomic dysfunction syndrome following bilateral percutaneous cervical cordotomy. *J. Neurosurg.* 39:168–180, 1974.
14. Gildenberg P.L., Lin P.M., Polakoff P.P., et al.: Anterior percutaneous cervical cordotomy: Determination of target point and calculation of angle of insertion. *J. Neurosurg.* 28:173–177, 1968.
15. Lin P.M., Gildenberg P.P., Polakoff P.P.: An anterior approach to percutaneous lower cervical cordotomy. *J. Neurosurg.* 25:553–560, 1966.
16. King R.B.: Anterior commissurotomy for intractable pain. *J. Neurosurg.* 47:7–11, 1977.
17. Broager B.: Commissural myelotomy. *Surg. Neurol.* 2:71–74, 1974.
18. Cook A.W., Kawakami Y.: Commissural myelotomy. *J. Neurosurg.* 47:1–6, 1977.
19. Lippert R.G., Hosobuchi Y., Nielson S.L.: Spinal commissurotomy. *Surg. Neurol.* 2:373–377, 1974.
20. Tew J.M., Tobler W.D., van Loveren H.: Percutaneous rhizotomy in the treatment of intractable facial pain (trigeminal, glossopharyngeal and vagus nerves), in Schmidek H.H., Sweet W.H. (eds.): *Operative Neurosurgical Techniques.* New York, Grune & Stratton, 1982, pp. 1083–1106.
21. Ori C., Salar G., Giron G.: Percutaneous glossopharyngeal thermocoagulation complicated by syncope and seizures. *Neurosurgery* 13:427–429, 1983.

22. van Loveren H., Tew J.M., Keller J.T.: A 10 year experience in the treatment of trigeminal neuralgia: Comparison of percutaneous stereotaxic rhizotomy and posterior fossa exploration. *J. Neurosurg.* 57:757–764, 1982.

23. Apfelbaum R.I.: Surgical management of disorders of the lower cranial nerves, in Schmidek H.H., Sweet W.H. (eds.): *Operative Neurosurgical Techniques.* New York, Grune & Stratton, 1982, pp. 1063–1082.

24. Nashold B.S., Crue B.L.: Stereotactic mesencephalotomy and trigeminal tractotomy, in Youmans J.R. (ed.): *Neurological Surgery,* ed. 2. Philadelphia, W.B. Saunders Co., 1982, pp. 3702–3716.

25. Bowsher D.: Role of the reticular formation in responses to noxious stimulation. *Pain* 2:361–378, 1976.

26. Nashold B.S., Wilson W.P., Slaughter D.G.: Sensations evoked by stimulation of the midbrain of man. *J. Neurosurg.* 30:14–24, 1969.

27. Amano K., Iseki H., Notani M., et al.: Rostral mesencephalic reticulotomy for pain relief: A report of 15 cases. *Acta Neurochir.* 30(suppl.):391–393, 1980.

28. Frank F., Tognetti F., Gaist G., et al.: Stereotaxic rostral mesencephalotomy in treatment of malignant faciothoracobrachial pain syndromes: A survey of 14 treated patients. *J. Neurosurg.* 56:807–811, 1982.

29. Nashold B.S., Wilson W.P., Slaughter D.G.: Stereotactic midbrain lesions for central dysesthesia and phantom pain: Preliminary report. *J. Neurosurg.* 30:116–126, 1969.

30. Torvik A.: Sensory, motor and reflex changes in two cases of intractable pain after stereotactic mesencephalic tractotomy. *J. Neurol. Neurosurg. Psychiatry* 22:299–305, 1959.

31. Gildenberg P.L.: Functional neurosurgery, in Schmidek H.H., Sweet W.H. (eds.): *Operative Neurosurgical Techniques.* New York, Grune & Stratton, 1982, pp. 993–1043.

32. Mark V.H., Ervin F.R., Hackett T.P.: Clinical aspects of stereotactic thalamotomy in the human: Part I. The treatment of chronic, severe pain. *Arch. Neurol.* 3:351–367, 1960.

33. McLaurin R.L.: Neurosurgical approaches to pain in cancer, in Lee J.F. (ed.): *Pain Management: Symposium on the Neurosurgical Treatment of Pain.* Baltimore, Williams & Wilkins Co., 1976, pp. 186–194.

34. Hurt R.W., Ballantine H.T.: Stereotactic anterior cingulate lesions for persistent pain: A report on 68 cases. *Clin. Neurosurg.* 21:334–351, 1974.

35. Foltz E.L.: Psychosurgical approach to chronic pain (cingulumotomy), in Lee J.F. (ed.): *Pain Management: Symposium on the Neurosurgical Treatment of Pain.* Baltimore, Williams & Wilkins Co., 1976, pp. 78–99.

36. Huggins C., Hodges C.V.: Studies on prostate cancer: The effects of castration, of estrogen, and of androgen injection on serum phosphatases in metastatic carcinoma of the prostate. *Cancer Res.* 1:293–297, 1941.

37. Tindall G.T., Christy J.H., Nixon D.W., et al.: Trans-sphenoidal hypophysectomy for pain in disseminated carcinoma of the breast and prostate gland, in Lee J.F. (ed.): *Pain Management: Symposium on the Neurosurgical Treatment of Pain.* Baltimore, Williams & Wilkins Co., 1976, pp. 172–185.

38. Tindall G.T., Nixon D.W., Christ J.H., et al.: Pain relief in metastatic cancer other than breast and prostate gland following transphenoidal hypophysectomy: A preliminary report. *J. Neurosurg.* 47:659–662, 1977.

39. Moricca G.: Pituitary neuroadenolysis in the treatment of intractable pain from cancer, in Lipton S. (ed.): *Persistent Pain: Modern Methods of Treatment.* London, Academic Press, 1977, pp. 149–173.

40. Levin A.B., Katz J., Benson R.C., et al.: Treatment of pain of diffuse metastatic cancer by stereotactic chemical hypophysectomy: Long term results and observations on mechanisms of action. *Neurosurgery* 6:258–262, 1980.

41. La Rossa J.T.: Strong M.S., Melby J.C.: Endocrinologically incomplete transethmoidal transphenoidal hypophysectomy with relief of bone pain of breast cancer. 298:1332–1335, 1978.

42. Leavens M.E., Hill C.S., Cech D.A., et al.: Intrathecal and intraventricular morphine for pain in cancer patients: Initial study. *J. Neurosurg.* 56:241–245, 1982.

43. Onofrio B.M., Yaksh T.L., Arnold P.G.: Continuous low-dose intrathecal morphine administration in the treatment of chronic pain of malignant origin. *Mayo Clin. Proc.* 56:516–520, 1981.

44. Babcock N.K., Nance P., Chapin J.W.: Respiratory arrest after intrathecal morphine. *JAMA* 245:1528, 1981.

45. Coombs D.W., Saunders R.L., Gaylor M.S., et al.: Relief of continuous chronic pain by intraspinal narcotics infusion via an implanted reservoir. *JAMA* 250:2336–2339, 1983.

46. Lazorthes Y., Siegfried J., Gouarderes C., et al.: Periventricular grey matter stimulation versus chronic intrathecal morphine in cancer pain. *Adv. Pain Res. Ther.* 5:467–475, 1983.

47. Poletti C.E., Schmidek H.H., Sweet W.H., et al.: Pain control with implantable systems for the long-term infusion of intraspinal opioids in man, in Schmidek H.H., Sweet W.H. (eds.): *Operative Neurosurgical Techniques.* New York, Grune & Stratton, 1982, pp. 1199–1212.

48. Greenberg H.S., Taren J., Ensminger W.D., et al.: Benefit from and tolerance to continuous intrathecal infusion of morphine for intractable cancer pain. *J. Neurosurg.* 57:360–364, 1982.

49. Chayen M.S., Rudick V., Borvine A.: Pain control with epidural injection of morphine, *Anesthesiology* 53:338–339, 1980.

50. Rawal N., Sjostrand U., Dahlstrom B.: Postoperative pain relief by epidural morphine. *Anesth. Analg.* 60:726–731, 1981.

40 / Chemonucleolysis

P. PRITHVI RAJ, M.D.

OF ANY CONSECUTIVE group of patients with radicular pain caused by disk displacement, 70% will spontaneously improve with time and conservative care and will require no further treatment.[1] Two months' elapsed time from the onset of the attack and at least 2 weeks of bed rest constitute adequate conservative care. During this time, the patient should show continual improvement, which means either that pain disappears or, if still present, is mild, intermittent, and tolerable. The patient should be able to return to work by the end of 2 months and, if the pain recurs, should lose less than 4 weeks' work per year as a result of these attacks. There should be progressively fewer physical findings.

Candidates for chemonucleolysis are selected from the 30% of patients that do not improve during this period of conservative management. For these patients, further conservative care is not indicated, but one can offer chemonucleolysis, epidural steroids, or surgery. A small percentage of this group may need immediate surgical decompression due to progressive neurologic changes.

INDICATIONS

Chemonucleolysis is indicated for patients who have not responded to adequate conservative care for proved disk disease (Table 40–1) and who are candidates for laminectomy and disk excision. One should restrict the use of chymopapain to the patient who has had unremitting symptoms for more than 60 days, has not responded to at least 2 weeks of bed rest, has radiculopathy with a significant decrease in straight leg raising, and has a corresponding positive myelogram and/or CT scan.

Intradiskal enzyme injection is presently done only by trained orthopedists and neurosurgeons with a special interest in spinal disorders. They should have some advanced instruction in the indications for and hands-on technique of chemonucleolysis and should be fully trained to manage patients who do not obtain relief.

There are no contraindications to the use of chymopapain in patients younger than 18 or older than 65. Young patients have more proteoglycans in the nucleus pulposus than older persons[2] and therefore theoretically should be better candidates for chymopapain.[3] Wiltse reported a 12% failure rate in patients in the second and third decades of life, compared to a 29% failure rate in patients in the fourth and fifth decades.[4] One would expect chymopapain to be more efficacious than collagenase in younger patients. Conversely, patients over 65 have more collagen in their disks;[5] therefore, collagenase should theoretically give better results in the older age group.

CONTRAINDICATIONS

Neurologic Deficit

Patients with major neurologic deficits should not be injected (Table 40–2). Paralysis of the anterior tibial, extensor communis, and peroneal muscles resulting in complete foot drop is one example of a major neurologic deficit; another example is paresis or paralysis of the gastrocnemius-soleus muscle group. Bilateral motor weakness with severe bilateral leg pain with or without sphincter dysfunction and a large central disk herniation is a contraindication to disk injection (cauda equina syndrome secondary to disk prolapse).[6] Symptoms of a neurogenic bowel or bladder (e.g., urinary hesitancy or

761

TABLE 40–1.—USUAL PHYSICAL FINDINGS IN PATIENTS WITH PROVED DISK DISPLACEMENT*

PHYSICAL FINDING	% OF PTS.
Painful crossed straight leg raising	97
Weakness	90
Asymmetric reflex	90
Sensory deficit	70

*From Hudgins P.W.: The predictive value of myelography in the diagnosis of ruptured lumbar discs. *J. Neurosurg.* 32:152,1970. Used by permission.

urgency, urinary retention, stress incontinence, loss of peroneal sensation and/or rectal tone, rectal incontinence) are contraindications to chemonucleolysis.

Patients with the above symptoms and signs usually have a complete or nearly complete myelographic block secondary to a large disk displacement. In the absence of the above symptoms, such blocks or a large disk noted on CT scan are relative contraindications to intradiskal injection.

Pregnancy

At present, pregnancy or suspected pregnancy is a contraindication to chemonucleolysis with either enzyme. The safety of this treatment during any phase of pregnancy remains to be determined in animal studies.

Previous Surgery

The indication for chemonucleolysis in patients who have undergone previous laminectomy and disk excision should be carefully determined by physicians experienced in evaluating and treating this group of individuals. The prognosis following repeated surgery for the relief of back pain is increasingly worse as the number of procedures increases.[7–9]

The patient with a recurrent herniated disk at the same level who had a pain-free interval longer than 6 months, the patient with sciatic pain in the opposite extremity from that previously relieved by surgery, or the patient with sciatic pain resulting from a disk herniation at a level other than the one previously excised should respond to chemonucleolysis.

One must be careful when injecting a disk space previously operated on. It is difficult to determine

TABLE 40–2.—CONTRAINDICATIONS TO CHEMONUCLEOLYSIS

With chymopapain
   History of allergy to papaya, meat tenderizer, or chymopapain
   Prior injection with chymopapain
With collagenase
   Exposure to burn ointment containing collagenase
   Previous serious wound infection
   Previous collagenase injection
Severe neurologic deficit
   Cauda equina syndrome
   Flail foot
   Gastrocnemius-soleus paralysis (poor pushoff)
   Gluteus paralysis (positive Trendelenburg's sign)
   Quadriceps paralysis
   Neurogenic bladder
   Neurogenic bowel
   Bilateral lower extremity paresis
   Progressive neurologic deficit
Coincidental diagnosis
   Pregnancy
   Ankylosing spondylitis
   Rheumatoid arthritis
   Poor general health (alcohol, medication, or drug abuse)
   Insulin-dependent diabetes mellitus
Differential diagnosis
   Suspicion of spinal cord tumor
   Spinal fluid protein level > 80 mg/dl
   Suspected disk space infection and/or
   Vertebral osteomyelitis
   Metastatic cancer
X-ray findings
   Complete or almost complete block on myelography
   Cervical disks
   Thoracic disks
   Spondylolisthesis (relative contraindication)
   Disk space inaccessible by lateral route
   Spinal stenosis
   Mechanical insufficiency (gas shadow in disk space, translation on stress films)
   Intrathecal and/or intravascular flow of contrast on diskography
Psychogenic regional pain disturbance associated with:
   Severe depression
   Hysterical symptoms and signs
   Psychosis
   Severe neurosis (hypochondriasis)

whether an indolent disk space infection exists. One cannot be sure whether the dura has been compromised by surgery, with the subsequent development of adhesions that would allow intradiskally injected substances to enter the subarachnoid space.

The most common reasons for failure of the first surgical procedure are unrecognized psychogenic causes, subsequent development of spinal stenosis, and foraminal entrapment. These conditions all respond poorly to chemonucleolysis.

PATIENT PREPARATION

To avoid the combined effects of myelography and enzyme injection, there should be an interval of at least 3 days between myelography and chemonucleolysis, if possible. The physician should conduct a thorough history and physical examination, consult with a psychologist, order laboratory studies, and perform myelography prior to deciding on chemonucleolysis. The physician should then discuss the diagnosis and the alternative modalities with the patient and the family.

The patient should not eat or drink after midnight the night before the procedure. Prior to the procedure, an intravenous (IV) line with an 18-gauge catheter is inserted in the arm and an infusion of 5% dextrose in lactated Ringer's solution is started. Preoperatively the patient is administered 100 mg of diphenhydramine (Benadryl) and 100 mg of hydrocortisone (Solu-Cortef) intramuscularly (IM).[1]

EQUIPMENT AND PHYSICAL FACILITIES

The following items should be available for every chemonucleolysis procedure:

Lead apron.
Fluoroscope.
Caps, gowns, masks.
Sterile gloves.
Tray containing preparation and draping materials.
Marking pen.
Centimeter ruler.
Lidocaine 1%, one new vial.
5-cc syringe with 18-gauge and 22-gauge needles for injection of lidocaine.
10-cc syringe with 18-gauge needle for Conray.
Conray-60 (60% iothalamate), one new vial.
3-cc syringes with 18-gauge needle for each disk to be injected.
Extension tubing with Luer-Lok connections.
Four 6-inch, 18-gauge needles with stylus.
Two 7-inch, 22-gauge needles with stylus.
Lead-impregnated surgical gloves.
Radiation monitoring badge.

Chemonucleolysis must be conducted where there is adequate fluoroscopy equipment to clearly visualize the disk space involved. Standby facilities for anesthesia and the appropriate resuscitative equipment are mandatory.

Chemonucleolysis can be performed in the operating room or in the radiology department, depending on the physician's preference and the facilities available.

PATIENT POSITION FOR CHEMONUCLEOLYSIS

The needle is inserted on the side of the radiculopathy—that is, patients with left-side sciatica are placed in the right lateral decubitus position and the needle is inserted on the left side. The tip of the needle should be placed within the disk space as close to the point of disk herniation as possible. During diskography, the extradural defect previously noted on the myelogram and/or CT scan is infiltrated with contrast material. One assumes that the subsequently injected enzyme will reach the offending disk material.[10]

The lateral decubitus position is preferred for ease of visualization of the disk space on the uniplanar fluoroscope. Some surgeons prefer to have the patient prone for this procedure.[11] They find it is more comfortable for the patient and that the extension of the hips rotates the ilium and lumbosacral spine into a lordotic position, which facilitates entry into the lumbosacral disk. The prone position requires adequate biplane fluoroscopy or a C-arm that can be rotated on a special table.[2] However, should a systemic reaction occur, it would take longer to rotate the patient to the supine position. With the patient prone, intra-abdominal pressure is increased and the visceral mass is forced posteriorly against the retroperitoneum.

ANESTHESIA

The preferred analgesic method for chemonucleolysis is local infiltration of 1% lidocaine or 0.5% bupivacaine into the skin and lumbar fascia. An anesthesiologist should be in attendance to monitor the patient's vital signs. Analgesia may be supplemented by administrating IV diazepam, 3–5 mg, and/or fentanyl, 50–150 μg. Occasionally one can supplement this sedation with 50% N_2O mixed with 50% O_2 by mask. The patient must be able to cooperate in flexing and extending the hips slightly or rotating the pelvis. The patient should also be able to inform of radiating leg pain if the needle irritates the nerve root.

The major reason for using local anesthesia is that

the patient can inform the physician of any immediate postinjection symptoms, which may herald the early onset of anaphylactic reaction. The earlier these reactions are recognized and treatment is instituted, the better the chance of avoiding severe progressive changes.[3] If general anesthesia is used, one should avoid agents such as halothane that increase cardiac excitability, especially with subsequent administration of adrenaline. One should also avoid curare, since it releases histamine.

TECHNIQUE

The iliac crest and the posterior superior iliac spine are found by palpation and marked. A mark is made just superior to the posterior superior iliac spine and iliac crest and 10 cm lateral to the tip of the spinous process of the third lumbar vertebra. At the mark, the subcutaneous tissue is infiltrated with a local anesthetic. A 6-inch, 18-gauge needle with a stylet is used. In some cases one may need an 8-inch, 22-gauge needle to pass through the 18-gauge needle for penetration into the narrow disk space.

A lead apron should be worn under a sterile gown and gloves. The needle is inserted at the site of the skin infiltration, at an angle of 45° to the sagittal plane of the body and 30° to the transverse plane, until the needle is stable. Three approaches are illustrated in Figure 40–1. The orientation of the spine on the fluoroscopy screen must be the same as the anatomical orientation of the patient on the table. Initially, the fluoroscopist needs to point out the disk space to be injected. The needle is aimed at that disk.

The angle of the needle is adjusted and the needle is further inserted to the level of the pars interarticularis. If continued insertion of the needle in the same direction will bring the tip to the superior posterolateral corner of the disk space, the insertion is continued. The bevel at this time should face directly laterally so that the needle tip can keep the needle snug against the superior facet process of the vertebra on which the disk rests—for example, the fifth lumbar superior facet for the fourth lumbar disk. If the bevel is pointed superiorly or inferiorly, the needle will be directed inferiorly or superiorly, respectively. If the facet joint capsule is irritated by penetration of the needle tip, the patient may experience localized back pain or referred pain to the buttocks. One should withdraw the needle and then redirect it. When the tip of the needle has reached the depth of the facet joints and pars interarticularis

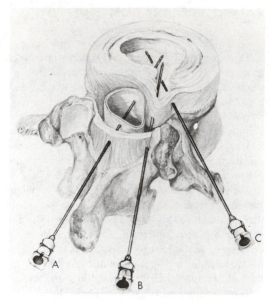

Fig 40–1.—Transdural, posterolateral, and lateral approaches to intradiskal injection: **A,** Lindblom's[31] transdural approach; **B,** Erlacher's[32] posterolateral approach; **C,** Edholm's[33] lateral approach. (From Brown.[18] Reproduced by permission.)

and the direction is correct, it is advanced a centimeter at a time and spot-checked with fluoroscopy. As the needle tip reaches the posterolateral and superior corner of the disk, a rubbery resistance is encountered.

Between the pars interarticularis and posterolateral corner of the disk, 1-cm advancement of the needle itself should correspond to a 0.5-cm advancement on the fluoroscope because of the angle of the needle. A 1-cm advancement of the needle with no change on the fluoroscope means that the angle is too large in the sagittal plane, and the needle may enter the spinal canal and penetrate the dura. On the other hand, a 1-cm advancement of the needle with a 1-cm advancement on the fluoroscope means that the angle of insertion is too shallow. Continued insertion of the needle at this angle will result in the needle passing anteriorly to the vertebral body (Fig 40–2).

When the needle touches the posterolateral corner of the disk, the patient may experience localized back pain or radiation into the buttocks. This is particularly true with a sensitive peripheral annulus fibrosus inflamed by a herniated disk.[12] If a rubbery resistance is felt, the needle can be inserted into the disk. The needle is advanced about 2 cm.

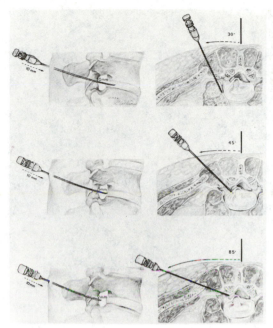

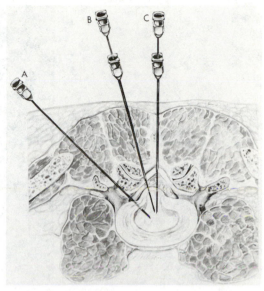

Fig 40–2.—Technique of chemonucleolysis: lateral *(left)* and transverse *(right)* views of the vertebral bodies. *Top views:* angle is too small in the sagittal plane. A 10-mm insertion of the needle would appear as a 10-mm change on the fluoroscopy screen. *Middle views:* when the angle is correct, a 10-mm insertion of the needle will appear as a 5-mm change on the fluoroscopy screen. *Bottom views:* angle is too large in the sagittal plane. A 10-mm insertion of the needle would appear as no change on the fluoroscopy screen. (From Brown.[18] Reproduced by permission.)

Fig 40–3.—Cross section of the lumbosacral disk with the two-needle technique: lateral *(A),* posterolateral *(B),* and median *(C)* approaches. Only the lateral approach is recommended. (From Brown.[18] Reproduced by permission.)

Occasionally it is difficult to insert an 18-gauge needle directly into the lumbosacral disk since the angle of approach is too acute. The difficulty usually arises when there is narrowing in the two lower lumbar disks. The disk narrowing, in conjunction with the fifth vertebra situated below the iliac crest, increases the angle of lateral approach. When this happens, one can use a two-needle technique (Fig 40–3). After the 18-gauge needle is inserted to the level of the superior lateral corner of the disk, the stylet is withdrawn and a 22-gauge, 8-inch needle, curved at the end, is inserted.

Once the needle tip is in the nucleus pulposus in the central portion of the disk, the bevel is turned superiorly. Lateral and anteroposterior (AP) x-ray films are taken. On the AP view, a line is drawn through the tips of the spinous processes (Fig 40–

4). The tip of the needle should be on this line. The disk space at the lumbosacral junction is seldom seen on the routine AP view due to the 15°–30° forward inclination of the lumbosacral disk. On the lateral view, an imaginary line is drawn through the center of the vetebral bodies and the sacrum (Fig 40–5), and the tip of the needle should lie on this line.

A 5-ml syringe and extension tubing filled with 60% iodothalamate (Conray-60) are then attached to the hub of the needle. There should be some resistance to injection. A severely degenerated disk that leaks has no resistance to injection. No more dye should be injected than is necessary to establish the diagnosis. An intact herniated disk will have moderate resistance and a normal disk will have a very high resistance with little flow of contrast. If a normal diskogram pattern appears, one should not force the injection since this may cause pressure necrosis in the cells of the nucleus pulposus. In the herniated disk, one injects enough contrast material to fill the area that corresponds to the extradural defect on the myelogram or CT scan. The patient may complain of reproduction of the usual leg pain at this point. If the dye leaks into the epidural space, one should stop injecting. Epidural leakage of dye occurs in

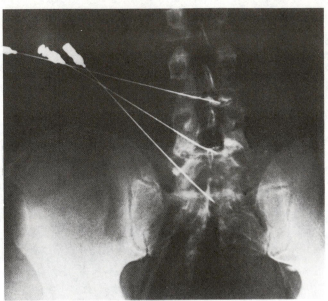

Fig 40–4.—Anteroposterior radiograph after needle insertion in the L2–3; L3–4, and L5–S1 disks. The tips of the needles are in line with the spinous processes when they are in the center of the disk. (From Brown.[18] Reproduced by permission.)

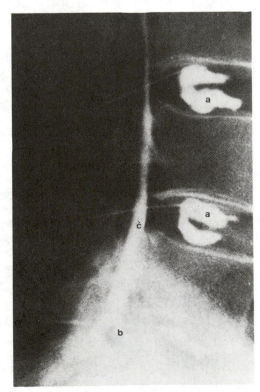

Fig 40–5.—Lateral radiograph showing a normal diskogram at the third and fourth lumbar interspace *(a)*, and an abnormal diskogram in the fifth lumbar interspace *(b)*, with leakage of contrast material posteriorly in the epidural space *(c)*. (From Brown.[18] Reproduced by permission.)

15%–25% of disks injected and is not a contraindication to chemonucleolysis. However, if the contrast runs from the disk space into the subdural or subarachnoid space and causes bilateral severe leg pain, one should suspect an intradural herniation. This is a rare occurrence but has been estimated to happen in one in 700 cases of disk displacement.[13] If this situation is suspected, neither chymopapain or collagenase should be injected, and the procedure should be abandoned.

Fifteen of 100 disks studied by cinefluoroscopy diskography performed on unfixed cadaver lumbar spines demonstrated an immediate flow of contrast from the intradiskal space into a subchondral vascular channel or into a vascular channel in the peripheral layers of the annulus fibrosus in a degenerated herniated disk.[14] The observation of rapid intravascular flow of x-ray contrast material at diskography and before chemonucleolysis is a relative contraindication to subsequent enzyme injection. The rapid flow of dye into the intravascular space at a low pressure would mean that a subsequent injection would take the same path and probably would not reach the offending disk herniation. A rapid intravascular injection of enzyme may contribute to the severity of an allergic reaction, should one occur.

The volume of injected contrast material should be noted. If there is an epidural leakage of contrast, the enzyme is injected in increments over a long period of time, 5–10 minutes, so that the enzyme flows slowly into the disk and has time to bind to the disk matrix substance. AP and lateral plain x-ray films should be taken for a permanent record. One should wait approximately 15 minutes prior to injecting the enzyme to rule out an allergic reaction to the contrast material.

To inject the fourth lumbar disk, one inserts the needle adjacent to the same insertion point for the lumbosacral disk, between 8 and 11 cm lateral to the point between the fourth and fifth spinous processes.

ENZYME INJECTION

Chymopapain is supplied in a lyophilized 20-mg vial containing 10,000 units and stored at −10° C. The enzyme is reconstituted with sterile water without additives. Five milliliters of sterile water are injected into the vial, and the contents are slowly dissolved in the water by rotating the vial gently. The vial should not be shaken, and bubbles should not form. The resulting mixture contains 4 mg (2,000 units) of chymopapain per milliliter. Between 4 and 12 mg (1–3 ml) of this mixture is injected into each disk space. Injection should be made slowly and smoothly to allow adequate flow and binding of the chymopapain to the substrate. The anesthesiologist should be alert to any symptoms of systemic allergic reaction. Thirty minutes after injection the patient can be taken to the recovery room. The patient is observed for another 30–60 minutes in the recovery room, after which he is returned to his room. In outpatient chemonucleolysis, the patient should be observed until all the effects of analgesics and sedatives have subsided, and later sent home with a reliable escort.

Collagenase is supplied in a vial containing slightly more than 1 ml of frozen enzyme suspension and should be stored at −15° to −20° C. Special instructions concerning dilution of the enzyme to the final solution, containing 600 units of collagenase per milliliter, come with each batch of vials. Between 300 and 600 units are injected per disk. At present, no more than two disks per patient are injected, i.e., 1,200 units per patient.

MANAGEMENT OF IMMEDIATE SYSTEMIC ALLERGIC REACTIONS

Anticipation of a reaction is essential. The patient should be optimally prepared and under only local anesthesia, to allow early recognition, and a large IV catheter should be in place.

Early recognition of the reaction is of paramount importance. There is some evidence that immediate recognition of a reaction and immediate administration of epinephrine and large volumes of IV fluids may alter the outcome by preventing catastrophic deterioration of the patient.

If the patient becomes anxious or develops tingling, itching, paresthesia, ''goose-flesh,'' hives, flush, wheezing, or stridor, in any combination, treatment is begun immediately. The patient may not have any cutaneous or respiratory symptoms but may instead develop hypotension, arrhythmias, loss of consciousness, or severe cardiovascular collapse.[15] The infusion of IV fluids is increased. One may administer 1–3 ml of a 1:10,000 solution of epinephrine IM or IV, depending on the severity of the reaction, and turn the patient supine. If the patient does not respond to the first dose of epinephrine and if a cardiac arrhythmia has not developed, the flow of IV fluids should be increased and epinephrine administered IV again. If wheezing and dyspnea develop, aminophylline, 250 mg in 500 cc of solution, should be administered over 15 minutes. Severe stridor as a result of laryngeal edema and dyspnea should be managed by placement of endotracheal tube and controlled ventilation.

When hypotension responds to epinephrine and IV fluid, additional diphenhydramine, 50–100 mg, and hydrocortisone, 10–200 mg IV, are indicated. When the condition is stabilized for at least 30 minutes, the patient may be taken to the recovery room. If the condition remains unstable, the patient should be transferred to an intensive care unit.

FAILURE OF CHEMONUCLEOLYSIS

Chemonucleolysis fails in 7%–30% of patients so treated,[16, 17] depending on the care taken in patient selection and attention to details of the technique. The average failure rate in one clinic is 15%.[18] Eight of 49 patients who were treated with chymopapain injection failed to obtain relief.

Failure to Relieve Sciatica

There are several reasons why an enzyme will fail to dissolve the displaced disk and relieve pressure on the neural elements. A common reason is failure of the enzyme to reach the offending disk material. The patient may have a sequestered fragment of disk in the spinal canal that cannot imbibe the intradiskally injected enzyme.

According to Bromley,[11] a sequestered fragment of disk in the spinal canal occurs in 13% of patients operated on for disk displacement. Another common reason for enzyme not reaching the offending disk material is that, on intradiskal injection, the fluid follows the path of least resistance, which in some instances may not be into the disk protrusion.[18] If, when dye is injected under fluoroscopy, the dye flows into the vertebral bodies, vascular channels, or an anterior lateral defect without properly filling the area corresponding to the disk protrusion seen on myelography and/or CT, one may anticipate this type of failure.[10]

Wrong Level

Injection of the enzyme at one level, chosen wrongly, will not affect the back pain even if the disk displacement was found at the adjacent level.

Routine multiple disk injections are not recommended. However, if a clinically significant disk displacement at more than one level is suspected, all levels suspected should be injected with dye to confirm the necessity for subsequent enzyme injection.

Failure of the Enzyme to Work

NOT ENOUGH ENZYME.—In a double-blind study, 1 ml containing 4 mg of chymopapain was not enough to effectively decompress the herniated disk.[11] The minimum effective intradiskal dose of collagenase has not been determined. However, an effective dose range of 500–600 units in a volume of 1–2 ml has produced disk narrowing.[2]

INACTIVE ENZYME.—Enzymes can be inactivated in transport or during storage. It is important to dilute chymopapain with sterile water without preservatives.[3] Alcohol should not be used to disinfect the vial prior to withdrawing the enzyme.[8]

MECHANICAL INSUFFICIENCY.—Mechanical insufficiency of the motion segment unit rarely develops as the result of chemonucleolysis. Dramatic disk space narrowing should result from collagenase injection. It remains to be determined whether collagenase injection will predispose to mechanical insufficiency of the motion segment unit. Conversely, it is possible that collagenase injection may prove to be an efficient method of stabilizing the intervertebral joint by stimulating narrowing and subsequent new collagen formation.

ACUTE FACET SYMPTOMS.—Following chemonucleolysis, transient leg pain on the side opposite to the original sciatica may occasionally develop. Affected patients may not have signs of nerve root irritation or compression. The referred leg pain probably occurs because of narrowing of the interspace, with subsequent subluxation of the facet joint processes, cartilaginous erosion, and reactive synovitis in the synovial facet joint capsule. Time, a lumbar support, and anti-inflammatory medication in conjunction with a graduated exercise program will help to alleviate leg pain that results from acute disk space narrowing. Referred pain of this nature usually resolves within 3 months of injection.

COMPLICATIONS

Complications from chemonucleolysis can be limited by excellent patient selection, preinjection rehabilitation, and careful attention to technique. Despite the best patient selection and technique, there will be a small percentage of unavoidable complications. Sensitivity reactions, although usually transient and not leading to permanent morbidity, are the most common of the unavoidable complications and potentially the most serious.

Sensitivity Reactions with Chymopapain

There were 201 sensitivity reactions in the first 13,700 patients treated with chymopapain (1.5%), of which 53 were mild, 52 were moderate, and 25 were severe immediate systemic reactions.[15] Two patients died.

The most recent statistics available are based on 40,000 patients injected with chymopapain. Four patients have died from anaphylaxis caused by chymopapain, an incidence of 0.01%.[18]

Postmorten Findings in Fatal Anaphylaxis

Edema of the airway in man is a feature of anaphylaxis unique to our species. Typical of autopsy findings in 43 patients reported by Delage and Irey[19] was distention of the lungs with laryngeal edema and pulmonary emphysema. The majority of the patients were young people treated with penicillin. These patients usually manifest respiratory distress followed by circulatory collapse. Occasionally, seizures, cyanosis, and gastrointestinal symptoms are the first signs of fatal anaphylaxis. The interval between injection and onset of the reaction was less than 20 minutes in 86% (37/43) of cases in which anaphylaxis resulted in death. The time from onset to death was 30 minutes in 14 of the 43 patients.

Case Reports of Nonfatal Anaphylaxis to Chymopapain

Nonfatal Anaphylaxis Under Anesthesia

An anaphylactic reaction to chymopapain during anesthesia was reported by Rajagopalan et al.[20] A 48-year-old woman was endotracheally intubated and anesthetized with general anesthesia using thiopental, nitrous oxide, and oxygen. An antihistamine (chlorpheniramine, 10 mg) and 100 mg of hydro-

cortisone IV were given after induction of anesthesia. Diskography was performed, and 10 minutes later 10,000 units of chymopapain was injected intradiskally. The patient was allowed to wake up at this stage and was extubated *15 minutes* after injection. A routine check of blood pressure showed an unobtainable pressure. Oxygen 100% was administered by mask and 800 ml of fluid was administered rapidly IV, along with methoxamine, 4 × 4 mg. One milliliter of 1:10,000 epinephrine solution was given IV after the electrocardiogram showed a normal pattern with a heart rate of 80 beats per minute. Immediately after receiving epinephrine, the patient had frequent premature ventricular contractions. Facial and periorbital edema and mild generalized bronchospasms developed. Fifteen minutes after the onset of the reaction, the patient's systolic blood pressure was 90 mm Hg, and although she was stuporous for several hours, she recovered completely within 10 hours.

Watts et al.[21] reported on four patients who had immediate systemic sensitivity reactions typical of anaphylaxis after chymopapain injections during general anesthesia. Following inducement of anesthesia with thiopental, the patients were paralyzed with succinylcholine and intubated. General anesthesia was maintained with halothane and oxygen. Diskography was performed at one to three levels with Renografin.

In the first patient, a 66-year-old man, hypotension developed within minutes after injection of 4 mg of chymopapain. He had a mild systemic reaction with a blood pressure of 70/50 mm Hg which responded immediately to 25 mg of IV ephedrine. Over the next 2 hours, additional doses of ephedrine were given to maintain normal blood pressure. The patient had received 100 mg of hydrocortisone and 50 mg of diphenhydramine IM before injection. He was receiving hydrocortisone at the time of the chymopapain injection. He had an uneventful recovery within 2 hours.

The second patient, a 60-year-old woman, had a cutaneous, petechiae-like eruption within minutes after 4 mg of chymopapain was injected. This would be classified as a mild systemic allergic reaction. She was treated with IV hydrocortisone, with no problem.

The third patient, a 25-year-old woman, had hypotension and generalized urticaria *within minutes* after injection of 4 mg of chymopapain into the L-4 disk and 4 mg into the L-5 disk. Hypotension and pulmonary wheezes developed and the patient was treated with hydrocortisone and epinephrine IV over the next few hours. She had not received preinjection steroids. After 4 hours her condition stabilized.

The fourth patient, a 32-year-old woman, had tachycardia and hypotension within *2 minutes* after injection of 4 mg of chymopapain. This was immediately treated with 25 mg of ephedrine IV. Within 3 minutes, her blood pressure was unobtainable; 0.3 ml of a 1:1,000 solution of epinephrine was given IV. Within minutes a previously unpalpable femoral pulse and carotid pulse were discernible. IV fluids were administered rapidly because no brachial pulse could be recorded. Over the next 2 hours, 4 L of balanced salt solution was given. Immediately after the hypotensive episode, the patient was placed on pure oxygen but remained comatose for 45 minutes. It was an hour before urinary output resumed. Two hours later, blood pressure had returned to 100/70 mm Hg. Twelve hours after injection of chymopapain, she became asymptomatic. She had received hydrocortisone and diphenhydramine IM as preoperative medications.

Reaction to Chemonucleolysis Under Local Anesthesia

There is a report of a 32-year-old man who, after diskography with Conray-60 at two levels, was injected with chymopapain at both levels. In *1 minute,* he developed severe back and bilateral leg pain and tingling in the arms, hands, feet, and perioral region, followed rapidly by pruritis and urticaria, perioral pallor, dyspnea, and stridor. One-half milliliter of 1:10,000 epinephrine solution was administered IV, along with several liters of Ringer's lactate. Within 10 minutes the patient had recovered, but he experienced headaches for several hours following the procedure. This patient had been premedicated one-half hour before the procedure with 50 mg of Benadryl and 100 mg of hydrocortisone IM and injected under local anesthesia with IV fluids running. In this case, a small dose of epinephrine, administered with 60 seconds of the onset of anaphylaxis, was sufficient to abort the attack. The reaction was rapidly recognized with the patient under local anesthesia.

PATHOPHYSIOLOGY OF ANAPHYLAXIS

Anaphylaxis in man is a systemic symptom complex resulting from antigen-antibody interaction.[22]

The patient must be exposed to the antigen at some time in the past so that IgE antibody is attached to the mast cells in the target organs (lung, gastrointestinal tract, and skin). With reinjection of antigen at various periods following sensitization, an antigen-antibody complex occurs on the surface of the mast cells, causing a massive release of the pharmacologic mediators: histamine, slow-reacting substance of anaphylaxis (SRS-A), serotonin, and bradykinin. These mediators then act on the target organs.

Mediators

Histamine, thought to be the major mediator of anaphylaxis in man, causes bronchial constriction and increases capillary permeability. SRS-A causes bronchial smooth muscle contraction in humans.[22] It is also responsible for increased vascular permeability. Bradykinin causes vasodilation, compounds the effects of histamine, increases capillary permeability, and is thought to be the primary substance in man responsible for the severe hypotension noted.

The mediators may cause a greatly variable response in different patients. The major targets in humans are smooth muscles, which, on contraction, may cause severe bronchiolar constriction, resulting in asphyxia, increased peripheral arterial resistance secondary to vasoconstriction, nausea and vomiting secondary to smooth muscle contraction in the bowel, and ''goose-flesh'' (cutis anserina) from contraction of the erector pili muscles in the skin.

The severe fall in arterial blood pressure is secondary to a decline in cardiac output and a loss of fluid from the intravascular space due to increased capillary permeability. Shock is due to reduced plasma volume, hemoconcentration, decreased cardiac output, reduced peripheral blood flow, and increased arterial constriction. It is very important to remember that hypotension is due to intravascular fluid loss, which in turn is due to increased capillary permeability.

Acute vascular collapse from anaphylaxis is secondary to cardiac arrhythmias, acute myocardial infarction, and vasomotor collapse. Direct cardiac anaphylaxis is secondary to the direct action of the chemical mediators on the myocardium and may be compounded by epinephrine, halothane, and preexisting heart disease.

Abnormal ECGs have been noted within 24 hours of the onset of systemic anaphylaxis in 6 of 14 patients.[23] None had preexisting heart disease. ECG changes may be the result of the direct effect of mediators on the myocardium and/or the compounding effects of epinephrine and anesthetic agents. Preexisting occult heart disease with superimposed stress may also be implicated when abnormal ECGs occur.

Prevention of Anaphylaxis

There are no reliable tests to predict whether a patient will experience an immediate systemic sensitivity reaction. Some reactions can be prevented by carefully noting a history of allergy to papaya, meat tenderizer containing papain, or previous injection with chymopapain. Previous allergic reaction to ointments containing collagenase or to a previous collagenase injection should also be sought in the history if this enzyme is to be given. Avoid injecting these patients.

In Wiltse et al.'s series of 1,200 patients,[24] the first 600 were not pretreated with antihistamines and steroids. There were seven serious allergic reactions. It remains to be determined whether the use of antihistamines and steroids as a prophylactic measure decreases the incidence and severity of anaphylactic reactions.

Kelly et al.[25] reported on 101 patients who had prior anaphylactoid reactions to contrast media and who were pretreated with prednisone and diphenhydramine 1 hour before a repeat diagnostic study with a contrast medium. Five of the 101 patients (5%) developed a systemic sensitivity reaction, characterized by mild urticaria and pruritis. There were no life-threatening reactions in this high-risk group of patients. In an earlier study of 115 patients, there was a 30% recurrence of serious anaphylactic reactions in patients who had had previous reactions to contrast media.[26] The data seem to suggest that antihistamines and hydrocortisone effectively reduce the risk of an anaphylactic reaction in the patient who has been presensitized with an antigen. That Kelly et al. found no significant life-threatening anaphylactic reactions in those patients, despite their previous systemic sensitivity reactions, is highly significant. There is evidence that pretreatment with steroids and antihistamines in Wiltse's series protected the patients against anaphylaxis. However, one should not be lulled into complacency when pretreatment has been given. Such precautions may give the patient an advantage, but early recognition of anaphylaxis and the administration of epinephrine and IV fluids are still essential.

H₁ and H₂ Antagonists for Anaphylaxis

One of the mediators of anaphylaxis, histamine, acts on two receptors, H_1 and H_2, both of which appear in the heart or on peripheral vasculature. Theoretically, the administration of an antagonist to both receptors may afford some protection against the cardiovascular effects of histamine release after anaphylactic reactions. Prospective double-blind studies have shown that administration of H_1 (diphenhydramine) and H_2 (cimetidine) protect patients from the hemodynamic effect of histamine release after IV administration of morphine.[27]

The use of cimetidine, 300 mg orally every 6 hours for 24 hours, and diphenhydramine (Benadryl), 50 mg orally every 6 hours for 24 hours, before injection of chymopapain is now advocated.[28] One must still be prepared to make an immediate diagnosis and administer adrenaline and large amounts of fluid, should an anaphylactic reaction occur. Pretreatment with cimetidine and diphenhydramine may be effective protection against the severe hemodynamic effects of a systemic allergic reaction.

Early Recognition of Anaphylaxis

McCulloch[29] treated 5,000 patients by injection with Discase and reported 15 acute severe anaphylactic reactions. The onset was varied: some patients had a precipitous fall in blood pressure followed by cutaneous manifestations; others had tingling, paresthesia, flush wheezing, and then a falling blood pressure. All the patients were injected under local anesthesia, with an anesthesiologist in attendance. McCulloch's experience with the successful management of anaphylaxis is probably the most extensive in the world. He emphasizes the importance of early recognition of symptoms and the immediate administration of epinephrine and IV fluids. None of his patients had permanent sequelae of immediate systemic sensitivity reactions to chymopapain.

COMPLICATIONS OTHER THAN ALLERGY

Neural Injury

Neural injury can be avoided by performing the procedure under local anesthesia and redirecting the needle when the patient complains of acute radicular pain. The nerve root or ganglion injured by needle penetrations is usually the one above the root or ganglion injured by disk displacement.

If causalgia or neuralgia develops from needle puncture, the only therapy is time and symptomatic treatment. Sympathetic block may help. The patient should be reassured that, in most instances, it will resolve.

Cardiovascular Complications

Avoidance of high-risk patients and the use of appropriate preinjection prophylaxis will help to decrease the incidence of these complications. A certain small incidence of cardiovascular complications, such as thromboembolic phenomena, cerebrovascular accidents, and myocardial infarctions, will occur during the course of treatment in any group of patients under stress. There are fewer of these complications with chemonucleolysis than with surgery, and if they do occur, they are more easily managed after chemonucleolysis than after surgery.

Neural Toxicity

Intrathecal Injection of Enzyme

Intrathecal injection of enzyme can be avoided if diskography is performed prior to enzyme injection. Although a case of intrathecal enzyme injection as the result of a preexisting intrathecal disk herniation has not been reported, it could occur, and one should pay attention to the contrast dye flow pattern before injecting enzyme. Enzyme should be injected via the lateral approach only, never by the posterolateral route, to avoid nerve root penetration and intrathecal injection.

If the patient complains of severe headache, back pain, and leg pain in conjunction with signs of increased intracranial pressure, an emergency spinal tap and repeated taps are in order to decrease the intrathecal cerebrospinal fluid pressure. An elevated cerebrospinal fluid pressure occurs secondary to hemorrhage.

Diskitis and Disk Space Infection

Most patients have some acute narrowing of the intervertebral disk following injection with either chymopapain or collagenase. After an initial period of 2–4 weeks of increased back pain, the patient should improve progressively between 4 and 7 weeks after injection. Increased pain accompanied by sleep disturbances and muscle spasm during this period should alert the physician to a possible disk space infection. Close adherence to proper injection technique should make this complication extremely rare. Early confirmation of the diagnosis can be made by a positive bone scan. Later in the course of the disease, after 2–3 weeks of increasing symptoms, the patient's x-ray films may show erosion of the bony end-plates of the vertebral bodies adjacent to the disk space in question. There may be an elevated sedimentation rate and white blood cell count, with a shift of the differential count to the left. A closed Craig needle biopsy, culture, sensitivity testing, and histologic study should be performed to confirm the diagnosis as soon as a disk space infection is suspected. Six weeks of specific IV antibiotic therapy, followed by 6 months of oral antibiotics, are indicated to eradicate this type of infection in an avascular space.[30]

SUMMARY

The object of chemonucleolysis is to inject the enzyme into the offending disk material by a percutaneous needle. The technique has evolved over the past 20 years to the point where it can be safely done on an outpatient basis with little anxiety, discomfort, or risk to the patient.[16] However, the surgeon should not be lulled into complacency by the seeming simplicity of this procedure.

The sequelae of this technique are the risks of disk space infection and nerve root injury, resulting in neuralgia or causalgia. The latter may be caused by needle penetration of the neural structures.[17] Close attention to detail can eliminate these and other technical complications. One must not forget the ever-present threat of an immediate, severe, life-threatening anaphylactic reaction.

REFERENCES

1. Pearce J., Moll J.M. II: Conservative treatment and natural history of acute lumbar disc lesions. *J. Neurol. Neurosurg. Psychiatry* 30:13, 1967.
2. Adams P., Eyre D., Muir H.: Biochemical aspects of development and aging of human lumbar intervertebral disks. *Rheumatol. Rehabil.* 16:22, 1977.
3. Nordby E.: Personal communication, August 1982.
4. Wiltse L.: Chemonucleolysis in ideal candidate for laminectomy. Personal communication, June 19, 1978.

5. Eyre D., Muir H.: Quantitative analysis of types I and II collagens in human intervertebral discs at various ages. *Acta Biochim. Biophys.*1:492:29, 1977.

6. Choudhury A.R., Taylor J.C.: Cauda equina syndrome in lumbar disc disease. *Acta Orthop. Scand.* 51:493, 1980.

7. Waddell G., Kummel E.G., Lotto W.N., et al.: Failed lumbar disc surgery and repeat surgery following industrial injuries. *J. Bone Joint Surg.* 61A:201, 1979.

8. Finnegan W.J., Fenlin J.M., Marvel J.P., et al.: Results of surgical intervention in the symptomatic multiply-operated back patient. *J. Bone Joint Surg.* 61A:1077, 1979.

9. Brown M.D.: Spinal surgery: A combined neurosurgical and orthopedic advanced course. University of Miami School of Medicine, Miami Beach, Florida, April 1982.

10. Brown M.D.: Chemoneucleolysis with discase: Technique, results, case reports. *Spine* 1:115, 1976; erratum, 1:116, 1976.

11. Bromley J.: Personal communication, August, 1982.

12. Smyth M.J., Wright W.W.: Sciatica and the intervertebral disc. *J. Bone Joint Surg* 40a:1401, 1958.

13. Blikra G.: Intradural herniated lumbar disc. *J. Neurosurg.* 31:676, 1969.

14. Lindahl S., Brown M., Irstam L., et al.: Roentgenologic grading of disc degeneration by discography. Paper presented to the International Society for the Study of the Lumbar Spine, Toronto, 1982.

15. McCulloch J.A.: Personal communication, August 1982.

16. Smith L.: Failures with chemonucleolysis. *Orthop. Clin. North Am.* 1:255, 1975.

17. McCulloch J.A.: Chemonucleolysis. *J. Bone Joint Surg.* 59:45, 1977.

18. Brown M.D.: *Intradiscal Therapy: Chymopapain or Collagenase.* Chicago, Year Book Medical Publishers, Inc., 1983.

19. Delage C., Irey N.: Anaphylactic deaths: A clinicopathologic study of 43 cases. *J. Forensic Sci.* 17:525, 1972.

20. Rajagopalan R., Tindal S., MacNab I.: Anaphylactic reactions to chymopapain during general anesthesia: A case report. *Anesth. Analg.* 53:191, 1974.

21. Watts C., Williams O.B., Goldstein G.: Sensitivity reactions to intradiscal injection of chymopapain during anesthesia. *Anesthesiology* 44:43, 1976.

22. Kelly J., Patterson R.: Anaphylaxis: Course, mechanism and treatment. *JAMA* 227:1431, 1974.

23. Hanashiro P.K., Weil M.H.: Anaphylactic shock in man. *Arch. Intern. Med.* 119:129, 1967.

24. Wiltse L.L., Widell E.H., Hansen A.Y.: Chymopapain chemonucleolysis in lumbar disc disease. *JAMA* 231:474, 1975.

25. Kelly J., Patterson R., Lieberman P., et al.: Radiographic contrast media studies in high-risk patients. *J. Allergy Clin. Immunol.* 62:181, 1978.

26. Fisher H.W., Doust V.L.: An evaluation of pretesting in the problem of serious and fatal reactions to excretory venography. *Radiology* 103:497, 1972.

27. Philbin D.M., Moss J., Akins C.W., et al.: The use of H_1 and H_2 histamine antagonists with morphine anesthesia: A double-blind study. *Anesthesiology* 55:292, 1981.

28. Schoning B., Lorenz W., Doenicke A.: Prophylaxis of anaphylactoid reactions to a polypeptidal plasma substitute by H_1 plus H_2 receptor antagonists: Synopsis of three randomized controlled trials. *Klin. Wochenschr.* 60:1048, 1982.

29. McCulloch J.S.: Personal communication, August 1982.

30. Digby J.M., Kersley J.B.: Pyogenic nontuberculous spinal infection. *J. Bone Joint Surg.* 61B:47, 1979.

31. Lindblom K.: Technique and results of diagnostic puncture and injection (discography) in the lumbar region. *Acta Orthop. Scand.* 20:315, 1950.

32. Erlacher P.R.: Nucleography. *J. Bone Joint Surg.* 34B:204, 1952.

33. Edholm P., Fernström I., Lindblom K.: Extradural lumbar disc puncture. *Acta Radiol. Diagn.* 6:322, 1967.

41 / Cryoanalgesia

P. PRITHVI RAJ, M.D.

CRYOANALGESIA IS A TECHNIQUE in which an extremly low temperature is used to achieve pain relief by blocking peripheral nerves or destroying nerve endings.

HISTORY

The beneficial effect of cold on inflamed and painful tissues was recorded by Hippocrates. In the 11th century A.D. an Anglo-Saxon monk suggested the use of cold to deaden the skin before scarification.[1] In 1812, Larre recognized that the limbs of soldiers that had been frozen by the Prussian snow could be amputated relatively painlessly.[2] In 1851, Arnott described the use of ice and salt mixtures at $-20°$ C to produce tumor regression, and also noted the anaesthetic effect.

Richardson introduced the ether spray in 1866 to obtain local analgesia by refrigeration. This was superseded in 1890 by the ethyl chloride spray, similar to what is in use today.[3] Thus "to freeze" became synonymous with "to numb."

Interest in the effects of cold on living tissue has increased considerably in the last 20 years as a result of the development of apparatus for the controlled maintenance of extremely low temperatures. In 1962 Cooper et al. described sophisticated apparatus that used liquid nitrogen to achieve a minimum temperature of $-196°$ C.[4] Later, Amoils developed a simple instrument that used carbon dioxide or nitrous oxide gas as the refrigerant and that achieved a minimum temperature of around $-70°$ C.[5]

The term cryoanalgesia was coined by Lloyd, Barnard, and Glynn to describe the destruction of peripheral nerves by extreme cold for pain relief.[6] The technique was introduced to destroy peripheral nerves as a means of relieving intractable pain that required prolonged somatic blockade. All other methods of peripheral nerve destruction, such as surgical neurectomy, crushing, or thermolysis, are associated with an unacceptable incidence of neuralgia. Certainly, somatic blockade by the injection of chemical neurolytes, such as phenol, has been shown morphologically to cause incomplete destruction of the nerve.[7] This may be the cause of the neuralgia that not uncommonly follows these injections or any other method of incomplete destruction of a peripheral nerve.[8] Cryolesions are associated with less fibrous tissue reaction and hence prevents neuralgia.[9]

THE EFFECT OF CRYOANALGESIA ON PERIPHERAL NERVES

The effects of cooling on peripheral nerve function have been extensively reported in the literature. Trendelenburg regarded cold as the most "gentle" form of nerve injury and used a temperature of approximately $-7°$ C to produce a degree of structural damage compatible with subsequent regeneration.[10] Blackwood and Russell confined their attentions to the clinical syndrome of "immersion foot" and studied nerve function after exposure to saline at 4° to 5° C.[11] The classic work of Denny-Brown and his colleagues clarified the pathologic changes that follow cold injury by exposing peripheral nerves to saline at $-4°$ to $+3°$ C, or to a CO_2 spray.[12]

When a controlled temperature of $-100°$ C is employed to produce a cryolesion, the axon below the level of injury and for a short distance above it does not survive (Fig 41–1). In more advanced third-degree injury there is also disorganization of the internal connective tissue components of the funiculus and, although the perineurium remains in-

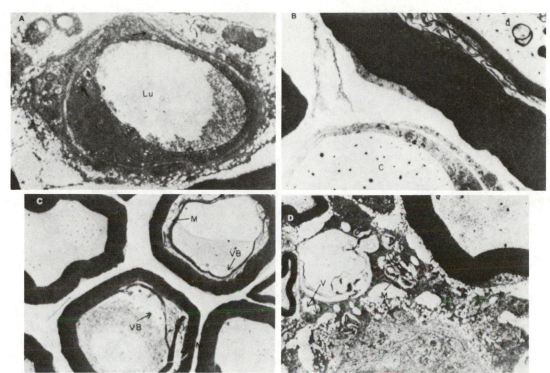

Fig 41–1.—A, effect of hypothermia on a peripheral nerve 1 hour after application. Electron micrograph shows the damage to the capillary lumen *(Lu)*. Note the cellular edema and endothelial residues *(arrows.)* **B,** effect of hypothermia 7 hours after application. Note accumulation of amorphous material in the axon *(a)* and the capillary lumen *(c)*. **C,** transverse section of several axons 7 hours after hypothermic injury. Note separation of myelin *(M)* and the numerous vesicular bodies *(VB)*. **D,** appearance 3 days after hypothermic injury. Phagocytic cells contain vacuoles of amorphous material *(V)*. Note also vacuolization of myelin *(M)*. (From Basbaum C.B.: Electrophysiological observations. *J. Neurocytol.* 2:171, 1973. Reproduced by permission.)

tact, the continuity of endoneurial tubes and Schwann cell complexes is destroyed. This has an adverse effect on nerve repair because of the inevitable intrafunicular fibrosis which diverts, delays, and distorts subsequent axon growth.

One of the properties of cryocoagulated tissue left in situ is its relatively inert pathobiologic behavior. This favors unimpeded regeneration of axons within their original endoneurial tubes, and then meticulous realignment with end organs.

The rate of axonal growth is more rapid after second-degree injury than after nerve suture. The prognosis of increasingly distal lesions improves in that muscle changes consequent on denervation have little time to develop before reinnervation occurs.

The actual mechanism of the cryoinjury remains speculative. Vascular stasis and ischemia provide a major contribution, but it is also possible that freezing may have a direct cryolytic effect on myeline and may disrupt the enzyme systems responsible for nerve sustenance. The ability of small nerves to obtain nutrition by direct diffusion further complicates the problem. Cryodestruction in other tissues is thought to be mediated predominantly through ischemia.[13, 14] Mobilization of a nerve will damage its nutrient arteries, but an effective collateral circulation is rapidly established. Experimental ligation of regional nutrient arteries over considerable lengths of a nerve trunk does not impair the structure and function of nerve fibers or their regeneration after crush injury.[15] In earlier experiments a normal response to stimulation was present after the nerve had been mobilized, indicating that a significant vascular insufficiency was not present before freezing.[16]

A number of workers have studied the functional

changes associated with cooling of sensory nerves[17, 18] and have demonstrated a variable susceptibility in different types of nerve fibers. While these observations cannot be completely explained in terms of fiber size,[19] Denny-Brown et al. reported that large and medium-sized myelinated fibers were selectively damaged by cooling, in contrast to fine nonmyelinated fibers, which were relatively resistant.[12] A selective response is unlikely after exposure to the lower temperatures used in cryotherapy, where an all-or-nothing lethal effect is anticipated. There is no evidence to suggest that the response of sensory nerves will differ significantly from that of their motor counterparts.

The crucial factor influencing the quality of regeneration is preservation of the intrafunicular connective tissue architecture, in particular the integrity of the individual endoneurial tubes.

INDICATIONS

Cryoanalgesia is indicated for postoperative or chronic pain. It is suitable for intercostal neurolysis, facial neurolysis, facet rhizolysis, sacral foraminal block, and somatic nerve root cryolesions. It has also been tried for neuroma pain, glossopharyngeal neuralgia, perineal pain, and coccydynia.

Postthoracotomy Pain

Intraoperative Intercostal Cryolysis

In the technique described by Nelson et al.,[20] intercostal cryolysis is performed intraoperatively at the conclusion of posterolateral or anterior thoracotomy. Five intercostal nerves adjacent to the incision site are identified about 2 cm lateral to the transverse process. These nerves are separated from the intercostal vessels and then frozen with the cryoprobe. The cryoprobe is maintained on the nerve until there is visible evidence of nerve frozen all round. The probe is thawed, and only then is it removed.

Nelson et al. compared narcotic administration in 38 patients in the first 5 postoperative days with or without intercostal cryolysis. The dosage of narcotics could be reduced by 20%–50% in patients that had undergone cryolysis. Furthermore, intercostal nerve freezing did not produce neuritis or neuromas on follow-up of up to 24 months. The technique gave sensory anesthesia approximately 4 inches wide which lasted for 6–8 months. Pain around the drainage tube site in the back and shoulder was not helped by intercostal cryolysis.

Katz et al. compared intercostal cryolysis with intercostal local anesthetic block and with no block in 24 patients.[21] The 15 patients who underwent cryotherapy had significantly less postoperative pain than the 9 patients who had local anesthetic blocks or no nerve block at all. In their study, nerve block with cryolysis lasted only up to 30 days. There were no adverse sequelae.

In the cryoanalgesia group the mean pain score was 2.8, compared to 6.0 in the noncryoanalgesia group, on a 10-point visual analogue scale administered 24 hours postoperatively. Pain relief in the cryoanalgesia group lasted for approximately 2–3 weeks.

Percutaneous Technique

In patients with chronic thoracic pain, open thoracotomy for cryolysis is unacceptable. In these patients a percutaneous technique can be utilized.

The skin is anesthetized with a local anesthetic and a large-bore needle is introduced through the skin to allow passage of a 14-gauge plastic cannula. The plastic cannula is introduced tangentially toward the intercostal nerve (Fig 41–2). When the cannula is at the nerve, the stylet is removed and the cryoprobe is introduced to a measured length such that the tip of the probe is 0.5 cm outside the cannula (Fig 41–3). The nerve stimulator of the cryoprobe can further confirm the approximation of probe to nerve. Two freeze-thaw cycles of 2 minutes each are used at a steady temperature of −60° C. Twelve patients were treated by the percutaneous

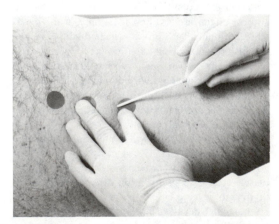

Fig 41–2.—A 14-gauge catheter is inserted for intercostal nerve freezing prior to insertion of the cryoprobe.

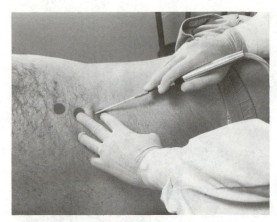

Fig 41–3.—A cryoprobe is inserted through the catheter on the intercostal nerve.

technique by Lloyd et al., who reported a median duration of pain relief of 14 days.[6]

Facial Pain

Bernard, Lloyd, and Glynn reported on 21 patients with intractable facial pain,[22] all of whom had failed to respond to medical or surgical treatment. The following nerves were involved: V_1 supraorbital and supratrochlear; V_2 infraorbital; and V_3 mental and lingual. The diagnoses in these patients were postherpetic neuralgia, neuralgia of unknown etiology, atypical facial neuralgia, tic douloureux, posttraumatic neuralgia, and cancer pain. All nerves were exposed prior to cryolysis.

In the postherpetic neuralgia patients, the median duration of pain relief was 38 days (range, 0–84 days). Sensory anesthesia was usually present for a prolonged period but did not correspond to pain relief. In the other patients the median duration of pain was 116 days, with a median sensory loss of up to 49 days.

Low Back Pain

Percutaneous Cryolysis of the Facet Nerve

Brechner studied the effect of percutaneous cryolysis of the nerves to the facet in patients with low back pain.[23] Her indications for facet neurolysis were the following: pain duration of more than 6 months, age between 25 and 55 years, no other medical or surgical alternatives available for low

back pain, radiation of pain to the buttocks and sciatic distribution, but not extending distally to the knee, and 75% pain relief with at least two previous nerve blocks with local anesthetics at that site.

Her technique is similar to that used for thermolysis by other workers.[24] The patient is placed in the prone position with a pillow under the iliac crest. The tips of the spinous processes are identified and a line is drawn running horizontally through them. At L-2, L-3, and L-4, a point 2½ inches lateral to the posterior tips of spinous processes is marked, and at L-5 and S-1, a point 3 inches lateral to the spinous process is marked (Fig 41–4). The needle is inserted through these points and perpendicular to the skin. As soon as the bone is encountered, fluoroscopy is used to confirm the location of the needle. Two milliliters of a local anesthetic is injected for diagnostic purposes. A 14-gauge Teflon catheter is then inserted at the same points. The stylet is removed and the cryoprobe is on the facet nerve, the characteristic low back pain is elicited. On the other hand, if the cryoprobe is on the spinal nerve, radicular pain is felt by the patient, and the needle is repositioned. Freeze-thaw cycles lasting 1 minute each are performed two to three times at two to three levels. The patient is encouraged to be active after the procedure.

There was 70% pain relief 1 hour after cryolysis. This relief lasted 1 week. Pain relief decreased to 50% at 3 weeks, and at 3 months the same intensity of low back pain was noticed as prior to facet cryolysis.

Glossopharyngeal Neuralgia

The glossopharyngeal nerve lies immediately subjacent to the tonsillar fossa. The painful and distressing condition of glossopharyngeal neuralgia can be treated by applying the probe to the tonsillar bed and freezing for 2 minutes, twice. This is a simple block to perform and has distinct advantages over the conventional injection of the glossopharyngeal nerve at a point just anterior to the tip of the mastoid process. Injection here may anesthetize the accessory vagus and hypoglossal nerves as well.

Perineal Pain

Perineal pain is a midline pain and therefore is difficult to block by intrathecal neurolytic agents without risking bladder and bowel dysfunction. Insertions of the cryoprobe through the sacral hiatus

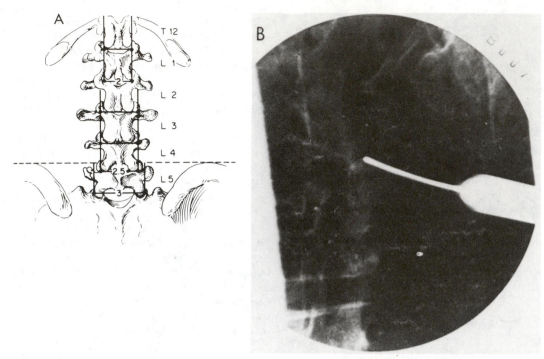

Fig 41–4.—A, landmarks for needle entry aimed toward the facet joints of the lower thoracolumbar area. **B,** radiograph confirming correct placement of the cryoprobe for facet denervation. (**B,** from Brechner.[23] Reproduced by permission.)

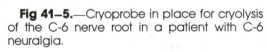

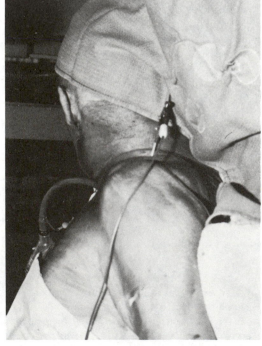

Fig 41–5.—Cryoprobe in place for cryolysis of the C-6 nerve root in a patient with C-6 neuralgia.

up to the level of the fourth sacral foramen can give good analgesia over the dorsal surface of the scrotum, perineum, and anus. Bladder dysfunction is not encountered, and analgesia usually lasts 6–8 weeks.

Coccydynia

This refers to pain in the coccygeal area, often resulting from a fall but occasionally idiopathic in origin. It can be treated by inserting the cryoprobe through the sacrococcygeal membrane into the sacral extradural canal at the level of the cornu, where the sacrococcygeal nerve escapes from the canal. Two cryolesions are made adjacent to each cornu, using two 1-minute freeze-thaw cycles. Other indications for cryoanalgesia include cervical nerve root lesion as shown in Figure 41–5.

TECHNIQUE OF CRYOANALGESIA

Patient Selection

Cryoanalgesia is indicated when a long-term reversible and peripheral nerve block is required and the nerve is accessible. The technique is very acceptable and has particular application in the treatment of intractable pain of any origin when intrathecal methods are contraindicated.

There is no absolute contraindication to cryoanalgesia except patient refusal.

This procedure is applicable to any situation where a "mixed" (i.e., motor and sensory function) nerve is involved. It is not advisable at present to freeze nerves with a large motor component (e.g., lumbar plexus) in view of the ensuing, albeit temporary, loss of function.

Preparation

The procedure is explained to the patient. During stimulation the patient will feel a pulse or beat that is not painful and is usually well accepted. The patient is told that the nerve will be frozen, resulting in numbness in the area supplied by the nerve. A few weeks following treatment, however, the numbness will wear off, and in a high proportion of cases the pain does not return for several months.

The procedure is normally performed as an outpatient procedure under local anesthesia. Some ap-

prehensive patients may require general anesthetic.

Radiography, particularly using image intensification, is a valuable addition to probe location but not essential in every case.

Procedure

Whichever site is chosen, accuracy of placement of the probe is essential. Where the nerve lies close to bone, as in the vertebral and sacral areas, use of an image intensifier may facilitate the procedure. The final positioning, however, is obtained by the use of the nerve stimulator. Exceptions are seen when the nerve is exposed and frozen under direct vision, i.e., for supraorbital and infraorbital blocks.

The skin is cleaned with an antiseptic solution and a wheal is raised with a local anesthetic solution. An introducer is used to create a tract for the probe, which is then passed through it in the direction of the nerve.

A 15–18-gauge cryoneedle is used to apply and maintain extreme cold. Blockade is based on the Joule-Thompson effect, with nitrous oxide used as the refrigerant gas. The Joule-Thompson effect occurs when gas at a pressure of about 700 pounds per inch is ejected through a nozzle; as the gas expands, it cools (Fig 41–6). Nitrous oxide cools to around $-70°$ C. The cold gas impinging on the inner surface of the needle tip absorbs heat from the surrounding tissue, and the warm gas is exhausted back up the needle and vented through a scavenging system. The Spembley-Lloyd cryoneedle incorporates a thermocouple to confirm the temperature achieved at the tip. In addition, there is an electrical connection at the tip of the probe connected to a peripheral nerve stimulator (Fig 41–7 and 41–8).

With the use of the nerve stimulator, and at a setting of 2–3 V, a muscle twitch will be obtained when the nerve is in reasonably close proximity. As the stimulation voltage is simultaneously lowered, the position of the probe is adjusted to maintain the

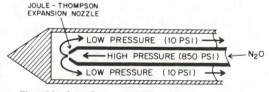

Fig 41–6.—Cross section of cryoprobe tip illustrating differences in pressure in the various compartments. (From Brechner.[23] Reproduced by permission.)

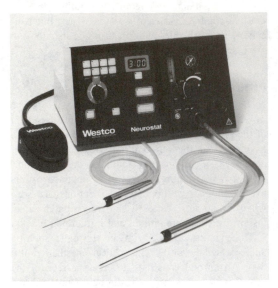

Fig 41–7.—Cryoanalgesia apparatus. (Courtesy of Westco Medical Corporation, San Diego, California.)

twitch response. It is important that the twitch be obtained with a minimum of stimulation. The nerve will then be lying adjacent to the probe tip. The probe must be carefully held in this position while freezing the nerve. The freeze control is set to freeze, and under normal operation the mode indicator should drop rapidly into the blue zone (freezing). The freeze should be timed for at least 2 minutes. The control is then set to the defrost position and the mode indicator will slowly move toward the red zone as the ice melts. As soon as the indicator is in the red zone, the freeze-thaw cycle is repeated

for an additional 2 minutes. When the indicator has once again returned to the red zone the probe may be withdrawn.

When purely sensory nerves (i.e., the articular nerve of Luschka, or cutaneous nerves) are frozen, it is not possible to elicit a muscle twitch. With the nerve stimulator in use, accurate placement is signaled by the referral of a tingling sensation and occasionally pain along the course of the nerve. Apart from a temporary exacerbation of the patient's pain, caused by stimulation of the nerve and abolished by freezing, these procedures should be painless. Use of the stimulator at a high rate setting gives the patient the experience of ''pressure'' on the nerve rather than discrete impulses, and this can assist in the accurate location of the probe tip, since low amplitudes can be used. If pain is produced by freezing and persists, it suggests that the probe is not sufficiently close to the nerve to cause destruction. The cryoprobe should then be reapplied.

Patient Reaction

Patients occasionally complain of burning, or bursting pain. Generally the patient reaction is excellent.

Post Application

Immediate pain relief is obtained and should last for a minimum of 3 weeks. Occasional areas of erythema are seen along the course of the treated nerve, but these are transient. A skin burn may occur if the neuroprobe is superficially placed and pro-

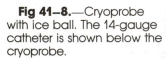

Fig 41–8.—Cryoprobe with ice ball. The 14-gauge catheter is shown below the cryoprobe.

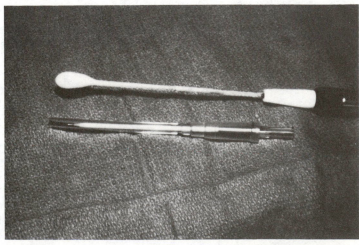

duces a large ice ball (e.g., intercostal block). This will heal, but the patient may be left with a small area of depigmentation for several months. Improved methods of insulation are overcoming this problem. Patients are usually seen in follow-up at 2, 6, and 12 weeks. Repeated treatments may be indicated. There is no evidence of permanent neurologic damage as a result of multiple treatments.

CLINICAL APPLICATIONS

The use of cyroanalgesia has limitations in that the duration of analgesia is determined by the time taken for normal regeneration of the peripheral nerve. Thus, the duration of pain relief is a function of the completeness of destruction of the peripheral nerve. The positioning of the needle is of paramount importance because the ice ball is of limited size and must incorporate the nerve to achieve complete destruction. The positioning of the needle is a function of the expertise of the clinician and the characteristics of the peripheral nerve to be frozen. The median duration of pain relief varies from about 2 weeks to about 5 months.[6, 22] Cryoanalgesia should not be used on mixed nerves unless there are extenuating circumstances because it will result in complete loss of function in the nerve, including paralysis of the muscles supplied by that nerve.

The most fruitful uses for cryoprobe blockade appear to be in special situations of postoperative and posttraumatic pain and for the medium-duration relief of chronic pain. Analgesia by intercostal block has been provided for patients undergoing thoracotomy; there was a significant reduction in the number of narcotic injections and the number of days a narcotic was required, compared to a control group.[25] The intercostal nerves can conveniently be blocked under direct vision at the end of the operative procedure. However, if access from the chest is limited, an external approach can be used. This approach may also be used for analgesia for fractured ribs. Three important points should be noted:

First, the cryoprobe should not be withdrawn until it has fully thawed; otherwise the surrounding tissue may adhere to the probe, and blood vessels and neural structures may be torn.

Second, great care should be exercised with cryoprobe blockade in the dural cuff region. It is possible for the cold lesion to extend to the spinal cord or for inadvertent thrombosis of a major "feeder artery" to result from the marked local reduction in temperature. Thus, in general, somatic blockade

should be carried out lateral to the paravertebral muscles unless it is necessary to block the posterior primary ramus.

Third, a major disadvantage of percutaneous use is that the freezing that occurs along the needle may result in full-thickness destruction of the skin. Following healing there is usually a depigmented scar. This can be prevented by heating the skin with an ordinary infrared lamp.

REFERENCES

1. Grattan J.H.G., Singer C.: *Anglo-Saxon Magic and Medicine.* Folcroft, Pa., Folcroft Library Editions, 1952.
2. Larre D.J.: *Surgical Memoirs of Campaigns of Russia, Germany and France,* Mercer J.C. (transl.). Philadelphia, Carey & Lea, 1832, p. 293.
3. Richardson B.W.: A new and ready mode of producing local anesthesia. *Medical Times and Gazette,* Feb. 3, 1866, pp. 115–117.
4. Cooper I.S., Grissman F., Johnson R.: Complete system for cryogenic surgery. *St. Barnab. Hosp. Med. Bull.* 1:11–16, 1962.
5. Amoils S.P.: The Joule Thompson cryoprobe. *Arch. Opthalmol.* 78:201–207, 1967.
6. Lloyd J.W., Barnard J.D.W., Glynn C.J.: Cryoanalgesia: A new approach to pain relief. *Lancet* 2:932, 1976.
7. Nathan P.W., Sears T.A., Smith M.C.: Effects of phenol solutions on nerve roots of the cat: An electrophysiological and histological study. *J. Neurol. Sci.* 2:7, 1965.
8. Melzack R., Wall P.D.: Pain mechanisms: A new theory. *Science* 150:971, 1965.
9. Whittaker D.K.: *An experimental study of the effects of cryosurgery on the oral mucous membrane,* thesis. Cardiff, University of Wales, 1973.
10. Trendelenburg W.: Langdauernde Nervenausschaltung mit sicherer Regenerationsfehigkeit. *Z. Ges. Exp. Med.* 5:371, 1916–1917; 7:251, 1918–1919.
11. Blackwood W., Russell H.: Experiments on the study of immersion foot. *Edinburgh Med. J.* 50:385, 1943.
12. Denny-Brown D., Adams R.D., Brenner E., et al.: The pathology of injury to nerve induced by cold. *J. Exp. Neuropath. Exp. Neurol.* 4:305, 1945.
13. Fraser J.D., Gill W.: Observations on ultra-frozen tissue. *Br. J. Surg.* 54:770, 1967.
14. Walder H.A.D.: *J. Cryosurg.* 1:306, 1968.
15. Blund M.J.: Ischemic degeneration of nerve fibers. *Arch. Neurol.* 2:528, 1960.
16. Carter D.C., Lee P.W.R., Gill W., et al.: The effect of cryosurgery on peripheral nerve function. *J. R. Coll. Surg. Edinb.* 17:1, 1972.
17. Gilliatt R.W., Whitteridge D.: Inspiratory vaso-constriction in patients after spinal injuries. *J. Physiol.* (London) 107:68, 1948.
18. Douglas W.W., Malcome J.L.: The effect of localized

cooling on conduction in cat nerves. *J. Physiol.* 130:53, 1973.

19. Blackwood W.: Studies in the pathology of human "immersion foot." *Br. J. Surg.* 31:329, 1944.

20. Nelson K.M., Vincent R.G., Bourke R.S., et al.: Intraoperative intercostal nerve freezing to prevent postthoracotomy pain. *Ann. Thorac. Surg.* 18(3):280–285, 1974.

21. Katz J., Nelson W., Forest R., et al.: Cryoanalgesia for post-thoracotomy pain. *Lancet* 3:512–513, 1980.

22. Bernard J.D.W., Lloyd J.W., Glynn C.J.: Cryosurgery in the management of intractable facial pain. *Br. J. Oral Surg.* 16:135, 1978–79.

23. Brechner T.: Percutaneous cryogenic neurolysis of the articular nerve of Luschka. *Reg. Anaesth.* 6:18–22, 1981.

24. Fox J.L., Rizolli H.V.: Identification of radiologic coordinates for the posterior articular nerve of Luschka in the lumbar spine. *Surg. Neurol.* 1:343–346, 1973.

25. Glynn C.J., Lloyd J.W., Bernard J.D.W.: Cryoanalgesia in the management of pain after thoracotomy. *Thorax* 35:325–327, 1980.

42 / Transcutaneous Electrical Nerve Stimulation

KATHY S. JOHNSON, R.N.

ALTHOUGH THE USE of transcutaneous electrical nerve stimulation (TENS) has become widespread only in recent years, the literature reveals that stimulation for relief of pain is actually quite ancient and has been used in various forms throughout the recorded history of medicine.

The present-day use of TENS began after the 1965 publication of Melzack and Wall's landmark paper, "Pain mechanisms: A new theory."[1] Two years later, it was found that external application of electrical stimulation was effective in relieving pain prior to surgical implantation of dorsal column electrodes. This led to the practical application of TENS as we know it today.[2]

TENS has now been shown to be effective in relieving both acute and chronic pain. Its use is expanding from pain control centers to emergency rooms, operating rooms, labor rooms, hospital floors, and practitioners' offices. There is a need for health professionals to become knowledgeable about and active with this noninvasive method of analgesia. Both nurses and physical therapists have been able to apply the technique well clinically. They play a key role as TENS specialists, educating and managing such patients. With proper knowledge, equipment, electrode placement, and setting, the patient can be taught to use a TENS unit at home. This gives the patient the ability to achieve maximum and prolonged pain relief via intermittent use, making adjustments as necessary.

PROPOSED MECHANISMS OF ACTION

Several theories have been proposed to explain why TENS is an effective mode of treatment for some pain syndromes. Two theories are generally accepted: the gate control theory and the endogenous opiate theory.

According to the gate control theory, stimulation of large myelinated A alpha fibers inhibits the transmission of pain impulses carried by the smaller unmyelinated C fibers and A delta fibers. This inhibition takes place at the level of the spinal cord in the substantia gelatinosa of the dorsal horn and in the higher CNS. These large myelinated A fibers have a low threshold for electrical stimulation and are therefore easily stimulated with a TENS unit.[3]

According to the endogenous opiate theory, the body produces endogenous opiods in response to certain types of electrical stimulation.[4] Endorphins have been known to produce analgesia by occupying the opiate receptor sites.

A third theory, the frequency-dependent conduction block theory, proposes that a pain-transmitting neuron can be rendered inactive or blocked by adjusting the frequency of the impulse so that it is delivered before all the ionic channels in that neuron respond. Since no action potential is generated by the neuron, pain sensation is not felt.[5]

Other theories proposed include modification of pain perception by the stimulation of afferent nerve fibers.[6] Physiologically, with the relief of pain, most TENS units probably also increase vascularity to the area of stimulation by producing localized vasodilation.[7, 8]

The placebo effect noted with the use of TENS has been a subject of study by many researchers. Evidently the placebo effect is minimal.[9] If it occurs, it will become evident during a trial of TENS.

THE NURSE'S ROLE

Because the use of TENS is becoming so wide-spread, the nurse's knowledge of and involvement in its application have become extremely important. Regardless of whether the nurse works in a hospital or an outpatient setting, she or he is bound to care for patients needing or already using TENS.

In most institutions, the physical therapist has the responsibility of TENS therapy. However, nurses have special abilities that allow them to assess and manage overall patient needs, including TENS therapy.

During both the evaluation and the treatment period, the nurse-patient relationship is enhanced as trust is developed, contributing to the success of TENS therapy. The nurse also serves an important role as an educator. Educational programs must be developed not only for the patient and family, but also for the physicians and other nursing staff on an ongoing basis.

The nurse considers all aspects of the patient—the biologic, psychological, social, and spiritual being. The nurse has the ability to assess these needs and can also act as patient manager by integrating the psychological and the physical treatment of the patient.

Continuity of care is established, as the nurse coordinates patient care. This is true of both the outpatient and the hospital setting, and especially in postoperative units, where the nurse observes the patient around the clock. In this role, the nurse becomes a vital component of the multidisciplinary approach to management of pain.

INDICATIONS FOR THE USE OF TENS

TENS has been demonstrated to be effective in relieving both acute and chronic pain. At times TENS alone may be sufficient to modulate pain, but it is often used in conjunction with more invasive forms of therapy to maintain relaxation and pain relief. Therefore, a multidisciplinary approach is of utmost importance in caring for the pain patient.

Chronic musculoskeletal pain, peripheral nerve injuries, phantom or stump pain, arthritis, carcinoma, postherpetic neuralgia, neuroma, sciatica, and chronic pancreatitis have all responded favorably to TENS treatment.[10–12] Pain of central origin and severe neuralgias rarely respond.[10] However, even in these cases a trial of TENS should be undertaken if indicated.

TENS has been beneficial for the following types of acute pain: strains, sprains, fractures, acute herpes zoster, incisional pain, paralytic ileus, and early labor.[11, 13–15]

Pain of psychogenic origin is unresponsive and is often aggravated. Patients who have previously undergone electroconvulsive therapy may be averse to TENS, as unpleasant associations may occur.

Factors that influence the effectiveness of TENS for each patient include the following:

The patient's environmental, cultural, and ethnic background.

Motivation to learn the proper application of TENS and comply with an evaluation and treatment regimen.

Cost.

Sensation perceived.

Type of TENS unit.

Electrode placement.

Skin resistance.

Parameters/modes of stimulation.

Patient/family education.

Past experience with TENS.

To ensure patient compliance, an individualized and positive but realistic approach to the patient's pain problem is necessary. Family education should be included in the teaching program whenever possible.

GOALS OF TENS THERAPY

The goals of TENS therapy as a single modality or in conjunction with other modalities are three-fold: a 50% increase in pain relief, a 50% increase in function, and a 50% decrease in pain medication. These results have been obtained in numerous studies and surveys conducted on both acute and chronic pain patients.[10, 11, 13, 16, 17]

EQUIPMENT

Units

At least 30 companies are manufacturing TENS units. Units may differ in size, shape, weight, durability, wave forms, ranges of parameters, modes and quality of stimulation, and number of control knobs (Fig 42–1). One should know not only the indications for the use of TENS, but also the quality and efficiency of the particular TENS unit prescribed. These considerations are imperative in organizing a TENS program.

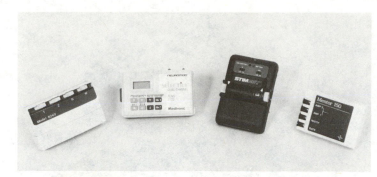

Fig 42–1.—Some examples of TENS units with varying modalities. *Left to right:* Tenzcare, Selectra, Stimset, and Mentor 150. (Courtesy of 3M Medical Products Division, St. Paul; Medtronic, Inc., Minneapolis; Codman & Shurtleff, Inc., Randolph, Massachusetts; and Mentor Corp., Minneapolis.)

Selection of the unit is individualized and based on a thorough TENS evaluation. For example, younger patients with a complicated pain problem may achieve best results with a unit that can deliver a spike or square wave and one that offers a selection for a variety of modes of stimulation such as conventional, burst, or modulation to match activity of different qualities of pain. In contrast, an elderly patient may achieve very good results with a unit that has preset parameters and can be easily used with minimum adjustment.

Wave Forms

Wave forms of TENS units are of two types, rectangular and spike. The rectangular wave form unit can be adjusted for amplitude and pulse width. The spike wave form unit has a fixed width and allows adjustments of amplitude only. These wave forms can be delivered as a monophasic (direct current) or a biphasic (alternating current). Direct current is not generally used in TENS as it can drive ions into the skin (ionotophoresis), leading to skin irritation and electrode decomposition.[18] With alternating current, the ions flow first in one direction, then in the opposite direction. This allows the electrolysis to be minimal and prevents skin irritation and electrode decomposition.

The biphasic alternating current has two phases, a dominant phase and a balancing phase. The dominant phase (active phase) has a greater amplitude and shorter pulse width. The current flows from the negative electrode to the positive electrode. In contrast, in the balancing phase, the current flows from the positive to the negative electrode. As neurons tend to depolarize more readily with the negative current, it is important that the TENS specialist be aware of the direction of the current. This allows more effective current flow into a special target area such as a trigger point.[18]

Electrodes

There are many types of electrodes. The choice of electrode must be individualized according to the age of the patient, area of pain, activity level, skin sensitivity, and assistance at home. Larger electrodes often require a higher pulse charge (width plus amplitude) to produce the same stimulation. Electrodes can be of the disposable or nondisposable type. Many nondisposable electrodes require the use of gel and tape.

Nondisposable Electrodes

Most nondisposable electrodes are made of carbonized silicone rubber (Fig 42–2). Carbon is very effective in the transmission of current. An aquaphilic gel is used to overcome skin resistance and to facilitate current transmission from the electrode.[12] This gel is evenly spread across the electrode to cover all edges. Failure to spread the gel evenly may result in a skin burn. After each use, these electrodes are easily cleaned with soap and water.

A major advantage of the nondisposable electrodes is that excellent skin contact can be achieved with proper taping. Current is evenly distributed over the skin area beneath the electrode. The taping also helps prevent the electrode from being pulled off by tight-fitting clothing. This is a consideration in selection for a very active person. Disadvantages include the time and manual dexterity needed to apply the gel and tape. Because motivation plays an important part in success with TENS, ease of application must be considered.

An allergic reaction producing contact dermatitis can result, usually from the tape. Hypoallergenic tape, gel, and electrodes (e.g., the karaya electrode) are available for those with sensitive skin.

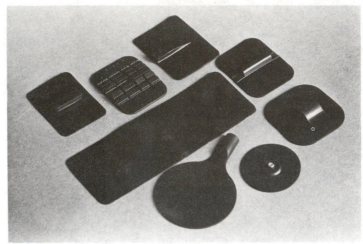

Fig 42–2.—Various nondisposable electrodes currently in use.

Disposable Electrodes

Pregelled disposable electrodes come in many styles and material (Fig 42–3). Many of these are reusable and can be used for 10–15 applications, others are used once and discarded. Some can be worn for up to 3 days by patients with no skin problems. Their main advantages are easy and quick application due to their self-adhering quality. The major complaints reported by patients using some of these disposable electrodes are that clothing easily pulls them off and they sometimes "fall apart," with the gel separating from the pad, especially during hot weather. Again, allergic reaction to these electrodes can occur, but is seen less frequently. Because cost is an important factor, some suppliers suggest that it is more economical to use disposable electrodes for multiple applications. To help assure adherence with any electrode, the skin should be cleansed prior to application. Tincture of benzoin or a thin layer of egg white can be applied to enhance adhesion.

ELECTRODE PLACEMENT

The choice of electrode site is a very important factor in the success of TENS. Sites are based on anatomy and physiology and depend on an awareness of the etiology, location, and character of the pain. Thus, thorough initial assessment and evaluation is extremely important, requiring time and patience.

In TENS, electrodes are placed on the skin di-

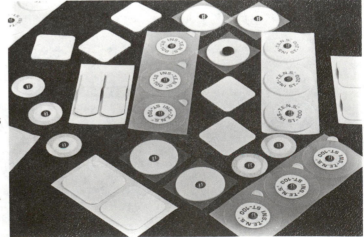

Fig 42–3.—Various disposable electrodes currently in use.

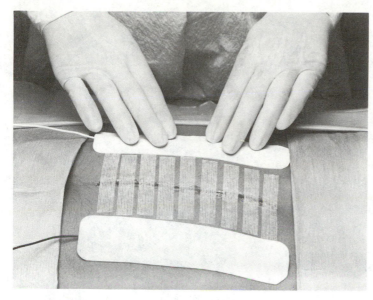

Fig 42–5.—Electrodes placed parallel to the incision. Electrodes should be placed in sterile fashion at the completion of surgery and should be part of the dressing of the incision. (Courtesy of 3M Medical Products Division, St. Paul.)

rectly over the area of pain (usually trigger points), within the dermatome where the pain is located, over myotomes, and over superficial peripheral nerves. Acupuncture points and motor points may also be used. These terms are defined in the following section. Mannheimer believes an optimal stimulation site requires that at least two of these entities exist at the same location.[19] There are a multitude of anatomical sites where more than one can be found (Fig 42–4, Plate 15).

Area of Pain

Electrodes are often placed over or surrounding an area of pain. These sites often lie within a dermatome or over a peripheral nerve. A very good example of this is postoperative incisional pain or an old incisional scar (Fig 42–5). Sterile electrodes are placed as close to the incision as possible, within about 1–6 cm of it. The electrode from each channel is then placed parallel to the incision, crossing over the incision or crisscrossing the incision. Another example is placement with upper back pain (Fig 42–6).

Dermatome Placement

A dermatome is a cutaneous region innervated by a particular spinal nerve through both of its rami.[20] A dermatome chart can be a useful tool in identify-

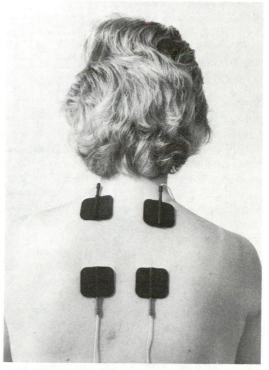

Fig 42–6.—Example of electrode placement for a patient with paravertebral pain in the upper back. The positive and negative electrodes could be placed ipsilaterally or in crisscross fashion.

ing these areas and also a good teaching aid for the patient. However, dermatome charts vary, as some dermatomes may overlap. Electrodes are placed in the area of pain going proximally along the dermatome to the spinal column. The use of dermatomes is very effective in areas of the trunk affecting the afferant nerve fibres.

As an example, a patient may complain of low back pain radiating down the posterior aspect of the right leg to the knee (Fig 42–7; see also Fig 42–4). After evaluation one may find the pain in the S-1 dermatome. After referral to a dermatome chart, the first channel may be placed at the posterior aspect of the thigh. Following the dermatome proximally, the second channel may be placed as near the vertebral column as the S-1 nerve exists. This method of selection is advantageous in that electrode sites can be easily rotated, thus decreasing the chance of skin irritation while still obtaining therapeutic results.

Myotome Placement

A myotome is a muscle group innervated by a single spinal segment. Effective electrode placement along a myotome can also be determined by referring to a chart.

Superficial Peripheral Nerve Placement

Peripheral nerves often become very superficial and are thus very good areas for electrode placement. It is beneficial in extremity pain distal to these nerves. For example, positioning over the common peroneal nerve as it crosses just below the head of the fibula is good for distal leg and foot pain. Placing electrodes over the supraorbital and infraorbital nerves can be effective in some facial pains (Fig 42–8).[12] In patients with headache, electrodes may be placed unilaterally over the supraorbital and superior occipital nerves.

Depending on electrode placement, stimulation of a peripheral nerve will also stimulate one or more dermatomes.[19] Distinguishing between the pain from a peripheral nerve injury and the pain from a nerve root lesion is important when choosing electrode sites. Electrodes should be placed proximal to the nerve injury. Placement distal to the nerve injury may result in a block of the input from the TENS unit and in increased pain.[19, 21, 22]

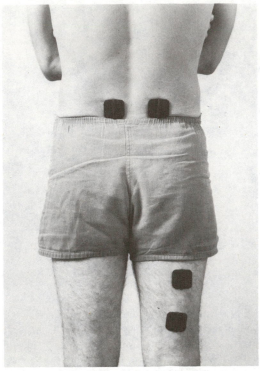

Fig 42–7.—Electrode placement for low back pain radiating to the posterior aspect of the right thigh. Electrode placement is based on the nerve distribution (sciatic nerve).

Acupuncture Point and Motor Point Placement

Acupuncture and motor points are sometimes chosen for electrode placement. These areas can be found by referring to appropriate charts (see Fig 42–4). Many acupuncture points are located over superficial branches of peripheral nerves,[23] which are particularly good locations. A motor point is the point at which a nerve enters the muscle. Both acupuncture and motor points may be effective areas for placement as they may be located on areas of lower skin resistance and higher density input to the CNS.[24]

Other Areas for Electrode Placement

Bilateral stimulation is extremely beneficial and can be used for unilateral pain conditions.[19] There can be a contralateral transmission from afferent nerves activated unilaterally by the TENS device.[25]

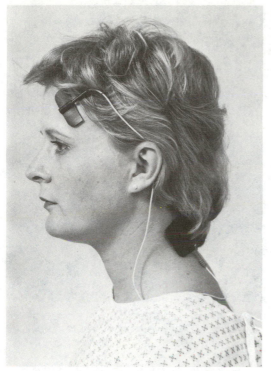

Fig 42–8.—Electrode placement over superficial peripheral nerves (supraorbital, supratrochlear nerves) and over the muscle configuration (trapezius) for tension headache.

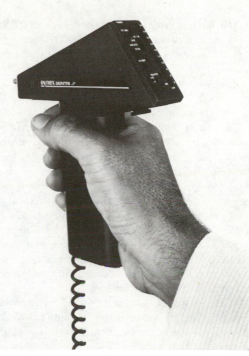

Fig 42–9.—A conductivity sensor probe used to determine electrode sites by locating areas of epidermal hyperconductivity. (Courtesy of LaJolla Technology, San Diego, California.)

This is very effective in the treatment of back pain.

If for some reason the painful region cannot be stimulated, for example because of a sensory problem, stimulation of the contralateral peripheral nerve or dermatome may be effective.[21, 26] This may be explained by reflex crossing at the spinal cord level[27] or between the cerebral hemispheres.[25, 28]

In some institutions a conductivity sensor probe is utilized to find sites for electrode placements (Fig 42–9). The purpose of this probe is to provide an accurate means of measuring epidermal hyperconductivity or areas of lowest resistance relative to surrounding tissue areas. If one uses these hyperconductive regions as sites for TENS electrode placement, the power dissipated by the underlying tissue is minimized.[29] The general regions where TENS therapy needs to be applied should be identified by routine methods of examination and diagnosis. The conductivity probe can then be used to pinpoint the optimal sites for electrode placement within proposed regions.[29]

When this particular sensor probe is used, the tip of the unit should be placed lightly on the skin in the selected region and the calibration button pushed. Pushing the calibration button causes the probe to measure the skin resistance at that point. After calibration, the probe tip should be lightly moved across the selected area; the skin resistance relative to the calibration point will be continually displayed. Any point that is clearly 40%–50% lower in resistance than surrounding tissue is the preferred electrode site.[29]

Areas to Avoid for Electrode Placement

Areas of insensitivity or hyperesthesia should be avoided in electrode placement.[10] Also, placement over bony prominences and hair-covered areas is not advisable because of the decrease in skin contact.

WAVE FORM PARAMETERS

The three parameters of current used in TENS units are rate, width, and amplitude. The rate regulates the number of electrical impulses delivered per second (pps). This can range from 2 to 200 pps and is most commonly 2–150 pps. The pulse width determines the duration of each impulse. It can be calibrated from 0 to 500 μsec, but a range of 50–250 μsec is most often used. The pulse width may be controlled by a separate dial or may be incorporated in the rate or amplitude control. The amplitude is the height of the pulse wave measured in milliamperes (mA). As the amplitude is increased, the height of the wave is increased. Most TENS units have two channels with amplitudes independent of each other. The total electrical energy (intensity) per pulse is determined by the amplitude and pulse width. Body weight, interelectrode distance, and the number of electrodes aid in determining the proper adjustment of these two settings.[30]

Various adjustments of these settings produce different sensations and can stimulate different nerve fibers as required for the particular pain problem under treatment.

MODES OF STIMULATION

Various control settings can be selected in TENS therapy. These include (1) the conventional mode, (2) a low rate, high width mode (acupuncture), (3) a burst mode, (4) a brief, intense mode, and (5) the modulation mode. Selection must be individualized for each patient and his pain problem to obtain optimal results with TENS therapy.

Conventional TENS Mode

The conventional mode is most frequently used (Fig 42–10). It has a wide range of effectiveness for acute and chronic pain. With this technique a high rate (> 10 pps, usually 80–100 pps) and low width (< 100 μsec) are used. Amplitude is set for comfort. To obtain best results with the conventional mode, the electrode placement should produce a tingling sensation throughout most of the pain distribution area. Stimulation occurs at the cutaneous level, affecting the sensory A alpha and A beta fibers.[30] This low-intensity mode of TENS acts pri-

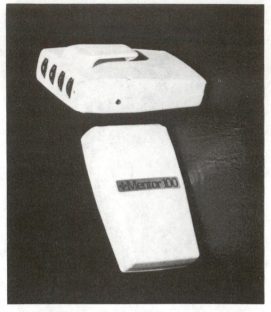

Fig 42–10.—Mentor 100 unit capable of delivering a conventional mode of TENS. (Courtesy of Mentor Corp., Minneapolis.)

marily according to the principles of the gate control theory.[31]

The following modes of TENS therapy are high-intensity forms of stimulation and are usually applied for shorter periods of time. Though these settings may be slightly uncomfortable themselves, antidromic inhibitory activity in the brain stem is triggered, thus blocking transmission of more powerful pain stimuli arising from other areas.[31] These settings are usually used for 15–45 minutes at most and only during acute flareups of chronic pain, for acute pain problems, or during painful procedures.

High Width, Low Rate (Acupuncture-like TENS) Mode

This setting is often the second mode of choice and is very effective for deep, aching chronic pain.[30] It is useful when previous nerve damage has occurred.[18] This mode stimulates the cutaneous, subcutaneous, and deep nerve fibers. A high width is used along with a low rate (< 10 pps, usually 2–4 pps) (Fig 42–11). The amplitude is adjusted to the point where muscle contraction is seen. Studies have shown that acupuncture-like TENS activates the production of endorphins.[4]

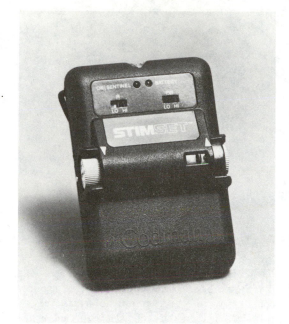

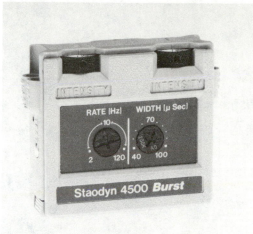

Fig 42–12.—Staodyn 4500 burst TENS unit capable of delivering a burst mode. (Courtesy of Staodyne, Longmont, Colorado.)

Fig 42–11.—Stimset TENS unit capable of delivering low-rate TENS. (Courtesy of Codman & Shurtleff, Inc., Randolph, Massachusetts.)

Burst Mode

Many TENS units have a burst component, a form of low-rate TENS (Fig 42–12). This is usually on the dial that regulates the rate. In this mode, a series or train of impulses (usually seven) occurring at a rate of 100 pps are delivered in bursts of two to four per second. Amplitude and pulse width vary but are usually high.[5] The burst mode can be used for acute, superficial pain with a low intensity or for chronic, deep pain with a high intensity. As used in the latter condition, the burst mode produces strong muscle contractions. It is usually more comfortable and often more effective than the single-pulsed low rate.

Brief Intense (High Rate, High Width, High Amplitude) Mode

This mode is best used during therapeutic procedures, for example joint mobilization, or when immediate pain relief is desired. The unit is adjusted to the above settings, with the pulse width greater than 200 μsec and the rate greater than 150 pps (Fig

42–13). The amplitude is adjusted to the highest level tolerated by the patient with muscle contraction or fasciculations. This mode stimulates the cutaneous and subcutaneous nerve fibers.

Modulation Mode

The modulation mode (Fig 42–14) is provided by a separate component in newer TENS units and is used in conjunction with the previous modes. In this mode the amplitude width, rate, or a combination are modulated, depending on the unit. For example, the width and rate alternate between low rate, high width and high rate, low width. This setting is unique in that the treatment alternates between superficial and deep stimulation. Some clinicians believe this setting may prevent adaptation to TENS.[18]

The duration of pain relief with TENS varies from the treatment time itself to several hours. Patients should have some relief of pain within 15–20 minutes after the unit is applied. If no relief is seen, a different setting, unit, or electrode placement should be tried. Evaluating the patient for a TENS unit requires much time and patience.

SIDE EFFECT AND CAUTIONS

Side effects from TENS, though minimal, include skin irritation and electrical burns.

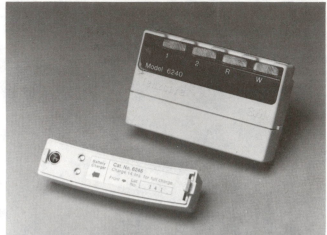

Fig 42–13.—Tenzcare TENS unit capable of delivering a brief intense mode. (Courtesy of 3M Medical Products Division, St. Paul.)

SKIN IRRITATION.—Units with a monophasic direct current may contribute more to skin irritation, especially at one electrode site (depending on the polarity). Therefore, positive/negative electrode sites should be rotated. With biphasic alternating current units this is usually not a problem. Skin ir-

ritation can also be avoided by good skin care. The skin should be cleansed prior to and after application. It may be necessary to try different types of electrodes, gel, and tape. If redness appears, application of an antacid to the area is often adequate. For a more serious skin reaction, the patient should seek a physician's opinion.

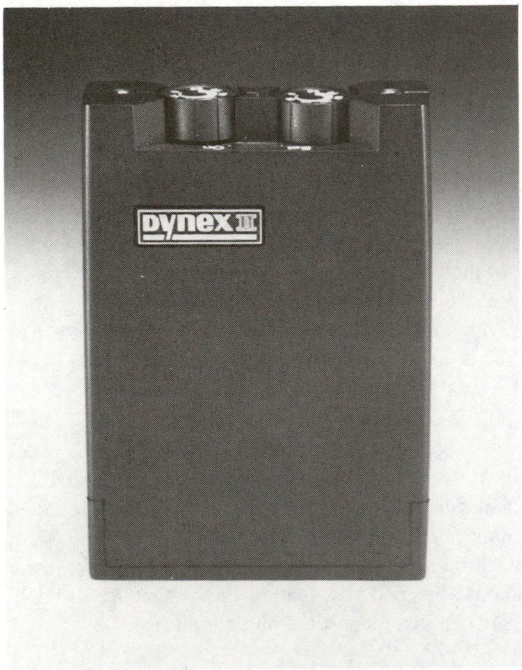

ELECTRICAL BURNS.—Electrical burns are rare. They can be prevented by using the proper amount of gel, covering the entire electrode surface, and making sure there are no bare wires.

No harmful side effects have been seen, but there are no scientific data to ascertain the safety of TENS at the following sites or with the following conditions: during pregnancy, in patients with cardiac pacemakers (especially demand type) or other internal electronic device, over the carotid sinuses, larynx, or trachea, or around the eye.[32] Some physicians object to the use of TENS over a malignant site, but others believe it will not increase the chances of metastasis.

Interference with an ECG monitor has been reported, along with interference on a fetal heart monitor when TENS was used during labor. Patients are advised to turn their units off while operating a microwave oven. With surgical implantation, electrodes should not be placed directly over the metal, as the metal may act as a conductor.[33] TENS units should be used with caution in an explosive environment. This may be an important consideration when using a TENS unit on a patient receiving oxygen.

Fig 42–14.—Dynex II TENS unit capable of providing a modulation mode. (Courtesy of LaJolla Technology, Inc., LaJolla, California.)

EXAMPLES OF APPLICATION AND ELECTRODE PLACEMENT

Acute Pain

Postoperative Pain

TENS can be extremely helpful in managing postoperative pain. The pain-free surgical patient is able to ambulate sooner and to cough more effectively, which decreases the chance of postoperative morbidity. For effective treatment, nurses should demonstrate TENS to the patient preoperatively, teaching its use and noting the settings comfortable to the patient. An important goal is for the patients to be in control of their own pain management. The orientation to the TENS unit will aid in achieving this goal.

A TENS unit that utilizes a wide range of parameters is preferred, as no single setting has been established to be effective for all postoperative patients. However, conventional TENS is often chosen.[33]

Electrodes should be sterile, hypoallergenic, adaptable to most incision lengths, and usable for 3–5 days.[33] One pair of electrodes can be placed parallel and as close as possible to the incision (1–6 cm) before the dressing is applied in the operating room (see Fig 42–5). The other pair can be placed following the appropriate dermatome paravertebrally. If the incision is longer than the electrode, the electrodes are placed nearer the proximal end of the incision.

The TENS unit should be turned on in the recovery room to the settings found comfortable during the preoperative session. The settings are adjusted as necessary when the patient is alert.[33] The unit is usually left on continuously during the first 24–48 hours postoperatively. After 48 hours, it can be used as required. The nurse should assure the patient that other modalities of postoperative analgesia are still available for them to use.

Labor Pain

As TENS has been demonstrated to be beneficial in various forms of acute pain, its use during labor and delivery has been investigated in recent years. It is most helpful during the early stages of labor.[15]

Electrodes are placed paravertebrally at the level of T10–L1 and S2–4 bilaterally (Fig 42–15). The intensity of the settings is increased as labor progresses. TENS has major advantages over other forms of analgesia in that it is noninvasive and is safe for the mother and the baby.[13] However, interference on the fetal heart monitor from the TENS unit has been reported.

Chronic Pain

TENS is an extremely important modality in the multidisciplinary approach to the chronic pain patient. With proper teaching, the patient can utilize various settings and modes as the need arises to control pain.

After a thorough assessment of the pain problem, proper electrode placement is determined. Conventional TENS is the mode most frequently used. Patients are usually instructed to use this setting for 2 hours on, 1 hour off, and off at bedtime, on a regular schedule. Not only does the skin need the 1-hour rest period, but the patient needs the rest to avoid building a tolerance to the unit with long-term use, as we see in our chronic pain patients. The prescribed schedule and settings may be modified over the course of treatment to accommodate the varying

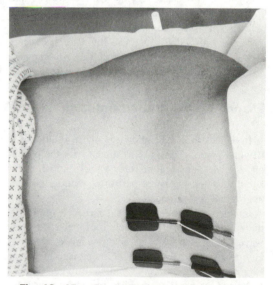

Fig 42–15.—Electrode placement for relief of pain during the first stage of labor. Electrodes are placed paravertebrally to cover the T-10, L-1, and S-2, S-4 dermatomes.

analgesia needs of the individual patient. For example, during an acute flare-up of the pain problem, the patient is taught to use a high-intensity mode such as the burst mode for 15–45 minutes. The length of time a chronic pain patient uses TENS varies, but often after approximately 1–6 months the patient can gradually be weaned off the unit, using it only on an as-needed basis.

TENS EVALUATION AND TRIAL

Assessment

Evaluation of the effectiveness of a TENS unit for each patient requires time and patience by both the nurse and the patient. The nurse should inform patients of the need for several trials before adequate and consistent relief is obtained, and should be prepared to support patients through this difficult period with adequate individualized teaching and encouragement. These interventions are vital to achieving the levels of patient participation and compliance required to make TENS therapy successful.

A minimum of three 1-hour sessions are necessary. Family members are encouraged to attend. During the first session a thorough evaluation that includes a physical examination and psychological assessment is necessary. This will aid in determining the patient's willingness and ability to learn and will also measure compliance. The patient's past experience with TENS may also influence his acceptance of a new trial. The goals of TENS therapy are stressed along with the benefits of self care.

Planning and Implementation

In the sessions that follow, the nurse should identify and plan the goals of treatment with the patient and family. Stressing the role of TENS in pain management as an integratal part of a multidisciplinary approach is essential.

Instructions are given on the theory of TENS therapy, along with the selection of electrode sites, wave forms, settings of parameters, mode selection, and proper times for use. The importance of proper skin care is emphasized. A simple form can be used to document sessions to aid in providing consistent continuity of care (Appendix 1 to this chapter).

Relief of pain should occur within 15–20 minutes after the unit is applied. If no relief is seen, a different setting, unit, or electrode placement is tried.

Evaluation

If the staff or the patient feels there has been no benefit from this modality, or the pain has been aggravated by it, TENS is discontinued. If there appears to be some relief of discomfort and pain, even if only for the time the unit is applied, the patient is given written instructions on the proper use of the device to reinforce what has been taught throughout the trial period (Appendix 2 to this chapter). A prescription for a 1-month trial on a rental basis is given and the patient is referred to a recommended, reliable supplier. The patient is reassured of the resources available for solving problems, including the physician, nurse, and supplier. Asking the patient to keep a pain relief log can be very helpful when he or she returns for reevaluation.

At the end of 1 month the patient is reevaluated. The impact of TENS on pain relief during daily activities can be established by asking the following questions:

What percentage of the pain has been relieved?

Is there an increase in activity?

Has there been a decrease in the amount of pain medication required? If so, how much?

The patients knowledge of how to use the unit is also assessed, including the ability to use alternative electrode placement, settings, modes, and duration of treatment to modify care as the need arises. Troubleshooting can also be done at this time. This may involve problems the patient is having with the equipment itself (e,.g., batteries, wires, electrodes, gel, tape, unit), or problems with settings, electrode placement, or skin irritation. The supplier is often very helpful with mechanical difficulties.

A follow-up system with the patient returning in 3 months, 6 months, and 1 year is encouraged. This is beneficial not only in assessing the amount of pain relief and troubleshooting for the patient, but also for gathering statistics, maintaining quality assurance, and evaluating units and suppliers.

REFERENCES

1. Melzack R., Wall P.: Pain mechanisms: A new theory. *Science* 150:971, 1965.
2. Shealy C.: Transcutaneous electroanalgesia. *Surg. Forum* 23:419–421, 1972.
3. Bloedel J., McCreery D.: Organization of peripheral and central pain pathways. *Surg. Neurol.* 4:65, 1975.
4. Sjolund B., Eriksson M.: Endorphins and analgesia produced by peripheral conditioning stimulation; in Bonica J.J., et al. (eds.): *Advances in Pain Research*

and Therapy. New York, Raven Press, 1979, vol. 3, pp. 587–591.

5. 3M:TENS: *How it works and when to use it*. St. Paul, Minnesota, 3M Corporation, 1983.

6. Long D., Carolan M.: Cutaneous afferent stimulation in the treatment of chronic pain. *Adv. Neurol.* 4:755–759, 1974.

7. McCaffery M.: Cutaneous stimulation, in *Nursing Management of the Patient With Pain*, ed. 2. Philadelphia, J.B. Lippincott Co., 1979, pp. 116–136.

8. Gilula M., Markovich S.: Holistic electrosleep: An electrophysiological equivalent of meditation of deep muscular relaxation. Paper presented at the Conference on Pain Management, Des Plaines, Ill., May 14–15, 1977.

9. Long D.: Cutaneous afferent stimulation for relief of chronic pain. *Congr. Neurol. Surg.* 21:257–268, 1974.

10. Long D.: The comparative efficacy of drugs vs. electrical modulation in the management of chronic pain, in LeRoy P.L. (ed.): *Current Concepts in the Management of Chronic Pain*. Chicago, Year Book Medical Publishers, 1977, pp. 53–71.

11. Shealy C.N.: Transcutaneous electrical stimulation for control of pain. *Clin. Neurosurg.* 21:269–277, 1974.

12. McDonnel D.: TENS in treating chronic pain. *AORN J.* 32:401–410, 1980.

13. Hymes A., et al.: Electrical surface stimulation for treatment and prevention of ileus and atelectasis. *Surg. Forum* 25:222–224, 1974.

14. Pike P.: Transcutaneous electrical stimulation. *Anesthesia* 33:165–171, 1978.

15. Stewart P.: Transcutaneous nerve stimulation as a method of analgesia in labour. *Anaesthesia* 34:361–364, 1979.

16. Doughterty R.: Transcutaneous electrical nerve stimulation: An alternative to drugs in the treatment of chronic pain. American Pain Society Conference, 1979.

17. Howell J.: Unpublished survey. University Hospital, Cincinnati, Ohio, 1983.

18. 3M:*TENS stimulators: Basic terms and features,* inservice slide presentation. St. Paul, Minnesota, 3M Corporation, 1983.

19. Mannheimer J.: Electrode placements for transcutaneous electrical nerve stimulation. *Phy. Ther.* 58:1455–1462, 1975.

20. Warwick R., Williams P.: *Gray's Anatomy,* ed. 35. Philadelphia, W.B. Saunders Co., 1973, pp. 1062–1064.

21. Long D.: Electrical stimulation for relief of pain from chronic nerve injury. *J. Neurosurg.* 39:718–722, 1973.

22. Meyer G., Fields H.: Causalgia treated by selective large fiber stimulation of peripheral nerves. *Brain* 95:163–168, 1972.

23. Gunn C., et al.: Acupuncture loci: A proposal for their classification according to their relationship to known neural structures. *Am. J. Clin. Med.* 4:183–195, 1976.

24. Roppel R., Mitchel F.: Skin points of anomalously low electrical resistance: Current voltage characteristics and relationship to peripheral stimulation therapies. *J. AOA* 74:877–878, 1975.

25. Picanza J., et al.: Pain suppression by peripheral nerve stimulation: Part I. Observation with transcutaneous stimuli. *Surg. Neurol.* 4:105–114, 1975.

26. Goodgold J.: *Anatomical Correlates of Clinical Electromyography*. Baltimore, Williams & Wilkens Co., 1974, pp. 57–151.

27. Sherrington C.: *Integrative Action of the Nervous System*. New Haven, Yale University Press, 1947.

28. Tien H.: Neurogenic interference theory of acupuncture anesthesia. *Am. J. Clin. Med.* 1:108–122, 1973.

29. La Jolla Technology: *Dynex sentri epidermal conductivity sensor*. La Jolla, 1983.

30. Biostim: *The theory of pain and the role of biostimulation*. Book 1. Princeton, Biostim, Inc., 1983, pp. 1–40.

31. Hachen H.: Psychological, neurophysiological, and therapeutic aspects of chronic pain: preliminary results with transcutaneous electrical stimulation. *Paraplegia* 15:353–367, 1977–1978.

32. FDA's Advisory Panel on Review of Neurological Devices: *Report on transcutaneous electrical nerve stimulation for pain relief*. Washington, D.C., FDA, 1976.

33. 3M: *TENS: The path to pain control. Managing postoperative pain with TENS,* in-service slide presentation. St. Paul, Minnesota, 3M Corporation, 1983.

Appendix 1

NURSING EVALUATION SHEET FOR TENS

Supplier: _____

Visit No.: _____

Unit:

Selectra _____   Orion _____   Stimburst _____

Comfort Wave _____   Staodyne _____   Tenzcare _____

Mentor _____   Spec II _____   Stimset _____

Dynex II _____   Epix _____   Other _____

Settings:

Continuous _____   Burst _____   Modulation _____   PW _____   Rate _____

Length of treatment: _____   *Instructions*

Quality of relief (%) _____   Dermatome theory & chart: _____

30-day trial: _____   Electrode placement: _____

Purchase: _____   Skin care: _____

Type of electrodes: _____   Dial settings: _____

RTC: _____   Theories: _____

Worker's Compensation: _____Yes _____No

Dates seen: _____   _____   _____   _____

Follow up: _____   _____   _____   _____

Comments: _____

_____

_____

_____ R.N.

_____ M.D.

Appendix 2

TENS INSTRUCTION SHEET UNIVERSITY OF CINCINNATI PAIN CONTROL CENTER

Skin Care

Remove electrodes at night. Wash skin well with soap and water. Dry, then apply lotion to the skin.

Do not leave machine on for longer than 2 hours at a time. Turn off for at least 1 hour in between "on" times to avoid muscle spasm and skin irritation.

Observe for signs of skin irritation:
Redness
Burning
Blisters
Rash
Swelling
Weeping
Itching
If skin irritation occurs:
1. Be sure you are not leaving the machine "on" longer than instructed.
2. Be sure the electrodes are left off the skin at least 6–8 hours or more every 24 hours.
3. Keep the area clean. If skin is only reddened, apply Maalox or Mylanta to reddened areas and move the electrodes to another site within your dermatome area.
4. If you develop a rash or open area on the skin, do not use your TENS unit until you have contacted your primary nurse.
5. If the electrode does not stick well, try applying a thin coat of raw egg white or Tincture of Benzoin liquid to the skin prior to placing the electrode on the skin. Tincture of Benzoin can be purchased over the counter at your drugstore.
6. If the wires you are using have pins to attach to the electrodes, make sure the pin is pushed completely in the electrode. Skin irritation can occur if the pin touches your skin when the unit is on. Take care not to bend wires sharply.

Electrode Care

If reusable/disposable electrodes are used, a small *amount of water on the electrode prior* to placing it on your skin is recommended. *DO NOT WASH DISPOSABLE ELECTRODES.*

If black reusable electrodes are used which require gel and tape for application to the skin, wash these daily with soap and water.

If the electrodes seem worn or crumbly, please call your supplier.

Electrode Placement

First, decide where to put the electrodes. If the painful area to be treated is very small, only two electrodes are necessary. If the area is larger, four or eight electrodes may be necessary.

The electrodes may be placed over the most tender points or along a dermatome pathway. Refer to your dermatome chart regarding electrode placement.

Equipment Care

Read your manual carefully before you operate your equipment at home.

If you have any problems with the equipment, please call your supplier.

Dial Settings

Your primary nurse will review with you the dial settings for the particular TENS unit found to be most helpful for your pain problem.

797

Usually, you need to preset the rate and pulse width on your unit. Then adjust the amps or channels to a comfortable level.

Your primary nurse has determined the following settings to be used at home:

Rate: _____
Pulse width: _____
Channel 1: _____
Channel 2: _____

Other notations to be made by the primary nurse:

_____

_____

Cautions

Do not place electrodes on or near eyes.

Do not place electrodes over the front or side of your neck.

If you have a pacemaker, do not use a TENS unit without your doctor's approval.

Wire Leads

Placement:

Do not place electrodes over a pregnant uterus.

Use TENS with caution if you are operating equipment or a moving vehicle.

Do not let anyone else use your TENS unit.

Using Your TENS

The machine should always be off when you are applying or removing electrodes, or when dial settings are changed.

Depending on the type of electrode used (disposable or reusable), place the electrode on the skin, attach the wires to the electrodes and then to the machine. NOTE: *Electrodes may be attached to the wires before applying to skin.* Your primary nurse will discuss with you the type of electrode you will be using—disposable or reusable.

Adjust dials to desired setting.

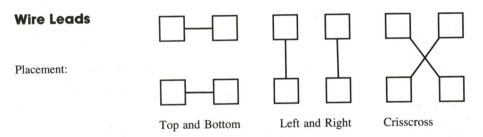

Top and Bottom   Left and Right   Crisscross

Again, should you have any questions, please call your primary nurse at the Pain Control Center.

43 / Acupuncture

P. PRITHVI RAJ, M.D.

THE TERM ACUPUNCTURE (acus = needle, puncture = puncture) is a European term coined in 1863 by the Dutch physician Willem Ten Rhyne, who introduced acupuncture to Europe. The oldest known book on acupuncture, the Nei Ching Suwen (The Yellow Emperor's Classic of Internal Disease), was probably written about the second or third century B.C. The practice of acupuncture must have been in existence for a considerable time.

Acupuncture is a traditional form of Chinese medicine and consists of inserting fine needles to the depth of a few millimeters at strategic points on the skin, known as acupuncture points. The acupuncture points are connected to each other by meridians. There are 14 meridians, of which two are unpaired and 12 are paired. Each meridian is classified as being either Yin or Yang and is further classified as belonging to one of the five elements. Thus, the Liver meridian is Yin and belongs to the element wood. Each meridian has a point on it corresponding to each of the five elements (Fig 43–1).

The acupuncture points are divided into six main classes: tonifying points, sedating points, source points, alarm points, associated points, and luo points. Their relations with each other are governed by three main laws: the "husband-wife," "mother-son," and "midnight-midday" laws.

The Chinese considered certain laws as basic to all their art, literature, philosophy and medicine. The most important are the principle of opposites and the law of the five elements. They divided the world into five elements, and all that existed was considered to belong to one or several of these elements. The elements were wood, fire, earth, metal, and water.

They believed there existed a dynamic balance of two opposing forces, Yin and Yang. When these forces were in harmony, all was well; if they became unbalanced, disease would result.

Yang is male, dominant and active; Yin is female, passive and restful. Hypertension, anxiety, and headaches are Yang diseases, whereas Yin is associated with conditions such as depression, lethargy, and obesity. Yin disease is treated by stimulating Yang, and vice versa. In modern terms Yang can be equated with the sympathetic division of the autonomic nervous system and Yin with the parasympathetic division.

THE ACUPUNCTURE POINT

Attempts at describing acupuncture points as anatomical entities have so far been less than convincing. These points have a functional electrical existence in that they are sites of low resistance and therefore high conductivity.[1] They are best detected by using a skin resistance meter. This meter lights an indicator bulb when the probe is placed on an area of low skin resistance. Melzack et al.[2] hypothesize that trigger points and acupuncture points for pain represent the same phenomenon. This does not appear to be likely, as trigger points have a physical existence whereas acupuncture points do not.

The most effective acupuncture points are often located where nerves enter muscle.[3] In classic Chinese acupuncture, points were recognized as having a rapid effect when stimulated on a point on the same meridian. Effective acupuncture can be practiced using the points alone.

Nakatani and Yamashita[4] state that the reason acupuncture points have low resistance is due to increased local sympathetic tone. This is supported by Wooley-Hart,[5] who found a direct connection between skin conductivity and local microcirculation.

799

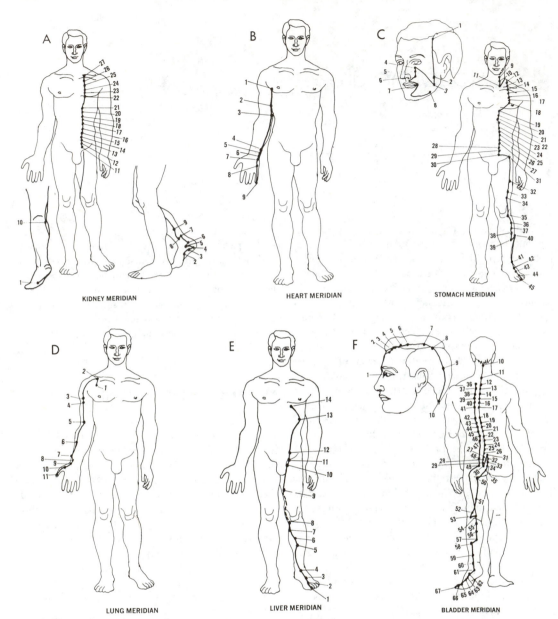

Fig 43–1.—The 14 acupuncture meridians. For a list of the acupuncture points (indicated by numbers), see Appendix 2 to this chapter. (From Duke M.: *Acupuncture: The Meridians of Ch'i.* New York, Pyramid House, 1972. Reproduced by permission.)

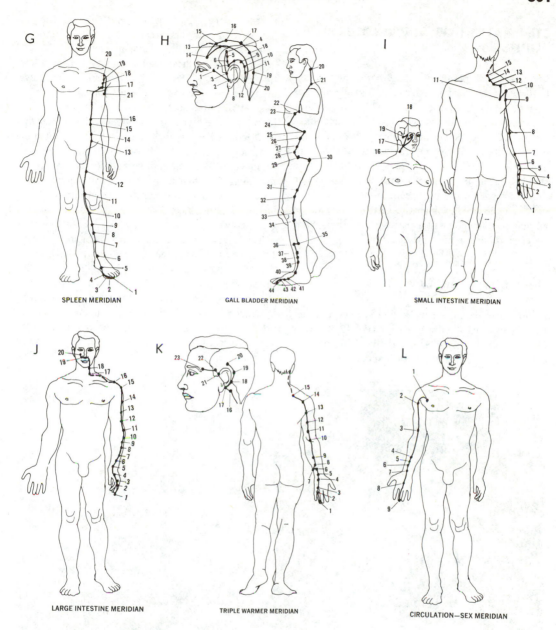

SPLEEN MERIDIAN

GALL BLADDER MERIDIAN

SMALL INTESTINE MERIDIAN

LARGE INTESTINE MERIDIAN

TRIPLE WARMER MERIDIAN

CIRCULATION—SEX MERIDIAN

STIMULATION OF ACUPUNCTURE POINTS

Acupuncture points are most commonly stimulated using solid stainless steel 30-gauge needles (Fig 43–2). I have used 30- or 32-gauge hollow stainless steel disposable needles and found them just as effective. Silver and gold needles are sometimes used. There are no convincing data to show that silver or gold needles are more effective than stainless steel. It is probable that polarity plays an important part in the therapeutic effect of acupuncture.[6, 7] Gold needles appear to shift the potential of an acupuncture point in a positive direction, while silver shifts it in a negative direction.[8]

Electro-acupuncture

In modern practice, acupuncture needles are often stimulated using a pulse generator (Fig 43–3). Most of the models in regular use deliver pulsed direct current with either a square or a spike wave at variable frequency, pulse width, and voltage. The sophisticated electro-acupuncture techniques are often more effective than manual acupuncture.

For pain relief, best results are obtained using low frequencies (2–4 Hz).[9, 10] The lower the frequency, the more time it takes to produce some of the beneficial effects of acupuncture and the longer these effects last. The higher the frequency, the shorter the time required to obtain beneficial effects, but they generally do not last.[11] Pulse width should not be set longer than 0.3 msec if stimulation is to be given for longer than half an hour, as tissue damage may result. Continuous nonpulsatile direct current stimulation will produce tissue damage if used longer than 15–30 sec.[11]

The safety of an electrical stimulator may be easily assessed by using the method outline by Omura.[9] Electro-acupuncture should not be applied across the precardia in a patient with a history of cardiac disease because of the danger of inducing fibrillation.

Other methods of stimulating acupuncture points are finger pressure Shiatsu, ultrasonics, flexible carbon surface electrodes, and lasers. None of these is any more effective than stainless steel needles. An-

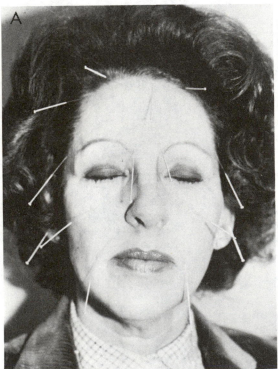
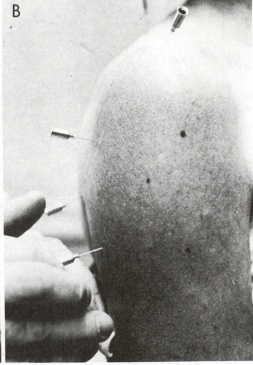

Fig 43–2.—Acupuncture needles. **A,** the traditional stainless steel needles, used here for migraine headache. **B,** hollow stainless steel needles.

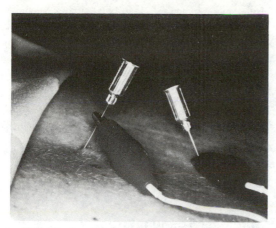

Fig 43–3.—Electro-acupuncture on a patient with low back pain.

algesia is not produced by subcutaneous injection of local anesthetic at the acupuncture points, but it is actually abolished by deep injection of local anesthetic at the acupuncture points.[12]

GENERAL EFFECTS OF ACUPUNCTURE

The classic sensation when the needle properly stimulates the point and is twirled is termed "Teh Chi" which means "obtaining Chi." This sensation is difficult if not impossible to get at nonacupuncture points. However, a therapeutic effect of some sort is nearly always obtained from nonacupuncture points, hence the concept of placebo acupuncture is meaningless. The effect is maximized by using an appropriate acupuncture point.[13]

The sensation of Teh-Chi is best described as a tingling, soreness, numbness, or heaviness. On obtaining Chi the "feel" on twirling the needle changes, and the experienced acupuncturist is often able to detect this without having to ask the patient what his subjective sensations are.

Acupuncture appears to have an ACTH-administration-like effect.[13] The white blood cell count may be raised if it was low prior to acupuncture and reduced if it was high, prior to acupuncture. The number of polymorphonuclear cells is increased, with a corresponding decrease in the number of lymphocytes, and in some cases acupuncture produces eosinopenia and basopenia.[13] The serum glucose level rises, pathologically increased serum lipid levels are reduced,[13, 14] serotonin is increased,[15] and an increase in indoleamine metabolism has been

found.[16] It has been shown that acupuncture increases endorphins in the body after approximately half an hour's stimulation.[17, 18] All of these changes are more or less point specific. Measurement of ACTH levels before and after acupuncture has not yet been carried out. An increase in brain blood flow, a lowering of blood pressure, and a delayed increase in gamma-globulins have also been noted.[13]

Attempts have been made to correlate hypnotizability with response to acupuncture. No significant correlation was found by Liao and Wan,[18] but Katz et al.[19] did find such a correlation. Goldberger and Tursky[20] found that acupuncture aimed at producing analgesia in an arm overcame countersuggestion given against the analgesia.

MECHANISM OF ACTION

The Gate Control Theory

The gate control theory of pain[21] appears to explain some of the effects of acupuncture. It certainly explains why pain relief may follow stimulation in the same dermatome as large fiber input inhibits small fiber input, as suggested by Head[22] and Zotterman.[23] It explains less well why stimulation of spinoreticular pathways by stimulating C fibers and A delta fibers produces better pain relief with acupuncture. It also does not explain why stimulation far from the site of pain may relieve that pain. However, it does provide some theoretical basis for the observed fact that classic acupuncture is often not successful at relieving pain in conditions characterized by large fiber destruction, e.g., postherpetic neuralgia, trigeminal neuralgia, causalgia, etc.[24]

Melzack[25] explains the long-term relief of pain with acupuncture by two mechanisms: first, a painful joint which is relieved of pain by appropriate stimulation becomes more mobile, and as this occurs, large fiber proprioceptive input is restored and thus the gate is closed. Second, pain may be learned centrally, and brief intense stimulation may break these memory traces.[25]

Endorphin Theory

Acupuncture has been shown to release endorphin and related compounds.[17, 18, 26] It has been assumed that these compounds are important in the use of acupuncture for the relief of pain. It is by no means certain that this is significant with the use of acupuncture for chronic pain relief.

It is interesting to note that acupuncture may increase ACTH secretion[13] and that ACTH is found in the anterior pituitary in the same cells as lipotropin. β-lipotropin is the parent substance for enorphins and enkephalins.[27] This may explain why systemic steroids depress the response to acupuncture by depressing ACTH secretion and β-lipotrophin secretion.

Bioelectric Phenomena

Recently the existence of a complete physiologic control system functioning in concert with, but separate from, the nervous system has been postulated.[28, 2] Much experimental evidence is presented suggesting that minute DC signals, such as the current of injury, may be the overt local expression of this system. These signals could be carried by way of neuralgia to a central integrating system and back out again to the response site. This glial system is compared to an analog computer using varying levels of DC as its signal; the nervous system is compared to a digital computer using action potential as its signal. They compare acupuncture points to booster amplifiers along the DC transmission lines, which correspond to the meridian pathways.[28] The lowered resistance at acupuncture points may partly be due to underlying glial cell DC activity. Clinical experience using acupuncture in conditions where pathology is known to affect the glial cells, such as multiple sclerosis, shows that acupuncture rarely has any effect. The bioelectric phenomena could explain why the results of acupuncture are often long-lasting, since stimulation of the glial system should stimulate healing processes.

Acupuncture appears to have a marked influence on the autonomic nervous system. It has been shown that acupuncture can prevent drug withdrawal syndrome, which is a parasympathetic crisis.

OTHER FORMS OF ACUPUNCTURE

Auricular Acupuncture

Auricular acupuncture has been developed by Nogier.[7] It is based on his hypothesis that there is a homunculus represented on the auricle (Fig 43–4). In its simplest possible terms, there is a knee point in the navicular fossa of the auricle which becomes reflexly tender if the ipsilateral and in some cases contralateral knee is painful. The tender auricular point is then found using a blunt probe and, on needling, the pain in the knee disappears in a substantial proportion of cases. This of course is a gross oversimplification of the method, as it has been developed into a complex branch of acupuncture in its own right by Nogier and his colleagues, and some anatomical and embryologic evidence has been produced to substantiate the basic theory.[29] The inser-

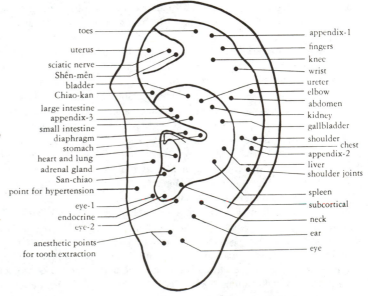

Fig 43–4.—Acupuncture points in auriculo therapy, as developed by Nogier.[7]

toes
uterus
sciatic nerve
Shên-mên
bladder
Chiao-kan
large intestine
appendix-3
small intestine
diaphragm
stomach
heart and lung
adrenal gland
San-chiao
point for hypertension
eye-1
endocrine
eye-2
anesthetic points
for tooth extraction

appendix-1
fingers
knee
wrist
ureter
elbow
abdomen
kidney
gallbladder
shoulder
chest
appendix-2
liver
shoulder joints
spleen
subcortical
neck
ear
eye

tion of a needle into the appropriate tender area on the pinna is almost always exquisitely painful; if it isn't the wrong point has been chosen. It is interesting to note that the pinna has been found to contain only free nerve endings and some specialized endings around hair follicles.[30]

Ryodoraku

This is a Japanese form of electro-acupuncture conceived by Nakatani. It is based on measuring the resistance at "Ryodo points" on each meridian and then either sedating or tonifying the meridian, depending on whether the resistance is above or below normal for that patient. In nearly all cases the points are the same as the classic source points, and the Ryodo points correspond more or less with acupuncture points. The information gained from measurement of the source points is much the same as that gained by the Chinese pulse diagnosis, i.e., each meridian is measured to determine if it is above or below normal. Successful treatment ends by making sure that all abnormal measurements have been corrected. Ryodoraku is therefore a modern version of Chinese acupuncture. It is precise, and once the basic techniques have been mastered, it is easy to use.

RESEARCH ON MECHANISMS OF ACUPUNCTURE ANALGESIA

Since 1973 there has been considerable research on the mechanisms of acupuncture analgesia. Perhaps the most exciting result was the finding that naloxone blocks acupuncture analgesia. This led to the hypothesis that acupuncture analgesia was mediated by endorphins.[17]

Mayer et al.,[29] studying acute laboratory-induced tooth pain in 20 human volunteers, produced acupuncture analgesia by manual twirling of needles in Hoku points over the first dorsal interosseous muscle of the hand. In a double-blind study they gave one group IV naloxone (0.8 mg) and another group IV saline. The saline-treated group showed acupuncture analgesia, while the naloxone-treated group showed no analgesia. One might argue that naloxone hyperalgesia simply subtracted from the analgesia of acupuncture. However, this is probably not the case, since some studies on acute laboratory-induced pain have shown that naloxone rarely produces hyperalgesia.[31]

The second naloxone study was carried out by Pomeranz and Chiu[17] in awake mice using the mouse squeak latency paradigm and electro-acupuncture in Hoku points. Numerous control groups were run to attempt to untangle some of the possible artifacts. The animals received electro-acupuncture alone; electro-acupuncture plus saline; electro-acupuncture plus naloxone (1 mg/kg IP); sham electro-acupuncture in a nonacupuncture point; naloxone alone; saline alone; or no treatment at all but just handling, restraint, and repeated pain testing. Naloxone completely blocked acupuncture analgesia, sham electro-acupuncture produced no effect, and naloxone alone produced very little hyperalgesia. Moreover, the results in mice and in humans proved first that acupuncture analgesia was not a psychological effect and second that acupuncture analgesia was truly blocked by naloxone. In another study, Cheng and Pomeranz[31] plotted a dose-response curve for naloxone and found that increasing doses produced increasing blockade. In a third study in anesthetized cats, Cheng and Pomeranz,[31] recording from lamina V cells, completely reversed the electro-acupuncture effects with 0.3 mg/kg naloxone IV.

Pomeranz and Paley[32] propose that acupuncture activates receptors in muscle and other peripheral structures which send afferent signals to the spinal cord via large myelinated A beta fibers. These synapse on spinal interneurons projecting via the anterolateral tract to higher brain centers. Shen et al.[33] have shown that lesions of the anterolateral tract abolish acupuncture analgesia. These primary afferents can also synapse on substantia gelatinosa cells in the spinal cord which produce segmental acupuncture analgesia by releasing enkephalins onto presynaptic opiate receptors located on terminals of nociceptive primary afferents. These enkephalins suppress the release of substance P and hence inhibit pain transmission. In contrast to this segmental acupuncture analgesia produced by short local circuits, there is a nonsegmental acupuncture analgesia produced by the ascending system which can end in two brain regions, the brain stem or the pituitary. In the brain stem there are two pathways: one goes through the periaqueductal gray and releases enkephalins and excites raphe cells by disinhibition of a second periaqueductal gray cell; the second pathway in the midbrain bypasses the enkephalin synapses to excite the raphe cells directly. By either route in the brain stem the raphe cells are excited and send descending inhibitory messages to the spinal cord via the dorsolateral funiculus (DLF), and serotinin is released to inhibit pain transmission in spinal cord nociceptive cells. The hypothalamic-pituitary pathway probably activates corticotrophin-releasing factor from the hypothalamus, to cause the release of ACTH and β-endorphin, possibly dynorphin, from the pituitary; the latter travels via the bloodstream to inhibit nociceptive cells, or travels via the reverse portal system into the CSF of the third ventricle to produce a direct effect on the thalamus and on the periaqueductal gray. In addition, β-endorphin cells in the arcuate nucleus of the hypothalamus might send analgesic signals to the periaqueductal gray to cause analgesia. There may be collaterals connecting the nociceptive pathway in the CNS which produce a negative feedback modulation of pain transmission in the spinal cord via the brain stem and the dorsolateral funiculus (DLF). This latter pathway is activated by intense, painful acupuncture, as shown by LeBars et al.[34] However, it should be emphasized that most of acupuncture analgesia is not painful, since A beta fiber stimulation is sufficient to produce analgesia. Toda et al.[35] have further shown that A beta stimulation in rats produces maximum analgesia, which is never augmented by recruiting A delta or C fibers.

SELECTION OF ACUPUNCTURE POINTS

The points of acupuncture are situated just below the skin in the subdermal fat. They are about 0.1 inch in diameter. There are certain basic rules for selection of acupuncture points. These rules are:

1. Select distal points according to the meridian channels. After selecting the involved meridian channel, one can select points distal to the elbow or knee joint or distal to the affected area. For example, if treatment is for headache, one can select points in the foot or hand. (See ''Headaches,'' in Appendix, this chapter.)

2. Select local points according to ''Ah-Shi'' or ''Trigger Points.''

3. Select points according to ''Back-Shu'' and the ''Front-Mu'' points. Usually ''Back-Shu'' points are for acute symptoms and ''Front-Mu'' points are for chronic symptoms. For example:

Acupuncture Point	Site of Visceral Pain
Bladder 18	Liver
Bladder 19	Gallbladder
Bladder 21	Stomach
Bladder 25	Colon
Bladder 27	Small intestine

4. Select points according to symptoms. For example:

Acupuncture Point	Symptoms
Large intestine 4; kidney 7	Hyper- or hypohydrosis
Large intestine 4, 11	Headache and facial pain
Kidney 1	Hypertension
Large intestine 4, 11; stomach 7, 44	Toothache
Gallbladder 34	Pain in the lungs, kidney, and intestine
Gallbladder 30, 34	Pain in the lower limb

5. One can choose acupuncture points on the opposite site of the pain; e.g., one can insert the needle at stomach 4, 6, 7 on the opposite side to be effective for facial paralysis.

Examples of selection of acupuncture points for shoulder girdle and buttock and extremity pain are illustrated in Figures 43–5 and 43–6.

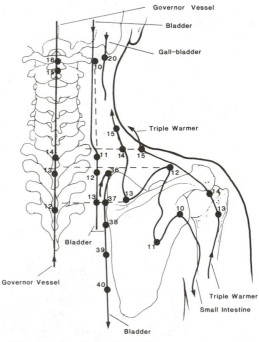

Fig 43–5.—Selection of acupuncture points for shoulder girdle and upper limb pain.

```
LOCAL POINTS              DISTAL POINTS
SI   10  11  12  13       SI    4   8
TW   13  14  16           LI    2   4   10
LI   13                   TW    4   6
B    37  38  39  40
```

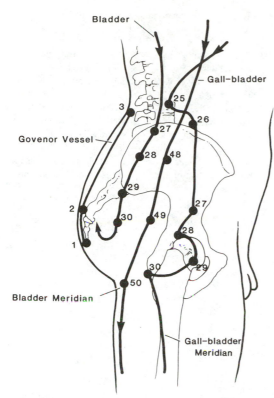

Fig 43–6.—Selection of acupuncture points for buttock and lower limb pain.

LOCAL POINTS

G	27	28	29	30	
B	28	49	50	29	39

DISTAL POINTS

B	60	54	50
S	41	42	34
G	32	35	

REFERENCES

1. Niboyet J.E.H.: La moindre resistance à l'electricite de surfaces punctiformes et de trajets cutanes concordant avec les "points" et "meridiens," bases de l'acupuncture. Thèse, Docteur ès Sciences, Paris, 1963.
2. Melzack R., Stillwell D.M., Fox E.J.: Trigger points and acupuncture points for pain: Correlations and implications *Pain* 3:3–23, 1977.
3. Gunn C.C.: Motor points and motor lines. *Am. J. Acupunc.* 6:55–58, 1978.
4. Nakatani Y., Yamashita K.: *Ryodoraku Acupunc.* Ryodoraku Research Institute, Tokyo, Japan, 1977.
5. Wooley-Hart A.: The role of the circulation in measurements of skin conductivity. *Br. J. Dermatol.* 87:213–226, 1972.
6. Becker R.O.: The significance of bioelectric potentials. *Bioelectrochem. Bioenerget.* 1:187–199, 1974b.
7. Nogier P.F.M., Bourdiol R.: Seminaire d'auriculomedecine. Lyon, France, June 1978.
8. Research Group of Acupuncture Anaesthesia, Peking Medical College: Effect of acupuncture on pain threshold of human skin. *Chin. Med. J.* 3:35, 1973.
9. Omura Y.: Electro-acupuncture: Its electro-physiological basis and criteria for effectiveness and safety. Part 1. *Acupunct. Electrother. Res.* 1:157–181, 1975.
10. Bossy J., Golewski G., Maurel J., et al.: Innervation and vascularization of the auricular correlated with the loci of auriculotherapy. *Acupunct. Electrother. Res.* 2:247–257, 1977.
11. Sinclair D.C.: *Cutaneous Sensation.* Oxford, Oxford University Press, 1967.
12. Omura Y.: Pathophysiology of acupuncture treatment: Effects of acupuncture treatment on cardiovascular and nervous systems. *Acupunct. Electrother. Res.* 1:51–142, 1976.
13. Kampik G.: Änderung erhöhter Serumlipide durch Akupunctur. *Akupunctur: Theorie and Praxis* 1:24–32, 1974.
14. The relation between acupuncture analgesia and neurotransmitters in rabbit brain. *Chin. Med. J.* 8:105, 1973.
15. Riederer P., Tenk H., Werner H., et al.: Manipulation of neurotransmitters by acupuncture. *J. Neurol Transm.* 37:81–94, 1975.
16. Pomeranz B.: Brain's opiates at work in acupuncture. *New Scient.* 73:12–13, 1975.
17. Pomeranz B., Chiu D.: Naloxone blockade of acupuncture analgesia: Endorphin implicated. *Life Sci.* 19:1757–1762, 1976.
18. Liao S.J., Wan K.K.: Patient hypnotizability and response to acupuncture treatments for pain relief. *Am. J. Acupunct.* 4:263–268, 1976.
19. Katz R.L., Kao C.Y., Spiegel H., et al.: Pain, acupuncture, hypnosis, in Bonica J. (ed.): *Pain Advances in Neurology.* New York, Raven Press, 1974, vol. 4, pp. 819–825.
20. Goldberger S.M., Tursky B.: Modulation of shock-elicited pain by acupuncture and suggestion. *Pain* 2:417–429, 1976.
21. Melzack R., Wall P.D.: Pain mechanisms a new theory. *Science* 150:971, 1965.
22. Head H.: *Studies in Neurology.* London, Kegan Paul, 1920.
23. Zotterman Y.: Tough, pain and tickling: An electrophysiological investigation on cutaneous sensory nerves. *J. Physiol. London* 95:1–28, 1939.
24. Levine J.D., Gormley J., Fields H.L.: Observations on the analgesic effects of needle puncture (acupuncture). *Pain* 2:149–159, 1976.
25. Melzack R.: *The Puzzle of Pain.* Penguin Modern Psychology, Penguin, Harmondsworth, England, 1973.
26. Reichmanis M., Becker R.O.: Relief of experimentally-induced pain by stimulation at acupuncture loci: A review. *Comp. Med. East West* 5:281–288, 1977.
27. Bowsher D.: Role of the reticular formation in response to noxious stimulation. *Pain* 2:361–378, 1976.
28. Becker R.O., Reichmanis M., Marino A.A., et al.:

Electrophysiological correlates of acupuncture points and meridians. *Psychoenerget. Syst.* 1:105–112, 1976.

29. Mayer D.J., Price D.D., Raffii A.: Antagonism of acupuncture analgesia in man by the narcotic antagonist naloxone. *Brain Res.* 121:368–373, 1977.

30. Goldstein A.: Endorphins and pain: A critical review, in Beers R.F. (ed.): *Mechanisms of Pain and Analgesic Compounds.* New York, Raven Press, 1979, pp. 249–262.

31. Cheng R., Pomeranz B.: Electroacupuncture analgesia is mediated in stereospecific opiate receptors and is reversed by antagonists of type I receptors. *Life Sci.* 26:631–639, 1969.

32. Pomeranz B., Paley D.: Electroacupuncture hypalge-

sia is mediated by afferent nerve impulses: An electrophysiological study in mice. *Exp. Neurol.* 66:398–402, 1979.

33. Shen E., Ma W.H., Lau C.: Involvement of descending inhibitions in the effect of acupuncture on the splanchnically evoked potential in the orbital cortex of the cat. *Sci. Sin.* 21:677–685, 1978.

34. Le Bars D., Dickenson A.H., Besson J.M.: Diffuse noxious inhibitory controls (DNIC): Lack of effect on non-convergent neurones, surpraspinal involvement and theoretical implications. *Pain* 6:305–327, 1979.

35. Toda K., Ichioka M., Suda H., et al.: Effects of electroacupuncture on the somatosensory evoked response in rat. *Exp. Neurol.* 64:898–904, 1979.

Appendix 1: List of Diseases and Symptoms Amenable to Acupuncture

ENUMERATED BELOW is a list of diseases and symptoms representative of ailments that are purported to respond well to acupuncture therapy. This list is selective and by no means complete. For each of the conditions mentioned, the common acupuncture points recommended for its treatment are listed. Also included are the ear points, whose usage, however, is optional.

Syncope

Main points. Jen-chung, Shao-shant. Strong stimulation is recommended. The patient should be in the Trendelenburg position.
Moxa heating. Pê-hui.

Upper Respiratory Infections

Main points. Fêng-ch'ih, Ho-ku.
Supplemental points. Yin-hsiang, T'ai-yang, Fêng-mên, Ta-ch'ui.

Asthma

Main points. Ch'uan-hsi, T'ien-t'u, Hsüan-chi, Tan-chung, Chiai-ch'uan.
Supplemental points. Ho-ku, Tsu-san-li.

Between the acute asthmatic episodes, any two to four of the main points along with the supplemental points may be used for treatment of the disease. Treatment is performed once daily and for a period of 7–10 days. For an acute attack, the main points Hsüan-chi and Tan-chung are used. Continuous twirling of the inserted needle for 2–5 minutes is recommended. If relief is not forthcoming, the main point Chiai-ch'uan is used in addition. This point is stimulated for 10–20 minutes.

Ear points. The point is located at the specific site for the lung.
Moxa heating. Ta-ch'ui, Fêng-mên, Fei-shu.

Heating is to be applied only between asthmatic attacks.

Cough

Main points. Fei-Shu, T'ien-t'u, Ch'ih-che, Lieh-ch'üeh, Ch'uan-hsi.

Rhinitis

Main points. Yin-t'ang, Ho-ku.
Supplemental points. Yin-hsiang.

Pharyngitis, Tonsillitis

Main points. T'ien-yung, Ho-ku.
Supplemental points. Shao-shang, Ch'ü-ch'ih.

Hypertension

Main points. Group I: Ch'ü-ch'ih, T'ai-ch'ung. Group 2: Fêng-ch'ih, Tsu-san-li.
Supplemental points. T'ai-yang, Yin-t'ang, I-fêng, Shên-mên.

The two main groups may be alternately used. For symptomatic relief, the supplemental points are added: for temporal headache, T'ai-yang; for frontal headache, Yin-t'ang; for tinnitus, I-fêng; and for insomnia, Shên-mên.

Ear points. The point is located at the specific site for the heart.

Gastralgia

Main points. Nei-kuan, Tsu-san-li.
Supplemental points. Chung-kuan, Wei-yü.
Ear points. The point is located at the specific site for the stomach. *Moxa heating.* Chung-kuan, Tsu-

san-li. Heating is performed only between attacks of pain.

Dyspepsia

Main points. Chung-kuan, T′ien-shu, Ch′i-hai, Tsu-san-li.

Supplemental points. P′i-yü, Shêng-yü, Nei-kuan, San-yin-chiao.

Ear points. These are located at the specific sites for the stomach, intestines, and gallbladder.

Moxa heating. Any of the above points may be used. For pediatric digestive disorders, the point Szǔ-fêng is used.

Constipation

Main points. Chih-kou, T′ien-shu.

Dysentery

Main points. Shang-chü-hsü, T′ien-shu.

Supplemental points. Nei-kuan, Kuan-yüan, Ch′ü-ch′ih.

Intermittent twirling for 30 minutes is recommended for the point Shang-chü′hsü. The supplemental points Nei-kuan for emesis and Ch′ü-ch′ih for fever are added as necessary. Treatment is performed one to three times a day.

Ear points. These are located at the sites designated for the small and large intestines.

Moxa heating. Chung-kuan, T′ien-shu, Ch′i-chung, Kuan-yüan.

Ileus (paralytic)

Main points. Tsu-san-li, Nei-kuan.

Ear points. The point is located at the specific site for the intestines.

Biliary Colic

Main points. Tanlangtien, Nei-kuan.

Ear points. These are located at the sites designated for the gallbladder and the liver.

Appendicitis

Main points. Lan-wei-hsüeh, Ch′ü-ch′ih, Nei-t′ing.

Supplemental points. T′ien-shu.

Intermittent twirling for 1–2 hours is recommended. Treatment is performed two to three times a day until the abdominal pain does not recur.

This treatment is not recommended when appendiceal rupture is suspected.

Impotence

Main points. Kuan-yüan, San-yin-chiao.

Supplemental points. Sheng-yu, Tsu-san-li.

Renal Colic

Main points. Shêng-yü, San-yin-chiao.

Supplemental points. Chih-shih, T′ai-ch′i.

Ear points. The point is located at the specific site for the urinary tract.

Urinary Tract Infections

Main points. Ts′ǔ-liao, San-yin-chiao, Chung-chi, Ch′ü-ch′üan.

Supplemental points. P′ang-k′uang-yü, Ch′ü-ch′ih.

Ear points. The point is located at the site designated for the urinary tract.

Headache

Frontal headache. The acupuncture points are Yin-t′ang, Tsuan-tsu, Ho-ku, T′ai-ch′ung.

Temporal headache. The acupuncture points are Fêng-ch′ih, T′ai-yang Szǔ-tsu-k′ung, Tsu-lin-ch′i, Chung-chu, Ho-ku.

Occipital headache. The acupuncture points are Fêng-ch′ih, T′ien-chu, Hou-ch′i, Shu-ku, Ho-ku.

Vertical headache. The acupuncture points are Pê-hui, Fêng-ch′ih, Ho-ku, T′ai-ch′ung.

Generalized headache. The acupuncture points are Fêng-ch′ih, Ho-ku Pê-hui, K′un-lun.

Toothache

Main points. Ho-ku.

Supplemental points. Chia-ch′ê, Hsia-kuan.

For toothache of the upper teeth, the supplemental point is Hsia-kuan; for the lower teeth, Chia-ch′ê.

Ear points. This point is located at the specific site for the cheek.

Tic Douloureux

Main points. Tsuan-tsu, Szǔ-pê, Hsia-kuan, Chia-ch'êng-chiang.
Supplemental points. Ho-ku, Nei-t'ing, T'ai-ch'ung, Tsu-san-li.
Ophthalmic branch: The point Tsuan-tsu is used.
Maxillary branch: The point Szǔ-pê is used.
Mandibular branch: The points Hsia-kuan and Chia-ch'êng-chiang are used.

Facial Nerve Paralysis

Main points. I-feng, Szu–pê, Yang-pê, Ti-ts'ang.
Supplemental points. Jen-chung, Chia-ch'êng-chiang, T'ai-yang, Ho-ku.

Amyotrophia

For the upper extremities. Chien-yü, Ch'ü-ch'ih, Lieh-ch'üeh, T'ai-yüan, Ho-ku.
For the lower extremities. Tsu-san-li, Fêng-shih, Huan-t'iao, Yang-lin-ch'üan, Chiai-ch'i, T'ai-yüan, Chüeh-ku, Fu-t'u.
The point Lieh-ch'üeh is specific for weakness of the wrist.

Hemiplegia

Main points. Chien-yü, Ch'ü-ch'ih, Wai-kuan, Ho-ku, Huan-t'iao, Fêng-shih, Yang-lin-ch'üan, Chüeh-ku, Lien-ch'üan.
Two to three of the main points from each afflicted extremity as well as the points Ch'ü-ch'ih and Yang-lin-ch'üan on the normal extremities are utilized in the treatment. The point Lien-ch'uan is specifically indicated for dysarthria.

Epilepsy

Main points. Hsin-yü, Fei-yü, P'i-yü, Ta-ch'ui.
Supplemental points. Tsu-san-li, Nei-kuan.

Insomnia

Main points. Shên-mên, San-yin-chiao.
Supplemental points. Nei-kaun, Yin-pê, T'ai-ch'i.

Neurasthenia

Main points. I-ming, Shên-mên, San-yin-chiao.
Supplemental points. T'ai-yang, Pê-hui, Nei-kuan, Chung-kuan, T'ien-shu, Kuan-yüan, Ts'ǔ-liao, Tsu-san-li.

Hysterical Behavior

Main points. Jen-chung, Nei-kuan, Ho-ku, T'ai-ch'i, San-yin-chiao.
This treatment is used in conjunction with orthodox psychiatric therapy.

Schizophrenia

Main points. Group 1: Jen-chung, Ho-ku, T'ai-ch'ung. Group 2: T'ai-yang, Nei-kuan, San-yin-chiao.
Supplemental points. Ya-mên, Ta-Ch'ui, T'ao-tao, T'ing-kung, Ching-ming.
Treatment is performed once or twice daily using the two groups of main points alternately. Best response is achieved by using all the points in the group simultaneously. Stimulation by twirling is maintained continuously or intermittently for one-half hour. A 26-gauge needle is used. If no response is noted in a week's time, supplemental points are added. As a rule, treatment is continued for a month on a daily basis, even after improvement is noted. Frequency of treatment can then be reduced to a weekly basis.

Pelvic Inflammatory Diseases, Menstrual Irregularities, and Cramps

Main points. Kuan-yüan, San-yin-chiao.
Supplemental points. Ch'i-ch'ung, Li-kou, Hsüeh-hai, Tsu-san-li, Yin-lin-ch'üan, P'i-yü, Kung-sun.
Ch'i-ch'ung and Li-kou are specific supplemental points for pelvic inflammatory diseases; Hsüeh-hai, Tsu-san-li, and Yin-lin-ch'üan for menstrual irregularities; and Kung-sun for menstrual cramps.
Ear points. Located at the specific sites for the uterus, the ovary, and the hormonal system.

Deafness and Mutism

Main points. Êrh-mên, T'ing-kung, T'ing-hui, Ya-mên, Lien-ch'üan.

Supplemental points. Ho-ku, Chung-chu, Wai-kuan.

For deafness, the main points Êrh-mên, T'ing-king, and T'ing-hui are used. When response is obtained, the points for mutism, Ya-mên and Lien-ch'üan, are added. In general, two or three of the main points, together with one of the supplemental points, are utilized. Performed once daily, the treatment is continued for 10 days. It is resumed after a rest period of 3–7 days. Intensive speech therapy is instituted as soon as the patient can hear.

Tinnitus

Main points. I-fêng, I-ming, T'ien-yu, Fêng-ch'ih.

Supplemental points. Chung-chu, Wai-kuan.

A combination of two main points and one supplemental point is used for each treatment.

Ménière's Disease

Main points. Fêng-ch'ih, Nei-kuan.

Supplemental points. Yifeng, T'ing-kung, Tsu-san-li, Chung-kuan.

The points Tsu-san-li and Chung-kuan are added to the main points when nausea is part of the symptomatology. If hearing is impaired, I-feng and T'ing-kung should also be used.

Lumbago

Main points. Pressure points.

Supplemental points. Hou-ch'i, Yin-mên.

Ear points. Located at the specific site for the spinal column.

Moxa heating. Same as acupuncture points.

Best results are obtained by simultaneous application of acupuncture and moxa heating.

Sciatica

Main points. Huan-t'iao, Yin-mên, Yang-lin-ch'üan pressure points.

Supplemental points. Shang-liao. Wei-chung, Ch'êng-san.

Ear points. Located at the specific sites for the spinal column, the kidney, and the point for the sciatic nerve.

Moxa heating. Same points as acupuncture points.

Best results are obtained by simultaneous application of acupuncture and moxa heating.

Painful Disorders, Hip

Main points. Huan-t'iao, Chü-liao.

Moxa heating. Same as acupuncture points.

Best results are obtained by simultaneous application of acupuncture and moxa heating.

Painful Disorders, Knee

Main points. Tupi, Liang-Ch'iu, Yang-lin-ch'üan pressure points.

Supplemental points. Wei-chung.

Moxa heating. Same as acupuncture points.

Best results are obtained by simultaneous application of acupuncture and moxa heating.

Painful Disorders, Ankle

Main points. Chieh-hsi, Ch'iu-hsü pressure points.

Supplemental points. Ching-ku.

Moxa heating. Same as acupuncture points.

Best results are obtained by simultaneous application of acupuncture and moxa heating.

Painful Disorders, Toe

Main points. Pa-fêng, Shang-pa-feng.

Moxa heating. Same as acupuncture points.

Best results are obtained by simultaneous application of acupuncture and moxa heating.

Painful Disorders, Heel and Sole of Foot

Main points. Pressure points.

Supplemental points. Ch'êng-san, T'ai-ch'i.

Moxa heating. Same as acupuncture points.

Best results are obtained by simultaneous application of acupuncture and moxa heating.

Painful Disorders, Shoulder

Main points. Chien-shu, Chien-liao, Nao-shu, T'ien-tsung, Chien-nei-lin, Chü-ku, pressure points.

Supplemental points. Ch'ü-yüan, Pi-nao, Yang-lin-ch'üan.

For subscapular bursitis, the main points to be used are T'ien-tsung, Nao-yü, and Chien-nei-lin.

For subacromial bursitis, the main points recommended are Chien-shu and Chien-liao.

For supraspinatus tendinitis, the main points are Chien-yü, and Chü-ku.

For tendinitis of the long head of the biceps muscle, pressure points are the main points.

In all of the above conditions, addition of the supplemental point, Yang-lin-ch'üan, is desirable.

Treatment is carried out every other day for a total of seven to ten treatments. If necessary, treatment may be resumed after a rest period of a week.

Best results are obtained by simultaneous application of acupuncture and moxa heating.

Ear points. They are located at the specific site for the shoulder.

Moxa heating. Same as the acupuncture points.

Painful Disorders, Elbow

Main points. Ch'ü-ch'ih, T'ien-ching, Chou-liao, pressure points.

Supplemental points. Yang-li-ch'üan.

Moxa heating. Same as the acupuncture points.

Best results are obtained by simultaneous application of acupuncture and moxa heating.

Pain Disorders, Wrist

Main points. Yang-ch'ih, Wai-kuan, pressure points.

Supplemental points. Yang-hsi, T'ai-yüan, Lieh-ch'üeh.

For deQuervain's disease (stenosing tenosynovitis over the radial styloid), the main points are the pressure points. The supplemental points are Yang-ch'i, T'ai-yüan, and Lieh-ch'üeh.

For median nerve compression at the wrist, the main points are Ta-lin, Shang-pa-hsieh, and Nei-kuan.

Moxa heating. Same as the acupuncture points.

Painful Disorders, Finger Joints

Main points. Pa-hsieh, Shang-pa-hsieh.

Ischemia of the Extremities

Main points. Ch'ü-ch'ih, and Shao-hai for upper extremities; Yang-lin-ch'üan and Yin-lin-ch'üan for the lower extremities.

Supplemental points. Shang-pa-hsieh for the upper extremities; Shang-pa-fêng for the lower extremities.

Moxa heating. Same as the acupuncture points.

This treatment is indicated for conditions such as intermittent claudication and Raynaud's disease.

Appendix 2: Index of Acupuncture Points*

A

Anmien 1	New Pt.
Anmien 2	New Pt.

C

Changchiang	GV-1
Changfeng	Spec Pt.
Changmen	LIV-13
Changyi	Spec Pt.
Chaohai	K-6
Chechin	G-23
Chengchi	S-1
Chengchiang	CV-24
Chengchieng	New Pt.
Chengchin	B-56
Chengfu	B-50
Chengku	Spec Pt.
Chengkuang	B-6
Chengling	G-18
Chengman	S-20
Chengming	Spec Pt.
Chengshan	B-57
Chengying	G-17
Chiache	S-6
Chiangchien	GV-18
Chianei	New Pt.
Chiangyin	New Pt.
Chiaohsin	K-8
Chiaoling	New Pt.
Chiaoyi	Spec Pt.
Chiaoyin	G-11
Chiapi	Spec Pt.
Chiching	New Pt.
Chuipang	
Chichupikuai	Spec Pt.
Chich'uan	H-1
Chichuan	Spec Pt.

Chichung	GV-6
Ch'ichung	Spec Pt.
Ch'ich'ung	S-30
Chiehchien	New Pt.
Chiehhehsueh	New Pt.
Chiehhsi	S-41
Chiehku	Spec Pt.
Chiencheng	SI-9
Chienchenghsueh	New Pt.
Chienchin	New Pt.
Chienching	G-21
Chienchungshu	SI-15
Chienfengshih	New Pt.
Chienhou yin chu	Spec Pt.
Chienhsi	New Pt.
Chienku	SI-2
Chienli	CV-11
Chienliao	T-14
CHIENMING	
(Head & neck region of the new acupuncture points.)	
Chienming 1	
Chienming 2	
Chienming 3	
Chienming 4	
Chienming 5	
Chienming	
(Upper limb region of the new acupuncture points.)	
Chiensanchen	
(Chienyu, Chienchien, Chienhou)	
Chienshih	P-5
Chienshu	Spec Pt.
Chienting	GV-21
Chientungtien	New Pt.
Chienwaishu	SI-14
Chienyu	LI-15
Chihai	CV-6
Chihaishu	B-24
Chihcheng	SI-7
Chihchien	New Pt.
Chihcuanchin	Spec Pt.
Chihping	New Pt.
Chihsia	New Pt.

*For a detailed description, read *An Explanatory Book of the Newest Illustrations of Acupuncture Points*, published by Hsiueh Hai Publisher, Inc., Taipei, Taiwan, 1973.

Chihhsieh	New Pt.	Chuchuehshu	Spec Pt.
Chihhsueh	Spec Pt.	Chuehpen	S-12
Chihjao	Spec Pt.	Chuehsun	T-20
Chihkou	T-6	Chuehyin	Spec Pt.
Chihli	New Pt.	Cheuhyinshu	B-14
Chihmo	T-18	Chuku	LI-16
Chihpien	B-49	Chuku	CV-2
Chihshih	B-47	Chuliao	G-29
Chihsueh	K-13	Chuliao	S-3
Chihtse	L-5	Chungchu	CV-3
Chihu	S-13	Chungchien	New Pt.
Chihyang	GV-9	Chungchu	T-3
Chihyin	B-67	Chungchu	K-15
Chimen	SP-11	Chungch'uan	Spec Pt.
Ch'imen	LIV-14	Chungchuan	New Pt.
Ch'imen	Spec Pt.	Chungchung	P-9
Chimo	LIV-12	Chungfeng	LIV-4
Chinchin, yuye	Spec Pt.	Chungfu	L-1
Chingchu	L-8	Chungku	Spec Pt.
Chingchung	Spec Pt.	Chungkui	Spec Pt.
Chingchung	New Pt.	Chungkung	Spec Pt.
Chinghsia	New Pt.	Chungliao	B-33
Chingku	B-64	Chunglushu	B-29
Chinglengyuan	T-11	Chungmen	SP-12
Ch'ingling	H-2	Chungshu	GV-7
Chingling	Spec Pt.	Chungting	CV-16
Chingmen	G-25	Chungtu	G-32
Chingming	B-1	Chungtu	LIV-6
Chinmen	B-63	Chungwan	CV-12
Chinso	GV-8	Chungyang	S-42
Chishe	S-11	Chuoyu	Spec Pt.
Chiuchi	Spec Pt.	Chupi	New Pt.
Chiuhou	Spec Pt.	Chupin	K-9
Chiuhsu	G-40	Ch'upin	G-7
Chiuneifan	New Pt.	Chutse	P-3
Chiutienfeng	Spec Pt.	Chuyangwei	Spec Pt.
Chiuwaifan 1	New Pt.	Chuyuan	SI-13
Chiuwaifan 2	New Pt.		
Chiuwei	CV-15	**E**	
Choujung	SP-20		
Chouliao	LI-12	Echung	Spec Pt.
Choushu	Spec Pt.	Erhchien	LI-2
Chuanchien	Spec Pt.	Erhchien	Spec Pt.
Chuanhsi	Spec Pt.	Erhhou chiangmo	Spec Pt.
Chuanliao	SI-18	Santiao	
Chuanshengtsu	Spec Pt.	(Three veins on the back of the auricle)	
Chucha	B-4	Erhmen	T-21
Chuchang	Spec Pt.	Erhpai	Spec Pt.
Chuche	Spec Pt.	Erhshanmen	Spec Pt.
Chuchih	LI-11		
Chuchuan	LIV-8	**F**	
Chuchueh	Spec Pt.	Feishu	B-13
Chuchueh	CV-14	Feiyang	B-58

Fengchih	G-20
Fengfu	GV-16
Fengkuan	Spec Pt.
Fenglung	S-40
Fengmen	B-12
Fengshih	G-31
Fengyen	Spec Pt.
Fengyen	Spec Pt.
Fuai	SP-16
Fuchieh	SP-14
Fufen	B-36
Fuhsi	B-52
Fuliu	K-7
Fupai	G-10
Fushe	SP-13
Futu	S-32
Futu	LI-18
Fuyang	B-59

H

Hanyen	G-4
Hengku	K-11
Hengwen	Spec Pt.
Heting	Spec Pt.
Hoku	LI-4
Holiao	LI-19
Holiao	T-22
Houchimen	Spec Pt.
Houchung	New Pt.
Houhsi	SI-3
Houhsuehhai	New Pt.
Houting	GV-19
Houtinghui	New Pt.
Houtinghsueh	New Pt.
Houtingkung	New Pt.
Houyangkuan	New Pt.
Houyeh	Spec Pt.
Hoyang	B-55
Hsiachingming	New Pt.
Hsiachishu	Spec Pt.
Hsiachuhsu	S-39
Hsiachui	Spec Pt.
Hsiafutu	New Pt.
Hsiahsi	G-43
Hsiakuan	S-7
Hsiakunlun	Spec Pt.
Hsialiao	B-34
Hsialien	LI-8
Hsiawan	CV-10
Hsiaochangshu	B-27
Hsiaochihchieh	Spec Pt.
Hsiaochihchien	Spec Pt.

Hsiaochihchien	Spec Pt.
Hsiaohai	SI-8
Hsiaokukung	Spec Pt.
Hsiaolo	T-12
Hsiapai	L-4
Hsiawenliu	Spec Pt.
Hsienku	S-43
Hsihsia	Spec Pt.
Hsikuan	LIV-7
Hsimen	P-4
Hsinfengshih	New Pt.
Hsinfutu	New Pt.
Hsingchien	LIV-2
Hsingfen	New Pt.
Hsinshih	Spec Pt.
Hsinshu	B-15
Hsinhui	GV-22
Hsishang	New Pt.
Hsiunghsiang	SP-19
Hsiwai	Spec Pt.
Hsiyangkuan	G-33
Hsiyen	Spec Pt.
Hsuanchi	CV-21
Hsuanchung	G-39
Hsuanli	G-6
Hsuanlu	G-5
Hsuanshu	GV-5
Hsuehchou	Spec Pt.
Hsuehhai	SP-10
Hsuehyatien	New Pt.
Huajoumen	S-24
Huakai	CV-20
Huanchung	Spec Pt.
Huangmen	B-46
Huangshu	K-16
Huantiao	G-30
Huato chiachi	Spec Pt.
(Hua To's vertebral point)	
Huitsung	T-7
Huiyang	B-35
Huijin	CV-1
Hungyin	Spec Pt.
Hunmen	B-42
Hunshe	Spec Pt.

J

Janku	K-2
Jenchung	GV-26
Jenying	S-9
Jihyueh	G-24
Juchung	S-17
Juken	S-18
Junghou	New Pt.

Taimo	G-26	Tsanchu	B-6		
Taipai	SP-3	Tsehsia	Spec Pt.		
Taiyang	Spec Pt.	Tsechien	Spec Pt.		
Taiyi	S-23	Tsengming 1	New Pt.		
Taiyinchiao	Spec Pt.	Tsengming 2	New Pt.		
Taiyuan	L-9	Tsengyin	New Pt.		
Takukung	Spec Pt.	Tsuchiaoyin	G-44		
Taling	P-7	Tsuchungping	Spec Pt.		
Talun	Spec Pt.	Tsuhsin	Spec Pt.		
Tanchuan	Spec Pt.	Tsulingchi	G-41		
Tanlangtien	Spec Pt.	Tsuluo	Spec Pt.		
Tanshu	B-19	Tsuming	Spec Pt.		
Taotao	GV-13	Tsunping	Spec Pt.		
Tapao	SP-21	Tsuoku	New Pt.		
Tatu	SP-2	Tsuoyi, Yuyi	Spec Pt.		
Tatun	LIV-1	Tsusanli	S-36		
Taying	S-5	Tsuyichung	New Pt.		
Tiaokou	S-38	Tuituan	GV-27		
Tiaoyueh	New Pt.	Tunchung	Spec Pt.		
Tichi	SP-8	Tungku (Bladder)	B-66		
Tichien	New Pt.	Tungku (Kidney)	K-20		
Tienchih	P-1	Tungli	H-5		
Tienching	T-10	Tungtien	B-7		
Tienchu	B-10	Tungtzuliao	G-1		
Tienchung	G-9	Tupi	S-35		
Tienchuan	P-2	Tushu	B-16		
Tienchuang	SI-16	Tzukung	CV-19		
Tienfu	L-3	Tzukung	Spec Pt.		
Tienhsi	SP-18	Tzuliao	B-32		
Tienjung	SI-17				
Tienliao	T-15				
Tienling	Spec Pt.		W		
Tienshu	S-25	Waichihli	New Pt.		
Tienting	LI-17	Waichinchin waiyuye	Spec Pt.		
Tient'ing	New Pt.	Waichiu	G-36		
Tientsung	SI-11	Waikuan	T-5		
Tientu	CV-22	Waihuaichien	Spec Pt.		
Tienyu	T-16	Wailaokung			
Tiho	Spec Pt.	Wailing	S-26		
Tingchuan	New Pt.	Waiming	New Pt.		
Tingchung	New Pt.	Waiszuman	Spec Pt.		
Tinghsueh	New Pt.	Waitingchuan	New Pt.		
Tinghui	G-2	Wanku (Gallbladder)	G-12		
Tingkung	SI-19	Wanku (Small Intestine)	SI-4		
Tingling	New Pt.	Wanli	New Pt.		
Tingmin	New Pt.	Weichung	B-54		
Tingshu	Spec Pt.	Weijehsueh	New Pt.		
Tingtou	Spec Pt.	Weile	New Pt.		
Titsang	S-1	Weiling	Spec Pt.		
Tituo	New Pt.	Weipao	Spec Pt.		
Tiwuhui	G-42	Weishang	New Pt.		
Toukuangming	Spec Pt.	Weishu (Bladder)	B-21		
Touwei	S-8	Weishu	New Pt.		

44 / Psychotherapy

THOMAS OXMAN, M.D.

PSYCHOLOGICAL INTERVENTIONS for the treatment of chronic pain come from a vast array of disciplines and theories. These approaches are frequently used in combination. For descriptive purposes, psychological treatment can be separated into four theoretical schools: (1) operant conditioning, (2) cognitive-behavioral, (3) psychophysiologic, and (4) psychodynamic.

OPERANT CONDITIONING

When the diagnostic workup reveals that environmental consequences are a major component of a patient's pain behavior, then management of those environmental consequences by operant conditioning may be of benefit. The methods of Fordyce have provided a significant and useful application of learning theory to chronic pain management.[1, 2] These methods were initially developed for use in an inpatient setting. In such an environment, the overall strategy is directed toward three goals simultaneously: (1) reducing positive reinforcement of pain behavior, (2) increasing positive reinforcement of well behavior, and (3) instructing and involving the patient's family and significant others to maintain the strategy after discharge. The first goal is usually the easiest; the last two are more difficult.

The treatment process begins by informing the patient and his family of the strategy. The therapist does not attempt to covertly change behavior. The nature of positive and negative reinforcement is explained. The patient is asked to keep a record for several days to weeks during which baseline data are collected regarding medication use, exercise and activity tolerance, and attention from others.

After the baseline data collection, if a significant amount of medication is being used, the prescription of it is changed from a pain-contingent to a strictly time-contingent basis. This decreases any accompanying attention the patient might obtain by asking for medicines and also decreases the need for a patient to focus on his pain to decide whether or not to take medication. Using the baseline data, the physician pinpoints the most painful activities of a patient's typical day and determines a regular schedule of medication given slightly *more* often than what was recorded during the baseline period. Medication is given whether or not a patient feels a need for it. With the patient's consent, medication is slowly reduced over a 6- to 8-week period while alternative therapies are being introduced.

A similar approach is applied to the patient's level of activity and exercise. Rest and attention from others often follow pain behavior produced by working to tolerance. Establishing a patient's exercise and activity limits creates a standard according to which the patient can be instructed to stop before reaching levels that are associated with pain. Rest and attention are no longer reinforcers for exercising to one's limits. In addition to gradually increasing exercise quotas, activities that were previously avoided because of pain can be reintroduced gradually in small achievable steps.

The most difficult step is preparing the patient, staff, and family to accept visible or audible signals of pain in as neutral a manner as possible and to provide extra positive attention for achieving well-behavior quotas. This is particularly difficult after discharge with respect to social reintegration. The family wants the patient to participate in recreational, social, and community activities, but patients who have suffered for more than 1–2 years may avoid such activities because of fear of embarrassment or awkwardness. Nevertheless, if introduced gradually, as with exercise, successful social experiences without embarrassment can lead to reintegration.

Operant conditioning programs have been reported to result in significant improvement that is maintained over time.[3] Nevertheless, patients accepted into these programs are from a very selected group: they have minimal obvious organic pathology, there has been identifiable reinforcement of pain behavior, the patients have a good psychosocial support system, and both patient and family are willing to participate.[2] Although the results will be less dramatic, it is still possible to use a less comprehensive operant conditioning approach in an outpatient setting and in patients who do not meet all of the above criteria. The following example illustrates such a use.

A 45-year-old married laborer incurred back and knee injuries in two separate work-related accidents at a warehouse. He was referred to the University of Cincinnati Pain Control Center 1 year after the last injury. At the time of initial examination he was on temporary total disability. He was taking hydrocodone with acetaminophen, carisoprodol with phenacetin and caffeine, and doxepin. Back examination revealed muscle spasm with trigger points. Arthroscopy of the knee revealed degenerative arthritis with osteophytes and possible neuroma.

The patient was begun on a multidisciplinary program of trigger point injections, physical therapy, transcutaneous electrical nerve stimulation, and behavioral evaluation. He was asked to keep a daily record of any changes in his pain. He was instructed to make six columns on lined paper and note the following: (1) date and time, (2) where he was, (3) whom he was with, (4) what he was doing, (5) pain rating (scale of 1 to 4), and (6) medications taken and other pain-relieving measures used. Analysis of 2 weeks of record-keeping revealed that he was taking the narcotic three to four times a day, especially on awakening and at bedtime. He was particularly likely to require narcotics if he stayed in bed too long in the morning, took long car rides, or sat on the patio watching his children. The records also revealed that he had very little social activity or regular exercise.

Based on these findings he was placed on a fixed time-contingent narcotic regimen and instructed to set his alarm to remind him not to stay in bed past 9:00 A.M. His wife was eager to attend his clinic appointments and helped in constructively discussing both his irritability and her frustration. She suggested he was irritated at their sons because of their superior physical abilities and frequent absences from the home. She was frustrated at their lack of social activity for the past year. A vacation was planned during which the patient was able to spend time with his sons at the beach. He was also able to gradually increase his exercise tolerance for walking. The change in environment and resulting improvement in mood led the patient to see the need for social reintegration. His wife was encouraged to be less demanding of social activity in return for their planning a series of short, nonthreatening outings twice a month. The patient was not embarrassed at the first of these outings and continues to follow the plan. Narcotics have been reduced; however, further knee surgery appears indicated.

A behavioral modification approach can also be used for the treatment of insomnia. This approach is especially indicated if bedtime has been identified as a cue for insomnia. The procedure of lying down in bed, turning off the light, and so forth can be associated with frustration, sleeplessness, and the expectation of nocturnal pain even if the pain has improved. If this process is occurring, the patient will often report that he sleeps better in a strange environment such as on a couch in the living room, in a hotel, or in a hospital.

The goal of a behavioral modification approach for insomnia is to associate the stimuli of the patient's bedroom with rapid sleep onset. The procedure for achieving this goal consists of seven steps.[4]

1. The patient should lie down in bed only when sleepy.
2. The bed should be used only for sleeping, not for reading or watching television. Sexual activity is the exception to this rule.
3. If the patient does not fall asleep quickly, he should get up and go to another room until sleepy again.
4. If the patient still does not fall asleep, then step 3 should be repeated.
5. The patient should get up at the same time each morning, regardless of the amount of sleep obtained. This helps establish a regular sleep-awake rhythm. An alarm should be used if necessary.
6. No naps during the day.
7. Three weeks may elapse before there is noticeable improvement. Accordingly, the time of sleep onset and the number of arisings can be graphed daily to help identify early and subtle improvement as an encouragement to continue with the plan.

COGNITIVE APPROACHES

Cognitive therapy is based on the premise that an individual's affect and behavior are largely determined by his subjective appraisal of events. Change of that appraisal is accomplished by one or more methods: (1) teaching coping strategies, (2) identifying negative thoughts and feelings associated with pain, (3) demonstrating the connection between the negative cognitions and pain, and (4) substituting adaptive, positive thoughts and feelings.[3] Coping strategies consist of several techniques such as education, imagery, distraction, relaxation training, and assertiveness training. Hypnosis and biofeedback are often part of such programs, although they may also be viewed as physiologic rather than cognitive approaches. Operant conditioning, too, has an implicit or explicit effect on attitude change and pain appraisal. Accordingly, the term cognitive-behavior therapy is often used.[3] The overall goal with respect to pain is to give the patient a new attitude and the feeling of being able to control the pain rather than being disabled by it.

As long ago as 1936 Chappell and Stevenson[5] reported that pain perception could be diminished by a three-part program: (1) providing information on the relationship of emotions or stress and pain physiology, (2) suggestion, and (3) directive instructions to stop negative habitual patterns of thinking.[5] A study by Egbert et al.[6] demonstrated that patients who were given preoperative reassurance, education, and relaxation training requested less postoperative narcotics and were discharged earlier than uninstructed controls. These two studies emphasize the common theme of making the patient an active participant to increase his sense of control.

As summarized by Turk,[7] direct instructions to the patient include several active coping strategies. Depending on the patient's proclivity and motivation, one or more should be practiced, and once the patient is skilled in their use, various strategies may be used in anticipation of or during increases in pain. For example, patients could enhance pain tolerance by (1) "somatization"—changing the mental label of pain (e.g., a certain feeling or an arm that has fallen asleep) and analyzing the sensation and bodily process; (2) "imaginative transformation of context"—acknowledging the pain but imagining it occurring in a fantasy (e.g., as an important spy shot escaping); (3) "imaginative inattention"—imagining oneself in a pleasant situation incompatible with pain (e.g., a pleasant day at the beach); (4) "imaginative transformation of the pain"—interpreting the pain sensations as trivial, unreal, or other than pain (e.g., numbness, tickling); or (5) "distraction"—focusing on physical characteristics of the environment or doing mental arithmetic. Such strategies have been validated primarily in experi-

mental pain. Nevertheless, Rybstein-Blinchek[8] recently used three of these strategies in 44 heterogeneous pain patients and reported greatest success with the "imaginative transformation of the pain." Further follow-up is necessary to see if the positive results are maintained over time and when the patient is no longer actively in therapy.

In addition to coping strategies for acute increases in pain, the long-term coping skills are of benefit. The physician should attempt to recognize those skills already employed by the patient and foster them. Denying or minimizing is probably an uncommon and generally maladaptive skill by the time a patient with chronic pain reaches the specialist. It is more appropriate to help the patient *seek appropriate information* regarding the pain. Usually this also requires that the patient accept the idea of permanently living with some degree of pain. Once this step is dealt with, a useful skill is to *set concrete limited goals*. This has already been discussed briefly with respect to activity and social reintegration using operant conditioning. Helping the patient to mentally *rehearse an alternative outcome* is appropriate if full or partial employment is not possible and if other activities must be relinquished and substituted. The request for *reassurance and support* can be provided through the doctor-patient relationship and patient groups. Finally, the importance of *finding a general purpose or meaning* of the pain and for life should not be minimized. Religious involvement or volunteer service may be of great benefit. In helping patients with these coping skills, the major tasks of the pain specialist are to be knowledgeable in providing or obtaining appropriate information, to recognize conflicting coping strategies in the family (e.g., the patient's setting concrete goals while the spouse is denying), and to recognize and manage emotional responses that are appropriate or inappropriate to the particular pain situation.[9]

Low self-esteem is common in chronic pain patients, and encouraging positive self-statements is a major key to the successful application of cognitive therapy. The therapist should inform the patient of this fact and state that he will frequently question and challenge the patient regarding any global automatic negative thoughts.[10] For example, chronic pain patients often expect the pain specialist to view them as "crazy" or as suffering "only psychogenic pain." The therapist might ask in the initial interview if the patient had any thoughts about coming for the evaluation. If such negative thoughts are revealed, the pain specialist can ask if those thoughts made the patient have any feelings such as anger, sadness, or anxiety. The therapist then uses this brief interchange to correct the negative thought by reassuring the patient of acceptance and to point out the connection between thought and affect. Similar experiences over time can teach the patient to question his own negative conclusions or predictions: "What is the basis for my conclusion? Are there other explanations? What do I really have to lose by going out socially?" The therapist also emphasizes the importance of the patient rewarding himself for improvement and the successful use of coping strategies.

Record-keeping used in operant conditioning or for monitoring any pain treatment provides another source for substituting positive, adaptive thoughts. This is illustrated by the following example, a continuation of the case discussed earlier:

The patient's 2-week pain diary revealed that he tended to become angry and experience more pain when interacting with his two sons. When we discussed this with him and his wife, it emerged that what bothered him was a feeling of inadequacy—he was no longer able to perform many physical activities with his sons. This led to the thought that he was not a good father. His wife pointed out the erroneous nature of this thought and its consequent affect. She also suggested that the thought was fueled by his overcompensating to make up for his own father's lack of involvement with him. Efforts by both patient and wife to keep these facts in mind made it possible for him to relate to his sons without becoming angry.

A different example is the headache diary used in the University of Cincinnati Headache Center. In this diary, patients score the severity of their headaches three times a day on a scale of 0 to 4. The daily scores are summed and placed on a monthly graph. As the frequency of headaches decreases with treatment the lines move lower on the graph, giving patients visible evidence of progress. Even if they are still having headaches, a positive feeling of progress is reinforced.

RELAXATION, HYPNOSIS, AND BIOFEEDBACK

One of the common objectives of these three modalities in pain management is to train the patient to self-induce a state that is incompatible with pain. The patient also can learn to identify early internal cues associated with tension in order to control its pain-exacerbating effect. There are many methods of relaxation training, but there is no definitive evidence that any one method is superior to another.[11] Training manuals or prepared audio tapes are available.[12–14]

Relaxation training has several major components.[15] Preparation begins with patient education and suggestion of positive results. Next, mental and muscular relaxation is enhanced by having the patient assume a comfortable position (usually in a cushioned reclining chair in a quiet room with soft lighting and a moderate temperature), wearing nonbinding clothing, and minimizing movement. Relaxation training is taught using a cognitive method such as by having the patient repeat (silently) words, sounds, or images, focus on his breathing, or focus on the difference in sensations from alternately contracted and relaxed muscle groups. While in the relaxed state, the patient may be encouraged to practice the active coping strategies discussed previously in the section on cognitive-behavioral approaches. Practice continues with the therapist as well as at home. Finally, the technique is used during exacerbation of pain or when a recurrence of pain is anticipated.

Hypnosis is one of the oldest methods of pain control. It is characterized by the common components of relaxation training.[3, 16] The same cognitive coping strategies used in relaxation training and other forms of cognitive therapy are also employed in hypnosis used for pain control; however, the relaxed state from hypnosis may make the images more vivid. For some patients this is due to the mystique of hypnosis, which reduces guilt from failure at other therapies, but for most people the vividness is directly related to their inherent capacity for suggestibility. Seventy percent of all males and females have been reported to be hypnotizable to some degree.[17] In 35% this capacity is minimal and in 5% it is maximal; the majority of people fall in the middle range. Although the capacity for hypnotizability adds greater vividness and impact to the coping strategies, sufficient motivation can compensate for the lack of hypnotizability. This emphasizes the falseness of the myth that only mentally weak or sick people are hypnotizable.[17] In fact, hypnosis should not be used in patients who fear losing control or being controlled, or whose hopes for a magical cure might be dashed by failure. Thus, hypnosis is contraindicated in patients with paranoid thinking of psychotic proportion or with severe depressive illness.

The type of hypnosis successfully used for

chronic pain control is more appropriately called self-hypnosis because, like relaxation training, it is an exercise which the patient must practice on his own. Hypnosis is not sleep or something projected upon the patient. Spiegel's method[17] makes use of a three-count system for entering and exiting from the relaxed state. At the count of 1, one thing is done, at 2, two things are done, and at 3, three things are done: (1) eyes gaze up, (2) eyelids are closed and a deep breath is taken, (3) patient exhales, eyes relax, and the body is imagined floating. While the body is "floating," a somatic sensation is suggested (initially by the therapist and subsequently by the patient), such as levitation of an arm or a sense of numbness, tingling, or warmth. The sensation is focused on as a marker for an altered state of awareness for meditation on one of the cognitive coping strategies. The self-induction is then reversed: (3) get ready, (2) with eyelids closed, eyes gaze up, (1) eyelids open slowly and eyes are relaxed. As an adjunct, the patient can be instructed to make a fist and then open it as a signal that the usual state of sensation and awareness have returned.

Several studies have shown that hypnosis can decrease the perception of experimental pain. Many case reports have suggested analgesic results of hypnosis in patients with cancer pain, headaches, neck and shoulder pain, and phantom limb pain. Nevertheless, there are few methodologically sound pain research studies of hypnosis.[3]

The use of biofeedback to control pain is based on the assumption that there is a disordered involuntary physiologic component of pain which a patient can learn to control and correct. The theoretical support for such an approach comes from a wide variety of animal experiments using operant conditioning but not necessarily studying pain. Miller[18] has performed and described many elegant studies which demonstrate that visceral somatomotor responses can be modified by the positive and negative rewards of learning. The addition of biofeedback to such modification refers to the use of instrumentation to amplify a physiologic response and transform it into visual or auditory signals. A needle, tone, or digital display provides immediate feedback to the patient.

Four types of biofeedback are currently being used with chronic pain patients. Electromyographic (EMG) feedback is employed for reducing muscle tension. Electroencephalographic (EEG) feedback is used to increase alpha wave brain activity, which is thought to be a sign of relaxation incompatible with pain. Skin temperature feedback is used to alter sympathetic nervous system–controlled dermal blood flow and hence temperature. Cephalic blood volume pulse feedback is used to control temporal artery pulsation in migraine headache.

The general clinical technique of biofeedback for pain is analogous to that of the other behavioral and cognitive approaches. Before beginning treatment, it is useful to provide the patient with a conceptual model of how and why biofeedback works. Part of this introduction includes the fact that biofeedback is something the patient does to himself rather than something the therapist does to the patient. Biofeedback procedures have rarely been used without relaxation training, operant conditioning, or cognitive-behavior therapy for chronic pain.[15, 19] The instrumentation can be of use in demonstrating the connection of thoughts and affect to pain. By observing the difference in the biofeedback signal before and after relaxation training, some patients become more convinced of the connection between mental states and pain. Currently there is no evidence as to which individuals will best respond to biofeedback. Similarly, there are insufficient data to suggest the optimum frequency of training or the type of signal.

Most research on the effectiveness of biofeedback for treatment of pain applies only to headaches. Many studies report positive benefits of biofeedback on tension and migraine headaches. Unfortunately, as has been pointed out in reviews of these studies,[20, 21] three major problems relating to experimental data and research design make it unclear what, if anything, biofeedback itself actually does. First, although frontalis muscle EMG feedback is associated with a reduction in the frequency or severity of tension headaches, there is no evidence that muscle tension is necessarily associated with tension headache[21–23] or that reduction of muscle tension at one site is generalizable to other sites.[20] Second, the value of finger temperature biofeedback per se for migraine headaches is problematic because of conflicting results, inadequate controls, the questioned generalizability of changes in finger vascular reactivity to cranial vessels, and the uncertain etiology of the migraine syndromes. Third, and most important, biofeedback is used in conjunction with other treatment methods, which makes isolation of its specific effects difficult or impossible. There is no evidence that biofeedback is any more efficacious than relaxation training without biofeedback. Nevertheless, biofeedback instrumentation is certainly more costly and more complex than what is required for relaxation training or hypnosis. For research purposes the collection of biofeedback data is valuable. For clinical use, more and better controlled research is required to determine the proper role of biofeedback in chronic pain management.

PSYCHOTHERAPY

The definition of psychotherapy is continuously changing. It varies from referring to psychoanalysis and its less intense derivative, psychodynamic psychotherapy, to any interaction between patients and health care professionals. Psychoanalysis and psychodynamic therapy, which make use of unconscious symbolic meanings and specific reference to the patient's thoughts and feelings about the therapist, are usually unsuitable for the management of chronic pain. Nevertheless, several therapeutic principles of psychotherapy overlap with the cognitive-behavioral approach and are relevant in treating the chronic pain patient.

Bruch[24] observed that a successful psychotherapist approaches each new patient as "a stranger whose anguish and problems are unprecedented and unique." The therapist must treat the patient in a special way based on the individual's particular situation as well as the therapist's catalogue of past therapeutic experiences. In psychotherapy this is achieved by (1) *listening* to the patient in such a manner that he feels understood, (2) *reformulating* what the patient says in order to clarify his situation and decrease the upset of uncertainty, and (3) *suggesting alternatives* which allow the patient to take control of his situation and feel less helpless. The three techniques of listening, reformulating, and suggesting alternatives are basic to all interactions between the physician and the patient. Attention to these techniques will increase a patient's participation and cooperation in any therapeutic plan.

Psychotherapeutic principles may be the most useful method of managing the predicament of patients with somatoform disorders. These patients usually do not accept or do well with referral to a mental health professional. It may become incumbent on the willing and understanding pain specialist to provide continued management of the somatoform patient. In doing so the pain specialist can prevent continuous frustrating referral and possible unnecessary surgery and drug abuse. Four basic principles should be kept in mind when treating the somatoform patient.[25-28] First, the treatment is aimed at the management and prevention of iatrogenic complications rather than at cure. One must

somehow convey to the patient that the physician is more interested in maintaining the doctor-patient relationship than in curing the pain. One of the most convincing methods of showing this interest is to offer the patient regular but reasonably spaced appointments or telephone contacts. These appointments need not be more than 15 minutes long. By establishing a series of regular appointments, the physician can also more readily end a visit by saying, "As we agreed, our time is up for today, but we can continue next time." Second, do not expect the patient to give up the symptom. Nevertheless, he may eventually *talk* less about it. A corollary of this is not to confront the patient with statements such as "There is nothing wrong with you" or "It is all in your head." Similarly, the patient should not be reassured. In fact it is occasionally useful to take a seemingly paradoxical position such as, "I don't know how you live with such pain." This can increase rapport with the patient if it is presented and accepted as a confirmation of his overall suffering. Third, the physician need do little more than listen during these visits. It is not necessary to ask regularly about the pain or other symptoms. To do so may unwittingly support the patient's denial of emotional conflict. Rather, when the patient does mention an affect or interpersonal relationship, the physician should gradually question and reinforce these statements. Eventually the patient may begin talking more about other aspects of his life than pain or other symptoms. This is a sign that the visits can slowly be spaced farther apart. Fourth, the use of drugs and procedures is to be minimized. If analgesic medication becomes necessary, it can be prescribed with a pessimistic attitude, such as, "I don't know how good this drug will be for your pain, but you can try it if you wish." On the contrary, if drugs are indicated, such as antidepressants after appropriate diagnosis, they should be given with an optimistic attitude but specific to the target symptom. For example, "This medicine will help you improve your mood and sleep so that you can better live with the pain."

Group psychotherapy may also complement cognitive-behavioral therapy. As with individual psychotherapy, there are several different theoretical approaches for conducting group therapy. These approaches range from a psychoanalytic model with no time limit and a passive therapist to a one-time session which is primarily educational and directed by a very active therapist. Many of the cognitive approaches, including relaxation training, can be conducted in a group format. Some patients are more accepting of these approaches in a group format, and the cost can certainly be reduced. Families or spouses can be involved, especially in the educational groups. For some specific problems such as low back pain or cancer, a support group of patients with the same symptom or illness can be of great benefit. In these groups, patients who have accepted and dealt with their illness can provide hope and encouragement to newer patients and their families.

SUMMARY

The mental health professions offer a vast array of disciplines relevant to chronic pain, including, among others, psychiatry, psychoanalysis, neuropharmacology, experimental psychology, and clinical psychology. Psychosomatic medicine provides a useful means for integrating these disciplines. When a biopsychosocial analysis of a patient's pain problem is made, selection of the most appropriate combination of therapies is facilitated. This selection can be enhanced in a multidisciplinary treatment setting where members of several different disciplines confer as a team to devise an individualized treatment plan with the patient. Two principles underlie the majority of treatment methods derived from these disciplines: patient education, and improving the patient's self-esteem. Scientific evidence for the superiority of any one treatment method is lacking. More rigorous research is needed on chronic pain and the specificity and indications for the various mental health therapies.

REFERENCES

1. Fordyce W.E., Fowler R.S., Lehmann J.F., et al.: Operant conditioning in the treatment of chronic pain. *Arch. Phys. Med. Rehabil.* 54:399–408, 1973.
2. Fordyce W.E.: Treating chronic pain by contingency management. *Adv. Neurol.* 4:583–589, 1974.
3. Turner J.A., Chapman C.R.: Psychological interventions for chronic pain: A critical review. II. Operant conditioning, hypnosis, and cognitive-behavioral therapy. *Pain* 12:23–46, 1982.
4. Hauri P.: Behavioral treatment of insomnia. *Med. Times* 107:36–47, 1979.
5. Chappell M.N., Stevenson T.I.: Group psychological training in some organic conditions. *Ment. Hygiene* 20:588–597, 1936.
6. Egbert L., Batit G., Welch C., et al.: Reduction of post-operative pain by encouragement and instruction. *N. Engl. J. Med.* 270:825–827, 1964.
7. Turk O.C.: Cognitive behavioral techniques in the management of pain, in Foreyt J.P., Rathjin D.P. (eds.): *Cognitive Behavior Therapy: Research and Applications.* New York, Plenum Press, 1978, pp. 199–232.
8. Rybstein-Blinchek E.: Effects of different cognitive strategies on chronic pain experience. *J. Behav. Med.* 2:93–101, 1979.
9. Moos R.H., Tsu V.D.: The crisis of physical illness: An overview, in Moos R.H. (ed.): *Coping with Physical Illness.* New York, Plenum Medical Book Co., 1977, pp. 3–21.
10. Beck A.T., Rush A.J., Shaw B.F., et al.: *Cognitive Therapy of Depression.* New York, Guilford Press, 1979, pp. 1–33, 61–86.
11. Taylor C.B.: Relaxation training and related techniques, in Agras W.S. (ed.): *Behavior Modification: Principles and Clinical Applications.* Boston, Little, Brown & Co., 1978.
12. Bernstein D.A., Borkovec T.D.: *Progressive Relaxation Training: A Manual for the Helping Professions.* Champaign, Ill., Research Press, 1973.
13. Benson H.: *The Relaxation Response.* New York, William Morrow, 1975.
14. Wolpe J., Lazarus A.A.: *Behavior Therapy Techniques.* London, Pergamon Press, 1966.
15. Pinkerton S.S., Hughes H., Weinrich W.W.: *Behavioral Medicine: Clinical Applications.* New York, John Wiley & Sons, 1982, pp. 90–106.
16. Spiegel D.: Hypnosis in the treatment of psychosomatic symptoms and pain. *Psychiatr. Ann.* 11:343–349, 1981.
17. Spiegel H., Spiegel D.: *Trance and Treatment: Clinical Uses of Hypnosis.* New York, Basic Books, 1978.
18. Miller N.E.: Fact and fancy about biofeedback and its clinical implications. *J.S.A.S. Catalog of Selected Documents in Psychology,* vol. 6. Washington D.C., American Psychological Association, 1976, p. 92.
19. Shapiro D., Surwit R.S.: Biofeedback, in Pomerleau O.F., Brady J.P. (eds.): *Behavioral Medicine: Theory and Practice.* Baltimore, Williams & Wilkins Co., 1979, pp. 45–73.
20. Turner J.A., Chapman C.R.: Psychological interventions for chronic pain: A critical review. I. Relaxation training and biofeedback. *Pain* 12:1–21, 1982.
21. Olton D.S., Noonberg A.: *Biofeedback: Clinical Applications in Behavioral Medicine.* Engle-Wood Cliffs, N.J., Prentice Hall, 1980, pp. 118–200.
22. Anderson C.D., Franks R.D.: Migraine and tension headache: Is there a physiological difference? *Headache* 21:63–71, 1981.
23. Tfelt-Hansen P., Lous I., Olesen J.: Prevalence and significance of muscle tenderness during common migraine attacks. *Headache* 21:49–54, 1981.
24. Bruch H.: *Learning Psychotherapy: Rationale and Ground Rules.* Cambridge, Mass., Harvard University Press, 1974.
25. Lowy F.H.: Management of the persistent somatizer, in Lipowski Z.J., Lipsitt D.R., Whybrow P.C. (eds.): *Psychosomatic Medicine: Current Trends and Clinical*

Applications. New York, Oxford University Press, 1977, pp. 510–522.

26. Brown H.N., Vaillant G.E.: Hypochondriasis. *Arch Intern. Med.* 141:723–726, 1981.

27. Aldrich C.K.: Severe, chronic hypochondriasis: I. A practical method of treatment. *Postgrad. Med.* 69:139–144, 1981.

28. Lipsitt D.R.: Medical and psychological characteristics of "crocks." *Psychiatry Med.* 1:15–25, 1970.

45 / Hypnosis

ROBERT E. PAWLICKI, Ph.D.
WILLIAM C. WESTER, II, Ed. D.

HYPNOSIS IS A UNIQUE and valuable tool in the treatment of chronic pain. It is difficult to think of another method as effective in creating comfort out of discomfort without the side effects frequently associated with techniques of pain control. What is the essence of this technique? When is it appropriate, and for whom? What are its limitations, and how does one become trained in its utilization?

Clinical hypnosis is an altered state of awareness in which the patient experiences increased suggestibility. The patient's conscious and unconscious mind is more likely to accept ideas uncritically. Briefly, the patient narrows his attention, while his mind is focused and receptive to therapeutic suggestion. This usually takes the form of the patient moving into a highly relaxed state. Erickson[1] defines hypnosis as essentially a communication of ideas and understanding to a patient in such a way that he will be more receptive to the suggestions, thereby becoming motivated to explore his own psychosomatic potentials to control psychological and physiologic responses and behavior.

Despite the popular view of hypnosis as a mystical and unusual experience, almost everyone has experienced some level of a hypnotic state at some time. Most of us can recall having been "mesmerized" by an absorbing book, film, or television program; many of us have driven long distances in which we "lost" an awareness of time and place. On those occasions we restricted our attention to the exclusion of stimulation around us, an experience that can be described as being in a hypnotic state. Similarly, a patient can learn to achieve, on his own volition, a narrowed attention with increased suggestibility for the therapeutic benefit. Clinically, the patient can enter into a hypnotic state with nothing to fear, for this is a safe procedure in which the experience is pleasant and usually refreshing.

Suggestive therapy, as hypnosis has been called, has been known for as long as we have had records. It is now recognized that earlier practices, such as incantation, the laying on of hands, animal magnetism, and so forth are most likely to have been effective through the use of a hypnotic method. The modern era of clinical hypnosis is ususasly dated from the time of Mesmer, about 1773, with the term hypnosis coined by James Braid, M.D. in approximately 1841. The American Medical Association approved the use of hypnosis as a therapeutic technique in 1958.

The growth of hypnosis has been limited by misconceptions held by laymen and professionals alike. For example, many individuals believe that hypnotized patients lose consciousness and control. This does not happen in hypnosis. Although hypnosis is an altered state of consciousness, the patient does not lose consciousness but is aware of everything at all times, perhaps in a heightened fashion. As well, since all hypnosis is self-hypnosis, the professional is actually acting as a facilitator, an agent, or a teacher to assist the patient in moving into a hypnotic state. The patient is in control, and if he wishes to terminate the hypnotic state, he may do so merely by opening his eyes or leaving the setting. Contrary to common belief, the patient retains basic control and will not spontaneously begin to reveal personal and intimate information. The patient may talk during the hypnotic session, and the professional may even utilize the conversation as part or a larger therapeutic intervention.

The range of problems for which hypnosis may be an appropriate therapeutic tool is extensive.

829

Within psychology, common areas of focus are the cessation of smoking, weight control, the treatment of phobias, depression, alcoholism, speech disorders, chronic pain, and self-esteem or ego strengthening, to name a few. The medical professional can utilize hypnosis within the framework of psychiatry, anesthesiology, surgery, the treatment of psychosomatic diseases, obstetrics/gynecology, control of bleeding, burn therapy, dermatology, and pain control. Examples from dentistry include reducing the fear of dental procedures, dental surgery, control of bruxism, bleeding, tongue biting, and saliva flow; for orthodontia; to reduce gagging, and to ease denture use and general oral hygiene.[2]

With such a range of uses for this powerful technique, the professional must make decisions concerning the appropriateness of the patient. The first step in reaching this decision is to take a complete history to determine contraindicating factors. Hypnosis is inappropriate in a patient with a physical illness, such as a severe heart dysfunction, where there may be danger in masking the disease. Additionally, patients with severe emotional disorders such as borderline psychosis or severe depression may not be appropriate candidates for hypnotherapy. It is apparent that the vast majority of patients are potential subjects for hypnotic treatment.

Among the best-known uses of hypnosis is for pain relief. Pain has been defined as a warning signal of threatened tissue damage, an integrated defense reaction, and/or a private experience of hurt.[3] As a significant subjective experience it is perhaps the factor that most frequently causes people to seek medical aid.[4] Acute pain has important survival characteristics, and the analgesic effect of hypnosis may be an excellent palliative to the acute pain problem.

There is good documentation that both experimental and clinical pain can be dramatically eliminated through hypnosis.[5, 6] Such pain relief, however, is usually shortlived.[7] The signal of chronic pain is maintained for longer than its informational value. The aching of low back pain, arthritis, or headache may be pointless in terms of survival after the patient has initiated appropriate treatment. Therefore, for lasting pain benefits to be achieved, hypnosis must be incorporated into a broader psychotherapeutic context. Chronic pain is a complex perception, emanating from many causative factors. To effectively utilize hypnosis for the chronic pain patient, a professional must have a clear understanding of the psychological state of the patient and the factors that may be maintaining the patient's pain.

Chronic pain nags, aggravates, and leads to a plethora of accompanying complications. In particular, chronic pain illustrates that pain is not a purely physical event. If it were, the same noxious stimuli should produce the same intensity and quality of pain in all individuals. Obviously such is not the case. This is because the pain is actually a composite of three different influencing factors: the emotional, the cognitive, and the physical. Melzack and Wall[8] call these contributions to pain the sensory/discriminatory aspect (physical sensations), the motivational/affective (emotional feelings), and the cognitive/evaluative (thoughts). Hypnosis, through its effect on thoughts and feelings, can profoundly alter the perception of pain.

As mentioned earlier, hypnosis is an altered state of awareness, usually accompanied by an intensified state of suggestibility and relaxation. How do these characteristics affect pain? Most likely the hypnotized patient experiences some benefit merely by entering a deep state of relaxation. We know that the chronic pain patient frequently experiences a stress/anxiety/pain syndrome that may exacerbate his or her experience of pain. Relaxation may short-circuit that cycle. Furthermore, the hypnotic state tends to shift the tension away from the pain as the patient reconceptualizes the pain itself or reconceptualizes the causes of the pain. For example, the pain can be visualized as resulting from a heroic event and thus made more palatable. In either event, the focus of attention shifts from the awful, debilitating, aversive characteristics to a neutral or perceived positive characteristic of the pain.

Medical treatment has been the most prevalent method of intervention for a variety of pain problems including such things as headache and low back pain. This treatment has basically consisted of pharmacologic interventions, since pain has been primarily perceived as a physiologic disorder. Both the demand for and the growth of pain control centers indicate, however, that the medical/pharmacologic approach is inadequate for a significant percentage of chronic pain patients. Hazardous side effects of medication, and research indicating the frequency of secondary psychological components of pain, precipitated a further search for psychologically based intervention procedures. This search has resulted in the increased utilization of biofeedback, relaxation training programs, and hypnosis as nondrug alternatives for the relief of pain.

Of the three interventions, hypnosis is particularly

useful; it is inexpensive, safe, nonaddictive, and each treatment usually has some success in pain reduction. After completing extensive laboratory research, Hilgard and Hilgard[6] noted that hypnosis is useful as a therapy for pain and can benefit suffering patients. The use of hypnosis for pain control and as an anesthesia is well documented.[8–10] Research in the early 1930s demonstrated that hypnotized subjects reacted less to painful stimuli than did nonhypnotized subjects. Clinically, there are a variety of strategies to facilitate the utilization of hypnosis to control pain. It is to these strategies that we now turn.

HYPNOTIC PAIN CONTROL STRATEGIES[11]

1. *Suggestions of deep relaxation* alone are frequently effective in pain control. Anxiety and pain are usually interrelated. Since anxiety is incompatible with relaxation, relaxation can break the pain cycle and reduce the level of pain.

2. *Direct suggestions of decreased pain* may be given—for example, "your unconscious mind will now help you to become more comfortable."

3. *Transfer of pain* from one part of the body to another where it is less disabling may help. For example, the pain in the shoulder may be transferred to a little finger, where it causes less suffering and disruption of the patient's daily routine.

4. *Transformation of pain sensations* into a sensation which is easier to tolerate, such as a feeling of warmth or tingling.

5. *Suggestions of numbness* by having the patient imagine an injection of lidocaine to the affected area.

6. *Dissociation* can be used to help the patient separate from his/her pain in a variety of ways. For example, a woman giving birth can be told to numb her body from the midline down or to imagine that part of her body being somewhere else and that she is watching the procedure.

7. *Distraction*. For example, recently a young girl cut her hand and was screaming hysterically. The physician said to her, "You have a really pretty color of blue blood." The girl stopped screaming, looked at her hand, and began to listen to the physician give other suggestions.

8. *Regression to a period before the onset of the pain* can help to control pain in a good subject.

9. *Distortion of time* is a useful method of making medical or dental procedures pass rapidly with less pain.

10. *"Switch" techniques* can be taught children and adults. The patient finds the switch in her/his brain (via imagery) that corresponds to the affected area and then turns that switch off. ˙

SELF-HYPNOSIS AND FACTORS DETERMINING THE PROBABILITY OF SUCCESS

Most experts in the field of hypnosis believe that all hypnosis is self-hypnosis and that patients can be taught to use hypnotic techniques on their own. It is much like learning to ski—first you need an instructor to teach you the basics. The hypnotherapist can show the patient the way, but then the patient must assume the responsibility for continued control of the pain. There are four determinants of one's ability to obtain relief with self-hypnosis:[12]

1. *Practice*. The patient must practice with a variety of hypnotic approaches, suggestions, and imagery. The first goal may be to ease tension followed by direct relief of pain.

2. *Motivation*. Motivation entails freeing oneself from the need to keep pain in one's life. The patient must look honestly at the place of pain in his/her life and try to understand why he might be holding onto pain.

3. *Fear of letting go of the pain*. The patient must realize that self-hypnosis only reduces unnecessary pain. The body's "alarm system" remains intact, and if further disease or degeneration takes place, the body will alert the patient. In the meantime, the patient could shut off the pain or turn it down to a more manageable level.

4. *Knowledge*. We create the feeling of pain in our brains. It serves our survival needs and we have the ultimate control over the pain.

It may be useful at this point to present two brief hypnotic treatment sequences which may be incorporated into a general therapeutic procedure of pain control.

BRIEF TREATMENT SEQUENCE[13]

Glove anesthesia technique (after an initial progressive relaxation procedure):

Now, I want you to imagine a brightly colored pail, filled with a sparkling blue liquid. This blue liquid is an extremely potent anesthesia. Place your hand inside the pail and feel your fingertips tingle as the anesthetic is quickly absorbed . . . [therapist continues until there is evidence of anesthesia in hand]. Continue to experience the numbness. In a little while I will ask you to gently place your hand on your head. This will give you the opportunity to transfer the feeling of numbness in your hand directly to your head, where you usually experience a headache. Now you can repeat the transfer process as many times as you want to or need to. After doing this you may be surprised to notice that you continue not only to feel relaxed and comfortable, but confident in your ability to achieve the goals you have set for yourself. [Patient is then asked to count from 1 to 10 and begin to alert himself.]

Size and shape sequence (after an initial progressive relaxation procedure):

Now that your body is completely relaxed, I want you to visualize any pain that has been present in your body. Give the pain a particular size and shape. Visualize its contours, its edges, and its placement in your body. You may even give it a color if you like. Notice the contrast between the pain area and the surrounding areas of your body. Notice exactly where the pain ends, and any differences you may see in the shading and color that are present in the pain area and not present in the surrounding nonpain areas. Now allow the size of your pain to grow gradually larger and larger until it is twice as big as it originally was. Once you can visualize your pain as twice its original size, slowly allow it to become smaller and smaller until it returns to its original size. After it has returned to its original size, slowly allow it to double in size once again. That's fine. Notice your pain, with all of its characteristics of color and shape, expands once again to double its size, just as it did a few seconds ago. This time, however, allow your pain to gradually shrink and shrink beyond its original size. Allow the color and shading of the nonpain areas to expand, taking over this space of the pain area. Allow your pain to diminish in size until it has finally disappeared. Allow its edges to move back, its contours to shrink to a tiny, tiny space until your mind's eye cannot see it any longer. When it has become so small that you cannot see it, notice the level of intensity of your pain. After doing this you may notice that you can repeat this process any time that you wish. You may also notice that on each occasion you proceed to implement this process you will continue to not only feel relaxed and comfortable, but also more and more confident in your ability to reduce the size and intensity of your pain. [Patient is then asked to count from 1 to 10 and begin to alert himself.]

FINDING OR BECOMING A QUALIFIED HYPNOTHERAPIST

The use of hypnosis for pain control is an effective therapeutic technique. Hypnosis should be viewed as an adjunct to all other medical or psychological treatments. For example, a lower dose of medication might be used in conjunction with hypnosis. Hypnosis should not be viewed as a panacea, and it should be used only when the professional has had appropriate training.

If one is interested in obtaining the services of a qualified psychologist or medical or dental practitioner who uses hypnosis, it may be useful to contact the state or professional societies. Major cities usually have professional associations that can direct parties to qualified professionals. As well, the Yellow Pages may carry listings of hypnotists or hypnotherapists. Two points to remember: First, select a professional who lists his or her advanced degrees. Confirmation of the appropriateness (or at least the lack of appropriateness) of the professional usually can be obtained from the local hypnosis society in larger cities. Second, examine whether the hypnotherapy is practiced within the broader context of the professional's expertise. Hypnosis is a tool to be used within those areas in which the professional has training and expertise and, because of the complex nature of chronic pain in particular, should be part of a larger therapeutic program.

For professionals who wish to become trained in the techniques of hypnosis, a major source of training is the American Society of Clinical Hypnosis. This professional organization, through its Education and Research Foundation, maintains a comprehensive schedule of training sessions in major cities across the country. These didactic and experiential training sessions, directed toward the psychologist and medical or dental practitioner, are provided at beginning, intermediate and advanced levels of expertise. For the chronic pain patient, and in the hands of a properly trained professional, hypnosis is a safe procedure with the potential of excellent benefits for the patient.

REFERENCES

1. Erickson M.H.: An introduction to the study and application of hypnosis for pain control, in Lassner J. (ed.): *Hypnosis and Psychosomatic Medicine*. New York, Springer-Verlag, 1968.
2. Wester W.C. II: *Questions and Answers About Clinical Hypnosis*. Columbus, Ohio, Psychological Publishing, Inc., 1982.

3. Sternbach R.A.: *Pain: A Psychophysical Analysis*. New York, Academic Press, 1968.

4. Ryan R.: *Headache and Head Pain*. St. Louis, C.V. Mosby Co., 1978.

5. Crasilneck H.B., Hall D.: *Clinical Hypnosis: Principles and Application*. New York, Grune & Stratton, 1975.

6. Hilgard E., Hilgard J.: *Hypnosis in the Relief of Pain*. Los Altos, Calif., William Kaufman, 1975.

7. Barbara J.: Incorporating hypnosis in the management of chronic pain, in Barbara J., Adrian C. (eds.): *Psychological Approaches to the Management of Pain*. New York, Brunner/Mazel, 1982.

8. Melzack R., Wall P.: Pain mechanisms: A new theory. *Science* 150:971–975, 1967.

9. Cheek D.B., LeCron L.M.: *Clinical Hypnotherapy*. New York, Grune & Stratton, 1968.

10. Crasilneck H.B., Hall J.A.: *Clinical Hypnosis: Principles and Applications*. New York, Grune & Stratton, 1975.

11. Haley J. (ed.): *Advanced Techniques of Hypnosis and Therapy: Selected Papers of Milton H. Erickson, M.D.* New York, Grune & Stratton, 1967.

12. Udolf R.U. *Handbook of Hypnosis for Professionals*. New York, Van Nostrant Reinhold Company, 1981.

13. Alman B.M., Lambrau P.T.: *Self Hypnosis: A Complete Manual for Health and Self-Change*. San Diego, International Health Publications, 1983.

46 / Biofeedback

ROBERT E. PAWLICKI, Ph.D.
CHRISTINE HOVANITZ, Ph.D.

COMPARED WITH most interventions to combat chronic pain, biofeedback is a relatively new phenomenon, yet the growth and utilization of this technique have been truly remarkable. Why has this procedure been so extensively utilized for chronic pain? What does biofeedback training involve? What are the conditions in which it is appropriately applied? Why does it work, and how does a professional become trained in its implementation? These are the questions this chapter addresses.

Biofeedback entails the use of instrumentation to demonstrate physiologic changes so that physical processes normally considered involuntary can be brought under voluntary control. The basic principles of biofeedback are as old as human observations of how we learn, for all effective and efficient learning involves some form of immediate feedback. In the simple example of learning to shoot an arrow toward a bull's-eye, with the knowledge of where the last arrow struck the target, an individual can make fine motor-muscular coordination adjustments to improve his ability to hit the target. Without such feedback or knowledge learning is very difficult indeed. Biofeedback gives the patient immediate and sensitive information about his biologic condition. The patient uses such information to learn to achieve control over bodily systems in order to enhance health. Some specialized instrumentation is required, although an instrument as simple as a hospital thermometer provides feedback to assist the patient in enhancing health. More sophisticated instrumentation, however, is usually required to provide immediate information on physiologic change, or biofeedback. The use of instrumentation in this latter manner is relatively new.

Until 1970 biofeedback training was primarily limited to laboratory experiments on lower animals. This animal research[1-3] provided convincing evidence that the autonomic nervous system, previously thought not to be under voluntary control, could be somewhat directed through the use of systematic feedback. At approximately the same time, researchers were working with human subjects to control a number of "involuntary" physiologic responses.[4-6] In each of these experiments the subjects were provided with information (feedback) they were not normally aware of. The instrumentation first measured physiologic response and signaled the subject whenever a tiny change occurred in the desired direction. Through such an arrangement, subjects soon learned to modify their targeted physiologic activities. Those techniques form the basis for what has become the field of biofeedback. Shortly thereafter, biofeedback training began to be adopted into regular practice in hospitals, clinics, and educational settings.

The range of disorders for which evidence is available of the clinical effectiveness of biofeedback is large and ever-expanding. Some of the more notable examples are spasmodic torticollis, neuromuscular re-education for hemiplegics, Raynaud's syndrome, heart rate conditioning, sensorimotor training for epileptic seizures, tension headaches, hypertension, migraine headaches, and muscle re-education.

Biofeedback techniques are particularly valuable for the treatment of chronic pain. There are three primary reasons for this assertion. First, while the list of problems suitable for treatment by biofeedback is extensive, the most frequent application of biofeedback involves the use of electromyography (EMG) equipment to assist the patient in reducing anxiety. Anxiety is common in the chronic pain population and frequently occurs as part of a stress/

anxiety/pain syndrome. Whether the pain is associated with headaches, the myofascial pain syndrome, or the many other pain syndromes amplified by anxiety, biofeedback provides a means by which a lower level of tension can be achieved in the patient's body, thereby interrupting the stress/anxiety/pain syndrome.

Second, biofeedback is particularly appropriate for the chronic pain patient because it emphasizes self-control. Probably the most common personality characteristic of chronic pain patients is a sense of dependency—a sense that the physical problem is out of their control and can only be appropriately managed by the medical professional. This tends to foster a feeling of insecurity and reliance on those around them. Biofeedback techniques encourage a reversal of such feelings and concomitant behaviors by allowing patients to take a major responsibility for their physical condition and improvement. This is in sharp contrast to the medical model with its focus on drugs, surgery, or other external controls. Indeed, the cognitive component of biofeedback may be just as important in altering the condition as any physical change that may occur.

Alteration of a patient's belief system concerning control over pain is often called cognitive restructuring and begins before actual biofeedback. In initiating biofeedback training, the appropriately trained professional establishes rapport, attempts to establish antecedents of the pain, searches for secondary gains, and examines the patient's usual response to stressful situations. In other words, behavioral analysis precedes the actual training, and it is during this period that the biofeedback therapist begins to assist the patient in adopting an attitude of self-control.

Third, chronic pain patients as a population are not psychologically minded. Rather, they exhibit a strong tendency to channel emotional difficulties into somatic concerns. Furthermore, they commonly regard mind and body as separate entities. Biofeedback training provides an excellent means of educating the patient in the mind/body relationship. For example, galvanic skin response equipment can easily be utilized to illustrate changes in the patient's tension level as a function of emotional variations. The demonstration of measureable changes as a result of the patient's recalling any emotionally distressing experience can assist the patient in recognizing the psychological contributions to the pain problem.

TYPES OF BIOFEEDBACK

Biofeedback techniques may be divided into two major branches; those intended to augment the process of relaxation and those intended to alter specific physiologic functions. This division roughly corresponds to the differentiation between cognitive and physiologic aspects of biofeedback treatment. Biofeedback for pain control may call on either or both of these kinds of techniques. The choice of technique depends on the nature and location of the pain complaint as well as on the patient's motivation.

Relaxation augmented by biofeedback is perhaps the most widely used procedure. The specific pathologic process underlying the pain need not be identified. As is true of the medical treatment of many disorders, the mechanism by which biofeedback of this type is frequently successful in reducing pain perception is not well understood. Two hypotheses have been advanced regarding its efficacy; biofeedback may raise the threshold of pain by adding a stimulus which competes for attention,[7] or relaxation may enhance the release of endorphins that modulate the perception of pain.[8] In any event, biofeedback-assisted relaxation involves providing the patient with information on his or her success at relaxation. Two techniques frequently used for this purpose are EMG and thermal measures. As the patient becomes more relaxed, muscle tension is reduced, and this reduction may be documented by EMG (Fig 46–1). During successful relaxation, a deactivation of the sympathetic nervous system occurs that reduces the constricting effect of the sympathetic nervous system on the peripheral blood vessels. With the increase in blood flow comes an increase in peripheral temperature. This may be assessed with a thermistor attached to the fingers so that the patient's success in raising (or lowering) his or her finger temperature may be provided. Biofeedback-augmented relaxation in this context is expressly for the purpose of pain reduction and is not intended to correct a pathologic disease process.

For certain disorders such as migraine or tension headache, torticollis, or Raynaud's disease, biofeedback for the purpose of altering abnormal physiologic processes has demonstrated significant success,[9] with improvement seen in both the pain symptoms and in the pathologic process. The techniques for this type of biofeedback may be the same as those previously mentioned (EMG or finger temperature measurement), although frequently they are

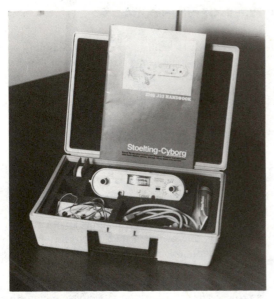

Fig 46–1.—Simple EMG apparatus.

not. For example, the treatment of a tension headache with biofeedback typically consists of EMG feedback assessed from the forehead (frontalis muscle) with the specific purpose of muscle tension reduction in that area; because muscle tension headaches are generally believed to result from chronically tense muscles of the head and neck,[10] a successful reduction of this tension should eliminate the disorder as well as the pain. Thus, although the equipment used is identical to that used in biofeedback-augmented relaxation, the effect on the patient will differ as a function of the particular disorder presented.

THE DECISION TO USE BIOFEEDBACK

The appropriateness of a patient for biofeedback is determined by the disease associated with the pain complaint and the predicted course of the disease, the documented success of biofeedback for that specific complaint, the success of alternative psychological and/or medical techniques and their potential side effects, the presence of severe psychopathology, and the willingness or motivation of the patient.

Because successful biofeedback often requires several weeks of training and application, the predicted course of the disease may dictate whether biofeedback treatment is practical. Biofeedback is not appropriate for psychotic patients. Perhaps the most difficult part of the decision, however, is the assessment of the patient's motivation. Successful biofeedback requires the patient's persistence during intervals of little progress, a relatively nonconflicted desire to improve, and a significant investment of time and energy.

It may be difficult to choose between relaxation treatment and relaxation augmented with biofeedback. Biofeedback may be included with relaxation training to document objectively the relationship between anxiety-producing thoughts and increased muscle tension. Biofeedback may also provide the patient with knowledge of small increments of improvement that could not be subjectively experienced. Especially for patients who are suspicious of psychological procedures, biofeedback may be an acceptable compromise. The decision to include biofeedback in a relaxation treatment program must take into account such drawbacks as expense, space and time requirements, and the patient's potential dependence on equipment for achieving a relaxed state.

PHYSICAL SETUP

As most biofeedback treatment requires a quiet setting free of interruption, and as most biofeedback equipment is both stationary and bulky, a room away from the main flow of traffic typically must be set aside for the sole use of biofeedback. Although not necessary, an adjacent room connected to the therapy room by a one-way mirror and intercom, and from which the therapist may control the biofeedback equipment, is useful.

Biofeedback equipment itself may be obtained from a variety of sources (see Appendix 2). Different biofeedback instruments vary greatly in sensitivity to physiologic changes, type of feedback (visual or auditory), and manner of data storage. Regardless of the complexity of equipment utilized, however, most systems have a basic structural similarity. All systems have some method of measuring the practical physiologic signal of interest by physical contact with the patient; for example, an EMG involves the placement of electrodes on the patient's skin where the underlying electrical activity is recorded (Fig 46–2). A thermistor, on the other hand, works as a transducer by changing its resistance as a function of temperature.

Once a potential is obtained, this signal is carried through a variety of devices designed to filter and amplify the original input. The final amplification of

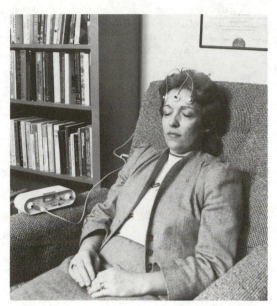

Fig 46–2.—Typical EMG biofeedback training.

the signal typically provides the voltage necessary to drive the recording device, which is often a polygraph. The patient may receive feedback regarding the physiologic response either directly from the polygraph or from an analogous visual or auditory display. Most biofeedback systems are able to assess simultaneously several different physiologic channels.

CONDUCTING THE BIOFEEDBACK SESSION

As in most behavioral therapies, a careful assessment with appropriate observation of self-monitoring of symptoms is completed prior to the initiation of treatment. (Details of the assessment procedures may be obtained from Olton and Noonberg[9] and Fischer-Williams et al.[7]) At the time of assessment a reasonable estimate of the probability of success is made that is based primarily on the type of physical disorder presented, and this information may be given to the patient to assist in his or her decision to undertake biofeedback. The length of total therapy as well as the length and frequency of the individual sessions is based also on the nature of the disorder, but this consideration includes such factors as inpatient/outpatient status and the ease of access to equipment, as well.

Each individual session typically involves a brief baseline assessment followed by a series of feedback trials. The precise mechanism by which patients learn voluntary control over typically "involuntary" physiologic processes is not well understood; outside of certain relaxation procedures, little or no direct verbal instruction beyond the statement of the final goal is given by the therapist.

UTILITY OF BIOFEEDBACK

The success rate of biofeedback in the treatment of various disorders is best estimated by examining controlled studies focusing on the specific disorder in question. The data for biofeedback treatment of migraine and tension headaches, for example, suggest an improvement/success rate of approximately 60%–70%.[10] Recent studies of Raynaud's disease indicate a 66.8% reduction in reported attacks.[11] Variables that influence the success rate in patients with the same physical complaints are poorly identified at present but are presumed to include such factors as compliance, course of disease, presence and magnitude of secondary gain associated with the pain complaint, and length of follow-up.

In spite of our lack of understanding concerning some of the mechanisms involved in the benefits derived from the use of biofeedback, this technique has many outstanding characteristics which encourage its use with chronic pain. As previously mentioned, biofeedback training can (1) be a catalyst in reducing anxiety and tension, (2) assist the patient in taking responsibility for some improvement in his pain problem, and (3) help the patient recognize the psychological contribution to the pain problem. Lastly, through muscle re-education the patient can make specific inroads in ameliorating the problem.

Given the benefits accruing from the utilization of biofeedback training, the question arises as to how one becomes knowledgeable and skilled in its utilization. The most straightforward procedure is to contact the Biofeedback Society of America (see Appendix II-B for the address of this organization) about the many professional training sessions presented around the country. In larger cities, local biofeedback societies may present training sessions. This information is sometimes available in the Yellow Pages. Additionally, it is important to realize that biofeedback is a tool that must be implemented in the context of a larger therapeutic setting. Thus, like other psychologically based interventions (e.g., hypnosis) biofeedback intervention for chronic pain should be embedded within a comprehensive treatment procedure. In this context, and utilized by a trained professional, biofeedback has much to offer the chronic pain patient.

REFERENCES

1. DiCara L., Miller N.E.: Instrumental learning of vasomotor responses by rats: Learning to respond differently in two ears. *Science* 159:1485–1486, 1968.
2. Miller N.E.: Learning of visceral and glandular responses. *Science* 163:434–445, 1969.
3. Miller N.E., DiCara L.: Instrumental learning of urine formation by rats: Changes in renal blood flow. *Am. J. Physiol.* 215:677–683, 1968.
4. Snyder C., Noble M.: Operant conditioning of vasoconstriction. *J. Exp. Psychol.* 77:263–268, 1968.
5. Brener J., Hothersall D.: Heart rate control under conditions of augmented sensory feedback. *Psychophysiology* 3:23–28, 1966.
6. Kamiya J.: Operant control of the EEG alpha rhythm and some of its reported effects in consciousness, in Tart C.T. (ed.): *Altered States of Consciousness.* New York, John Wiley & Sons, Inc., 1969, pp. 507–517.
7. Fischer-Williams M., Nigl A.J., Sovine D.L.: *A Textbook of Biological Feedback.* New York, Human Sciences Press, 1981.
8. Basbaum A.I., Fields H.L.: Endogenous pain control mechanisms: Review and hypothesis. *Ann. Neurol.* 4:451–452, 1978.
9. Olton D.S., Noonberg A.R.: *Biofeedback: Clinical Applications in Behavioral Medicine.* Englewood Heights, New Jersey, Prentice-Hall, Inc., 1980.
10. Adams H.E., Feuerstein M., Fowler J.L.: Migraine headache: Review of parameters, etiology, and intervention. *Psychol. Bull.* 87:217–237, 1980.
11. Freedman R.R., Ianni P., Wenig P.: Behavioral treatment of Raynaud's disease. *J. Consult. Clin. Psychol.* 51:539–549, 1983.

47 / Physical Therapy

VICKIE M. FAIRCHILD, B.S., L.P.T.
LYNNE M. SALERNO, B.S., L.P.T.
STACY L. WEDDING, B.S., L.P.T.
ELLIOTT WEINBERG, B.S., L.P.T.

PHYSICAL THERAPY plays a key role in the management of patients with acute and chronic pain in a pain control center. The objectives of physical therapy are (1) to evaluate and prevent disability, (2) to restore function, (3) to promote healing, and (4) to help the patient adapt to permanent disability.

In the treatment of acute pain one often focuses on the specific pathology to reduce or eliminate pain. On the other hand, in the treatment of chronic pain the physical therapist must interact with specialists from multiple disciplines for total patient care. The elimination or reduction of pain can be accomplished through the following modalities:

Heat
  Superficial
    Hydrocollator pack
    Paraffin bath
    Hydrotherapy
    Contrast bath
  Deep
    Shortwave diathermy
    Microwave diathermy
    Ultrasound
Cryotherapy
  Cold pack
  Ice massage
  Ethyl chloride
Electrical stimulation
  Alternating and direct current
  Iontophoresis
  High-voltage galvanic stimulation
  Transcutaneous elecrical nerve stimulation
Massage
  Soft tissue mobilization

Effleurage (stroking)
    Superficial
    Deep
  Pétrissage (kneeding)
  Fricton
  Tapotement (percussion)
  Vibration
Traction
  Intermittent
  Static
  Manual
  Positional
Mobilization
Exercise
  Passive
  Active assisted
  Active
  Active resistive
    Isometric
    Isotonic
    Isokinetic
Other techniques
  Endurance
  Desensitization
  Breathing
  Relaxation
  Proprioceptive neuromuscular facilitation
  Coordination

Individualizing the patient's physical therapy begins with a thorough evaluation. The evaluation consists of a detailed interview to obtain baseline information regarding the patient's mental status, pain, daily activities, vocation, and medical and surgical history. After the history is taken, the following features are evaluated: gait, posture, range of motion, joint mobility, flexibility, muscle strength, coordination, sensation, reflexes, and skin condition. From the subjective and objective evaluation, individualized goals for physical therapy are set. These goals are then incorporated into the overall multidisciplinary management plan.

The remainder of this chapter discusses the various physical therapy modalities and techniques available for treating the pain patient.

HEAT

Therapeutic effect can be provided by superficial or deep heat. Heat produces both general and local physiologic effects. General effects include an elevated body temperature, pulse rate, and respiratory frequency rate and a decreased blood pressure. Local effects include analgesia, relaxation, relief of muscle spasm, consensual effect, and an increase in local tissue temperature, tissue metabolism, circulation, sweating, and vasodilation. Secondarily, these general and local effects increase the oxygen supply to the tissues and eliminate the tissues' waste products. The extent of the physiologic response depends on the extent of area treated, the duration and frequency of treatment, the skin thickness, the intensity of the heat source, the body's ability to dissipate heat, and the difference between skin temperature and heat source temperature.

Superficial Heat

Hydrocollator Packs

Hydrocollator packs are applied to an area for local physiologic effects. The heat is maintained within the moist heat pack approximately 20–30 minutes. Hydrocollator packs should be used cautiously or not at all in patients with loss of or diminished sensation, open lesions, or inflamed joints.

Paraffin bath

The paraffin bath (Fig 47–1) is a combination of mineral oil and wax which is maintained at a temperature of 126° F. The paraffin bath softens the skin, produces an intense erythema, and makes the cutaneous and other soft tissues more supple. The

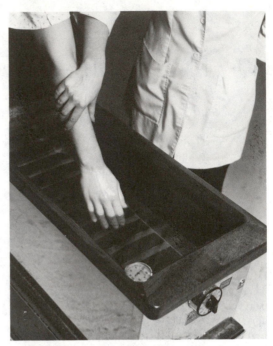

Fig 47–1.—The dip paraffin bath is a source of full contact thermal heat.

paraffin bath should be used cautiously or not at all in patients with circulatory impairments, open lesions, malignancies, skin infections, or sensory deficits.

Hydrotherapy

Hydrotherapy is a means of applying a moist heat evenly to completely cover the area being treated. Hydrotherapy for pain patients is provided through whirlpools and swimming programs. In whirlpools, an electric turbine agitates the water, producing mechanical effects along with the effects of the water (Fig 47–2). These mechanical effects are gentle massage, debridement, relief of pain, and relaxation of muscle spasm. Swimming programs provide a range of benefits to pain patients, such as endurance, coordination, strengthening, and relaxation. Water helps to eliminate the effects of gravity through its buoyant qualities while also providing resistance to exercise. Hydrotherapy should be used cautiously or not at all in patients with infections with edema, skin rashes, or peripheral vascular disease, and patients in whom an increase in systemic temperature is undesirable.

deep heat modalities used for therapeutic purposes are shortwave diathermy, microwave diathermy, and ultrasound. All of these deep heat sources utilize heating by conversion.

Diathermy

"Diathermy may be defined as the generation of heat produced due to the resistance offered by the body tissues with a passage of high-frequency electric current."[1] The energy of shortwave diathermy is transferred into the deeper tissue layers by a high-frequency current, whereas microwave diathermy energy is propagated by means of electromagnetic radiation. "Under optimal conditions, shortwave diathermy will cause a significant tissue temperature rise (TTR) to a depth of 3 cm, whereas microwave diathermy will cause a TTR of 5 cm."[1] The frequencies of shortwave diathermy are rigorously controlled to comply with the tolerances specified by the Federal Communications Commission. The wavelengths corresponding to the allowed frequencies are 22, 11, and 7.5 meters.[2] Shortwave diathermy utilizes four types of electrodes: (1) pads and cuffs, (2) air-spaced plates, (3) drum, and (4) induction field cable. Microwave diathermy, however, offers only one main type electrode which can be beamed to only one surface.

Contraindications to diathermy include the general contraindications to heat, as well as treatment over a pregnant uterus, severely edematous areas, ischemic tissues, malignancies, thrombophlebitis, and hemorrhagic diathesis. Precaution should be taken over areas with sensory impairment and in debilitated patients. Special care must be taken when using diathermy around the eyes. Microwave diathermy definitely should not be used around the eyes. Shortwave diathermy may be used, but cautiously; contact lenses must be removed.

Ultrasound

Ultrasound utilizes heating by conversion through the use of high-frequency acoustic vibration which penetrates into the deeper tissue layers.[2] Therapeutic ultrasound uses ultrasonic waves consisting of mechanical vibrations of 700,000–1,000,000 cycles per second. The wavelength is 0.15 cm. The effects from ultrasound are thermal, nonthermal, and biophysical. In recent years there has been a great deal of research on the effects of and indications for the

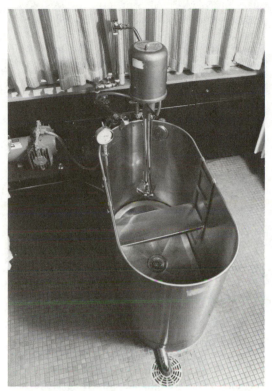

Fig 47–2.—Whirlpools provide pain relief and promote relaxation, thereby increasing circulation and range of motion. In addition, water is a comfortable medium for exercise.

Contrast Baths

Contrast baths entail immersing the extremities first in hot water (105° F) and then in cold water (55° F). The extremity or part is first immersed in hot water for 3–8 minutes and then rapidly immersed in cold water for 1–3 minutes (3:1 time ratio of hot to cold water immersion), ending with final immersion in the hot water. Contrast baths greatly stimulate the peripheral circulation in the extremities without causing any kind of vascular impairment. The treatment has also been effective in reducing edema due to sprains and strains in the extremities. Contraindications are acute sensory loss, Berger's disease, and Raynaud's phenomenon.

Deep Heat

Deep heat provides some benefits that cannot be attained with superficial heat. The three types of clinical use of ultrasound, which vary considerably. The thermal effects have been found to include (1) an increase in peripheral arterial blood flow, (2) an increase in permeability of biologic membranes and a change in membrane potentials, (3) alteration of conduction velocity in peripheral nerves and the production of temporary blocks, (4) alteration of spinal reflexes, and (5) elevation of the pain threshold. The clinical nonthermal effect of ultrasound is the acceleration of diffusion processes across biologic membranes. The biophysical response of ultrasonic energy in tissues depends mainly on two factors, absorption characteristics of the biologic media and reflection of ultrasonic energy at tissue interfaces.[2] All general contraindications to heat therapy should be observed carefully. Ultrasound should not be applied to the eye, over the spinal cord following laminectomy, over the thoracic area where pacemakers are implanted, or over the pregnant uterus. Similarly, ultrasound should not be used in patients with vascular insufficiency, over a treatable malignancy, over healing fractures, or near growth centers of bone until bone growth is essentially complete.

Phonophoresis

Phonophoresis is the movement of substances due to radiation pressure changes caused by transmission of high-frequency sound waves through the couplant into tissues. Significant amounts of medication can be recovered 10 cm deep in the skin after 5 minutes of exposure with the stationary procedure. The technique of phonophoresis minimizes the pain increase immediately following intra-articular or intramuscular injection.[1] Phonophoresis is superior to iontophoresis, as the substances can be driven deeper into the tissues. There is little possibility of skin irritation or burns, and the driven compound does not dissociate into ionized fragments.

CRYOTHERAPY

Heat has been used for the relief of pain for a long time. However, in recent years cold has become increasingly popular and is now used in the form of baths, ice packs, vapocoolant sprays, and ice massage. The initial reaction to cold is vasoconstriction, within 3–5 minutes, followed by a period of vasodilation. After this period of vasodilation, the vessels again become sensitive to the constrictor effect of cold. Cryotherapy usually takes 10–20 minutes. After the ice packs are removed, the skin temperature increases to 25° C for at least 1 hour.[2] Sensory impulses are diminished with local application of extreme cold, and the technique can therefore be effective in promoting muscle relaxation in patients with muscle spasm. Indications for the therapeutic use of cryotherapy are edema, inflammation, strains, and contusions. Raynaud's phenomenon is a contraindication.

ELECTRICAL STIMULATION

Therapeutic electrical stimulation, when properly used and controlled, approximates natural physiologic impulses. The effectiveness of an electrical stimulus depends on its intensity, wave form, and the duration of its effective period.[3] Electrical stimulation utilizes (1) low-frequency alternating currents, also referred to as faradic current (this involves a directional change in the flow of ions), and (2) direct current, also referred to as galvanic, which involves a unidirectional flow of ions. Frequencies range from 0.5 to 3,000 Hz. The frequency used depends on the patient response, the condition being treated, the clinician's preference, and the type of unit used. The physiologic effects of electrical stimulation are also determining factors.[3]

Iontophoresis

Iontophoresis is the process of transferring ions of a topical agent into the body by an electromotive force, usually a direct current. The advantage of this technique is that it allows a relatively large amount of a drug to be delivered subdermally and to deeper structures. The main disadvantage of iontophoresis is the occurrence of skin burns or excessive destruction of the mucous membranes; however, such effects are always due to excessive density of current. Another disadvantage is the difficulty in estimating the dosage delivered.

The clinical application of an electrical current is primarily dependent on the state of innervation of the muscle. The only way a denervated muscle can be adequately contracted is by using a current with impulses of sufficient duration to correspond with the chronaxie (10–100 msec) and a frequency that corresponds to the frequency of tetanus (3–10 pulses/second). Direct current provides these features to stimulate a denervated muscle.

Normal innervated muscle responds to both alternating and direct current. Alternating current is more comfortable and has less of a bite to it. Stimulation of a normal muscle or atrophied muscle, secondary to immobilization, can be done as a form of passive exercise and is a therapeutic adjunct during muscle re-education.

Electrical stimulation is beneficial in the treatment of acute and chronic pain. Due to the facilitation of increased blood supply to the injured tissues, the rate of repair may be stimulated. Relaxation is obtained in skeletal muscles with spasms associated with pain through inhibition. In addition, providing relaxation can increase the range of motion. Spastic muscles resulting from upper motor neuron lesions can be inhibited with electrical stimulation by causing sufficient contractions of the involved muscle groups so that fatigue results. The agonistic muscle group can then be simulated to provide muscle re-education and active isolated movement if this is desired.

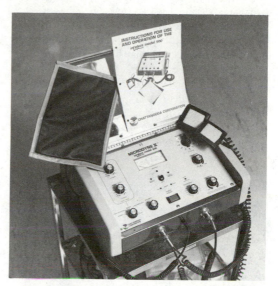

Fig 47–3.—High-voltage galvanic stimulation is commonly used in physical therapy and is a valuable treatment mode in a pain control center.

High-voltage Galvanic Stimulation

High-voltage galvanic stimulation through high-voltage, high peak current (HVHPC) generators has been used to reduce pain, increase joint mobility, improve peripheral circulation, hasten tissue healing, decrease muscle spasms, and reduce edema (Fig 47–3). High-voltage galvanic stimulation is sometimes preferable to low-voltage direct current because it penetrates deeper and provides a stronger contraction with less pain during stimulation. With deeper penetration, HVHPC generators can be placed farther from the motor point and can indirectly stimulate sympathetic nerves and the smooth muscle of blood vessels.[4] The HVHPC generators have a voltage exceeding 150 V with a maximal peak current of 300–400 mamp. The stimulation is delivered via direct current, with variations available in the pulse rate (frequency) and pulse duration. The pulse rate usually "ranges between 50–75 μsec and permits selective stimulation of predominantly sensory and motor axons and much less stimulation of pain conduction nerve fibers."[4]

Electrical Stimulation

Recently, electrical stimulation has been tried for scoliosis, temporomandibular joint dysfunction, nonunion bone fracture, and stress incontinence. Although it is not a new treatment technique, the psychological benefits of electrical stimulation may be of importance and should not be overlooked.

Three major contraindications to electrical stimulation are (1) unstable cardiac pathology (the modality inteferes with demand-type pacemakers and may cause arrhythmias), (2) phlebothrombosis or thrombophlebitis, and (3) skin disorders.

MASSAGE

Massage is a modality whereby the tissues of the body are systematically and scientifically manipulated by the hands for therapeutic purposes. Over the centuries, massage has been used by both man and animal. The oldest written record of massage comes from the Chinese.[2]

The effects of massage may be mechanical or reflexive. Reflexive effects are produced in the skin by stimulation of the peripheral receptors and transmission of impulses via the spinal cord to the cerebral cortex. This produces sensations of pleasure or relaxation. Some authors state that the increase in blood flow is probably through the sympathetic modulation by the reflex mechanism, rather than by local mechanical effect.[5] The mechanical effects of massage, however, may assist the circulatory and lymphatic systems and stretch the adhesions between muscle fibers and fascia.

The common techniques of massage are (1) *stroking* or *effleurage,* which may be superficial or deep; this is the rhythmical movement of hands over body parts, maintaining constant pressure through the stroke; (2) *kneading* or *pétrissage,* which consists of manipulation of skin and muscle, with particular attention given to the configuration of soft tissue structures; (3) *friction massage,* which involves circular movements directed to a specific area of the underlying soft tissues; and (4) *percussion* or *tapotement* movements, or rapidly alternating movements performed to produce stimulation. Hacking, clapping, beating, and vibration are examples of percussive methods.

Massage is useful in any condition in which the relief of pain, reduction of adhesions, reduction of swelling, or relaxation of muscle tissue are indicated. Massage should be used cautiously or not at all in patients with infections, malignancies, acute circulatory disorders, and certain skin diseases.

TRACTION

Cervical and lumbar traction has been used for musculoskeletal dysfunction and diskogenic and degenerative diseases. Methods of traction currently available are *intermittent, static, gravitational,* and *positional.* The purpose of traction is to distract the vertebrae, thereby separating the facets and opening the foramina. It can also be used to relax muscle spasms. Currently there is a debate in the literature over the effects of traction on skeletal and soft tissues and the intensity and direction of force that must be applied to the cervical and lumbar spine.

Lumbar Traction

When lumbar traction is indicated, an initial consideration is to determine the approach. *Intermittent* traction allows variable hold/relax cycles to be instituted by mechanical or manual forces in variable positions; these cycles incorporate the components of trunk range of motion. The coefficient of friction of a patient's body on a surface is such that any force less than 25% of the body weight is incapable of producing traction in the lumbar spine.[6] A *vertical distraction device* employing strong mechanical traction forces has demonstrated up to 2.5 mm widening of lumbar intervertebral joint spaces.[7] Physical therapy units utilize traction units (e.g., split-sliding table) that reduce the friction coefficient. Treatment usually lasts 20–30 minutes, and the

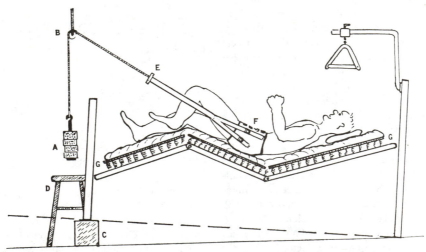

Fig 47–4.—Pelvic traction with the patient in a semi-Fowler position. The patient wears a pelvic band; the pull acts to flex the lumbar spine. *A,* weights, usually 20 lb, are used to apply traction. *B,* overhead pulley is placed so that the pull tilts or lifts the pelvis. *C,* 10-inch block elevates foot of the bed. *D,* stool supports weights when they are temporarily disengaged. *E,* spreader bar separates lateral straps pulling on the pelvic band around the patient's pelvis. *F,* pelvic band with buckles to permit easy detachment by the patient. *G,* split board between mattress and box springs prevents sagging. (From Cailliet.[8] Reproduced by permission.)

force ranges from 25% to 50% or more of the patient's body weight, depending on the patient's tolerance. *Static traction* employs continuous traction forces (Fig 47–4). Cailliet recommends 4-hour durations. This is usually well tolerated. As the vertical angle is increased the duration of traction is also increased.[8] *Gravitational lumbar traction* combines gravity and the patient's lower body weight to overcome friction between the body and hospital bed (Fig 47–5). This produces lumbar distraction. Traction begins at 35° of tilt for reducing frictional resistance. The angle of traction is progressively increased at regular intervals.[9] Treatment times vary, and traction is used intermittently over a period of time. In *positional traction* the patient assumes specific postures to open the vertebral articulations. The patient remains in a given position for a prescribed period of time to relieve stress to specific structures and decrease pain.

Cervical Traction

Cervical traction employs intermittent, static, and positional techniques. *Intermittent traction* elongates the neck and straightens the cervical lordosis. This opens the posterior articulations, widens the intervertebral foramina, disengages the facet surfaces, and elongates the posterior group of muscles and ligaments.[10] *Static traction* provides the added advantage of immobilization of the cervical spine. Manual traction is very useful and often advantageous over mechanical traction as it affords greater control of the position of the head and provides specific grading and duration of the force applied. In one study, manual traction of 300 pounds doubled the intervertebral disk spaces. A minimum vertebral traction force of 25 pounds is necessary to straighten the cervical lordosis.[10] Besides the amount of force applied, the angle of pull and the position of the head are important. Particular attention should be directed to the type of harness used to minimize stress on the temporomandibular joint and to direct most of the force posteriorly.

Home traction units are available for both lumbar and cervical spine dysfunctions; however, cervical traction units are more widely used. As with the lumbar spine, positional traction is beneficial in treating cervical spine dysfunction and controlling pain.

Contraindications to the use of traction are acute trauma, malignancy, hemorrhage, acute inflammation or inflammatory disease, and acute lumbago.[7]

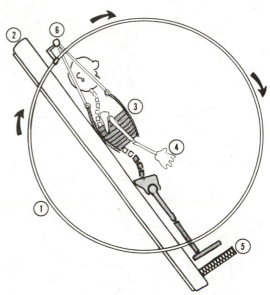

Fig 47–5.—Gravity lumbar traction: *(1)* lumbar traction applied in a hospital setting with a circular bed; *(2)* mattress with bedboard within a Stryker Circ-O-Lectric bed; *(3)* chest harness with lower straps under the rib cage and upper straps firmly grasping the rib cage; *(4)* bed manually controlled by the patient; *(5)* footplate several inches below patient's feet for security; *(6)* snap ring attached to bed frame. (From Cailliet.[8] Reproduced by permission.)

Traction should be used cautiously in patients with neurologic deficits.

MOBILIZATION

Mobilization entails therapeutic maneuvers applied to a dysfunctional joint to restore its arthrokinematics (Fig 47–6).[11] Arthrokinematics includes active and passive and accessory movements (joint play and component motions). Mobilization involves only the accessory movements. Joint play, as defined by Paris, is movement not under voluntary control that occurs in response to an outside force.[11] It is assessed in grades 0–6 (ankylosed to unstable). An example of joint play is the forward glide of the tibia and fibula on the talus during heel strike. Component motions are motions that take place in a joint complex or related joint to facilitate a particular active motion—for example, the spreading of the tibia and fibula to accommodate the wider anterior talus.

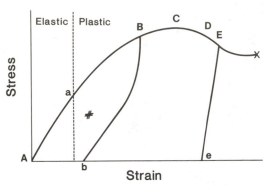

Fig 47–6.—Stress-strain curve; *A*, point of initiation; *a*, end of elastic range; *B*, moderate mobilizing force; *b*, achievable lengthening point of *B*; *c*, optimal stress; *D*, necking; *E*, maximal mobilizing force; *e*, achievable lengthening point of *E*; *X*, point of tissue destruction; *#*, hysteresis loop (heat).

Mobilization techniques are most effective when performed at the necking point.[12]

Indications and contraindications vary according to the experience and expertise of the therapist and the technique used. Mobilization can be used to reduce pain, reduce muscle guarding, or produce a mechanical effect. It is contraindicated in patients with a malignancy, tuberculosis, osteomyelitis, active osteoporosis, fractures, ruptured ligaments, acute arthritis in any form, or disk prolapse with severe neurologic changes. Precaution is indicated for disk prolapse with herniation but without neu-

rologic changes, spondylosis, spondylolisthesis, hypermobility, and scoliosis. It is relatively contraindicated in patients with upper respiratory tract infection, ligament laxity, during pregnancy, and in patients in poor general health.

Techniques of Mobilization

The three main types of mobilization are distraction (traction), nonthrust (articulation), and thrust (manipulation). Distraction is the separation of two articular surfaces in the long axis extension. Nonthrust mobilization incorporates oscillation of the joint within the limits of an accessory motion or oscillation stretch of the joint at the end of its accessory range of motion. Thrust is a sudden, high-velocity, short-amplitude motion delivered at the physiologic limits of an accessory range of motion.

There are different approaches to treatment with mobilization, which may be based on relieving nerve root pressure, relieving pain, or normalizing joint mobility (Fig 47–7). The techniques followed usually are those described by Cyriax, Kaltenborn, Maign, Maitland, Mennell, and Paris.

EXERCISE

Therapeutic exercise may be defined as structured and controlled body movements to correct an impairment, improve musculoskeletal function, or maintain a state of well-being. Exercise may vary

Fig 47–7.—Spinal mobilization in the lumbar area. First, one upper and one lower extremity are flexed and partially dangling over the plinth. Second, one upper extremity and trunk are rotated as a unit by the therapist, with manual pressure applied at the desired level.

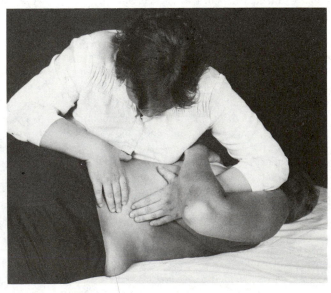

from a highly selected activity, restricted to specific muscles or regions of the body, to overall conditioning, incorporating anaerobics and aerobics. To plan a therapeutic exercise program, the physical therapist must know gross human anatomy, kinesiology, physiology, neuroanatomy, and neurophysiology.[2]

The objective of therapeutic exercise is to increase muscle strength, elasticity, circulation, range of motion, and endurance. In addition, therapeutic exercise is indicated to improve coordination and body awareness (posture, kinesthesia, proprioception). The prescription of an exercise program to produce a desired objective is just as specific as, and often more involved than, the prescription of a drug. An adequate and effective program of therapeutic exercise requires that the prescription be modified as the patient's condition changes.[2] The therapeutic exercise program includes any combination of passive, active assisted, active, and resistive exercises.

Passive Exercise

Passive exercise is joint motion within the unrestricted, normal range of the joint that is produced entirely by an external force (manual or mechanical) and without coordinated voluntary muscle contraction by the patient (Fig 47–8). The primary benefits of passive exercise are to maintain existing joint and soft tissue range of motion, minimize potential for the development of contractures, maintain mechanical elasticity of soft tissue, assist with the maintenance of circulation, and provide sensory and proprioceptive stimulation. There are limitations to passive exercises. It will not prevent muscle atrophy

or increase muscle strength or endurance, and it may be difficult to apply when the muscle is innervated or when pain is present.

Active Assisted Exercise

Active assisted exercise is a means of muscular contraction which is supplemented by an external force (manual or mechanical). The external force may be provided by the therapist, pulleys, a shoulder wheel, or antigravity slings. Active assisted exercise is designed to initiate independent active muscle contraction. This can be of great psychological benefit to the patient as it decreases the fear of moving a painful body part.

Active Exercise

Active exercise entails voluntary muscle contraction by the patient to move the joint through the available range of motion without assistance from an external force. Active exercise facilitates circulation greater than that achieved with passive exercise, maintains soft tissue flexibility, decreases the potential for the development of muscle atrophy, and improves coordination and kinesthetic responses.

Active Resistive Exercise

Resistive exercise incorporates three basic types of active exercise; isometric, isotonic, and isoki-

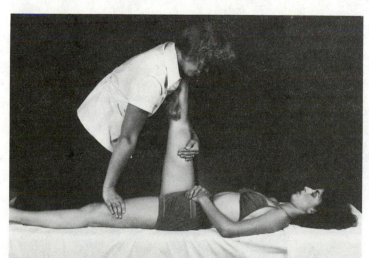

Fig 47–8.—Passive exercise for stretching the hamstring. In passive exercise, manipulation is provided by external forces. In this exercise, care is taken to maintain the opposite leg flat on the plinth.

netic. Benefits obtained from resistive exercise are increased strength, increased power, hypertrophy of muscle fibers, and cardiovascular conditioning.

Isometric Exercise

An isometric contraction is one in which there is increased muscle tension without change in the length of the muscle.[13] It is achieved by pushing against an immovable object, against manual resistance provided by the therapist, or by holding a given weight in a static position. The program can be modified by varying the intensity, number of repetitions, frequency (days per week), and duration (number of weeks). Hettinger and Muller showed that in order to gain strength using an isometric contraction, the isometric tension must exceed 67% of the marginal contractile force of the muscle. Rose, using the method of Hettinger and Muller, showed that a brief maximal resistance exercise (the greatest amount of weight that can be maintained for 5 seconds) performed once a day resulted in improved muscle strength ranging from 82% to 162% over a period of 39–90 days.[2] Strength will develop only at the angle of contraction. Therefore, various angles may be employed in an isometric strengthening exercise program. Isometrics, in addition to increasing strength, can be used to gain muscle control and prevent adhesions.

Isotonic Exercise

Isotonic exercise is the contraction of muscle fibers with a decrease in muscle fiber length, without a change in muscle tension.[14] To achieve the maximal strength and muscle hypertrophy from isotonic exercise, maximal effort at maximal tension is required.[2] Isotonic exercise includes both concentric and eccentric muscle contractions which provide strengthening to the exercised muscles. Klausen et al.[15] suggest that exercises involving eccentric contraction presents vastly different physiologic responses than concentric. In eccentric contractions, the body is capable of producing higher muscle tensions while maintaining the same levels of oxygen consumption and circulatory and pulmonary stress as during concentric exercise. Some studies indicate the eccentric contractions produce greater tension (greater than 40%); however, other studies show the contrary. Muscle soreness may be more pronounced with eccentric contractions.[16] In designing a rehabil-

itation program both isotonic contractions are used based on the patient's needs and limitations.

Delorme's progressive resistive exercise program consists of the 10 repetition maximum (R.M.). The program is initiated with one-half the 10 R.M., then three-quarters the 10 R.M., and then the full 10 R.M. Oxford, concerned with fatigue and recovery, suggests using regressive resistive exercise beginning with the full 10 R.M., then three-quarters 10 R.M., and then one-half to the full 10 R.M.[21] Rose utilizes lifting a maximum weight one time daily and holding it isometrically at the end of range of motion. This has been termed brief maximal resistive exercise.[2]

Isokinetic Exercise

Recent studies indicate that isokinetic exercise is advantageous in rehabilitation when compared to isotonic exercise. Strength, coordination, and endurance can be increased if concentric contractions are performed at a controlled rate. Variations in muscle strength throughout the range of motion can be determined with the use of isokinetic machinery.

Isokinetic exercise is an active, voluntary muscle contraction which moves a body segment through the available range of motion while the speed is kept constant. One objective means of measuring isokinetic performance by a trained professional is through the use of the Cybex machine (Fig 47–9). A major advantage of using the Cybex machine is that variable speeds and angular velocities may be selected (isometric contraction at a given joint position) 36 revolutions per minute (rpm). Once these features are determined, they are kept constant throughout the patient's use.

Different areas of a patient's muscular performance can be determined on the Cybex. Different types of power (the rate of doing work) are low, high, instantaneous, and average, with varying loads and speeds. Endurance is another feature that can be determined by quantifying fatigue rates in the musculature as a result of repetitive, maximum effort, reciprocal contractions. The true presence of weakness, pain, or irritation is indicated by the slope, shape, peak and specific values of the torque developed dynamically at each point in the range of motion. The Cybex is also useful in comparing strengths of body parts. This is used in pain patients for objective measurement of their present muscular state and to indicate progress in the rehabilitation program.

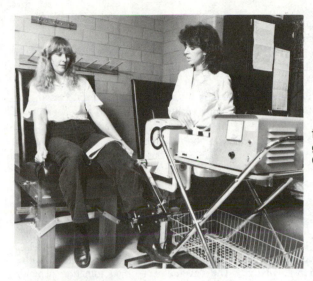

Fig 47–9.—Isokinetic exercises for the quadriceps and hamstring muscle groups performed with the aid of the Cybex machine.

OTHER TECHNIQUES OF THERAPEUTIC EXERCISE

These techniques include endurance activities, desensitization, breathing, relaxation, proprioceptive neuromuscular facilitation, and coordination. These techniques may be used individually or in conjunction with any of the previously discussed modalities.

Endurance

Endurance activities are defined as low weight, high repetition movements of a particular muscle or muscle group, performed over a prolonged period of time, to improve overall body condition. Muscular endurance is related to muscular strength, circulation, local metabolism, fatigue, and motivation to carry on the activity.[2] Walking is a very useful therapeutic exercise to improve endurance for most chronic pain patients. The distance of ambulation is a good objective measurement of progress. Endurance exercises may also include an aquatic program with various types of swimming strokes and weighted activities.

Desensitization

Desensitization is used to reduce hyperesthesia, such as in reflex sympathetic dystrophies, neuralgias, or nerve entrapments. The rationale behind de-

sensitization is to provide higher tolerance for tactile stimulation and/or temperature changes. Tactile stimuli may include air current, light touch, or deep touch. Treatment is generally initiated by the use of noninvasive stimuli. Ice massage, TENS, and friction massage have been found clinically beneficial when used in conjunction with desensitization treatment.

Breathing

Breathing exercises promote deep breathing, rib cage flexibility, chest wall muscle relaxation, and increased vital capacity. Breathing exercises may be indicated in patients with musculoskeletal pain in the cervical, thoracic, or chest wall areas, as well as in patients with chronic obstructive pulmonary disease, scoliosis, neuromuscular disorders, and following thoracic surgery. Types of breathing exercises include diaphragmatic, chest wall stretching, segmental, and postural.

Relaxation

An important part of the patient's home exercise program is the use of relaxation exercises. The goal is to teach the patient to become aware of the difference between the contractile state of a muscle and the resting state. Relaxation training is a progressive technique. Breath control is an essential aspect of this technique and is achieved through coordination of diaphragmatic and intercostal breathing. The patient is made aware of muscular tension by focusing on large muscle masses such as the biceps or quadriceps muscles. The patient is instructed to maximally contract then maximally relax this muscle and continue this process with progressively smaller contractions until fully controlled relaxation is achieved. Another technique focuses on the body parts instead of individual muscle masses. The selective relaxation of muscles helps avoid pain due to prolonged muscle tension.

Proprioceptive Neuromuscular Facilitation

Proprioceptive neuromuscular facilitation is used to promote or hasten the response of the neuromuscular mechanism of the proprioceptors.[17] Diagonal facilitatory patterns of movement are utilized because of their functional correlation with movement (Fig 47–10). Proprioceptive neuromuscular facilitation is a valuable treatment tool because of its universal application in numerous neuromuscular impairments and because it may be performed utilizing any level in the developmental sequence. The primary principles are as follows:[17]

1. Use of the developmental sequence for treatment of patients of all ages, emphasizing proximal-distal and cephalad-caudal progression in movements.
2. Use of sensory and tactile stimulation to increase proprioceptive awareness.
3. Use of coordinated movement proceeding distally to proximally, utilizing a timed sequence of movement.
4. Use of isotonic contractions to encourage movement and isometric contractions to encourage stability and postural sustenance.
5. Use of primitive to complex activities, depending on the patient's abilities.
6. Use of stronger components of a total pattern to augment the weaker components.
7. Use of the patient's abilities to lessen his inabilities.
8. Use of repetitions of coordinated movement to increase strength and endurance and to adjust the rate of movement. Resistance is graded according to the needs and abilities of the patient.

Proprioceptive neuromuscular facilitation utilizes total patterns of movement, specific patterns of facilitation, and techniques for hastening motor learning.

Coordination

Coordination entails the combined activities of a number of muscles in the smooth patterns (of movement) seen under normal conditions.[2] The chronic pain patient is often unable to perform certain coordinated movements. Even though the accomplishment of the movement is perceived by the CNS, the coordinated motion of the component parts is not achieved. The CNS does not perceive all the activities that are occurring or the speed of reaction required to elicit the number of highly selective responses necessary for coordinated motion. There is, therefore, a subconscious reflex mechanism in the brain which responds with multiple pathways to initiate activities simultaneously and allows us to carry the multimuscular activities we perform continually.[18] The development of coordination depends on multiple repetitions of a precisely performed pattern of movement. Control of the coordinated activity is monitored through feedback from sensory stimuli, primarily proprioceptive; however, visual and tactile stimuli play a role as well.

As a particular activity is performed over and over again, a pathway is formed, an engram. An engram is formed through appropriate proprioceptor feedback which is integrated in the cerebellum and then transmitted to the automatic monitory center. The more precise the pattern of movement, the better will be the eventual engram. This is why complex movements must be broken into simplified parts and the simple patterns of movement mastered first before one proceeds to more complicated activity.

The Frenkel exercises used in the treatment of ataxia can also be applied for coordination movements. These exercises allow the use of other stimuli when proprioception is impaired. They utilize total patterns of movement, righting reflexes and stabilization techniques while stressing prime movers. Proprioceptive neuromuscular facilitation patterns can be used to develop coordination; they have the added advantage of incorporating muscle strengthening through manual resistance and gravity resistance through the use of weighted activities.

Besides repetition, precision, and perpetual practice, factors such as inhibition and time must be considered when developing coordination. There must be inhibition of undesired activity. The training of coordination requires progressive selective inhibition during increasing effort so that a capacity for inhibition increases and greater effort can be ex-

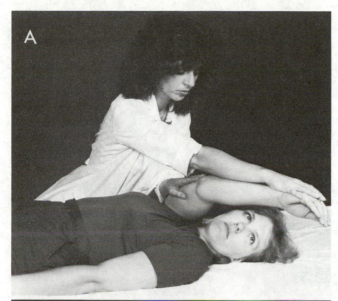

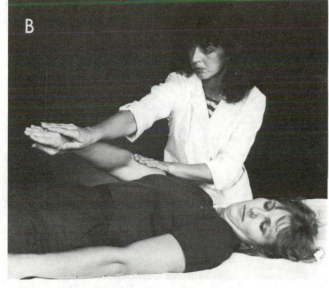

Fig 47–10.—Proprioceptive neuromuscular facilitation for the upper extremity. **A,** movement from a position of shoulder flexion, ER (external rotation), shoulder horizontal adduction elbow extension, supination of the wrist, and finger extension to a position of shoulder extension, IR (internal rotation). **B,** adduction, elbow extension, pronation of the wrist, and finger flexion.

erted without loss of coordination. There is, however, a progressive decline in ability to control motion during the period of inactivity.

It is the role of the physical therapist to evaluate the pain patient thoroughly and consider the indication of various modalities at his or her disposal. The individualized physical therapy program is then designed, taking into consideration the programs outlined by other specialties. Once the program is started, it becomes the responsibility of the physical therapist to monitor that the patient is following the program as outlined, to change the program as the

need arises, to keep the other specialists informed of the patient's progress, and finally to predict the outcome of that program. It is our experience that prolonged pain relief and ability to cope with intractable pain are best achieved with an active physical therapy program and least achieved when such programs are abandoned.

REFERENCES

1. Griffin J., Karselis T.: *Physical Agents for Physical Therapist*. Springfield, Ill. Charles C Thomas, Publisher, 1978, p. 108.

2. Ellwood, Kottke, Krusen, Frank: *Handbook of Physical Medicine and Rehabilitation*. Philadelphia, W.B. Saunders Co., 1971, pp. 279–280.

3. Shriven W.J.: *Manual of Electrotherapy*. Philadelphia, Lea & Febiger, 1975, p. 142.

4. Alon G.: *High Voltage Galvanic Stimulation*. Chattanooga, Tenn., Chattanooga Corporation, 1981, pp. 1–3.

5. Manwell E., Moor F., Muench G., et al.: *Manual of Hydrotherapy and Massage*. California, Pacific Press, 1964, pp. 132–133.

6. Swezy R.L.: *Arthritis: Rational Therapy and Rehabilitation*. Philadelphia, W.B. Saunders Co., 1978, p. 140.

7. Cyriax J.: *Textbook of Orthopaedic Medicine. Vol. 1: Diagnosis of Soft Tissue Lesions*. New York, Bailliere Tindall Publishers, 1978, p. 495.

8. Cailliet R.: *Low Back Pain Syndrome*. Philadelphia, F.A. Davis Co., 1981, p. 92.

9. Owdenhoven R.: Gravitational lumbar traction. *Arch. Phys. Med. Rehabil.* 510, 1978.

10. Cailliet R.: *Neck and Arm Pain*. Philadelphia, F.A. Davis Co., 1981, p. 124.

11. Paris S.: Mobilization of the spine. *J. Am. Phys. Ther. Assoc.* 59:989, 1979.

12. Paris S.: The spine etiology and treatment of dysfunction including joint mobilization. Course given by Stanley V. Paris, 1979.

13. *Taber's Cyclopedic Medical Dictionary*. Philadelphia, F.A. Davis Co., 1973, p. I-53.

14. *Blakiston's Gould Medical Dictionary,* ed. 4. New York, McGraw-Hill Book Co., 1979, p. 709.

15. Klausen K., Knuttgen H.G., Paediatri A., et al.: Exercise with concentric and eccentric muscle contractions. *Scand. Suppl.* 45:217, 1971.

16. Adamcyk K.O., Johnson B.L., Stromme B., et al.: A comparison of concentric and eccentic muscle training. *Med. Sci. Sports* 8(1):35–38, 1976.

17. Knott M., Voss D.: *Proprioceptive Neuromuscular Facilitation Patterns and Techniques,* ed. 2. New York, Harper & Row Publishers, 1968, p. 4.

18. Easton J.K.M., Ozell A.T., Burrill C.: The training of coordination. *Arch. Phys. Med. Rehabil.* 59:567, 1978.

PART VII

Appendices

Appendix I / Formulas

WILLIAM MEISSNER, R. Ph.

Appendix I-A / Analgesic Solutions

BROMPTON COCKTAIL

Ingredients/Materials

One 2000-ml graduated flask
One 1-gallon plastic jug
Morphine sulfate
Cocaine flakes
Simple syrup
Chloroform water
Ethyl alcohol 95%

Manufacturing Procedure

1. Dissolve morphine and cocaine in about 100 ml of chloroform water.
2. Place this solution in the 2,000-ml graduated flask.
3. Add simple syrup and mix.
4. Add ethyl alcohol and mix.
5. Pour this liquid into the plastic gallon jug.
6. Measure the remaining chloroform water in the graduated flask (approx. 1,800 ml).
7. Add it to the gallon jug along with the rest of the solution and mix well.

Each 5 ml of the resulting solution contains 5 mg of morphine and 2.5 mg of cocaine.

Expiration: 6 months

MODIFIED BROMPTON COCKTAIL

Ingredients/Materials

Morphine sulfate solution: 10 mg/5 ml (1,900 ml)
　　　　　Cocaine tabs: 135 mg　　(1,890 ml)
　　　　　Sterile water: qs　　(3,840 ml)

Procedure

Dissolve cocaine tabs in small amount of water. Add morphine solution, then add sufficient quantity of water to make 3,840 ml.

Each 5 ml of the resulting solution contains 5 mg of morphine and 2.5 mg of cocaine.

Expiration: 6 months

Appendix I-B / Bupivacaine

PREPARATION OF BUPIVACAINE FOR CONTINUOUS PERINEURAL INFUSION

Route: Extravascular infusion (*do not give intravenously*)

Concentration: 0.125%–0.75%

Rate: Usually 6–10 ml/hour, but may be as high as 15 ml/hour

Volume: 250 cc. This is a 24-hour supply for most patients. Some patients with two catheters will need two bottles per 24-hour period.

Dilutions: Bupivacaine may be mixed with 0.9% sodium chloride. No other solution should be used in this procedure. If the final concentration ordered is commercially available, just draw up the ampules into an evacuated bottle. (Filter through a 5μ filter needle.) If the concentration must be made up, for example 0.125%, use 0.9% NACI to dilute whatever percentage solution is available. Make the final volume 250 ml.

Label format (if commercially available strength):
  Patient's name and room number
  Bupivacaine 0.25% 250 cc
  Not to be given IV. Use with an infusion pump.
  Rate: Titrate per physician's orders
  Bottle No.:
  Prepared by:

BUPIVACAINE-MEPERIDINE SOLUTION FOR EPIDURAL INFUSION

Ingredients/Materials

Bupivacaine (% specified by physician)
Meperidine (% specified by physician)
Empty sterilized IV bag

Manufacturing Procedure

All procedures are to be done under a laminar flow hood.

1. Draw up desired amount of bupivacaine.
3. Draw up desired amount of meperidine.
3. Draw up desired amount of normal saline.

Example: 0.2% marcaine with 0.1% meperidine 300 ml is ordered.
  Draw up 300 mg of meperidine.
  Draw up 600 mg of bupivacaine.
  Add sufficient quantity of normal saline to make 300 ml.

  If 0.25% bupivacaine solution is used:
  Draw up 240 ml of Marcaine.
  Draw up 3 ml of meperidine.
  Draw up 57 ml of saline.

  If 0.5% bupivacaine solution is used:
  Draw up 120 ml of Marcaine.
  Draw up 3 ml of meperidine.
  Draw up 177 ml of saline.

  If 0.75% bupivacaine solution is used:
  Draw up 80 ml of Marcaine.
  Draw up 3 ml of meperidine.
  Draw up 217 ml of saline.

Label

Special Notes

Send with 0.22-μ Millex GS filter.
Bupivacaine can also be mixed with morphine usually as bupivacaine 0.0625% with morphine as 0.01% in 300 ml saline solution.

Expiration: 24 hours

Appendix I-C / Neurolytic Solutions

PHENOL IN GLYCERIN OR SALINE

Ingredients/Materials

Millex FG 0.2-μ filter (acid-stable)
10 ml of ethanol (95% of 100%)
12-ml plastic syringe
5-ml glass syringe and needle
35-ml plastic syringe
Phenol 89%
Glycerin
Sodium chloride 0.9% (preservative-free)
Plastic glove
30-ml empty sterile vial

Manufacturing Procedure

1. Draw up 10 ml of ethanol in the 12-ml plastic syringe. Remove needle, attach 0.2-μ Millex FG (acid-stable) filter to syringe, and push ethanol through the filter onto a 4 × 4 gauze pad. Set aside, keeping the filter sterile. Discard the gauze pad.

2. With gloves on, draw up 5 ml of phenol into the glass syringe. Remove needle and attach 0.2-μ filter which has been prepared with ethanol, taking care to keep hub of syringe dry during the change. (If the hub is wet, the filter may come off when pressure is applied.) Attach the needle and slowly push 2 or 3 ml of phenol into empty glass container and discard. (This eliminates the ethanol residue in the filter.) Push slowly to avoid breaking the filter membrane.

3. Transfer the required amount of phenol for the percentage required into the empty 30-ml sterile vial, via the filter. Remember to do so slowly.

3%	1 ml of phenol 89%
6%	2 ml of phenol 89%
8%	2.7 ml of phenol 89%
10%	3.3 ml of phenol 89%
12%	4.1 ml of phenol 89%

4. Draw up a sufficient quantity of glycerin or saline to bring final volume to 30 ml and place in 30-ml sterile vial along with phenol.

5. Mix thoroughly and autoclave at 250° C for 20–30 minutes.

Expiration: 30 days

12% PHENOL IN RENOGRAFIN

Ingredients/Materials

Millex FG 0.2-μ filter (acid-stable), cat. No. SLFG025LS
10 ml of ethanol (95% or 100%)
12-ml syringe (plastic)
5-ml syringe (glass) and needle
35-ml syringe (plastic)
Phenol 89%
MD-76 Renografin
Plastic gloves
30-ml empty sterile vial
Foil

Manufacturing Procedure

1. Draw up 10 ml of ethanol in 12-cc plastic syringe, remove needle, attach 0.2-μ Millex-FG (acid-stable) filter to syringe, and push ethanol through the filter onto a 4×4 inch dry gauze pad. Set aside, keeping filter sterile. Discard gauze pad.

2. With gloves on, draw up 5 ml of phenol into glass syringe. Remove needle and attach the 0.2-μ filter which has been prepared with ethanol, taking care to keep the hub of the syringe dry during the change. (If the hub is wet, the filter may come off when pressure is applied.) Attach the needle and *slowly* push 0.9 cc of phenol into empty glass container and discard. This eliminates the ethanol residue in the filter. Push slowly to avoid breaking the filter membrane.

3. Now transfer the proper amount of phenol into the empty 30-ml vial, via the filter. Remember to do so slowly.

3%	1 ml of phenol 89%
6%	2 ml of phenol 89%
8%	2.7 ml of phenol 89%
10%	3.3 ml of phenol 89%
12%	4.1 ml of phenol 89%

4. Draw up appropriate amount of Renografin and place in 30-ml vial along with the measured amount of phenol to make the desired concentration of phenol.

5. Wrap vial in foil and attach label to vial.

Label

Special Notes

Protect from light.

Expiration: 30 days

PHENOL IN AMIPAQUE

Ingredients/Materials

Millex FG 0.2-μ filter (acid-stable)
10 ml of ethanol (95% or 100%)
12-ml plastic syringe
5-ml glass syringe and needle
35-ml plastic syringe
Phenol 89%
Amipaque, 6.75 gm
Diluent
Plastic gloves
30-ml empty sterile vial

Manufacturing Procedure

1. Draw up 10 ml of ethanol in 12-ml plastic syringe. Remove needle. Attach 0.2 μ Millex-FG (acid-stable) filter to syringe and push ethanol through the filter onto a 4 × 4 gauze pad. Set aside, keeping the filter sterile. Discard the gauze pad.

2. With gloves on, draw up 5 ml of phenol into the glass syringe. Remove needle and attach 0.2 μ filter which has been prepared with ethanol, taking care to keep hub of syringe dry during the change. (If the hub is wet, then filter may come off when pressure is applied). Attach the needle and slowly push 2 or 3 ml of phenol into the empty glass container and discard. This eliminates the ethanol residue in the filter. Push slowly to avoid breaking the filter membrane.

3. Transfer proper amount of phenol, depending on percentage needed, into the empty 30-ml vial via the filter. Remember to do so slowly.

3%	1 ml phenol 89%
6%	2 ml phenol 89%
8%	2.7 ml phenol 89%
10%	3.3 ml phenol 89%
12%	4.1 ml phenol 89%

4. Reconstitute Amipaque, 6.75 gm, in vial with 11.7 ml of diluent contained in package to yield a 220 mg/ml concentration. Add appropriate amount of Amipaque to phenol so that final volume is 30 ml.

5. Wrap vial in foil and attach label on vial.

Expiration: 30 days

Appendix II / Equipment

P. PRITHVI RAJ, M.D.
K. JOHNSON, R.N.

Appendix II-A / TENS Units

K. JOHNSON, R.N.

ADDRESSES OF TENS MANUFACTURERS IN THE UNITED STATES (Partial List)

Biostim
Clarksville Rd. and Everett Drive
P.O. Box 3138
Princeton, NJ 08540

Codman/Stimtech
Codman & Shurtleff, Inc.
Randolph, Mass. 02368

Empi, Inc.
261 S. Commerce Circle
Fridley, MN 55432

LaJolla Technology, Inc.
11578 Sorrento Valley Road
San Diego, CA 92121

3M/Medical Products Division
3M Center Bldg. 225–55
St. Paul, MN 55144

Medical Devices, Inc.
833 Third St. SW
St. Paul, MN 55112

Medtronic, Inc.
6951 Central Avenue
P.O. Box 1250
Minneapolis, MN 55440

Mentor
1499 W. River Road North
Minneapolis, MN 55411

Staodyn
Box 1379
Longmont, CO 80501

Neuromedics, Inc.
1027 Dixie Drive
Clute, TX 77531

COMPARISON CHART—TENS UNITS

Manufacturer:	**Biostim**	**Biostim**
Unit:	Biomod (Fig A1)	Recovery Mate (for postoperative use) (Fig A2)
Physical Characteristics		
Dimensions	8.5 × 6.0 × 2.5 cm	2.8 × 2.8 × 7.4 cm
Weight	125 gm	115 gm
Channels	Dual	Single—modular; up to four is practical
Electrical Characteristics		
Power source	Nonrechargeable or rechargeable	High-density lithium battery
Constant current	Yes	Yes
Wave form	Square*	Square*
Pulse width (μsec)	40–220 adjustable, continuous	Standard: 135, fixed Modulation: 135 + 30% modulation
Pulse rate (pulses/ sec)	Standard: 3–150 Burst: 2 bps Modulation: automatically varies pulse width and rate every second	Preset: 65 pps, 30% modulation
Output (mamp)	0–80 (500 ohms)	0–60 (500 ohms)
Burst mode	Yes	No
Modulation mode	Yes; pulse rate and pulse width	Yes; pulse rate and pulse width
Safety Features		
Color-coded leads	Yes	Yes
Knob protector	Yes	Yes
Sentinel	"Startle guard"	"Startle guard"
On/off indicator	Yes	Yes
Low battery indicator	LED light dims	LED light dims
Battery Recharge Time	As per battery manufacturer's specs; usually 4–12 hr	N.A.
Unit Warranty	Lifetime	Disposable

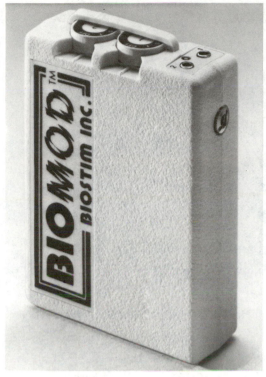

Fig A1.—Biostim Biomod unit.

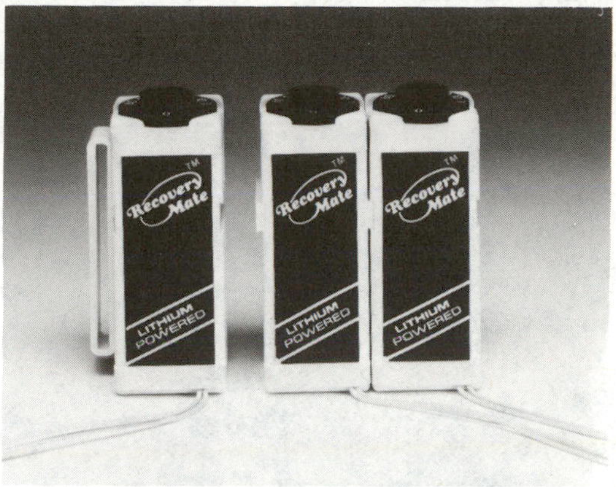

Fig A2.—Biostim Recovery Mate unit.

Manufacturer:	Codman/Stimtech	Codman/Stimtech
Unit:	EPC/Dual (postoperative) (Fig A3)	Stimburst (Fig A4)

Physical Characteristics

Dimensions	9.4 × 6.3 × 3.5 cm	6.8 × 7.3 × 3 cm
Weight	175 gm with battery	165 gm with battery
Channels	Dual	Dual

Electrical Characteristics

Power source	Nonrechargeable: 9-V alkaline	Rechargeable battery pack
Constant current	Yes	Yes
Wave form	Square*	Square*
Pulse width (μsec)	170 fixed	50–250
Pulse rate (pulses/ second)	80 fixed	3–150
		Burst: 7 pulses of 150 pps at intervals of 0.5 sec
Output (mamp)	0–50 (500 ohms)	0–50 (500 ohms)
Burst mode	No	Yes
Modulation mode	No	No

Safety Features

Color-coded leads	No—polarity Yes—channels	
Knob protector	?	No
Sentinel	Yes	Yes
On/off indicator	Yes	Yes
Low battery indicator	Yes	Yes

Battery Recharge Time	NA	5 hr
Unit Warranty	1 yr	2 yr

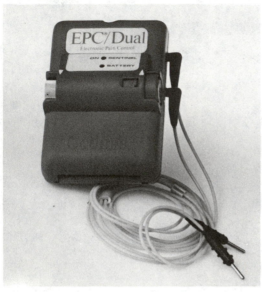

Fig A3.—Codman/Stimtech EPC/Dual unit.

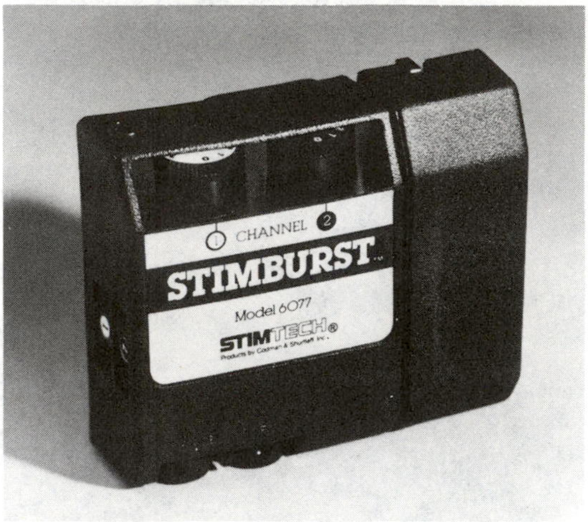

Fig A4.—Codman/Stimtech Stimburst unit.

Manufacturer:	Codman/Stimtech
Unit:	Stimset (Fig A5)

Physical Characteristics

Dimensions	9.5 cm × 6.4 × 3.5 cm
Weight	166 gm with battery
Channels	Dual

Electrical Characteristics

Power source	Nonrechargeable: 9 V
Constant current	Yes
Wave form	Square*
Pulse width (μsec)	Lo: 50, fixed
	Hi: 200, fixed
Pulse rate (pulses/ sec)	Lo: 3
	Hi: 80
Output (mamp)	0–50 (500 ohms)
Burst mode	No
Modulation mode	No

Safety Features

Color-coded leads	No—polarity
	Yes—channels
Knob protector	No
Sentinel	Yes
On/off indicator	Yes
Low battery indicator	Yes

Battery Recharge Time	N.A.
Unit Warranty	2 yr

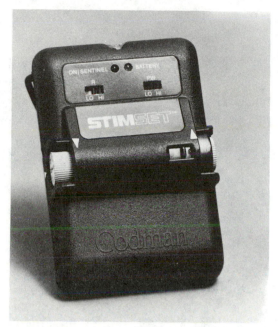

Fig A5.—Codman/Stimtech Stimset unit.

Manufacturer:	Empi, Inc.
Unit:	Epix (Fig A6)

Physical Characteristics

Dimensions	9.1 × 6.3 × 2.1 cm
Weight	70 gm with battery
Channels	Dual

Electrical Characteristics

Power source	Rechargeable: 9 V
	Nonrechargeable: 9 V alkaline
Constant current	Yes
Wave form	Voltage source square
	Current source spike
Pulse width (μsec)	Square: 0–330 at 50% amp. and max. pulse width
	Spike: 200 at 50% amp.
Pulse rate (pulses/ sec)	2–100
Output (mamp)	0–50 mA (1,000 ohms)
	0–50 V (1,000 ohms)
Burst mode	Yes
Modulation mode	Yes: pulse rate and/or amplitude

Safety Features

Color-coded leads	Yes
Knob protector	Yes

Sentinel	No	
On/off indicator	Yes	
Low battery indicator	Yes	
Battery Recharge Time	Approx. 12 hr	
Unit Warranty	3 yr	

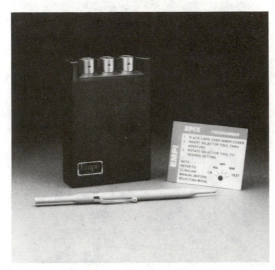

Fig A6.—Empi, Inc. Epix unit.

Manufacturer:	3M	3M
Unit:	Tenzcare 6242 (Fig A7)	Tenzcare 6240 (Fig A8)
Physical Characteristics		
Dimensions	9 × 5.7 × 2.2 cm	6.9 × 11.0 × 2.4 cm
Weight	135 gm	170 gm
Channels	Dual	Dual
Electrical Characteristics		
Power source	Rechargeable, nonrechargeable—4-N type	Disposable
Constant current	Yes	Yes
Wave form	Square*	Square*
Pulse width (μsec)	30–200 adjustable, continuous	Low: 50
		High: 200
Pulse rate (pulses/sec)	4–185	Low: 3
		High: 100
Output (mamp)	Low: 0–70 mA (500 ohms test load)	0–85 (500 ohms)
Burst	High: 0–55 mA (1,000 ohms test load)	
Burst mode	Yes	No
Modulation mode	Yes: pulse width, pulse rate	No
Safety Features		
Color-coded leads	No	Yes
Knob protector	Yes	Yes
Sentinel	Yes	No

On/off indicator	Yes	Yes
Low battery indicator	Yes—low battery cutoff	Yes
Battery Recharge Time	14 hr	N.A.
Unit Warranty	2 yr	2 yr

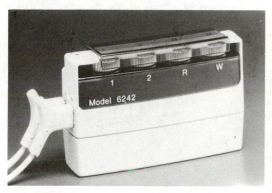

Fig A7.—3M Tenzcare 6242 unit.

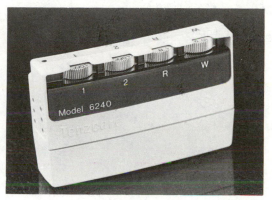

Fig A8.—3m Tenzcare 6240 unit.

| **Manufacturer:** | Medical Devices Inc. | Medical Devices Inc. |
| **Unit:** | Spec IIs | Postoperative |

Physical Characteristics

Dimensions	7.5 × 5.3 × 1.7 cm	7.5 × 5.3 × 1.7 cm
Weight	51 gm	51 gm
Channels	Dual: amplitude, pulse rate, and pulse width isolated	Dual: amplitude, pulse rate, and pulse width isolated

Electrical Characteristics

Power source	Rechargeable, disposable	Rechargeable, disposable
Constant current	Yes	Yes
Wave form	Square*	Square*
Pulse width (μsec)	35–200	35–200
Pulse rate (pulses/ sec)	2/18–120	2/18–120
Output (mamp)	0–60 (± 20%, 500 ohm)	0–60 (± 20%, 500 ohm)
Burst mode	No	No
Modulation mode	No	No

Safety Features

Color-coded leads	No	No
Knob protector	Yes	Yes
Sentinel	No	No
On/off indicator	Yes	Yes
Low battery indicator	Yes	Yes
Battery Recharge Time	8–24 hr (large) 8–19 hr (small)	8–24 hr (large) 8–19 hr (small)
Unit Warranty	2 yr	2 yr

Manufacturer:	Medical Devices Inc.	Medtronics
Unit:	Spec IISX (Fig A9)	Comfort-Burst (Fig A10)

Physical Characteristics

Dimensions	8.5 × 5.3 × 1.7 cm	4.5 × 8.4 × 1.9 cm
Weight	63 gm	75 gm with battery
Channels	Dual	Dual

Electrical Characteristics

Power source	Rechargeable, nonrechargeable (AA, AAA batteries)	Rechargeable
Constant current	Yes	Yes
Wave form	Square*	Spike*
Pulse width (μsec)	35–200	80, fixed (500 ohms)
Pulse rate (pulses/ sec)	2/18–120	Standard: 85
		Burst: 3 bps (7 ppb)
Output (mamp)	0–55	0–75
	(± 20% 500 ohms)	(100–1000)
Burst mode	Yes: cycled	Yes
Modulation mode	Yes: pulse rate and/or pulse width	No

Safety Features

Color-coded leads	No	Yes
Knob protector	Yes	Recessed
Sentinel	No	No
On/off indicator	Yes	Yes
Low battery indicator	Yes	No

Battery Recharge Time	8–24 hr (large) 8–19 hr (small)	12–14 hr

Unit Warranty	2 yr	2 yr

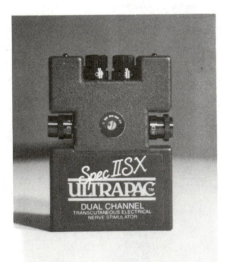

Fig A9.—Medical Devices Spec IISX unit.

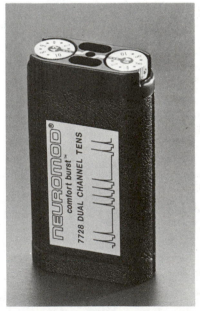

Fig A10.—Medtronics Comfort-Burst unit.

Manufacturer:	Medtronic	Medtronic
Unit:	Comfortwave (Fig A11)	Selectra (Fig A12)

Physical Characteristics

Dimensions	6 × 9.3 × 2.8 cm	6 × 9.3 × 2.8 cm
Weight	180 gm	180 gm
Channels	Dual	Dual

Electrical Characteristics

Power source	Rechargeable:
	  nickel cadmium
	Nonrechargeable:
	  AAA alkaline
		Rechargeable:
		  nickel cadmium
		Nonrechargeable:
		  AAA alkaline

Constant current	Yes	Yes
Wave form	Square*	Selectable: Spike* or square
Pulse width (μsec)	50–250, adjustable	Square: 50–250, adjustable Spike: 80, fixed (500 ohms)
Pulse rate (pulses/ sec)	85 pps, fixed Lo rate: 2 bps, 7 ppb	Standard: 2–99 Burst: 2 bps, 7 ppb (square, spike) Burst: 85, fixed
Output (mamp)	0–50	Square: alkaline, 0–60 Rechargeable: 20–50 Spike: alkaline, 0–150 Rechargeable: 0–80 (200–1,000 ohms)
Burst mode	Yes	Yes
Modulation mode	Yes: pulse rate and/or pulse width	No

Safety Features

Color-coded leads	Yes	Yes
Knob protector	Yes	Yes
Sentinel	No	No
On/off indicator	Yes	Yes
Low battery indicator	No	No

Battery Recharge **Time**	6–8 hr	6–8 hr
Unit Warranty	2 yr	2 yr

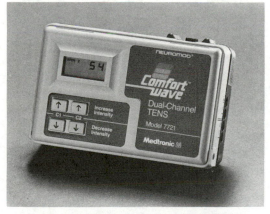

Fig A11.—Medtronic Comfortwave unit.

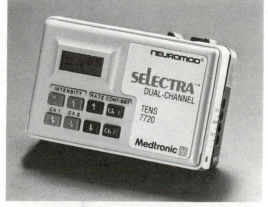

Fig A12.—Medtronic Selectra unit.

Manufacturer:	Mentor	Mentor
Unit:	100 (Fig A13)	150 (Fig A14)

Physical Characteristics

Dimensions	10.7 × 6.5 × 2.3 cm	7.6 × 5.6 × 1.8 cm
Weight	200 gm	100 gm
Channels	Dual	Dual

Electrical Characteristics

Power source	Rechargeable: AA nickel cadmium Nonrechargeable	Rechargeable: N nickel cadmium Nonrechargeable
Constant current	Yes	Yes
Wave form	Square	Square
Pulse width (μsec)	50–500	60–160
Pulse rate (pulses/sec)	2–200	Standard: 2–150, adjustable Burst: 2 bps
Output (mamp)	0–65 (500 ohms)	0–60 (500 ohms)
Burst mode	No	Yes
Modulation mode	No	No

Safety Features

Color-coded leads	No	No
Knob protector	No	Recessed
Sentinel	No	No
On/off indicator	Yes	Yes
Low battery indicator	No	No

Battery Recharge Time	8–12 hr	6 hr
Unit Warranty	2 yr	2 yr

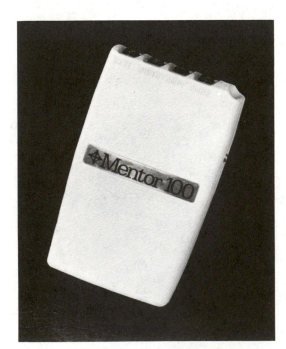

Fig A13.—Mentor 100 unit.

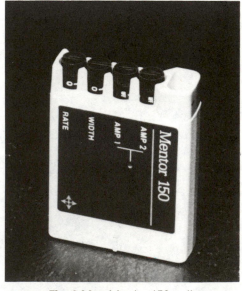

Fig A14.—Mentor 150 unit.

Manufacturer: Neuromedics

Unit: Orion (Fig A15)

Physical Characteristics
Dimensions   7.62 cm × 4.57 × 1.68 cm
Weight   117.5 gm with battery pack
Channels   Dual

Electrical Characteristics
Power source   Rechargeable, nonrechargeable
Constant current
Wave form   Spike
Pulse width (μsec)   20, fixed
Pulse rate (pulses/   3–100, adjustable
    sec)   Burst: conventional, 1 pps; low, 7 pps
Output (mamp)   0–150
Burst mode   Yes
Modulation mode   Yes: rate, amplitude

Safety Features
Color-coded leads   Yes
Knob protector   Yes
Sentinel   No
On/off indicator   Yes
Low battery indicator   Yes

Battery Recharge   16 hr
    Time

Unit Warranty   Lifetime

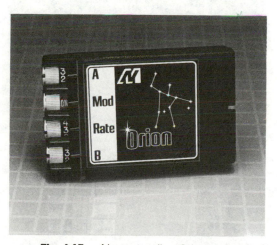

Fig A15.—Neuromedics Orion unit.

Manufacturer: Staodyn   Staodyn

Unit: 4500 Burst (dual)   4500 Modulation (Fig A16)
                           2300 Burst (single)

Physical Characteristics
Dimensions   6.3 × 6.0 × 1.9 cm   6.3 × 6.0 × 1.9 cm
Weight   88 gm with battery   88 gm with battery

Channels	4500—dual 2300—single	Dual

Electrical Characteristics

Power source	Rechargeable: AA Nonrechargeable: AA	Rechargeable: AA Nonrechargeable: AA
Constant current	No	No
Wave form	Square*	Square*
Pulse width (μsec)	40–100	40–100
Pulse rate (pulses/ sec)	4500: 2–120 2300: 2–120	2–140
Output (mamp)	6–70 (500 ohms)	6–75 (500 ohms)
Burst mode	Yes	No
Modulation mode	No	Yes

Safety Features

Color-coded leads	Yes	Yes
Knob protector	Yes	Yes
Sentinel	No	No
On/off indicator	Yes	Yes
Low battery indicator	Yes	Yes

Battery Recharge Time	18 hr, Ni-Cad 90 hr, alkaline	18 hr, Ni-Cad 90 hr, alkaline

Unit Warranty	Lifetime	Lifetime

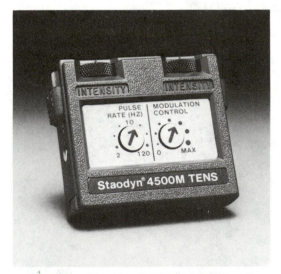

Fig A16.—Staodyn 4500 Modulation unit.

Manufacturer:	Staodyn
Unit:	4500 (Fig A17)

Physical Characteristics

Dimensions	6.3 × 6.0 × 1.9 cm
Weight	88 gm with battery
Channels	Dual

Electrical Characteristics

Power source	Rechargeable: AA
	Nonrechargeable: AA
Constant current	No
Wave form	Square*
Pulse width (μsec)	40–100
Pulse rate (pulses/ sec)	2–140
Output (mamp)	6–70 (500 ohms)
Burst mode	No
Modulation mode	No

Safety Features

Color-coded leads	Yes
Knob protector	Yes
Sentinel	No
On/off indicator	Yes
Low battery indicator	Yes

Battery Recharge Time	18 hr, Ni-Cad
	90 hr, alkaline

Unit Warranty	Lifetime

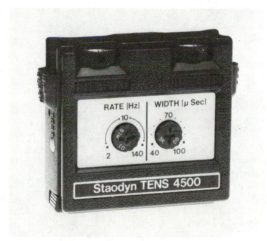

Fig A17.—Staodyn 4500 unit.

Manufacturer:	LTI
Unit:	Dynex II

Physical Characteristics:

Dimensions	6.4 × 8.9 × 2.2 cm
Weight	114 gms
Channels	Dual

Electrical Characteristics

Power source	Rechargeable
	Nonrechargeable: 9 V alkaline
Constant current	Yes
Wave form	Square*
Pulse width (μsec)	40–200 adjustable, continuous
Pulse rate (pulses/ sec)	2–110

Output (mamp)	0–60 (1,500 ohms)
Burst mode	Yes
Modulation mode	Yes: pulse width

Safety Features

Color-coded leads	Yes
Knob protector	Yes
Sentinel	No
On/off indicator	Yes
Low battery indicator	Yes

Battery Recharge Time	9 hr

Unit Warranty	2 yr

*Zero net D/C component.

Appendix II-B / Biofeedback

ROBERT E. PAWLICKI, Ph.D.

A BRIEF LISTING OF SUPPLIES OF BIOFEEDBACK EQUIPMENT SUPPLIERS

Stoelting-Cyborg
1350 S. Kostner Ave.
Chicago, IL 60623

Tel. (312) 522-7777

Stoelting-Cyborg supplies a modern computer-based biofeedback system capable of assessing multiple psychophysiologic channels as well as handling complex statistics and data manipulations (Fig A18).

Thought Technology, Ltd.
2180 Belgrave Ave.
Montreal, Quebec H4A 2L8

Tel. (514) 489-8251

Thought Technology offers relatively inexpensive GSR, EMG, and heart rate portable monitors.

Lafayette Instrument Co.
P.O. Box 5729
Lafayette, IN 47905

Tel. (317) 423-1505

Lafayette Instruments offers an extensive supply of equipment including single and multiple channel, stationary and portable biofeedback instruments. Most equipment involves polygraph display.

Autogenic Systems Inc.
Dept. MA-3
802 Allston Way
Berkeley, CA 94710

Tel. (415) 548-6056

Autogenics supplies a popular line of instrumentation and will provide complete service, including equipment setup and training of technicians.

Self Regulation Systems, Inc.
15521 N.E. 90th St.
Redmond, WA 98052

Tel. (206) 882-1101

Self Regulation Systems supplies a computer-based biofeedback system capable of data analysis and graphic display.

For a more extensive listing of biofeedback supplies, see Alton & Noonberg, *Biofeedback: Clinical Application in Behavioral Medicine*. Englewood Cliffs, N.J., Prentice-Hall, Inc, 1980.

FOR INFORMATION ON STANDARDS AND EDUCATION, RELATED TO THE PRACTICE OF BIOFEEDBACK

Biofeedback Society of America
4301 Owens Street
Wheat Ridge, CO 80033

Tel. (303) 420-2889

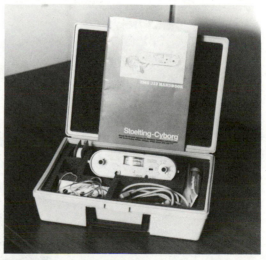

Fig A18.—Stoelting-Cyborg biofeedback apparatus.

Appendix II-C / Peripheral Nerve Stimulators

P. PRITHVI RAJ, M.D.

ADDRESSES OF MANUFACTURERS OF NERVE STIMULATORS IN USA (Partial List)

Bard Inc.
Westmount, IL 60559
(Fig A19)

Output Inc.
Portland, Oregon

Dupaco
1740 LaCosta Meadow
San Marcos, CA 92069
(Fig A20)

Anesthesia Associates
581 N. Twin Oaks
P.O. Box 1105
San Marcos, CA 92069

Professional Instruments
416 Pickering Street
P.O. Box 38245
Houston, TX 77088

Neuro Technology
Houston, Texas (Fig A21)

Burroughs Welcome
Research Triangle Park
North Carolina 27709

Nerve Finder
Regional Master Corp.
P.O. Box 431832
Miami, FL 33143

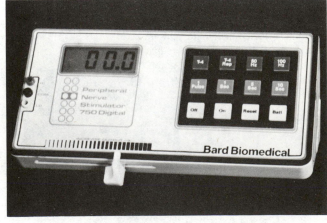

Fig A19.—Bard Biomedical 750 digital peripheral nerve stimulator.

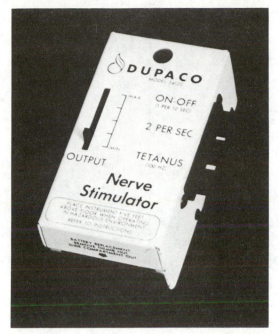

Fig A20.—Dupaco peripheral nerve stimulator.

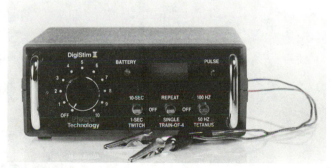

Fig A21.—Neuro Technology DigiStim II peripheral nerve stimulator.

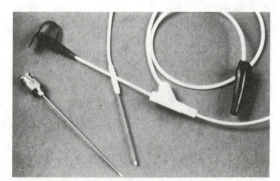

Fig A22.—Sheathed and unsheathed needles of a peripheral nerve stimulation unit.

TABLE A1.—PERFORMANCE OF COMMERCIALLY AVAILABLE NERVE STIMULATORS

MANUFACTURER	CONSTANT CURRENT	LINEARITY	METER POLARITY*	PULSE WIDTH (μsec)	PULSE INTERVAL	HIGH AND LOW OUTPUT	BATTERY INDICATOR	MAX. OUTPUT AT 2,000 OHMS (mamp)
Output Dupaco	++	Poor		200	1 Hz			28
	+	Good		500	2 Hz			19.5
Bard	High ++ Low ++	Good	Yes	200	1 Hz	Yes	Yes	High: 4.3 Low: 17.5
Anaesthesia Associates	++	Fair		500	5 Hz		Yes	21.5
Professional Instruments	++	Poor		150	1 Hz			
Neuro Technology	High ++ Low +++	Good	Yes	200	1 Hz	Yes	Yes	High: 66 Low: 22
Burroughs-Welcome	++	Poor		†	1 Hz			25
Nerve Finder	+++	Poor	Yes	1,000	1 Hz		Yes	15

*None of the instruments tested had the ideal labeling of "needle" and "grounding."
†Hyperbolic pulse.

Appendix II-D / Epidural Nerve Stimulators

P. PRITHVI RAJ, M.D.

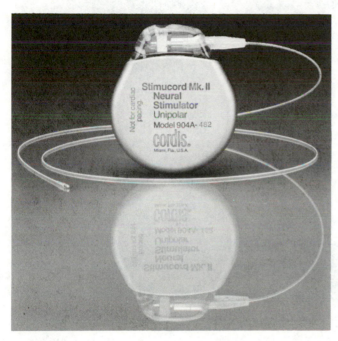

Fig A23.—Cordis Stimucord Mack II unipolar epidural nerve stimulator. (Courtesy of Cordis Corporation, Miami, Fla.)

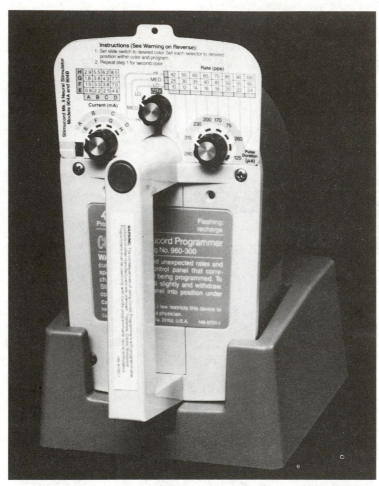

Fig A24.—Programmer for Cordis Stimucord Mark II epidural nerve stimulator. (Courtesy of Cordis Corporation, Miami, Fla.)

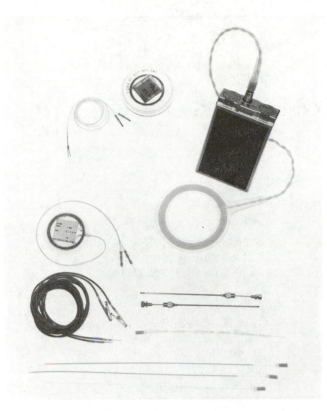

Fig A25.—Avery percutaneous electrical stimulator. Figure also shows transmitter, antenna, receiver, electrodes, and accessories. (Courtesy of Avery Laboratories, Inc., Farmingdale, N.Y.)

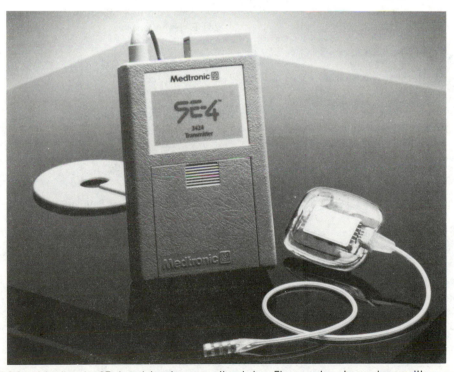

Fig A26.—Medtronic SE-4 epidural nerve stimulator. Figure also shows transmitter, receiver, and antenna.

Appendix III / Pain Clinics*

UNITED STATES

Alabama

Shelby Anesthesia Services
Shelby Memorial Hospital
Alabaster, AL 35020

Anniston Pain Clinic
1029 Christine
Anniston, AL 36201

Brookwood Medical Center
Pain Management Center
Brookwood Drive
Birmingham, AL

University of Alabama in Birmingham Pain Center
1813 6th Ave., South
Birmingham, AL 35294

Arizona

St. Joseph's Hospital Pain Center
350 W. Thomas Road
Phoenix, AZ 85013

Scottsdale Memorial Hospital
7200 E. Osborn Road
Scottsdale, AZ 85251

Jack L. Marteney, D.D.S., Ltd.
5747 E. 5th St.
Tucson, AZ 85711

University of Arizona Hospital
Pain Clinic
Tucson, AZ 85724

Veteran's Hospital
South 6th
Tucson, AZ 85723

Arkansas

Southwestern Human Services Institute, Inc.
324 W. Pershing Blvd.
North Little Rock, AR 72114

California

Beverly Hills Pain and Stress Control Center
8920 Wilshire Blvd., Suite 525
Beverly Hills, CA 90211

Biofeedback Medical Clinic
18370 Burbank Blvd.
Tarzana, CA 91356

Bay Area Pain Rehabilitation Center
281 E. Hamilton Ave.
Campbell, CA 95008

Norman Fischer, D.D.S
22030 Sherman Way, No. 204
Canoga Park, CA 91303

Rancho Los Amigos Hospital
Downey, Calif.

City of Hope Pain Center
1500 E. Duarte Road
Duarte, CA 91010

North Coast Clinic for Pain and Stress
  Management
2773 Harris Ave.
Eureka, CA 95501

Pain Treatment Center
Scripps Clinic Medical Institutions
10666 N. Torrey Pines Road
La Jolla, CA 92037

Pain Control Center
Loma Linda University Medical Center
Loma Linda, CA 92350

---

*Partial listing.

Pain Therapy and Evaluation Unit
Jerry L. Pettis Memorial Veterans Hospital
Loma Linda, CA 92354

Pain Management Program
VA Medical Center
5901 East 7th St.
Long Beach, CA 90822

UCLA Center for Health Science
Pain Management Clinic
10833 Le Conte
Los Angeles, CA 90024

Center for Integral Medicine
1900 Avenue of the Stars, Suite 2440
Los Angeles, CA 90067

Pain Diagnostics and Rehabilitation Institute
2210 W. 3rd St.
Los Angeles, CA 90057

UCLA Pain Control Unit
Franz Hall A181
UCLA Hospital and Clinics
Los Angeles, Calif.

Louis W. Lewis, M.D.
443 W. 22nd Street
Merced, CA 95340

Hoag Memorial Hospital-Presbyterian
301 Newport Boulevard
Newport Beach, CA 92660

Lawrence Pain Control Group
7535 Laurel Canyon Boulevard
North Hollywood, CA 91605

Providence Hospital
30th and Summit St.
Oakland, CA 94609

University of California at, Irvine Medical Center
101 City Drive South
Orange, Calif.

Los Medanos Community Hospital
550 School St.
Pittsburg, CA 94565

University of California at Davis School of
    Medicine
4301 X St.
Professional Building, Room 253
Sacramento, CA 95817

San Bernardino Community Hospital
Pain Management Center
SBCM 1500 W. 17th St.
San Bernardino, CA 92411

Chronic Pain Program
Sharp Rehabilitation Center
7901 Frost St.
San Diego, CA 92007

Mercy Hospital and Medical Center
4077 Fifth Avenue
San Diego, CA 92103

Pain Unit, VA Medical Center
3350 La Jolla Drive
San Diego, CA 92161

Department of Neurosurgery
Univ. of California Medical Center
San Francisco, CA

Saint Francis Memorial Hospital
900 Hyde St.
San Francisco, CA 94109

St. Mary's
450 Stanyan
San Francisco, CA 94117

Department of Anesthesia Nerve Block Clinic
University of California
San Francisco, CA 94143

The San Jose Orthopedic Pain Center
2512 Samaritan Court, Suite G
San Jose, CA 95124

Cox Pain Center
2066 Chorro Street
San Luis Obispo, CA 93401

Joel E. Berger, D.D.S.
1183 Los Angeles Ave.
Simi Valley, CA 93065

Harbor General Pain Clinic
Harbor UCLA Medical Center
1000 W. Carson St.
Torrance, CA 90509

Southwest Surgical Clinic
Multispecialty Outpatient Surgical Services
4201 Torrance Blvd., Suite No. 240
Torrance, CA 90503

Walnut Creek Hospital
175 La Casa Vista
Walnut Creek, CA 94598

Colorado

Boulder Memorial Hospital
Pain Control Center
311 Mapleton Ave.
Boulder, CO 80203

Colorado Pain Rehabilitation and Counseling
Center
1660 S. Albion St. No. 309
Denver, CO 80222

Denver Pain and Stress Control Center
2045 Franklin St.
Denver, CO 80205

University of Colorado Medical Center
Pain Clinic
4200 E. 9th Ave.
Box B113
Denver, CO 80262

Connecticut

Pain Clinic
Greenwich Hospital
Greenwich, CT 06830

Research Institute of Acupuncture and Chinese
Medicine
Route 188 and N. Benson Road
Middlebury, CT 06762

Arthur Taub, M.D., Ph.D.
Pain Clinic
60 Temple St.
New Haven, CT 06510

VA Medical Center
West Spring St.
West Haven, CT 06516

Delaware

Delaware Pain Center
249 E. Main St.
Newark, Delaware 19711

District of Columbia

Georgetown University Medical Center
3800 Reservoir Road
Washington, D.C. 20007

Greater Southeast Community Hospital Pain Center
1310 Southern Avenue, S.E.
Washington, D.C. 20032

Florida

Fort Lauderdale Pain Control Center
1925 North East 45th St.
Suite 226
Fort Lauderdale, FL 33308

University of Florida
College of Dentistry Pain Clinic
Box J16
J. Hillis Miller Health Center
Gainesville, FL 32610

Miami Pain Control Center
7000 S.W. 62nd Ave.
Suite 234
Miami, Florida 33134

Miami Heart Institute
4701 N. Meridian Ave.
Miami Beach, FL 33139

Pain Treatment Center
Baptist Hospital of Miami
8900 North Kendall Drive
Miami, FL 33176

The Pain Center
Mount Sinai Medical Center
4300 Alton Road
Miami Beach, FL 33140

University of Miami School of Medicine
Dept. of Neurological Surgery
Miami, FL 33101

Institute for Physical and Behavioral Medicine
12550 Biscayne Boulevard, No. 700
North Miami, FL 33181

Medical Center Clinic
8333 No. Davis Highway
Pensacola, FL 32504

Pain Clinic
U.S. Naval Aerospace Regional Medical Center
Pensacola, FL 32512

Hubert Rutland Hospital
5115 58th Ave.
St. Petersburg, FL

Georgia

Atlanta Pain Control and Rehabilitation Center
17 Prescott St., NE
Atlanta, GA 30308

Emory University Pain Control Center
Center for Rehabilitation Medicine
1441 Clifton Road, N.E.
Atlanta, GA 30322

Georgia Baptist Hospital
300 Boulevard
Atlanta, GA 30312

The Pain Rehabilitation and Biofeedback Center of
    West Georgia, Inc.
8954 Hospital Drive, Suite 100-C
Douglasville, GA 30134

Hawaii

St. Francis Hospital Pain Study Unit
2230 Liliha Street
Honolulu, HI 96817

Illinois

Southern Illinois University
School of Dental Medicine
2800 College Avenue
Alton, IL 62002

B.R.A.I.N.S. Labs
Biofeedback Re-Education and Integrative
    Neurophysiology
2010 South Arlington Heights Road
Arlington Heights, IL 60005

Chicago Osteopathic Hospital
5200 South Ellis Ave.
Chicago, IL 60615

Diamond Headache Clinic
5252 N. Western
Chicago, IL 60625

Illinois Masonic Medical Center
836 West Wellington
Chicago, IL 60657

Low Back and Pain Clinic
Rehabilitation Institute of Chicago
345 E. Superior St.
Chicago, IL 60611

Pain Control Clinic
1825 West Harrison St.
Chicago, IL 60612

Temporomandibular Joint and Facial Pain Research
    Center
801 So. Paulina
University of Illinois Medical Center
Chicago, IL 60612

Rush Pain Center
1725 West Harrison St.
Suite 262
Chicago, IL 60090

Navy Regional Medical Center
Great Lakes, IL 60088

The Pain Treatment Center
Lake Forest Hospital
660 Westmoreland
Lake Forest, IL 60045

Foster G. McGraw Hospital of Loyola University
2160 South 1st Ave.
Maywood, IL 60153

Methodist Medical Center
Pain Management Clinic
221 N.E. Glen Oak
Peoria, IL 61636

Peoria Pain Control
Medical Arts Building, No. 101
1101 Main St.
Peoria, IL 61606

R.C. Balagot, M.D. and Assoc.
4332 W. Oakton
Skokie, IL 60076

Marianjoy Rehabilitation Hospital
Pain Center
26 W. 171 Roosevelt Road
Wheaton, IL 60187

Indiana

Elkhart General Hospital
Elkhart, IN 46514

St. Mary Medical Center
Pain Control Center
540 Tyler
Gary, IN 46402

Community Hospital Rehabilitation Center for Pain
1500 N. Ritter Ave.
Indianapolis, IN 46219

Pain Clinic
Mercy Hospital
Mason City, IN 50401

St. Joseph's Hospital Pain Control Unit
811 E. Madison
P.O. Box 1935
South Bend, IN 46634

Kansas

Kansas University Medical Center
3900 Rainbow Boulevard
Kansas City, KS 66103

Pain Clinic of Wichita, P.A.
3243 East Murdock, Suite 401
Wichita, KS 67208

Kentucky

Louisville Pain Clinic
326 Medical Towers South
Louisville, KY 40202

University of Louisville
Oral Diagnosis-Facial Pain Clinic
Health Sciences Center
501 S. Preston St.
Louisville, KY 40232

Louisiana

Hotel Dieu Pain Rehabilitation Unit
2021 Perdido St.
New Orleans, LA 70112

L.S.U. Medical Center
Oro-Facial Pain Unit
1100 Florida Ave.
New Orleans, LA 70119

Pain Clinic and Acupuncture Institute of New
  Orleans
401 Robert E. Lee Blvd.
New Orleans, LA 70124

Shreveport Pain and Rehabilitation Center
1128 Louisiana St.
Shreveport, LA 71101

Maine

Osteopathic Hospital of Maine
335 Brighton Ave.
Portland, ME 04102

Massachusetts

Baystate Medical Center
759 Chestnut St.
Springfield, MA 01106

New England Rehabilitation Hospital
Rehabilitation Way
Woburn, MA 01801

University of Massachusetts
  Medical Center
55 Lake Ave.
Worcester, MA 01605

Anesthesia Pain Service
Massachusetts General Hospital
Fruit St.
Boston, MA 02114

Boston Pain Unit
Massachusetts Rehabilitation Hospital
125 Nashua St.
Boston, MA

Tufts University School of Medicine
New England Medical Center Hospital
171 Harrison Ave.
Boston, MA 02111

Brockton Hospital Pain Clinic
680 Centre St.
Brockton, MA 02402

Maryland

Myo-Oral Facial Pain Clinic (MOFP)
666 W. Baltimore St.
University of Maryland
Baltimore, MD 21201

Sinia Hospital of Baltimore
2401 W. Belvedere Ave.
Baltimore, MD 21215

Pain Treatment Center
The Johns Hopkins Hospital
601 N. Broadway
Baltimore, MD 21205

Theratec Treatment Center
Village of Cross Keys
Suite 262
Baltimore, MD 21210

National Institutes of Health
  Clinic Center
Bethesda, MD 20014

Neurobiology and Anesthesiology Branch
National Institute of Dental Research
National Institute of Health
Bethesda, MD 20205

Associated Pain Consultants
8808 Cameron St.
Silver Springs, MD 20910

Fairland Pain Clinic
13616 Colefair Drive
Silver Springs, MD 20904

Metropolitan Pain Control Center
8808 Cameron St.
Silver Springs, MD 20910

Mensana Clinic
Greenspring Valley Road
Stevenson, MD 21153

Michigan

Biofeedback Institute of Michigan
555 S. 14 Mile Road
Clawson, MI 48017

Sinai Hospital Pain Clinic
6767 W. Outer Drive
Detroit, MI 48235

University of Detroit
School of Dentistry
2985 E. Jefferson Ave.
Detroit, MI 48207

Chronic Pain and Holistic Health Center, Inc.
3006 Waters Building
Grand Rapids, MI 49503

Ingham Medical Center Pain Clinic
401 W. Greenlawn
Lansing, MI 48910

Pain and Stress Management Program
Psychological Evaluation and Treatment Center
15209 W. Michigan Ave.
Marshall, MI 49068

Pain Research and Control Institute
22401 Foster Winter Drive
Southfield, MI 48075

Barry N. Tilds, D.D.S., P.C.
35101 Dodge Park
Sterling Heights, MI 48077

Minnesota

Minneapolis Pain Control Center
Southdale Medical Building
Suite 621
6545 France Avenue S.
Edina, MN 55435

6681
6681 Country Club Drive
Golden Valley, MN 55427

Golden Valley Health Center
4101 Golden Valley Road
Golden Valley, MN 55422

Acupuncture and Pain Clinic
Hibbing General Hospital
2015 Fourth Ave. E.
Hibbing, MN 55746

Pain Clinic of St. Joseph's Hospital
324 Garden Blvd.
Mankato, MN 56001

Low Back Clinic and Department of
 Neuroaugmentive Surgery
Sister Kenny Institute
2545 Chicago Ave.
Minneapolis, MN 55404

Metropolitan Medical Center
800 S. 8th St.
Minneapolis, MN 55404

Midwest Pain Center
6490 Excelsior Blvd.
Minneapolis, MN 55426

Minneapolis Pain Clinic
Pain Rehabilitation Program
4225 Golden Valley Road
Minneapolis, MN 55422

Mount Sinai Hospital Acupuncture Clinic
2215 Park Avenue South
Minneapolis, MN 55404

Parkview Treatment Center
3705 Park Center Blvd.
Minneapolis, MN 55416

University of Minnesota Hospitals
Neurosurgery Department
420 Delaware
Minneapolis, MN 55455

Mayo Clinic—St. Mary's Hospital
Rochester, MN 55901

Mayo Pain Clinic and Pain Management Center
200 2nd St. SW
Rochester, MN 55901

St. Paul Pain Control Center
Doctors Professional Building
Suite 325
280 N. Smith Ave.
St. Paul, MN 55102

St. Paul Ramsey Hospital and Medical Center
640 Jackson St.
St. Paul, MN 55101

Mississippi

The UMC Multidisciplinary Pain Clinic
University of Miss. Medical Center
2500 N. State Street
Jackson, MS 39216

Missouri

St. Francis Medical Center
Cape Grandeau, MO 63701

Ellis Fischel State Cancer Hospital
115 Business Loop 70 West
Columbia, MO 65201

Harry S. Truman Memorial
Veterans Hospital
800 Stadium Blvd.
Columbia, MO 65201

Charles E. Still Osteopathic Hospital
1125 S. Madison St.
Jefferson City, MO 65101

Montana

Missoula Pain Clinic
Missoula Rehabilitation Center
2829 Fort Missoula Road
Missoula, MT 59801

Nebraska

Nebraska Pain Management Center
University of Nebraska Hospital and Clinic
42 and Dewey Ave.
Omaha, NE 68105

Pain Clinic
7701 Pacific St.
Suite 123
Omaha, NE 68124

New Jersey

John Ort, M.D.
21 Holster Road
Clifton, NJ 07013

Northeast Pain Control Center
No. 1 Racetrack Road
East Brunswick, NJ

New Jersey College of Medicine and Dentistry,
Dental School
100 Bergen St.
Newark, NJ 07103

Temporomandibular Joint and Headache Pain
Center
New Jersey College of Dentistry
100 Bergen St.
Newark, NJ

St. Mary's Hospital
135 So. Center St.
Orange, NJ 07050

Pain Clinic, St. Joseph's Hospital
703 Main St.
Paterson, NJ 07012

Delaware Valley Physical Therapy Associates
1520 Pennington Road
Trenton, NJ 08618

C.N.S. and Pain Management Institute of
Pennsylvania
769 Northfield Ave.
West Orange, NJ 07052

Oncology and Hematology Associates
603 North Broad
Woodbury, NJ 08086

New Hampshire

Dartmouth Hitchcock Medical Center
Hanover, NH 03755

New Mexico

Lovelace Medical Center
5200-5400 Gibson Blvd.
Albequerque, NM 87108

New York

Lourdes Hospital
169 Riverside Drive
Binghamton, NY 13905

Acupuncture Clinic at Diagnostic and Treatment
Center
Albert Einstein College of Medicine
1165 Morris Park Ave.
Bronx, NY 10461

Montefiore Hospital Headache Unit
111 East 210th St.
Bronx, NY 10467

Kingsbrook Jewish Medical Center
86 East 49th St.
Brooklyn, NY 11203

Pain Therapy Center
Maimonides Medical Center
4802 10 Ave.
Brooklyn, NY 11219

Parsons Acupuncture Clinic
25 - 14 Parsons Blvd.
Flushing, NY 11354

Andrew A. Fischer, M.D., P.C
17 Wooley Lane East
Great Neck, NY 11021

Facial Pain Group
Department of Dentistry
Queens Hospital Center
82-86 164th St.
Jamaica, NY 11432

Duane H. Tucker, D.O.
1133 Colvin Blvd.
Kenmore, NY 14223

Nassau County Medical Center
2201 Hempstead Turnpike
East Meadow
Nassau, NY

Columbia-Presbyterian Medical Center Pain
  Treatment Center
622 W. 168 St.
New York, NY 10032

David B. Kriser
Oro-Facial Pain Center
N.Y.U. College of Dentistry
421 First Ave.
New York, NY 10010

Facial Pain Clinic
Columbia University School of Oral and Dental
  Surgery
630 West 168th St.
New York, NY 10032

Hospital for Joint Diseases
1919 Madison Ave.
New York, NY 10035

Institute of Rehabilitation Medicine
400 E. 34th St.
New York, NY 10016

Memorial Sloan Kettering Cancer Center
1275 York Ave.
New York, NY 10021

New York Hospital Pain Clinic
525 E. 68th St.
New York, NY 10021

Pain Consultation Service
Department of Anesthesiology
530 First Ave., Suite 3E
New York, NY 10016

St. Luke's Hospital
TMJ Facial Pain Clinic
421 West 113th Str. and Amsterdam Ave.
New York, NY 10025

St. Vincent's Hospital, NYC
153 West 11th St.
New York, NY 10012

Veterans Administration Medical Center
130 W. Kingsbridge Road
New York, NY 10468

Phelps Memorial Hospital Pain Clinic
North Broadway
North Tarrytown, NY 10591

Family Practice Center
840 Humboldt Parkway
Snyder, NY 14211

Upstate Medical Center
State University Hospital
750 E. Adams St.
Syracuse, NY 13210

Pain Clinic
Westchester County Medical Center
Valhalla, NY

North Carolina

UNC Pain Center
NCMH Box 106
NC Memorial Hospital
Chapel Hill, NC 27514

Duke Pain Clinic
Box 3094
Duke University Medical Center
Durham, NC 27710

North Dakota

T.N.I. Pain Clinic
700 First Ave. South
Fargo, ND 58102

Ohio

Yale S. Palchick
3455 Granger Road
Akron, OH 44313

Pain Relief Center
University of Cincinnati Medical Center
Goodman St.
Cincinnati, OH 45267

Ohio Pain and Stress Treatment Center
1460 W. Lane Ave.
Columbus, OH 43221

Miami Valley Hospital
One Wyoming St.
Dayton, OH 45409

Elyria Pain and Respiratory Clinic
436 East River St.
Elyria, OH 44035

Maumee Valley Physical Therapy
    Associates, Inc.
6005 Monclova Road
Maumee, OH 43537

Medical College of Ohio Hospital
Caller Service No. 10008
Toledo, OH 43699

Wadsworth Pain Clinic
195 Wadsworth Road
Wadsworth, OH 44281

Youngstown Osteopathic Hospital
1319 Florencedale
Youngstown, OH 44505

Rehabilitation and Pain Clinic, Inc.
727 Market St.
Zanesville, OH 43701

Oklahoma

Thomas L. Ashcraft, M.D.
2325 S. Harvard
Tulsa, OK 74114

Oregon

Sacred Heart General Hospital
1200 Alder St.
Eugene, OR 97401

Northwest Pain Center
10615 S.E. Cherry Blossom Drive
Suite 170
Portland, OR 97216

Pain Evaluation Clinic of Good Samaritan Hospital
1120 N.W. 20th Ave., Suite 105
Portland, OR 97209

Pennsylvania

Pain Clinic
Charles Cole Memorial Hospital
Coudersport, PA 16915

Pain Clinic at DuBois Hospital
DuBois, PA 15801

Pain Clinic
Delaware County Memorial Hospital
Drexel Hill, PA 19026

Polyclinic Medical Center
3rd St. and Polyclinic Ave.
Harrisburg, PA 17110

Pain Control Center
1086 Franklin St.
Johnstown, PA 15905

Allegheny Valley Hospital
1300 Carlisle St.
Natrona Heights, PA 15065

Citizens General Hospital
651 4th Ave.
New Kensington, PA 15068

Peckville Pain Clinic
144 Main St.
Peckville, PA 18452

Pain Control Center of Temple University
Temple University Hospital
3401 N. Broad St.
Philadelphia, PA 19140

TMJ and Facial Pain Clinic
University of Pennsylvania School of Dental
    Medicine
4001 Spruce St.
Philadelphia, PA 19104

Thomas Jefferson University Hospital
111 S. 11th St.
Philadelphia, PA 19107

Pain Control Clinic
Room 9408
DeSoto at O'Hara St.
Presbyterian University Hospital
Pittsburgh, PA 15213

Shadyside Hospital
5230 Centre Ave.
Pittsburgh, PA 15232

VA Hospital
University Drive C
Pittsburgh, PA 15240

Low Back Pain Clinic
Crozer-Chester Medical Center
Upland, Chester, Pennsylvania 19013

Puerto Rico

San Juan Pain Clinic
461 Calle 6
Ext. San Agustin
Rio Piedras, Puerto Rico

South Carolina

Department of Anesthesiology
Medical University of S.C.
Charleston, SC 29403

V.A. Medical Center
Garner's Ferry Road
Columbia, SC 29201

South Dakota

St. Joseph's Hospital Pain Clinic
Lewiston, SD 83501

Tennessee

Faculty Medical Practice Corp.
Pain Clinic
66 N. Pauline
Memphis, TN 38105

Texas

Dallas Rehabilitation Institute
7850 Brookhollow Road
Dallas, TX 75235

Texas Neurological Institute
7777 Forest Lane, Suite 2420
Dallas, TX 75230

Veterans Administration Hospital
4500 S. Lancaster
Dallas, TX 75216

Metroplex Dolorology Center
1650 W. Magnolia, Suite 103
Fort Worth, TX 76104

University of Texas Medical Branch
John Sealy Hospital
Suite 2A
Galveston, TX 77550

University of Texas Medical Branch (Galveston)
8th and Mechanic St.
Galveston, TX 77550

Medical Center Del Oro Hospital
8081 Greenbriar
Houston, TX 77054

Pain Control and Biofeedback Clinic
Department of Anesthesiology
Baylor College of Medicine
Texas Medical Center
Houston, TX 77030

Chronic Pain Treatment Program of B.C.M. at The
   Methodist Hospital
6516 Bertner Blvd.
Houston, TX 77030

University of Texas Medical School
Anesthesia Pain Clinic
6431 Fannin St.
Houston, TX 77030

University of Texas Pain Clinic
Hermann Hospital
1203 Ross Sterling Ave.
Houston, TX 77030

Wilford Hall USAF Medical Center
Lackland AFB, TX 78236

Texas Tech University School of Medicine
3601 4th St.
Health Sciences Center Hospital
Lubbock, TX 79430

North Texas Back Institute
3901 West 15th St.
Plano, TX 75075

Anesthesia Pain Clinic
4499 Medical Suite 306
San Antonio, TX 78229

A. Murphy V.A. Hospital
7400 Merton Minter Blvd.
San Antonio, TX 78284

University of Texas Health Science Center
Anesthesia Pain Clinic
7703 Floyd Curl Drive
San Antonio, TX 78284

Villa Rosa Rehabilitation Center
5115 Medical Drive
San Antonio, TX 78229

Scott and White Clinic
Scott and White Hospital
2401 South 31st St.
Temple, TX 76501

Hohf Clinic and Hospital, Inc.
1404 E. Hiller
Victoria, TX 77901

Utah

W. Lynn Richards, M.D.
480 South 400 East
Bountiful, UT 84010

Rehabilitation Center
McKay-Dee Hospital
3939 Harrison Blvd.
Ogden, UT 84409

Salt Lake Pain Clinic
508 E.S. Temple, Suite A16
Salt Lake City, UT 84103

Virginia

University of Virginia Pain Center
Box 293
University of Virginia Medical Center
Charlottesville, VA 22908

Pain Control Clinic, Dibrell Hall
115 South Main St.
Danville, VA 24541

National Capital Center for Craniofacial Pain
803 West Broad St.
Falls Church, VA 22046

Medical College of Virginia Department of
  Anesthesiology
Pain Clinic
P.O. Box 785
MCV Station
Richmond, VA 23298

MCV/VCU Temporomandibular Joint and Facial
  Pain Center
Box 637 Medical College of Virginia
Richmond, VA 23298

Medical College of Virginia
Comprehensive Center
1200 E. Broad St.
Richmond, VA 23298

Veterans Administration Medical Center
Richmond, VA 23249

Washington

Whatcom-Skagit Pain Clinic
3401 Byron Ave.
Bellingham, WA 98225

Chronic Genito-Urinary System Pain Clinic (for
  Women)
University Hospital
1959 N.E. Pacific
Seattle, WA 98195

Northgate Pain Clinic
Anders E. Sola, M.D.
120 Northgate Plaza
Room 340
Seattle, WA 98125

Swedish Hospital Pain Clinic
702 Summit Ave.
Seattle, WA 98104

Mason Clinic Pain Clinic
1100 Ninth Ave.
P.O. Box 900
Seattle, WA 98040

University of Washington Pain Clinic
1959 N.E. Pacific St.
Seattle, WA 98195

Sacred Heart Medical Center
W. 101 8th Ave.
Spokane, WA 99204

West Virginia

Appalachian Regional Hospital and Veterans
  Hospital of Marshall University, S.M.
Beckley, WV 25801

West Virginia University Pain Clinic
West Virginia University Medical Center
Morgantown, WV 26506

H. J. Thomas Memorial Hospital
4605 MacCorkle Ave. S.W.
South Charleston, WV 25309

Wisconsin

Pain and Health Rehabilitation Center
Rt. 2, Welsh Coulee
LaCrosse, WI 54601

University of Wisconsin
Clinical Science Center
600 Highland Ave.
Madison, WI 53792

Chronic Rehabilitation Program
Mt. Sinai Medical Center
950 N. 12th St.
Milwaukee, WI 53233

Curative Rehabilitation Center
9001 W. Watertown Plank Road
Milwaukee, WI 53226

Milwaukee County Medical Complex
Pain Clinic
8700 W. Wisconsin Ave.
Milwaukee, WI 53226

Veterans Administration
Medical Center
5000 West National Ave.
Wood, WI 53193

ARGENTINA

Hospital Durand
Division de Anesthesiologia
Seccion de Dolor
Avenida Diaz Velez 5044
1404 Buenos Aires
Argentina

AUSTRALIA

Pain Clinic
Royal Adelaide Hospital
Adelaide, South Australia 5000

Royal Prince Alfred Hospital Pain Clinic
Missendon Road
Camperdown, NSW, Australia 2050

Sir Charles Gardner Hospital
Sherton Park
Perth, Western Australia 6009

Pain Unit
Flinders Medical Centre
Adelaide, South Australia, Australia 5042

The Prince of Wales Hospital Pain Clinic
High Street
Randwick, N.S.W., Australia 2031

The Pain Clinic
St. Vincent's Hospital
Victoria Street, Darlinghurst
Sydney, N.S.W., Australia 2010

AUSTRIA

University Klinik für Neurochirurgie
A-8036
Graz
Austria

Ludwig Boltzmann Acupuncture Institute
Mariannengasse 10
Austria

BELGIUM

Clinique de la Douleur
I Heger Bordet St.
Brussels, Belgium B 1000

Department of Anesthesiology
Academic Hospital
De Pintelaan 135
B-9000 Ghent, Belgium

Eemheid Voor Pijntherapie
35 Capucienenvoer
Leuven, Belgium 3000

Neurosurgery Department
St. Vincentiusziekenhuis
St. Vincentiusplein 1
9000 Gent
Oost-Vlaanderen, Belgium 9000

Hospital D'Ougree
Pain Clinic Dpt.
Rue G. Trasenster
Ougree, Belgium B4200

BRAZIL

Jony Andrade Sobrinho
Manoel Bandeira St.
Judiai Sao Paulo, Brazil 13200

CANADA

Headache Research Unit
Ambulatory Care Centre
University of Calgary Medical School
Calgary, Alberta, Canada T2N 1N4

Department of Psychiatry
University of Alberta
Edmonton, Alberta, Canada T6G 2G3

Victoria General Hospital Pain Clinic
Tower Road
Halifax, Nova Scotia, Canada B3H 2YD

Pain Clinic
Hamilton Civic Hospital
Barton Street Unit
237 Barton Street
E. Hamilton, Ontario, Canada L8 L2X2

McMaster U. Pain Clinic
1200 Main St. W.
McMaster U. Medical Centre-2F
Hamilton, Ontario, Canada L85 4J9

University Hospital
P.O. Box 5339
Postal Station A
London, Ontario, Canada N6A 5A5

Victoria Hospital Pain Clinic
375 South St.
London, Ontario, Canada N6A 4G5

St. Joseph's Hospital Pain Clinic
Grosvenor St.
London, Ontario, Canada N6G 123

London Psychiatric Hospital
850 Highbury Ave.
London, Ontario, Canada N6A 4H1

Pain Management Unit
Department of Anesthesia
687 Pine Ave. W.
Montreal, Quebec, Canada H3A 1A1

Montreal Neurological Institute
3801 University St.
Montreal, Quebec, Canada H3A 2B4

Montreal General Hospital
Montreal, Quebec, Canada

Hotel-Dieu of Montreal
Pain Clinic
3820 St. Urbin
Montreal, Canada H2W 2TB

Royal Ottawa Hospital
1145 Carling Ave.
Ottawa, Ontario, Canada K17 7K4

St. Josephs Hospital
Peterborough, Ontario, Canada K9H 7B6

Centre Hospitalier de L'Universite Laval
2705 Boul. Laurier
Ste.-Foy Que. 10e, No. 2209
Quebec (Ste-Foy) Canada G1V 4G2

Hospital St. Josef de Rimouski
150 Rue Rouleau
Rimouski, Quebec, Canada

Pain Management Service
(Satellite of Saskatoon Clinic)
Plains Health Centre
Regina, Saskatoon, Canada S4S 5W9

Pain Management Service
University Hospital
Saskatoon, Sask., Canada S7N 0W8

Rosedale Pain Treatment Center
600 Sherbourne Street
Toronto, Ontario, Canada M4Y 1W4

The Wellesley Hospital Pain Study Group
160 Wellesley St. East
Toronto, Ontario, Canada

Neurosurgical Division
Department of Surgery
Toronto General Hospital
101 College St.
Toronto, Ontario, Canada

Smythe Pain Clinic
121 University Wing
Toronto General Hospital
Toronto, Ontario, Canada M5G 1L7

Maxwell Anesthetic Service
202, 805 West Broadway
Vancouver, BC, Canada V5Z 1K1

North York Pain Clinic
1333 Sheppard Ave. East
Willowdale, Ontario, Canada

Berkely Clinic
1273 Ovellette Ave.
Windsor, Ontario, Canada N8X 1J3

General Centre Health Science
700 William St.
Winnipeg, Manitoba, Canada R3E 0Z3

CZECHOSLOVAKIA

Bulovka Hospital
2 Budinova
Praha 8
Liben, Czechoslovakia CS-180 81

DENMARK

Margrethe Knudsen
Anaesth. In Ch.
Sygehuset, Horsens
Sundvej 32
8766 Horsens
Denmark

ENGLAND

Pain Relief Unit
Abingdon Hospital
Abingdon, Oxfordshire, England

Pain Relief Clinic
Royal United Hospital
Bath, Avon, England

Pain Relief Clinic
Royal Infirmary
Blackburn, Lancashire, England

Bradford Area Pain Relief Clinic
Royal Infirmary
Duckworth Lane
Bradford, West Yorkshire
United Kingdom BD9 6RJ

Macmillan Unit
Christ Church Hospital
Christchurch, Dorset, England

Hastings Pain Clinic
Royal East Sussex Hospital
Cambridge Road
Hastings, East Sussex, England TN 36 IER

Pain Relief Service
General Infirmary at Leeds
Great George St.
Leeds, W. Yorkshire, England LS1 3EX

Liverpool Dental Hospital
Pembroke Place
Liverpool, United Kingdom L69 3BX

North West Regional Pain Relief Centre
Hope Hospital
Eccles Old Road
Manchester, England

Pain Relief Clinic
Royal Victoria Infirmary
Wolfson Unit of Clinic Pharmacology
Newcastle upon Tyne, England NE1 4LP

Centre for Pain Relief
Department of Medical and Surgical Neurology
Walton Hospital
Rice Lane
Liverpool, United Kingdom

Dr. J. N. Kenyon
21 Aigburth Drive
Sefton Park
Liverpool, England L17 4JQ

Hallamshire Hospital
Glossor Road
Sheffield, S Yorks
England S10 2JF

Eric Angel Pain Clinic
Freedom Fields Hospital
Plymouth, Devon, United Kingdom

National Hospital for Nervous Diseases
Queen Square
London, W C 1 England

St. Christopher's Hospice
51–53 Lawrie Park Road
Sydenham, London, England 6 DZ

United Norwich Hospitals
Pain Relief Service
Norwich, Norfolk, England

Southampton Pain Clinic
Royal South Hants Hospital
Eanshawe Street
Southampton, Hampshire, England

FINLAND

Department of Anesthesiology and Department of
Neurosurgery
University of Central Hospital
90220 Oulu 22
Finland

Pain Center
34 Palomaentie
Tampere, Finland SF-33230

FRANCE

Centre Oscar Lambret
B.P. 3569
59020 Lille Cedex
France

Centre Hospitalier de Mont Morency
17 Rue du Docteur Millet
Montmorency
Val D'Oise, France 95160

Centre Paul Lamarque
34033 Montpellier
Cedex, France

Consultation de Reflexotherapie
Centre Hospitalier Regional et Universitaire
B.P. 26–30006
Nimes, France

Hospital Saint-Antoine
184, Rue du Faubourg Saint-Antoine
Paris, France 75012

Clinique Universitaire de Neurochiburgie
Hopital Purpan (Place Baylac) Toulouse, France
31052

WEST GERMANY

Neurochirurgische Universitatsklinik
110 Im Neuenheimer Field
6900 Heidelberg
West Germany

Schmerzambulanz der Univ. Frauenklinik
4–14 Pulsstrasse
1000 Berlin
19 West Germany

Schmerzambulanz
Kreis Krankenhaus
4A Krankenhaus Str.
D-8765 Erlenbach
West Germany

Bezirkskrankenhaus Gunzburg
Akaidemsches Krankenhaus für die Universität
Ulm
Schmerzambulanz
D-8870 Gunzburg
West Germany

Interdisciplinary Pain Clinic
University Hospital
L Langenbeckstrabe
65 Mainz
West Germany

Klinikum Minden (Anesthesia)
6 Mismarckstr.
Minden
NRW W. Germany 4950

Red Cross Krankenhaus
Manigua
Neuromedizinisches Institut.
Scheffeleck
Neiderrader Landstrasse 58
Frankfurt am Main
West Germany 6000

Anaesthesie Abteilung
Kreiskraukeuhaus
1 Osswald
8130-Starnberg, West Germany

Neurosurgical Clinic
Krhs. Bethesda
1 Hainstr. 35
56 Wuppertal 1
West Germany

HOLLAND

St. Hippolytusziekenhuis
Reinier de Graedweg 11
Delft, Holland 2625AD

Lukas Ziekenhuis
31 Albert Schweitzerlaan
Apeldoorn, Holland 7300DS

CHINA

University of Hong Kong
Faculty of Medicine
Physiology Department
5 Sassoon Road
Hong Kong

ISRAEL

Rambain Medical Center
Batgalim
Haifa, Israel

Dept. of Biomedical Engineering
Technion
Israel Institute of Technology
Haifa, Israel

Clinic for Spinal Disorders
Hadassah University Hospital
Mt. Scopus
Jerusalem, Israel

Pain Clinic
Hadassah University Hospital
Ein Karem
Jerusalem, Israel

ITALY

Major Comprehensive Pain Center
Reparto di Analgesia
Ospedale Generale Regionale
Ancona, Italia 60100

Centro De Terapia del Dolore
26 Via Michele Coppino
Cuneo, Italy 12100

Centro do Algologia
Clinica Medica
85 Viale Morgani
Firenze, Italy I-50134

Dept. of Anesthesiology
Ospedale Civile
Pz. S. Agostino
Modena, Italy 41100

Istituto di Neurochirurgia
Dell' Universita
Di Padova
Via Giustiniani 2
Padova, Italy 35100

Neurosurgical Clinic
University of Pavia
Piazzale Golgi
Pavia, Italy 27100

Instituti Ospedaliere DiPietra Ligure
Pietra Ligure, Italy 17027

Istituto Regina Elena per lo Studio e la Cura del
    Tumori
(National Cancer Institute, Regina Elena)
291 Viale Regina Elena
Rome Italy 00161

Ist. Neurochirursia
Universita' Cattolica
1 Larso A. Semelli
Rome, Italy 00158

Centro Cefalee Dell' Universita
3 Via Genova
Ospedale S. Giovanni
Torino, Italy 10126

Giuseppe Franchi M.D.
Reparto di Rianimazione e di Terapia del Dolore
Ospedale Civile Maggiore di Verona
Verona, Italy 37025

JAPAN

Pain Clinic in Aizuchuo Hospital
181–1 Tsurga
Aizuwakamatsu-shi
Fukushimaken, Japan 965

Amomori Prefectural Central Hospital
1–2–24 Nagashima, Aomori
Aomori-ken, Japan 030

Pain Clinic
Department of Anesthesiology
Osaka Medical College
7 Dagikumachi 2chome
Takatsuki
Osaka, Japan 569

Neurosurgical Pain Clinic
Department of Neurosurgery
University of Tokyo Hospital
7–3–1 Hongo
Tunkyo-ku, Tokyo Japan

Pain Clinic
Fukuoka University Hospital
34 Nanakuma Nishiku
Eukuoka, Japan 814

Department of Anesthesiology
Kyushu University
3–1–1 Maedashi, Higashiku
Eukuoka, Japan

Department of Anesthesiology
Gifu University Hospital
40 Tukasamachi
Gifu, Japan

Department of Anesthesiology
Hirosaki Univ. Sch. Med.
53 Honcho
Hirosaka, Aomori-ken
Japan

Pain Clinic
Kanazawa University School of Medicine
13–1 Takara-Machi
Kanazawa city
Ishikawa-Ken, Japan 920

Neurosurgery Clinic
Saitama Cancer Center
818 Komuro
In-a-machi, Saitama, Japan 362

Outpatient Clinic of Department of Anesthesiology
Kumamoto University Medical School
1–1–1 Honjo Machi
Kumamoto, Japan 860

Pain Clinic
Tottori Kosei Hospital
343 Shimotanaka
Kurayoshi, Tottori Prefecture, Japan

Department of Anesthesiology
Gunma University Hospital
3 Chyome Showa-machi
Maebashi, Gunma, Japan 371

Department of Neurosurgery
Faculty of Medicine
Shinshu University
Asahi 3–1–1
Matsumoto, Japan

Pain Clinic
1–757 Asahimach
Niigata, Japan 951

Clinic of Dental Anesthesiology
Osaka University Dental Hospital
4–3–48 Keta-ku Nakanoshiona
Osaka City, Japan

EHIME University School of Medicine
Department of Anesthesiology
Shigenobu, EHIME-ken, Japan 791–02

Pain Clinic
Department of Anesthesia
Tokyo University Hospital
7–3–1 Hongo
Bunkyo-ku
Tokyo, Japan 113

Department of Neurosurgery
Kinki University Medical School
Sayama-Cho, Minami-Kawachi-Gun
Osaka, Japan 589

Pain Clinic
Department of Anesthesiology
Showa University Hospital
1–5–8 Hatanodai Hospital
Shinagawa-ku, Tokyo, Japan 142

Department of Neurosurgery
Neurological Inst.
Tokyo Women's Medical College
10 Kawada-cho
Shinjuku-ku, Tokyo, Japan 162

Pain Clinic
Surugadai Nihon University Hospital
1–8–13 Kanda-Surugadai
Chiyoda-ku
Tokyo, Japan 101

Yamagata University Hospital
Zao-Ida
Yamagata, Japan 990–23

Tottori University Hospital
36–1 Nishimachi
Yonago, Tottori-ken, Japan 683

MEXICO

Instituto Nacional de la Nutricion
Ave. San Fernando y San Buenaventure
Tlalpan
Mexico Distrito Federal, Mexico 22

NEW ZEALAND

Auckland Pain Clinic
Auckland Hospital
Park Road
Auckland-3, New Zealand

Pain Clinic
Middlemore Hospital
Otahuhu
Auckland 6, New Zealand

Dunedin Pain Relief Clinic
Dunedin Public Hospital
Great King Street
Dunedin, Otago, New Zealand

Pain Clinic
Palmerston North Hospital
Palmerston North, Monawata
New Zealand

NIGERIA

Pain Clinic
University College Hospital
Ibadan, Oyo, Nigeria

Acupuncture and Pain Relief Clinic of 'Luth'
Lagos University Teaching Hospital
Lagos, Nigeria PMB 12003

NORWAY

Department of Neurology
Akershus Central Hospital
University of Oslo
N 1474 Nordbyhagen, Norway

PHILLIPINES

Phillipine General Hospital
Taft Avenue
Manila, Phillipines

POLAND

Poradnia Leczenia Bolu
15 A Kopernika
Krakow, Poland 31–501

Pain Centre
1 a Banacha Street
Warsaw, Poland 02–907

Pain Clinic
Integrated Health Care Complex
16, Kozielska Str.
44–100 Gliwice, Poland

SPAIN

Ciudad Sanitaria ''1° de Octobre''
Carretera de Andalucia Km 5
Madrid, Spain

SWEDEN

Department of Anesthesiology
Centralsjukhuset
S-65185
Karlstad, Sweden

37 Lasarettsgatan
Smartmottagnin, Lasarettet
S-59100 Motala, Sweden

Low Back Unit
Department of Orthopedics, Surgery
Huddinge University Hospital
S 141 86 Huddinge
Stockholm, Sweden

Anders Bjelle, M.D.
Department of Rheumatology
University Hospital S-90185
Uned, Sweden

Modality Orientated Pain Center
Central Hospital
Vasteras, Sweden

Department of Anesthesiology
Centralsjukyuset
S-65185 Karlstad Sweden

Smartmottagningen
Sandvikens Sjukhus
811 00 Sandviken, Sweden

SWITZERLAND

Schmerzklinik Kirschgarten
30 Hirschgaesslein
4051 Basel, Switzerland

Medical Department Lory, Inselspital
3010 Berne Inselspital, Berne
Berne, Switzerland

Schmerzzentrum, Kantonsspital Liestal
Kantonsspital Liestal
CH4410 Liestal, Switzerland

THAILAND

Siriraj Hospital
Banmgkok, Thailand

THE NETHERLANDS

Gronigen Pain Centre
University Hospital
Clinic of Psychiatry
Oostersingle 59
Groningen, The Netherlands

University Hospital
Leiden, The Netherlands

TURKEY

Bilge Kadriye, M.D.
Profesorlersitesia
Blok Katz Daires
Istanbul, Etiler, Turkey

WALES

Pain Clinic
Bangor
Gwyneed
Wales, U.K.

YUGOSLAVIA

Pain Clinic of the Institute of
Clinical Neurophysiology
7 Zaloska
Ljubljana, Yugoslavia 61105

Appendix IV / Educational Material

ROBERT E. PAWLICKI, M.D.
P. PRITHVI RAJ, M.D.

FILMS ON CHRONIC PAIN: ANNOTATED BIBLIOGRAPHY

Carron, Harold. *Evaluation of the Chronic Pain Patient*
Pain Clinic, Department of Anesthesiology, University of Virginia Medical Center, Charlottesville, Virginia

Carron describes various aspects of the chronic pain experience, including the meaning of pain, past pain experience, ethnic and cultural implications, and the psychological makeup of the patient. He differentiates between acute and chronic pain, making seven comparisons. In the evaluation of the chronic pain patient, Carron cites nine components of the assessment process: pain history, social history, occupational history, drug history, psychological history, physical examination, special studies, psychological testing, and psychological interview. He proposes criteria for evaluating each component and specifies the information that must be obtained before a treatment regimen can be formulated.

Carron, Harold. *Your Pain: How to Manage It*
Pain Management Center, Department of Anesthesiology, University of Virginia Medical Center, Charlottesville, Virginia

Carron and associates provide material designed to answer patients' questions about pain and its treatment. The distinction is made between acute and chronic pain. Acute pain is associated with tissue damage, is time-limited, and may be treated in a straightforward manner. Chronic pain presents a complicated picture. It may not be associated with tissue damage and may result in muscle weakness, medication dependency, "doctor shopping,"

depression, irritability, social isolation, and financial problems. Therefore, chronic pain requires a different treatment approach. It may not be possible to eliminate chronic pain immediately or totally, but the following goals are stressed: a decrease in the frequency and intensity of the pain, a decrease in the amount of analgesic medications taken, an increase in the patient's knowledge of pain and factors that influence it, improved patient functioning despite the pain, cessation of "doctor shopping," and development of the patient's ability to cope more effectively with any new or remaining pain. To accomplish these goals, a multidisciplinary treatment approach is presented that includes medical interventions, psychological strategies, physical therapy, and patient and family involvement. It is stressed that the patient is an active participant in any treatment.

Claves, John. *Hypnotic Control of Low Back Pain*

Claves addresses the myths and utility of hypnosis in this interesting presentation. A patient with chronic low pain describes her condition and explains how hypnotherapy has helped to regain and maintain aspects of functional living. Claves' technique for hypnotherapy is then demonstrated on this patient. Very informative.

Melzack, Ronald. *Psychosocial Aspects of Chronic Pain*

Melzack gives a dynamic and articulate 1-hour lecture outlining the active components of acupuncture and how these components may be found in other cultures worldwide. He dispells the myths and stereotypes of acupuncture and focuses on the use of intense sensory input to decrease pain as a key ingredient in acupuncture-induced analgesia. Through slides and films he shows cross-cultural examples of "hyperstimulation analgesia," including the practice of "cupping" and an East African practice known as trepanation. Melzack then integrates trigger points, acupuncture site, and referred pain with the above in a discussion of his gate control theory of pain. Finally, he discusses memory traces to account for the long-acting analgesia that results from the brief duration of hyperstimulation analgesia. Highly recommended for the professional as an introduction to Melzack's work. Some graphic footage.

Murphy, Maryann. *Pain-Tension Cycle*
Harmarville Rehabilitation Center, 1981 (20 minutes)

A basic and informative presentation for the layman which elaborates on the factors involved in the relationship between pain and tension. The narration begins with a role-played first-hand account of how pain and tension exacerbate each other over time, followed by a brief lecture clarifying this relationship. The commentary focuses on how increased muscle tension can create more pain, how pain medications may actually worsen the problem, and how focusing on oneself, pain, and psychosocial concerns can increase distress and pain. A good film for patient viewing.

NBC News. *Pain! Where Does It Hurt the Most?*
Edwin Newman, narrator, 1972

This program, intended for the layperson, addresses the problem of chronic pain and the methods used in treatment. By following patients with a variety of pain problems such as low back pain, phantom limb pain, pain during childbirth, and burns,

the viewer learns the distinction between acute and chronic pain. Experts such as Sternback and Fordyce demonstrate operant pain treatment, hypnosis, acupuncture, and surgical interventions. This program is an excellent introduction and may prepare patients/clients for a more advanced presentation of pain treatment.

Sternbach, Richard. *Psycho-Social Aspects of Chronic Pain*
Pain Clinic, Department of Anesthesiology, Scripps Clinic, La Jolla, Calif.

This is an informative presentation given by a leader in the behavioral management of chronic pain. Sternbach explains the differences in signs and treatment of acute and chronic pain and addresses the implications for rehabilitative need in the latter. He also touches on the chemical and electrical treatments used in the management of chronic pain and ends the presentation by expressing the necessity for health care professionals to take a parallel (physical and behavioral), multidisciplinary approach to this growing problem

Toomy, Timothy C., and Dorothy M. Larkin. *Pain Intervention via Relaxation Technique*
Pain Clinic and Burn Center, University of Virginia Medical Center, Charlottesville, Virginia

This presentation illustrates the usefulness of relaxation therapy in the painful dressing changes of a young girl who has third-degree burns over most of her body. Since the girl must undergo frequent dressing changes to prevent infection and promote wound healing, general anesthesia and narcotics clearly are not indicated. Relaxation therapy is demonstrated by Toomy and Larkin, and the dressings are changed successfully without pain. Implications for the use of relaxation therapy in the treatment of chronic pain are discussed.

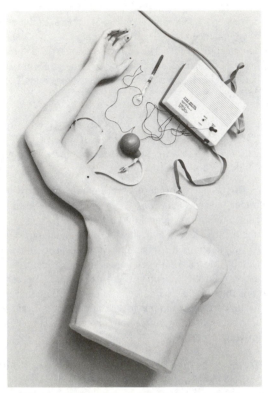

Fig A27.—American Society of Regional Anesthesia brachial plexus model (Nasco, Fort Atkinson, Wis.).

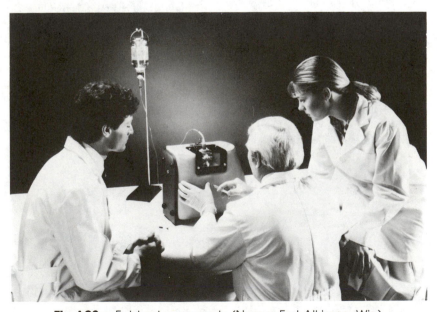

Fig A28.—Epidural mannequin (Nasco, Fort Atkinson, Wis.).

Index